Essentials of Nursing Informatics

Notice

Medicine is an ever-changing science. As new research and clinical experience broaden our knowledge, changes in treatment and drug therapy are required. The authors and the publisher of this work have checked with sources believed to be reliable in their efforts to provide information that is complete and generally in accord with the standards accepted at the time of publication. However, in view of the possibility of human error or changes in medical sciences, neither the authors nor the publisher nor any other party who has been involved in the preparation or publication of this work warrants that the information contained herein is in every respect accurate or complete, and they disclaim all responsibility for any errors or omissions or for the results obtained from use of the information contained in this work. Readers are encouraged to confirm the information contained herein with other sources. For example and in particular, readers are advised to check the product information sheet included in the package of each drug they plan to administer to be certain that the information contained in this work is accurate and that changes have not been made in the recommended dose or in the contraindications for administration. This recommendation is of particular importance in connection with new or infrequently used drugs.

Essentials of Nursing Informatics

FIFTH EDITION

Virginia K. Saba, EdD, RN, FAAN, FACMI

CEO and President
SabaCare, Inc.
Arlington, Virginia
Distinguished Scholar, Adjunct
Georgetown University
Washington, District of Columbia
Professor, Adjunct
Uniformed Services University
Bethesda, Maryland

Kathleen A. McCormick, PhD, RN, FAAN, FACMI, FHIMSS

Senior Principal Scientist/Vice President
SAIC-Frederick
Rockville, Maryland

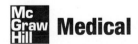

New York • Chicago • San Francisco • Lisbon • London Madrid • Mexico City
Milan • New Delhi • San Juan • Seoul • Singapore • Sydney • Toronto

The McGraw-Hill Companies

Essentials of Nursing Informatics, Fifth Edition

This book was written by Kathleen A. McCormick in her private capacity. No official support or endorsement by Science Applications International Corporation-Frederick (SAIC-F) is intended or should be inferred.

1 2 3 4 5 6 7 8 9 0   DOC/DOC   15 14 13 12 11

ISBN 978-0-07-174371-6
MHID 0-07-174371-5

This book was set in Berling Roman by Thomson Digital.
The editors were Joseph Morita and Peter J. Boyle.
The production supervisor was Sherri Souffrance.
Project management was provided by Aakriti Kathuria, Thomson Digital.
The designer was Mary McKeon; the cover designer was Elizabeth Pisacreta.
RR Donnelley was the printer and binder.

This book is printed on acid-free paper.

Library of Congress Cataloging-in-Publication Data
Essentials of nursing informatics / [edited by] Virginia K. Saba, Kathleen A. McCormick. — 5th ed.
      p. ; cm.
   Includes bibliographical references and index.
   ISBN-13: 978-0-07-174371-6 (pbk. : alk. paper)
   ISBN-10: 0-07-174371-5 (pbk. : alk. paper)
   1. Nursing--Data processing. 2. Computers. 3. Information storage and retrieval systems—
Nursing. I. Saba, Virginia K. II. McCormick, Kathleen Ann.
   [DNLM: 1. Nursing Informatics. WY 26.5]
   RT50.5.S23 2011
   610.730285—dc22
                                         2011014335

McGraw-Hill books are available at special quantity discounts to use as premiums and sales promotions, or for use in corporate training programs. To contact a representative please e-mail us at bulksales@mcgraw-hill.com.

CONTENTS

CONTRIBUTORS

Gregory L. Alexander, PhD, MHA, RN
Assistant Professor
Sinclair School of Nursing
University of Missouri
Columbia, Missouri
Chapter 8: Human Factors

Patricia E. Allen, RN, EdD, CNE, ANEF
Professor and Director
Center for Innovation in Nursing Education
Texas Tech University Health Sciences Center
School of Nursing
Lubbock, Texas
*Chapter 37: Initiation and Management of Accessible,
Effective Online Learning*

Ida M. Androwich, PhD, RN-BC, FAAN
Professor and Program Director
Health Systems Management Program
Niehoff School of Nursing
Loyola University/Chicago
Maywood, Illinois
*Chapter 28: Incorporating Evidence: Use of Computer-based
Clinical Decision Support Systems for Health Professionals*

Myrna L. Armstrong, EdD, RN, FAAN
Professor and Regional Dean
Texas Tech University Health Sciences Center
Anita Thigpen Perry School of Nursing
Highland Lakes Campus
Marble Falls, Texas
*Chapter 37: Initiation and Management of Accessible,
Effective Online Learning*

Dixie B. Baker, PhD
Senior Vice President
Science Applications International Corporation
Chief Technology Officer
Health Solutions
Redondo Beach, California
*Chapter 17: Trustworthy Systems for Safe and Private
Healthcare*

Suzanne Bakken, RN, DNSc, FAAN, FACMI
Alumni Professor of Nursing
Professor of Biomedical Informatics
Columbia University
New York, New York
Chapter 12: Advanced Terminological Approaches in Nursing

Khadija Bakrim, MEd
Instructional Designer
Texas Tech University Health Sciences Center
School of Nursing
Lubbock, Texas
*Chapter 37: Initiation and Management of Accessible
Effective Online Learning*

Emily B. Barey, RN, MSN
Director
Nursing Informatics
Epic Systems Corporation
Verona, Wisconsin
Chapter 20: Computerized Provider Order Entry

Mary Lee Barron, PhD, RN, APRN, FNP-BC
Associate Professor and Director
Master's Degree
Doctor of Nursing Practice Program
St. Louis, Missouri
*Chapter 30: Internet Tools for Patient Care in
Advanced Practice*

Amy J. Barton, PhD, RN
Associate Professor
College of Nursing
University of Colorado
Anschutz Medical Campus
Aurora, Colorado
Chapter 38: Innovations in E-Health

Carol J. Bickford, PhD, RN-BC
Senior Policy Fellow
Department of Nursing Practice and Policy
American Nurses Association
Silver Spring, Maryland
Chapter 11: The Practice Specialty of Nursing Informatics

Derryl E. Block, PhD, MPH, RN
University of Wisconsin Green Bay
Green Bay, Wisconsin
Chapter 34: Public Health Practice Applications

Enola Boyd, EdD, MS
Instructional Designer
Texas Tech University Health Sciences Center
Anita Thigpen Perry School of Nursing
Lubbock, Texas
Chapter 37: Initiation and Management of Accessible, Effective Online Learning

Robyn Carr, RGON
Director, Informatics Project Contracting
IPC and Associates
Waikato, New Zealand
Chapter 47: Pacific Rim Perspectives

Heather Carter-Templeton, MSN, RN
Nursing Instructor
Capstone College of Nursing
Tuscaloosa, Alabama
Chapter 26: Translation of Evidence Into Nursing Practice

Marian Celli, MS, RN, BC, FHIMSS
Beacon Consulting
Nokesville, Viginia
Chapter 6: System Life Cycle: Implementation and Evaluation

Kathleen G. Charters, PhD, RN, CPHIMS, CNE
Clinical Information Systems Specialist
Creative Computing Solutions, Inc.
Rockville, Maryland
Chapter 10: Mobile Computing Platforms

Thomas R. Clancy, PhD, MBA, RN
Clinical Professor and Director
Faculty Practice and Business Development
University of Minnesota School of Nursing
Minneapolis, Minnesota
Chapter 23 Planning, Design and Implementation of Information Technology in Complex Healthcare Systems
Chapter 24: The Integration of Complex Systems Theory Into Six Sigma Methods of Performance Improvement: A Case Study

Helen R. Connors, PhD, RN, DrPS (Hon), FAAN
Associate Dean for Integrated Technologies
Executive Director
Kansas University Center for Health Informatics
E. Jean M. Hill Endowed Professor
University of Kansas
Kansas City, Kansas
Chapter 41: A Paradigm Shift in Simulation: Experiential Learning in Second Life

Mical DeBrow, PhD, RN
Practice Director
Siemens Healthcare
Malvern, Pennsylvania
Chapter 25: Workflow and Healthcare Process Management

Connie White Delaney, PhD, RN, FAAN, FACMI
Professor and Dean
School of Nursing Academic Health Center
Director, Biomedical Health Informatics
Associate Director, CTSI-BMI
Acting Director, Institute for Health Informatics
University of Minnesota, School of Nursing
Minneapolis, Minnesota
Chapter 13: Nursing Minimum Data Set Systems

Cathy Delmain, RN
Senior Clinical Analyst
Health Services
Siemens Healthcare
Malvern, Pennsylvania
Chapter 31: IT for the Rural Healthcare Market

Marina Douglas, MS, RN
Principal, Beacon Healtcare Consulting
Nokesville, Virginia
Chapter 6: System Life Cycle: Implementation and Evaluation

Patricia C. Dykes, DNSc, MA, RN
Corporate Manager
Nursing Informatics and Research
Clinical Informatics Research and Development
Partners Healthcare
Wellesley, Maryland
Chapter 7: Healthcare Project Management

Laketa Entzminger
Medical Student
Saint Louis University
School of Medicine
St. Louis, Missouri
Chapter 30: Internet Tools for Patient Care in Advanced Practice

W. Scott Erdley, DNS, RN
Associate Professor
Wegmans School of Nursing
St. John Fisher College
Rochester, New York
Chapter 9: Open Source and Free Software

Ann Patricia Farrell, BSN, RN
Principal, Farrell Associates
San Francisco, California
Chapter 21: Electonic Health Record Vendor Applications

Veronica D. Feeg, PhD, RN, FAAN
Professor
Division of Nursing
Assistant Dean for Research and Scholarly Practice
Associate Dean for the PhD Program
Molloy College
Rockville Centre, New York
Chapter 43: Computer Use in Nursing Research

Barbara B. Frink, PhD, RN, FAAN
Lecturer and Adjunct Associate Professor
University of Pennsylvania School of Nursing
Philadelphia, Pennsylvania
Lecturer and Associate Faculty
Johns Hopkins University School of Nursing
Baltimore, Maryland
Vice President
Clinical Excellence and Informatics
Main Line Health System
Bryn Mawr, Pennsylvania
Chapter 39: Consumer and Patient Use of Computers for Health

Judy D. Gibson, MSN, RN
Centers for Disease Control and Prevention
Atlanta, Georgia
Chapter 34: Public Health Practice Applications

Matthew C. Grissinger, RPh, FISMP, FASCP
Director
Error Reporting Programs
Institute for Safe Medication Practices
Clinical Analyst
Pennsylvania Patient Safety Authority
Horsham, Pennsylvania
Chapter 22: The Role of Technology in the Medication-Use Process

Thomasine D. Guberski, PhD, CRNP
Associate Professor
Department of Organizational Systems
and Adult Health
University of Maryland School of Medicine
Baltimore, Maryland
Chapter 10: Mobile Computing Platforms

Paul D. Guillory, BSN, RN
Clinical Applications Coordinator
Clinical Informatics Service Department
Department of Veterans Affairs
Pacific Island Healthcare System
Honolulu, Hawaii
*Chapter 36: Web 2.0 and Its Impact on Healthcare
Education and Practice*

Nora Hammell, MN, RN
Director
Nursing Policy
Canadian Nurses Association
Ottawa, Ontario, Canada
Chapter 45: Nursing Informatics in Canada

Kathryn J. Hannah, PhD, RN
Health Informatics Advisor
Canadian Nurses Association
Ottawa, Ontario, Canada
Adjunct Professor
Department of Biomedical Informatics
School of Medicine
University of Utah
Salt Lake City, Utah
Chapter 45: Nursing Informatics in Canada

Nicholas R. Hardiker, PhD, RN
Reader
School of Nursing and Midwifery
University of Salford
Salford, United Kingdom
Chapter 12: Advanced Terminological Approaches in Nursing

**Michelle Honey, PhD, RN, MPhil (Nursing),
FCNA(NZ)**
Senior Lecturer
University of Auckland
School of Nursing
Auckland, New Zealand
Chapter 47: Pacific Rim Perspectives

Evelyn J. S. Hovenga, PhD, RN, FACS, FACHI
CEO, Professor and Director eHealth Education
Pty Ltd and RSC Training
Adjunct Professor, Victoria University, Melbourne
Melbourne, Victoria & Rockhampton, Queensland,
Australia
Chapter 47: Pacific Rim Perspectives

Kathleen M. Hunter, PhD, RN-BC
Specialization Coordinator
Nursing Informatics
School of Nursing
Walden University
Minneapolis, Minnesota
Chapter 11: The Practice Specialty of Nursing Informatics

Elizabeth Johnson, MS, FHIMSS, CPHIMS, RN-C
Vice President
Applied Clinical Informatics
Tenet Healthcare Corporation
Dallas, Texas
Chapter 16: Nursing Informatics and Healthcare Policy

Virpi Jylhä, PT, MSc
Researcher
Department of Health and Social Management
University of Eastern Finland
Kuopio, Finland
Chapter 46: Nursing Informatics in Europe

Tae Youn Kim, PhD, RN
Assistant Professor
College of Nursing
University of Wisconsin–Milwaukee
Milwaukee, Wisconsin
Chapter 12: Advanced Terminological Approaches in Nursing

Margaret Ross Kraft, PhD, RN
Assistant Professor
Niehoff School of Nursing, Loyola
University of Chicago
Maywood, Illinois
*Chapter 28: Incorporating Evidence: Use of Computer-based
Clinical Decision Support Systems for Health Professionals*

Darlene Lacy, PhD, RN, BC
Assistant Professor
Texas Tech University Health Sciences Center
Anita Thigpen Perry School of Nursing
Highland Lakes Campus
Marble Falls, Texas
Chapter 37: Initiation and Management of Accessible,
Effective Online Learning

Gail E. Latimer, MSN, RN, FACHE, FAAN
Vice President and Chief Nursing Officer
Siemens Medical Solutions, Inc. USA
Health Services
Malvern, Pennsylvania
Part 5: Continuum of Care Information Technology Systems
Chapter 1: Overview of Computers and Nursing

Mary Ann Lavin, ScD, RN, APRN, FAAN
Associate Professor and Director
Clinical Services, Casa de Salud
Saint Louis University School of Nursing
St. Louis, Missouri
Chapter 30: Internet Tools for Patient Care in
Advanced Practice

June Levy, MLS
General Manager
Cinahl Information Systems
Glendale, California
Chapter 44: Information Literacy and Computerized
Information Resources

Susan H. Lundquist, RN, BSN
Director
Patient Care Solutions Health Services
Siemens Healthcare
Malvern, Pennsylvania
Chapter 31: IT for the Rural Healthcare Market

Michelle Mandrack, RN, MSN
Director
Consulting Services
Institute for Safe Medication Practices
Horsham, Pennsylvania
Chapter 22: The Role of Technology in the
Medication-Use Process

Heimar F. Marin, PhD, RN, FACMI
Professor and Director
Graduate Program in Health Informatics
Universidade Federal de São Paulo
São Paulo, Brazil
Chapter 49: Nursing Informatics in South America

Cynthia M. Mascara, MSN, MBA, RN
Principal Consultant
Clinical Outcomes
Siemens Healthcare
Malvern, Pennsylvania
Chapter 25: Workflow and Healthcare
Process Management

Kathleen A. McCormick, PhD, RN, FAAN,
FACMI, FHIMSS
Senior Principal Scientist/Vice President
SAIC-F
Rockville, Maryland
Part 3: Informatics Theory
Part 4: Current Issues in Informatics
Part 9: The Future of Informatics
Chapter 1: Overview of Computers and Nursing
Chapter 26: Translation of Evidence Into Nursing Practice
Chapter 51: Future Directions

Mary L. McHugh, PhD, RN
Professor and Dean
School of Nursing
American University of Health Science
Signal Hill, California
Chapter 4: Computer System Basics

Lynn McQueen, DrPH, MS, MPA, RN
Office of Rural Health
Department of Veterans Affairs
Washington, DC
Chapter 26: Translation of Evidence Into Nursing Practice

Bernadette Melnyk, PhD, RN, CPNP/PMHNP, FNAP, FAAN
Dean and Distinguished Foundation Professor in Nursing
Arizona State University College of Nursing and Health Innovation
Phoenix, Arizona
Chapter 27: Evidence-Based Practice

Susan Meyer RN (B.SocSc(Nurs); Dip Paediatrics)
IT Manager
Addington Hospital
Durban, South Africa
Chapter 50: Nursing Informatics in South Africa

Jennifer V. Moore, MHA
Principal, Healthcare Information Consultants, LLC
Baltimore, Maryland
Chapter 19: Home Health: The Missing Ingredient in Healthcare Reform

Jacqueline Moss, PhD, RN
Associate Professor and Assistant Dean for Clinical Simulation and Technology
University of Alabama at Birmingham
School of Nursing
Birmingham, Alabama
Chapter 14: Overview of the Clinical Care Classifications System: A National Nursing Standard Coded Terminology

Judy Murphy, RN, FACMI, FHIMSS
Vice President
Information Services
Aurora Healthcare
Milwaukee, Wisconsin
Chapter 7: Healthcare Project Management
Chapter 16: Nursing Informatics and Healthcare Policy

Peter J. Murray, PhD, RN, FBCS, CITP
Executive Director
International Medical Informatics Association
Lincoln, United Kingdom
Chapter 9: Open Source and Free Software

Lynn M. Nagle, PhD, RN
Assistant Professor
Lawrence S. Bloomberg Faculty of Nursing
University of Toronto
Toronto, Ontario, Canada
Chapter 45: Nursing Informatics in Canada

Eun-Shim Nahm, PhD, RN, FAAN
Associate Professor and Program Director
Nursing Informatics
Department of Organizational Systems and Adult Health
University of Maryland
School of Nursing
Baltimore, Maryland
Chapter 40: Nursing Curriculum Reform and Healthcare Information Technology

Susan K. Newbold, PhD, RN-BC, FAAN, FHIMSS
Consultant
Franklin, Tennessee
Part 8: International Perspectives
Chapter 1: Overview of Computers and Nursing
Chapter 32: Ambulatory Care Information Systems

Marilyn M. Nielsen, RN-BC, BSN, MS
Clinical Informatics
Centura Health
Littleton Adventist Hospital
Littleton, Colorado
Chapter 38: Innovations in E-Health

Kay Lynn Olmsted, RN, MSN, FNP-BC
Doctor of Nursing Practice
Georgia Southern University
Statesboro, Georgia
Chapter 36: Web 2.0 and Its Impact on Healthcare Education and Practice

Hyeoun-Ae Park, PhD
College of Nursing
Seoul National University
Seoul, Republic of Korea
Chapter 48: Asian Perspectives

Diane S. Pravikoff, PhD, RN, FAAN
Director of Research/Professional Liaison
Cinahl Information Systems
Glendale, California
*Chapter 44: Information Literacy and Computerized
Information Resources*

Susan J. Quinn, EdD, MBA, RN, CNI
Director
Penn Care at Home
University of Pennsylvania Health System
Philadelphia, Pennsylvania
Mentor, Thomas Edison State College
Trenton, New Jersey
Chapter 33: Overview of Post Acute Services

Janise Richards, PhD, MPH, MS
Centers for Disease Control and Preventions
Division of Global HIV/AIDS
Epidemiology and Strategic Information Branch
Health Informatics Team
Atlanta, Georgia
Chapter 34: Public Health Practice Applications

Theresa A. Rienzo, RN, MS, MLIS
Associate Librarian Reference Services
Nursing and Allied Health Divisions
Molloy College
Rockville Centre, New York
Chapter 43: Computer Use in Nursing Research

Virginia K. Saba, EdD, RN, FAAN, FACMI
CEO and President
SabaCare, Inc.
Arlington, Virginia
Distinguished Scholar, Adjunct
Georgetown University
Washington, DC
Professor, Adjunct
Uniformed Services University
Bethesda, Maryland
Part 1: Computers and Nursing
Part 3: Informatics Theory
Part 7: Research Applications
Chapter 1: Overview of Computers and Nursing
Chapter 2: Historical Perspectives of Nursing Informatics
*Chapter 14: Overview of the Clinical Care
Classifications System*
*Appendix A: Clinical Care Classification (CCC) System
Version 2.0*

Kaija Saranto, PhD, RN, RNT
Professor
Department of Health and Social Management
University of Eastern Finland
Kuopio, Finland
Chapter 46: Nursing Informatics in Europe

Andrea Schmid-Mazzoccoli, PhD, RN, MSN, MBA
Chief Nurse Executive
Senior Vice President
Center for Clinical Excellence
Bon Secours Health System
Baltimore, Maryland
Chapter 29: The Magnet Model

Joanne M. Seasholtz, PhD, RN, MSN, MBA, FACHE
Principal Consultant
Siemens Medical Solutions
Malvern, Pennsylvania
Chapter 27: Evidence-based Practice

Joyce Sensmeier, MS, RN-BC, CPHIMS, FHIMSS
Vice President
Informatics Healthcare Information and
Management Systems Society
Chicago, Illinois
Chapter 15: Health Data Standards: Development,
Harmonization, and Interoperability

Diane J. Skiba, PhD
Professor and Healthcare Informatics Coordinator
College of Nursing
University of Colorado
Anschutz Medical Campus
Aurora, Colorado
Part 6: Educational Applications
Chapter 1: Overview of Computers and Nursing
Chapter 36: Web 2.0 and Its Impact on Healthcare
Education and Practice

Capt. Lynn A. Slepski, PhD, RN, CCNS
United States Public Health Service
Senior Public Health Advisor
Department of Transportation
Washington,DC
Chapter 35: Informatics Solutions for Emergency
Planning and Response

M. Kathleen Smith, MScEd, RN-BC, FHIMSS
Managing Partner
Informatics Consulting and Continuing
Education, LLC
Gaithersburg, Maryland
Part 2: Computer Systems
Chapter 1: Overview of Computers and Nursing
Chapter 5: Systems Life Cycle: Planning and Analysis

Arunkumar Srinivasan, MS
Computer Scientist
Division of Notifiable Disease Surveillance
Office of Surveillance Epidemiology and Laboratory
Services
Atlanta, Georgia
Chapter 34: Public Health Practice Applications

Annelle Tanner, RN, MSN, EdD
Regional Coordinator
Fetal and Infant Mortality Review and Reduction
Louisiana Office of Public Health
Maternal Child Health
Alexandria, Louisiana
Chapter 44: Information Literacy and Computerized
Information Resources

Kaarina Tanttu, PhD, MNSc
Director of Nursing
Bureau of Nursing Care
Hospital District of Southwest Finland
University Hospital of Turku
Turku, Finland
Chapter 46: Nursing Informatics in Europe

Sheryl L. Taylor, BSN, RN
Vienna, Virginia
Chapter 21: Electonic Health Record Vendor Applications

Patricia A. Trangenstein, PhD, RN, BC
Vanderbilt University
School of Nursing
Frist Nursing Informatics Center
Nashville, Tennessee
Chapter 41: A Paradigm Shift in Simulation: Experiential
Learning in Second Life

Michelle R. Troseth, MSN, RN, DPNAP
Executive Vice President
Chief Professional Practice Officer
CPM Resource Center/Elsevier
Grand Rapids, Michigan
Chapter 42: The TIGER Initiative

Denise D. Tyler, MSN/MBA RN-BC
Clinical Specialist
Information Systems
Kaweah Delta Healthcare District
Visalia, California
Chapter 5: Systems Life Cycle: Planning and Analysis

Irene van Middelkoop, Hons BA (Cur)
CAPRISA
University of KwaZulu-Natal
Durban, South Africa
Chapter 50: Nursing Informatics in South Africa

Amy M. Walker, MS, RN, CPHQ, FACHE, NEA-BC
Healthcare IT Strategist and CEO
Optimize IT Consulting LLC
Washington, District of Columbia
Chapter 18: Shaping Nursing Informatics Through the Public Policy Process

Judith J. Warren, PhD, RN, BC, FAAN, FACMI
Christine A. Hartley Centennial Professor
School of Nursing
Director of Nursing Informatics
Kansas University Center for Health Informatics
University of Kansas
Kansas City, Kansas
Chapter 41: A Paradigm Shift in Simulation: Experiential Learning in Second Life

Charlotte A. Weaver, PhD, RN, MPH, FHIMSS
Chief Clinical Officer and Senior Vice President
Gentiva Health Services
Atlanta, Georgia
Chapter 19: Home Health: The Missing Ingredient in Healthcare Reform

Elizabeth Weiner, PhD, RN-BC, FACMI, FAAN
Senior Associate Dean for Informatics
Centennial Independence Foundation
Professor of Nursing
Professor of Biomedical Informatics
Vanderbilt University
Nashville, Tennessee
Chapter 35: Informatics Solutions for Emergency Planning and Response

Lucy A. Westbrooke, RN, DipNg, PG Dip Bus (Health Informatics)
Information Management Consultant
Information Management and Technology
Auckland District Health Board
Auckland, New Zealand
Chapter 47: Pacific Rim Perspectives

Bonnie L. Westra, PhD, RN, FAAN
Associate Professor
University of Minnesota
School of Nursing
Minneapolis Minnesota
Chapter 2: Historical Perspective of Nursing Informatics
Chapter 13 Nursing Minimum Data Set Systems

Luann Whittenburg, PhD, RN
United States Delegate
American National Standards Institute Technical Advisory Group
Vice-Convenor
International Organization for Sandardization
Technical Committee: Health Informatics (ISO/TC215)
Washington, District of Columbia
Chapter 14: Overview of the Clinical Care Classifications System: A National Nursing Standard Coded Terminology

Marisa L. Wilson, DNSc, MHSc, RN-BC
Assistant Professor
Department of Organizational Systems and Adult Health
Division of Nursing Informatics
University of Maryland
School of Nursing
Baltimore, Maryland
Chapter 40: Nursing Curriculum Reform and Healthcare Information Technology

Patricia B. Wise, RN, MS, MA
COL (USA retired)
Vice President
Healthcare Information and Management Systems
Society
Chicago, Illinois
Chapter 3: Electronic Health Records From a Historical Perspective

Rita D. Zielstorff, RN, MS, FAAN, FACMI
Independent Consultant
Clinical Informatics
North Andover, Massachusetts
Chapter 39: Consumer and Patient Use of Computers for Health

The New Era of Healthcare Delivery

Healthcare in the United States (and other countries in the industrialized world) continues to experience increases in costs that outpace the rate of inflation. Invariably these increases do not bring commensurate improvements in care quality and reliability.

This imbalance has been present for many years. However, concerns about these problems recently have evolved from anxiety to alarm.

A significant federal government deficit accompanied by growing demands for Medicare services. States struggling with increases in Medicaid costs at a time of falling tax revenues. Businesses worried about remaining competitive in a global economy and a lingering recession. Individuals struggling with unemployment, shrunken retirement plans, and underwater mortgages. These factors are creating a perfect storm of pressure to "finally fix" the healthcare system.

The recently passed Patient Protection and Affordable Care Act (PPACA) ushers in an era of broad health insurance coverage and the first wave of substantial healthcare payment reform. The private sector has also unleashed a new and complementary wave of changes in provider reimbursement approaches.

While quite diverse, all of these payment reform efforts have several characteristics:

- Providers will be asked to measure and report the quality, safety, and efficiency of care delivered.
- A significant portion of reimbursement will be based on these measures; providers will face material financial risk if their care is deemed to be substandard.
- Reimbursement is evolving to include concepts such as episodes and bundles; concepts that reimburse based on the holistic care of a patient, be it a single payment for hip replacement surgery and rehabilitation care or a single payment for all care delivered to a diabetic over the course of a year.
- Regardless of care performance the amount reimbursed for a care episode, for example, will be progressively decreased.

- Greater transparency of provider quality scores and costs will be required enabling purchasers of care and consumers to make more informed choices as they seek care.
- Efforts will be made to compare the effectiveness of new treatments over current treatments; treatments that fail to demonstrate increased effectiveness will not be reimbursed.
- Provider organizations will be asked to become accountable for the care of populations of patients with these providers establishing new care arrangements such as Accountable Care Organizations and Patient Centered Medical Homes.

While these payment reform efforts are still emerging, because of the shift from anxiety to alarm, they are likely to cause major change in the healthcare industry. This change may result in the most significant upheaval in the United States healthcare system in over 40 years.

In the background of this set of sweeping changes is the realization that significant reimbursement change represents the most potent form of "disruptive innovation" in healthcare.

It is difficult to be certain about the impact of these changes on the healthcare system in the decade ahead. There are dozens of new approaches to reimbursement and their effectiveness at a national scale or across all populations is unclear. Moreover, it is not possible to attempt to transform the largest and most complex sector of any economy and have a complete understanding of the mature forms of the new healthcare system. We are in for a decade of experimentation, chaos, and uncertainty.

While the future form of the country's healthcare system is unclear there is reasonable certainty regarding the major health information system applications that will be necessary in the new era.

- An integrated electronic health record (EHR) that spans inpatient, outpatient, and emergency department care
- A revenue cycle system that also spans this care continuum and is well integrated with the EHR

- Workflow engines that help improve the performance of core clinical processes (e.g., patient discharge, chronic disease management, and infection management) and rules engines that critique a specific clinician decision (e.g., drug-drug interaction checking after the entry of a medication order)
- Business intelligence and care analytics technologies that enable providers to measure the quality, safety, and efficiency of their care and understand the resulting reimbursement ramifications
- Interoperability technologies that enable providers to exchange clinical data, care plans, and care events (such as an unplanned emergency room visit) with other providers as they jointly manage the care of patient
- Patient-facing technologies such as the personal health record and online patient communities that assist patients in managing their own care

For a provider to thrive in the decade ahead and achieve the level of care delivery that will become the new standard they must implement and use a solid foundation of health information technology. It is not possible to achieve necessary levels of care process performance, conform to evidence-based healthcare, or manage increasingly complex reimbursement arrangements without such a foundation.

The federal government understood the need for this foundation when it passed the HITECH Act of 2009 that provided financial incentives for hospitals and eligible professionals if they could demonstrate that they were meaningful users of EHRs. In effect the government, as the largest purchaser of healthcare in the world, was saying clinicians must use the technology to enter orders, document care delivered, and exchange data with other providers if they are to succeed in addressing the changes introduced by the PPACA.

The nursing community has always been the backbone of care delivery. The community must be active, thoughtful, and vigorous contributors to reshaping the healthcare system. They must also be skilled and effective in their application of information technology to improve care. To a large degree the future of healthcare depends on the domain of nursing informatics being well integrated with and practiced by the nursing community.

I applaud the editors and authors of the fifth edition of *Essentials of Nursing Informatics*. This book could not be more timely and important.

John Glaser, PhD, FACMI, FCHIME, FHIMSS
CEO, Siemens Health Services
Siemens Healthcare

The year 2010 will be marked as a watershed year in advancing electronic health records (EHR) in the United States. On the heels of the landmark Health Information Technology for Economic and Clinical Health Act, or HITECH, passed in 2009, U.S. healthcare began responding to the promise of financial incentives for meeting the first of a progressively more rigorous series of tests of the "meaningful use" of health information technology. In essence the escalating requirements progress from attestation to structural measures of certified health records being present in hospital and office environments in Stage I to process measures of their use in Stage II to outcome requirements for demonstrating improved healthcare performance in Stage III. The three stages must be achieved by the end of 2014 not only to realize maximum incentive payments, but to avoid financial penalty.

A substantial focus of meaningful use is directed toward advancing computerized provider order entry (CPOE), specifically practitioner order entry. Two observations on this focus are necessary: First, CPOE is critical to the delivery of real-time, context sensitive decision support. Beyond safeguards against placing orders that are contraindicated (such as for medications to which the patient is allergic), decision support, order sets, cost information, and real-time evidence delivery can help improve the effectiveness and efficiency of clinical decision making. These "conversations" really cannot be intermediated by clerical personnel. Thus, the intended progression from structure to process to outcome, in this regard, evolves from deploying technology for CPOE to broad use of CPOE with decision support to reporting improved care outcomes because of its use.

The second observation is that the focus, while not excluding nurse practitioners and other nonphysician clinicians with prescriptive authority, is physician focused. As chair of the Health IT Standards Committee for the U.S. Department of Health and Human Services' Office of the National Coordinator for Health Information Technology, I have received many expressions of concern that nurses felt left out. The reason that Congress legislated HITECH and Meaningful Use as they did is, frankly, not a badge of honor for physicians. We physicians are categorically behind nurses in the use of health information technology in care environments.

It is both likely and necessary that the experience that the nursing profession has gathered in the robust use of EHR and related technologies in daily practice will be essential to completing adoption among all clinicians and in advancing the field of biomedical informatics. That this is the fifth edition of *Essentials of Nursing Informatics* is testament to this rich and productive history. Similarly, it is also testament to the ascension of the field of nursing informatics and to the key role of the discipline in advancing science and value-driven healthcare, not only in the United States, but globally.

There is much work to be done in the United States. As of 2010, only about 3.8 percent of U.S. hospitals use advanced clinical information systems with CPOE and real-time clinical decision support at the HIMSS Stage 6 or 7 (HIMSS, 2010). Most U.S. hospitals are still at Stage 4 or below and have substantial work in their efforts to meet meaningful use requirements. In contract, innovations in EHR for the relatively less complex office practice environment include friendlier user interface and the increasing availability of easier to manage Web-based applications. These innovations have accelerated implementation. In 2010, HITECH's promised incentives spawned a doubling of use of EHRs in medical offices, from about 27 percent in 2008 to 49 percent by late 2010. HITECH also requires national identification and adoption of interoperability standards that will facilitate secure, private, and appropriate transmission of health information among not only providers, payers, and other authorized parties but also importantly with patients. The envisioned end product is a nationwide network that will support exchange of clinical and administrative health information.

While the promise for patients not having to fill out another clipboard of the same information provided at their last health encounter is enticing, the ability to inform care over time and across environments improves safety, quality, and efficiency. As U.S. healthcare implements reform, the demands for delivering and demonstrating value will increase. Value will be realized first at the transactional level, and information continuity will diminish waste from duplication. Breeches in safety are not only harmful but are a source of waste as well, both in human and financial terms. The potential for information systems to link the unique circumstances of a patient to the evidence that has been demonstrated to provide the best outcomes will also drive value.

The informatics nurses' role, however, is ultimately transformative. While nurses who specialize in informatics are at the center of creating information continuity across time and geography, they are even more central to redefining how teams operate, how each clinician can interact with other professionals in an informed manner and interact with patients and their families with the information required for therapeutically rich conversation. The disciplines that are the focus of this book will be cornerstones of team-based care that allows each health professional to practice at the top of his or her license and that includes the patient or their proxy as an informed member of the care team.

Therein, the greatest contributions of nursing informatics will be found. The mantra of the nursing informatics is moving *from data to information to knowledge to wisdom*. In the near term, nursing informatics will help the other health professions automate the generation of information that can drive both the knowledge development that underpins a learning health system and the application of that knowledge that is required for evidence-based practice. More profoundly, the early adopter advantage enjoyed by nurses in the adoption of health information technology positions nursing informatics to help realize wisdom that will inform the challenges in health and care.

Jonathan B. Perlin, MD, PhD, MSHA, FACP, FACMI
President, Clinical Services and Chief Medical Officer
HCA / Hospital Corporation of America
&
Chair, Health Information Technology Standards Committee, Office of the National Coordinator for Health Information Technology,
U.S. Department of Health and Human Services
Adjunct Professor of Medicine and Biomedical Informatics,
Vanderbilt University
Adjunct Professor of Health Administration,
Virginia Commonwealth University

In 2010 the United States entered a new decade of electronic health records (EHR) as declared by the President of the United States and endorsed by the Secretary of U.S. Department of Health and Human Services. The American Recovery and Reinvestment Act of 2009, which includes funding for the Health Information Technology for Economic and Clinical Health Act (HITECH) from which the Meaningful Use program comes, is rapidly resharing the funding and implementation of the EHR in the United States. The Patient Protection and Affordable Care Act (PPACA) is a federal statute that was signed into law in 2010. This law and the Healthcare and Education Reconciliation Act of 2010 focus on the reform of the private health insurance and prescription drug coverage. These new legislations will necessarily impact nursing informatics and the nursing profession.

The fifth edition of *Essentials of Nursing Informatics* addresses this new landscape by introducing four new section editors and many new authors who discuss concepts important to the implementation of the legislation. They explore the technology, practice, and social behavioral phenomena that are now often called "Health 2.0," in which consumers use the Internet to publish information on their own healthcare experiences. The movement of information onto "the cloud," grid platforms, and large networks is commonly referred to as Web 2.0. The linkage of these networks is driving Open Source tools, platforms, software, codes, and standards. Using this new online environment only for patient care without educating healthcare professionals and demonstrating effectiveness and efficiency would be meaningless. Disseminating this information through web technology, publications, workshops, weekend immersions, collaboration, and meetings provides a complement to traditional academic teaching.

The earliest personalized health projects tackled breast cancer screening epidemiology and sharing of the best clinical trials to treat and cure women. For example, armies of women have been created in part by establishing networks; infrastructures; linkages; services to end-users; standards; security; ethical, legal and regulatory policies; and social networks supported by large economic investments.

The patient exists at home, in rural communities, in ambulatory care environments, in acute care hospitals, in nursing homes, and in hospices—an entire continuum of care—and this continuum is the essence of transformational health. Underlying this transformation is the "rapid learning healthcare system," driven by information technology, that incorporates scientific evidence to improve quality, reduce errors, and inspire new research studies. Central to moving patients from these different environments is an information system infrastructure that features *interoperability* (allowing computer systems to talk to each other) and *intergratability* (allowing computers to understand each other). The new HITECH environment must also establish trust that health information technology (HIT) can preserve patients' privacy and confidentiality. The mandate for standards has become a mantra from the authors. The standards are critical so that national and international networks can be formed to coordinate care and establish the effectiveness of disease diagnosis, treatment, and cures.

The abundance of evidence demands user and software services or systems, decision support tools, and frameworks for harmonizing data. The new HIT enables clinicians to have access to electronic data, feedback on their performance measured by evidence, and continuous monitoring at the point of care (when the episode of care is occurring).

In summary, the payment and delivery processes can be continuously evaluated only when public and private payers contribute toward the data supporting the patient in whatever environment he/she is receiving care, when incentives are aligned to evidence-based principles, and when support for self-management is available to the patient, or consumer. The ultimate incentive for use comes from governance policies that integrate theory with practice into meaningful use. New theories of management expand our previous concepts into an understanding of how to implement these systems, and understanding and managing the workflows and complex environments. New models of governance and policy requirements are needed for the technical environments. Efficient resource utilization and scheduling patients are needed to facilitate movement from one environment the patient resides in to another. The simplest use case becomes complex when a patient who sees clinician A in location A travels to location B for the winter and sees clinician B. Moving prescriptions from pharmacy A to pharmacy B requires the same standards, integration, interoperability, and monitoring of adverse reactions and drug interactions at each pharmacy, and should not be dependent on dealing with the same pharmacy chain. Similarly, this scenario should not require that the patient seek a clinician in the same network in location A as in location B.

The purpose of this book is to provide the new and innovative technologies for the nursing informatician as well as the nurse at the bedside. This book is dedicated toward helping nurses prepare for "meaningful use" patient care requirements in this electronic age.

ACKNOWLEDGMENTS

As we initiated this book we experienced many family events in addition to the professional growth of the editors and section editors. In this preface we would like to share with you a glimpse of some of the family events that were occurring.

Virginia has served as the 'mother' of the book's family' for the five editions. She saw the need for the first edition which is the reason it was initially prepared, and why it still exists. In fact, the book represents the educational aspect of her career in nursing informatics. She collaborated with Kathleen as a major force in the book's evolution. She considers most of the authors to be her extended family. Her involvement with her other family—sister Bernice, nieces Tisha and Caroline, and nephews Richard and Robin—kept her occupied with their problems and joys as well as provided the support she needed working on this edition.

On a happy note, when we signed the contract with McGraw-Hill, Kathleen's daughter-in-law and son announced that her pregnancy and the birth of their first grandson would cover the same 9 months that the book was in gestation. At the time that the book was being delivered to the publisher, the birth of Simon Francis occurred. The father of the baby, Francis Jr., was only six years old when the first edition was published. Kathleen's youngest son, Christopher, now 24, was not even born when the first edition was released. Throughout the life of this book, the McCormick men have had to share their wife/mother on weekends and holidays with chapter reviews, writing, and editing. They have also shared in the fun travelling locally, nationally, and internationally to have reunions with many of the book authors. It has been a wonderful journey to see the McCormick men embrace some of the authors of this book as their confidants.

A book is a family affair from many other perspectives—that means rolling up your sleeves and helping. Oftentimes, when I called the Newbold house, I spoke with Susan's husband because Susan was off working. One father took care of the 3-year-old twins (Cara and Skye), 6-year-old Beth, and 17-year-old Julia so that author/mother Lynn could work on her chapter. Finalizing the chapter, husband Hal also hired the graphic artist for a book illustration. At a local book night out party, the husbands/sons voted on the pyramid or circular format for a figure.

As Kathleen Smith said in her communication to the readers, "It has been a pleasure working with these experts in their field of nursing informatics."

As one of the authors put it, the content of the book is coming along fine, but "life keeps getting in my way." During this book production, a section editor lost her father; and another author was caring for her dying father. During book production some authors were unable to meet their contract obligations to write a chapter because of family stresses or tragedies.

Writing and editing a book has been a life-changing experience for the authors, editors, and our families. During this past year, Gail E. Latimer has experienced two family weddings, Mark to Meredith and Tara to Tom. Her family shares in the experience and she knows Brad and Mark are eager to read the final book. As Gail said, "My only disappointment is that my father is not alive to experience my dream come true. I dedicate the Continuum of Care Information Systems to him."

Diane Skiba would like to thank her family and friends for their support and understanding as she worked evenings and weekends on the education section. She is thankful for the privilege to mentor her two coauthors Paul D. Guillory and Kay Lynn Olmsted. Both are graduate students who managed to carve out time in their busy lives to start the journey of scholarly writing. She would also like to acknowledge all her graduate students who challenge her each and every day to be a better teacher and scholar.

We have never met Joe Morita or Midge Haramis, the New York McGraw-Hill editor and administrative coordinator for this book, but they seem a very important part of our family. They were the correspondents with all of the authors, assuring contracts were in place and material was kept organized for book production and marketing. Our family was extended during production to include Peter Boyle, Sherri Souffrance, and Aakriti Kathuria and Anand Kumar from Thomson Digital; and during marketing to include the able support from Deborah Cruz and Mary McKeon for her beautiful tanzanite colored design.

Computers and Nursing

Virginia K. Saba • Kathleen A. McCormick

Overview of Computers and Nursing

Virginia K. Saba / Kathleen A. McCormick / M. Kathleen Smith /
Gail E. Latimer / Diane J. Skiba / Susan K. Newbold

• OBJECTIVES

1. Provide an overview and introduction to each of the new sections in the 5th edition.
2. Describe the new concepts of nursing informatics technologies and information technology.
3. Identify the current concepts in informatics theory and the current issues in informatics.
4. Define the multiple uses of nursing informatics through the continuum of care.
5. Specify new applications in education and research.
6. Describe a scenario for a personalized health future.

• KEY WORDS

Standards and Policies
Nursing Informatics
Systems Life Cycle
Workflow
Continuum of Care
2nd Life
e-Health Research
International Perspectives
Personalized Future
e-Learning
Information Literacy

The welcome of four new section editors brings the 5th edition of *Essentials of Nursing Informatics* into a new era. Four section editors who are shaping nursing informatics were invited to join book editors, Virginia K. Saba and Kathleen A. McCormick to shape content for the 5th edition. After a market scan of the book was done by several leading nurses in informatics, Kathleen Smith was invited to be a section editor to bring new perspectives on system life cycle and human factors. Her invaluable guidance in developing the content comes from her experience in the Weekend Immersion in Nursing Informatics Courses that are offered nationally. The chapter Systems Life Cycle has been expanded to two chapters; and the chapters Human Factors and Healthcare Project Management have been added to this section. Gail Latimer developed the core content for the new perspectives on information technology applications. From her global perspective in nursing executive leadership and corporate America, she broadened the applications into areas that were previously uncovered in previous editions. She brings new content for CPOE, Magnet, TIGER, Rural Health, Workflow, Complex Systems Theory, as well as updates on Enterprise Applications. She expanded the content in Continuum of Care, Evidence from a broadened theoretical framework, and the applications perspective. Diane Skiba has crafted the educational section defining second life, distance education, e-learning in the information age, and innovations in e-Health. The section on research focusses on research applications, information literacy, and computerized resources. Susan Newbold represents the American Medical Informatics Association on the International Medical Informatics Association Nursing Informatics Special Interest Group. She has not only brought the readers updates from five continents/countries (South American, Canada, Europe, Asia, Australia, and New Zealand), but also brought in a new welcomed continent, Africa.

Some general impressions of the content and concepts discussed in the 5th edition are the multiple authors who refer to the Institute of Medicine landmark books *To Err Is Human* and *Crossing the Quality Chasm*. Other common references were in healthcare, IT, quality and education, the influence of the health reform legislation (*Patient Protection and Affordable Care Act* [Public Law No. 111-148] American Recovery and Reinvestment Act of 2009, and *Health Information Technology for Economic and Clinical Health Act*), and the quality and depth of understanding that nurse with a focus on the three stages of meaningful use experts have in the content areas of their respective chapters. The majority of authors who had chapters in the 4th edition did not update their chapters, but completely rewrote them since there was so much new information. The authors found it difficult in this edition to stay to their recommended page limits. The majority exceeded our expectations of chapter content and page count. Because of life circumstances or busy schedules, some authors were unable to meet commitments for the 5th edition, but we hope that they will continue to contribute through the literature in journals and future editions.

PART 1: COMPUTERS AND NURSING (VIRGINIA K. SABA)

Historical Perspective of Nursing Informatics

This section is introduced with the chapter on nursing informatics (NI) history by Virginia Saba and Bonnie

Westra who updated a similar chapter in the 4th edition. They reviewed whether the highlighted events, activities, and initiatives were critical in NI history and, if so, included them again in this chapter. A new section was added describing the NI pioneer history project which was initiated in 2004. They highlight the major history project activities, including (1) the contacting of the original 145 nurses who shaped the NI specialty; (2) the collection, storage, and indexing of their archival documents at the National Library of Medicine's history collection; (3) the lessons learned from the videotaping of 33 NI pioneers; and (4) other information, such as the Web address of where the videotapes are stored and can be viewed. They conclude the chapter with an updated and revised table on Landmark Events in Computers and Nursing.

The Davies Award for Excellence given by the Healthcare Information and Management Systems Society was updated by Patricia Wise. She describes the criterion for becoming a Davies Award winner, which marks technological innovation as well as evidence of achieving quality, reduced errors and costs, and improved outcomes of care. This chapter updates the new awardees and their recognized achievements.

PART 2: COMPUTER SYSTEMS (M. KATHLEEN SMITH)

Chapter 4, Computer Systems Basics, by Mary McHugh provides the key concepts of Computer Hardware and Software needed by today's student and user from an educator's point of view. This chapter has combined three chapters from the 4th edition (Hardware, Software, and Data Processing). She provides strategies used to permit users to store and retrieve data as well as process the data into whatever products are desired. Data is broadly described in relation to computerized information systems. The basics in this chapter set the stage for the remainder of the section.

In Chapter 5, Kathleen Smith and Denise Tyler discuss the Systems Life Cycle phases of planning, systems analysis and design, systems selection, and the first seven steps of the 14 Steps of Implementation. Careful planning, strong executive support, and early involvement of staff are key to successful implementation or upgrade of a clinical information system.

Marina Douglas and Marian Celli discuss the last seven steps of the 14 Steps of Implementation. The Informatics Nurse role is well suited to have an active and often lead role in clinical systems/electronic health record implementations. Steps 8 to 14 build on the planning and analysis discussed in Chapter 5.

Attempting to implement or upgrade a system without reviewing and completing the tasks associated with each of the 14 steps generally results in system failure in one or more of the following areas: (1) A clinical information system does not meet the stated goal of the project. (2) There is failure to gain end user acceptance. (3) Expenditures exceed budget. (4) Anticipated benefits are unrealized.

In Chapter 7, Judy Murphy and Patricia Dykes describe how healthcare project management augments the Systems Life Cycle chapters, as it outlines the project management phases, called *Process Groups*, used to organize and structure the Systems Life Cycle in order to successfully complete all the implementation steps of a project. The project management process groups progress from initiation activities to planning activities, executing activities, monitoring and controlling activities, and closing activities.

In Chapter 8, Human Factors, Gregory Alexander discusses the significant role informatics nurses are playing in understanding the complex interactions between human–machine systems as they are implemented. After completing his doctoral dissertation on this subject, Greg is the ultimate expert in discerning the literature on human factors. He succinctly provides an enormous human factors reference base for all nurses pursuing information technology. Understanding human factors enables nurses to recognize how work is performed and to develop human–machine systems that support the work of the organization, and facilitates implementing usable clinical information systems.

Peter Murray and Scott Erdley comprehensively define Open Source and Free Software (OSS/FS) explaining their differences and similarities in Chapter 9. The chapter also introduces some particular applications, operating systems, and licensing issues. Some commonly available and healthcare-specific applications are introduced with examples. Also some organizations working to explore the use of OSS/FS within healthcare and nursing with some additional resources are introduced. This chapter is filled with Websites to retrieve OSS/FS.

Kathleen Charters and Thomasine Guberski describe Mobile Computing Platforms, providing current technologies for use in the healthcare field. The chapter provides a detailed description of a variety of devices and highlights how mobile devices are being used for healthcare information systems. The authors describe how the trend of mobile devices continues to expand to include wireless connectivity. It introduces the reader to the next generation of computing in healthcare and nursing informatics.

PART 3: INFORMATICS THEORY (VIRGINIA K. SABA)

The section on informatics theory provides an update on theoretical views on NI as a distinct nursing specialty. Chapter 11 by Katheen Hunter and Carol Bickford on NI theory highlights the new information and models presented in the 2008 American Nurses Association's (ANA) updated *Nursing Informatics: Scope and Standards of Practice*. They address the pertinent core concepts, definitions, and interrelationships, including the functional areas and latest certification requirements. They list and provide a brief description of the 12 recognized nursing terminologies by the ANA.

The chapter on advanced terminology, prepared by Nicholas Hardiker, Suzanne Bakken, and Tae-Youn Kim, focuses on providing the background necessary to understand recent approaches to solving the vocabulary problem, including examples.

The chapter is followed with a chapter by Connie Delaney and Bonnie Westra on the nursing minimum data sets—NMDS, i-NMDS, and NMMDS—which are being used nationally and internationally. They provide a synthesis of historical, current, and future NMDS systems and how they can increase nursing data and information capacity to drive knowledge building for the profession and contribute to the standards supportive of the electronic health record.

The section ends with a chapter by Virginia Saba, Jacqueline Moss, and Luann Whittenburg who provide an overview of the Clinical Care Classification (CCC) System. They address how the CCC System is being used in nursing practice, education, and research, including a brief description of the CCC Costing Method that is currently being tested. A copy of the CCC System in presented in Appendix A.

PART 4: CURRENT ISSUES IN INFORMATICS (KATHLEEN A. MCCORMICK)

The 5th edition is timely in that the policies for Health IT are incentivized and the nursing profession has been a part of shaping those policies. The importance of standards nationally and globally is described by Joyce Sensmeier in Chapter 15. She clearly delineates the importance of the standards harmonization of information for system interoperability. She introduces new standards that are a global, multidisciplinary consortium to support the acquisition, exchange, submission, and archiving of clinical research data and metadata, such as the Clinical Data Interchange Standards Consortium and the National Information Exchange Model, interoperability frameworks which enable information sharing among organizations.

As Judy Murphy and Elizabeth Johnson state in Chapter 16, "Today, [nurses] constitute the largest single group of healthcare professionals, including experts who serve on national committees and participate in interoperability initiatives focused on policy, standards and terminology development, standards harmonization, and adoption." In their excellent chapter, Judy and Elizabeth discuss the significant impact of federal legislation on the use of health information technology. Whether nurses are in IT or administrative positions or practice, they should read the updates on policy from these national leaders shaping policy.

A trust framework is shaped by Dixie Baker, who served on the Office of the National Coordinator standards committee. Chapter 17 identifies the seven layers of protection essential for establishing and maintaining trust in a healthcare enterprise and explains the role trust plays in Health Information Technology adoption, quality, and safety. The seven layers include risk management, information assurance policy, physical safeguards, operational safeguards, architectural safeguards, security technology safeguards, and usability features. She relates how these Health Information Portability Accountability Act and American Recovery and Reinvestment Act of 2009 provisions relate to this framework and the implications for the nursing profession.

A challenge comes from identifying the multiple levels of policy that the nursing profession is engaged in to assure not only the advancement of informatics but also the educational and public policy implications. In Chapter 18, Amy Walker clearly defines the multiple communities that coexist in shaping policy and recommends collaboration, cross education, and information resource sharing to fully advance the healthcare provided by nurses to the American public. She provides a framework for nurses engaged in policy formulation to utilize.

In Chapter 19, Charlotte Weaver and Jennifer Moore focuses on the health policy issues of home health agencies, such as their lack of a power base, funding, and resources. They address the home health policies in relation to the U.S. federal reimbursement schemes, including a comparison of similar policies in other countries. Also, they highlight health reform legislation and how the American Recovery and Reinvestment Act of 2009 is opening the door to include the emphasis on home healthcare.

PART 5: CONTINUUM OF CARE INFORMATION TECHNOLOGY SYSTEMS (GAIL E. LATIMER)

As with the transformation planned for American healthcare, the section Practice Application from the 4th edition has transformed in the 5th edition to the section Continuum of Care Information Technology Systems. This new section was revised to reflect the Healthcare industry and initiatives, concepts, and solutions needed to support the change. Readers will experience the new continuum of care and environment of health from episode to episode of care delivery models. Their knowledge will expand as case studies and best practices are addressed to create new cultures and environments, theories, and applications.

The United States has experience an unprecedented period with Healthcare reform. Information Technology plays a critical role in the transformation, in that the U.S. government has instituted laws and financial rewards around the rich adoption of information technology. Hence, authors will reference the American Recovery and Reinvestment Act of 2009 and the "interim final rule." At the time of this edition's publication, several areas of the final rules have not been defined, so the authors have provided Websites for your reference.

This newly created section, Part 5, begins with a comprehensive, detailed chapter addressing consideration on implementing computerized provider order entry (CPOE). Emily Barey's chapter on CPOE is a must read to all considering meaningful use, no matter if the health system is considering going for the reward (money).

In Chapter 21, Ann Farrell and Sheryl Taylor were very busy surveying the major IT vendors to update their chapter. They have expanded their survey to include evidence-based clinical content and standardized terminology. Note the care flow diagram has been updated.

Matthew Grissinger and Michelle Mandrack provide a comprehensive chapter evaluating the role technology can play in safe medication practice. Patient safety is a core value for all clinicians and in all environments were care is provided.

New leadership styles and problem solving techniques are needed for the newly transformed health environment. Thomas Clancy's overview of a complex adaptive system and case study is sure to shift your thinking and provide topics for team discussion. Future leaders must embrace the principles of Complexity Theory for todays and future success. These chapters are followed by Chapter 25 where Mical DeBrow and Cynthia Mascara describe how workflow and healthcare process management can help support a more efficient, safer, and cost-effective information flow. One example of an advanced workflow technology system embedded within a healthcare information system is described in their chapter.

Several chapters describe the evidence perspective of healthcare. Chapter 26, by Lynn McQueen, Health Carter-Templeton, and Kathleen McCormick, is a broad framework of the many types of evidence being discussed from research and practice. This comprehensive chapter describes case studies that demonstrate the use of evidence in improving healthcare. In Chapter 27, Joanne Seasholtz and Bernadette Melnyk focus on the information technology supporting evidence with a focus on improving quality of care. They discuss how different vendors approach incorporating evidence in their information systems. The chapter by Ida Androwich and Margaret Kraft focuses on computerized decision support systems designed to support decision-making activities. They stress why such systems use an enormous amount of data to facilitate decision processes on the delivery and management of patient care.

Magnet-designated hospitals have demonstrated nursing excellence through successful shared governance structures and cultures of professional practice and benchmarking metrics. IT plays a critical role in all five components of the ANCC Magnet Model. Andrea Schmid-Mazzoccoli, a Magnet surveyor, provided a comprehensive overview of the new Magnet Model in Chapter 29. Health systems around the globe look to regulatory standards and the Institute of Safe Medicine Practice for best practice to ensure a culture of safety.

The Continuum of Care section ends with a shift to where healthcare is delivered, not the hospitals but the community. Researchers hypothesize that there will not be enough physicians to meet the demands of the baby boomers. Mary Ann Lavin, Laketa Entzminger, and Mary Lee Barron address the role technology will play to support advanced practice. Susan Lundquist's and Cathy Delmain's new chapter on the rural market opens a whole new perspective on healthcare in rural and critical access hospitals. Adoption of Ambulatory Care Systems and demonstrating meaningful use are critical components of U.S. healthcare reform. In Chapter 32, Susan Newhold highlights information systems in ambulatory care settings. Susan provides an overview of the role technology plays and the need for sharing data, and an overview of all aspects of ambulatory care that impact on the required IT, such as where clients are treated, benefits for nurses, implementation, and resources. She

extensively list the organizations involved in ambulatory care information systems.

Susan Quinn shares a perspective of the post acute environment, defined as services provided in the community, not in a facility. She addresses the main drivers of reimbursement, terminology, and interoperability. She wraps up Chapter 33 with future trends.

The last two chapters are a sign of the new healthcare world—Public Health and Emergency Planning and Response. A new chapter on practice applications in public health by Judy Gibson, Janise Richards, Arunkumar Srinivasan, and Derryl Block brings an aspect to the continuum of care that is sometimes overlooked. They provide an overview of applications in informatics, describe legislation that has affected public health information systems, and provide examples of electronic data exchange between clinical care and public health. They also introduce the emerging role of the public health nurse informatician and how it differs from the role of the public health nurse. These authors address the trends and surveillance needed in a new world of healthcare and prevention. While Betsy Weiner and Lynn Slepski shift our thinking to responses to manmade and natural challenges and the role an electronic health record can play in supporting people in a time of need.

Revising this section and working with these exceptional content experts was an enlightening experience. The authors and I will feel we have achieved success if after reading this new section we can change your paradigms and thinking.

PART 6: EDUCATIONAL APPLICATIONS (DIANE SKIBA)

The Internet has changed the way we work, the way we learn, the way we play, and now even the way we receive healthcare. As of June 2010, there were over 1.9 billion users worldwide (http://www.internetworld stats.com/stats.htm). Although the Internet has been around for many years, the introduction of the World Wide Web allowed "everyday" users to access information and knowledge from around the globe. The Web allows users to not only find the information and knowledge one needs but now with Web 2.0 tools allows one to create, interact, and publish their own information and knowledge.

Many have written that the Internet and the Web, like the personal computer, are disruptive innovations (http://www.claytonchristensen.com/disruptive_innovation.html). This term, introduced by Clayton Christensen, refers to an innovation that challenges the current established product or service and provides a less expensive alternative, thus allowing more consumers access to this product or service. In this section, the reader will learn how disruptive innovations in healthcare and education are changing the delivery and access to these services. You will also get a glimpse of other technologies associated with social media and mobile applications that may ultimately push what John Doerr calls the third wave of disruptive innovations (http://www.kpcb.com/team/doerr).

Chapter 36, Web 2.0 and Its Impact on Healthcare Education and Practice, by Diane Skiba, Paul Guillory, and Kay Lynn Olmstead, provides a foundation for the examination of disruptive innovations. This chapter describes the evolution of the Internet and the Web with a particular emphasis on Web 2.0 and its associated tools. In the second iteration of the Web, the dynamics have changed from a dissemination platform to one that is collaborative, interactive, user-generated, and supportive of the wisdom of the crowd concept. The chapter examines the use of Web 2.0 tools, especially social software such as communication, social writing, social bookmarking, and social networking tools, in both education and healthcare. There is no doubt many of these tools are disruptive to the current methods of education and healthcare delivery.

Chapter 37, by Patricia Allen, Khadija Bakrim, Darlene Lacy, Enola Boyd, and Myrna Armstrong, focuses on the delivery of cost-effective, high-quality education at a distance. The chapter traces the history of distance education and provides a current snapshot of online education. Although the market demand for online education continues to increase, the authors noted that there is still some skepticism related to quality. The chapter tackles the quality issues from both student and faculty perspectives, as well as challenges related to effectiveness and intellectual property.

Marilyn Nielsen and Amy Barton's Chapter 38 explores the concept of healthcare at a distance. This chapter examines the evolution of e-Health and how it is distinctive from telemedicine and telehealth. They describe the potential disruptive innovation of mobile health and its various applications. Numerous examples are given on how e-Health applications are transforming healthcare, education, and research. The chapter also contains an examination of the challenges as e-Health evolves and changes the way healthcare is delivered. The chapter concludes with an e-Health case study.

In Chapter 39, Rita Zielstorff and Barbara Frink examine the use of computers by consumers and patients for healthcare. This comprehensive review of the consumer engagement in their healthcare not only examines consumer use of a variety of tools but also demonstrates the potential of disruptive innovations and their impact on healthcare. The chapter identifies the major challenges of consumer and patient computing, such as privacy and security, the digital divide, quality of health information, impact on patient-provider relationships, and potential solutions. The authors also address the role of the informatics specialists in consumer and patient computing and potential research areas for further investigation. There is an extensive list of resources and readings at the conclusion of the chapter.

Equipped with a solid foundation of the current and potential tools shaping the delivery of healthcare education and practice, it is important to examine the impact on nursing education in general as well as the education of informatics specialists. Chapter 40, by Eun-Shim Nahm and Marisa Wilson, describes how the convergences of driving forces, such as federal initiatives, technology advances, and consumer engagement, are influencing the transformation of informatics education. The chapter addresses the need for informatics competencies for various levels of nursing education and for nursing faculty.

Judith Warren, Helen Connors, and Patricia Trangenstein, in Chapter 41, describe an innovative approach to provide immersive educational environments to teach nurses, in particular nursing informatics students. In the chapter, they not only describe the pedagogy of using simulations and Second Life in health professional education but also examine the various strategies for educating students in Second Life. Faculty and administration considerations for the use of Second Life in education are explored. The chapter contains images of the University of Kansas Medical Center Island in Second Life.

In the concluding chapter in this section by Michelle Troseth, she describes the evolution of the Technology Informatics Guiding Education Reform (TIGER) Initiative since its inception in 2004. This grassroots effort has made significant use of intellectual and social capital across nursing organizations and professionals to promote what all current and future nurses need the necessary knowledge and skills to practice in an ever-increasing technology-rich and consumer-centric healthcare environment.

PART 7: RESEARCH APPLICATIONS (VIRGINIA K. SABA)

The section on research applications addresses two major aspects of computer use in nursing research—research applications and information literacy and computerized resources. The first chapter, by Veronica Feeg and Theresa Rienzo, provides an overview of the software applications related to the stages of the research process; how computers facilitate the work of the research in both quantitative and qualitative aspects; and computer research use for the major healthcare categories. They provide an excellent step by step overview of the research process, starting with proposal, implementation, analyses, and dissemination.

This second chapter in this section, by Diane Pravikoff, June Levy, and Annelle Tanner, provides information about electronic resources that are easily available and accessible and that can assist nurses in maintaining and enhancing their professional practices. They identify the resources that aid the nurse in keeping current with the published literature and information sources for nursing practice, research, and/or education. The findings of a national study of computerized information literacy are provided, which had indicated the lack of nursing knowledge and competency in this field. They provide an extensive list of electronic resources with their Web addresses.

PART 8: INTERNATIONAL PERSPECTIVES (SUSAN K. NEWBOLD)

The excellent integration of evidence into research to measure outcomes is especially informative in the chapter on Canada, by Lynn Nagle, Kathryn Hannah, and Nora Hammell, where their Information Highway is described. Heimar Marin updates the policies, education, and practice in South America.

The changes going on in Europe are defined by Kaija Saranto, Virpi Jylhä, and Kaarina Tanttu. This chapter is an intricate look at each of the member states in the European Union and the e-Health initiatives and comparative data on the continent. They update the use of nursing terminologies in Europe, give examples of nursing informatics education throughout Europe, and examples of cooperation among National Nurses' Associations working together to advance nursing practice, quality care, workforce issues, and nursing informatics competencies. In addition, they describe national demonstrations for documenting nursing in electronic health records with an example of using meaningful use data from structured data. Future developments include the expansion of more sophisticated data acquisition, statistical analysis, and tools for reporting benchmarks at organizational and national levels.

Coordinating the Pacific Rim and including Australia, New Zealand, and Hong Kong is a comprehensive

update from Evelyn Hovenga, Michelle Honey, Lucy Westbrooke, and Robyn Carr. The Asia perspective is described by Hyeoun-Ae Park who coordinated Korea, Japan, and Taiwan. This chapter updates the use of nursing terminology in Asia and describes the expansion of ubiquitous computing in Korea such as the "smart digital home," "health management and health promotion using U-IT technology for the underprivileged population," "Ubiquitous home healthcare for the elderly", and the "u-City project."

Finally, for the first time, the continent of Africa is represented in a chapter by Irene van Middelkoop and Susan Meyer. For newcomers, they have clearly articulated formation of nursing informatics in South Africa, the problems of implementing computerization in a resource constrained environment, the barriers to forming a nursing informatics specialty, and the emergence of how nurses are using technology and standards. This is especially significant in that Africa was the host country to MEDINFO in 2010.

PART 9: THE FUTURE OF INFORMATICS (KATHLEEN A. MCCORMICK)

While we have one chapter on the future, as noted by Kathleen McCormick, all of the chapters point to a future in nursing informatics. We witness in version 5.0 the focus on the patient in this edition but recognize that the individual patient is a part of an enterprise of healthcare environments. To explain individual health, the information has to be translated from large population studies, evidence, through information systems that are interoperable and integrate data, and services to ultimately improve patient quality and safety. The dependencies on the activities in different environments lead to a broader understanding of the total patient clinical care and the component of their health as participants in a population, and the target of improved quality and safety. The concept of access has expanded to include the ability to aggregate individual data through patient matching of age, gender, ethnicity, health condition, genotype, and those who do or do not respond to treatments. The adaptive clinical trial is introduced as a new method to accommodate this new personalized health paradigm. The next level of matching is to providers who have similar types of patients. The final level is to match patients to improve access, quality of care, outcomes, and report notifiable diseases in surveillance networks. The essential goal is to be able to contribute, encrypt or deidentify information, aggregate or group data in a technically secure environment, and reprocess or reuse patient data. Data have the potential to go from environments to regional, national, and global exchanges.

SUMMARY

In summary, the variations in use of computer technology in nursing practice have expanded both in the United States and internationally. This book, like the IT community IS *GLOBAL*. It describes our shared challenges, successes, and requirements for going forward together as we utilize information technology to improve the quality of care to patients in diverse environments, improve patient safety and the effectiveness of patient care, and utilize evidence in delivering care. We have so much to learn from each other in the implementations of technology toward nursing care. The global network of nursing in informatics can be declared a victory for the "army of nursing informatics." It has been a privilege to work with the individual authors and new section editors in bringing this 5th edition to the readers. We hope you enjoy reading these chapters as much as we have.

Historical Perspectives of Nursing Informatics

Virginia K. Saba / Bonnie L. Westra

- ## OBJECTIVES
  1. Identify a brief historical perspective of nursing informatics.
  2. Explore lessons learned from the pioneers in nursing informatics.
  3. List the major landmark events and milestones of nursing informatics.

- ## KEY WORDS
  computer literacy
  computer systems
  data standards
  information systems
  Internet
  nursing informatics

OVERVIEW

The importance of computer and health information technology (HIT) as an essential tool in the delivery of contemporary healthcare is indisputable. Computerization affects all aspects of healthcare delivery including provision of care, education of healthcare providers, scientific research required for advancing healthcare delivery, administration of healthcare delivery services, reimbursement for care, and the legal and ethical implications involved in healthcare provision. Modern healthcare consumers use computers, various technologies, and processes associated with them in a multitude of healthcare activities.

Health information technology is an all-encompassing term referring to any technology that captures, processes, and stores health information. Initially HIT primarily referred to computer systems. However, with the vast expansion of technology, nurses have supported the consumers to evolve to a consumer-centric healthcare system. HIT now refers to multidisciplinary use of technology, including use by consumers and public health professionals. Over the history of nursing informatics, there has been a shift from the use of mainframe computers with dumb terminals in which nursing documentation was largely ignored toward the use of multiple technologies including wireless, handheld, and mobile computers; radio-frequency technologies; and interoperable electronic health records that support continuity of care across healthcare settings and information systems.

Computers in nursing are used to manage patient care information, monitor quality, and evaluate outcomes. Computers and networks are now used for communicating (sending and receiving) data and messages via the Internet, accessing resources, and interacting with patients on the Web. Nurses are increasingly involved with systems used for planning, budgeting, and policy making for patient care services as well as enhancing nursing education and distance learning with new media modalities. Computers are also used to support nursing research, test new systems, design new knowledge databases, and advance the role of nursing in the healthcare industry.

This chapter is an updated and revised version of the chapter "Historical Perspectives of Nursing and the Computer" published in the 4th edition, *Essentials of for Nursing Informatics* (Saba & Erdley, 2006). In this chapter the significant events influencing nursing informatics are analyzed according to (1) **six time periods**; (2) a synthesis of lessons learned from 33 videotaped interviews with **nursing informatics pioneers**; 3) **standards initiatives** including nursing practice and education, nursing content, and confidentiality and security standards; (4) **healthcare data standards organizations;** (5) **significant landmark events**; and (6) a table with **major landmark milestones** listing those events that influenced the introduction of computers into the nursing profession including the key "computer/informatics" nurse that directed the activity.

MAJOR HISTORICAL PERSPECTIVES OF NURSING AND COMPUTERS

Six Time Periods

Prior to the 1960s. Computers were first developed in the late 1930s to early 1940s, but use in the healthcare industry occurred in the 1950's. During this time, there were only a few experts who formed a cadre of pioneers that attempted to adapt computers to healthcare and nursing. At this time the nursing profession was also undergoing major changes. The image of nursing was evolving, the number of nurses increasing, and nursing practices and services were expanding in scope, autonomy, and complexity from physicians' handmaidens to professional status. These events provided the impetus for the profession to embrace computers.

Computers were initially used in healthcare facilities for basic office administrative and financial accounting functions. These early computers used punch cards to store data and card readers to read computer programs, sort, and prepare data for processing. They were linked together and operated by paper tape and used teletypewriters to print their output. As computer technology advanced, the healthcare technologies also advanced.

1960s. During the 1960s the uses of computer technology in healthcare settings began to be questioned.

Questions such as "Why use computers?" and "What should be computerized?" were discussed. Nursing practice standards were reviewed, and nursing resources were analyzed. Studies were conducted to determine how computer technology could be utilized effectively in the healthcare industry and what areas of nursing should be automated. The nurses' station in the hospital was viewed as the hub of information exchange, the most appropriate center for the development of the computer applications.

By the mid-1960s, clinical practice presented nurses with new opportunities for computer use. Increasingly complex patient care requirements and the proliferation of intensive care units required that nurses become super users of computer technology as nurses monitored patients' status via cardiac monitors and instituted treatment regimens through ventilators and other computerized devices. A significant increase in time spent by nurses documenting patient care, in some cases estimated at 40% (Wolkodoff, 1963; Sherman, 1965), as well as a noted rise in medication administration errors prompted the need to investigate emerging hospital computer information systems.

1970s. During the late 1960s through the 1970s, hospitals began developing computer-based information systems which initially focused on physician order entry and results reporting; pharmacy, laboratory, and radiology reports; information for financial and managerial purposes; physiologic monitoring systems in the intensive care units; and a few systems started to include care planning, decision support, and interdisciplinary problem lists. While the content contained in early hospital information systems frequently was not specific to nursing practice, several systems provided nurses with a foundation on which to base future nurse information systems (Blackmon et al., 1982; Collen, 1995; Ozbolt & Bakken, 2003; Romano, McCormick, & McNeely, 1982). Regardless of the focus, which remained primarily medical practice, nurses often were involved in implementing HIT systems.

Interest in computers and nursing also emerged in public and home health and education during the 1960s to 1970s. Automation in public health agencies began as a result of pressure to standardize data collection procedures and provide statewide reports on the activities and health of the public (Parker, Ausman, & Overdovitz, 1965). In the 1970s, conferences sponsored by the Division of Nursing, Public Health Service, and the National League for Nursing helped public and home health nurses understand the importance of nursing data, the relationship to Medicare and Medicaid requirements, and the usefulness of computers for capturing and aggregating information. Additional government-sponsored conferences focused on education about computers for nurses (Public Health Service, 1976). At the same time that hospitals and public health embarked on investigating computers and nursing, the opportunity to improve education with computer technology also began. Bitzer (1966) reported on one of the first uses of a computerized teaching system called PLATO, as an alternative to traditional classroom education.

The early nursing networks, which were conceived at health informatics organizational meetings, helped to expand nursing awareness of computers and the impact HIT could have on practice. The state of technology initially limited opportunities for nurses to contribute to the HIT design, but as technology evolved toward the later part of the 1970s and as nurses provided workshops nationally, nurses gained confidence that they could use computers to improve practice. The National League of Nursing, Public Health Services, the US Army Nurse Corps, and several University Schools of Nursing provided educational conferences and workshops on the state-of-the-art regarding computer technology and its influence on nursing. During this time, the Clinical Center at the National Institutes of Health implemented one of the earliest clinical information systems in nursing practice.

1980s. The field of informatics emerged in the healthcare industry and nursing in the 1980s. Technology challenged creative professionals and the use of computers in nursing became revolutionary. As computer systems were implemented, the needs of nursing took on a cause-and-effect modality; that is, as new computer technologies emerged and as computer architecture advanced, the need for nursing software evolved. It became apparent that the nursing profession needed to update its practice standards and determine its data standards, vocabularies, and classification schemes that could be coded for the computer-based patient record systems.

During this period, many mainframe health information systems (HISs) emerged with nursing subsystems. These systems documented several aspects of the patient record; namely, provider order entry emulating the Kardex, results reporting, vital signs, and other systems documented narrative nursing notes using word-processing software packages. Discharge planning systems were developed and used as referrals to community, public, and home healthcare facilities in the continuum of care.

In the 1980s, the microcomputer or personal computer (PC) emerged. This revolutionary technology made computers more accessible, affordable, and usable by nurses and other healthcare providers. PCs brought computing power to the workplace and, more importantly, to the point of care. PCs served as dumb terminals linked to the mainframe computers and as stand-alone systems (workstations). The PCs were user-friendly and allowed nurses to design and program their own applications

Nurses began presenting at multidisciplinary conferences and formed their own working groups within HIT organizations. There were significant changes in reimbursement and healthcare legislation that increased the demand in healthcare facilities to collect, analyze, and disseminate aggregated clinical information. As medical informatics evolved, nursing began focusing on what was unique about nursing within the context of informatics. Resolutions were passed by the American Nurses Association (ANA) to form a Council on Computer Applications in Nursing (CCAN). Nursing informatics newsletters, journals, and books started to be published.

1990s. By the 1990s, large integrated healthcare delivery systems evolved, further creating the need for information across organizations within these large systems to standardize processes, control costs, and assure quality of care (Shortliffe, Perreault, Wiederhold, & Pagan, 2003). Improvements in networks and the growth of the Web allowed organizations to connect more effectively and increased access to information that supported practice. Advances in relational databases, client-server architectures, and new programming methods created the opportunity for better application development at lower costs. Legislative activity in the mid 1990s paved the way for electronic health records through the Health Insurance Portability and Accountability Act (HIPAA) of 1996 (public-law 104-191), emphasizing standardized transactions, and privacy and security of patient-identifiable information (Gallagher, 2010). The complexity of technology, workflow analysis, and regulations shaped new roles for nursing.

In 1992, the ANA recognized nursing informatics as a specialty with a separate scope of practice, standards, and certification examination (ANA, 2001, 2008). Numerous local, national, and international organizations provided a forum for networking and continuing education for nurses involved with informatics (Sackett & Erdley, 2002). The demand for nursing informatics (NI) expertise increased in the healthcare industry and other settings where nurses functioned, and the technology revolution continued to impact the nursing profession.

The need for computer-based nursing practice standards, data standards, nursing minimum data sets, and national databases emerged concurrent with the need for a unified nursing language, including nomenclatures, vocabularies, taxonomies, and classification schemes (Westra, Delaney, Konicek & Keenan, 2008). Nurse administrators demanded that the HIT include nursing care protocols and nurse educators continued to require use of innovative technologies for all levels and types of nursing and patient education. Also, nurse researchers required knowledge representation, decision support, and expert systems based on standards that allowed for aggregated data (Bakken, 2006).

Technology rapidly changed in the 1990s, increasing its use within and across nursing units, as well as across healthcare facilities. PCs continued to get smaller and notebooks were becoming affordable, increasing the volume of computers available for nurses to use. Linking computers through networks both within hospitals and health systems as well as across systems facilitated the flow of patient information to provide better care. Additionally, the Internet began providing access to information and knowledge databases to be integrated into bedside systems. By 1995, the Internet had moved into the mainstream social milieu with electronic mail (e-mail), file transfer protocol (FTP), Gopher, Telnet, and World Wide Web (WWW) protocols, which greatly enhanced its usability and user-friendliness (Saba, 1996; Sparks, 1996). The Internet also was used for high-performance computing and communication (HPCC) or the "information super-highway." It facilitated data exchange between computerized patient record systems across facilities and settings and over time. The Web became integral for information systems and the means for nurses to browse the Internet and search worldwide resources (Nicoll, 1998; Saba, 1995).

Post 2000. A 'C' change occurred in the new millennium as more and more health information became digitalized and newer technologies emerged. With the 2004 Executive Order 13335 establishing the Office of the National Coordinator (ONC) for Health Information Technology and calling for all healthcare providers to adopt interoperable electronic health records (EHRs) by 2014, the use of EHRs exploded. The challenge for nurses became the design of systems to support their workflow as well as the integration of information from multiple sources to support the knowledge work of nurses. In late 2000, as hospitals became "paperless" they now began employing new nurses who had never charted on paper.

Technological developments that influence healthcare and nursing include data capture and data sharing technologies. Wireless point of care, regional database projects, and increased IT solutions proliferated in healthcare environments, but predominately in hospitals and large healthcare systems. The use of bar coding and radio-frequency identification (RFID) emerged as a useful technology to match patients with the right medications to improve patient safety. RFID also is emerging to help nurses find equipment, or scan patients to assure all surgical equipment is removed from inside patients before surgical sites are closed (Westra, 2009). Smaller mobile devices with wireless or internet access such as notebooks, tablet PCs, personal digital assistants (PDAs), and smart cellular telephones increased access to information for nurses within hospitals and in the community. The development and subsequent refinement of voice over Internet protocol (VoIP) today provides inexpensive voice communication for healthcare organizations.

The Internet also provided a means for development of clinical applications. Databases for EHRs could be hosted remotely on the Internet, decreasing costs of implementing EHRs. Remote monitoring of multiple critical care units from a single site increased access for safe and effective cardiac care (Rajecki, 2008). Home healthcare has also increasingly partnered with information technology for the provision of patient care. Telehealth applications, a recognized specialty for nursing since the late 1990s, provided a means for nurses to monitor patients at home and support specialty consultation in rural and underserved areas.

A combination of the economic recession along with the escalating cost of healthcare resulted in the American Recovery and Reinvestment Act of 2009 (ARRA) providing Health Information Technology for Economic and Clinical Health (HITECH) funding to select and implement EHRs, support health information exchange, enhance community- and university-based informatics education, and support leading edge research to improve the use of HIT (Gallagher, 2010). The billions of dollars invested are intended to move the health industry forward toward complete digitalization of health information. Meanwhile the Centers for Medicare and Medicaid Services (CMS) have increased reimbursement for 'meaningful use' of EHRs through 2015 and then penalize eligible providers and facilities who do not meet 'meaningful use' criteria by that date. Nurses are involved with all phases from implementation of systems, assuring meaningful use of EHRs, and evolving health policy affecting EHR systems.

Another impact of the escalating cost of healthcare is a shift toward a consumer-centric healthcare system. Consumers are encouraged to be active partners in managing their own health. A variety of technologies have evolved to enable consumers to have access to their health information and choose whether to share this across healthcare providers and settings. Personal health records multiplied as either stand-alone systems or those tethered to EHRs. Consumers are increasing in health information literacy as they demand to become more involved in managing their own health.

NURSING INFORMATICS PIONEERS

History Project

Beginning in 2004, the rich stories of pioneers in nursing informatics were captured through a project sponsored by the American Medical Informatics Association Nursing Informatics Working Group (AMIA-NIWG). The AMIA-NIWG History Committee developed an evolving list of pioneers and contributors to the history of nursing informatics. Pioneers were defined as those who "opened up" a new area in nursing informatics and provided a sustained contribution to the specialty (Westra & Newbold, 2006; Newbold & Westra, 2009). Through multiple contacts and review of the literature, the list grew to 145 pioneers and contributors who shaped nursing informatics since the 1950s. Initially, each identified pioneer was contacted to submit their nonpublished documents and/or historical materials to the National Library of Medicine's (NLM) to be indexed and archived for the Nursing Informatics History Collection. Approximately 25 pioneers submitted historical materials that were cataloged with a brief description.

Currently, the cataloged document descriptions can be searched online: www.nlm.nih.gov/hmd/manuscripts/accessions.html. The documents can be viewed by visiting the NLM. Eventually each archived document will be indexed and available online in the NI History Collection. Also from the original list, a convenience sample of pioneers was interviewed over a 4-year period at various nursing informatics meetings. Videotaped stories from thirty-three pioneers were recorded and are now available on the AMIA website: www.amia.org/niwg-history-page.

Videotaped Interviews. The AMIA Nursing Informatics History page contains a wealth of information. The 33 videotaped interviews are divided into two libraries. The full interviews are available in Library 1: Nursing Informatics Pioneers. For each pioneer, a picture, short biographical sketch, transcript of the interview, and MP3 audio file are included in addition to the videotaped interview. In Library 2: Themes from Interviews, selected segments from the interviews are shared for easy comparison across the pioneers. The themes include:

- Nursing informatics—what it is, present, future, what nursing brings to the table
- Significant events that have shaped the field of nursing informatics
- Pioneers' paths—careers that lead up to involvement in (nursing) informatics
- When they first considered themselves informatics nurses
- Pioneers' first involvement—earliest events they recall
- Informatics—its value, pioneers' realizations of the value of informatics, how they came to understand the value of informatics
- Demographic of pioneers including names, educational backgrounds, current positions
- Personal aspirations and accomplishments, overall vision that guided the pioneers' work, people the pioneer collaborated with to accomplish their visions and goals
- Pioneers' lessons learned that they would like to pass on

The website also provides "use cases" for ideas about how to use the information for teaching and learning more about the pioneers. These resources are particularly useful for courses in informatics, leadership, and research. They also are useful for nurses in the workforce who want to learn more about nursing informatics history.

Backgrounds. The early pioneers came from a variety of backgrounds as nursing education in nursing informatics didn't exist in the 1960s. Almost all of the pioneers were educated as nurses, though a few were not. A limited number of pioneers had additional education in computer science, engineering, epidemiology, and biostatistics. Others were involved with anthropology, philosophy, physiology, and public health. Their career paths varied considerably. Some nursing faculty saw technology as a way to improve education. Others worked in clinical settings and were involved in "roll-outs" of information systems. Often these systems weren't designed to improve nursing work, but the pioneers had a vision that technology could make nursing practice better. Other pioneers gained experience through research projects or working for software vendors. The commonality for all the pioneers is they saw various problems and inefficiencies in nursing and they had a burning desire to use technology to "make things better."

Lessons Learned. What are some of the lessons learned from the pioneers? Pioneers by definition are nurses who forged into the unknown and had a vision of what was possible, even if they didn't know how to get there. One of the pioneers advised, "Don't be afraid to take on something that you've never done before. You can learn how to do it. The trick is in finding out who knows it and picking their brain and if necessary, cornering them and making them teach you!" Another said, "Just do it, rise above it [barriers], and go for it… you are a professional, and…you have to be an advocate for yourself and the patient." Many of the pioneers described the importance of mentors, someone who would teach them about informatics or computer technology, but it was still up to them to apply their new knowledge to improve nursing. Mentors were invaluable by listening, exchanging ideas, connecting to others, and supporting new directions. Networking was another strong theme for pioneers. Belonging to professional organizations, especially interprofessional organizations, was key for success. At meetings, the pioneers networked and exchanged ideas, learning from others what worked and, more importantly, what didn't work. They emphasized the importance of attending social functions at organizational meetings to develop solid relationships so they could call on colleagues later to further network and exchange ideas.

Accomplishments. The nursing informatics pioneers described many accomplishments. Early work for many of the pioneers focused on *terminology development*, which means standardizing the terms used by nursing to describe care of patients. While early terminology work began in the 1970s with the North American Nursing Diagnoses Association, the Omaha System, the Clinical Care Classification (CCC) System, the Nursing Minimum Data Set (NMDS), and the Nursing Management Minimum Data Set (NMMDS) in the 1980s provided the framework for the documentation of the essential data elements to explain not only care of patients but the context of care. Other pioneers focused on implementing information systems, care plan functionality, and decision-making rules in information systems to support the cognitive work of nurses. As nursing informatics grew, there was a focus

on identifying informatics competencies to educate the next generation of nurses.

Nursing informatics did not occur in a vacuum; a major effort was made to promote the inclusion of nurses in organizations affecting health policy decisions such as the National Committee on Vital and Health Statistics (NCVHS), American National Standards Institute (ANSI), Health Level 7 (HL7), and more recently the ONC for Health Information Technology Policy and Standards Committees. The nursing pioneers influenced the evolution of informatics as a specialty from granular-level data through health policy and funding to shape this evolving and highly visible specialty in nursing.

Standards Initiatives

The third significant historic perspective concerns standards initiatives focusing on nursing practice standards, nursing content standards, and confidentiality and security standards as well as federal legislation that impacts the use of computers for nursing. These standards have influenced the nursing profession and its need for computer systems with appropriate content or terminologies. Legislative acts during the early stages significantly influenced the use of computers to collect federally required data, carry out reimbursement, measure quality, and evaluate outcomes. This section only highlights briefly the critical initiatives "to set the stage" for more information in other chapters of this book.

Nursing Practice and Education Standards. Nursing practice standards have been developed and recommended by the ANA, the official professional nursing organization. The ANA published *Nursing Scope & Standards of Practice* (ANA, 2004) that focused not only on the organizing principles of clinical nursing practice but also on the standards of professional performance. The six phases of the nursing process serve as the conceptual framework for the documentation of nursing practice. The updated *Nursing Informatics Scope & Standards of Practice* (ANA, 2008) builds on clinical practice standards, outlining further the importance for implementing standardized content to support nursing practice by specialists in nursing informatics. The American Association of Colleges of Nursing (AACN), which accredits nursing education programs, revised *The Essentials for Doctoral Education for Advanced Nursing Practice* (AACN, 2006) and *The Essentials of Baccalaureate Education for Professional Nursing Practice* (AACN, 2008) to require the use of computers and informatics for both baccalaureate and graduate education. These new requirements for informatics competencies prepare nurses to use HIT successfully and to contribute to the ongoing design of technologies that support the cognitive work of nurses.

Nursing Content Standards. The nursing process elements in EHRs are essential for the exchange of nursing information across information systems and settings. The original data elements and the historic details of nursing data standards are described in the third edition of this book. Standardization of healthcare data began in 1893 with the *List of International Causes of Death* (World Health Organization, 1992) for the reporting of morbidity cases worldwide, however the standardizing of nursing data has a history beginning in 1973 (Westra et al., 2008). Prior to that time nursing theorists proposed concepts, activities, tasks, goals, and so forth, as well as frameworks as a theoretical foundation for the practice of nursing, which could not be processed by computer. Since 1973 several nursing organizations, educational institutions, and vendors developed nursing data sets, classifications, or terminologies for the documentation of nursing practice. These nursing terminologies were developed at different times by different organizations or universities. They vary in content (representing one or more nursing process data elements), most appropriate setting for use, and level of access in the public domain.

Currently, the ANA has recognized 12 nursing terminologies. (See Chapter 11 *The Practice Specialty of Nursing Informatics* for their descriptions). The ANA is also responsible for determining whether the terminology met the criteria, 6 of which have been included in the National Library of Medicine's (NLM) Metathesaurus of the Unified Medical Language System (UMLS) (Humphreys & Lindberg, 1992; Saba, 1998) and in the Systematized Nomenclature of Medicine—Clinical Terms (SNOMED-CT).

Of the 12 terminologies recognized by the ANA, 3 are reference terminologies that include multiple nursing terminologies: SNOMED-CT, Logical Observation Identifiers Names and Codes (LOINC), and the International Classification of Nursing Practice (ICNP). One of the exciting advances for nursing is the recent recognition of the ICNP as one of the WHO's Family of Disease & Health Related Classifications, equivalent to the ICD-10 (WHO, 1992). This worldwide recognition is a watershed event for recognition that nursing terms are important to describe health and healthcare in HITs. Currently, ICNP and SNOMED-CT, as reference terminologies, are collaborating, meaning that the ICNP terms are being incorporated into SNOMED-CT (International Council of Nursing, 2010). This does not preclude using the CCC System (See Chapter 14: *Overview of the CCC System and Appendix A*) as an interface terminology for the actual point-of-care documentation and linking with SNOMED-CT for the mapping across settings.

Confidentiality and Security Standards. Increasing access through the electronic capture and exchange of information raised concerns about the privacy and security of personal health information (PHI). Provisions for strengthening the original HIPAA legislation were included in the 2009 HITECH Act (Gallagher, 2010). Greater emphasis was placed on patient consent, more organizations handling PHI were included in the legislation, and penalties were increased for security breaches.

Heath Care Data Standards Organizations

It is believed that there are a large number of standards organizations that influence healthcare data and content as well as the architecture, functional requirements, and certification of EHRs. Only a few key organizations that impact health information technology (HIT) Systems are described here. (Also see Chapter 15: *Health Data Standards Development*).

American National Standards Institute. The American National Standards Institute (ANSI) is the leading U.S. organization for coordinating and promoting voluntary consensus standards in healthcare. ANSI, founded in 1918, is a private nonprofit membership organization established to coordinate and approve voluntary consensus standards efforts in the United States (ANSI-2008). ANSI combined with the Healthcare Informatics Standards Board (HISB) to form ANSI-HISB to fulfill a request by the European standards coordinating organization (CEN TC/251) to represent the U.S. standards effort. Thus, the ANSI-HISB organization acted as one, linking to the two major organizations in Europe, the European Standardization Committee (CEN) and International Standards Organization (ISO).

In 2005 the ANSI-HISB was integrated with the ONC Healthcare Information Technology Standards Panel (HITSP) to successfully serve the Office of the National Coordinator of Health Informatics and Technology as a coordinating body to facilitate and promote the development and use of national and international healthcare information standards (ANSI, 2008).

The new HITSP, guided by ANSI, brought together a cross section of public and private sector interests: vendors, clinicians, academia, consumers, federal health agencies including the Military Health System and the VA Health Administration, and several standards development organizations (SDOs) to examine and participate in developing principles and strategy for U.S. health standards selection. The HITSP mission was to determine a widely accepted and useful set of standards to enable widespread interoperability among healthcare software applications and support a local, regional, and national health information network for the United States.

Early in the standards review process ANSI HITSP recognized that an interoperable nursing terminology standard was needed for meeting the clinical healthcare documentation provided for nursing care of patients. The CCC System was the first national nursing standard accepted by Health and Human Services (HHS) for the information exchange of health data in the EHR through the ONC and HITSP Biosurveillance Technical Committee. The Secretary of HHS adopted the first set of approximately 55 standards including the CCC System in 2007 and 2008.

American Society for Testing and Materials. The American Society for Testing and Materials (ASTM) E-31 Committee on Healthcare Informatics is an accredited committee that develops standards for health information and health information systems designed to assist vendors, users, and anyone interested in systematizing health information (Cendrowska et al., 1999; Hammond, 1994).

Health Level Seven. Health Level Seven (HL7) is an organization accredited by the ANSI, which was created to develop standards for the electronic interchange of clinical, financial, and administrative information among independent healthcare–oriented information systems. It grew out of efforts that involved multiple vendors to initiate open HISs (Agency for Healthcare Policy & Research, 1999; Fitzmaurice, 1995; Hammond, 1994; Van Bemmel & Mussen, 1997).

SNOMED International. SNOMED International, know as the International Health Technology Standards Development Organization (IHTSDO) since 2007, is another organization that serves as an umbrella for the structured nomenclatures, and its merger with the Read Codes from the National Health Service in the United Kingdom formed in 1999. Since the existing medical and disease condition nomenclatures are already indexed, the newly named SNOMED-CT also serves as the coding strategy and has become a national standard for the EHR, aspects of which are integrated into the UMLS and are available to the public. In 2006, the IHTSDO was formed and acquired the rights to SNOMED-CT to expand use to the global community. The overarching vision was to harmonize terms in SNOMED with international terms. While nurses are involved in many levels of the organization, a very active nursing special interest group specifically attends to the nursing terminologies.

National Committee on Vital and Health Statistics. The National Committee on Vital and Health Statistics (NCVHS), founded in 1949, established a Workgroup on Computer-Based Patient Records to help the Department of Health and Human Services investigate and approve healthcare standards for the federal government to use to implement federal legislation (Chute, Cohen, & Campbell, 1996). The Committee evaluated and recognized medical, nursing, and other health profession nomenclatures for HHS to implement the HIPAA of 1996 (NCVHS, 1996). The NCVHS workgroup on Computer-Based Patient Records prepared a report for HHS recommending standards to implement the HIPAA legislation. They proposed standards for the electronic transmission of federally mandated reimbursement for Medicare and Medicaid patient services. They also recommended that the selected transaction and code sets primarily focus on privacy and security for the EHR.

The newly named Standards Subcommittee, established in 2000, was involved in several other federal and national initiatives such as the Patient Medical Record Information (PMRI), which was the second phase of the HIPAA legislation. The Standards Subcommittee was also involved in several other initiatives such as the development of the proposal for e-Prescribing under the Medicare Prescription Drug Improvement and Modernization Act of 2003; the Technical Framework for the Nationwide Health Information Network; the Concept Paper: Toward Enhanced Information Capacities for Health; and initial hearings on Meaningful Use in April 2009 before ONC appointed the two HIT committees.

Consolidated Health Informatics Initiative. The Consolidated Health Informatics Initiative (CHII) was established to review the existing portfolio of clinical vocabulary and messaging standards in order to support and enable federal agencies to build interoperable federal health data systems. Twenty federal departments and agencies including HHS, Veterans Affairs (VA), Department of Defense/Health Affairs (DoD/HA), Social Security Administration (SSA), General Services Administration (GSA), and the National Institute of Standards and Technology (NIST) were active in the CHII governance process that required all federal agencies to incorporate the adopted CHII standards into individual agency health information enterprise architecture (EA) that would be used to build health data systems or modify existing ones. The CHII initiative outreached to the private sector through the NCVHS.

Integrating the Healthcare Enterprise (IHE) International. In 1998, the Health Information Management and Systems Society (HIMSS) and Radiological Society of North America (RSNA) began cooperative efforts to promote interoperability among imaging and information systems. The IHE working groups with industry representatives, standards experts, and others formed the IHE Planning and Technical Committees to design profiles for 'edge to edge' sharing of information (e.g., from application to application, system to system, and setting to setting) across multiple healthcare enterprises (www.ihe.net/About/ihe_faq.cfm).

The IHE approach supports the use of existing standards in an integrated manner including defining configuration choices when necessary. The initiative defines a technical framework for the implementation of established messaging standards to acieve specfic clinical goals.. IHE strives to accelerate the process for defining, testing, and implementing standards-based interoperability among EHR systems.

LANDMARK EVENTS IN NURSING AND COMPUTERS

Major Milestones

Computers were introduced into the nursing profession over 40 years ago. Major milestones of nursing are interwoven with the advancement of computer and information technologies, the increased need for nursing data, development of nursing applications, and changes making the nursing profession an autonomous discipline.

The landmark events are also categorized and described in the chapter "Historical Perspectives of Nursing and the Computer" (Saba, & Erdley, 2006) published in the fourth edition of *Essentials of Nursing Informatics*. In this edition, the major landmark milestones table has been updated in Table 2.1. The

milestone events are listed in chronological order including for the first time, the key NI pioneer or expert involved in the event as well as the first time a key event occurred, which may be ongoing. Many other events may have occurred but this table represents the most complete history of the NI movement.

There are currently several key events in which the NI community participates, and many of them are held annually. The conferences, symposia, institutes, and workshops provide an opportunity for nursing informatics novices and experts to network and share their experiences. They also provide the latest information, newest exhibits, and demonstrations on this changing field.

SUMMARY

Computers, and subsequently information technology, emerged during the past 5 decades in the healthcare industry. Hospitals began to use computers as tools to update paper-based patient records. Computer systems in healthcare settings provided the information management capabilities needed to assess, document, process, and communicate patient care. As a result, the "human-machine" interaction of nursing and computers has become a new and lasting symbiotic relationship (Blum, 1990; Collen, 1994; Kemeny, 1972).

The history of informatics from the perspective of the pioneers was briefly described in this chapter. The complete video, audio, and transcripts can be found on the AMIA website (www.amia.org/niwg-history-page). Over the last 50 years, nurses have used and contributed to the evolving HIT technologies for the improved practice of nursing.

Innumerable organizations sprang up in an attempt to set standards for nursing practice and education, standardize the terminologies, create standard structures for EHRs, and attempt to create uniformity for the electronic exchange of information. This chapter highlighted a few key organizations.

The last section focused on landmark events in nursing and computers, including major milestones in national and international conferences, symposia, workshops, and organizational initiatives contributing to the computer literacy of nurses Table 2.2. The success of the conferences and the appearance of nursing articles, journals, books, and other literature on this topic demonstrated the intense interest nurses had in learning more about computers and information technologies. These advances confirmed the status of NI as a new ANA specialty in nursing and provided the stimulus to transform nursing in the 21st century.

TABLE 2.1	Landmark Events in Computers and Nursing		
Year(s)	Title	Sponsor(s)	Coordinator/Chair/NI Representative(s)
1973	First Invitational Conference: Management Information Systems (MISs) for Public and Community Health Agencies	National League for Nursing (NLN) & Division of Nursing, Public Health Service (DN/PHS), Arlington, VA	Goldie Levenson (NLN) Virginia K. Saba (DN/PHS)
1974 to 1975	Five Workshops on MISs for Public and Community Health Agencies	NLN & DN/PHS, selected US cities	Goldie Levenson (NLN) Virginia K. Saba (DN/PHS)
1976	State-of-the-Art Conference on Management for Public and Community Health Agencies	NLN & DN/PHS, Washington, DC	Goldie Levenson (NLN) Virginia K. Saba (DN/PHS)
1977	First Research: State-of-the-Art Conference on Nursing Information Systems	University of Illinois College of Nursing, Chicago, IL	Harriet H. Werley Margaret Grier
1977	First undergraduate academic course in Computers & Nursing	The State University of New York at Buffalo, Buffalo, NY	Judith Ronald (SUNY, Buffalo)
1979	First Military Conference on Computers in Nursing	TRIMIS Army Nurse Consultant Team, Walter Reed Hospital, Washington, DC	Dorothy Pocklington (ANC) Linda Guttman (ANC)
1980	First Workshop on Computer Usage in Healthcare	University of Akron, School of Nursing, Continuing Education Department, Akron, OH	Virginia Newbern (UA/SON) Dorothy Pocklington (TRIMIS Army) Virginia K. Saba (DN/PHS)
1980	First computer textbook: *Computers in Nursing*	Nursing Resources, Boston, MA	Rita Zielstorff, Editor
1981	First Special Interest Group Meeting on Computers in Nursing	Annual SCAMC Conference Event, Washington, DC	Virginia K. Saba, Chair (DN/PHS)
1981	First nursing papers at Fifth Annual Symposium on Computer Applications in Medical Care (SCAMC)	Annual SCAMC Conference Sessions, Washington, DC	Virginia K. Saba (DN/PHS) Coralee Farlee (NCHSR)
1981 to 1984	Four National Conferences on Computer Technology and Nursing	NIH Clinical Center, TRIMIS Army Nurse Consultant Team, & DN/PHS NIH Campus, Bethesda, MD	Virginia K. Saba (DN/PHS) Ruth Carlsen & Carol Romano (CC/NIH) Dorothy Pocklington & Carolyn Tindal (TRIMIS Army)
1981	Early academic course on Computers in Nursing (NIH/CC)	Foundation for Advanced Education in Sciences (FAES) at NIH, Bethesda, MD	Virginia K. Saba (DN/PHS) Kathleen A. McCormick (NIH/PHS)
1982	Study Group on Nursing Information Systems	University Hospitals of Cleveland, Case Western Reserve University, & National Center for Health Services Research (NCHSR/PHS), Cleveland, OH	Mary Kiley Gerry Weston (NCHSR)

Year	Event	Location	Person(s)
1982 to present	Initiated Annual International Nursing Computer Technology Conference	Rutgers, State University of New Jersey, College of Nursing, CE Department, selected cities	Gayle Pearson (Rutgers), Jean Arnold (Rutgers)
1982	First International Workshop: The Impact of Computers on Nursing	London Hospital, UK & IFIP-IMIA, Harrogate, UK	Maureen Scholes (UK), Barry Barber (UK)
1982	First Newsletter: *Computers in Nursing*	School of Nursing, University of Texas at Austin, Austin TX	Gary Hales (UT)
1982 & 1984	Two Boston University (BU) Workshops on Computers and Nursing	Boston University School of Nursing, Boston, MA	Diane Skiba
1982	PLATO IV CAI Educational Network System	University of Illinois School of Nursing, Chicago, IL	Pat Tymchyshyn
1983 to present (Every 3 Years)	Initiated nursing papers at MED-INFO World Congress on Medical Informatics, International Medical Informatics Association (IMIA)	1983—Amsterdam, NL; 1986—Washington, DC, USA; 1989—Singapore, Malasia; 1992—Geneva, Switzerland; 1995—Vancouver, Canada; 1998—Seoul, South Korea; 2001—London, UK; 2004—San Francisco, CA; 2007—Brisbane, AU; 2010—Capetown, SA	Elly Pluyter-Wenting, First Nursing Chair
1983	Second Annual Joint SCAMC Congress & IMIA Conference	SCAMC & IMIA, San Francisco, CA & Baltimore, MD	Virginia K. Saba Nursing, Chair
1983	Early Workshop on Computers in Nursing	University of Texas at Austin, Austin, TX	Susan Grobe
1983	First Hospital Workshop on Computers in Nursing Practice	St. Agnes Hospital for HEC, Baltimore, MD	Susan Newbold
1983	First Nursing Model for Patient Care	TRIMIS Program Office, Washington, DC	Karen Rieder (NNC), Dena Nortan (NNC)
1983 to present (every 3 years)	Initiated International Symposium on Nursing Use of Computers & Information Science, IMIA Working Group 8 on Nursing Informatics (IMIA/NI-8); Renamed IMIA Nursing Informatics, Special Interest Group (IMIA/NI-SIG)	1983—Amsterdam, Netherlands; 1985—Calgary, Canada; 1988—Dublin, Ireland; 1991—Melbourne, Australia; 1994—San Antonio, TX, USA; 1997—Stockholm, Sweden; 2000—Auckland, New Zealand; 2003—Rio de Janeiro, Brazil; 2006—Seoul, Korea; 2009—Helsinki, Finland; 2012—Montreal, Canada	1983—Maureen Scholes, First Chair; 1985—Kathryn J. Hannah & Evelyn J. Guillemin; 1988—Noel Daley & Maureen Scholes; 1991—Evelyn S. Hovenga & Joan Edgecumbe; 1994—Susan Grobe & Virginia K. Saba; 1997—Ulla Gerdin & Marianne Tallberg; 2000—Robyn Carr & Paula Rocha; 2003—Heimar Marin & Eduardo Marques; 2006—Hueoun-Ae Park; 2009—Anneli Ensio & Kaija Saranto; 2012—Patricia Abbott

(continued)

TABLE 2.1	Landmark Events in Computers and Nursing *(continued)*		
Year(s)	**Title**	**Sponsor(s)**	**Coordinator/Chair/NI Representative(s)**
1984	American Nursing Association (ANA) initiated First Council on Computer Applications in Nursing (CCAN)	ANA	Harriet Werley, Chair
1984	First Seminar on Microcomputers for Nurses	University of California at San Francisco, College of Nursing, San Francisco, CA	William Holzemer, Chair
1984	First nursing computer journal: *Computers in Nursing CIN, Renamed Computers, Informatics, Nursing*	JB Lippincott, Philadelphia, PA	Gary Hales
1984 to 1995	First *Directory of Educational Software for Nursing*	Christine Bolwell & National League for Nursing (NLN)	Christine Bolwell
1985	NLN initiated First National Forum on Computers in Healthcare and Nursing	National League for Nursing, New York City, NY	Susan Grobe, First Chair (UT)
1985	First Annual Seminar on Computers and Nursing Practice	NYU Medical Center, NY, NY	Patsy Marr (NYU) Janet Kelly (NYU)
1985	First Invitational Conference: Nursing Minimum Data Set (NMDS) Conference	University of Illinois School of Nursing, Chicago, IL	Harriet Werley Norma Lang
1985	Early academic course: Essentials of Computers, in undergraduate and graduate programs	Georgetown University School of Nursing, Washington, DC	Virginia K. Saba
1985 to 1990	Early 5-year Project: Continuing Nursing Education in Computer Technology, Focus: Nursing Faculty	Southern Regional Education Board (SREB), Atlanta, GA	Eula Aiken (SREB)
1985	First Test Authoring Program (TAP)	Addison-Wesley Publishing, NY, NY	William Holzemer (UCSF)
1986	Two early Microcomputer Institutes for Nurses	Georgetown University, School of Nursing, Washington, DC, & University of Southwest Louisiana Nursing Department, Lafayette, LA	Virginia K. Saba (GU/SON) Dorothy Pocklington (USL) Diane Skiba (BU)
1986	Established first nurse educators's newsletter: *Micro World*	Christine Bolwell & Stewart Publishing, Alexandria, VA	Christine Bolwell
1987	Initiated & created Interactive Videodisc Software Programs	American Journal of Nursing, NY, NY	Mary Ann Rizzolo
1987	International Working Group Task Force on Education	IMIA/NI Working Group-8 & Swedish Federation, Stockholm, Sweden	Ulla Gerdin (NI)- Kristina Janson Jelger & Hans Peterson (Swedish Federation)

Year	Event	Organization/Location	Person
1987	Videodisc for Health Conference: *Interactive Healthcare Conference*	Stewart Publishing, Alexandria, VA	Scott Stewart, Publisher
1988	Recommendation #3: "Support Automated Information Systems."	National Commission on Nursing Implementation Project (NCNIP), Secretary's Commission on Nursing Shortage	Vivian DeBack, Chair
1988	Priority Expert Panel E: Nursing Informatics Task Force	National Center for Nursing Research, NIH, Bethesda, MD	Judy Ozbolt, Chair
1989	Invitational Conference: Nursing Information Systems, Washington, DC	National Commission on Nursing Implementation Project (NCNIP), ANA, NLN, & NIS Industry	Vivian DeBack, Chair
1989 & 1991 to Present	Initiated 1st graduate programs with specialty in Nursing Informatics, Master's & Doctorate	University of Maryland School of Nursing, Baltimore, MD	Barbara Heller, Dean Program Chairs: Carol Gassert, Patricia Abbott, Kathleen Charters, Judy Ozbolt, & Eun-Shim Nahm
1989	ICN Resolution Initiated Project: International Classification of Nursing Practice (ICNP)	International Council of Nurses Conference, Seoul, Korea	Fadwa Affra
1990 to 1995	Annual Nurse Scholars Program	HBO & HealthQuest Corp.	Roy Simpson (HBO) Diane Skiba (BU) Judith Ronald (SUNY Buffalo)
1990	Invitational Conference: State-of-the-Art of Information Systems	NCNIP, Orlando, FL	Vivian DeBack, Chair
1990	Renamed ANA Steering Committee on Databases to Support Nursing Practice	ANA, Washington, DC	Norma Lang, Chair
1990	Task Force on Nursing Information Systems	NCNIP, ANA, NLN, NIS Industry Task Force, Project Hope, VA	Vivian DeBack, Chair
1991 to 2001	Annual European Summer Institute	International Nursing Informatics Experts	Jos Aarts
1991	First Nursing Informatics Listserv	University of Massachusetts, Amherst, MA	Gordon Larrivee
1991	Formation of Combined Annual SCAMC Special Nursing Informatics Working Group & AMIA NIWIG	AMIA/SCAMC Sponsors, Washington, DC	Judy Ozbolt, First Chair
1991 & 1992	Two WHO Workshops on Nursing Informatics	World Health Organization & US PHS, Washington, DC, & Geneva, Switzerland	Marian Hirschfield, (WHO) Carol Romano (PHS)
1991 to Present	Initiated Annual Summer Institute in Nursing and Healthcare Informatics (SINI)	University of Maryland School of Nursing (SON), Baltimore, MD	Program Chairs: Carol Gassert, Mary Etta Mills, Judy Ozbolt, & Marissa Wilson
1992	ANA approved Nursing Informatics as a new Nursing Specialty	ANA Database Steering Committee, Washington, DC	Norma Lang, Chair

(continued)

TABLE 2.1	Landmark Events in Computers and Nursing *(continued)*		
Year(s)	**Title**	**Sponsor(s)**	**Coordinator/Chair/NI Representative(s)**
1992	Formation of Virginia Henderson International Nursing Library (INL)	Sigma Theta Tau International Honor Society, Indianapolis, IN	Judith Graves, Director
1992	ANA recognized 4 nursing terminologies: CCC System (HHCC), OMAHA System, NANDA, & NIC	ANA Database Steering Committee, Washington, DC	Norma Lang, Chair
1992	Read Clinical Thesaurus added nursing terms in UMLS	Read Codes Clinical Terms, Version 3	Ann Casey (UK)
1992	Nursing Minimum Data Set Conference	Canadian Nurses Association, Edmonton, Alberta, Canada	Phyllis Giovannetti, Chair
1993	Four ANA-'Recognized' Nursing Terminologies Integrated into UMLS	ANA Database Steering Committee & NLM	Norma Lang, Chair Betsy Humphreys (NLM)
1993	Initiated Virginia Henderson Electronic Library Online via Internet	Sigma Theta Tau International Honor Society, Indianapolis, IN	Carol Hudgings, Director
1993	Initiated AJN Network Online via Internet	American Journal of Nursing Company, NY, NY	Mary Ann Rizzolo, Director
1993	ANC Postgraduate course: Computer Applications for Nursing	Army Nurse Corps, Washington, DC	Army Nurse Corps (ANC)
1993	Formation of Nursing Informatics Fellowship Program	Partners Healthcare Systems, Wellesley, MA	Rita Zielstorff, Director
1993	Alpha Version Working Paper of ICNP	International Council of Nurses, Geneva, Switzerland	Fadwa Affara,
1993	Formed Denver Free-Net	University of Colorado Health Sciences Center, Denver, CO	Diane Skiba
1993	Priority Expert Panel E: Nursing Informatics Report: Nursing Informatics: Enhancing Patient Care	National Center for Nursing Research, (NCNR/NIH), Bethesda, MD	Judy Ozbolt, Chair
1994	ANA-NET Online	American Nurses Association, Washington, DC	Kathy Milholland
1994	Four Nursing Educators Workshops	Southern Council on Collegiate Regional Education & University of Maryland, Washington, DC; Baltimore, MD; Atlanta, GA; Augusta, GA	Eula Aiken (SREB), Mary Etta Mills (UMD)
1994	Next Generation Clinical Information Systems Conference	Tri-Council for Nursing and Kellogg Foundation, Washington, DC	Sheila Ryan, Chair

Year	Event	Organization/Location	People
1995	First International NI Teleconference: Three Countries Linked Together	International NI Experts: NI, U.S.A; HIS, Australia; NI, New Zealand	Sue Sparks (USA); Evelyn Hovenga (AU); Robyn Carr (NZ)
1995	First Combined NYU Hospital & NYU SON: Programs on Nursing Informatics & Patient Care: A New Era	NYU School of Nursing & NYU Medical Center, NY, NY	Barbara Carty, Chair; Janet Kelly, Co-Chair
1995	First Weekend Immersion in NI (WINI)	CARING Group, Warrenton, VA	Susan Newbold (CARING); Carol Bickfod (ANA); Kathleen Smith (USN Retired)
1995	First CPRI Davies Recognition Awards of Excellence Symposium	Computer-Based Patient Record Institute, Los Angeles, CA	Intermountain Healthcare, Salt Lake City, UT; Columbia Presbyterian MC, NY, NY; Department of Veterans Affairs, Washington, DC
1995	Initiated CARING Web site	CARING	Susan Newbold (CARING)
1996	ANA established Nursing Information & Data Set Evaluation Center (NISDEC)	ANA Database Steering Committee, Washington, DC	Rita Zielstorff, Chair; Connie Delaney, Co-Chair
1996 to 1999	Nightingale Project-Health Telematics Education, 3 Workshops & 2 International Conferences	University of Athens, Greece, & European Union	John Mantas, Chair (Greece); Arie Hasman, Co-Chair (Netherlands)
1996	Initiated TELENURSE Project	Danish Institute for Health & Nursing Research & European Union	Randi Mortensen, Director; Gunnar Nielsen, Co-Director
1996	First Harriet Werley Award for Best Nursing Informatics Paper at AMIA	AMIA-NI Working Group (NIWG), Washington, DC	Rita Zielstorff (MGH Computer Lab)
1997	Invitational National Nursing Informatics Workgroup	National Advisory Council on Nurse Education & Practice & DN/PHS	Carol Gassert, Chair
1997	ANA published NIDSEC Standards and Scoring Guidelines	ANA Database Steering Committee	Rita Zielstorff, Chair; Connie Delaney, Co-Chair
1997	National Database of Nursing Quality Indicators (NDNQI®) launchec	American Nurses Association, Washington, DC	Nancy Dunton, PI
1998	Initiated NursingCenter.Com Web site	JB Lippincott, NY, NY	Maryanne Rizzalo, Director
1999	Beta Version of ICNP published	International Council of Nurses, Geneva, Switzerland	Fadwa Affara
1999 to 2008	Annual Summer Nursing Vocabulary Summit	Vanderbilt University, Nashville, TN	Judy Ozbolt, Chair

(continued)

TABLE 2.1	Landmark Events in Computers and Nursing *(continued)*		
Year(s)	Title	Sponsor(s)	Coordinator/Chair/NI Representative(s)
1999	Convergent Terminology Group for Nursing	SNOMED/RT International, Northbrook, IL	Suzanne Bakken, Chair (NYU), Debra Konichek
1999	Inaugural Virtual Graduation: Post-Masters ANP Certificate Program	GSN, Uniformed Services University VA TeleConference Network, Bethesda, MD Eight Nationwide VA MCs	Faye Abdellah (USU Dean) Virginia Saba (USU-PI) Charlotte Beason (VA)
1999	First meeting: Nursing Data Standards Project for Central Organization (PAHO) & Brazil	Pan American Health Organization (PAHO), Washington, DC	Roberto Rodriquez (PAHO) Heimar Marin (Brazil)
2000	ICNP Programme Office established	International Council of Nurses, Geneva, Switzerland	Amy Coenen, Director
2000	Computer-Based Patient Record Institute (CPRI) 2000 Conference	CPRI, Los Angeles, CA	Virginia Saba, Nursing Chair
2001	AMIA Nursing Informatics Leaders	University of Wisconsin, Madison, WI Columbia University, NY, NY	Pattie Brennan, President Suzanne Bakken, Program Chair
2002	ICNP Strategic Advisory Group Established	ICN, Geneva Switzerland	Amy Coenen, Director
2002	Conference on Strategy for Health IT and eHealth Vendors	Medical Records Institute (MRI), Boston, MA	Peter Waegemann, President
2002	AAN Conference: Using Innovative Technology	American Academy of Nursing, Washington, DC	Margaret McClure, Chair Linda Bolton, Co-Chair Nellie O'Gara, Co-Chair
2002	Initiated AAN Expert Panel on Nursing Informatics	American Academy of Nursing Annual Conference, Naples, FL	Virginia Saba, Chair Ida Androwich, Co-Chair
2003	Finnish Nursing Informatics Symposium	Finnish Nurses Assoc (FNA) & Siemens Medical Solutions, Helsinki, Finland	Kaija Saranto (FN) Anneli Ensio (FN) Rosemary Kennedy (Siemens)
2003	First ISO-approved nursing standard: Integrated Reference Terminology Model for Nursing	IMIA/NI-SIG & ICN, Oslo, Norway	Virginia Saba (NI/SIG), Chair (NI/SIG) Kathleen McCormick, Co-Chair (NIWG) Amy Coenen, Co-Chair (ICN) Evelyn Hovenga, Co-Chair (NI/SIG) Susanne Bakken, Chair, Tech. Group
2004	First ICN Research & Development Centre	Deutschsprachige ICNP Freiburg, Germany	Peter Koenig, Director
2004 to Present	Initiated Annual Nursing Informatics Symposium at HIMSS Conference & Exhibition	HIMSS Annual Conference, Orlando, FL	Joyce Seisemeier, Chair

Date	Event	Organization	People
2004	Initial formation of Alliance for Nursing Informatics	AMIA/ HIMSS	Connie Delaney, Chair; Joyce Sensemeier, Co-Chair
2004 to 2012	First nurse on NCVHS Standards Subcommittee	NCVHS, Washington, DC	Judy Warren, KUMC
2004	Office of the National Coordinator for Health Information Technology (ONC) established	National coordinators	First Coordinator: Dr. David Brailer; Dr. Robert Kolodner; Dr. David Blumenthal
2004	Technology Informatics Guiding Education Reform (TIGER)—Phase I	National members; Online teleconferences	Marion Ball, Chair; Diane Skiba, Co-Chair
2006	First TIGER Summit	100 representatives from 70 organizations, held at USU, Bethesda, MD	Marion Ball, Chair; Diane Skiba, Co-Chair
2005, 2003, & 2009	ICNP Version 1.0, Version 1.1, & Version 2	ICN	Amy Coenen, Director
2006 & 2008	Symposium on Nursing Informatics	Brazil Medical Informatics Society	Heimar Marin, Chair
2007 to 2008	First National Nursing Terminology Standard: Clinical Care Classification (CCC) System	ANSI-HTISP; Bio-surveillance Committee recommended & HHS approved	Virginia K. Saba & Colleagues, Developers
2009 to present	American Recovery and Reinvestment Act of 2009—Health Information Technology for Economic and Clinical Health (HITECH); ONC formed 2 national committees, each with 1 nurse	Health Policy Committee & Health Standards Committee	Connie Delaney (UMN); Judy Murphy (Aurora Health Systems)
2009	ICNP recognized by WHO	ICN & WHO, Geneva, Switzerland	Amy Coenen, Director
2010	Doctor of Nursing Informatics Program specialty formed	University of Minnesota, Minneapolis, MN	Connie Delaney, Dean; Bonnie Westra, Chair
2010	American Nursing Informatics Association (ANIA) & CARING merged	ANIA & CARING	Victoria Bradley, First President

TABLE 2.2	Major Events for Nursing Informatics Community

Conferences and Workshops

- AMIA Annual Symposium:
  - NI Workshop
  - NI Working Group (NIWG)
  - Harriet Werley Award
  - Virginia K. Saba Award
- HIMSS Annual Conference & Exhibition
  - NI Symposium
  - NI Task Force
  - Nursing Informatics Leadership Award
- Annual Summer Institute in Nursing Informatics (SINI) at University of Maryland
- Annual Rutgers State University of New Jersey College of Nursing: Nursing & Computer Technology Conference 'Outstanding Contribution in Field of NI Award'
- Annual American Academy of Nursing (Annual)
  - Panel of NI Experts
- Sigma Theta Tau International: BiAnnual Conference
  - Virginia K. Saba NI Leadership Award
  - Technology Award
- Nursing Informatics Special Interest Group of the International Medical Informatics Association (IMIA/NI-SIG): Tri-Annual Conference
- International Medical Informatics Association (IMIA): Triennial Congress
  - Nursing Papers

Professional Councils

- American Nurses Association (ANA)
  a. Certification
  b. Committee
- National League for Nursing
- American Academy of Nursing
  a. Expert Panel of Nursing Informatics

Certification

- ANA
- HIMSS

REFERENCES

Agency for Healthcare Policy and Research. (1999). *Current activities of selected healthcare informatics standards organizations: A compilation.* Rockville, MD: AHCPR, U.S. DHHS.

American Association of Colleges of Nursing. (2006, October). *The essentials of doctoral education for advanced nursing practice.* Retrieved from http://www.aacn.nche.edu/education/essentials.htm.

American Association of Colleges of Nursing. (2008, October 20). *The essentials of baccalaureate education for professional nursing practice.* Retrieved from http://www.aacn.nche.edu/education/essentials.htm.

American National Standards Institute (2008). *United States Standards Strategy: A revision of the National Standards Strategy for the United States.* Retrieved from http://www.ansi.org.

American Nurses Association. (2001). *Scope and standards of nursing informatics practice.* Washington, DC: ANA.

American Nurses Association. (2004). *Standards for clinical nursing practice.* Washington, DC: ANA

American Association of Nurses. (2008). *Nursing informatics: Scope & standards of practice.* Washington, DC: ANA.

Bakken S. (2006). Informatics for patient safety: A nursing research perspective. *Annual Review of Nursing Research, 24,* 219–254.

Bitzer, M. (1966). Clinical nursing instruction via the Plato simulated laboratory. *Nursing Research, 15*(2), 144–150.

Blackmon, P. W., Mario, C. A., Aukward, R. K., Bresnahan, R. E., Carlisle, R. G., Goldenberg, & Patterson, J. T. (1982). *Evaluation of the medical information system at the NIH clinical center. Vol 1, Summary of findings and recommendations.* Springfield, VA: NTIS (Publication No. 82-190083).

Blum, B. I. (1990). Medical informatics in the United States, 1950–1975. In B. Blum & K. Duncan (Eds.), *A History of Medical Informatics* (pp. xvii–xxx). Reading, MA: Addison-Wesley.

Cendrowska, T. J., Amatayakul, M., & Tessier, C. (1999). Standards in healthcare: Meeting industry's needs by using ASTM standards. In *Proceedings of the 1999 annual HISS conference: Volume 3* (pp. 433–442). Chicago, IL: HIMSS Publications.

Chute, C. G., Cohen, S. P., and Campbell, K. E. (1996). The content coverage of clinical classifications. *Journal of the American Medical Informatics Association, 3,* 224–233.

Collen, M. F. (1994). The origins of informatics. *Journal of the American Medical Informatics Association, 1*(2), 91–107.

Collen, M. F. (1995). *A history of medical informatics in the United States 1950 to 1990.* Bethesda, MD: American Medical Informatics Association.

Department of Health and Human Services (HHS). (2006, December 19). Presidential Initiatives: Consolidated Health Informatics. Retrieved from http://www.hhs.gov/healthit/chiinitiative.html.

Department of Health and Human Services (HHS), National Committee of Vital and Health Statistics (NCVHS). Retrieved from http://www.ncvhs.hhs.gov.

Fitzmaurice, M. J. (1995). Computer-based patient records. In J. Bronzino (Ed.), *Biomedical engineering handbook* (1st Ed.) (pp. 2623–2634). Boca Raton, FL: CRC Press.

Gallagher, L. A. (2010). Revising HIPAA. *Nursing Management, 41*(4), 34–40.

Hammond, W. E. (1994). The role of standards in creating a health information infrastructure. *International Journal of Bio-Medical Computing 34,* 29–44.

Humphreys, B. L., & Lindberg, D. A. B. (1992). The unified medical language system project: A distributed experiment in improving access to biomedical information. In K. C. Lun, P. DeGoulet, T. E. Piemme, & O. Reinhoff (Eds.), *MEDINFO 92: Proceedings of the Seventh World Congress of Medical Informatics* (pp. 1496–1500), Amsterdam: North-Holland.

International Council of Nursing & International Health Terminology Standards Development Organisation. (2010, June). Harmonization [Press Release]. *ICN Bulletin,* (p. 2).

Kemeny, J. G. (1972). *Man and the computer.* New York: Charles Scribner.

National Committee on Vital and Health Statistics (NCVHS). (1996). *Report: Core healthcare data elements.* Washington, DC: GPO (Pub No. 1996-1722-677/82345).

Newbold, S., & Westra, B. (2009). American Medical Informatics Nursing Informatics History Committee Update, *CIN: Computers, Informatics, Nursing, 27,* 263–265.

Nicoll, L. H. (1998). *Computers in Nursing's: Nurses' Guide to the Internet* (2nd ed.) New York: Lippincott.

Ozbolt, J. G., & Bakken, S. (2003). Patient-care systems. In E.H. Shortliffe, L. E. Perreault, G. Wiederhold, & L. M. Pagan (Eds.) *Medical informatics computer applications in healthcare and biomedicine series: Health informatics* (2nd ed.) (pp. 421–442). New York: Springer.

Parker, M. Ausman, R. K., & Ovedovitz, I. (1965). Automation of public health nurse reports. *Public Health Reports, 80,* 526–528.

Public Health Service (1976). *State of the art in management information systems for public health/community health agencies. Report of the conference.* New York: National League of Nursing.

Rajecki, R. (2008). eICU: Big brother, great friend: Remote monitoring of patients is a boon for nurses, patients, and families. *RN, 71*(11): 36–39.

Romano, C., McCormick, K., & McNeely, L. D. (1982). Nursing documentation: A model for a computerized data base. *Advances in Nursing Science, 4*(2), 43–56.

Saba, V. K. (1995). A new nursing vision: The information highway. *Nursing Leadership Forum, 1*(2), 44–51.

Saba, V. K. (1996). Developing a home page for the World Wide Web. *American Journal of Infection Control 24,* 468–470.

Saba, V. K. (1998). Nursing information technology: Classifications and management. In J. Mantas (Ed.), *Advances in Health Education: A Nightingale Perspective.* Amsterdam: IOS Press.

Saba, V. K., & Erdley, W. S. (2006). Historical perspectives of nursing and the computer. In V. K. Saba & K. A. McCormick (Eds.) , *Essentials of nursing informatics,* (4th ed.) (pp. 9–28). New York: McGraw-Hill.

Sackett, K. M. & Erdley, W. S. (2002). The history of healthcare informatics. In S. Englebardt & R. Nelson (Eds.), *Healthcare informatics: an interdisciplinary approach* (pp. 453–476). St. Louis, MO: Mosby.

Sherman, R. (1965). Computer system clears up errors, lets nurses get back to nursing. *Hospital Topics, 43*(10), 44–46.

Shortliffe, L. E. Perreault, G. Wiederhold, & L. M. Pagan (Eds.) (2003). Medical informatics computer applications in healthcare and biomedicine (2nd Ed). New York: Springer.

Sparks, S. (1996). Use of the Internet for infection control and epidemiology. *American Journal of Infection Control 24,* 435–439.

Van Bemmel, J. H., & Musen, M. A. (Eds.) (1997). *Handbook of medical informatics.* Germany: Springer-Verlag.

Westra, B. L. (2009). Radio frequency identification—Will it reach a tipping point in healthcare? *American Journal of Nursing, 109*(3), 34–36

Westra B. L., & Newbold S. K. (2006). American Medical Informatics Association Nursing Informatics History Committee. *CIN: Computers, Informatics, Nursing, 24*:113–116.

Westra, B. L., Delaney, C. W., Konicek, D., & Keenan, G. (2008). Nursing standards to support the electronic health record. *Nursing Outlook, 56,* 258–266.e1

Wolkodoff, P.E. (1963). A central electronic computer speeds patient information. *Hospital Management, 96,* 82–84.

World Health Organization (1992.). ICD-10: International statistical classification of diseases and health related problems. Geneva: WHO.

Electronic Health Records From a Historical Perspective

Patricia B. Wise

- OBJECTIVES
    1. Describe the evolution of computer-based patient records to electronic health records.
    2. Describe the Nicholas E. Davies Program.
    3. Name the 4 critical sections of the Davies application.
    4. Describe how the Davies Award process leads the nation in identification of value derived from electronic health records.

- KEY WORDS

    CPR project evaluation criteria
    electronic health record
    Nicholas E. Davies Award of Excellence
    Organizational Davies
    Ambulatory Care Davies
    Public Health Davies

HISTORICAL PERSPECTIVE

The journey from paper to electronic collection of personal medical information has been difficult. In 1989, the Institute of Medicine (IOM) of the National Academy of Sciences convened a committee and asked the question, "Why is healthcare still predominantly using paper-based records when so many new computer-based information technologies are emerging?" (Dick, 1991). The same question can still be asked today. Rather than turn to computer scientists to answer the question, the IOM invited representatives of major stakeholders in healthcare and asked them to define the problem, identify issues, and outline a path forward. Two major conclusions resulted from the committee's deliberations. Firstly, the computer-based patient record (CPR) is an essential technology for healthcare and is an integral tool for all professionals. Secondly, the committee after hearing from numerous stakeholders recognized that there was no national coordination or champion for CPRs. As a result, the IOM committee recommended the creation of an independent institute to provide national leadership. The Computer-Based Patient Record Institute (CPRI) was created and given the mission to initiate and coordinate the urgently needed activities to develop, deploy, and routinely use CPRs to achieve improved outcomes in healthcare quality, cost, and access.

As described by the IOM, a CPR is "an electronic patient record that resides in a system designated to support users through the availability of complete and accurate data, practitioner reminders and alerts, clinical decision support systems, links to bodies of medical knowledge, and other aids" (Dick, 1991). Over the years, the electronic records have been referred to by a number of terms including electronic medical record, electronic patient record, electronic health record, computerized patient records, ambulatory medical record, and computer-based medical record. This varied terminology did little to provide a technical framework to advance the development of these systems.

Introduction to Davies

CPRI, founded in 1992, was a unique organization representing all stakeholders in healthcare focusing on clinical applications of information technology. A CPRI Work Group on CPR Systems Evaluation developed the CPR Project Evaluation Criteria in 1993. These criteria, drawn together with input from national experts and volunteer members, formed the basis of a self-assessment that could be used by organizations and outside reviewers to measure and evaluate the accomplishments of CPR projects. The 4 major areas of the initial criteria—management, functionality, technology, and impact—provided a framework through which to view an implementation of computerized records. The criteria also provided the foundation for the Nicholas E. Davies Award of Excellence Program.

The Davies Program, named for Dr. Nicholas E. Davies, an Atlanta-based physician, President-elect of the American College of Physicians, and a member of the IOM committee on Improving the Patient Record was killed in a plane crash just as the IOM report on CPRs was being released. Modeled after the Baldridge Award, this program is intended to award and bring to national attention excellence in the implementation and derived value of electronic health records (EHRs). The program is founded on the belief that healthcare organizations benefit when collective experiences and lessons learned are shared. Now in its 16th year, the Davies Program has had 6 criteria revisions and seen its terminology updated from the computerized patient record, to the electronic medical record (EMR), and to today's electronic health record (EHR). CPRI merged with HOST in 2000, followed by a consolidation of CPRI-HOST with Healthcare Information and Management Systems Society (HIMSS) in 2002. Throughout the various transitions the program has survived and flourished. Today, under HIMSS management, the Davies Award of Excellence is offered in 4 categories: Organizational or Acute Care, first offered in 1995; Ambulatory Care, started in 2003; Public Health, initiated in 2004; and Community Health Organizations (CHO), first presented in 2008. More than 65 recipients

across the 4 tracks have shared their award-winning journeys and lessons learned (Table 3.1).

Throughout the years much has remained the same in organizations that have successfully implemented electronic records while at the same time differences have been noted. This chapter will look at the characteristics of winning organizations that have prevailed over time, while exploring the changing technologies and speed of implementation.

WHAT'S THE SAME?

How They Define the Effort

The 27 Organizational Davies winners located throughout the country, started and completed their implementations at different times, in different departments of their facilities, and under different types of leadership. On the surface it would appear they have little in common. However, a closer look reveals that these organizations have much in common. Leadership in healthcare does start at the top. Solid, committed executive leadership does make things happen. No Davies winner has achieved a full and successful implementation of their EHR without the vision and support of all of the organization's top leaders as well as supervisors and managers. Prior to the onset of effort, the winning organizations have clearly made the EHR a key component of their strategic vision. Recognized organizations know and understand that healthcare is an information business. Leadership is required to select appropriate vendors, plan the implementation, and corral the support of staff including clinician champions. A recent winner, MultiCare of Tacoma, Washington indicated that operational leadership was essential in identifying specific key stakeholders and securing their engagement. Calling it "engagement from the top down," all hospital executives and administrators rounded daily, walking the floors and providing encouragement (MultiCare, 2009). This level of hands-on engagement enforced for the leadership, as well as the employees, what the implementation and "go live" meant for the organization. A first-year winner, the Veteran's Health Administration (VHA) whose mission is to provide high-quality healthcare for America's veterans, made the development of an EHR a major long-term goal (Curtis, 1995). Their EHR continues today to support the care excellence provided to the nation's warriors. Brigham & Women's Hospital (BWH), a 1996 winner, decided in 1989 to redevelop their information systems, moving the computer from its role as a reporter of requested facts to an integral tool in the healthcare

TABLE 3.1	Nicholas E. Davies Award Winners

ORGANIZATIONAL

2009
MultiCare

2008
Eastern Maine Medical Center

2007
Allina Hospitals & Clinics

2006
Center For Behavioral Health
Generations+/Northern Manhattan Health Network

2005
Citizens Memorial Healthcare

2004
Evanston Northwestern Healthcare

2003
Cincinnati Children's Hospital Medical Center

2002
Maimonides Medical Center
Queens Health Network

2001
The University of Illinois at Chicago Medical Center
Ohio State University Health System
Heritage Behavioral Health Center, Inc.

2000
Harvard Vanguard Medical Associates
VA Puget Sound Healthcare System

1999
The Queen's Medical Center
Kaiser Permanente Rocky Mountain Region

1998
Northwestern Memorial Hospital
Kaiser-Permanente Northwest

1997
Kaiser-Permanente of Ohio
North Mississippi Health Services
Regenstrief Institute for Healthcare

1996
Brigham and Women's Hospital
Group Health Cooperative of Puget Sound

1995
Intermountain Healthcare
Columbia Presbyterian Medical Center
Department of Veterans Affairs

AMBULATORY

2009
Virginia Women's Center

2008
Cardiology Consultants of Philadelphia (CCP)
Oklahoma Arthritis Center (OAC), P.C.
Palm Beach Obstetrics & Gynecology PA

2007
Valdez Family Clinic
Village Health Partners (formerly Family Medical
    Specialists of Texas)

2006
Alpenglow Medical, PLLC
Cardiology of Tulsa (COT)
Piedmont Physicians Group (PPG 775)

2005
Southeast Texas Medical Associates
Sports Medicine & Orthopedic Specialists
Wayne Obstetrics and Gynecology

2004
Old Harding Pediatric Associates
Pediatrics @ the Basin
North Fulton Family Medicine
Riverpoint Pediatrics

2003
Cooper Pediatrics
Evans Medical Group
Roswell Pediatric Center

PUBLIC HEALTH

2009
Boston Public Health Commission, Infectious Disease Bureau
    Boston Syndromic Surveillance System (B-SYNSS)
Denver Public Health, Denver Public Health Information
    Service (DPH-IS)

2008
Cherokee Indian Hospital Authority (CIHA), Resource Patient
    Management System (RPMS) Electronic Health Record (EHR)
New Jersey Department of Health and Senior Services (NJDHSS),
    Communicable Disease Reporting and Surveillance System
    (CDRSS)

(continued)

TABLE 3.1	Nicholas E. Davies Award Winners *(continued)*
PUBLIC HEALTH (continued)	
2007 Illinois—National Electronic Disease Surveillance System (I-NEDSS) • INEDSS—Manage Tuberculosis Business Rules • I-NEDSS Manage Tuberculosis Case Institute for Family Health **2006** Texas Department of State Health Services (DSHS) Behavioral Health Integrated Provider System (BHIPS), a Web-Based Electronic Health Record (EHR)	New York State Environmental Public Health Tracking Network (NYS EPHTN) Data Exchange System. **2005** Indian Health Service Clinical Reporting System North Carolina Disease Event Tracking and Epidemiologic Collection Tool (NC-DETECT) **2004** Utah Statewide Immunization Information System (USIIS) – Utah Department of Health South Dakota Electronic Vital Records and Screening System Pennsylvania's National Electronic Disease Reporting System (PA-NEDSS)
COMMUNITY HEALTH ORGANIZATION	
2009 Urban Health Plan Heart of Texas	**2008** Columbia Basin Health Association Community Health Access Network (CHAN) New York Children's Health Project (NYCHP) White River Rural Health Center, Inc.

process. The BWH vision encompassed the establishment of a new technical platform that would serve as the base to provide the processing power and scalability envisioned for the future (Teich, 1996). More recently, Maimonides Medical Center located in Brooklyn, New York turned to the EHR in response to managed competition. In 1996, in New York's deregulated reimbursement system, Maimonides' goal to expand rapidly into an integrated delivery system placed the EHR at the core of its new business model. At the time this vision seemed remote since Maimonides was still dependent on 1960s legacy keypunch-based mainframes (Beltran, 2002). Maimonides Chief Executive Officer (CEO) Stanley Brezenoff and Chief Operating Officer (COO) Pamela Brier backed their vision with commitment of one-third of the medical center's capital budget for 7 years to realize the goal (Beltran, 2002). As Harvard Vanguard was formed in 1997 the vision encompassed a multisite, multispecialty group practice whose EHRs linked to its practice management system (Crowell, 2000).

The EHR implementation in all winning organizations was a clear part of the strategic vision and defined by remarkably similar organizational goals and objectives. Eastern Maine Medical Center, a 2008 Davies recipient, defines the organization's "pillar" goals for community, finance, quality, people, growth, and service (Hartz, 2008). The Veterans Affairs (VA) Puget Sound Healthcare System (VA Puget Sound), a 2000 Davies

winner, delineated several key objectives: improving the accessibility and availability of clinical information, support of integrated care delivery across 2 different sites, and maximizing improvements in quality care through the use of order entry and order checks and reminders (Payne, 2000). Strikingly similar were the project objectives of Queens Health Network, Queens, New York, a 2002 winner, which were shared by all the medical staff and administration. Those included improved quality of patient care through timely access to patient information, improved documentation of clinical data throughout the continuum of care, and the integration of clinical information from a variety of legacy systems (Carr, 2002). The 2003 Davies winner, Cincinnati Children's Hospital Medical Center (CCHMC), made optimizing patient safety and consistency in care the top two strategic objectives that took precedence in the planning, design, and implementation of their EHR (Jacobs, 2003).

How Is the Effort Organized?

The implementation of an EHR is a daunting effort. An organization-wide strategic effort needs to be governed by defined structure, oversight, and project leadership. Planning for an EHR involves numerous committees; the more input planners receive, the more buy-in they achieve from management and staff. If every department is appropriately represented, implementation can proceed more smoothly as concerns and challenges are aired in a timely fashion. For Eastern Maine Medical Center the governance structure for technology projects has evolved through the years with active participation for overall business case analysis from the project management office. This group is responsible for putting into action all the planning, execution, and control of all project activities. The team is made up of workgroups for transformation of care, culture, and technology (Hartz, 2008). The planning process requires the skills of financial and operational administrators as well as clinicians from all departments working closely with information technology professionals. Project leaders do not necessarily come from the Information Services department. For Allina Hospitals and Clinics of Minneapolis, MN, who received the Davies Award in 2007, a new governance structure was necessary to undertake a project of the magnitude represented in an EHR implementation. For the majority of their implementation, approximately 250 full-time employees, most of whom had other positions within Allina, served on one of 7 committees guiding the technology deployment. Success with implementation requires integrating the system with the business of care delivery (Allina, 2007). Owners of the business, the clinicians, must be directly involved and engaged throughout the planning and implementation cycles. Nurses need to participate in design review, serve as champions, and provide local resources to ensure the planned implementation will enhance their ability to care for the patient. Centralized planning is desired, however Davies winners that have rolled out implementations across multiple sites have repeatedly advised that all implementation is local and local clinicians must be engaged in order to achieve success.

Many Davies applicants described similar evolutions in the governance of the EHR system implementation. Throughout each phase there was representation of key stakeholders. Nurses, physicians and clinical support staff led the needs analysis effort to ensure clinical quality. Due to the technologies involved, the selection process or design phase required input from not only clinicians but also from information system specialists. The contract negotiation phase was guided by hospital administration and information systems personnel with close oversight of the financial, technical, and legal implications. The early portion of system implementation, usually consisting of hardware and software installations, was led by personnel from information systems.

The VA Puget Sound formed a Steering Committee whose members included the Chiefs of Medicine, Surgery, Nursing, Mental Health and Ambulatory Care. In turn, each department nominated members for 2 special groups of users, Clinical Users and Super Users. The Clinical Champions were approximately 20 physicians, nurses, and other allied health professionals who were advocates of the project and willing to lead discussions and provide presentations and education sessions for other members of their profession. Super Users were a larger group whose members received more training and worked closely with the developers in planning system changes and improvements. The Super Users additionally served as local resources for their colleagues, answering questions, and providing on-the-spot training (Payne, 2000). A consistent characteristic of winning organizations is the customer service and constant consideration of the impact of the system on the end user. Consider the needs not only of large clinical departments but also those of small niche services. Consider the impact to patient care not only during the busiest hours, but also during weekend and nighttime hours. No EHR implementation can be successful without the buy-in from the clinicians throughout the facility, in all departments and on all shifts. Another characteristic of Davies winners has been the active pursuit of feedback from all users. Winning organizations have employed a user-inclusive design for feedback or have developed "help" buttons that allow clinicians to instantly communicate frustrations or suggestions for design improvements.

Change Management

No EHR implementation will be successful without deliberate, carefully designed, clinician involved proactive change management. To maximize success, it must be recognized that the forthcoming implementation will bring about a culture of change. The positive effect of this upcoming change must be echoed by medical, nursing, and administrative leadership. At the outset of their EHR implementation, MultiCare committed not to simply build the system around the existing processes. Their approach to future state workflow design was focused on eliminating waste and gaining maximum value from the new systems' capabilities (MultiCare, 2009). This was made possible through the collaboration between subject matter experts, system analysts, and clinicians as well as their vendor counterparts. New systems necessitate new standard operating procedures. Their approach focused on establishing operational ownership, fostering staff involvement, producing effective and timely communication, developing super user and physician champion networks, and providing complete just-in-time training (MultiCare, 2009). New policies and procedures must be considered, written, and tested before "go live."

CASE STUDY: A MULTICARE CONNECT WORKFLOW WALKTHROUGH AND TUNNEL TOURS

In 2007 and 2008, the MultiCare Connect project team hosted events called Workflow Walkthroughs and Tunnel Tours. The Workflow Walkthroughs were a chance for employees throughout the health system to see how MultiCare Connect worked in a day of the life of a patient. Members of the project team wrote and performed the "day in the life" experience: highlighting how the patient entered the health system through the emergency department, was moved to inpatient, and what happened after the patient was discharged. In 2007, the theme was "The Great Treasure Hunt." The event featured keynote speakers from the executive team, large group scenarios, and breakout sessions for individual departments. In 2008, the theme was "Telling the Patient's Story," and again featured the group scenario and breakout sessions. In addition, participants were able to visit an area of the hospital where key workflows were printed out in Visio format and shown end-to-end on the walls. Subject matter experts hosted the Tunnel Tours and were available to answer questions and show the workflows in greater detail on their laptops. A similar Tunnel Tour ran in 2007 as a standalone event. The Tunnel Tours also provided opportunities for the clinical staff to call out areas of the workflows that didn't match their daily practice or identify areas for improvement to conform to best practice standards (Multicare, 2009).

At CCHMC, several weeks of live implementation planning preceded the arrival of the EHR in any patient unit. Clinical advocates from the respective units performed usability tests. In the case of CCHMC, these tests revealed that the time it took to perform the frequent documentation of various clinical data, such as vital signs, was unacceptable. Consequently, CCHMC pursued a critical care documentation system that allowed for multiple close interval entries (Jacobs, 2003).

Strong end-user support for new systems was a key factor for success. Ohio State University Health System (OSUHS) treated this as an organizational effort and responsibility. All available personnel were required to support each phase. Roving support personnel termed "red coats" responded to user calls for help around the clock (Ahmed, 2001). Just-in-time training was organized by specialty or department at Maimonides Medical Center. All system documentation was deployed prior to implementation, including test plans, training manuals, user manuals, system specifications, and pocket reference guides for physicians. Development of downtime procedures and user access policies were included in all the system training (Beltran, 2002).

Maimonides, as well as other Davies winners, learned early on that process redesign was required to achieve the desired efficiency and results. It was necessary to achieve agreement from physicians and nurses on standard orders, practice protocols, and decision support rules in order to see measurable improvements in patient outcomes (Beltran, 2002). Getting clinicians to use an EHR as part of their day-to-day work is one of the most significant hurdles that had to be overcome by successful Davies applicants. Maimonides, a 2002 winner, decided not to call their clinician classes *training*. Instead, announcements featured an educational offering designed to show physicians and nurses how to navigate the Internet and the Maimonides intranet. After completing this 2-hour introductory-level class, caregivers eagerly signed up for the next level. Their self-perceived stigma about not knowing how to use a PC and perform simple navigation had been alleviated (Beltran, 2002). At the University of Illinois at Chicago Medical Center (UICMC) extensive efforts were made from the onset to establish that the EHR was "owned" by clinicians and not the Information Technology Department. The priorities for implementation became driven by what the clinicians believed would generate the most value, both for themselves and their patients (Keeler, 2001).

Queens Health Network (QHN) noted in their application that resistance at all levels of the organization to the EHR was being confronted and transformed. At a steering committee meeting, one chief of service complained that the business of an academic medical center was to teach physicians to practice medicine, not to practice typing. This was challenged by a counterpart who asserted that the skills required of any 21st century healthcare personnel, including nurses and physicians, must include mastery of the computer (Carr, 2002). Clinicians at all levels and from all departments must become partners in the technology process.

At some point in the planning for the EHR implementation all Davies winners came to the realization that electronic media are intrinsically different from paper. Electronic media are interactive. The term *hard copy* illustrates the difference; paper is tangible and static, electronic information is fluid and reactive. Manual paper processes cannot simply be transferred to electronic media. An institutional EHR implementation forces an examination of the underlying work processes. The EHR will act as a catalyst for the development of clinical practice standards across services and departments from one campus to another within the organization. Although the Queens Health Network delivers more babies than any other provider in Queens, clinical practices between providers, and even from site to site, differed despite adherence to nationally recognized practice standards. At Queens it took an extensive discussion among several clinicians to define the algorithm to electronically calculate the estimated date of confinement, with each caregiver having a slightly different and preferred methodology, backed by academic resources, to obtain this date (Carr, 2002).

IMPACT TO VALUE

Davies applications have utilized the term *soft return on investment* (ROI) for clinical variables promulgated by EHRs in such areas as patient safety, process improvement, legible documentation, and regulatory compliance. In their written applications, Davies Award winners offer detailed analysis in these categories, though they do not always include hard statistical data that proves their business cases. Documenting the impact of an EHR is very difficult at best; impossible for some organizations. Unlike the many industrial companies that practice Six Sigma principles, a process-improvement protocol requiring reams of data, healthcare providers face many challenges in quantifying every aspect of their practice. The system impacts an organization in subtle ways, such as avoidance of a medication error, and directly through nonduplication of an ordered test. Still, soft ROI carries great importance for healthcare institutions. Reducing errors through clinical decision support saves lives. Having access to a patient's medical record at the moment it is needed is invaluable. Citizen's Memorial Healthcare, the first rural and community hospital to win a Davies, stated in their 2005 application that patient safety was impacted by "eliminating handwriting/transcription errors by requiring completeness of orders through clinical decision support, and by providing access to clinical information and a patient medical history" (Citizens Memorial Healthcare, 2005).

Throughout this past decade of Davies winners, the application process has included a documentation of impact and value to the implementing organization. Value has never been assumed and winning applicants justified their clinical systems. Winners highlighted their successes based on value to the care processes. From 1995–2001 applicants were asked to provide examples of impact derived for the organization from the EHR. As applications were evaluated great emphasis was placed on the organization's ability to demonstrate positive impact. Davies applicants were encouraged to provide quantitative examples of benefits that had been obtained against costs that had been incurred to help guide and direct expecta-

tions in other settings. Organizations with long standing EHR efforts were not exempt. Dr. Clem McDonald from Regenstrief described "the unremitting pressure to show value" (McDonald, 1997). Organizations with a research orientation such as Intermountain Healthcare, Brigham, and Regenstrief demonstrated proof of value through research and publications. These early Davies winners have contributed significantly to the body of research on the power and importance of clinical decision support to improve the process of healthcare and patient safety (McDonald, 1997).

During the first years of the Davies program, all winning organizations cited improvements in care documentation. Quality-of-care enhancements through avoidance of medication error, increased appropriateness of care interventions, and compliance with managed care and disease management protocols were obtained by all organizations. Additional quality impact was noted in improved continuity of care as medical records and plans of care were available in detail for on-call residents or weekend triage nurses.

Organizations applying for the Davies Award in 2002 and beyond faced revised criteria in which the impact section had been changed to value. Healthcare facilities were expected to document the business case of the EHR. Maimonides faced an uphill battle as the organization moved toward an EHR. Before 1996, technology investments at Maimonides had not provided measurable results. No ROI could be documented. The perception was that technology offered little or no value. MMC realized that traditional cost-benefit justifications did not fully measure the value of clinical applications. What dollar amount was equal to improved patient outcome and satisfaction, increased efficiencies in the delivery of care, and accurate immediate access to patient and care information? Since metrics are needed to measure success, an interdisciplinary team was created prior to each technology initiative to identify benchmarks and savings to be realized from the new initiative (Beltran, 2002).

Maimonides used Eclipsys' strategic investment model to measure the business value of its projects. This computer model aligns business goals with the appropriate technology solution. The model then provides balanced decision-making criteria including tangible and intangible benefits and risks. The resulting analysis provides net present value, internal rate of return, payback periods, and ROI for each system (Beltran, 2002). Using this model, Maimonides has since 1996, realized a 9.4% ROI, a 3.84-year payback, and positive net cash flow by year 4. Capital reimbursements, grant awards, and partial revenue from the medical center's length of stay reduction have also partially contributed to this ROI.

Additional ROI was achieved in the radiology department, where picture archiving communication systems (PACS) and voice recognition have produced savings of over $10.5 million over 5 years from savings in film, film jackets, and transcription (Beltran, 2002).

The Queens Health Network and Medical Board were cognizant that the value of the EHR technology must be demonstrated. They determined that for their organization's success, the business case would be measured by the improvement of processes that impact patient care: improved access to patient information, complete legible clinical documentation, and timely and accurate patient data at point of service. Process improvements were measured by analyzing different tools, their actions, and effect on patient care. One example of this was the nutritional screening tools with decision support that were made available for nurses and other clinicians in ambulatory care (Carr, 2002).

Online documentation by physicians and nurse practitioners has clearly enhanced the value of the Queens EHR. Queens Hospital Center, a component of the QHN, reported a 50% decrease in the number of pharmacist interventions in medication orders in the ambulatory setting because of system alerts, and improved legibility and completeness of prescriptions. At Elmhurst Hospital, an acute care facility of QHN, the completion in the EHR of patient problem lists, orders and referrals for mammography, Pap smears, and diabetic retinal examinations had reached 100% by 1999 (Carr, 2002). Three months prior and six months after EHR implementation, QHN measured compliance with the Joint Commission on Accreditation of Healthcare Organizations (JCAHO)-mandated summary list that included patient diagnoses, procedures, allergies and adverse drug reactions, and patient medications. All elements of the summary list were required to be complete in order for compliance to be achieved for any individual record. Implementation of the EHR led to noteworthy and sustainable improvements with a jump from 3.7% (three months prior to EHR) to 100% (six months after conversion from paper to electronic records) (Carr, 2002).

The 2003 Organizational Davies winner, CCHMC, also centered the business justification on process improvement as the driver for technological change. Immediately after successful EHR implementation, the institution began to see significant benefits in targeted processes (Jacobs, 2003). In recent years, CCHMC believed patient safety was a cornerstone of quality. Through institutional committees such as Medication Safety, Patient Safety, and Risk Management, deficiencies in the area of patient safety had been noted. These deficiencies at times were related to inconsistency of care between providers.

TABLE 3.2	MultiCare Realized Significant Improvements in Patient Safety and Quality of Care (MultiCare, 2009)

- 13% decrease in the use of unsafe abbreviations
- 13% decrease in adverse drug reactions within the first 2.5 months of implementing computerized physician order entry (CPOE)
- 24% reduction from the time a STAT med is ordered to the time it is verified by pharmacy
- 27% increase in documentation of the plan of care by at least 2 disciplines
- 45% reduction from the time a routine medication is ordered to the time it is verified by pharmacy
- 75% of orders are entered directly by physicians
- Estimated 108 lives saved among diabetic patients
- Mean laboratory order turnaround time reduced by 30%
- Median imaging order turnaround time reduced by an average of 50%

Though not unique to CCHMC, problems with poorly or illegibly written orders were commonplace. The CCHMC formulary lists 3,770 medications. Of these, 470 were designated "high alert" due to their narrow window for therapeutic use or widespread frequency. Prior to EHR implementation, age-adjusted dose range checking limits were established for all 470 high-alert medications to include minimum and maximum single doses, maximum total daily doses, and minimum and maximum frequencies. As a result of the EHR implementation clinicians at CCHMC now generate complete, unambiguous, legible orders that include clinician contact name and pager number on all orders (Jacobs, 2003).

Table 3.2 is a summary of the benefits of the EHR at MultiCare, 2009.

Still Expensive

A commonalty shared by all Davies Organizational winners is the cost of their EHR implementation: expensive. This trait continues even today. Speaking with the individuals who provide care in Davies Award–winning organizations one repeatedly hears that the EHR has paid for itself time and again in patient safety, improved quality outcomes, and provider satisfaction. Over the years of the Davies Program, organization after organization has set aside multiple millions from their capital budgets to finance the cost of the infrastructure, hardware, and software all needed for an EHR implementation. Difficult to calculate but consistently present are the employee hours lost from patient care for the planning process, design phase, testing, and educational needs all required to support a successful implementation.

Focus on Decision Support

The functionality of an EHR is the result of the data it captures and the assistance it provides to all members of the healthcare team. An integral component of the EHR is its ability to offer clinical support in the provider's decision-making process. Previously, computerized systems delivered results reporting and reviewing. The pioneering visionaries recognized the value of real-time alerting, reminding, and protocol support. Davies winners have consistently recognized that decision support takes 2 forms. The first can be seen in applications that are designed to facilitate best practices through evidence-based clinical practice guidelines, electronic order protocols, electronic order defaults, and allowable order-specific elements. The second type of decision support is found in alerts and reminders that warn clinicians about patient variables (MultiCare, 2009).

Eastern Maine Medical Center identified 5 broad categories of clinical decision tools (CDS) used in their organization (Hartz, 2008) (Table 3.3).

A multidisciplinary team at Ohio State University Health System developed guidelines that were incorporated into order protocols and then into provider order entry (POE). In addition more than 400 electronic order protocols that address safety, quality, standardization, and cost with embedded alerts and reminders are also available in POE (Ahmed, 2001). At Maimonides, the power of advanced knowledge-based prompting and decision support can be seen in the Perinatal EHR, which capitalized on bedside workstations to deliver real-time point-of-care decision support. Since 99% of perinatal data can be entered via structured database fields rather than using free text, the ability of the system to analyze and assess is greatly enhanced. The system continuously assesses recorded documentation and generates menus automatically tailored to the current clinical situation (Beltran, 2002).

WHAT'S DIFFERENT?

Where Winners Obtained Systems

In the first years of the Davies, winning organizations had spent years in the development of their award-winning

TABLE 3.3	Category of CDS Tool, Description of Functionality, Value and Effectiveness (Hartz, 2008)	
Category of CDS Tool	**Description of Functionality**	**Value and Effectiveness**
Groups of predefined orders (Evidence-based care sets)	Evidence-based order sets, clinical pathways serve as a starting point for disease-specific orders. Allows providers to select all relevant orders for a specific diagnosis.	Promotes consistent standards of care based on best practices.
Order checking with reference database	Medication orders are verified for drug allergy, drug-drug interactions and contraindications, and therapeutic duplication checking using reference database or rules engine. This database is updated monthly.	Information available to the provider at time of order entry facilitates best decision thereby reducing medication errors.
Complex orders with specialized tools	Templates and tools are available to use, such as dosing calculator, taper dosing, sliding scale, custom TPN, etc.	Help and guide clinicians with complex dosing or medication administration.
Order-relevant patient data display	Automatic display of patient-specific information related to the intervention being ordered, e.g., color-coded laboratory data displayed in flow sheets indicating normal or abnormal laboratory data.	Facilitates review of patient information to determine best course of action, drug choice, timing, dosing, and other interventions.
Rules-based prompting and alerts	Synchronous and asynchronous alerts and reminders such as dose-range checking and medication renewal alerts.	Notifies clinicians of potential adjustments needed to drug therapy based on medications ordered and most recent lab data.

systems. The three organizations honored in the first year of the program all developed their own systems. Intermountain Healthcare (IHC) in Utah was the practice site for a visionary group of clinicians and scientists. Around 1965 they began experimenting with the process of applying computer technology to the provision of care. From these early experiments came the creation of an integrated, rules-based, patient-centered information system entitled HELP (Health Evaluation through Logical Processing) (Grandia, 1995). Throughout the late 1970s and early 1980s the HELP system was expanded until 1985 when it became apparent that an enterprise-wide clinical information system was needed. A 5-year budget of $50 million was set aside for the creation of this system, which was based on the creation of an enterprise-wide data repository fed by IHC's clinical, financial, and managed care plan systems.

Columbia-Presbyterian Medical Center received a first-year award for their Clinical Information System (CIS), which was built as a central hub that enabled clinical systems on disparate platforms to share patient data. The hub consisted of a series of concentric layers handling a variety of requests from the various client applications to either store or retrieve data (Johnson, 1995). Network integration was accomplished by establishing connectivity to the token ring or Ethernet (Johnson, 1995).

Also honored in the first year of the Davies program was the Veteran Health Administration (VHA) for a computer-based patient record that was based on the Decentralized Hospital Computer Program (DHCP), a comprehensive system covering medical management, fiscal, and clinical functions. The DHCP served as the fundamental information system for the VHA's medical care network supporting 171 medical centers, 450 outpatient clinics, and 131 nursing homes (Curtis, 1995). As part of their commitment to provide high-quality healthcare to the veterans of the United States, a major goal of this system was to share and exchange data, first throughout the VHA, then with other federally-based healthcare facilities, and finally with private sector organizations (Curtis, 1995). Despite funding at $1.2 billion for a 12-year life cycle from 1983 to 1994, there was no major electronic medical record acquisition in VHA. Due to the necessity of keeping all options open for future growth, the VHA considered it vital to maintain a high degree of both vendor and platform independence. Consequently, systems procurements for the DHCP were open acquisitions with requests for proposals (RFP) written in terms of generic performance requirements, with the result that most major hardware vendors were represented in the various incremental procurements (Curtis, 1995).

Second-year award winner, Brigham & Women's Hospital (BWH) developed Brigham Integrated Computing System (BICS) with the help and participation of a large number of their clinicians. These clinicians spent a portion of their time on system development and the remainder on clinical practice (Teich, 1996). This project was an ambitious redevelopment of the hospital's information system that dated back to 1989. One of the project's goals was to change the computer's role in the healthcare process. Instead of assuming the traditional computer role of results reporting, the computer would become an active partner in promoting optimal quality of care, reducing adverse events, and reducing costs (Teich, 1996). For more than 20 years, Harvard Vanguard Medical Associates had utilized an automated medical record system (AMRS) that had become outdated. This Boston-based clinician-led multispecialty group practice, a sixth-year Davies winner, tried self-development, and then co-development, before implementing their current system, which was purchased from a vendor (Crowell, 2000).

All winners since 2000 have implemented commercially sold, multicomponent systems procured from a variety of vendors. Maimonides chose multiple vendors when implementing their system. This modified best of breed approach, met physician and departmental needs while conforming to the medical center's interfacing, hardware, software, and operating standards.

The technology employed in the system affects the ability to meet user expectations, including a wide variety of functional and organizational needs, reliability, response time, and scalability. The Davies program has shown that there is no single best technology solution. Awardees have been successful using a wide range of approaches in implementing systems. Over the years these have included several cases of completely homegrown systems based on different technology platforms, a mainframe-based vendor solution, homegrown systems with commercially procured document imaging, homegrown results management integrated with a commercially purchased clinical system, and complete purchase from a vendor of an electronic medical record (Metzger, 1999).

TIME TO GET THERE

As more healthcare organizations purchase commercially available EHRs the timeline from initial planning, through purchase, training, and successful implementation shortens. For early Davies winners like the VHA, Brigham & Women's, and Regenstrief Institute for Healthcare (1997 Davies winner) the EHR was part of a strategic plan that took more than a decade to realize. The Regenstrief Institute was founded in 1969 in Indianapolis, Indiana on the belief that industrial engineering principles could be applied to healthcare. Under the leadership of Clement McDonald the vision of a longitudinal, integrated acute and ambulatory care record that provided information for clinical decision support and other applications developed over 3 decades (McDonald, 1997). At North Mississippi Health Services (NMHS) development started in the late 1970s when the Information Services Department and a consultant interviewed users to determine needs and wants for the most far reaching medical system available. By the end of 1997 the clinical information stored in their EHR was available at approximately 120 different locations within their healthcare delivery system. The 2 winners of the 2001 Davies Award, the University of Illinois at Chicago Medical Center (UICMC) and the Ohio State University Health System (OSUHS) each spent 7 years in the planning and implementation of their commercially procured systems (Keeler, 2001). Cincinnati Children's Hospital Medical Center placed the development of a robust information technology infrastructure in their 1995 organizational strategic plan. The following years saw a dramatic increase in the development of the Information Services Department and accompanying increase in network infrastructure to support the vigorous development and implementation of clinical systems (Jacobs, 2003). By March 2000, CCHMC had completed the implementation of an enterprise-wide PACS system, and by December 2002 the EHR was implemented on 13 inpatient care units (Jacobs, 2003).

Recent winners have shortened the timeline to less than 3 years from acquisition to enterprise-wide implementation. The practice of deriving value from the EHR is never complete. Organizations are utilizing their databases to study best practices and seek new ways to improve population health. Clinical outcomes are compared and contrasted at the clinician level. The journey envisioned decades ago continues across the country.

EXTERNAL AGENDA

Factors external to healthcare organizations helped to accelerate the timeline for adoption of EHRs. In 1993, the driving force for developing an Advanced Clinical Information System at Queens's Medical Center in Honolulu, Hawaii was the onset of healthcare reform and managed care. Survival of Queens necessitated a seamless integrated healthcare system. Clinical and administrative leaders of Queens convened a planning committee from which emerged the vision held by all physicians, nurses, and allied health professionals that a computer-based patient record was essential to improve care (Davis, 1999). The EHR at UICMC was initially developed to mitigate concerns that the organization's legacy patient care information system was not Year 2000 (Y2K) compliant (Keller, 2001). For Heritage Behavioral Health Center of Decatur, Illinois the impetus was felt in the mid-1990s when competition for service contracts increased. Heritage found itself poorly prepared with an outdated back-office system. An agency-wide, point-of-service information system would give the organization a competitive edge in quality-based effective clinical services. The focal point of this information system was to be an EHR that supported the delivery of care (Willkinson, 2001). The EHR at Queen's Health Network in Queens, New York was seen as key to the strategic position of Queens in the competitive healthcare marketplace of New York City. The EHR was viewed as essential to the development of an effective infrastructure from which to support the reorganization of care, design of quality measures, streamlined reporting processes, and the cornerstone of evidence-based medicine to improve management of chronic disease (Carr, 2002).

Today the focus is on obtaining "meaningful use." The American Recovery and Reinvestment Act (ARRA) of 2009, was signed into law by President Obama in February, 2009. The ARRA aims to stimulate the economy through investments in infrastructure, unemployment benefits, transportation, education, and healthcare. It includes over $20 billion to aid in the development of a robust information technology (IT) infrastructure for healthcare and to assist providers and other entities in adopting and using health IT. Congress designed the legislation to improve US healthcare through the development of a solid health information infrastructure, while simultaneously stimulating the economy through new investment and job growth. Specifically, there are 5 broad goals: (1) improve quality, safety, efficiency, and reduce health disparities; (2) engage patients and families; (3) improve care coordination; (4) ensure adequate privacy and security protections for personal health information; and (5) improve population and public health. *Meaningful use of certified EHR technologies* is a term used in the ARRA. It is clearly defined by CMS in a "Notice of Proposed Rulemaking" (NPRM) as the use of health IT to further the 5 broad goals of the ARRA, and to further the goal of information exchange among health professionals.

Certified technology is also a term created in ARRA, meaning a qualified EHR that has been properly certified as meeting the standards adopted under section 3004 of the Public Health Service Act. Providers can earn a Medicare or Medicaid incentive payment(s) by demonstrating meaningful use of certified EHR technology. The billions of dollars spent incentivizing healthcare organizations is spurring acquisition at a previously unachieved pace across the nation.

TECHNOLOGY

The technology behind each EHR affects its ability to meet user demands for rapid response, system reliability, future growth, and customization. Since the inception of the Davies award, new technologies have emerged and are being incorporated into the systems being employed today. The technology used by any Davies winner is difficult to precisely replicate due to data capture. The unique interfaces, user agreements, cultural changes, workflow revisions, and window and menu customizations tend to make each EHR unique.

Document imaging systems have been incorporated into many EHRs as a key component of the transition strategy to move an organization from a paper-based to an electronic system. First seen in the earliest Davies winners as a means to organize paper components of the medical chart, these systems have emerged as a key technology to capture paper originating from outside the system and stray clinical documentation.

A picture archiving and communication system (PACS) has been deployed with a great degree of user acceptance and satisfaction in Davies winners during the last decade. This technology makes diagnostic-quality images available wherever high-resolution monitors are found: emergency rooms, intensive care units, and ambulatory surgeries.

At Queens in New York, users are issued an electronic key at training and must chose a password that is changed every 3 months. Both the physical device (key) and electronic password are required to sign onto the system every time. This process, taking about 5 seconds, requires the use of a plastic key that contains encrypted user file and security access information (Carr, 2002).

Wireless technology was noted in a 1999 winner, Queens of Hawaii. Mobile wireless workstations in the intensive care units (ICU) were integral to improving team function. Wireless ICU workstations that could be wheeled about and used in the patients' rooms improved clinician efficiency and the quality of patient care (Davis, 1999). Today, wireless technology is ubiquitous in Davies organizations. Mobile computing extends to the clinician's palm.

Hardware for the EHR has seen significant changes over the past decade. Intermountain Healthcare, a first-year Davies winner, initiated their system on serial terminals that were migrated to Intel-286–based personal computers. Today, high-speed work stations with flat panel monitors help manage workflow and clinical communications in all recent Davies winners. Fiber optic cables facilitate communications within and to remote locations of the organization.

SUMMARY

The Nicholas E. Davies Program, founded by CPRI in 1991 and now managed by HIMSS, reflects the nation's journey from paper-based to electronic capture of medical data. A review of award-receiving applications reveals that despite great advances in technology, there is no substitute for top-down leadership and the involvement of clinicians in all aspects of system acquisition, implementation, and movement to quality outcomes.

REFERENCES

Ahmed A., Teater P., Bentley T. D. (2001). The design and implementation of a computerized patient record at the Ohio State University health system: A success story. *Proceedings of the Seventh Annual Nicholas E. Davies CPR Recognition Symposium.* Chicago, IL: HIMSS.

Allina Hospitals and Clinics. (2007). *HIMSS Davies Organizational Award application.* Retrieved from http://www.himss.org/content/files/davies/2007/org/DaviesAwardApplication%20Allina_revised.pdf.

Beltran J., Cassera F., Daurio N., Davidson S., Evanzia J., Fielding M., et al. (2002). Maimonides Medical Center makes a quantum leap with advanced computerized patient record technology. *Proceedings of the Eighth Annual Nicholas E. Davies EMR Symposium.* Chicago, IL: HIMSS.

Carr D. M. (2002). Queens Health Network healthcare information system: A model for electronic physician order entry. *Proceedings of the Eighth Annual Nicholas E. Davies EMR Symposium.* Chicago, IL: HIMSS.

Citizens Memorial Healthcare. (2005). *Davies Organizational Award application.* Retrieved from http://www.himss.org/content/files/davies/2005/CMH_FULL_APPLICATION.pdf.

Crowell, M., Lopez, R., Cochran, D., Packer M., Beraha N., Wetmore B., et al. (2000). The Journey to a CPR in a Large Multi-Specialty Group Practice. *Proceedings of the Sixth Annual Nicholas E. Davies CPR Recognition Symposium.* Bethesda, MD: CPRI-HOST.

Curtis, C. (1995). A computer-based patient record emerging from the public sector: The decentralized hospital computer program. *Proceedings of the First Annual Nicholas E. Davies CPR Recognition Symposium.* Bethesda, MD: CPRI.

Davis D., Moriyama R., Tiwanak G., Morse L., Sailo C., (1999). Clinical performance improvement with an advanced Clinical Information System at the Queen's Medical Center. *Proceedings of the Fifth Annual Nicholas E. Davies CPR Recognition Symposium.* Bethesda, MD: CPRI.

Dick, R. S., Steen, E. B. (Eds.). (1991). The computer-based patient record: An essential technology for healthcare. Institute of Medicine. Washington, D.C.: National Academy Press.

Grandia, L., Pryor, T., Wilson, D., Gardner R., Haur, P., Huff S., et al. (1995). Building a Computer-based Patient Record System in Evolving integrated Health System. *Proceedings of the First Annual Nicholas E. Davies CPR Recognition Symposium.* Bethesda, MD: CPRI.

Hartz, E. (2008). EMMC patient first initiatives: Transformation of patient care. *HIMSS Davies Award Application.* Retrieved from http://www.himss.org/davies/docs/Organizational/EasternMaineMedical_application.pdf.

Jacobs B., Lykowski G., Mahoney, D., Goodiienc M., Price T., Speight M., et al. (2003). Improving the Quality and Safety of Care through implementation of an integrating Clinical Informatics System. *Proceedings of the Ninth Annual Nicholas E. Davies EMR Recognition Symposium.* Chicago, IL: HIMSS.

Johnson S., Forman B., Cimino J., Bripesak G., Sengupta S., Sideli R., (1995). A Technological Perspective on the Computer-based Patient Record. *Proceedings of the First Annual Nicholas E. Davies CPR Recognition Symposium.* Bethesda, MD: CPRI.

Keeler, J. (2001). The Gemini project: University of Illinois at Chicago Medical Center. *Proceedings of the Seventh Annual Nicholas E. Davies CPR Recognition Symposium.* Chicago, IL: HIMSS.

McDonald, C., Tierney W., Overhage J. M., Dexte P., Takesue, B., Abernathy G. (1997). The three legged stool: Regenstrief Institute for Healthcare. *Proceedings of the Third Annual Nicholas E. Davies CPR Recognition Symposium.* Bethesda, MD: CPRI.

Metzger J., Simpson N., Underwood C. (1999). Lessons from the First four years. *Proceedings of the Fifth Annual Nicholas E. Davies CPR Recognition Symposium.* Bethesda, MD: CPRI.

MultiCare Davies Application. (2009). *HIMSS Davies Organizational Award Application.* Retrieved from http://www.himss.org/davies/docs/2009_RecipientApplications/MultiCareConnectHIMSSDaviesManuscript.pdf.

Payne, T. H., Torell, J., Hoey, P. (2000). Implementation of the computerized patient record system and other clinical computing applications at the VA Puget Sound healthcare system. *Proceedings of the Sixth Annual Nicholas E. Davies CPR Recognition Symposium.* Bethesda, MD: CPRI-HOST.

Teich J. M., Glaser J. P., Beckley R. F., Arrnow M., Bates D. W., Kuperman G. J., et al. (1996). Toward Cost Effective Quality Care: The Brigham Integrated Computing Experience. *Proceedings of the Second Annual Nicholas E. Davies CPR Recognition Symposium.* Bethesda, MD: CPRI.

Wilkinson, G. (2001). Award for Behavioral Health: Heritage Behavioral Health Center, Inc. *Proceedings of the Seventh Annual Nicholas E. Davies CPR Recognition Symposium.* Chicago, IL: HIMSS.

PART 2

Computer Systems

M. Kathleen Smith

Computer System Basics

Mary L. McHugh

• OBJECTIVES

1. List the key hardware components of a computer and the four basic operations of the central processing unit.
2. Describe how power is measured for computers.
3. Describe common computer input, output, and storage devices.
4. Define the difference between computer software and computer hardware.
5. List the categories of programming languages and identify at least one example of each.
6. Identify the five defining attributes of a system and define the meaning of each.
7. Describe the relationship between data to wisdom continuum and database systems.
8. Describe the purpose, structures, and functions of database management systems.
9. Outline the life cycle of a database system.
10. Explain concepts and issues related to data warehouses in healthcare.

• KEY WORDS

information systems
computer science
software
hardware
systems
database
data warehouse

INTRODUCTION

This chapter presents the basics of computer systems and data processing. The basics consist of computer hardware, software, and the strategies used to permit users to store and retrieve data and process it into whatever products are desired. In this context, the word *data* is broadly defined as all the data that users enter into a computer. Because of the changes in knowledge and user needs, this chapter provides the basic information that one should know about the computer and combines four chapters: computer hardware, software, data processing, and computer systems, previously published in the 4th edition.

Note: This chapter includes sections from a previous edition written by Ramona Nelson.

HARDWARE

Computer **hardware** is defined as all of the physical components of the machine itself. The basic hardware of a computer includes the electronic circuits, microchips, processors, and the motherboard itself inside the computer housing. In addition, hardware typically includes devices that are peripheral to the main computer box such as input and output devices, including the keyboard, mouse, printer, fax, and storage components such as the internal hard drive and any external storage drives, including the number of Universal Serial Bus (USB) drives that can be plugged in, card readers, other drives, and so on. Typically, computer systems are composed of many different component parts that enable the user to communicate with the computer and with other computers to produce work. The group of required and optional hardware items that are linked together to make up a computer system is called its configuration. When computers are sold, many of the key components are placed inside a rigid plastic housing or case, which is called the **box**. What can typically be seen from the outside is the box (Fig. 4.1) containing the internal components, and the peripherals such as a keyboard, mouse, speakers, monitor, and printer.

A computer is a machine that uses electronic components and instructions to the components to perform calculations and repetitive and complex procedures, process text, and manipulate data and signals. Computer technology has evolved from huge electronic calculators developed with military funding during World War II to palm and tablet-sized information-processing machines

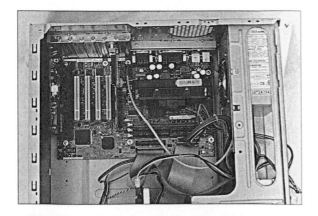

• **FIGURE 4.1.** Computer box with components loaded. (Reproduced, with permission, from Rosenthal M. (1999). *Build Your Own PC* (p. 82). New York, NY: McGraw-Hill.)

available to virtually everybody. Today, computer processors are encountered in most areas of people's lives. From the grocery store to the movie theater; from infusion pumps to physiologic monitors; from the bedside alarm clock to the automobile accelerator, computer processors are employed so widely that the late 20th and early 21st century can accurately be described as the beginning of the information age.

Computer hardware advanced rapidly during the late 1900s and into the first decade of the 2000s. These advances did not bypass the healthcare industry. Computers have allowed fantastic changes in the practice of radiology and imaging, allowing noninvasive visualization of the human body that heretofore could only be performed in surgery, if at all (Gettman & Blute, 2007). Computer technology has revolutionized many surgeries such that invasion and peripheral tissue damage is minimized. It has allowed surgeons to insert endoscopy tools that allow for both visualization and precise removal of diseased tissues, leaving healthy tissues minimally damaged and the patient unscarred (Marescaux et al., 2007; Gumbs et al., 2009). Virtual reality programs in surgery have greatly enhanced the scope and complexity of surgeries that are now amenable to endoscopic approaches (Linte et al., 2008).As a result, massive damage to skin, subcutaneous tissues, muscles, and organs have been eliminated from many procedures. Today, millions of patients who formerly would have needed weeks in the hospital for recovery are now able to be released from the hospital the same day as their surgery or in a day or two at most.

Computers are now pervasive throughout the healthcare industry. Their applications are expected to continue to expand and thereby improve the quality of healthcare while at the same time reducing some costs. Most important, the applications of computers to healthcare will greatly expand the diagnostic and therapeutic abilities of practitioners and broaden the options available to recipients of healthcare. Additionally, telemedicine is now being used to reduce the impact of distance and location on accessibility and availability of healthcare (McConnochie et al., 2009). None of these changes could have happened without tremendous advances in the machinery, the hardware, of computers.

This chapter covers various aspects of computer hardware: components and their functions and classes of computers and their characteristics and types. It also highlights the functional components of the computer and describes the devices and media used to communicate, store, and process data. Major topics addressed include basic computer concepts and classes and types of computers, components, and computer communications. To understand how a computer processes data, it is necessary to examine the component parts and devices that comprise computer hardware.

COMPUTER HARDWARE FUNDAMENTALS

The box of any computer contains a **motherboard** (Fig. 4.2). The motherboard is a thin, flat sheet made of a firm, nonconducting material on which the internal components—printed circuits, chips, slots, and so on—of the computer are mounted. The motherboard is made of a **dielectric** or nonconducting plastic material, and the electric conductions are etched or soldered onto the bottom of the board. The motherboard has holes or perforations through which components can be affixed (Fig. 4.3). Typically, one side looks like a maze of soldered metal trails with sharp projections (which are the attachments of the chips and other components affixed to the motherboard). On one side can be seen the microchips, wiring, and slots for adding components. The specific design of the components—especially the central processing unit (CPU) and other microprocessors—is called the computer's architecture.

A computer has four basic components, although most have many more add-on components. At its most basic, a computer must consist of a CPU, input and output controllers, and storage media.

Memory includes the locations of the computer's internal or main working storage. Memory consists of registers (a small number of very high-speed memory locations), random access memory (RAM), which is the main storage area in which the computer places the programs and data it is working on, and cache (a small memory storage area holding recently accessed data).

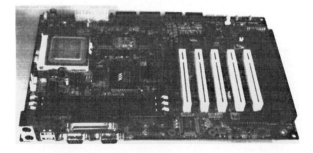

• **FIGURE 4.2.** Motherboard with CPU, chips, and slots. (Reproduced, with permission, from Pilgrim A. (2000). *Build Your Own Pentium III PC* (p. 34). New York, NY: McGraw-Hill.)

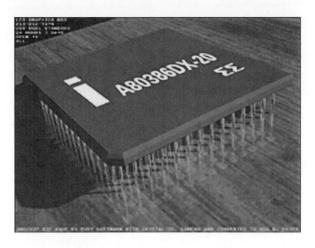

• **FIGURE 4.3.** CPU chip attached to motherboard. (Courtesy of James C. Miller.)

Memory

There are two types of memory in the main memory of a computer. They are read-only memory (ROM) and RAM.

Read-Only Memory. ROM is a form of permanent storage. This means that data and programs in ROM can only be read by the computer, and cannot be erased or altered. ROM generally contains the programs, called firmware, used by the control unit of the CPU to oversee computer functions. In microcomputers, this may also include the software programs used to translate the computer's high-level programming languages into machine language (binary code). ROM storage is not erased when the computer is turned off.

Random Access Memory. RAM refers to working memory used for primary storage. It is volatile (changeable) and used as temporary storage. RAM can be accessed, used, changed, and written on repeatedly. It contains data and instructions that are stored and processed by computer programs called applications programs. RAM is the work area available to the CPU for all processing applications. The computer programs, which are stored on media such as a Digital Versatile Disc (DVD), on the hard drive, or on USB flash drives (also known as jump drives), are not permanent parts of the computer itself. They are loaded when needed, and they can be altered. The contents of RAM are lost whenever the power to the computer is turned off.

Input and Output

To do work, the computer must have a way of receiving commands and data from the outside and a way of reporting out its work. The motherboard has slots and circuit boards that allow the CPU to communicate with the outside world. Input and output devices are wired to a **controller** that is plugged into the slots or circuit boards of the computer. Some devices can serve as both input and output devices. Such devices as the hard drive on which most of the programs people use as well as their personal data are stored, the disk drives, DVDs and CDs on which people store most of their personal data, and more recently, the USB flash drives, serve to both receive and send information to the computer.

Input Devices. These devices allow the computer to receive information from the outside world. The most common input devices are the keyboard and mouse. Others commonly seen on nursing workstations include the touch screen, light pen, voice, and scanner. A touch screen is actually both an input and output device combined. Electronics allow the computer to "sense" when a particular part of the screen is pressed or touched. A light pen is a device attached to the computer that has special software that allows the computer to sense when the light pen is focused on a particular part of the screen. For both the touch screen and light pen, software interprets the meaning of that screen location to the program. Voice systems allow the nurse to speak into a microphone to record data. Many other input devices exist. Some devices are used for security and can detect users' fingerprints, retinal prints, voiceprints, or other personally unique physical characteristics that identify users who have clearance to use the system. In healthcare computing, some medical devices serve as input devices. For example, the electrodes placed on a patient's body provide input into the computerized physiologic monitors.

Output Devices. These devices allow the computer to report its results to the external world. Output can be in the form of text, data files, sound, graphics, or signals to other devices. The most obvious output devices are the monitor (display screen), printer, USB flash drive, and read/write CDs and DVDs.

Storage Media

Storage includes the main memory but also external devices on which programs and data are stored. The most common storage device is the computer's hard drive. Other common media include external hard drives,

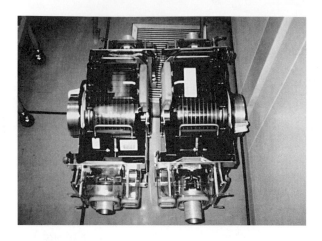

• **FIGURE 4.4.** Hard disk platters from an IBM mainframe computer. (Courtesy of Akos Varga.)

flash drives, and read/write DVDs and CDs. The hard drive and diskettes are magnetic storage media. DVDs and CD-ROMs are a form of optical storage. Optical media are read by a laser "eye" rather than a magnet.

Hard Drive. The hard drive is a peripheral that has very high speed and high density (Fig. 4.4). That is, it is a very fast means of storing and retrieving data as well as having a large storage capacity in comparison with the other types of storage.

CD-ROM and DVD. CD-ROMs and DVDs are rigid disks that hold a higher density of information and have higher speed (Fig. 4.5). Until the late 1990s, CD-ROMs were strictly input devices. However, new technology developed by Philips Corporation permitted the development of a new type of CD that could be written on by the user. These are called CD-RWs.

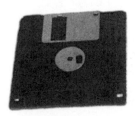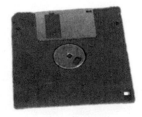

• **FIGURE 4.5.** Diskette with write protect slot. (Reproduced, with permission, from Pilgrim A. (2000). *Build Your Own Pentium III PC* (p. 165). New York, NY: McGraw-Hill.)

USB Flash Drive. As demands for higher and higher density transportable storage rise, the popularity of the USB disk has also risen. A USB flash drive is actually a form of a small, removable hard drive that is inserted into the USB port of the computer. There are many names for it, including pen drive, jump drive, thistle drive, pocket drive, and so forth. This is a device that can store 4 gigabytes (GB) for about $10 to 128 GB for under $300. It is highly reliable and small enough to transport comfortably in a pants pocket. The device plugs into one of the computer box's USB ports and instead of saving to hard drive or CD-ROM or floppy, the user simply saves to the flash drive. Since the flash drive can store so much data in a package so much smaller than a CD or DVD, the convenience makes it worth the higher price to many users. Of course, as its popularity increases, prices drop.

Other Output Devices. As computers became more standard in offices during the 1990s, more and more corporate and individual information was stored solely on computers. Even when paper backup copies were kept, loss of information on the hard drive was usually inconvenient at the least and a disaster at worst. Diskettes could not store large amounts of data, so people began to search for economical and speedy ways to backup the information on their hard drive.

Computer Power

The terms **bits** and **bytes** refer to how the machine stores information at the lowest, or "closest to machine registers and memory," level. Computers do not process information as words or numbers. They handle information in bytes. A byte is made up of 8 bits.

Bits and Bytes

A bit (**bi**nary dig**it**) is a unit of data in the binary numbering system. Binary means two, so a bit can assume one of two positions. Effectively, a bit is an ON/OFF switch—ON equals the value of 1 and OFF equals 0. Bits are grouped into collections of 8, which then function as a unit. That unit describes a single character in the computer, such as the letter A or the number 3, and is called a byte. A byte looks something like this:

0	0	0	0	1	1	0	0

There are 255 different combinations of 0 and 1 in an 8-character (or 1-byte) unit. That forms the basic limit to the number of characters that can be directly expressed in the computer. Thus, the basic character set hardwired into most personal computers (PCs) contains 255 characters. In the early days of PCs, this was a problem because it severely limited the images that could be produced. However, with the advent of graphics cards and additional character sets and graphics that the new technology allowed, virtually any image can be produced on a computer screen or printed on a printer. Even without graphics cards, additional character sets can be created by means of programming techniques. The size of a variety of computer functions and components is measured by how many bytes they can handle or store at one time (Table 4.1).

TABLE 4.1	Meaning of Storage Size Terms		
Number of Bytes	**Term**	**Formula**	**Approximate Size in Typed Pages or Other Comparison**
1,024	1 kilobyte (K)	$2^{10} \approx 1,000$	One-third of a single-spaced typed page
1,048,576	1 megabyte (M or MB)	$2^{20} \approx 1,024^2$	600-page paperback book
1,073,741,824	1 gigabyte (G or GB)	$2^{30} \approx 1,024^3$	Approximately 1 billion bytes or an encyclopedia
1,099,511,627,776	1 terabyte (T or TB)	$2^{40} \approx 1,024^4$	Approximately 1 trillion bytes
1,125,899,906,842,624	1 petabyte (PB)	$2^{50} \approx 1,024^5$	None available
1,152,921,504,606,846,976	1 exabyte (EB)	$2^{60} \approx 1,024^6$	About 10 to the 18th power bytes
1,180,591,620,717,411,303,424	1 zettabyte (ZB)	$2^{70} \approx 1,024^7$	None available
1,208,925,819,614,629,174,706,176	1 yottabyte (YB)	$2^{80} \approx 1,024^8$	None available

≈means approximately equals.

Main memory, which includes the ROM on the motherboard in today's computers, is very large as compared with that of just a few years ago. Since the size of memory is an important factor in the amount of work a computer can handle, large main memory is another key measure in the power of a computer. In the mid 1970s, the PCs on the market were typically sold with a main memory of between 48 and 64 K. By 2010, the size of main memory in computers sold to the public had risen exponentially and most computers were advertised with between 1 and 8 GB of main memory and computers with 20 GB or more of main memory were available.

Another important selling point of a computer is the size of the hard drive that is installed in the box. The first hard drives sold for microcomputers in the 1970s were external devices that stored about 1,500 K. At that time, home computers were not sold with internal hard drives. When the user turned on the computer, they had to be sure the operating system (OS) diskette was in the disk drive, or the computer could not work. This architecture severely limited the size and functionality of programs. Therefore, consumer demand for hard drives was such that their size grew exponentially while at the same time the cost of hard drive storage decreased exponentially. By late 1999, home computers typically sold had between 6 and 20 GB of space on the hard drive; and in 2010 the typical laptop computer was sold with a 300 to 500 GB hard drive, and desktops often came with hard drives that offered a terabyte or more of storage. Applications programs have become so large that both the main memory and especially the hard drive storage space have had to increase exponentially.

Computer Speed

Earlier in the discussion about the CPU, it was noted that the basic operations of the CPU are called cycles, and the four types of cycles, or operations of a CPU, include: fetch, decode, execute, and store. It takes time for the computer to perform each of these functions or cycles. The CPU speed is measured in cycles per second which are called the clock speed of the computer. One million cycles per second is called 1 megahertz (MHz) and a billion cycles per second is called 1 gigahertz (GHz). CPU speeds are very fast, and today's computers perform many billions of cycles per second. For example, the original IBM PC introduced in 1981 had a clock speed of 4.77 MHz (4.77 million cycles per second). In 2010, home computers commonly had from 1.8 to 3 GHz speeds. In general, the higher the clock speed possessed by the CPU, the faster and (in one dimension)

the more powerful the computer. However, clock rate can be misleading, since different kinds of processors may perform a different amount of work in one cycle. For example, general purpose computers are known as complex instruction set computers (CISCs) and their processors are prepared to perform a large number of different instruction sets. Therefore, a cycle in a CISC computer may take longer than that for a specialized type of computer called a reduced instruction set computer (RISC). Nonetheless, clock speed is one important measure of the power of a computer.

The computer is generally described in terms of several major characteristics that have been generally explained—automatic, electronic, and general purpose—as well as in terms of speed, reliability, and storage capacity. The computer is **automatic** because it is self-instructed; that is, it automatically processes data using computer programs called software. The computer is **electronic** because it uses microelectronic components etched on silicon chips for its circuitry. This means that its basic building blocks are microminiaturized. The computers discussed so far are **general purpose** machines, because the user can program them to process all types of problems and can solve any problem that can be broken down into a set of logical sequential instructions. Special purpose machines designed to do only a very few different types of tasks have also been developed. An example of a special-use computer is the RISC computer described above. The computer is also characterized by its **speed** and split-second processing of large amounts of data, its **reliability** due to the silicon circuitry, and its ability to **store** large amounts of data that can be retrieved quickly.

The computer is also described by its **architecture**, which refers to the design of the individual hardware components and to the microprocessors used. A key characteristic of a computer is its hardware platform, or simply, its platform. The two main types of platform in the commercial PC market are the IBM (typically called the IBM/Microsoft platform) and the Apple Macintosh platform. The two are not compatible, and without a translator, one computer cannot read the other's media.

COMPUTER SOFTWARE

Software is the general term applied to the instructions that direct the computer's hardware to perform work. It is distinguished from hardware by its conceptual rather than physical nature. Hardware consists of physical components, whereas software consists of instructions communicated electronically to the hardware. Software is needed for two purposes. First, computers do not directly understand human language, and software is needed to translate instructions created in human language into machine language. At the machine level, computers can understand only binary numbers, not English or any other human language.

Second, packaged or stored software is needed to make the computer an economical work tool. Users could create their own software every time they needed to use the computer. However, writing software instructions (programming) is extremely difficult, timeconsuming, and, for most people, tedious. It is much more practical and economical for one highly skilled person or programming team to develop programs that many other people can buy and use to do common tasks. Software is supplied as organized instruction sets called programs, or more typically as a set of related programs called a package.

For example, several prominent software companies sell their own version of a package of programs that are typically needed to support an office computer, including a word processing program, a spreadsheet program, a graphics program, and sometimes a database manager. Programs translate operations the user needs into language and instructions that the computer can understand. By itself, computer hardware is merely a collection of printed circuits, plastic, metal, and wires. Without software, hardware is nonfunctional.

BRIEF HISTORY OF COMPUTER PROGRAMMING AND SOFTWARE

The idea of having computer programs stored on a hard drive and brought into memory at the user's command has its roots in the 1800s, long before the first true computer was invented. Augusta Ada Byron, Countess of Lovelace (1815–1852), a mathematician and co-researcher with Charles Babbage (1792–1871), first described the concept of a stored computer program. Babbage was a late nineteenth-century mathematician and inventor. He invented (but never built) a device that he named the "analytical machine." Babbage's son finally built his machine in 1910 but was never able to make it work reliably (Fig. 4.6). However, the concept of a machine that could perform mathematical functions stimulated the thinking of other scientists and mathematicians about how to build such a machine and how instructions could be communicated to the machine. In her writings about Babbage's concept of an analytical engine, Countess Lovelace theorized the use

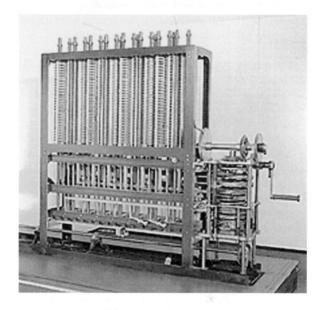

• **FIGURE 4.6.** Babbage's analytic machine.

of automatic repetitious arithmetic steps that the analytical engine would follow to solve a problem, namely, the "loop concept." This concept gave her the title of the "first programmer" in computer history. However, it was John von Neumann (1903–1957) who proposed that both data and instructions could be stored in the computer and that the instructions could be automatically carried out. The stored program concept was subsequently implemented as a major concept in the evolution of the computer.

Programs often require data as input. Today, people take for granted that computers will process huge amounts of data; however, it was not always feasible to handle large datasets. In the case of management of very large collections of data, necessity was truly the mother of invention. As part of the development of the new nation, America's founders decreed that a census of the population be taken every 10 years, the first of which commenced on August 2, 1790. The order was more difficult to carry out than anticipated. It took over 9 months to gather and process the 1790 census information, and there were only about 3.8 million people in the United States at the time. There were simply no machines to help with data collection or collation—they had not been invented yet! By the 1860 census, it was apparent that the manual methods of processing the census were inadequate. Unless the number of questions was severely limited, it would take more than 10 years to process the 10-year census data. Some type of machine was needed if the constitutional requirement for a census was to be fulfilled successfully.

Ultimately, the development of data processing machines was taken from the field of textiles. Jacquard blouses, so popular in women's better clothing stores, were made possible by an invention of a weaver from France, Joseph Jacquard (Delve, 2007). Jacquard invented the Jacquard loom, a device that used blocks of wood with holes drilled in such a way that the threads to be woven into cloth could form a "program," or set of machine instructions, to the loom (Fig. 4.7). The instructions varied the way the cloth was worked by the loom so that a particular design (such as flowers or birds) would be produced in the fabric; that is, the weave produced images without changing the thread color or type.

In 1881, Herman Hollerith (1860–1929), a 19-year-old graduate of the Columbia School of Mines, was employed as a special agent by the U.S. Census Bureau.

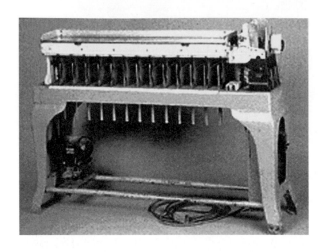

• **FIGURE 4.8.** Hollerith's counting machine.

Recognizing the problem with trying to process such massive amounts of data, Hollerith used Jacquard's idea but developed a machine that could read punched cards and tabulate the results. In 1884, Hollerith patented his machine and punched-card system (Fig. 4.8). Hollerith's ideas were so successful that he formed a company called Tabulating Machine. Eventually, after several changes of ownership and name changes, the company became International Business Machines, more popularly known as IBM. The punched-card method of entering programs (software) and data into computers continued to be promoted until 1984 when IBM discontinued selling its card puncher (IBM, 2010). In the rare computing center, some punched-card use continues even in 2010 (da Cruz, 2010; Whittle, 2010). After the mid to late 1980s, keypunch machines and punched-card readers were withdrawn from most computer centers.

In any history of computer programming, a remarkable woman known as "The Mother of Computing" should be acknowledged. Rear Admiral Grace Murray Hopper was born in New York in 1906 (Beyer, 2009). She obtained a degree in mathematics and physics, Phi Beta Kappa from Vassar in 1928, and her PhD in mathematics in 1934. In 1941, she offered her services to her country by enlisting in the U.S. Naval Reserve. On active duty throughout World War II, she was assigned to the Bureau of Ordinance Computation at Harvard University, where she worked with the first digital mainframe computers, the Mark I, and its successor, the Mark II. Dr. Hopper was perhaps the world's most expert programmer of early computers. During her long career,

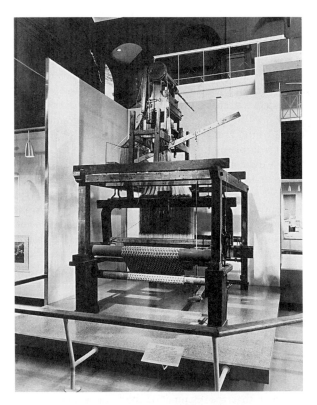

• **FIGURE 4.7.** The Jacquard loom. (Smithsonian Institution Photo No. 45599.)

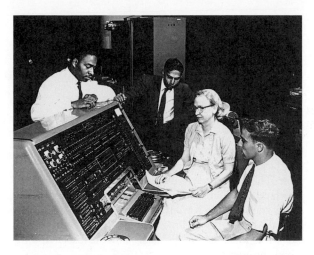

• **FIGURE 4.9.** Rear Admiral Grace Hopper, PhD, and colleagues. (Smithsonian Institution Photo No. 83.4878.)

she greatly advanced the power of computers through her innovations in computer programming and program languages (Fig. 4.9). She is said to have written the third program ever on the Mark I, which was the first large-scale, digital computer in history. In 1946, the navy returned Hopper to inactive duty, but they recalled her to active duty in 1967 during the Vietnam War. Her brilliance with computers was considered irreplaceable by the military, and she continued to serve her country until she retired a second time in 1986 at the age of 79. Throughout her career, she developed many of the concepts and mathematical foundations of computer programming science.

A major activity in program testing is **debugging**, which means checking the program to ensure that it is free of error. This term was coined by Grace Hopper. In 1945, when working at Harvard on the Mark II computer, her program crashed. On examination of the computer, she discovered that a moth caught in the machine had caused the crash (Beyer, 2009). To correct the problem and get the system working again, she "debugged" the computer. As a result, the term was used to refer to any correction of a computer programming error.

Admiral Hopper was widely known not only for her accomplishments in computer programming language development but also for her extraordinary vision and wit. She was the early force behind the idea that computer programming languages should become more like the English language. She recognized that obscure assembly and machine-like programming languages limited access to the computer and therefore the utility

of the machines. Her work on programming languages in the early 1950s formed the foundation for the first truly English-like language, the **CO**mmon**B**usiness-**O**riented **L**anguage (COBOL). COBOL was considered the first "universal" programming language and is still used in many older (legacy) business applications. In an age when the focus was on bigger rather than on more friendly computers, she quipped, "In pioneer days they used oxen for heavy pulling, and when one ox couldn't budge a log, they didn't try to grow a larger ox. We shouldn't be trying for bigger computers, but for more systems of computers" (Beyer, 2009). She recognized that a better approach would be to have many computers working independently and together so that more work could be accomplished. Today, the Internet, the network of networks, might be viewed as the realization of Grace Hopper's early vision of computing. It is appropriate that this section be closed with another of her quotes: "Life was simple before World War II. After that, we had systems" (Beyer, 2009).

TYPES OF SOFTWARE

There are two basic types of software: system software and applications software. System software "boots up" (starts up and initializes) the computer system; controls input, output, and storage; and controls the operations of the application software. Applications software includes the various programs that users require to perform day-to-day tasks. They are the programs that support the actual work of the user. Some users claim a third type of software called utility programs. These are programs that are used to help maintain the system, clean up unwanted programs, protect the system against virus attacks, access the World Wide Web (WWW), and the like. Sometimes it can get confusing as to whether programs are utility programs or system software because system software packages today usually include a variety of utility programs with the basic system software packages.

System Software

System software consists of a variety of programs that control the individual computer and make the user's application programs work well with the hardware. System software consists of a variety of programs that initialize, or boot up, the computer when it is first turned on and thereafter control all the functions of the computer hardware and applications software. System software helps speed up the computer's processing, expands the power of the computer by creating cache memory, reduces the amount of confusion when multiple programs are running together, "cleans up" the hard drive so that storage is managed efficiently, and performs other such system management tasks.

Basic Input/Output System. The first level of system control is handled by the basic input/output system (BIOS) stored on a ROM chip on the motherboard. The software on the BIOS chip is the first part of the computer to function when the system is turned on. It first searches for an OS and loads it into the RAM. Given that the BIOS consists of a set of instructions permanently burned onto a computer chip, it is truly a combination of hardware and software. Programs on chips are often called firmware, because they straddle the line between hardware and software. For this reason, many computer engineers make a distinction between firmware and software. From that perspective, the OS is actually the first level of system software.

Operating Systems. OSs are actual software, loaded from the hard drive into RAM as soon as the computer is turned on. While the firmware cannot be upgraded without changing the hardware chip, the OS can be upgraded or entirely changed through software. The user simply deletes OS files from the hard drive and installs a new OS from a CD-ROM or floppy diskettes or perhaps downloads it from a Website. Most users purchase a computer with the OS already installed on the hard drive. However, the OS can be purchased separately and installed by the user. OSs handle the connection between the CPU and peripherals. (The connection between the CPU and a peripheral or a user is called an interface.) The OS manages the interfaces to peripheral hardware, schedules tasks, allocates storage in memory and on disks, and provides an interface between the machine and the user.

One of the most critical tasks (from the user's perspective) performed by the OS involves the management of storage. In the early computers, there were no OSs. Every program had to explicitly tell the CPU exactly where in RAM to locate the lines of program code and data to be used during processing. That meant the user had to keep track of thousands of memory locations, and be sure to avoid writing one line of code over another active line of code. Also, the programmer had to be careful that output of one part of processing did not accidentally get written over output from another part of processing. As can be imagined, the need for management of storage consumed a great deal of time and programming code, and it produced many errors in

programs. Since those errors had to be discovered and corrected before the program would run correctly, the lack of an OS made programming enormously time-consuming and tedious. In comparison, programming today—while still a difficult and time-consuming task—is much more efficient.

User Interfaces

Disk Operating System. The OS also provides a basic interface between the user and the hardware and software. There are two types of OS user interface: the interface provided by a disk operating system (DOS) and a graphical user interface (GUI) provided by OSs such as Microsoft Windows. Essentially, DOS OSs present a blank screen to the user, and the user submits typed commands.

DOS OSs were first designed for mainframe computers and replicated the procedures programmers used under manual OSs. They were an extension of the move away from dependency on human operators and tedious memory allocation programming requirements. When OSs were first developed for mainframes, they permitted tremendous advances in productivity in the computer department. However, just about everybody associated with the computer department at that time was a programmer. They all knew the syntax (wording and sequencing of commands). Thus, the need to type in long, non–English-like commands was not viewed as a great burden.

As computers became more popular and their applications became more useful to the general population, the need to learn DOS's obscure syntax became a real issue in office and home computing. Business people, office support personnel, and home users may have wanted to use computers for document preparation, financial management tasks, games, and other personal applications; however, they very much did not want to learn programming. Unfortunately, some programming skills had to be acquired to use the DOS interface effectively. During the late 1970s and early 1980s, a great proportion of the potential market for PCs was lost because of people's extreme resistance to using systems with such a poor user interface.

Graphical User Interface. In 1979, Steve Jobs of Apple Computers made a strategic decision to abandon the DOS interface and move to a GUI system for a new product to be called the Macintosh. The idea came as a result of his visit to the Xerox laboratory, where he saw the GUI that had been developed for a system that never really succeeded in the popular computer market.

In 1984, the Macintosh with the first commercially available GUI was introduced. This was the "computer for everybody," and the PC market exploded. Although the GUI did not eliminate the need for users to spend time learning new programs, it did bring closer to reality the ideal that computers could become "self-teaching" devices. People could begin to use computers with minimal training, using built-in tutorials and online answers to common questions. Bill Gates, founder and CEO of the Microsoft Corporation, quickly recognized the need to provide a GUI product and immediately began development of Windows, the GUI for the IBM PC platform. The popularity of GUIs is a function of their use of pictures rather than typed narrative commands.

A GUI OS supports use of graphic images called icons to represent commands to the computer. Each icon image is designed to look like the physical representation of the operation the user wishes to employ. For example, a small image of a printer is used to symbolize the command to print a page or document. Rather than typing in commands such as PRINT FILE, the user simply clicks the mouse button on the printer icon, and the print command is executed.

There are far too many commands needed for running most application programs for all commands to be represented by icons. Therefore, GUI OSs also support the operation of **menus**. Similar to menus in restaurants, the GUI menu provides a narrative list of common commands, or operations that the computer can execute. Rather than typing out a command, the user simply clicks the mouse button on the menu item desired, and the command represented by that menu word is executed. In complex programs that have hundreds or thousands of commands, the GUI supports **nested menus**.

Nested menus are submenus and sub-submenus; that is, the user clicks on a menu item, and instead of executing a command, the computer presents another menu of choices. (The submenu is fit, or nested, inside the main menu.) Clicking on a menu choice on a submenu might bring forth yet another menu. The process proceeds until the actual operation to be executed is listed. The nested menu format permits a virtually unlimited number of command options to be presented to the user, who never needs to remember the proper wording and order of a command in order to execute it.

Utility Programs. In addition to the operating system, there are a variety of other system programs available to the user. Some are called **utility** programs and are designed to enhance the functions of the OS or perhaps to add facilities that the basic OS does not offer. These include programs that provide algorithms (formulae) for efficiently sorting a large set of numbers or character-based items, copying files or parts of files, security programs, and the like.

Language Translation Utilities. People and computers do not speak the same language. At the machine level, computers only understand binary. Human beings do not speak binary. Consequently, it is very difficult to write a program in the machine's language. Translation programs are needed to convert instructions written in an English-like language into binary. These types of translation programs are called **assemblers**, **compilers**, or **interpreters**. Originally, they were all machine-dependent; that is, a compiler written for an IBM 360 mainframe computer could not work on a Hitachi mainframe computer. Even worse, a program written to work with one compiler could not work on a computer with a different compiler, even if the programming language was the same. With the advent of portable translators, that limitation has been at least partially overcome. Translation programs today are often 90% or more portable among different computer platforms. However, when buying a compiler, one still needs to purchase the version that has been customized to the user's computer platform.

The World Wide Web and Web Browsers. The WWW is a sort of network system utility program for the Internet. It provides a protocol for document transfer across the Internet. A Web browser is a utility program that allows the user to access the Web and the materials available through the Web. Prior to the advent of the WWW, commands to access and transfer documents throughout the Internet required users to know the command syntax of the Unix OS. While Unix is still the OS of the Internet, its command language is about as obscure to the average reader as machine language.

The Internet is a system of data and voice lines routed through dedicated servers to create a network of networks; that is, it consists of linkages that allow users from one computer network to access the documents and files available on another network. The trick in developing a network is figuring out how to make documents stored on one platform available to networks that use entirely different platforms. Early in the development of computer communications, utility programs called file transfer protocols (FTPs) were developed to allow files to be ported from one computer to another and from one network to another.

While the original Internet was an extremely useful system to programmers and scientists who could

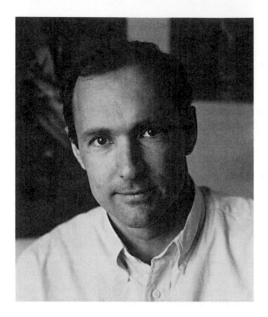

• **FIGURE 4.10.** Tim Berners-Lee. (Courtesy Donna Coveney/MIT.)

construct commands in the Unix syntax, it was time-consuming to use. In 1989, Tim Berners-Lee, a scientist at CERN, Switzerland's laboratory for particle physics, originated the idea of having a protocol that would be standard for all documents and sites on the Internet (Berners-Lee & Fischetti, 2000) (Fig. 4.10). In this way, use of the Internet would be greatly facilitated not only for programmers, but for just about everybody who might want to use it. In August 1991, CERN released the first WWW software.

Berners-Lee conceived the WWW as a system utility program that requires all users to adhere to a standard set of text retrieval protocols (ie, a standard command syntax for transfer of text from one computer to another). This set of protocols is called the Hypertext Transfer Protocol (HTTP). "Hypertext" refers to the facility that permits a standard text-linking command to be incorporated into documents. Text linking occurs when content in one document refers to another document, and the user can click on the linking text and have the protocol automatically move the user from the first document to the linked document (Berners-Lee & Fischetti, 2000). The WWW also needed to have a standard addressing system, so that every document would have only one address. This addressing system is called the Uniform Resource Locator (URL). Finally, it needed a way to have documents formatted so that colors, fonts, spacing, tables, and images could be cre-

ated and transmitted across the Internet. The language developed for the Internet is called HTML, which stands for Hypertext Markup Language. HTML allows document creators to format their text.

Although the WWW was an enormous advance, it still lacked one utility necessary to making the Web a household tool for everyone; it lacked a user-friendly GUI. This problem was addressed through the release of Mosaic, a GUI interface for the Web developed by the National Center for Supercomputing Applications (NCSA) at the University of Illinois at Urbana-Champaign. Mosaic was largely developed by Marc Anderson who later founded Netscape, one of the two most popular Web browsers.

Applications Software

Applications software includes the various programs people use to do work, process data, play games, communicate with others, or watch multimedia programs on a computer. Unlike system and utility programs, they are written by or for system users. When the user orders the OS to run an application program, the OS transfers the program from the hard drive, diskette, or CD-ROM into RAM and executes it.

Application programs are written in a particular programming language. Then the program is "compiled" (or translated) into machine language so the computer can understand the instructions and execute the program. Originally, programs were written for a specific computer and could only run on that machine. However, the science of programming languages and their translation eventually advanced to the point that programs today can generally be "ported" (or transferred) across many machines. This advance permitted programmers to develop programs that could be used on a class of machines, such as the IBM type or Macintosh (the two are still generally incompatible). This advance opened a whole new industry, since programs could be marketed as off-the-shelf software packages.

Programming Languages

A programming language is a means of communicating with the computer. Actually, of course, the only language a CPU can understand is binary or machine language. While it is certainly possible for programmers to learn to use binary—some highly sensitive defense applications are still written in machine language—the language is painfully tedious and inefficient use of human resources, and its programs are virtually impossible to update and debug. Since the invention of computers, users have longed for a machine that could accept instructions in everyday human language. Although that goal largely eludes programmers, applications such as office support programs (i.e. word processors, spread sheets, presentation graphics applications and the like) have become much easier to use with graphical user interface based commands.

Generations and Levels of Programming Languages

Programming languages are divided into five generations, or sometimes into three levels. The term level refers to how close the language is to the actual machine. The first level includes the first two generations of programming languages: machine language and assembly language. The second level includes the next two generations: high-level procedural and nonprocedural languages. The third level (and fifth generation) is natural language.

The low-level languages are machinelike. Machine language is, of course, binary. It consists of strings of 0s and 1s and can be directly understood by the computer. However, it is difficult to use and to edit.

Machine Language. Machine language is the true language of the computer. Any program must be translated into machine language before the computer can execute it. The machine language consists only of the binary numbers 1 and 0, representing the **ON** and **OFF** electrical impulses. All data—numbers, letters, and symbols—are represented by combinations of binary digits. For example, the number 3 is represented by 8binary numbers (00000011), and 6 is represented by 00000110. Traditionally, machine languages are machinedependent, which means that each model of computer has its own unique machine language.

Assembler Language. Assembler language is far more like the English language, but it is still very close to machine language. One command in machine language is a single instruction to the processor. Assembler language instructions have a one-to-one correspondence with a machine language instruction. Assembler language is still used a great deal by system programmers and whenever application programmers wish to manipulate functions at the machine level. As can be seen from Figure 4.11, assembly language, while more English-like than machine language, is extremely obscure to the nonprogrammer.

Third-Generation Languages. Third-generation languages include the procedural languages and were the beginning of the second level in programming languages. Procedural languages require the programmer to specify both what the computer is to do and the procedure for how to do it. These languages are far more English-like than assembly

```
PRINT_ASCII PROC
        MOV DL, 00h
        DL MOV CX, 255
PRINT_LOOP:
        CALL WRITE_CHAR
        INC DL
        LOOP PRINT_LOOP
        MOV AH, 4Ch
        INT 21h ;21h
PRINT ASCII        ENDP
```

• **FIGURE 4.11.** Assembler language lines of code.

and machine language. However, a great deal of study is required to learn to use these languages. The programmer must learn the words the language recognizes, and must use those words in a rigid style and sequence. A single comma or letter out of place will cause the program to fail or crash. The style and sequence of a language are called its syntax. FORTRAN and COBOL are examples of early third-generation languages.

A third-generation language written specifically for use in healthcare settings was MUMPS (Massachusetts General Hospital Utility Multi-Programming System). MUMPS was originally developed to support medical records applications at Massachusetts General. MUMPS offers powerful tools to support database management systems; this is particularly useful in any setting in which many users have to access the same databases at the same time. Therefore, MUMPS is now found in many different industries such as banks, travel agencies, stock exchanges, and of course, other hospitals. Originally, MUMPS was both a language and a full OS; however, today most installations load MUMPS on top of their own computer's OS.

Today, the most popular computer language for writing new OSs and other system programs is called C. (It was named after an earlier prototype program called simply B.)

Two important late third-generation languages are increasing in importance as the importance of the Internet grows. They include the visual programming languages and Java. Java was developed by Sun Microsystems to be a relatively simple language that would provide the portability across differing computer platforms and the security needed for use on a huge, public network like the Internet. The world community of software developers and Internet content providers has warmly received Java. Java programming skills are critical for any serious Web developer.

Visual Programming Languages. As the popularity of GUI technology grew, several languages were developed to facilitate program development in graphics-based environments. Microsoft Corporation has marketed two very popular such programs: Visual BASIC (Beginners' All-purpose Symbolic Instruction Code) and Visual C++. These programs and their cousins marketed by other companies have been used for a variety of applications, especially those that allow users to interact with electronic companies through the Internet.

Fourth-Generation Languages. Fourth-generation languages are specialized application programs that require more involvement of the user in directing the program to do the necessary work. Some people in the computer industry do not consider these to be programming languages. Procedural languages include programs such as spreadsheets, statistical analysis programs, and database query languages. The difference between these languages and the earlier generation languages is that the user specifies *what* the program is to do, but not *how* the program is to perform the task. The how is already programmed by the manufacturer of the language program. For example, to perform a chi-square calculation in FORTRAN, the user must specify each step involved in carrying out the formula for a chi-square and the data on which the operations are to be performed. In Statistical Package for Social Sciences (SPSS), a statistical analysis program, the user enters a command (from a menu of commands) that tells the computer to compute a chi-square statistic on a particular datasheet. The formula for chi-square is already part of the SPSS program; the user does not have to tell SPSS how to calculate the chi-square.

Fifth-Generation Languages. Fifth-generation or third-level languages are called natural language. In these types of programs, the user tells the machine what to do in the user's own natural language or through use of a set of very English-like commands. Ideally, voice recognition technology is integrated with the language so that voice commands are recognized and executed. True fifth-generation languages are emerging. True natural language recognition, in which any user could give understandable commands to the computer in his or her own word style and accent is being performed at the beginning of the twenty-first century. However, natural language systems are clearly in the future of personal computing. The great difficulty is, of course, how to reliably translate natural, spoken human language into a language the computer can understand.

To prepare a translation program for a natural language requires several levels of analysis. First, the sentences need to be broken down to identify the subject's words and relate them to the underlying constituents of speech (ie, parsed). The next level is called semantic analysis, whereby the grammar of each word in the sentence is analyzed. It attempts to recognize the action described and the object of the action. There are several computer programs that translate natural languages based on basic rules of English. They generally are specially written programs designed to interact with databases on a specific topic. By limiting the programs to querying the database, it is possible to process the natural language terms.

COMMON SOFTWARE PACKAGES FOR MICROCOMPUTERS

The most common package sold with computers is a standard office package. The standard office package includes a wordprocessing program, a spreadsheet program, a presentation graphics program, and some form of database management system. The two most commonly used programs are an e-mail system and a word processor. In fact, some people purchase a computer with only an OS, word processor, and an Internet browser, and sign up for their e-mail account and use little else. Another very common product is a desktop publisher. Most of these common programs have to be written in two versions: one for the IBM PC platform and one for the Macintosh. Typically, software packages are sold on DVDs, although some are available on flash drives and many software companies are now marketing their products through the Internet and customers download the software directly through the Internet from the vendor's Website.

SOFTWARE PACKAGE OWNERSHIP RIGHTS

Protecting ownership rights in software has presented a challenge to the computer software industry. A program sold to one customer can be installed on a very large number of machines. This practice obviously seriously harms the profitability of software development. If programs were sold outright, users would have every right to distribute them as they wished; however, the industry could not survive in such market conditions. As a result, the software industry has followed an ownership model more similar to that of the book publishing industry than to the model used by vendors of most commercial products.

When most commercial products like furniture or appliances are sold, the buyer can use the product or resell it or loan it to a friend if so desired. The product sold is a physical product that can be used only by one customer at a time. Copying the product is not feasible. However, intellectual property is quite a different proposition: what is sold is the idea. The medium on which the idea is stored is not the product. However, when the PC industry was new, people buying software viewed their purchase as the physical diskette on which the intellectual property was stored. Software was expensive, but the diskettes were cheap. Therefore, groups of friends would often pool money to purchase one copy of the software and make copies for everyone in the group. This, of course, enraged the software vendors.

As a result, copyright laws were extended to software so that only the original purchaser was legally empowered to install the program on his or her computer. Any other installations were considered illegal copies, and such copies were called pirate copies. Purchasers of software do not buy full rights to the software. They purchase only a license to use the software. Individually purchased software is licensed to one and only one computer. An exception can be made if the individual has both a desktop and a laptop. Fair use allows the purchaser to install the software on all the machines he or she personally owns—provided the computers are for that user's personal use only. Companies that have multiple computers that are used by many employees must purchase a separate copy for each machine, or more typically, they purchase a "site license." A site license is a way of buying in bulk, so to speak. The company and software vendor agree on how many machines the software may be used on, and a special fee is paid for the number of copies to be used. Additional machines over the number agreed on require either an increase in the allowable sites—and payment of the higher sitelicense fee, or separate copies of the software may be purchased. What is not permitted, and is, in fact, a form of theft, is to install more copies of the software than were paid for.

COMMON SOFTWARE USEFUL TO NURSES

In most hospitals, software used by nurses are based in a Hospital Information System (HIS). The HIS is a multipurpose program, designed to support many applications in hospitals and their associated clinics. The components nurses use most includes admission, discharge, and transfer (ADT) systems that help with patient tracking, medication administration record (MAR) software, laboratory systems that are used to order laboratory tests and receive the results. Increasingly, hospitals have added charting software that computerizes at least some parts of the nursing record. In addition, quality and safety groups such as the Leapfrog group consider a computer physician order entry (CPOE) system to be so important that they list it as a separate item on their quality checklist. Additionally, nurses may have the support of computer-based systems for laboratory and radiology orders and results reporting, a computerized patient acuity system used to help with nurse staff allocation, and perhaps there may be a hospital e-mail system used for at least some hospital communications. Increasingly, nurses are finding that they are able to build regional, national, and international networks with their nursing colleagues with the use of chat rooms, bulletin boards, and listservs on the Internet. Given that many people have personal digital assistants (PDAs) as part of their cellular phone, nurses may download software onto their PDA to assist them with patient care. Such programs include drug guides, medical dictionaries, and consult guides for a variety of patient populations and clinical problems (eg, pediatric pocket consultation, toxicology guide, guide to clinical procedures, etc.).

Some nursing applications include a handy "**dashboard**," which is an application that provides a sort of a menu of options from which the nurse can choose. Typically, dashboards provide the nurse a quick way to order common output from certain (or all) screens, or may provide some kind of alert that a task is due to be performed.

COMPUTER SYSTEMS

Every functioning computer is a system; that is, it is a complex entity, consisting of an organized set of interconnected components or factors that function together as a unit to accomplish results that one part alone could not. At a minimum, a computer must have at least four components to function. These minimum components are a power source, a CPU, a peripheral to allow input, and a peripheral to permit output. Of course, computers typically have more than four components. Computer system may refer to a single machine (and its peripherals) that is unconnected to any other computer. However, most healthcare professionals use computer systems consisting of multiple, interconnected computers that function to facilitate the work of groups of providers and their support people in a system called a

network. The greatest range of functionality is realized when computers are connected to other computers in a network or, as with the Internet, a system of networks in which any computer can communicate with any other computer.

Common types of computer networks are point to point, local area network (LAN), wide area network (WAN), and metropolitan area networks (MAN). A point-to-point network is a very small network in which all parts of the system are directly connected via wires or wireless (typically provided by a router in a single building). LANs, WANs, and MANs are sequentially larger and given the number of users, they require communications architecture to ensure all users on the network are served. If the network capacity is too small, some users will experience very long waits or perhaps the system will crash from overload (ie, stop working and have to be restarted).

Computer networks must allocate time and memory space to many users, and so must have a way to organize usage of the network resources so that all users are served. There are a variety of allocation strategies for high-level communication in networks. The most common are token ring (developed by IBM), star (also called multipoint; all communications go through a single hub computer), bus (in which all computers are connected to a single line), and tree. For very large networks, backbone communication technology is increasingly used.

The use of systems in computer technology is based on system theory. System theory and its subset, network theory, provide the basis for understanding how the power of individual computers has been greatly enhanced through the process of linking multiple computers into a single system and multiple computer systems into networks.

SYSTEM THEORY

System theory provides the conceptual basis for understanding complex entities that consist of multiple interrelated parts working together to achieve a desired result. Such entities are called **systems**. A system, by its nature, is not random; it is orderly and predictable in its functioning. If a system begins to exhibit unpredictable behavior, one of two conditions pertains. Either the system is malfunctioning for some reason internal or external to the system itself, or the observer does not fully understand the system and thus a proper result is misinterpreted as incorrect (unpredicted). The key concepts of system theory are parts, interaction (among the parts), interdependency (among the parts), input, output, processing, feedback, and control. The primary propositions of the theory are the following:

1. A system takes in input on which to perform processes.

2. The processes performed by a system on input result in system output.

3. The processes in a system are subject to control forces.

4. Feedback is the key mechanism of control in a system.

5. A system's parts interact in such a way that the parts are interdependent with respect to the system's processes.

6. Impingement on one part in a system will produce effects on the system's processes and may produce distortions on other parts of the system. A corollary to this proposition is the following:

    a. Distortion in one part of a system may be a symptom of a problem in another component. (This is called a secondary malfunction.)

    b. Thus, correction of a malfunctioning part will correct the system functioning only if the malfunction was a primary malfunction and not a secondary malfunction.

7. Effects on the system's processing function will affect the system's output.

8. A system is more than the sum of its parts. Thus, while a system can be broken down into its component parts, if this is done, the system no longer exists. Corollaries to this proposition are the following:

    a. The functioning of a system is different than the functioning of its separate parts.

    b. The output of each separate part, even if combined, does not equal the output of the system.

    c. When combined into a system, the component parts form an entirely new entity.

SYSTEM ELEMENTS

A system consists of the following 6elements: the system's set of interdependent parts, input to the system, system processes, output of the system, system control, and feedback.

Interdependent Parts

The most defining attribute of a system is that its parts interact to conduct some process. Without the interaction, the system process could not occur. Therefore, in the production of the system's process, the parts are interdependent. Each acting alone could not perform the system's process. In computer systems, the process involves mathematical, logical, or data transfer operations requiring interaction among the CPU, RAM, and ROM chips and the motherboard's power source.

Input

Input is any factor from the external environment that is taken into the system. Input in a computer system may serve to initiate system functioning, as when the machine is turned on and the OS is loaded into RAM. It may consist of data that the system is to process. In living systems, input may consist of energy from the Sun, nourishment, or stimulation, or it might be information needed to survive, function, or enjoy life. However, by itself, input is just inert substance or data. The system must act on input if it is to get use from it.

Process

Process is the activity of the system. A system performs process on its inputs to produce outputs, or create some sort of result. (Survival is the result of the processes of a living system.) Process in a computer system can be seen in the example of a presentation graphics system. The hardware, software, and peripherals constitute the interdependent parts. The commands entered by the user, the numerical data for a graphic, and the alphanumeric characters used for title, labels, and notations on the graph constitute the input. The system sends the translated data and commands to the CPU, which performs the ordered operations (processes) on the input to create a graphic image (eg, pie graph and bar graph). Then the graphic package further processes the instructions to produce whatever output is ordered by the user of the system.

Output

Output is any product or waste produced as a result of system process. Not all processes produce a visible, external product. (The result of life processes may be homeostasis, energy, movement, or feedback within the living system.) However, in many of the systems people work with, such as manufacturing systems, the purpose of the system is to produce output. For example, the output of the manufacturing process at Ford Motor Company is composed of automobiles, trucks, and specialty vehicles. For computer systems, output is the reason the system was created or purchased. Typical computer system output includes electronic data transmission from the main memory to a hard or floppy disk, paper reports, or data transmissions (such as information exchange through the Internet).

For example, many users today have word processing and presentation graphics program packages. The output from the presentation graphics system might be an electronic file stored on the hard drive or on a portable floppy disk. It might be an image printed in either black and white or color on a piece of paper or a transparency; or it might be that same image printed onto color 35-mm film for processing into a color slide. Output from a word processor is usually a professionally formatted and printed text document.

Control

Control refers to any component or activity that serves to prevent or correct problems or errors in the system's input, process, or output. A system must function within rules and procedures that keep it functioning smoothly. These rules and procedures constitute a system's **control** operations. Process means activity. Activity must have some beginning and end point, or else the system goes out of control. Cancers are an example of an out-of-control function in a person's body. Cells that need to regrow as part of healing from injury must stop growing once repair is accomplished. When cells continue to grow without control, the result is eventually fatal. Control is an essential function of any system.

In computer systems, a variety of control facilities exist within the OS. Most application programs also incorporate control functions to help the user avoid erroneous results. Control in computers functions by checking, validating, and verifying input and output data and by checking for and flagging certain conditions during processing. An example of a processing error is division by zero. Such an operation is impossible, and whenever such a problem is detected, processing is terminated and an appropriate error message is displayed on the screen or printout.

A good application program will have special programming that creates "error traps" to detect certain kinds of errors. For example, most word processor programs automatically detect words that are misspelled. In such a program, the concept, "misspelled" means that the word has no match in the word processor's dictionary and therefore is not recognized by the program. The user is notified that the system does not recognize the word (by a change in color of the word on the screen, by underlining, or in some other way). Data entry programs for some statistical analysis programs may detect impossible values. The way they do this is that during creation of the data entry screen, the developer identifies upper and lower numerical limits or acceptable/unacceptable characters for the type of data to be stored in that variable. Any value that does not fit the defined acceptable codes is considered an out-of-range value. Then any time a data entry person enters an out-of-range value, processing stops, and a warning message is issued.

Feedback

Feedback is output from one part of a system process that serves as input to another part of a system process. Feedback is a special case of control. Feedback within a system is typically used as part of a system's self-regulation function. For example, in human beings, body temperature is regulated by a feedback system. A falling core temperature stimulates temperature-sensitive neurons in the hypothalamus. In response, the hypothalamus (in conjunction with certain higher brain centers) activates a number of temperature response mechanisms, most obviously the shivering response. Shivering consists of rapid muscle movements—and muscle movement produces heat. The heat is disseminated and raises the body temperature; that, in turn, changes the sensations to the hypothalamus temperature-sensing neurons. (This is a much-simplified picture and only a small part of the temperature-regulatory feedback system in a human being.)

In a computer system, feedback components are important functions of the OS and utility programs. The user will experience the results of feedback if a save command orders the system to store a file on a diskette that is already full. The OS checks the diskette, and the discovery of a full condition initiates a subroutine (small program module used repeatedly). The subroutine stops the processing and issues a message to the user that the command has failed because the disk is full.

A clinical computing example of feedback is the ventilation rate in a mechanical ventilator set at demand. The processor in the ventilator detects its own activity, and based on the timing of the last activity, it initiates or does not initiate another breath. That is, it has a timer that keeps track of the most recent breath taken by (or delivered to) a patient. The ventilator is set to deliver a breath if a certain amount of time has elapsed since the last breath. If the patient's breathing rate is such that each breath is taken prior to the deadline, the system does not initiate forced inspiration. Otherwise, the machine initiates a breath. In this way, the ventilator controls the rate at which it delivers breaths to the patient—neither too fast nor too slow for optimal oxygenation.

INFORMATION SYSTEMS

An information system (IS) is the collection and integration of various pieces of hardware and software and the human resources that meet the data collection, storage, processing, and report generation needs of an organization. For most large healthcare organizations, the software requirements are varied and complex. The hardware must always be purchased to fit the software requirements. As a result, most large organizations must retain a sophisticated IS department to construct, maintain, and interface the various—and sometimes incompatible—hardware and software necessary to support the work of the organization. When an organization is so large and its computing requirements so diverse that the organization simply cannot obtain a single system to meet all its needs, the result is usually a hodge-podge of incompatible software and hardware platforms. The IS department must program and maintain the software interfaces that let the systems work together. The key pieces of an information system are the hardware, software, and the database or databases in which the organization's data are stored.

Information System Types

Information systemsare found almost everywhere in healthcare, including hospitals, clinics, community health agencies, research facilities, and educational institutions. Their configuration, power, and functions vary widely depending on how they are used and the type of work performed in the organization. There is a wide range of IS in healthcare facilities that provide different functions. They have different titles/names, which overlap depending on the context in which they are used. The major ones to be described include management information systems (MIS), bibliographic retrieval systems, stand-alone systems, transaction systems, physiologic monitoring systems, decision support systems, and expert systems.

Management Information Systems. An MIS provides managers information about their business operations. A MIS is defined as an organized system for managing the flow of information in an organization in a timely manner. Its primary use is assisting in the decision-making processes. The MIS in a healthcare facility may be integrated with a large, HIS, or it might be a stand-alone system. Most MIS systems have programs that support strategic planning, management control, and operations support.

Strategic planning refers to the policy decisions made by the top-level team of administrators. Strategic planning is the work that seeks to position the organization with respect to its customers and competitors. The management control function refers to the program and personnel decisions made by middle-level managers, supervisors, and head nurses. They need information to measure performance standards and to control, plan, and allocate resources. The operations control support functions provide data and information to the first line managers. For example, unit managers need information on the state of the unit budget, on occupancy and workload, and on overtime hours spent. They need information on incident reports, infection rates, and other clinical indicators of care quality. They need the type of information that helps them manage the unit in such a way that patient care is effectively and efficiently carried out.

A healthcare MIS typically provides information that can be used to generate the balance sheet and cash flow reports, help the finance department gather information for other financial reports, and track inpatient occupancy rates by unit or department, clinic visits, procedures, and so forth. It also usually has programs that will allow management to analyze trends in the data and project future business given current trends and other assumptions. However, most MIS databases supplement internal data with data from external, local, regional, and national databases. Many organizations join private organizations that share buying power and information useful to management.

Increasingly, healthcare organizations are joining each other into private consortia. The purpose is the collection of information from all members so that averages and ranges of performance data can be used for benchmarking purposes. The University Hospital Consortium in Oakbrook, Illinois, is one such organization. Hospital consortia provide their members with a variety of reports that supplement, and sometimes help managers interpret, their own internal organizational data.

Bibliographic Retrieval Systems. A bibliographic retrieval system is a retrieval system that generally refers to bibliographic data, document information, or literature. Such a system is primarily used to store and retrieve data and not to conduct any computations per se. The textual data are input and stored and are available for retrieval in a user-friendly format that is easy to read and understand. The system is designed to provide bibliographic data on journal articles, books, monographs, and textual reports. It generally contains the full citations, keywords, abstracts, and other pertinent facts on the documents in the database. An example of a bibliographic retrieval system is PubMed, developed and published by the National Library of Medicine (NLM). The NLM made PubMed available free online to anyone who wishes to use it. PubMed may be accessed at www.nlm.nih.gov. Unfortunately, many of the journal articles one finds on PubMed are not available full text unless the user has access to a medical library's MEDLINE with Full Text. Another useful search engine for finding health-related resources is www.googlescholar.com.

Stand-Alone, Dedicated, or Turnkey Systems. A stand-alone system is a special purpose system. It is developed for a single application or set of functions. A patient classification system is an example of a stand-alone system. Most stand-alone systems are described by their purpose, such as a pharmacy or laboratory system or an imaging system in the radiology department. Until recently, most turnkey systems ran on a microcomputer or PC. However, during the 1990s, most vendors of large HIS changed their design strategy. Formerly, most vendors deliberately designed their systems to be unique rather than easily integrated with other systems. Due to customer demand and the realization that a hospital's needs were simply too large for any one vendor to support completely, most HIS vendors made real efforts to make their products more friendly or compatible with other products. Advances in networking science have also changed the technology available for transporting information across different products and platforms. Eventually, most organizations should be able to freely move their data from one system to another electronically.

Transaction Systems. A transaction system is used to process predefined transactions and produce predefined reports. It is designed for repeated operations using a fixed list. From this list, displayed on a computer terminal, a user selects the names of transactions to be processed. A computer program is written so that it can be used repeatedly to process the same type of transactions and generate the same type of reports or products. The computer programs and the list of transactions are retained in storage and retrieved as needed.

An inventory system is an example of a transaction system. It is used to monitor the distribution of items as well as to update and reorder supplies. These kinds of operations are repetitious and always processed in the same manner. A standard list of items is initially developed. Inventory systems usually have information about vendors and prices, track inventory, and can generate automatic reorders when stock on hand drops below a certain level. Typically, inventory control systems produce a set of management reports that helps management keep track of which items are increasing in demand so they can take advantage of volume discounts. The transactions can also be summarized and reports developed to produce monthly bills, prepare order vouchers, and summarize the inventory status for any given time period. In this type of system, the computer program is specifically written to process the transactions (raw data). Grocery store scanners are linked to a transaction-based inventory control system.

Pharmacy, laboratory, and admission/discharge/transfer systems are also forms of transaction systems. Transaction systems can also be designed to process routine medical or nursing orders and permit clinicians to update the orders in real time. This activity is done to ensure that the orders once entered are current in the system. The updating of medical and nursing orders can also be summarized for documenting care plans, change of shift reports, discharge summary, quality review, research studies, and so forth.

Physiologic Monitoring Systems. Physiologic monitoring systems are widely used in hospital patient care units, in surgery, and more and more commonly, in private homes. The heart monitor was one of the first physiologic monitors used by nurses. Primarily due to the heart monitor, survival rates for hospitalized myocardial infarction patients increased by about 30% in the early 1970s. In the labor and delivery unit, mothers' uterine contractions and fetal heart rate are routinely monitored so that complications can be recognized and addressed without delay. Brain waves are monitored in seizure and sleep disorders units. Intraventricular pressure is monitored in neurologic intensive care units for patients at great risk of cerebral aneurysm rupture.

All of these devices are a form of an oscilloscope. An oscilloscope is an electronic device that senses electric impulses and converts them into waveforms on a monitor screen. On the screen, the impulses are represented by a light cursor (a point on the screen that is bright as compared with the darker background). The cursor moves from left to right across the screen at a timed rate (ie, moves a defined number of centimeters across the screen per second). When the monitor is not connected, the cursor travels at the bottom edge of the usable screen

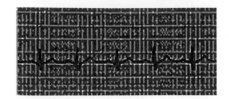

• **FIGURE 4.12.** An ECG.

in a straight line, and this line is called the **baseline**. The strength of the impulse deflects the cursor vertically. Thus, when a positive or negative impulse occurs in the human body being monitored, the cursor is deflected up or down from the baseline. As the impulse ebbs, the cursor returns to the baseline (Fig. 4.12).

Physiologic monitoring systems are being used more frequently to measure and monitor continuous automatic physiologic findings such as heart rate, blood pressure, and other vital signs. Monitoring systems provide alarms to detect significant abnormal findings when personnel are needed to provide patient care and save lives.

Decision Support Systems. A decision support system is a computer system that supports some aspect of the human decision-making process. Decision support systems work with the user to support, but not replace, human judgment in a decision-making situation. Decision-making systems also exist, and these tend to be closed systems that function on internal feedback loops. Decision support systems may model the decision process. This type of system guides the user in a highly structured approach that helps identify the salient components of the problem.

Certain types of analytic modeling systems may also be considered as decision support systems. Business and engineering applications for decision support include linear programming, computer simulation modeling, trend analysis, and forecasting. Although some merely consider these tools to be analysis tools, others consider them to be decision support systems, since they are used to analyze the outcomes of a variety of possible decisions. Still another form of decision support system is an **optimization** program. Optimization programs take all the information about a problem situation and generate a variety of possible solutions. Then each solution is **implemented** (usually simulated in a computer), and the results of the implementation for each solution are compared. Then the optimization program selects the best solutions based on the outcomes. In an optimization problem, several variables exist such that as one improves, another deteriorates. The difficulty is in producing a solution that jointly maximizes the benefits while minimizing the negative consequences. Nurse staffing is a good example of an optimization problem. If high levels of nursing hours are provided, costs of idle time rise. As staffing levels are lowered, more and more patient care needs are neglected. Since both nurse supply and patient acuity vary, however, a perfect staffing level does not exist, so the real challenge is to determine the optimal staffing level for an organization. Other decision support systems provide expert advice to the user.

Expert Systems. An expert system is a computer system containing the information and decision-making strategies of an expert to assist nonexperts in decisionmaking. An expert system is designed for users to simulate the cause and effect reasoning that an expert would use if confronted with the same situation in a real live environment.

The heart of an expert system has two parts: (1) a knowledge base containing facts and data pertinent to the problem area and (2) an inference engine programmed to replicate the reasoning and decision-making strategies of expert clinicians. The format for decisionmaking allows the *What if?—then* construct of logic. This approach is used to draw inferences about the problem posed by the user so that a solution or possible solutions to the problem can be provided. The inference system is based on a method of reasoning that can be either inductive or deductive. Expert systems can be used for assisting practitioners to implement clinical practice guidelines.

Artificial Intelligence Systems. An artificial intelligence (AI) system is a system that attempts to model human reasoning processes. The field is concerned with symbolic inference and knowledge representation. Symbolic inference is concerned with deriving new knowledge from known facts and the use of logical inference. An example of an inference rule is *if A > B and B > C, then A must be greater than C.* Knowledge representation is the field concerned with devising ways to represent and use abstract knowledge and then store those representations and use rules in a computer system. Once abstract phenomena can be represented, and the rules about how to combine facts about phenomena can be determined and programmed into the computer, then new facts can be added as they are discovered. Then the computer can replicate the human process of developing new knowledge by combining new facts with existing knowledge patterns to generate new facts and understandings.

A true AI system can also track the accuracy of its predictions and judgments and alter its own decision-making rules, based on new knowledge it generates for itself. This capacity replicates the human power to reason under conditions of uncertainty. AI is a subject that sheds light on the nature of thinking by simulating the process of reasoning. Programs have been devised to solve typical mental problems in an effort to demonstrate that the reasoning process follows a systematic series of rules.

Pattern recognition and problem solving are important aspects of AI. People have longed for computers that they could talk with rather than having to rely on slow and inconvenient methods of data entry such as typing. Unfortunately, understanding natural human language has proven to be a most difficult task, requiring a much higher degree of intelligence than simple serial processing.

Natural Language Systems. A natural language system is a system that can understand and process commands given in the user's own natural, spoken language. It does not require the user to learn a special vocabulary, syntax, and set of programming rules and instructions. Natural language requires the computer to understand a wide range of words, speech styles (accents), syntax, and sentence structures. Some computer programs are marketed to accept and process natural language input. They consist of relatively crude matching technique methods to process the input. The newer natural language systems are used to recognize and process human speech (voice) and/or handwriting.

HOSPITAL INFORMATION SYSTEMS

An HIS, sometimes called a medical information system (MIS) or patient care system (PCS), provides support for a wide variety of both administrative and clinical functions. The purpose of an HIS is to manage information needed to facilitate daily hospital operations by all healthcare personnel. Administrators manage financial budgets and establish charges for services; physicians diagnose, treat, and evaluate patient conditions; nurses assess, plan, and provide patient care; other personnel provide ancillary services; and a variety of other personnel support the delivery of patient care services.

An HIS is usually a large package of programs, and it is often purchased from a single vendor. While the hospital may own programs that were not supplied by the HIS vendor, the difficulties of integrating programs from multiple vendors can greatly raise the cost of operating the HIS department. Therefore, most hospitals try to keep the number of different products to a minimum.

HIS Configurations

An HIS can use several different computer system configurations. The most common configuration uses a mainframe computer with hardwired terminals or workstations. Users are able to work directly with the mainframe through an interactive interface and real-time processing. Another, and increasingly popular, configuration employs a LAN. The HIS software is either on the mainframe or on a network server. Users access the HIS through their office PC and the network connections.

Many HIS configurations consist of multiple separate systems that are either linked through a network or, in some cases, may not be electronically linked at all. Many hospitals' configurations include dedicated IS for special purposes, such as nurse staffing, pharmacy, or laboratory systems.

Program Modules Available in an HIS

Programs typically offered in an HIS include a wide variety of administrative applications (modules) such as admission and discharge, patient tracking, finance, payroll, billing, budgeting support, inventory, and management reporting programs. Clinical support programs are increasingly being viewed as critically important modules in an HIS. As a result, vendors have increased the number and quality of the clinical support tools available in commercial HIS packages.

Administrative applications refer to the support of the administrative functions of patient care. They generally include budgeting and payroll, cost accounting, patient billing, inventory control, bed census, and medical records. These are the same systems that are available in almost any MIS. For nursing administration, a variety of administrative support systems are available commercially as part of an HIS, as partially integrated systems, or as completely stand-alone systems. Patient classification systems are one of the most popular modules for nursing administration. These systems support the process of assigning nursing staff to units and patients. They function by evaluating the acuity of patients in a particular unit and determining the number of nurses needed to care for that group of patients. Many of these modules can produce a variety of specialized operations reports. Other supports for upper and middle management include staff scheduling and budget support modules.

Semiclinical Modules

Two modules in a HIS support both administrative and clinical operations. These are the ADT and order entry systems. The ADT module monitors and sometimes controls the flow of patients in a hospital from admission to discharge. The ADT module may automatically prepare the midnight census and activity reports. Admissions and discharges constitute the hospital's patient census, which is a key factor in billing and future planning for how to best deploy hospital resources.

Another semiclinical module is the order-entry-results-reporting (OE) module. OE is almost always available in a HIS. Order entry means that staff can enter laboratory, pharmacy, and radiology orders online. Results reporting means that the lab, pharmacy, and radiology can enter the results into the computer system and have those results available to the nursing unit. Some are paperless systems in which all results are reported and posted to the chart electronically. Others may post the results online, but paper reports are still generated and manually posted to the patient chart.

Clinical Support Modules

Charting Systems. Support for nurse charting is highly variable. However, during the 1990s, most vendors greatly upgraded their clinical record products and most vendors now offer some form of online charting. Usually included are the medication administration reports, admission assessment, shift assessments, special assessments (eg, neurologic assessments and labor records), at least some elements of the nursing care plan (such as nursing diagnosis and interventions), vital signs records, wound care, and hygienic care records. Some provision is usually made for online progress notes.

Unfortunately, there is still a major stumbling block to computerizing the record of nursing care. The lack of a universally implemented standard nursing language continues to impede both the development effort and the market success of the systems that are available. Worse, for the profession of nursing, it impedes efforts of nurses to document the outcomes—and therefore the value of nursing care. This problem is not a function of lack of nursing nomenclatures. The American Nurses Association has recognized such nomenclatures as the Clinical Classification System developed by Dr. Virginia Saba (see Chapter 14: CCC System), the Nursing Intervention Classification/Nursing Outcomes Classification (NIC/NOC), North America Nursing Diagnosis Association (NANDA), and the Omaha system.

POINT-OF-SERVICE SYSTEMS

A point-of-service (POS) or point-of-care system is a special type of clinical system. A POS system uses a hand-held or bedside PC to ensure that data are entered at the point at which they are collected. In other types of clinical systems, the placement of workstations may create a problem for nurses. Typically, workstations have been located at the nurses' station, or in a separate physician's charting room; however, patient data are not collected at those locations. This situation forces the nurse to note information on a scrap sheet and later transcribe it to the computer record. This approach produces several suboptimal conditions. First, it is costly to record the same data twice. Second, there is a certain amount of error whenever data are transcribed from one place to another. Third, there is a greater potential that the scrap sheet and the data it contains could be lost or misplaced. Fourth, if the scrap sheet is lost, there is a potential for compromise of patient confidentiality. Fifth, there is always a delay between the time data are collected and the time those data show up on the chart. Finally, the remote workstation approach virtually guarantees idle nursing time because only one person can use the workstation at a time, and there is always competition for access to the workstations. POS systems eliminate all of these problems.

A POS system is designed to save time by recording critical clinical data such as patient assessment, drug administration, vital signs, and so forth, as they are administered by the provider of the service. It also provides immediate access to key patient information to all care providers involved with the patient. It can retrieve the patient's care plan, latest vital signs, or medication administered. A POS system is generally installed in a direct patient care unit, such as the intensive or critical care units, but can be also found in patient care units in a facility where an HIS is installed.

LABORATORY, PHARMACY, AND RADIOLOGY MODULES

Laboratory, pharmacy, and radiology support programs are needed by all hospitals. A typical laboratory system, for example, includes a laboratory test request, generates the specimen labels, tracks the specimen through the various laboratory stages, generates the results, and communicates the findings to patient's medical record. Pharmacy systems track medication orders and changes in orders. They often have drug interaction warning programs, dosage calculators, and other supports for the pharmacy function. They generally include a computer-stored database of the Physicians' DeskReference (PDR), which provides a knowledge base for the pharmacists. Radiology systems are usually separate products developed by companies that specialize in diagnostic computer imaging systems. Ideally, they can be linked with the HIS in such a way that the pictures (digitized versions of the radiographic studies) and radiologist report can be viewed at the bedside or unit workstation.

The purpose of any information system is to process data and information to support human knowledge and decision making. Professional nurses are knowledge workers because their primary value is interpretation of clinical data and information, and the clinical judgments and decisions they make based on that knowledge. As clinical information and knowledge become increasingly voluminous and complex, nurses will progressively depend more and more upon computer information support systems.

DEFINING DATA, DATABASES, INFORMATION, AND INFORMATION SYSTEMS

Data are raw, uninterrupted facts without meaning. For example, the following series of numbers are data, but have no meaning: 98, 116, 58, 68, 18. Reordered and explained as vital signs they have meaning and are therefore *information*: 98.0, 58, 18, 116/68. The nurse knows these data provide information on a person's basic condition. However, there is little the nurse can do with this information because in order to interpret the data so that it becomes *knowledge*, the nurse must be able to fit it into a *pattern* of prior knowledge about vital signs in order to interpret the information. If the nurse knows these vital signs were collected as part of a sports physical for a high school athlete, then the knowledge the nurse has of how to interpret vital signs is available to put the information into context. Context and pattern knowledge allow the nurse to understand the meaning and importance of those data and to make decisions about nursing actions with regard to the information. While data by themselves are meaningless, information and knowledge, by definition are meaningful. When the nurse makes good decisions on the basis of the knowledge, he or she exhibits *wisdom*.

For data to be placed in context so that information is produced, the data must be processed. This means that the data are organized so that patterns and relationships between the data can be identified. When the user understands the patterns and relationships in the data, knowledge results. Finally, the knowledge is used as the basis for making clinical judgments and decisions and choosing nursing actions to implement. When the results of the nursing actions are beneficial, the nurse has demonstrated wisdom. The "data to information to knowledge to wisdom" progression is predicated on the existence of accurate, pertinent, and properly organized data. There are several approaches to organizing data.

Some common approaches include sorting, classifying, summarizing, and calculating. For example, students will often take all of their notes and handouts from their nursing classes and organize them into folders. The folders can be located on a personal computer, placed in a box, deposited in a file cabinet, or stored in some other media. Each folder is used for a different topic. The data in the folders can be organized by nursing problems, interventions, medical diseases, cell biology, or drugs, to name but a few classifications for the information. Sometimes it is difficult to decide which folder the notes should be stored in. Students may make a copy of the notes and store it in both folders or may put the notes in one folder and a cross-reference note in the other folder. In the process of organizing the data/information a database has been created.

Another common example of a database is a checkbook used to store everyday financial data. Each number by itself means nothing; however, if the owner of the checkbook is careful to capture each entry and correctly calculates as money moves in and out of the account, the final number will summarize the current status of the checking account. This information can be very meaningful to the owner of the checkbook. If these same data are captured in a money management software package, a number of reports can be generated from these dates.

A database is an organized collection of related data. Placing notes in folders and folders in file cabinets is one example of creating a database; however, a database can be organized and stored in many different formats. A common paper example is the phone book. A much more complex example can be a patient's medical record. Each of these databases can be used to store data and to search for information. The possibility of finding information in these databases depends on several factors. Four of the most important are the following:

1. How the data are named (indexed) and organized
2. The size and complexity of the database
3. The type of data within the database
4. The methodology or tools used to search the database

The systematic approach used to name, organize, and store data in a database has a major impact on how easy it is to find information in the database. The phone book is organized alphabetically by name. This makes it very easy to find a phone number if you know the person's name and very difficult to find a person's name if you start with the phone number. A large database can be more difficult to search than a small database. The size of a database is determined not only by the amount of data in the database, but also by the number and complexity of the relationships between the data. For example, the phone book may be for a large city and require two volumes, while the patient's chart may reflect an overnight observational visit at the hospital. While the phone book may be larger, there are a minimum number of relationships between the data. Data in the patient's chart can be organized in an infinite number of ways. A wide range of caregivers will see different relationships and reach different conclusions from reading the same chart.

Information systems are used to process data and produce information. The term information system is often used to refer to computer systems, but this is only one type of information system. There are manual information systems as well as human information systems. The most effective and complex information system is the human brain. People are constantly taking in data and processing that data to produce meaning.

Types of Data

When developing automated database systems, each data element is defined. As part of this process, the data are classified. There are two primary approaches to classifying data in a database system. First, they are classified in terms of how these data will be used by the user. This is sometimes referred to as the conceptual view of the data. For example, the data may be classified as financial data, patient data, or human resource data. The conceptual view of the data has a major impact on how the data are indexed. Second, data are classified by their computerized data type. For example, data can be numbers or letters or a combination of both. This classification is used to build the physical database within the computer system. It identifies the number of spaces needed to capture each data element and the specific functions that can be performed on these data.

Computer-based Data Types. Alphanumeric data include letters and numbers in any combination; however, the numbers in an alphanumeric field cannot perform numeric function. For example, an address is alphanumeric data that may include both numbers and letters. A social security number is an example of alphanumeric data made up of numbers. It makes no logical sense to add or perform any other numerical functions on either addresses or social security numbers. The number of spaces that can be used for an alphanumeric field must be identified for the computer system. Memo is a specific type of alphanumeric data with increased spaces and decreased indexing options.

Numeric data are used to perform numeric functions including adding, subtracting, multiplying, and dividing. There are several different formats as well as types of numeric data. The number of digits after the decimal or the presence of commas in a number are examples of format options. Numeric data can be long integer, currency, or scientific.

Date and time are special types of numeric data with which certain numeric functions are appropriate. For example, two dates could be subtracted to determine how many days, months, and/or years are between the two dates. However, it would not make sense to add together several different dates.

Logic data are data limited to two options. Some examples include YES or NO, TRUE or FALSE, 1 or 2, and ON or OFF.

Conceptual Data Types. Conceptual data types reflect how users view the data. These can be based on the source of the data. For example, the lab produces lab data, and the x-ray department produces image data. Conceptual data can also be based on the event that the data are attempting to capture. Assessment data, intervention data, and outcome data are examples of data that reflect event capturing.

One of the major advantages of an automated information system is that each of these data elements can be captured once and used many times by different users for different purposes. For example, a patient with diabetes mellitus has an elevated blood sugar level. This datum may be used by the physician to adjust the patient's insulin dose and used by the nurse in a patient education program. These basic data elements can also be aggregated and summarized to produce new data and information that may be used by a different set of users. This is referred to as "data collected once, used many times." Figure 4.13 gives an excellent example of this concept.

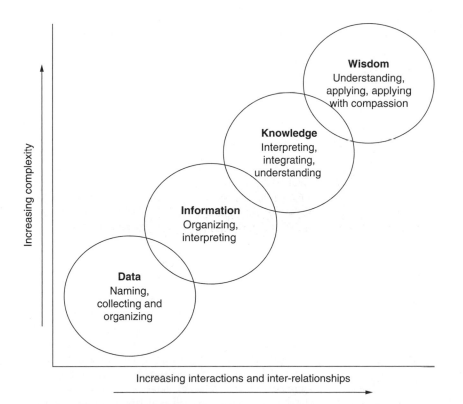

• **FIGURE 4.13.** The Nelson data to wisdom continuum. (Reprinted with permission from Englebardt, S. and Nelson, R. (2002). *Healthcare Informatics: An Interdisciplinary Approach*. Figure 1–4, p. 13, Elsevier.)

Structural or Physical Data Models

The physical data model includes each of the data elements and the relationship between the data elements, as they will be physically stored on the computer. There are four primary approaches to the development of a physical data model. These are hierarchical, network, relational, and objectoriented. The initial database models were hierarchical and network. The relational and objectoriented are much more common today.

Hierarchical. Hierarchical databases have been compared to inverted trees. All access to data starts at the top of the hierarchy or at the root. The table at the root will have pointers called branches that will point to tables with data that relate hierarchically to the root. Each table is referred to as a node. For example, a master index might include pointers to each patient's record node. Each of the patient record nodes could include pointers to lab data, radiology data, and medication data for that patient. The patient record nodes are called parent nodes, while the lab, medication, and radiology nodes are called child nodes. In a hierarchical model, a parent node may have several children nodes, but each child node can only have one parent node. Figure 4.14 demonstrates a hierarchical model and the related terminology.

Hierarchical models are very effective at representing one-to-many relationships; however, they have some disadvantages. Many data relationships do not fit the one-to-many model. Remember the class notes that were put in two folders. In addition, if the data relationships change, this can require significant redesign of the database.

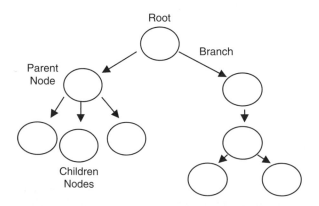

• **FIGURE 4.14.** Hierarchical database model.

Network Model. Network models developed from hierarchical models. In a network model, the child node is not limited to one parent. This makes it possible for a network model to represent many-to-many relationships; however, the presence of multiple links between data does make it more difficult if data relationships change and redesign is needed.

Relational Database Models. Relational database models consist of a series of files set up as tables. Each column represents an attribute, and each row is a record. Another name for a row is tuple. The intersection of the row and the column is a cell. The datum in the cell is the manifestation of the attribute for that record. Each cell may contain only one attribute. The datum must be atomic or broken down into its smallest format. For example, a blood pressure reading would be broken down into the systolic and the diastolic reading. Because of this limitation, the relationships represented are linear and only relate one data element to another.

A relational database joins any two or more files and generates a new file from the records that meet the matching search criteria. Figure 4.15 includes two related tables: Table A and Table B. Both tables include the patient's ID number. This is the common field by which the tables can be joined. By joining these two tables, it is possible to create a new table that identifies all patients who have a diagnosis of cerebral vascular accident (CVA). For example, Table C is created by the DBMC in response to the query, "List all patients with a diagnosis of CVA."

While a relational database consists of multiple tables, it is possible to build a simple database with one table. This type of database is a flat file. An Excel spreadsheet is an example of a flat file. This approach is good if you have a relativity small amount of data and simple questions. For example, Excel can be used to calculate grades, convert the final number grades to letter grades, and then fill in a table with the number of A, B, C, D, and F's.

Object-oriented Model. An object-oriented database was developed because the relational model has a limited ability to deal with binary large objects or BLOBs. BLOBs are complex data types such as images, sounds, spreadsheets, or text messages. They are large nonatomic data with parts and subparts that are not easily represented in a rational database. In object-oriented databases the entity as well as attributes of the entity are stored with the object. An object can store other objects as well. In the object-oriented model, the data definition includes both the object and its attributes. For example,

Table A

ID	L-NAME	F-NAME	SEX	B-DATE
12	Smith	Tom	M	01-23-73
14	Brown	Robert	M	02-01-77
13	Jones	Mary Lou	F	12-12-54
15	Yurick	Edward	M	04-04-38

Table B

ID	DX-1	DX-2	DX-3	DX-4
12	MI	CVA	GLACOMA	PVD
14	CVA	HEPATITIS C	COLITIS	UTI
13	DIABETES M	ANGINA	CVA	GOUT
15	CERF	AMENIA	GLACOMA	PEPTIC ULCER

Table C

ID	L-NAME	F-NAME	DX-1	DX-2	DX-3
12	Smith	Tom		CVA	
14	Brown	Robert	CVA		
13	Jones	Mary Lou			CVA

• **FIGURE 4.15.** Relational database.

amoxicillin is an antibiotic. All antibiotics have certain attributes or actions. Because amoxicillin is an antibiotic, it can be stored in the object antibiotic and inherit the attributes that are true of all antibiotics. The ability to handle nonatomic complex data and inheritance attributes are major advantages in healthcare computing.

DATABASE LIFE CYCLE++++

The development and use of a DBMS follow a systematic process called the life cycle of a database system. The number of steps used to describe this process can vary from one author to another. In this chapter, the life cycle process will be described in five steps. While the process of developing a DBMS moves forward through these steps, there is a recursive pattern to the development. Each step in the process provides the developer(s) with new insights. As these new insights occur, it is sometimes necessary to make modifications in previously completed steps of the process.

Initiation

Initiation occurs when a need or problem is identified and the development of a DBMS is seen as a potential solution. This initial assessment looks at what is the need, what are the current approaches, and what are the poten-

tial options for dealing with the need. For example, the staff development department in a home health agency may want to automate their staff education records. The current approach is to maintain an index card for each staff member. The index card lists all the programs attended by the individual staff member. When the card gets full, a second card is stapled to the first card. When the department needed to know how many total hours of staff development education had been provided monthly by each branch office for the last year, the department was required to pay staff several hours of overtime to review the cards and collect these data. The department had a computer with a DBMS software program; however, no one in the department knew how to use the program or structure the data for a database program. A decision was made to request assistance in designing a database from the information services department. The nurse who organized most of the reports for the department attended in-service classes and worked with the database administrator from the information services department. Now the staff development department was ready to start planning for their automated DBMS.

Planning and Analysis

This step begins with an assessment of the users view and the development of the conceptual model. What are all the information needs of the department and how is the information used? This includes the internal and external uses of information. External needs for information come from outside the department. What are all the reports that the department produces? What are the requests for information that the department has been unable to fill? What information would the department like to report but has not reported because it is too difficult or time-consuming to collect the data? Internally what information does the department use in planning and/or developing educational programs? How does the department evaluate the quality of individual programs or its overall performance? How does the department evaluate the performance of individual faculty? By understanding the informational needs of the department, it is possible to identify data and the data relationships that will need to be captured in the DBMS. Diagrams and narrative reports will be used to describe the data elements, their attributes, and the overall ideal information flow in the conceptual model. A well-developed conceptual model based on a careful assessment of the user's needs will be a major advantage for the database administrator. The conceptual model provides the framework for the physical model developed by the database administrator.

Detailed Systems Design

The detailed systems design begins with the selection of the physical model: hierarchical, network, relational, or objectoriented. Using the physical model, each table and the relationships between the tables are developed. At this point, the data entry screens and the format for all output reports will be carefully designed. The users in the department must validate the data entry screens and output formats. It is often helpful to use prototypes and screen shoots to get user input during this stage. Revisions are to be expected.

Implementation

Implementation includes training the users, testing the system, developing a procedure manual for use of the system, piloting the DBMS, and finally going live. The procedure manual outlines the rules for how the system is used in day-to-day operations. For example, what is the procedure for recording attendance at individual classes, and when is the attendance data to be provided to the data entry clerk? In going live with a database system, one of the difficult decisions is how much previous data must be loaded into the DBMS. The initial request that stimulated the development of the DBMS

would have required at least 1 year of previous data to be loaded into the automated database system.

Evaluation and Maintenance

When a new database system has been installed, the developers and the users can be very anxious to immediately evaluate the system. Initial or early evaluations may have limited value. It will take a few weeks or even months for users to adjust their work routines to this new approach to information management. The first evaluations should be informal and focus more on troubleshooting specific problems. Once the system is up and running and users have adjusted to the new information processing procedure, they will have a whole new appreciation of the value of a DBMS. At this point, a number of requests for new options can be expected.

THE DEVELOPMENT OF DATA WAREHOUSES

In the late 1980s and early 1990s, a number of changes stimulated the development of the data warehouse concept. Computer systems became much more powerful. Database theory and products were much more sophisticated. Users were becoming computerliterate and developing more requirements. A core of healthcare informatics leaders had developed. The move away from fee-for-service to managed care created a new set of information needs. While systems were still used to track charges for services, they also needed to assist analysts to calculate the actual cost of providing health services. Historical data within the computer systems took on a new value. Analyzing historical data for the institution required that data from each of the systems be collected and stored in a common storage system called a data warehouse.

A data warehouse is defined as a large collection of data imported from several different systems within one database. The source of the data includes not only internal data from the institution but can also include data from external sources. For example, data related to standards of practice could be imported into a data warehouse and used to analyze how the institution achieved a variety of goals related to these standards. Smaller collections of data are referred to as data marts. A data mart might be developed with the historical data of a department or a small group of departments. A data mart can also be developed by exporting a subset of the data from the data warehouse.

Purposes of a Data Warehouse

The development of a data warehouse requires a great deal of time, energy, and money. An organization's decision to develop a data warehouse is based on several goals and purposes. Because of its integrated nature a data warehouse spares users from the need to learn several different applications. For example, a warehouse no longer requires healthcare providers to access the lab reporting system to see lab work and use a different application with a different interface to view radiology results. When users are viewing several different applications there are several different "versions of the truth." These can result from looking at the database at different times as well as the use of different definitions. For example, the payroll database may show a different number of nurses on staff than the automated staffing system. That is because the payroll would include nurses in administrative positions; however, the staffing system may only include the nurses assigned to patient care.

These types of definitions are decided in building the warehouse and provide a more consistent approach to making decisions based on the data. A data warehouse makes it possible to separate the analytical and operational processing. With this separation the architectural design of the data warehouse is designed to support decisional information needs. The user can slice and dice the data from different angles and at different levels of detail.

Functions of a Data Warehouse

The management of a data warehouse requires three types of programs. First the data warehouse must be able to extract data from the various computer systems and import that data into the data warehouse. This is a key point for nursing. If nursing data are not in the various computer systems or do not exist in any standardized format, they cannot be extracted and imported into the data warehouse. Nursing data are not limited to the data that nurses generate but include all the data that nurses use for client care, administration, research, and education.

Furthermore, the data definitions that were established in the original computer systems must now be revised so that the data from the different systems can be integrated. For example, does the data definition for patient problem(s) include all problems identified by all professional caregivers, or is it limited to the medical diagnosis?

Second, the data warehouse must function as a database able to store and process all of the data in the database. This includes the ability to aggregate the data and process the aggregated data. For example, the operational database systems used to manage the institution on a day-to-day basis do not usually offer the opportunity to look at data over time, yet a data warehouse supports integration of data and the analysis of trends over time. The individual data elements that are imported into the warehouse are referred to as primary data. The aggregate data produced by the warehouse database system are referred to as secondary data or derived data.

Third, the data warehouse must be able to deliver the data in the warehouse back to the users in the form of information.

Information from a data warehouse can be used for decision support systems for both managers and direct care givers. It can support clinical and administrative research, education, quality improvement, infection control, and a myriad of other decision-making activities in healthcare institutions. The data hospitals collect are already used to support planning, marketing and project management as well as reporting to accreditation and regulatory agencies. Having it in a data warehouse would greatly improve the efficiency of developing reports. The advent of data warehouses promises to convert clinical information from a wasted resource, available only by individual patient, into a resource that can be used for clinical effectiveness review, clinical research, and a source of new discovery. In these ways, clinical data will ultimately benefit all people through improvement in clinical care.

SUMMARY

In this chapter the basics of computer hardware and software are presented. A very brief history of computing is provided so that the reader will understand "where we have been and where we are now." People often assume that computers should be able to solve all their work-related problems, but understanding the state of the art will assist in realistic planning for computer system design and utilization. Readers are introduced to software, which is the set of commands given to a computer to tell it how to do work. Computers are systems, and to understand how computer systems fit into clinical systems and support the work of nurses, the reader is provided with a brief introduction to systems theory. Information systems in general and hospital information systems in particular are the computer applications nurses are most likely to work with in hospitals and clinics. An introduction to such systems is presented. Finally, the reader is provided with an introduction to data, data models, the lifecycle of a database management system and with a very brief overview of data warehouses.

REFERENCES

Berners-Lee, T., & Fischetti, M. (2000). *Weaving the web: The origin, design, and ultimate destiny of the World Wide Web by its inventor.* San Francisco, CA: Harper Books.

Beyer, S. (2009). *Grace Hopper and the invention of the information age.* Cambridge, MA:MIT Press.

da Cruz, F. (2010). *IBM punch cards. Columbia University computing history.* Retrieved July 8, 2010, from http://www.columbia.edu/acis/history/cards.html

Delve, J. (2007). Joseph Marie Jacquard: Inventor of the Jacquard loom. *IEEE:Annals of the History of Computing,* 29(4), 98–102.

Gettman, M., & Blute, M. (2007). Transvesicalperitoneoscopy: Initial clinical evaluation of the bladder as a portal for natural orifice translumenal endoscopic surgery. *Mayo Clinic Proceedings,* 82(7), 843–845.

Gumbs, A., Fowler, D., Milone, L., Evanko, J., Ude, A., Stevens, P., & Bessler, M. (2009). Transvaginal natural orifice translumenal endoscopic surgery cholecystectomy: Early evolution of the technique. *Annals of Surgery,* 29(6), 908–912.

IBM Archives. (2010). *IBM 29 card punch. IBM Archives.* Retrieved July 10, 2010 from http://www-03.ibm.com/ibm/history/exhibits/vintage/vintage_4506VV4002.html

Linte, C., Moore, J., Wiles, A., Wedlake, C., & Peters, T. (2008). Virtual reality-enhanced ultrasound guidance: A novel technique for intracardiac interventions. *Computer Aided Surgery,* 13(2), 82–94.

Marescaux, B., Dallemagne, B., Perretta, S., Wattiez, A., Mutter, D., & Coumaros, D. (2007). Surgery without scars. *Archives of Surgery,* 142(9): 823–826.

McConnochie, K., Wood, N., Herendeen, N., Ng, P., Noyes, K., Wang, H., & Roghmann, K. (2009). Acute illness care patterns change with use of telemedicine. *Pediatrics,* 123(6), e989–e995.

Whittle, D. (2010) Is AID stuck using IBM punched cards? *AID Watch.* June 29, 2010. Retrieved July 7, 2010 from http://aidwatchers.com/2010/06/is-aid-stuck-using-ibm-punch-cards/

5

Systems Life Cycle: Planning and Analysis

M. Kathleen Smith / Denise D. Tyler

- ## OBJECTIVES
  1. Compare the systems life cycle with the nursing process.
  2. Discuss the elements of a systems life cycle analysis.
  3. Describe an information systems selection process.
  4. Describe the elements of implementation planning.
  5. Discuss the first 7 steps of the 14-step implementation process.

- ## KEY WORDS
  nursing process
  systems development life cycle
  project management process
  systems initiation
  systems planning
  systems analysis
  systems selection

INTRODUCTION

Aspects of information system software have been in healthcare institutions for over 30 years. There is an ongoing need to install new applications or replace existing software in a clinical setting. Clinical implementation projects are initiated for a variety of reasons. Some of the reasons may include standardizing care, increasing safety, decreasing pharmacy and emergency expenditures, and increasing medication safety. Adoption of an electronic health record (EHR) or a single component like barcode medication administration (BCMA) requires a major change in the organization, and major commitment from the staff and leaders of the organization (Gay, 2006). Billions of dollars have been provided by the federal government for meaningful use of certified health information technology products for providers and hospitals in Medicare and Medicaid incentive plans. This funding is part of the American Recovery and Reinvestment Act of 2009 (ARRA). Healthcare providers, hospitals, and physicians' offices are working diligently to install or upgrade health information technology products that are certified, standardized, and meaningful in their use (Murphy, 2009; Hoehn, 2010). For a description of the Stage 1 Meaningful Use Criteria refer to www.himss.org/content/files/HIE_MU_Matrix033110.pdf. For information about the Certification Commission for Health Information Technology (CCHIT) see www.cchit.org/

Nurses are a vital part of a team to lead and install or upgrade an EHR. In addition to having a strong clinical background, nurses are schooled in the scientific nursing process. They use this process of assessment, diagnosis, outcomes/planning, implementation, and evaluation in a variety of settings and areas. According to the American Nurses Association (ANA) (www.nursingworld.org/EspeciallyForYou/StudentNurses/Thenursingprocess.aspx) it is one of the common threads uniting nurses across the healthcare setting.

Nursing informatics is the nursing specialty practice that "integrates nursing science, computer science, and information science to manage and communicate data, information, knowledge, and wisdom in nursing practice" (ANA 2008, p. 1). The standards of nursing informatics practice include:

Standard 1. Assessment

Standard 2. Problem and issues identification

Standard 3. Outcomes identification

Standard 4. Planning

Standard 5. Implementation

 Standard 5a. Coordination of activities

 Standard 5b. Health teaching and health promotion and education

 Standard 5c. Consultation

Standard 6. Evaluation (ANA, 2008, pp. 65–73).

The systems development life cycle (SDLC) contains five phases: initiatation, analysis, design, implementation, and continuous improvement or support. These five phases closely parallel the project management phases: project initiation, project planning, project execution, project control, and project closing.

Nurses find that the standards of nursing informatics practice, the SDLC process used to develop and install an information system, and the project management process (PMP) are very similar to the nursing process. Figure 5.1 provides a comparison of the nursing process with the nursing informatics standards of practice,

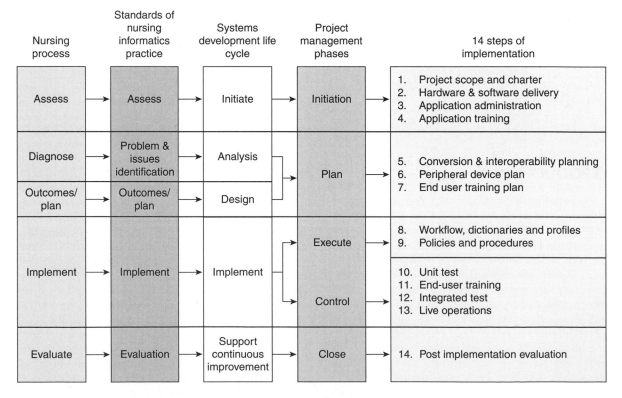

**Standard processes supporting
14 steps of implementation**

Nursing process	Standards of nursing informatics practice	Systems development life cycle	Project management phases	14 steps of implementation
Assess	Assess	Initiate	Initiation	1. Project scope and charter 2. Hardware & software delivery 3. Application administration 4. Application training
Diagnose	Problem & issues identification	Analysis	Plan	5. Conversion & interoperability planning 6. Peripheral device plan 7. End user training plan
Outcomes/ plan	Outcomes/ plan	Design		
Implement	Implement	Implement	Execute	8. Workflow, dictionaries and profiles 9. Policies and procedures
			Control	10. Unit test 11. End-user training 12. Integrated test 13. Live operations
Evaluate	Evaluation	Support continuous improvement	Close	14. Post implementation evaluation

• **FIGURE 5.1.** Standard processes supporting the 14 steps of implementation.

the SDLC, the PMP and the standard processes supporting the 14 steps of implementation. All of these methodologies impact clinical system implementations and upgrades. One of the reasons that nurses are valuable members or leaders of the team implementing a clinical system is the ability to integrate the nursing process and the standards of nursing informatics practice with the SDLC and PMP. The informatics nurse uses the strong nursing background with the business management applications during the system life cycle.

This chapter will discuss the systems life cycle phases of planning, systems analysis and deign, and systems selection along with the first 7 steps of the 14-step implementation process. See Table 5.1 for a description of these first 7 steps. The final 7 steps of the 14-step implementation process will be discussed in Chapter 6. Project management is discussed in detail in Chapter 7.

SYSTEMS LIFE CYCLE: PLANNING AND ANALYSIS

Systems Planning

Planning starts with a vision of what is required. The corporate governance develops vision and mission statements along with strategic goals, objectives, and policy guidelines. These documents drive the decision to install or upgrade the clinical information system in the institution. Planning for system implementation is similar to the planning phase in the nursing process. It involves interdisciplinary collaboration to develop a strategy, prioritization, documentation, communication, and selection of appropriate interventions. The vision needs to be developed in a collaborative, interdisciplinary manner that includes staff and leadership with representation by both the business side and clinical side of the organization.

Strategic Planning

The strategic plan serves as a formal document outlining the organization's plans and priorities. It also serves as a statement of the organization's commitment to information technology. The vision in the plan needs to be broad enough to be adaptable and allow for growth, but detailed enough to provide a vision to guide the implementation and growth of technology. Technology has become so pervasive within hospitals that it is hard to imagine a major decision being made by a hospital that would not have technological ramifications (Ward, 2010).

Many organizations have a separate strategic plan for technology. This reflects the growing recognition of the importance of technology to healthcare. Other organizations include technology in their organizational strategic plan, with the belief that technology is a vital component of the organization's planning for the future. Whether the organization has separate strategic plans that complement each other or the two are interwoven into one document is not as important as the recognition that implementing technology is strategically significant.

The strategic plan can be a general, long-term vision spanning 2 to 10 years or a combination of the vision and plan, including goals and timelines. It should provide a vision of how technology can assist in meeting the organization's overall mission and vision statements. A short-term vision is necessary in the early stages of implementing technology to serve as a map and inspiration to keep affected parties engaged and to prevent the loss of momentum.

Systems Analysis

Systems analysis is a formal inquiry to identify a better course of action and make an informed decision about the best course of action. One of the initial steps of systems analysis is reviewing workflow and processes (Smith, 2000). What changes may impact workflow and processes and what improvements can be made? A combination of interviews, observations, and meetings are techniques that can be utilized to identify organizational needs. Meetings with stakeholders including management and end users can help identify what they expect the system to do, as well as gaps and other changes. Dennis, Wixom, and Roth (2009) note that the fact-finding process during the analysis phase is a crucial step that creates the foundation of the new system.

Along with the all-important workflow analysis done by interdisciplinary teams that involves a high percentage of end users, this phase also includes the analysis of network and security systems. The system must be compliant with the Health Insurance Portability and Accountability Act (HIPAA) enacted in 1996 (Department of Health and Human Services, 2009). Networks, including wireless networks, must be extensively tested to verify that they are operating sufficiently during high usage times. This includes testing the wireless cart, barcode scanner, and communication devices in any area they might be utilized. Do not forget to involve staff caring for patients and unit leaders when determining possible locations for use. An example of this is the go-live of a barcoding medication administration (BCMA) system that did not test hall beds used during high census times. It almost never fails that high census numbers follow go-lives, no matter what the normal census activity is for the time period.

Reporting requirements must also be evaluated and specifications developed. If examples were obtained during site visits, use them in conjunction with the model reports supplied by the vendor when appropriate. Careful evaluation of current reports should be done during this phase to prevent missing reports or duplicating unused reports. This should involve those who really use the reports, including end users, managers, and executives. Determining how changes are made to the system will affect reports. Developing a change management process and communication tool early will prevent problems later in the implementation and after the system is live.

Gap Analysis. A gap analysis requires comparing the current tools used in the workflow with the new workflow and tools available in the new computer application; any gaps are identified and documented. The significance of each gap must then be evaluated. Gaps may need to be resolved or addressed before the system can be implemented. This is an opportunity to improve the workflow or eliminate steps that do not add value, or anything in between. In order to perform a meaningful gap analysis, the staff participating *must* understand the current systems and processes. Performing a thorough and accurate gap analysis can help minimize scope creep later in the project, and help ensure adequate resources are devoted to each issue. In many implementations scope creep and delays are a result of poorly documented gaps.

Risk Analysis. A risk analysis needs to be done at the beginning of a project and continue throughout the process. This is similar to an assessment (e.g., what are the real and potential risks and problems, and what is the plan to prevent them?). Early identification of risks during projects improves with time and experience, similar to the early identification of patient problems and potential problems made by the expert nurse. Similarly, early identification can help minimize problems and improve outcomes. Careful planning for potential problems can assist the newer nurse in informatics, just as it does in the clinical area.

SYSTEMS SELECTION

The systems selection is a critical and complex step. Organizational strategic planning should be developed before vendor selection. Deciding on what vendors to consider will be affected by organizational decisions

about using a best-of-breed versus a single-vendor approach, or a hybrid of both philosophies. Selecting a clinical system is an expensive, far-reaching undertaking. Understanding a vendor's level of stability and long-term vision for business and product development is critical. The most attractive, or "best"-appearing, product today may not be the best fit in the future if the vendor's vision is not harmonious with the organization. Consider the vendor selection process as a long-term relationship, not a short-term date. Table 5.1 presents suggested vendor selection criteria with weighting for use during the systems selection process.

Have a firm understanding of the project before starting vendor selection; this is a good time to develop or to review the strategic plan. Know the organization's problems, priorities, and desired outcomes. Find the vendor that is the best fit for the organization. Know the departments affected, the scope of the project, and the reasons for embarking on the project: Is it to replace a legacy system, to improve reporting, decrease errors, or meet regulatory requirements?

Tell the vendor(s) what is wanted and expected. Don't change the project to fit the vendor's application. What can the vendor do for the organization? The right vendor should not only be able to meet and exceed expectations but also demonstrate things they can do that the organization had not identified. McCoy, Bomentre, and Crous (2006) recommend defining success in advance to help keep the focus on what has been deemed important to the organization. They go on to stress the importance of pre- and post-implementation metrics to help ensure the project deliverables are in line with expectations. Developing a detailed request for proposal (RFP) that is distributed to potential vendors is a practice used by many organizations to fully describe the organization's vision and goals.

Doing a business review of the vendor's stability, customer satisfaction, and product offerings is important. Understanding the vendor's long-term goals for product development and support are also critical. Systems must be supported for both day-to-day usage and growth to meet the ever-changing needs of healthcare providers.

Things to consider include the following:

- Vendor's long-term goals: Will they continue developing the product or are they devoting more time and money to a new or different application?
- Vendor's financial viability: If the vendor is publicly traded, how is their stock doing? What percentage do they devote to research and development (R&D)? Have they had recent layoffs?

TABLE 5.1	Vendor Selection Criteria

Vendor Selection Criteria

Criteria	Weighting
Demonstrate clinical functionality	20%
Interoperability	15%
Acquisition and implementation cost	10%
Hardware platform and technical requirements	10%
Implementability	15%
CCHIT certification	10%
Vendor partnership and ongoing viability	10%
Future vision	10%

Vendor Selection Criteria Weighting with Samples of Details

Criteria	Weighting
Demonstrate Clinical Functionality	20%

Ease of use
Number of clicks to enter an assessment
Screen design and appearance
Does it make sense?
Will it be easy to train/education on how to use?
Will it be easy to remember?
Are the displays easy to read?
How quickly does the system open?
How quickly do the screens open/change
How are requests for enhancements handled? What is the average number done a year?
What kind of peer-to-peer support and education is offered?

Interoperability 15%
What can it easily interface (and who has done it)?
Is this standard or is there an add-on cost for interfaces?
Do they partner with an evidence-based content provider?

Acquisition and Implementation Cost 10%
What does the contract include?
Is there a minimal skill for vendor staff?
What staffing have other customers required for implementation?
What staffing have other customers required for ongoing support?
What hardware is recommended?

Hardware Platform and Technical Requirements 10%
Do you have staff who can support this?
Does this include scalability and redundancy?
How much downtime is required for this application?
How often are upgrades applied?
What kind of downtime is associated with upgrades?
What kind of testing and problems are associated with upgrades?

Implementability 15%
Ask to see sample documentation and project plans for implementations and upgrades.
Is the system easy to configure and customize?
Are the reports customizable?
Do you have access to the data?
How difficult is it to set up printing and security?
How easy is it to convert your current data?

(continued)

TABLE 5.1	Vendor Selection Criteria *(continued)*
Vendor Selection Criteria Weighting with Samples of Details	
CCHIT Certification Is this product certified? Are other products by the vendor certified?	10%
Vendor Stability and On-going Viability What has the stock activity been compared with other vendors? Have they had recent layoffs? How many? What kind? What is the average employee tenure? How many implementations has the company had in the last year? Do they have a basic end-user education plan that you as a customer can modify to fit your needs?	10%
Future Vision and Vendor Partnership Does the vendor "fit" with your organization? Does your staff feel comfortable with the vendor's staff? Does their product suite and development plans align with current and future needs? Compare the vision and mission of the vendor with your organization? Do they complement each other? Are there gaps? Is the vendor comfortable with allowing private dialogue on site visits?	10%

- Vendor staff qualifications: What qualifications and experience does their staff have? Specifically ask about staff involved in product development, implementation, and support. (Hint: Once the vendor has been selected, ask for resumes and the right to interview and approve staff involved on the project). Consider including minimum staff qualifications in the contract.

Another consideration for vendor selection is the stability of the application itself. What is the platform, and who is the staff required to support it? What do other customers say about the product? Asking for information on electronic lists, such as ANIA-CARING, is an excellent way to find out what the positives and negatives are from current customers. This feedback can also assist in developing questions and in some cases with negotiating the contract.

Once the search is narrowed down the next step includes viewing demonstrations and performing site visits. Develop a list for each application under consideration and include a way to score each topic. Establish a team to evaluate applications. This team can assist in developing tools for demonstrations and site visits.

End-User Involvement in the Selection

No matter what application or products are under consideration, the selection team should include end users. The staff, or end users selected, need to be well rounded, well respected, and should include staff who are not "techie." One thing to consider when evaluating

a clinical system is its ease of use: Can a member of your team—not the most computer-savvy person—sit down and figure out how to navigate the system without any prompting? Do the screens flow well? Do they make sense? Are they consistent? Is the same design, including commands, used between modules? Is the system easy to learn and remember?

Other questions for the vendor and current customers include: How many sites are live with the version of the application under consideration? What kind of input do customers have in product development and prioritizing changes and enhancements? How is this input obtained: formally, informally, or a combination? Is the customer input regularly requested and affected?

Business Case Foundation

Historically, the return on investment (ROI) for many clinical applications may be fuzzy, or related to more intangible measurements such as improved outcomes and a decreased length of stay. Institutions implemented clinical systems because they recognized that improved care and improved outcomes made good business sense, and it was the right thing to do. Now, with the availability meaningful use and ARRA funds there will also be a tangible ROI. Looking at the timeline for the meaningful use funds, many institutions are pushing for faster implementations and/or considering reprioritizing their purchase and implementation of applications. When developing a timeline around ARRA funds, many institutions look at the payout only and do not include possible gained or lost interest, which can be significant.

Business Process Review

The business process is intimately tied to clinical workflow. Improving clinical practice, streamlining and improving the accuracy of documentation, and decreasing duplication can improve clinical practice and workflow. When appropriate, linking documentation directly to charging can improve clinical practice, further decrease duplicative efforts, improve the accuracy of charge capture, decrease the volume of charges that are written off due to lack of documentation, and decrease missing charges. This may not significantly impact the actual reimbursement, but will affect the contracted rates, the amount of time spent auditing, and decrease write-offs.

Requirements Analysis: A Step to Identify Functional Specifications

The requirement analysis circles back to the short- and long-term goals for the computer system. It is an interdisciplinary, multilevel analysis, or assessment, that needs to be done in preparation for the system selection. It should be tied into the strategic plan of the organization. System requirements also need to include usability to ensure a system that will be successfully implemented. Performing a requirements analysis necessitates collecting data on the current workflow, which is best done by a combination of observation and interviews. Using interviews alone is not sufficient since not all activities are done consciously, and may not always be in line with formal policies. The requirements analysis should include how the system is expected to work, and allows validation that the technology is performing as intended (TIGER Usability Report, 2009). This documentation can then be used after the system selection during the implementation process, and after implementation it can be used as part of the post-implementation metrics to determine success.

System requirements analysis needs to include the ability to set up the system. The ability to customize a system is usually important, but beware of a system that requires a complete rebuild to meet your needs; there are times when this may be necessary to meet the needs of specialty areas, but should not be required for the majority of areas. Along with screen and workflow design, consider other requirements such as capacities to create and customize reports, integrate with existing systems, set up alerts, and use basic functions like uploading tools. Imagine manually adding the doctor master files and room and bed files into a system because there is no upload tool for this function. This is not as inconceivable as it sounds; an example of this scenario is included in the TIGER Usability Report (2009).

Vendor Analysis: A Step to Vendor Selection

Developing a request for information (RFI) or a request for proposal (RFP) can be a daunting task. If there is no expertise on site, consider utilizing an outside consultant with experience assisting similar organizations. Other tools and companies that can assist with providing information about the vendor companies of interest include:

- The US Department of Health and Human Services, Health Resources and Services Administration (HRSA) has an extensive Web resource describing the selection guidelines for an EHR. It describes the vendor analysis and selection process through the use of an RFI or RFP. The December 2008 guide also includes information on vendors with CCHIT certification. This information can be found at www.hrsa.gov/healthit/ehrguidelines.htm.

- Another rich resource is the Health Information and Management Systems Society (HIMSS) Web site: www.himss.org/ASP/GoogleSearch.asp?q=vendor+selection&client=default_frontend&output=xml_no_dtd&proxystylesheet=default_frontend&site=Production_collection.

- HIMSS Analytics provides innovative research and informed decisions about healthcare data relating to information technology processes. For more information, visit www.himssanalytics.org/.

- KLAS provides research about healthcare technology solutions. It provides information for healthcare information technology vendors and providers. For more information and to purchase a report, visit www.klasresearch.com/.

Site Visit

Once the vendor selection has been narrowed to the top 3 to 5 vendors, it's time to make site visits to like institutions that have the vendors' products up and running. Site visits can be virtual, on-site, or a combination of both. Having virtual site visits, like phone interviews, can allow more people to "see" the system and talk to the staff on the site. This can be an effective step in the selection process. However, as with hiring staff, a phone interview is rarely the last step, and is usually followed by a traditional site visit. Deciding who should go on site visits can be difficult. Too large a group may limit what you can do and where you can go, but an adequate "entourage" must go to all sites to ensure that the right people are at the table to provide input for the decision-making process.

Preparing staff for the visit includes reviewing questions to ask and specific details to observe. Developing a check list or tool to document observations can help prepare staff, keep them focused on the priorities they had agreed on, and minimize bias. Ask the hosts for significant lessons learned, things they would do again, and things they would do differently. Document this; many of these lessons apply to any vendor!

Contract Negotiation

Begin contract development and negotiation during the sales process (McDowel, Wahl, & Michelson, 2003). Know what you are paying for. Do not bundle services with software and equipment. Your people and/or third party consultants should do the analysis for hardware, etc.; the vendor can advise based on their experience but should not be the only point of knowledge. Do not base the timeline on what works for the vendor; again, plan and be prepared.

Pay based on deliverables. The final (and biggest chunk) of the amount due should be based on first usage of a working system (in production and live, not a test system). Be very specific about the deliverables (delivered and working). Add penalties for delays caused by the vendor (9 out of 10 delays are caused by the customer). Include expectations for support during the implementation, go-live, and post go-live. Things that are not standard may be included based on feedback from current customers. Learning from their wins and less than positive experiences can minimize your issues. When possible, include timelines for vendor support. If the product is purchased because of a specific feature, and the vendor cannot support implementing this feature for a lengthy period of time, disillusionment and frustration can result. This can be costly in obtaining buy-in for future implementations.

Insist on quality consultants, require experience, and insist on resumes, interviews and final approval. If there is a large team of consultants, having one or two newer, hard-working, bright members may be acceptable as long as key members with experience complement them, but having less knowledgeable consultants in key positions should not be accepted. Consider contracting for third party consultants if the vendor cannot meet minimum requirements and include this in the contract. The role of the vendor's project manager (PM) is vital to the project's success (Tyler, 2001). They need to know the product and the good resources and consultants (by name). They need to have excellent communication and team-building skills, and should be well liked and respected. The length of engagement of the PM may extend past the project. This longer-term relationship can be very positive, as long as the roles of customer and vendor stay clearly defined and the PM maintains his or her objectivity and edge.

Expense Management

When negotiating rates, include a rate for what the vendor will charge. Include guidelines for travel (commercial airlines, no first class, more economical hotels, reservations made within a specific period ahead of time, minimum time on site [e.g., three 8-hour days]). Consider requiring approval for travel booked at the last minute or for less than the specified time as well as the maximum billable hours per week.

Ensure that there is an internal plan to budget for staff time along with management and information technology (IT) time, this is necessary for staff involvement in the selection and design of the system. Education and support during the go-live event must also be included when budgeting. System design does not stop when the system is stable and in place. Long-term involvement by end users needs to be maintained for changes, upgrades, and optimization of the system.

14 STEPS OF IMPLEMENTATION

Once the vendor and system has been selected, it is time to start the implementation process. One project team sometimes does the system selection process and a different team accomplishes the system implementation. Some organizations use the same team for the entire systems life cycle. The 14 steps of implementation also use the SDLC process of initiation, analysis, design, implementation, and evaluation. Refer again to Figure 5.1 and Table 5.2 to identify the first 7 steps of implementation. In the 14 steps of implementation, steps 1 through 4 are a part of initiating or assessing how to install an EHR. Steps 5 through 7 start the planning process for implementing the EHR. The last 7 steps are described in Chapter 6. Implementation planning establishes the functional and technical specifications for the upgraded or new EHR. The project manager and project team leaders ensure that all steps are planned, executed, and tracked (Douglas & Celli, 2006).

Step 1. Project Scope and Charter

The first step is to establish the project charter and scope. The project charter defines the scope, objectives, participants for a project, and the governance of the project. It establishes the authority assigned to the

TABLE 5.2	Steps 1 to 7 of the 14-Step Clinical Implementation Plan

Step 1. Project Administration

Project Governance
Project Steering Committee
Project Plan
Project Resources
Project Planning and the Nursing Process
Project Status Meetings
Systems Management Support
Executive Sponsor
Roles

Step 2. Hardware and Software Delivery
Technical Environment
Loading the New Software
Downtime Planning

Step 3. Application Administration
Ongoing Technical and Information System Support
   for the Applications
Daily and Nightly Maintenance Procedures

Step 4. Application Training
Team Leader Training
Vendor Training

Step 5. Conversions and Interoperability Plan
Conversion Planning
Interface or Interoperability Planning
 Data Dictionary Build

Step 6. Peripheral Device Plan
Peripheral Device Selection Criteria
Prepare User Areas

Step 7. End-User Training: Planning
Super Users
Role-Based Assignment
Training and Education Plans

project manager. The purpose of the project charter is to document the reasons for undertaking the project, the objectives and constraints of the project, the directions concerning the solution, and the identities of the main stakeholders.

Project Governance. The term *project governance* is often used in IT projects. Project governance is similar to the project charter as it identifies the scope of the project, the executive sponsor of the project, and the business and clinical champions for the project (Kraatz, 2010). Whitten and Bentley (2007) use the term project initiation to establish the project scope, goals, timelines,

budget, and project evaluation criteria. Planning for the project evaluation, conducted in step 14, will be started now. The project governance document describes the "who, what, when, where, and why" and possibly the "how" of the project. The primary stakeholders and project team include program managers, project managers, systems owners, systems analysts, and clinical champions (Kraatz, 2010). Often, the clinical information systems (CIS) steering committee includes the primary stakeholders and representatives from the legal department and health information management (HIM) department (Douglas & Celli, 2006). Project Coordination and planning meetings are scheduled to keep the project on time and within budget. These meetings discuss the development, design, and implementation of the CIS, and identify cross-departmental dependencies.

Planning a project is similar to planning a wedding. Identify a general date. Set the go-live date after developing the schedule for delivery of the project hardware (computers, monitors, mobile carts, handheld devices, Ethernet wiring and/or wireless routers, servers, tape backup systems, etc.) and the project software. A timeline or plan cannot be developed without a date. Each step is vital; avoid duplicating the story about the poor site that had servers and mainframe computers delivered prior to completion of the building planned to house the equipment.

Project Steering Committee. The project steering committee (PSC) owns the business case and drives the project at a high level. This group agrees upon the scope of the project and the funding. It establishes the responsibilities of the project director and provides guidance and direction to the project director. This group resolves cross-departmental issues and boundaries and identifies policy issues for consideration and resolution. The PSC reviews the project status; approves milestones, changes, and exceptions; and finally approves closure of the project. Membership includes the project sponsor, project lead, project manager, project director, program director, and other stakeholders. The project charter should:

- Contain a statement of the purpose of the project.
- Identify the executive sponsor and charter owner.
- Describe the committee membership and responsibilities.
- Identify the time commitment and meeting schedule.
- Establish the boundaries, ground rules, and administrative housekeeping.
- Identify the deliverables, and project timeline.

TABLE 5.3	Project Charter Contents
Name, version, date, approval	
Purpose	
Description	
Goals and objectives	
Scope	
Critical success factors	
Assumptions	
Constraints	
Charter owner	
Membership	
Meeting commitment (e.g., monthly meetings)	
Responsibilities	
Boundaries	
Ground rules	
Administrative housekeeping	
Deliverables	

See Table 5.3 for the project charter contents. For additional information on the development of a project scope and charter, please see Chapter 7 and the following Internet resources:

www.brighthub.com/office/project-management/
articles/5159.aspx

www.projectconnections.com/knowhow/subsets/
project-plans.html?gclid=CNuP1aCilqICFch_
5Qod2i45DQ

Project Plan. The project plan serves as a map, a timeline, and a resource guide. The primary uses of the project plan are to document planning assumptions and decisions, facilitate communication among stakeholders, and document the approved scope, cost, and schedule baselines. Inadequate or incorrect project requirements are the most common cause of project failures (Lewis, 2001). During the system selection process, ask to see examples of project plans and ask other customers about their experiences with the vendor's plans. The plan should be detailed, complete, and easy to adapt to the specific needs of the customer's site. A good project plan is a valuable tool. A bad project plan can be a more painful project than the actual project itself. One resource for developing a project plan is the Project Management Institute's PMBOK® (Project Management Institute).

Project Resources. Identifying resources is part of the project plan. The vendor should be able to assist with the job descriptions, and the PM can identify staff that can function in these roles. Resources can be the biggest

asset in a project and the biggest risk. Losing a key person can seriously impact a project, so a backup plan for these individuals should be part of the risk assessment and project plan.

Project Planning and the Nursing Process. The reason nurses who are organized leaders in the clinical arena adapt so well to project management is the similarities of project planning to the nursing process. Figure 5.1 illustrates the way the two complement each other. Nurses are also taught to work collaboratively with other disciplines, to interact and lead teams from their first clinical day in nursing school. As they grow as professionals, they develop and hone these skills, which include leadership, organization, and problem solving.

Project Status Meetings. Status meetings need to be a priority and scheduled regularly with attendance as an expectation. They may be daily, weekly, or monthly depending on the need for updates and reassessment and may last for half an hour to an hour. Status meetings include documentation of key elements that need to be addressed, issues that need more time or resources to complete, and problems that need escalating. These meetings are important for resource allocation and team building, and should include application (clinical and non-clinical), hardware, and technical updates. Do not leave testing plans or training to the last minute; they should be included on the status meeting agenda(s) from the beginning.

Status meetings need to include a log of issues— things that are going well and things that are not going well. Many plans include a green, yellow, or red status for each key section. This is a visual guide for upper management to assist in identifying areas at risk for delays and may need more resources, senior-level attention, or both. See Table 5.4 for a suggested agenda for project status meetings.

Develop and maintain an issues log. Identify the responsible vendor and on-site person responsible for these issues. This issues log should be maintained in a central location and include the type of issue and the recommended "fix". Another key tool to maintain is a document that tracks task completion (with a timeline, a risk assessment log, and a system change request log). A log of change requests will be used to prioritize what needs to be done pre-live and what can wait till after the go-live.

This chapter assumes the following:

• A commercial off the shelf (COTS) system will be used for this project.

TABLE 5.4	Project Status Meeting Agenda
Team Updates	Status/Tasks/Risks
Orders	
Documentation	
Interfaces	
Other application	
Reports	
Education	
Network	
Hardware	
Integrated test plan	
Action Items	
Tickets with Vendor	
Report to Senior Management	
Exit Criteria	
Post–Go-Live Tasks	

- A nursing informatics specialist will be used as a project leader during the implementation of the COTS software.
- The budget determination and tracking will be done by the program manager or project manager.
- Traditional system testing (simultaneous testing of hardware, software, networks, and applications) on prescribed servers and network bandwidth to maintain desired response time (screen-to-screen flips, database update) will have been done by the vendor.

Systems Management Support. Management of all levels must support the project from selection through post-live support and optimization. While executive-level support is important, having the upper-level management or directors and the unit-level management understand and support the process is crucial. Their support is critical initially to ensure staff involvement, and later to support system development, or optimization, and use.

Executive Sponsor. Whether the chief nursing officer (CNO) is the executive sponsor for a clinical selection and implementation or not, he/she must understand and support the process. The CNO must, if necessary:

- Insist that all other levels of management be involved and supportive.
- Ensure that the clinical leadership understands and buys into the value of technology.
- Ensure that all levels of staff are provided with the education and training they need to support the implementation of clinical systems.

- Insist that appropriate time for staff involvement in all stages from selection to post-implementation optimization is an organizational priority.
- Insist that time is allotted for adequate training and education and that it is a priority to ensure adequate staffing to support all go-live events.

The CNO needs to start emphasizing this list before and during the budget process, and must insist that it is appropriated even if it was not included when the budget was finalized. While the CNO does not need to be involved in the daily workings, he/she does need to be able to clearly communicate the goals of the project to executive leadership and staff.

Roles. Titles may vary, but several functions are fundamental. The role of a PM is integral. The PM is both the backbone and heart of the project. The PM must be organized and needs to see the big picture and still manage the details. Depending on the size and scope of the project, the PM may have project leads that are specialists in managing specific teams or details.

The size and number of teams is also dependent on the applications being implemented. For clinical applications, all areas affected must be represented and an interdisciplinary team is the ideal medium for developing collaboration and understanding between departments. A mix of end users or staff and different levels of management and leadership can lead to a highly functioning team that can work together to select, design, implement, and optimize any system.

Management must be represented on teams without overwhelming them. They must also hold staff accountable for representing their areas in the meetings and bringing decisions back to the staff they are representing for feedback. They should ask for their representatives to report on the status and decisions made, as well as feedback requested at staff meetings and on any staff communication tools.

Vendor representation can be invaluable in meetings; they know the product and should have experience in implementing systems that allows them to ask questions about the current workflow and the vision for the future workflow. This can lead to a collaborative effort to design and implement a system that works for the customer, so the customer will in turn provide positive feedback when asked about the vendor—a win-win situation.

For major products, try to have less than 50% of the build done by the vendor or outside consultants. More than this can result in challenges supporting the system post go-live. Put the best staff on the important projects to ensure success. Include leaders with experience managing and marketing change and change management.

Staff, or end users, must participate in all aspects of system selection and design. Their feedback is invaluable in all aspects of the system life cycle. Staff selected for this role must be content experts who are respected by their peers. Using staff as super users is an excellent way for staff to support their peers during education and go-live support. These staff should ideally be scheduled as extra staff, with no clinical assignment for the first few days of the go-live. For larger installations, technical experts, both vendor and IT staff, need to be on site and available 24 × 7 to offer support, problem solve, and make rounds on units to provide extra support in addition to the super users. One indication of excellent education is cutting back on this support sooner than planned (Tyler & Robertson, 2009). This is a sign to the organization and positively affects the budget.

Step 2. Hardware and Software Delivery

Early in the planning process, a technical plan for the hardware type and the kind and number of workstations must be determined for the type and location of software applications. A strong technical manager and team are required for this work. This group must work closely with clinicians in the area and the clinical project leads to determine the following:

- Amount and locations of hardware (e.g., mainframes, personal computers, tablets, and personal digital assistants [PDA])
- Amount and locations of the peripherals used with the hardware (e.g., mouse, printers, monitors, and scanners)
- Software to be used on each application (e.g., Will the hardware have access to the internet, use word processing and spreadsheet applications, require use of a camera, or a barcode scanner?)
- Interfaces used to transmit data from one application to another (involve the interface team and application leads in these decisions)
- Method to convert data from a legacy system to the new system (Douglas & Celli, 2006; Hebda & Czar, 2009).

Technical Environment. In addition to the types of hardware used for the project, the team must determine the location and functionailty of the electricity (plugs and circuits), the number and location of hardware platforms that must be connected to the emergency backup generator, and the functionailty, location, and strength of a wireless network, when needed. The technical environment must provide the state-of-the-art technology for optimal performance of the EHR.

The team must also consider the location and type of data backup, from location of storage of the backup (on site or off site), size of the backup units (servers and tape backups), size of the room or building to store the servers, network, and backup systems), and the management of the technical equipment. (Will this require additional personnel, or will this function be outsourced?) Will the type of network or backbone (ring, star, hub, etc.) affect the way software is loaded and operates? Will a wide area network (WAN), a local area network (LAN), or a metropolitan area network (MAN) be used? If so, consider how this technology affects software and hardware performance and requirements.

Loading the New Software. The technical manager determines the technical specifications and operational detail for the new or upgraded EHR. The detailed procedures to maintain the software on a daily, weekly, and monthly basis are specified. The operations plan should include the following:

- Schedule for routine maintenance
- Plans for operations during systems failure (e.g., a power outage)
- Downtime plans
- Procedures for recovering data after a planned and unplanned downtime
- System change control policies
- Procedures for identifying, tracking, testing, and applying software fixes and upgrades (Douglas & Celli, 2006).

Downtime Planning. When the system goes down, it is critical to coordinate when to start using downtime forms. One major consideration is how (or whether) to "back-enter" data that was collected during the downtime. While having information available in the clinical system is important, the time spent back-entering may not be the best option for clinicians. There is no right or wrong answer, but the plan must be clear and achievable. If the policy and plan require back-entry of all information, but that is not possible or realistic, the resulting gap is larger than the gap created by not having the information available. One option is to document in the clinical system the time period that information is not available. If the paper documentation is scanned into the document imaging system and available via a link then the potential problems with information residing in multiple systems is minimized.

Trying to match electronic documentation to the downtime form is not realistic due to maintenance and difficulty of transposing electronic documentation onto paper. The downtime forms must include all required information in a format that can be quickly learned and utilized. If the downtime form requires extensive training to be used, it is too complicated. It needs to be similar to a disaster record, which, in effect, it is.

Step 3. Application Administration

Ongoing Technical and Information System Support for the Applications. Evaluating the current system's software and hardware support (if in place) and whether it is adequate to support new applications is critical. Will 24 × 7 help desk support be provided? Is current staffing adequate (both numbers and skills sets)? Support may be on site or outsourced. If the help desk support is outsourced, where will the support be located? Will a different level of support be provided for physicians and clinicians than for other personnel in the institution? Will the information support staff and clinical analysis be required to take on-call shifts to assist clinical personnel? If so, establish policies on overtime pay and benefits.

Daily and Nightly Maintenance Procedures. Many systems require daily, weekly, or monthly maintenance or backup. This may be done and scheduled by the vendor or the site. If the software requires daily or nightly scheduled maintenance the least disruptive time of the day to perform maintenance should be determined. Early commercial or banking modules for maintenance put the information system offline for several hours when the bank wasn't open. That model does not work for a hospital information system that provides services 24 × 7. Will there be a redundant system to keep the computers online continuously? Where, for how long, and in what format will backups be stored? Be sure to plan for all these considerations prior to implementing the information system.

Step 4. Application Training

Team Leader Training. Key personnel for the implementation project will need education and training, and possibly certification, in using the applications that will be installed in the institution. Training for project leads and project managers should begin as soon as possible after the vendor has been selected. Team or project leads need a solid understanding of the application in order to lead the customization required for the institution. Be sure to budget for this training requirement.

Vendor Training. The locations and styles of training may differ significantly between vendors. Some require vendor-based training with follow up. Others provide options for hospital- or vendor-based training with expert consults to reinforce and supplement training. Training may be on site or at the vendor's location. If on-site education is selected, then clear expectations about interruptions from work need to be established. Regardless of the method or location, training is critical for the success of the project and should be a priority for hospital administration.

Step 5. Conversion and Interoperability Planning

Conversion Planning. As more facilities are converting from older, mainframe systems to new technology, data conversion becomes an increasingly important issue. Tools to aid in the conversion can be complicated, time consuming, and prone to problems. Talking to other customers who have done similar conversion can help plan for the process and avoid issues. Do not depend only on the vendor for this information! Ensure that the staff responsible for the conversion understands the conversion tools. Staff that understand the new system, the old system, and the conversion tools used in the process will be able to more successfully ensure clean data is converted, and will be able to develop better tools for post-conversion quality assessment (QA).

Interface or Interoperability Planning. Lack of system integration can result in duplicate entries and lead to missing important details about patients. This can lead not only to dissatisfaction with the system, but can contribute to errors when delivering patient care. Talking to other customers about integration and including written requirements in the contract can minimize surprises and problems. Problems with integration are one of the most common causes of delays in the implementation timeline. Testing needs to be done early and often. Some "star" interface analysts actually become familiar with applications and enter orders or look for order status updates (OSU) and results themselves before turning the testing over to other analysts. This level of analyst is extremely valuable because they can troubleshoot early and extremely effectively. One hint when working with applications and interfaces is, if there is any doubt at all that a change may affect an interface, involve the interface analyst and test.

Data Dictionary Build. The data dictionary, often call metadata, is information about the what and where of data in the database. This is often a table of tables containing a list of tables in the database, as well as a description of the fields in the tables (Kennedy, 2002). The metadata describes the meaning, relationships, origins, and formats. A data dictionary is necessary for the database management system to access the data. Now is the time to build the data dictionary and describe the terms used within the database.

Step 6. Peripheral Device Plan

Peripheral Device Selection Criteria. The selection of peripheral devices is one of the most important parts of an implementation. The technical staff needs to first evaluate tools for usability, battery life, stability, functionality and compatibility with the systems, and the ability of the organization to support and maintaining the equipment. Then options need to be provided to end users. The use of a pilot unit for decisions on equipment may be valuable, but the pilot unit needs to be similar to the units it will be evaluating for; having a unit that is unique in its setup, workflow, and/or staffing is not appropriate for decisions that will affect other areas.

Prepare User Areas. When using wireless technology, testing is critical. The system must be tested in any area where it might be used, and during both peak and non-peak times. Problems must be quickly identified and resolved or mobile devices will not be trusted or utilized. In-room devices must be tested for all possible scenarios to make sure the device is easy to reach, stable, and ergonomically appropriate. Involving experts in ergonomics, such as employee health nurses or occupational therapists, can assist in this stage of design.

Establishing a timeline for the deployment of peripheral devices is essential. Don't forget the space and time to stage the equipment, including dealing with boxes and Styrofoam, labeling and inventorying each piece of equipment, and ensuring that the peripheral devices connect to the intended computers, notebooks, or PDAs.

Step 7. End-User Training Plan

The planning for end-user training begins as the system selection begins. Establish a manager and training team for the information system education and training process. Determine the type of training to provide. What are the pros and cons of classroom training versus computer-based training (CBT) or web-based training? What are the policies for attending and completing the training? What is the length of time for application training? Do employees need basic computer literacy (using a mouse, searching the Internet, "netiquette" education)? What are the policies for employees who fail to attend or complete the required training? Establish a budget that includes clinical coverage for employees attending the training. Will the physicians be paid to attend training classes? Will employees be compensated to complete training modules away from the institution?

Super Users. Super users are often members of the selection and/or design team. They are unit-based personnel who are skilled in the use of the clinical software, understand how to use the system, and more importantly, can explain how to operate the system to new users. They not only assist in the planning and execution of training and education of the software, they work on the unit, know the other personnel on the unit, and can quickly show other unit personnel how to accomplish tasks in the software environment.

Role-Based Assignment. Access to specific functions in the EHR is usually assigned based on the role of the employee and the security policies of the organization. For example, a nurses' aide cannot enter a doctor's order. Registered nurses can be allowed to enter orders in a variety of settings, depending on the policies of the institution. A nurse can enter verbal orders from a physician, and in some cases can enter a series of orders based on an established protocol. Only certain personnel are authorized access to sensitive health information (e.g., HIV results). Planning and defining access to the EHR should start as soon as the system is selected. Also plan what data are displayed and how data is tailored to fit the workflow of different roles.

Training and Education Plans. Orchestrating the education for a major system implementation can be complicated, challenging, and extremely rewarding. It must be well planned and organized. Scheduling can be a nightmare, so it needs to be thoroughly considered, constructed, and automated. Staff should be able to sign up online, and managers should receive automated reports on who has signed up and attended (and who has not).

Marketing and all levels of management must communicate and reinforce the importance of attending education. Ideally, staff who do not attend education should not be allowed to work. Likewise, class attendance must be treated with the same significance as scheduled work; "no shows" should not be tolerated and a plan for discipline should be clearly defined and communicated.

Just as organizations going from paper to technology need to plan for education on computer skills as well as system education, organizations that are moving from older technology to systems with a windows look and feel also need to plan for a change in how staff interact with the computer, and assist staff with mouse and windows skills.

The education should be consistently delivered, and should reinforce appropriate use of the system and workflow. Having all levels of management, especially upper management, understand and communicate clearly and frequently why the change is necessary for the organization will help with change management, and with receptivity to education. Using scripts for delivery and standard scenarios for the hands-on portions of education can help provide consistency and help with the comfort level of staff doing the education. Testing should not only provide documentation of competency, but should also reinforce important aspects of the new system.

Systems testing must be completed so no major changes are made after education has started. Having the increased volume of staff and end users may result in suggestions for system changes, these changes must be prioritized. There may be a small number of changes that need to be made to improve the system and decrease problems during go-live, other changes may be added to the post–go-live optimization. Other suggestions may not fit with the overall vision of how the system will be used, or may be impractical or impossible. Part of the planning needs to include responding to these suggestions in a timely and respectful manner.

CONCLUSION

This chapter discussed the beginning of the systems development life cycle: project planning, systems analysis, systems selection, and the first 7 steps of the 14-steps implementation process. Careful planning, strong executive support, and early involvement of staff are key to a successful implementation or upgrade of a clinical information system.

REFERENCES

American Nurses Association. NursingWorld. (2011). *The Nursing Process: A Common Thread Amongst All Nurses.* Retrieved from http://www.nursingworld.org/EspeciallyForYou/StudentNurses/Thenursingprocess.aspx.

Dennis, A., Wixom, B. H., & Roth, R. M. (2009). *System Analysis and Design* (4th ed.). Hoboken, NJ: John Wiley & Sons

Department of Health and Human Services. (2009). *Health information privacy.* Retrieved from http://www.hhs.gov/0cr/privacy/hipaa/understanding/index.html.

Douglas, M., & Celli, M. (2006). Implementing and upgrading clinical information systems. In V. Saba, & K. McCormick. (Eds.) *Essentials of nursing informatics* (4th Ed.) (pp. 291–310). NY, NY: McGraw-Hill.

Gay, T. L. (2006). A case study on computerized physician order entry. Retrieved from http://web3.streamhoster.com/mtc/blueprint12_19_06.pdf.

Hebda, T., & Czar, P. (2009). *Handbook of informatics for nurses & healthcare professionals.* (4th Ed.). Upper Saddle River, NJ: Prentice Hall.

Hoehn, B. J. (2010). Meaningful use: What does it mean for healthcare organizations? *Journal of Healthcare Information Management, 24*(1), 10–12.

Kennedy, M. (2002). Supporting administrative decision making. In S. Englebardt, R. Nelson. (Eds.) *Healthcare informatics: An interdisciplinary approach.* St. Louis, MO: C.V. Mosby.

Kraatz, A. S., Lyons, C. M., & Tomkinson, J. (2010). Strategy and governance for successful implementation of an enterprise-wide ambulatory EMR: Overcoming the challenges, complexities and culture. *Journal of Healthcare Information Management, 24*(2), 34–40.

Lewis, J. P. (2001). Project planning scheduling & controlling. (3rd ed.) San Francisco, CA: McGraw Hill.

McCoy, M. J., Bomentre, B. J., & Crous, K. (2006). Speaking of EHRs: Parsing EHR systems and the start of IT projects. *Journal of AHIMA 77*(4), 24–28.

McDowell, S. W., Wahl, R, & Michelson, J. (2003). Herding cats: The challenges of EMR vendor selection. *Journal of AHIMA 17*(3), 63–71.

Healthcare Information and Management Systems Society. (2010). Meaningful Use, Certification Criteria and Standards, and HHS Certification Process. Retrieved from http://www.himss.org/EconomicStimulus.

Murphy, J. (2009). Meaningful use for nursing: Six themes regarding the definition for meaningful use. *Journal of Healthcare Information Management, 23*(4), 9–11.

American Nurses Association. (2008). *Nursing informatics: Scope and standards of practice.* (2008). Silver Spring, MD: ANA.

Project Management Institute. (2011). Retrieved from http://www.pmi.org/Pages/default.aspx.

Smith, K. (2000). Needs assessment. In M. Brady & M. Hassett (Eds.), *Clinical informatics.* Chicago, IL: HIMSS Guidebook Series.

The Tiger Initiative. (2009). Designing usable clinical information systems: Recommendations from the TIGER usability and clinical application cesign collaborative. Retrieved from http://www.tigersummit.com/Competencies_New_B949.html.

Tyler, D. (2001). Lessons learned: During a big bang conversion at a 530 bed healthcare system. *Caring Newsletter, 16*(4), 5–6.

Tyler, D., & Robertson, C. (2009, August). Mission education: Providing personalized education for over 2000 users. *Presentation at Siemens Innovations*. Philadelphia PA.

Ward, M. (2010, April). Why a detailed IT plan should be part of your organization's strategy. *Healthcare Financial Management*, Available from http://findarticles.com/p/articles/mi_m3257/is_4_64/ai_n53301510/pg_5/?tag=content;col1 Retrieved March 15, 2011, 108–110.

Whitten, J. L., & Bentley, L. D. (2007). *Systems analysis and design methods*. Boston, MA: McGraw-Hill/Irwin.

6

System Life Cycle: Implementation and Evaluation

Marina Douglas / Marian Celli

- OBJECTIVES
  1. Describe 2 steps of a 14-step implementation methdology.
  2. Describe the focus of the 2 major testing steps: step 10, unit testing, and step 12, integrated testing.
  3. Describe the nurse informaticist role in the testing process.
  4. Describe 3 elements of a go-live plan.

- KEY WORDS

  commercial off the shelf (COTS) system
  implementation approach
  system maintenance
  unit test
  integrated test
  data mapping and conversion
  intraoperability
  data dictionary

INTRODUCTION

There are numerous constructs for implementing clinical systems. Figure 6.1 displays the steps of 4 frequently used constructs in relation to each other, providing support to the 14-step implementation process described first in Chapter 5 and described further in this chapter. The informatics nurse is well suited to have an active, often lead, role in clinical systems and electronic health record (EHR) implementations. In providing positive and direct patient care, the nurse conducts frequent assessments of not only patients and their families, but the dynamics of their disease states, their environments, and their assigned health-care teams. Such requirements exist for leading and/or participating in a clinical systems implementation project. (Douglas, 2000).

The successful implementation of an EHR requires blending theory and experience to attain a successful project outcome. In reality, implementation projects are rarely "text book" in nature. It is the front line, hands-on experience acquired from lessons learned over time, which require sifting and sorting constructs and theories, and the ability to skillfully apply this knowledge at a particular moment during the clinical information system (CIS) or EHR project that will ultimately ensure success.

The extremely high visibility and cost of CIS and EHR implementations warrants the best balancing of

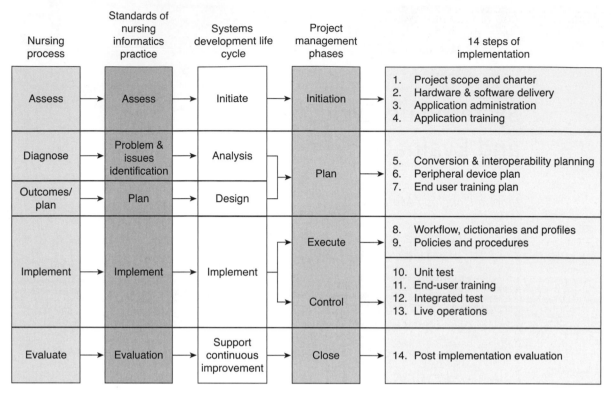

Nursing process	Standards of nursing informatics practice	Systems development life cycle	Project management phases	14 steps of implementation
Assess	Assess	Initiate	Initiation	1. Project scope and charter 2. Hardware & software delivery 3. Application administration 4. Application training
Diagnose	Problem & issues identification	Analysis	Plan	5. Conversion & interoperability planning 6. Peripheral device plan 7. End user training plan
Outcomes/ plan	Plan	Design		
Implement	Implement	Implement	Execute	8. Workflow, dictionaries and profiles 9. Policies and procedures
			Control	10. Unit test 11. End-user training 12. Integrated test 13. Live operations
Evaluate	Evaluation	Support continuous improvement	Close	14. Post implementation evaluation

• **FIGURE 6.1.** Standard processes supporting the 14 Steps of implementation.

academics and hands-on experience. The 14 steps of implementation have developed over a long history of healthcare systems implementation projects and frequent visits to the academic world for review. The steps are listed in Figure 6.2; this chapter will focus on steps 8 through 14 (see Chapter 5 for a discussion of steps 1 through 7). Steps 8 through 14 build on the assessments and planning initiated in the earlier steps. Regardless of the size or type of system, any CIS or single-application design, implementation, or upgrade must address the 14 steps of implementation. Figure 6.3 provides a more detailed view of the tasks associated with steps 8 through 14.

Attempting to implement or upgrade a system without reviewing and completing the tasks associated with each of the 14 steps generally results in system failure in one or more of the following areas:

- CIS does not meet the stated goal of the project.
- There is failure to gain end-user acceptance.

Clinical Systems 14 Step Implementation Methodology
Step #1   Project Administration
Step #2   Hardware and Software Delivery
Step #3   Application Administration
Step #4   Application Training
Step #5   Conversions And Interoperability Plan
Step #6   Peripheral Device Plan
Step #7   End User Training - Planning
Step #8   Workflow, Dictionaries & Profiles
Step #9   Policies & Procedures
Step #10 Unit Testing
Step #11 End User Training - Execution
Step #12 Integrated System Testing
Step #13 Live Operations
Step #14 Post Live Evaluation

• **FIGURE 6.2.** Clinical Systems 14 Step Implementation Process.

CLINICAL SYSTEMS 14 STEP IMPLEMENTATION METHODOLOGY
Details Steps 8 - 14
Step# 1 Project Adminitration
Step# 2 Hardware and Software Delivery
Step# 3 Application Administration
Step# 4 Application Training
Step# 5 Conversions and Interoperability Plan
Step# 6 Peripheral Device Plan
Step# 7 End User Training - Planning
Step# 8 Workflow, Dictionaries & Profiles
Workflow Document
Design Dictionaries and Screens
Roles Based Access
Complete Data Dictionaries
Step# 9 Policies & Procedures
IS Policies & Procedures
Department Policies & Procedures
Complete Polices & Procedures
Step# 10 Unit Testing
Verify Dictionary Completion
Prepare Test Plans
Establish Issue Tracking mechanism
Establish Testing Area and Test Data
Conduct Unit Testing
Approve for Integrated Testing
Step# 11 End User Training - Execution
Verify Completion of Workflow Document, Policies and Procedures
Execute Training Plan
Step# 12 Integrated System Testing
Testing Planning and Preparations
Conduct Integrated Testing
Go - No Go Decision
Detailed Cut Over Plan
Approve for Live Use
Step# 13 Live Operations
Live Event Preparation
Develop Go Live Plan -
Establish Command Center
Prepare System for GO-Live
Execute Go Live Plan
Step# 14 Post Live Evaluation
Monitor/Evaluate Clinical Operations
Post Live Benchmark data
Project Evaluation
Close Implementation Project

• **FIGURE 6.3.** Details of Steps 8 Through 14.

- Expenditures exceed budget.
- Anticipated benefits are unrealized.

Step 8. Workflow, Data Dictionaries, and Profiles

There are 3 major tasks within step 8:

1. Create the workflow document.
2. Build the data dictionaries.
3. Establish and build role-based user profiles.

Workflow Document. The workflow document builds on the scope document developed in step 1 and takes into account the features and functions of the new system. It collects information on the current workflow in all of the departments affected by the new system and is used to determine how processes will be supported by the automated system. It assimilates the data into logical sequencing of tasks and subtasks performed by the end users for each goal or problem area. Departmental standards of care, ordering patterns, procedures, operating manuals, reports (routine and regulatory), and forms used in day-to-day operations are collected (often referred to as the as-is state). Individual data elements required by clinicians in each department are identified and analyzed for continuity and duplication. The workflow document includes the following:

- A list of assumptions about the process or work effort
- A list of the major tasks performed by the user
- A list of the subtasks and steps the user accomplishes
- A detailed outline of:
  - The determination of optional or required status for each task
  - The frequency of the task being performed
  - The criticality and important factors of the tasks and subtasks
  - The order of the subtasks
- The number and frequency of alternate scenarios available to the end user to accomplish a particular task

There are multiple sources of data for completing a workflow document. These include the following:

- Written documents, forms, and flow sheets
- Policy and procedure manuals
- Questionnaires
- Interviews with key stakeholders
- Observations of work processes

The workflow *to-be* state evolves from discussions, interviews, and review of the workflow as-is processes. The to-be workflow state then becomes the roadmap for designing and building the new system (see Chapter 5 for a discussion on workflow). With a thorough understanding of the workflow, dictionary responses can be determined.

Data Dictionary Build. A data dictionary (sometimes called a table or file) is a repository of the allowable responses entered into a specific field in a system. (For example: System field = user type, the associated data dictionary lists the types of users allowable for processing by the system [e.g., RN, LPN, MD, Lab Tech].) The tasks of collecting and entering the responses into the new system comprise the data dictionary build. The sources of responses are varied, many having been collected in earlier tasks. Utilizing the forms (i.e., reports collected during the workflow tasks), potential responses are reviewed and entered into the data dictionaries as data elements. Data elements evaluated during step 5, conversion and interoperability planning, are also reviewed and entered into the system to ensure needed data will be available for all departments and disparate systems.

As entries are made into the data dictionaries, team members should review the impact of the format and display of those entries as seen from the end user's perspective. In some instances, the entries of a data dictionary are displayed in different sorts, either facilitating end-user entry or creating unnecessary stumbling blocks. Therefore, it is helpful to enter a few responses into each dictionary and review the entries from the end user's perspective before completely loading each dictionary

Data standards from both within the institution (e.g., allowable abbreviations) and best practices from outside agencies (e.g., Center for Medicare and Medicaid Services, Institute for Healthcare Improvement, National Data Standards, American Standard Testing Methods) are considered. The data dictionaries can be built by team members, vendors, or consultants.

Once population of the data dictionaries has begun, routine technical backups and testing of the restore functions must begin to prevent data and time losses.

Role-Based User Profiles. The use of role-based access control is required by a number of regulatory bodies within the federal government and industry regulatory groups. With the passage of the Health Information

Portability and Accountability Act (HIPAA) (Center for Medicare/Medicaid, 2010) in particular, organizations are required to limit access to a patient's written and electronic personal health information (PHI) by healthcare workers to a "need-to-know" basis. The permissions to perform certain operations, and therefore have access to a patient's PHI, are assigned to specific roles. Members of staff (or other system users) are assigned particular roles, and through those role assignments acquire permissions to perform particular system functions. Since users are not assigned permissions directly, but only acquire them through their role (or roles), management of individual user access becomes a matter of assigning appropriate roles to the user; this simplifies common operations, such as adding a user or changing a user's department.

The first step in this task is to determine the roles and permissions of the role within an institution. For example, an RN role allows the initiation of a care plan, while the LPN role allows only the updating of a care plan (Ferraiolo, Kuhn, & Sandhu, 2007).

Step 9. Policies and Procedures

All policies and procedures must reflect current practice. Those policies affected by the automation must be revised to reflect the new practice. Additional policies and procedures may be required in response to automation. For example, consider IT policy for making changes and downtime procedures. This can be a time-consuming endeavor and should be completed prior to unit testing and end-user training so new changes reflecting the use of the new automated system can be taught and tested prior to activation of the new system.

Step 10. Unit Testing

In this step, unit testing, 3 key tasks are accomplished.

- Development and execution of unit test scripts and scenarios
- Establishment of an issue tracking mechanism
- Review of unit testing results

An early form of unit testing begins with the entry of responses into dictionaries. As entries are made, team members test to see how the entries support the needed workflow. The formal unit test focuses on how the new system supports departmental operations and workflow. The unit test plan outlines the departments to be tested, the number of testing days, location, and resources needed. In addition, it outlines the information to be

tested, all required reports, outcomes analysis, issue tracking, and resolution processes. This can be complex when testing a clinical provider order entry (CPOE) application where time sensitive orders, co-signatures, roles-based access, modification to orders, requisition generation, results reporting and corrected results must be tested. Individual test scripts, or scenarios, are developed reflecting department workflow; the scripts are role-based. The scripts outline processes to be tested and closely track all requirements of the scope and workflow documents. Although time consuming, development of detailed unit test scripts is a valuable task as these scripts become the foundation for the development of the integrated test scripts described in step 12. Nursing informaticists are well suited to this task. They frequently have delivered direct patient care requiring knowledge of key nursing and ancillary departmental processes, and are thereby familiar with overall hospital care coordination. They also possess knowledge of the automated system and application processes impacting clinical information and patient care.

Unit test scripts are executed, the results are reviewed by the department and the project team, corrections are made, and the scripts are retested before the final sign off by departmental users. The signoff verifies that the system supports the individual department's workflow. If feasible, resources from the Help Desk can be a part of unit testing; this adds to their knowledge of the system and is helpful when they field calls from end users.

Issue Tracking. An issue tracking mechanism and process is a fundamental tool for managing an implementation. The tracking mechanism can be as sophisticated as a software application specially designed to track IT issues or as simple as a spreadsheet. Procedural and training concerns identified during workflow review, technical interfacing or conversion concerns, as well as computer program errors are entered into the issue tracking mechanism. Basic data elements to be tracked are listed below:

- Issue number
- Issue priority (critical, high, medium, low, future)
- Application affected
- Description of issue
- Software pathway taken
- Role of user
- Date issue submitted
- Person submitting issue
- Technical assigned to

- Status (entered, assigned, in-progress, testing, retest, complete, moved to live, live retest, closed)
- Resolution (programmatic, procedural, training)
- Resolution description
- Testing team

Definition of Priority. The definition of the priorities will be a significant factor in allocating programming resources to fix or develop program code prior to activating the new system. Defining terms and obtaining agreement from the project team members during this step and before initiating testing is highly advised. Often-used priorities and definitions are:

Critical Issues impacting clinical processing for which there is no workaround, or without which patient safety is compromised and or regulatory requirements will not be met

High Issues impacting clinical processing or training for which significant effort or workaround will be required to complete a task or process

Medium Issues impacting clinical process or training for which a workaround exists

Low Issues with minimal impact to clinical processing, though if a workaround available would provide improved workflow

Frequent review and quick resolution of issues provides a large benefit to the project. The list of open issues and recently closed issues are benchmarks for the project's progress. The issue tracking must be up-to-date, as it will be the roadmap to keep the system fine-tuned and functioning in support of the end user. Some organizations choose to use the current Help Desk mechanism or system.

Note: As the system becomes individualized for the healthcare institution, the technical team may do a concurrent volume test. A volume test is done to ensure the system can process the anticipated number of data transactions and volume of end users on the system during peak times of use on a typical day. In some instances, the acceptable length of response time (often measured as time elapsed from the request for a screen change to the next screen) and/or the time elapsed to save entered data is stipulated in the contract with the vendor. For example, screen-to-screen response time may be required to perform at a subsecond rate for 18 out of 20 reviewed screen change requests measured during peak system use.

Step 11. End-User Training: Execution

The end-user training plan developed in step 7 is operationalized in step 11. Training end users to use the system properly is essential to the successful adoption and assimilation of the new system into the organization. A CIS will function only as well as its users understand its operation and the operations streamline their work. Key concerns often addressed by the technical staff prior to training include room availability, readiness of the application software, and the training domain (directory). Room readiness ensures sufficient power, network access, appropriate workstations, and functional printers. Some sites use the soon-to-be production workstations to accommodate the large-scale training effort prior to implementation. The training domain (directory) must include the most recent version of all required software. There is significant complexity in building the training database for an orders/results or CPOE training program. Time-sensitive orders, results, future orders, and so on require setup prior to training classes. It is helpful if the technical team in conjunction with the end-user trainers create a baseline training database. The training database snapshot affords the ability to reset the domain (directory) to the baseline data after each training session, saving significant setup time and facilitating standardization of training examples in the system. The ongoing maintenance of the training domain is necessary to support new-user orientation and system upgrades.

Training Material. Typical training documents will include the actual training manuals, training aids (if used), online computer-based training programs, quick reference guides, participant sign-in sheets, evaluation forms, blank issue lists, and copies of policies and procedures affected by the new system. Key policies, such as scheduled and unscheduled downtime and Help Desk assistance, are incorporated into training. Some healthcare facilities require all end users to successfully complete training as a requirement prior to receiving their logon to the new system.

Step 12. Integrated Testing

Integrated testing is complex and challenging, as it reflects how the new system will work in day-to-day operations of the organization. It requires attention to detail in building upon the unit test scripts to develop integrated test scripts. The integrated test period tests interaction among departments affected by the new system, the coordination of resources representing all departments carrying out the test scripts, as well as the tracking and thoughtful evaluation of issues arising during the test period. It is not unusual to have a small committee of project team members charged with organizing this resource-intensive testing period.

Three important tasks accomplished in step 12 are:

- Execution and evaluation of integrated testing
- The institution's decision to move forward with the planned Go-Live date or halt implementation (also known as the Go - No Go decision)
- The development of a detailed cutover plan

Prerequisites. Completion of the prerequisites for the initiation of step 12, integrated testing, is crucial. These include completion of all data dictionaries, successful unit testing, resolution of critical issues discovered in unit testing, and completion of interface unit testing. Once prerequisite tasks are completed, the system is deemed "frozen" and integrated testing can begin. To thoroughly test system integration, it is imperative to test the impact of dictionary and program changes as they move through all disparate applications and systems. Therefore, making changes to data dictionaries or program code is not permitted during rounds of integrated testing. At the end of each round of integrated testing, issues uncovered are reviewed and issue resolution is determined. Any and all fixes and changes must be made in accordance with the change management plan and thoroughly retested. This change management plan is often co-managed by members from the technical team, clinical team, and quality assurance department.

Integrated Testing. The integrated testing plan outlines each system and interface affected by the new system and tests the departmental functions in an integrated manner, mimicking the anticipated real-time use of the system. In particular, integrated testing focuses on interfaced data from disparate systems ensuring it is appropriately reaching its target destinations in its desired format. The focus of unit testing is limited to departmental function, whereas integrated testing ensures all departments and systems are functioning together as outlined in the project scope and workflow documents. Building on the unit test script created in step 10, the integrated test scripts must reflect the business and clinical practices, and data flow throughout the organization. The integrated testing plan determines the number of testing days, the location, and resources (e.g., people, technical support, hardware, and software) needed. In addition, it outlines the information to be tested across disparate systems as well as the review of all reports required for operational and administrative functions.

For example, the already implemented medical records system must receive patient demographic data from the new system. All fields passed in the medical records interface must be tested in 4 specific modes. The acronym CRUD is helpful to remember; test the creation of new data passing to disparate systems, the ability to review the data in online displays of both the registration system and the legacy medical records system, transmitting data updates, and deletion of data in one system and its impact on other systems and applications. The downtime plan for use during the cutover period (see Cutover Plan later in this chapter) is thoroughly tested during this step, ensuring all departments and teams are aware of their tasks and the impact of those tasks on other departments involved in the plan. When completed, integrated testing scenarios are approved by a representative of each affected system and department indicating the testing has been completed and their department will function as detailed in the project scope and workflow documents.

Note: There are those who advocate a parallel testing period. It is our experience that parallel testing (i.e., entering data in the old system while also entering this exact data in the new system, with a thorough review of discrepancies) results primarily in a test of the abilities of the project teams to enter the same data in two systems, and less about the functionality of the new system. Concentrating on creating and carrying out a thoroughly considered and executed integrated testing period accomplishes the same goal with all project team efforts concentrated on the new system and processes.

Securing the needed resources for integrated testing can be daunting, as all affected systems are being tested in a near real-time representation of a patient's encounter. If feasible, resources from the Help Desk can be part of integrated testing; this adds to their knowledge of the system and is beneficial when they field calls from end users.

Issue Tracking and Resolution during Integrated Testing. As described in step 10, unit testing, the effective use of an issue tracking system is imperative. Collection and review of issues discovered during testing will require attention to detail, the ability to test and recreate scenarios, determine the cause and remedy, assign a priority, and determine the amount of time likely needed to fix the problem. Applying and adhering to issue resolution criteria during integrated testing is often a source of conflict. Establishing integrated testing criteria with the project team prior to unit testing is highly recommended, as discussed above. During integrated testing, the software change management plan is adhered to. Based on the number and priority of issues uncovered during testing, the team may decide only those issues categorized as critical and potentially high should be addressed prior to the Go-Live date. The number of critical issues remaining at the end of integrated testing can impact the Go-Live timeframe.

Go – No Go Decision. At the completion of integrated testing, the organization makes a formal decision to proceed or postpone activation of the new system. Often referred to as the Go – No Go decision, members from the steering committee, project team, and technical staff review the outstanding issues from both the unit testing and integrated testing. Objective criteria established in step 1, project scope and charter; step 7, end-user training: planning; step 10, unit testing; and step 12 integrated testing for the new system's acceptable level of functionality are reviewed. Areas specifically reviewed are the status of:

- Project scope document
- Application software
- System hardware
- Networks
- End-user training
- Conversion programs
- Interface programs
- Issues list: priority, status, and number of open issues

Members of the steering committee, in consultation with the project manager, technical manager, and selected project team leaders, evaluate the available data. With all in order, the organization moves toward the activation of the new systems (the Go Live). If major concerns still exist, an alternate Go-Live date may need to be considered.

Cutover Plan. The cutover plan provides the detailed steps required for each department to accomplish a seamless transition from the old system to the new system. The cutover plan is data driven based on the requirements of the departments and the technical team. The length of time between the initiation of the cutover plan and the move to processing on the new system, the Go Live, is often dependent on the amount of data to be converted from the old system to the new system. The technical manager plays an integral role in determining this plan.

Here is a technical example: Hospital A has 3.4 million patient demographic records in the legacy master patient index, which they are planning to convert programmatically to the new system. There are 254 data elements for each record to be converted. Unit testing of the conversion program indicates 200,000 records can be converted per hour requiring a minimum of 17 hours to complete the conversion. The cutover plan must account for this period of time when neither the legacy system nor the new system are fully functional.

Here is a procedural example: Between the hours of 11 PM and 6 AM, all in-patient and emergency registrations are completed by the emergency room staff. The master patient index conversion will impact their ability to register emergency patients during the cutover period. A process and procedure to register and assign medical records and account numbers during this time, as well as to enter registrations into the new system at the appropriate time, is required to ensure that delivery of patient care is not impacted.

Figure 6.4 provides a template for development of a detailed cutover plan indicating both the tasks to be accomplished, the expected time frame to complete the task, the party responsible for completing the task, and the person to whom the handoff to initiate the next task will be. Testing of communication channels during the cutover period during the integrated testing period will prove invaluable during the actual cutover period.

Step 13. Live Operations

The 4 key tasks within step 13 (lucky 13) are:

- Developing the Go-Live plan
- Establishing a command center
- First productive use of the new system: the Go Live
- Resolution of issues arising during the first 1 to 3 weeks of processing on the new system

Few, if any, healthcare organizations have the luxury to stop operations during an implementation (Lorenzi, Novak, Weiss, Gadd, & Unertl, 2008). The Go-Live plan encompasses the cutover plan (data driven) and the plan for the facility to continue to operate (people and processes) during this period. Staffing, patient care delivery, and support of the end user during the Go-Live period are detailed within the Go-Live plan

The command center is set up and ready to coordinate all issues, concerns, and Go-Live Help Desk functions. The command center has a sufficient number of phone lines and beepers to support the move to the live production environment. For a period of time, this will include 24 hours-per-day operations. Often, the representatives and consultants of the new software company

DONE	DATE	START TIME	TARGET END TIME	SEQUENCE	TASK DESCRIPTION	TASK DEPENDENCY	RESP PERSON	HANDOFF CONTACT	COMMENTS
	2-Nov	8:30	30-Nov	SMS-1	Change profile PRFDT to 29 days. Continue changing this profile (minus one day) on a daily basis until 11/30 when it is set to 1.	None			All areas that enter orders. To prevent future orders to be placed in legacy system with start date greater that conversion date.
	30-Nov	12:00	23:00	CAI-1	Review/Final configuration changes	None			
	30-Nov				CHECKPOINT CONFERENCE CALL	Scheduled	ALL		
	30-Nov	14:00	16:00	MD-1	Order rewrites by physicians. Nursing staff will hold on to any orders which can be held until 02:00	None			6 a.m. Lab draws should not wait until 2 p.m. Enter when orders are rewritten. WE ARE NOT REWRITING MEDICATION ORDERS!
	30-Nov	14:00	16:00	Nursing-1	Enter orders for 6 A.M. Lab draw in legacy system	Legacy Lab Up	Nurses Staff		
	30-Nov	18:00	0:00	Nursing-2	Validation of Allergies (including food allerg(ies) and patient factors data on Go-Live patient factor validation checklist		Nurses Only	Hand off validation Checklist	Go-Live patient factor validation form checklist created help with this.

• FIGURE 6.4. Sample cutover plan.

are on site to assist with Go-Live support and staffing of the command center. The advantages of having a designated command center include close proximity of clinical, administrative, technical, and vendor team members to quickly assess and prioritize issues. This close proximity also allows rapid communications and trending of problems in near real time during the first days of the new system's use.

Team members, trainers, and super users serve as resources to the end users on a 24-hour basis during Go Live, often for a period of 1 to 2 weeks.

The coordination of all activities requires a cohesive team effort. Communication among the team members is foundational; end users are informed of the sequence of events, the expected time frames for each event, and the channels established for reporting and resolving issues.

Daily meetings of key team members to review issues and chart the progress of the new system are held. Decisions affecting the Go Live are made in a timely manner and require a thoughtful and thorough approach when changes to procedures and computer programs are contemplated. The executive team and senior management group are kept as up to date as the end users. The goal of most clinical implementations is to improve the delivery of information to the end user, a method for improving the delivery of patient care. The end user's suggestions and issues, therefore, must be tracked and resolved. Providing timely follow up to issues and suggestions will be critical to the success of the new system. Often, the informatics nurses are responsible for this follow-up.

It is highly recommended to have all end-user logins, passwords, and system printers tested 5 to 7 days before the Go-Live date. Requests for login and password support comprise the largest number of calls to the command center during the first few weeks of a new system's use. Clinical and departmental managers are in the best position to ensure that all staff have logged into the new system and have the appropriate role for their job requirements. Login issues are followed closely by printer issues (e.g., printer offline, printer settings incorrect, output expected to print at a location doesn't print) during the first weeks of a new system. The hardware team members can best troubleshoot issues when they have been given a script outlining one or two functions resulting in a printed output. Assuring these two areas are addressed completely prior to Go Live will dramatically lessen the anxiety of the end users, as well as eliminate a large number of calls to the command center during the Go-Live period.

With an organized and thorough integrated testing period, the actual first productive use of the system and subsequent days of the Go-Live period are likely to be a boring nonevent. Feedback from the end users and administrative staff will help determine how long the command center will need to be staffed on a 24-hour basis.

Step 14. Post Go Live Evaluation

The important tasks of the Post Go Live evaluation are:

- Collection of post-live success criteria
- Completion of a system and project evaluation including the results of the success criteria
- Transitioning end-user support from the command center to the Help Desk
- Closure of the project

During this step, the system is evaluated to determine whether it has accomplished the project scope document's stated objectives. It involves a comparison of the working system with its functional requirements to determine how well the requirements are met, to determine possibilities for growth and improvement, and to preserve the lessons learned from the implementation project for future efforts. The Post Go Live evaluation describes and assesses, in detail, the new system's performance. Utilizing the criteria established in step 1, the evaluation process summarizes the entire system, identifying both the strengths and weaknesses of the implementation process. Comparison of the pre- and post-implementation success criteria data provide quantitative data regarding the successes of the new system. The evaluation often leads to system revisions and, ultimately, a better system.

To evaluate an implemented hospital information system, many principles are important. One authority suggests evaluating duplication of efforts and data entry, fragmentation, misplaced work, complexity, bottlenecks, review and approval processes, error reporting via the issue tracking mechanism, or the amount of reworking of content, movement, wait time, delays, setup, low-importance outputs, and unimportant outputs.

This evaluation component becomes a continuous phase in total quality management. The system is assessed to determine whether it continues to meet the needs of the users. The totally implemented system will require continuous evaluation to determine if upgrading is appropriate and/or what enhancements could be added to the current system. Formal evaluations generally take place no less than every 6 months and routinely every 2 to 4 years after the system has been implemented. An outside evaluation team can conduct the formal evaluation to increase the objectivity level of the findings. Informal evaluations are done on a weekly basis.

Other approaches to evaluating the functional performance of a system exist. The Clinical Information System Evaluation Scale (Gugerty, Mranda, & Rook, 2006) describes a 37-item measurement tool for assessing staff satisfaction with a CIS. Investigating such functions as administrative control, medical and nursing orders, charting and documentation, and retrieval and management reports are used to assess system benefits. Each of these areas is evaluated through time observations, work sampling, operational audits, and surveys (Nahm, 2007). The system's functional performance can be assessed by examining nurses' morale and nursing department operations.

Documentation of care must be assessed if patient care benefits are to be evaluated. The following questions should be asked:

- Does the system assist in improving the documentation of patient care in the patient record?
- Does the system reduce patient care costs?
- Does the system prevent errors and save lives?
- Evaluating nurses' morale requires appraising nurses' satisfaction with the system. The following questions may be considered useful:
  ○ Does the system facilitate nurses' documentation of patient care?
  ○ Does it reduce the time spent in such documentation?
  ○ Is it easy to use?
  ○ Is it readily accessible?
  ○ Do the display screens have an easy-to-use design?
  ○ Do the displays capture patient care?
  ○ Does the system enhance the work situation and contribute to work satisfaction?

Evaluating departmental benefits requires determining if the CIS helps improve administrative activities. The following questions must be answered:

- Does the new system enhance the goals of the department?
- Does it improve department efficiency?

- Does it help reduce the range of administrative activities?
- Does it reduce clerical work?

Other criteria are necessary to evaluate technical performance; these include reliability, maintainability, use, response time, accessibility, availability, and flexibility to meet changing needs. These areas are examined from several different points, including the technical performance of the software as well as hardware performance. The following questions must be answered:

- Is the system accurate and reliable?
- Is it easy to maintain at a reasonable cost?
- Is it flexible?
- Is the information consistent?
- Is the information timely?
- Is it responsive to users' needs?
- Do users find interaction with the system satisfactory?
- Are input devices accessible and generally available to users?

Implementation of a clinical system is a project; by definition a project has a beginning, a middle, and an end (Lewis, 2007; Project Management Institute, 2010). Transitioning the end-user support functions from the command center to the Help Desk, and submission of the Post Go Live evaluation to the steering committee are particularly important events in determining the end of an implementation project and the beginning of the maintenance and growth phases of the new system.

SUMMARY

A clinical information system or new clinical application implementation project can be a large undertaking for healthcare organizations both in terms of financial costs and resources. The 2009 passage of the American Recovery and Reinvestment Act (ARRA) affords healthcare organizations moving toward automated clinical information systems significant financial incentives if activation of the automated system results in a high level of system use by clinicians (also termed *meaningful use*) (US Health and Human Services, 2010). The amount of incentives available to an organization is greatest when implementations are completed in 2010 and 2011 (ARRA, 2009; US Health and Human Services, 2010). Successful implementations in the near term will provide organizations both financial assistance as well as ongoing clinical information support. This chapter presents steps 8 through 14 of a comprehensive implementation process tailored specifically for clinical systems.

REFERENCES

111th Congress. (2009). *American Recovery and Reinvestment Act 2009*. Retrieved from http://www.hhs.gov/news/press/2009pres/12/20091230a.html, http://www.recovery.gov/News/press/Pages/20100212_HHS_HealthIT.aspx, & http://www.hhs.gov/news/press/2010pres/02/20100212a.html.

Center for Medicare/Medicaid Services. (1996). *Health information portability and accuntability act of 1996 (HIPPA)*. Retrieved from http://www.cms.gov/HIPAAGenInfo/01_Overview.asp.

Douglas, M. (2000). Butterflies, bonsai, & Buonarroti: Images for the nurse analyst. In M. Ball, K. Hannah, S. Newbold, & J. Douglas (Eds.), *Nursing informatics: Where caring and technology meet* (pp 69–79). New York: Springer-Verlag,.

Gugerty, B., Mranda, M., & Rook, D. (2006). The clinical information system implementation evaluation scale. *Student Heath Technology Informatics*, *122*, 621–625.

Ferraiolo, D., Kuhn, R., & Sandhu, R. (2007). RBAC standard rationale: Comments on a critique of the ANSI standard on role based access control. *IEEE Security & Privacy*, *5*(6), 51–53.

Lewis, J. (2007). *Fundamentals of project management* (p. 11). New York: ADCOM.

Lorenzi, N., & Riley, R. (2000). Managing change. *Journal of the American Medical Informatics Association*, *7*(2), 116–124.

Naham,E., Vaydia, V., Ho, D., Scharf, B., & Seagull, J. (2007). Outcomes assessment. *Nursing Outlook*, *55*(6), 282–288.

Project Management Institute. (2010). Retrieved from http://www.pmi.org.

SUGGESTED READINGS

Aarts, J., Doorewaard, H., & Berg, M. (2004). Understanding implementation: The case of a computerized physician order entry system in a large Dutch university medical center. *Journal of the American Medical Informatics Association*, *11*(3): 207–216.

American Nurses Association. (2008). *The scope of practice for nursing informatics*. Washington, D. C.: American Nurse Publishing.

ASTM E1384. (2007). *Standard practice for content and structure of the electronic health record (EHR)*. West Conshohocken, PA: ASTM International. doi:10.1520/E1384-07.

Ash, J., Fournier, M., Stavri P., & Dykstra, R. (2003). Principles for a successful computerized physician order entry implementation. *American Medical Informatics Association Symposium Proceedings* (pp. 36–40).

Ash, J., Anderson, J., Gorman, P., Zielstorff, R., Norcross, N., Pettit, J. & Yao, P. (2000). Managing change: Analysis of a hypothetical case. *Journal of the American Medical Informatics Association*, *7*(2), 125–134.

Augustine, J. (2004). System redesign and IT implementation. *Advance for health information executives*, *8*(1), 41–43.

Balas, E., Austin, S., Mitchell, J., Ewigman, B., Bopp, K., and Brown, G, et al., (1996). The clinical value of computerized information services. *Archives of Family Medicine*, *5*(3), 271–278.

Bauer, J. (2004). Why CPOE must become SOP. *Journal of Healthcare Information Management*, *18*(1), 9–10.

Briggs, B. (2003). CPOE: Order from chaos. *Health Data Management*, February 2003. Retrieved from archive at www.HealthDataManagement.com.

California Healthcare Foundation, (2002). *Computerized physician order entry: Cost benefits and challenges: A case study approach* (pp. 28–36). Long Beach, CA: First Consulting Group.

Ciotti, V., & Bogutski, B. (1994). 10 commandments: Negotiating HIS contracts. *Healthcare Informatics*, *11*(7), 16–20.

Clayton, P., Sideli, R., & Sengupta, S. (1992). Open architecture and integrated information at Columbia-Presbyterian Medical Center. *MD Computing*, *9*(5), 297–303.

Convey, S. (1992). *The seven healthy habits of highly effective people: Restoring the character ethic* (pp. 95–144). New York: Fireside.

Cook, R. (1998). Do we need this? *Modern Physician*, *3*(10), 35–58.

Dick, R., & Steen, E. (Eds.). (1991). *The computer-based record: An essential technology for healthcare*. Washington, D. C.: National Academy Press.

Fitzgerald, J., Fitzgerald, A., & Satllings, W. (1981). *Fundamentals of systems analysis* (2nd ed.). New York: John Wiley & Sons.

Gause, D., & Weinberg, G. (1989). *Exploring requirements: Quality before design*. New York: Dorset House Publishing.

Ginsburg, D. A., & Browning, S. J. (1989). Selecting automated patient care systems. In V. K. Saba, K. A. Rider, & D. B. Pocklington (Eds.) (pp. 229–237), *Nursing and computers: An anthology*. New York: Springer-Verlag.

Kaplan, B. (1997). Addressing organizational issues into the evaluation of medical systems. *Journal of the American Medical Informatics Association*, *4*(2), 94–101.

Lorenzi, N, Novak, L, Weiss, J, Gadd, C, & Unertl, K. (2008). Crossing the implementation chasm. *Journal of the American Medical Informatics Association*, *15*(3), 290–296.

Peitzman, L. (2004). Addressing physician resistance to technology. *Advance for Health Information Executives, 8*(5), 69–70.

Protti, D., & Peel, V. (1998). Critical success factors for evolving a hospital toward an electronic patient record system: A case study of two different sites. *Journal of Healthcare Information Management, 12*(4), 29–37.

Schooler, R. & Dotson, T. (2004). Rolling out the CIS. *Advance for Health Information Executives, 8*(2), 63–70.

Sengstack, P., & Gugerty, B. (2004). CPOE systems: success factors and implementation issues. *Journal of Healthcare Information Management, 18*(1), 36–45.

Yourdon, E. (1989). *Modern structures analysis.* Englewood Cliffs, NJ: Yourdon Press.

7

Healthcare Project Management

Judy Murphy / Patricia C. Dykes

• OBJECTIVES

1. Describe the 5 process groups in project management methodology, and identify key inputs and outputs for each.
2. Illustrate the "triple constraint" relationship between scope, cost, and time, and how it can impact project quality.
3. Explain how a clinical system project is initiated and the role of the project charter.
4. Identify 5 techniques that will positively impact the quality, efficiency, and effectiveness of a clinical system implementation.

• KEY WORDS

project management
project methodology
health information technology
process groups
triple constraint

INTRODUCTION

It's difficult to read a newspaper, magazine, or Web page today without somehow hearing about the impact of information technology (IT). Information in all forms is traveling faster and being shared by more individuals than ever before. Think of how quickly you can use the Internet to buy just about anything, make an airline reservation, or book a hotel room anywhere in the world. Consider how fast you can share photos or video clips with your family and friends. This ubiquitous use of technology is permeating the healthcare industry as well, and the future of many organizations may depend on their ability to harness the power of IT, particularly in the area of electronic health records (EHRs) and health information exchange.

Good project management is needed in order to accomplish the work, facilitate the change, and deliver the improvements made possible by health IT implementation. Project management is not a new concept; it has been practiced for hundreds of years, as any large undertaking requires a set of objectives, a plan, coordination, the management of resources, and the ability to manage change. Today, however, project management has become more formal with a specified body of knowledge, and many healthcare organizations have adopted the project-oriented approach as a technique to define and execute on their strategic goals and objectives.

Good project managers for health IT projects are in high demand. Colleges have responded by establishing courses in project management and making them part of the health informatics curriculums for continuing education, certificate, and degree programs. This chapter offers a high-level look at the methodology behind project management in order to provide a framework for the development of project management skills, structure for the implementation work processes, and organization of the projects' tasks.

CHAPTER OVERVIEW

This chapter augments the Systems Life Cycle chapter, as it outlines the project management phases, called *process groups*, used to organize and structure the systems life cycle in order to successfully complete all the implementation steps of a project. The overview section will provide an introduction to project management and background information on project definitions, as well as a discussion of important skills for project managers. Each subsequent section will review 1 of the 5 project management process groups. The last section will describe some additional considerations for health IT projects, such as governance and positioning of project management in the healthcare organization.

What Is a Project?

There are many different definitions of what a project is, but they all have the same components: a project is temporary, has a defined beginning and end, and is managed according to time, budget, and scope. Kerzner defines a project as, "A temporary endeavor undertaken to create a unique product, service, or result. Has a specific objective, defined start and end dates, funding limitations, consumes resources (human, equipment, materials) and is generally multifunctional or cross-organizational in nature." (Kerzner, 2006, p. 2) The Project Management Institute (PMI) defines a project as follows, "A project is a *temporary* endeavor undertaken to create a *unique* product or service. *Temporary* means that every project has a definite beginning and a definite end. *Unique* means that the product or service is different in some distinguishing way from all other products or services." (PMI, 2004, p. 4) Schwalbe goes on to differentiate a project from operations in the following way: "Operations work is done to sustain the business. Projects are different from operations in that they end when the objectives have been reached or the project has been terminated." (Schwalbe, 2010, p. 4)

What Is Project Management?

Project management is facilitation of the planning, scheduling, monitoring and controlling of all work that must be done to meet the project objectives. PMI states that "project management is the application of knowledge, skills, tools and techniques to project activities to meet project requirements." (PMI, 2004, p. 7) It is a systematic process for implementing systems on time, within budget, and in line with customer expectations of quality. Project managers must not only strive to meet specific scope, time, cost, and quality project goals, they must also facilitate the entire process to meet the needs and expectations of the people involved in or affected by project activities.

Introduction to the 5 Process Groups

The project management process groups progress from initiation activities to planning activities, executing activities, monitoring and controlling activities, and closing activities. Each of these will be described in detail in ensuing sections of this chapter. However, it is important to note here that these groups are integrated and not linear in nature, so that decisions and actions taken in one group can affect another. Figure 7.1 shows the 5 groups and how they relate to each other in terms of typical level of activity, time, and overlap. Of course, the level of activity and length of each process group varies for each project (Schwalbe, 2006).

Project Management Knowledge Areas

The project management knowledge areas describe the key competencies that project managers must develop and use during each of the process groups. Each of these competencies has specific tools and techniques associated with it, some of which will be elaborated in following sections of this chapter. Table 7.1 shows the 9 knowledge areas of project management. The 4 core areas of project management (bolded in the table) are project scope, time, cost, and quality management. These are considered core, as they lead to specific project objectives. The 4 facilitating knowledge areas of project management are human resources, communication, risk, and procurement management. These are considered facilitating, as they are the processes through which the project objectives are achieved. The ninth knowledge area, project integration management, is an overarching function that affects and is affected by all of the other knowledge areas. Project managers must have knowledge and skills in all of these 9 areas.

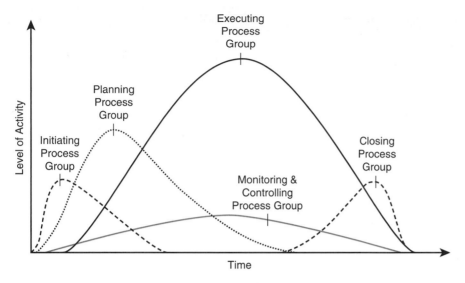

• **FIGURE 7.1.** Level of activity and overlap of process groups over time. (Adapted from Schwalbe, K. (2006). *Information Technology Project Management*, (4th ed.) (p. 73). United States: Thomson Course Technology.)

INITIATING PROCESS GROUP

The initiating process group (IPG) is defined by the PMI as follows, "those processes performed to authorize and define the scope of a new phase or project or that can result in the continuation of halted project work" (PMI, 2004, p. 352). The purpose of the IPG is to formally define a project including the business need, key stakeholders, and project goals. A clear definition of the business case is critical for defining the scope of the

TABLE 7.1	Knowledge Areas Used in Each Process Group*				
Knowledge Area	**Project Management Process Group**				
	Initiating	Planning	Executing	Monitoring & controlling	Closing
Project integration management	X	X	X	X	X
Project scope management		X		X	
Project time management		X		X	
Project cost management		X		X	
Project quality management		X	X	X	
Project human resource management		X	X	X	
Project communications management		X	X	X	
Project risk management		X		X	
Project procurement management		X	X	X	X

*Bold indicates the 4 core knowledge areas.
Adapted from Schwalbe, K. (2010). *Information technology project management*, (6th ed.) (pp. 83–84). United States, Boston: Course Technology, Cengage Learning.

TABLE 7.2	Tools to Support the Initiating Process Group	
SWOT Analysis	**Stakeholder Analysis**	**Value-Risk Assessment**
Method for identifying potential strengths and weaknesses of the project team or organization relative to a proposed project and the potential opportunities and threats inherent in conducting a project.	Documents important information about stakeholders that makes explicit their support, level of influence on a project, and strategies for managing relationships to ensure project success (Figure 7.1).	Tool that supports objective rating of a project using pre-established criteria that are consistent with the mission, vision, and values of an organization.

project and for identifying the opportunity associated with completing the project. The business case includes the potential risks associated with completing or not completing the project at a given point in time. The work completed throughout the IPG builds a foundation for buy-in and commitment from the project sponsors and establishes understanding of associated challenges. The IPG is characterized by information gathering and research that leads to full disclosure of both the benefits and the costs associated with a given project. Historical information is assembled during the IPG to identify related projects or earlier attempts at similar projects. Historical information provides insight into challenges associated with the project and buy-in from stakeholders. The IPG may lead to formal project selection or it may culminate in a decision to forgo or postpone a project.

The set of work completed in the IPG is often done directly for a business sponsor and may be accomplished without a formal project team in place. During the IPG the goals of the proposed project are analyzed to determine the project scope and associated time, costs, and resource requirements. Key stakeholders are identified and may be engaged in defining the project scope, articulating the business case, and developing a shared vision for the project deliverables. The inputs needed to support the work of the IPG include tools and information that support the knowledge area of project integration management. "Project integration management includes the processes and activities needed to identify, define, combine, unify and coordinate the various processes and project management activities within the project management process groups" (PMI, 2004, p. 77). Sound integration management contributes to a solid understanding of whether the project is a good match for the organization and if so, how the project fits into the organizational mission and vision. The involvement of stakeholders in the process of project integration management is fundamental to their engagement in the project and involvement in defining

and working toward project success. Informational inputs such as the sponsor's description of the project, the organizational strategic plan, the published organizational mission, and historical information on related projects support the integration work of the IPG. Examples of tools and techniques that facilitate completing the information gathering, research, and related analyses required during the IPG include the strengths, weaknesses, opportunities, and threats (SWOT) analysis, stakeholder analysis, and the value-risk assessment (see Table 7.2 and Figure 7.2).

Tangible outputs of the IPG include the completed project charter that formally defines the project including the business case, key stakeholders, project constraints, and assumptions. The project charter includes signatures of the project sponsors and team members, indicating a shared vision for the project and formal approval to move forward with planning the project. The outputs from the IPG are used to inform project planning and reused during project closure to facilitate evaluation of the project deliverables.

PLANNING PROCESS GROUP

The planning process group (PPG) is often the most difficult and unappreciated process in project management, yet it is one of the most important and should not be rushed. This is the phase where decisions are made on how to complete the project and accomplish the goals and objectives defined in the initiating process group. The project plan is created with the main purpose of guiding the project execution phase. To that end, the plan must be realistic and specific; a fair amount of time and effort needs to be spent and people knowledgeable about the work need to help plan the work. The *project plan* also provides structure for the project monitoring and controlling process, as it creates the baseline to which the work is measured against as it is completed.

Step 1: List stakeholders and assign code. Classify stakeholders according to influence level

Stakeholder analysis coding key	
Code/Name	Influence level
A.	(H)
B.	(H)
C.	(H)
D.	(H)
E.	(H)
F.	(H)
G.	(H)
H.	(H)
I.	(M)
J.	(H)
K.	(L)
L.	(L)
M.	(H)
N.	(H)

Step 2: Identify sources and causes of resistance and strategies for overcoming

Source of resistance	Causes of resistance	Strategies for overcoming resistance
Technical	• Lack of coding skills • Lack of documentation skills • Lack of understanding • Inadequate tools to support skill level	• Education & training • Use of dissemination tool (Marketing w/"on call", mox, email, ect...) • Involve staff in tool development to support new skills
Political	• Job responsibility • Scope • Territoriality	• Clarify responsibility • Disseminate "elevator speech" • Involving stakeholders • Past successes
Cultural	• Ingrained departmental • Resistance to change • "If it ain't broke...	• Education & training • Involve staff in tool development to support new skills

Step 3: Plot strategies for managing stakeholders

Stakeholder analysis: *outpatient oncology care: improving the reimbursement process*

Names/influence level	Strongly against (-2)	Moderately against (-1)	Neutral (0)	Moderately supportive (+1)	Strongly supportive (+2)	Strategies for overcoming resistance
A. (H)					X	
B. (H)					X	
C. (H)					X	
D. (H)					X	
E. (H)					X	
F. (H)					X	
G. (H)					X	
H. (H)					X	
I. (M)					X	
J. (H)					X	
K. (L)			X			
L. (L)			X			
M. (H)					X	
N. (H)			X (C)	√		(4,8)
O. (M)			X (P)		√	(1,2,7)
P. (M)			X (P)		√	(2,4,7)
Q. (L)		X (C,T)	√			(2,3,4)
R. (H)	X		√			(7)
S. (H)			X			
T. (H)				X		
U. (H)			X			
V. (H)			(P,C,V)		√	(2,3,4)
W. (H)					X	
X. (H)				X		
Y. (L)				X		
Z. (L)				X		
AA. (L)				X		

1. Use of dissemination tool (Marketing w/"on call",mox,email,ect...)	2. Clarify responsiblity	3. Education & training
4. Involve staff in tool development to support new skills	5. Disseminate "elevator speech"	6. Past successes
7. Involving stakeholders		

• **FIGURE 7.2.** Stakeholder analysis.

TABLE 7.3	Planning Process Group Tools and Techniques
Scope statement	Defines the boundaries of the project work; often developed directly from: • Voice of the customer • Project charter • SWOT analysis (strengths, weaknesses, opportunities and threats • Stakeholder analysis • Value-risk assessment.
Project charter	Describes the high-level scope, time, and cost goals for the project objectives and success criteria, a general approach to accomplishing the project goals, and the roles and responsibilities of project stakeholders.
RACI chart	Helps define the roles and responsibilities of project teams and team members; shows who is: • Responsible: Completes the task • Accountable: Signs off on the task • Consulted: Has information necessary to complete the task • Informed: Needs to be notified of task status or results
Work breakdown structure (WBS)	Displays the project graphically, subdivided into manageable work activities, including the relationship of each task to other tasks, the allocation of responsibility, the resources required, and the time allocated.
Risk register	Prioritizes the list of project risks, often including a plan for risk avoidance and risk mitigation strategies.

During the initiating phase, a lot of information was collected to define the project, including the scope document and project charter, which provide validation and approval for the project. During the planning phase, the approach to accomplish the project is defined to an appropriate level of detail. This includes defining the necessary tasks and activities in order to estimate the resources, schedule, and budget. Failure to adequately plan greatly reduces the project's chances of successfully accomplishing its goals (Schwalbe, 2010).

Project planning generally consists of the following steps:

- Define project scope
- Refine project objectives
- Define all required deliverables
- Create framework for project schedules
- Select the project team
- Create the work breakdown structure
- Identify the activities needed to complete the deliverables
- Sequence the activities and define the critical path activities
- Estimate the resource requirements for the activities
- Identify required skills and resources
- Estimate work effort and time and cost for activities
- Develop the schedule

- Develop the budget
- Complete risk analysis and avoidance
- Create communication plan
- Gain formal approval to begin work

Some of the tools and techniques employed during the PPG are listed in Table 7.3. One of the most important is the work breakdown structure (WBS). Projects are organized and understood by breaking them into a hierarchy, with progressively smaller pieces until they are a collection of defined "work packages" that include tasks. The WBS is used as the outline to provide a framework for organizing and managing the work. The deliverable of this phase is a comprehensive project plan that is approved by the sponsor(s) and shared with the project team in a project kick-off meeting (Houston, 2007).

EXECUTING PROCESS GROUP

The executing process group (EPG) is defined by the PMI as follows, "Those processes performed to complete the work defined in the project management plan to accomplish the project's objectives defined in the project scope statement" (PMI, 2004, p. 360). The EPG is characterized by carrying out the work of the project and associated activities defined by the project plan to meet project requirements. During the EPG the project team follows the project plan and each team member contributes to the ongoing progress of the plan. Project deliverables are managed during the

TABLE 7.4	Executing Process Group Tools and Techniques
Project meetings	Gathering of project team for the purpose of advancing the work of the project. All participants have a predefined role; action items and decisions are tracked and formally communicated.
Gantt chart	Tracks and communicates project tasks, resources, and milestones against time over the course of a project. (Many of the Web references at the end of the chapter contain links to sample Gantt charts.)
Request for proposal	Used to solicit proposals from prospective vendors.
Issue log	Provides a means to prioritize and track items that represent a degree of risk to meeting project deliverables.
Progress reports	Keeps project team informed of project status, milestones to date, and areas of concern.

EPG by careful tracking of scope, time, and resource use with ongoing updates made to the project plan and timeline to reflect progress made. The key responsibilities of the project manager during the EPG are integration of the project team and activities to keep the work of the project moving toward the milestones established during the project planning phase. Clear communication and effective management of project resources are essential. The inputs needed to support the work of the EPG include tools and information that facilitate assimilation of the following knowledge areas into project efforts (PMI, 2004; Schwalbe, 2006):

- Integration management: Coordination of project resources and activities to complete the project on time, within budget, and in accordance with the project scope defined by the customer.

- Quality management: Monitoring of project performance to ensure that the deliverables will satisfy the quality requirements specified by the customer.

- Human resource management: Enhancing and motivating performance of project team members to ensure effective use of human resources to advance project deliverables.

- Communication management: Distribution of information in a complete and timely fashion to ensure all stakeholders are informed and miscommunication channels are minimized.

- Procurement management: Obtaining goods and services from outside an organization including identifying and selecting vendors and managing contracts.

As noted above, the inputs needed to support the work of the EPG include tools and information that promote clear communication, control the work, and manage project resources. Some common tools employed during the EPG are described in Table 7.4.

The tools and techniques used during the EPG and associated documentation facilitate completion of project work and provide a means to identify and track ongoing activities against the project plan. Variances may arise during project execution and may trigger an evaluation and a replanning of activities. Deliverables produced through use of the EPG input tools and techniques are then used as outputs to inform the work conducted over subsequent process group phases. For example, during the EPG, the Gantt chart provides a means to monitor whether the project is on schedule and for managing dependencies between tasks. This same tool is useful in monitoring and controlling process groups (MCPG) where the Gantt chart is used to proactively identify when remedial action is needed and to ensure that project milestones are met in accordance with the project plan.

MONITORING AND CONTROLLING PROCESS GROUP

The purpose of the MCPG is to observe project execution so that issues and potential problems can be identified in a timely manner and corrective action can be taken when necessary to control execution of the project. It is the process of measuring progress toward project objectives, monitoring deviation from the plan, and taking corrective action to ensure progress matches the plan. The MCPG is performed throughout the life of the project across all phases, and provides feedback between project phases (PMI, 2004).

The project manager facilitates project control by measuring actual performance against the planned or estimated performance from the project plan in the areas of scope, resources, budget, and time. The key benefits of project control are that when project performance is observed and measured regularly, variance to the plan can be identified and mitigated quickly to minimize delays and avoid cost overruns. Estimates say that 80% of healthcare projects fail; one-third are never completed, and

TABLE 7.5	Monitoring and Controlling Process Group Tools and Techniques
Project management methodology	Follow a methodology that describes not only what to do in managing a project, but how to do it.
Project management information systems	Hundreds of project management software products are available on the market today, and many organizations are moving toward powerful enterprise project management systems that are accessible via the Internet.
Time reporting tools	Ability to enter and track project effort by resource and against the project tasks.
Progress reports	Answers the questions: • How are my projects doing overall? • Are my projects on schedule? • Are my estimates accurate? • Are my resources properly utilized?

most are over budget, behind schedule, or go live with reduced scope (Kitzmiller, 2006). The reasons for these failures vary, but project control can help improve on-time, on-budget, and in-scope delivery of projects. During the control phase, the project manager needs to support the project team with frequent checks and recognition of the completion of incremental work efforts. This way, the project manager can adapt the work as needed. Project managers also need to work with the project sponsors to identify the risks of keeping on time and on budget versus modifying the schedule or scope to better meet the organization's need for the project (Houston, 2007).

The Triple Constraint

Every project is constrained in some way by scope, cost, and time. These limitations are known as the triple constraint. They are often competing constraints that need to be balanced by the project manager throughout the project's life cycle. Scope refers to the work that needs to be done to accomplish the project goals. Cost is the resources required to complete the project. Time is the duration of the project. A modification to the project will impact 1 or more of the 3 constraints, and often requires tradeoffs among them. For example, if there is an increase in scope, either cost or time, or both, will need to be increased as well. Or in another example, if time is decreased when a deadline is moved up, either scope will need to decrease or cost (resources) will need to increase. It is a balancing act.

The tools and techniques employed during the MCPG are described in Table 7.5.

CLOSING PROCESS GROUP

The closing process group (CPG) is defined by the PMI as follows, "Those processes performed to formally terminate all activities of a project or phase and transfer the completed product to others or close a cancelled project" (PMI, 2004, p.354). The goal of the CPG is to finalize all project activities and to formally close the project. During the CPG the project goals and objectives set during the IPG are compared with deliverables and analyzed to determine the project's success. Key stakeholders are engaged with evaluating the degree to which project deliverables were met. The inputs needed to support the work of the CPG include the outputs from earlier process group phases and the tools and information that support the knowledge areas of project integration and procurement management (PMI, 2004; Schwalbe, 2006).

- Integration management: Coordination of project closure activities including formal documentation of project deliverables and formal transfer of ongoing activities from the project team to established operational resources.

- Procurement management: Coordination of formal contract closure procedures including resolution of open issues and documentation of the archival of information to inform future projects.

Some common tools employed during the CPG are described in Table 7.6.

The tools and techniques used during the CPG and associated documentation facilitate project closure and provide a means to identify lessons learned. Moreover, these tools and techniques are used to document best practices including updates to the organization's project management toolbox (Milosevic, 2003). During the CPG, standard tools available to the project team to support best practices are identified and made available to support application of best practices in future projects. Including a formal step for adapting the project management toolbox during the CPG ensures that the toolbox remains pertinent and continues to support

TABLE 7.6	Closing Process Group Tools and Techniques
Post-implementation survey	Provides an opportunity for project stakeholders to evaluate the project from multiple perspectives including product effectiveness, management of the triple constraint, communication management, and overall performance of the project team.
Post-mortem review document	Provides a means to document the formal project evaluation and summarizes the plusses and deltas associated with a given project. Facilitates discussion related to lessons learned that can be applied to future projects.
Project closeout checklist	Used to ensure that agreed upon features of project closure are completed related to the following: post-implementation review, administrative closeout procedures, and formal acknowledgement of the project team.

best practices relative to the types of projects typically conducted within an organization.

OTHER CONSIDERATIONS

Project Governance

There is no question that successful projects are owned and sponsored by the leaders and staff that will be making the practice change and will be benefiting by the change. So in the ideal scenario, the governance committee(s) are led by top business and clinical leaders, with membership built on broad representation from key business and clinical departments. In addition to evaluating and ranking the technology project proposals brought to them, they take responsibility for generating an overall roadmap to use to compare each proposal against. They set guiding principles for concepts like integration versus best-of-breed systems. They consider where the organization needs to be going and what practice and care changes are required, then solicit proposals from the strategic business units who are responsible for making those changes. In other words, they don't just see themselves as "governing" the project selection process, but rather as "driving" the implementation of projects that support strategic initiatives and deliver strategic value. It may seem like a nuance, but consider that these are not governance committees that pick IT projects, but rather are governance committees that allocate IT resources to strategic projects (Murphy, 2009).

Skills Needed for Project Managers

There is general agreement that good project managers need to have both people skills and leadership skills. Here is one skills list that describes the many facets of the project manager's role:

- Communication skills: Listens, persuades
- Organizational skills: Plans, sets goals, analyzes

- Team-building skills: Shows empathy, motivates, promotes esprit de corps
- Leadership skills: Sets examples, provides vision (big picture), delegates, positive, energetic
- Coping skills: Flexible, creative, patient, persistent
- Technology skills: Experience, project knowledge

Project Management Office

There are different ways to position project mangers in a healthcare organization. Some have them in the IT department, some have them in the clinical department, others have them in an informatics department, and still others have matrix roles. Many have now created a project management office to provide best practices and support for managing all projects in an organization. The office can also provide education, coaching, and mentoring, as well as project management resources. With the federal incentives for health IT, the industry has begun the challenging task of implementing EHR system projects to demonstrate meaningful use. With this increase in projects, there is an increased demand for good project mangers and consistent project management methodology for completing projects.

Project Management Institute

The Project Management Institute (PMI) was founded in 1969 by a group of project managers and is considered to be the leading professional organization for project managers worldwide (PMI, 2010). The primary goal of the PMI is "to advance the practice, science and profession of project management throughout the world in a conscientious and proactive manner so that organizations everywhere will embrace, value and utilize project management and then attribute their successes to it" (PMI, 2010). The PMI publishes the Guide to the *Project Management Body of Knowledge (PMBOK® Guide)* which is a collection of consensus-based standards and best practices. The *PMBOK® Guide* is currently in its fourth edition and has been adopted by the American National Standards Institute (ANSI) (PMI, 2010).

Project Management Professionals

The PMI offers multiple levels of credentialing to assist project professionals with advancing their careers in project, program, and portfolio management. PMI credentials are available related to many aspects of project management including program management, scheduling, and risk management. PMI membership is not required for credentialing (PMI, 2010). In addition to meeting a set of published prerequisite requirements, PMI credentialing requires that candidates successfully pass a credentialing exam. Complete information about PMI credentials and the credentialing process can be accessed from the PMI Web site (www.pmi.org).

Project Management Resources on the Web

Many Web-based resources exist to support project management best practices. A recent search using the key words "project management resources" on a popular search engine returned over 70 million results. A list of validated Web-based resources is included in the Resource List at end of this chapter.

SUMMARY

Today, as so often in history, healthcare resources are limited. Yet there are many varied and complex healthcare technology projects demanding resources. So how does one ensure that healthcare dollars and clinician time are spent wisely on projects that guarantee patient-driven outcomes? In addition to selecting and funding the projects wisely, the authors believe that good project management minimizes risk and enhances success. We further contend that clinicians, and particularly nurses, are excellent candidates, once trained in project management techniques, to be good project managers. Executive management should support, and maybe even demand, project management training for the organization's clinical IT project team leaders.

Nursing informatics has been evolving since its inception some 25 years ago. More often than ever, project management skills are being included in training and formal education programs. And, increasingly, informatics nurses are stepping up to the plate and taking on key roles in the planning, selection, implementation,

and evaluation of the critical clinical systems needed in healthcare today. We hope that we have provided a glimpse into the skills that will enable this to happen. Good project management holds part of the key to consistent success with EHR system implementations in healthcare today.

REFERENCES

Houston, M., & Bove, L. (2007). *Project management for healthcare informatics.* New York: Springer.

Kerzner, H., & Saladis, F. (2006). *Project management workbook and PMP/CAPM exam study guide* (9th ed.). Hoboken, NJ: John Wiley & Sons, Inc.

Kitzmiller, R., Hunt, E., & Sproat, S. B. (2006). Adopting best practices: Agility moves from software development to healthcare project management. *Computers, Informatics, Nursing, 24*(2), 75–82, quiz 83–74.

Milosevic, D. Z. (2003). *Project management toolbox.* Hoboken, NJ: John Wiley & Sons, Inc.

Murphy, J. (2009). The best IT project is not an IT project: Nursing informatics commentary. *Journal of Healthcare Information Management, 23*(1), 6–8.

Project Management Institute. (2004). *A guide to the project management body of knowledge* (3rd ed.). Newton Square, PA: Project Management Institute, Inc.

Project Management Institute. (2010). Retrieved from http://www.pmi.org/Pages/default.aspx.

Schwalbe, K. (2006). *Information technology project management* (4th ed.). United States, Boston: Thomson Course Technology.

Schwalbe, K. (2010). *Information technology project management,* (6th ed.). United States: Course Technology, Cengage Learning.

OTHER RESOURCES

Books

Cleland, D., & Ireland, L. (2007). *Project management strategic design and implementation* (5th ed.). New York: McGraw-Hill.

DeCarlo, D. (2004). *Extreme project management.* Hoboken, NJ: Jossey-Bass.

Kendrick, T. (2000). *The project management tool kit.* Washington, DC: American Management Association.

Kerzner, H. (2006). *Project management: A systems approach to planning, scheduling and controlling.* (9th ed.). Hoboken, NJ: John Wiley & Sons, Inc.

Lewis, J. P. (2001). *Project Planning, Scheduling, and Control.* (3rd ed). New York: McGraw-Hill.

Lowenthal, J. N. (2002). *Six sigma project management: A pocket guide.* Milwaukee, WI: ASQ Quality Press.

Manas, J. (2006). *Napoleon on project management: Timeless lessons in planning, execution and leadership*. Nashville, TN: Thomas Nelson.

Murphy, J., & Gugerty, B. (2006). Nurses in Project Management Roles. In C.A. Weaver, C. W. Delaney, P. Weber, & R. L. Carr (Eds.), *Nursing and informatics for the 21st century: An international look at practice, trends and the future* (145–154). Chicago: HIMSS Press.

Project Management Institute. (2008). *A guide to the project management body of knowledge* (4th ed.). Newton Square, PA: Project Management Institute, Inc.

Web Sites

Agile Project Leadership Network. (25 June, 2010). *Organization to connect, develop and support great project leaders*. Retrieved from http://apln.org.

Cornell University. (25 June, 2010). *Cornell project management methodology (CPMM)*. Retrieved from https://confluence.cornell.edu/display/CITPMO/Cornell+Project+Management+Methodology+%28CPMM%29.

Gantthead.com. The online community for IT Project Managers (25 June, 2010). *Extreme project management report*. Retrieved from http://www.gantthead.com/extreme-project-management.

Lewis Institute. (25 June, 2010). *Lewis project management systems*. Retrieved from http://www.lewisinstitute.com.

Musser, J. (25 June, 2010). *Project reference*. Retrieved from http://www.projectreference.com.

Standish Group. (25 June, 2010). *The extreme chaos report*. Retrieved from http://www.standishgroup.com/sample research/index.php.

State of New York. (25 June, 2010). *Project management*. Retrieved from http://www.oft.state.ny.us/pmmp/guidebook2/managementguide/mgtguide.pdf.

University of Texas. (25 June, 2010). *Build vs. buy methodology*. Retrieved from http://www.utexas.edu/its/archive/eis/buybuild/methods/discussion/index.html.

Bright Hub. (25 June, 2010). *Free project management forms & templates you can download*. Retrieved from http://www.brighthub.com/office/project-management/articles/26131.aspx#ixzz0rs5TNOvf.

Journal Articles

Becker, J., & Rhodes, H. (2007). Enterprise project management is key to success: Addressing the people, process and technology dimensions of healthcare. *Journal of Healthcare Information Management, 21*(3), 61–66.

Belassi, W., & Tukel, O. I. (1996). A new framework for determining critical success/failure factors in projects. *International Journal of Project Management, 14*(3), 141–151.

Chaiken, P. B., Christian, E. C., & Johnson, L. (2007). Quality and efficiency successes leveraging IT and new processes. *Journal of Healthcare Information Management, 21*(1), 48–53.

Corfield, L. (2008). Project management skills prove invaluable. *Health Estate, 62*(8), 19–20.

Hartman, F., & Ashrafi, R. (2002). Project management in the information systems and information technologies industries. *Project Management Journal, 33*(3), 5–15.

James, D., Kretzing, J. E., & Stabile, M. E. (2007). Showing "what right looks like"—How to improve performance through a paradigm shift around implementation thinking. *Journal of Healthcare Information Management, 21*(1), 54–61.

Jiang, J., Chen, E., & Klien, G. (2002). The importance of building a foundation for user involvement in information system projects. *Project Management Journal, 33*(1), 20–26.

Jiang, J., Klien, G., & Balloun, J. (1996). Ranking of system implementation success factors. *Project Management Journal, 27*(4), 49–53.

Lang R. D. (2005). IT project management in healthcare: Improving the odds for success. *Journal of Healthcare Information Management, 19*(1), 2–4.

Loo, R. (2003). Project management: A core competency for professional nurses and nurse managers. *Journal of Nursing Staff Development, 19*(4), 187–193; discussion 194.

Sa Couto, J. (2008). Project management can help to reduce costs and improve quality in healthcare services. *Journal of Evaluation in Clinical Practice, 14*(1), 48–52.

Shellenbarger, T. (2009). Time and project management tips for educators. *Journal of Continuing Education in Nursing, 40*(7), 292–293.

Wolff, P. (2003). Is your organization project management savvy? *Journal of Healthcare Information Management, 17*(1), 50–54.

Human Factors

Gregory L. Alexander

- OBJECTIVES
  1. Compare beginning frameworks for human factors approaches in nursing.
  2. Illustrate the properties of human factors systems and subsystems.
  3. Apply human factors systems and subsystems in healthcare.
  4. Propose how human factors approaches can improve human performance and outcomes in healthcare.

- KEY WORDS

  human factors
  patient care
  information technology
  patient safety
  system design

INTRODUCTION

Healthcare is a complex technological industry prone to accidents that result in disability or death. For example, consider the following scenarios: a nurse giving a 10cc intravenous injection of potassium chloride from a bottle with a green label when she thought she was injecting 10cc of normal saline flush from a bottle with a nearly identical green colored label; the connection of a feeding tube to an intravenous catheter; or, a unit of whole blood being hung and infused intravenously with an incompatible secondary fluid after many iterations of staff confirming the correct blood type and patient (Alexander & Stone, 2000; Simmons & Graves, 2008). One of the greatest contributors to these accidents and others in complex organizations is human error (Reason, 1990). However, implying that accidents are caused by human error does not mean that humans should be assigned blame, because most accidents result from system failures (Berwick, 1991). System failures pose the greatest threat to safety because they have been built into system processes and may have been present long before any active errors occurred (Reason, 1995). Human factors experts attempt to understand interactions between humans and different elements of the system to improve design, implementation, and safe use of system components. This chapter provides important information for nurses and other providers engaged in human factors efforts to improve healthcare systems and processes. The purpose of this chapter is to elevate nurses' levels of understanding about using human factors approaches to evaluate system performance, to facilitate the infusion of human factors concepts into nursing by identifying properties of human factors systems, and to describe how human factors evaluation can lead to improved performance and outcomes in nurse-led systems.

BEGINNING FRAMEWORKS FOR HUMAN FACTORS EVALUATION IN NURSING

The term *human factors* has been defined a number of ways by a number of experts (see Table 8.1). In healthcare, human factors experts attempt to understand the interrelationships between humans, the tools they use (i.e., information technology), the environments in which they live and work, and the tasks they perform (Staggers, 2003; Weinger, Pantiskas, Wiklund, & Carstensen, 1998; Staggers, 1991). Approaches used by human factors experts include the systematic application of information about human characteristics and behavior for the design of tools people use, methods for their use, and the design of the environments people live and work in (Johnson & Barach, 2007). The goal of a human factors approach in nurse-led systems is to optimize the interactions between nurses and the tools they use to perform their jobs, minimize error, maximize efficiency, optimize well-being, and improve quality of life (Staggers, 2002).

Early pioneers in nursing informatics set the stage for the development of nursing information systems and the use of these systems in storing information, knowledge development, and growth of technology in caregiving activities (Werley & Grier, 1981; Schwirian, 1986; Graves & Corcoran, 1989; Turley, 1996). These early models had several limitations including a lack of environmental and task-oriented elements, conceptual differences across frameworks, and a lack of time dimensions. Subsequently, nursing frameworks were proposed to assist in understanding the dynamic interactions that occur between nurses, information technology, and enabling elements that optimize a user's ability to process information via computers (Staggers & Parks, 1993). These became the early foundations for incorporating human factors approaches into the design of information technologies used by nurses. However, there were still limitations identified in these early models because they did not explicitly make the patient part of the model and they didn't define the context or include all elements of the metaparadigm or nursing (Effken, 2003). Effken (2003) proposed the informatics

TABLE 8.1	Human Factors Definitions		
Author	**Year**	**Human Factors Definition**	
McCormick & Sanders	1982	The systematic application of relevant information about human abilities, characteristics, behaviors, and motivations to the execution of functions.	
Kantowitz & Sorkin	1983	The discipline that tries to optimize the relationship between technology and the human.	
Meister D	1989	HF is the study of how humans accomplish work-related tasks in the context of human–machine–system operation and how behavioral and nonbehavioral variables affect that accomplishment. Human factors is also the application of behavioral principles for the design, development, testing, and operation of equipment and systems.	
Weinger & Englund.	1990	Refers to the designing of equipment, machines, or systems to accommodate the characteristics, expectations, and behaviors of the humans who use them in their everyday working and living environments.	
Staggers	1991	Optimal match between humans, their environments, technology, and the task at hand.	
Traub	1996	The application of scientific information about human beings (and scientific methods of acquiring such information) to the problems of design. Human factors is not: (1) just applying checklists and guidelines; (2) using oneself as the model for designing things; (3) just common sense; or (4) a styling exercise.	
Sawyer	1996	Is a discipline that seeks to improve human performance in the use of equipment by means of hardware and software design that is compatible with the abilities of the user population.	
Hasler	1996	(1) An applied science focused on minimizing human errors and optimizing performance where human beings interface with a device. (2) HF engineering, also known as ergonomics, is the study of the physical characteristics and limitations of humans, which can be further subdivided into physical and anatomic characteristics.	

TABLE 8.1	Human Factors Definitions *(continued)*		
Author	**Year**	**Human Factors Definition**	
Weinger, Pantiskas, Wiklund, & Carstensen	1998	Human factors is the study of the interrelationships between humans, the tools they use, and the environments in which they live and work.	
Welch	1998	Improvement in efficiency, safety, and user satisfaction.	
Rogers, Lamson, & Rousseau	2000	A general tenet of human factors design is that safety should be ensured through design of the system. If a potential hazard cannot be designed out, then it should be guarded against. If guarding against the hazard is not possible, then an adequate warning system should be developed.	
Lin, Vicente & Doyle	2001	This discipline focuses on the interaction between technology, people, and their work context. Human factors has sometimes been narrowly associated with Human Computer Interaction design guidelines.	
Weinger & Slagle	2002	Techniques to extract detailed information about system performance and risks to safety	
Wears & Perry	2002	The study of how human beings interact with their environment for useful purposes. The study of factors that make work easy or hard.	
Gosbee	2002	(1) The discipline that uses methods and concepts to understand and build systems that are more efficient, comfortable, and safe. (2) A discipline concerned with the design of tools, machines, and systems that take into account human capabilities, limitations, and characteristics. (3) Ergonomics, usability engineering, and user-centred design are considered synonymous.	
Bates & Gawande	2003	Principles of design using human factors suggest it is important to make warnings that are more serious look different than those that are less serious.	
Nemeth	2004	The development and application of knowledge about human physiology and behavior in the operational environment.	
Potter, Boxerman, Wolf, Marshall, Grayson, Sledge, & Evanoff	2004	The study of human beings and their interactions with products, environments, and equipment in performing tasks and activities	
Boston-Fleischhauer.	2008	The discipline that studies human capabilities and limitations and applies that knowledge to the design of safe, effective, and comfortable products, processes, and systems for the human beings involved.	

Bates, D. W., & Gawande, A. A. (2003). Improving safety with information technology. *New England Journal of Medicine, 348*, 2526–2534.

Boston-Fleischhauer, C. (2008). Enhancing healthcare process design with human factors engineering and reliability science, part 1: Setting the context. *Journal of Nursing Administration, 38*, 27–32.

Gosbee, J. (2002). Human factors in engineering and patient safety. *Quality and Safety in Healthcare, 11*, 352–354.

Kantowitz, B. H., & Sorkin, R. D. (1983). *Human factors: Understanding people--system relationships*. New York: John Wiley & Sons, Inc.

Lin, L., Vicente, K. J., & Doyle, D. J. (2001). Patient safety, potential adverse drug events, and medical device design: A human factors engineering approach. *Journal of Biomedical Informatics, 34*, 274–284.

McCormick, E. & Sanders, M. S. (1982). *Human factors in engineering and design*. (5th ed.) New York: McGraw-Hill Book Company.

Meister, D. (1989). *Conceptual aspects of human factors*. Baltimore: The Johns Hopkins University Press.

Rogers, W. A., Lamson, N., & Rousseau, G. K. (2000). Warning research: An integrative perspective. *Human Factors, 42*, 102–139.

Sawyer, D. (1996). Do it by design: An introduction to human factors in medical devices. Retrieved from http://www.fda.gov/cdrh/humfac/doitpdf.pdf.

Traub, P. (1996). Optimising human factors integration in system design. *Engineering Management Journal, April*, 93–98.

Wears, R. L., & Perry, S. J. (2002). Human factors and ergonomics in the emergency department. *Annals of Emergency Medicine, 40*, 206–212.

Weinger, M. B., & Slagle, J. (2002). Human factors research in anesthesia patient safety: Techniques to elucidate factors affecting clinical task performance and decision making. *Journal of the American Medical Informatics Association, 9*, S58–S63.

Welch, D. L. (1998). Human factors engineering. Human factors in the healthcare facility. *Biomedical Instrumentation & Technology, 32*(3), 311–316.

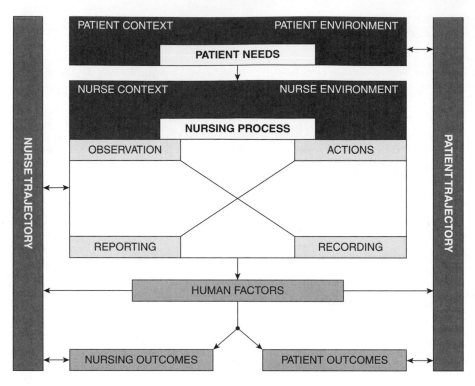

• **FIGURE 8.1.** Alexander's nurse-patient trajectory framework.

research organizing model, which emphasized all elements of the metaparadigm of nursing including the system, nurse, patient, and health. Later, Alexander's Nurse-Patient Trajectory Framework was proposed (Alexander, 2007). Alexander's framework (see Figure 8.1) utilizes nursing process theory, human factors, nursing, and patient trajectories as components of a framework that can be used to evaluate patient care systems. The framework specifically emphasizes the use of human factors approaches to link patient care processes, nurse and patient trajectories, and nursing and patient outcomes. The remainder of this chapter will focus on the concepts underlying human factors within Alexander's Nurse-Patient Trajectory Framework.

PROPERTIES OF HUMAN FACTORS SYSTEMS

A system is defined as any organized collection of elements that interacts to achieve desired outcomes (Nemeth, 2004). In human factors models, human-machine systems have been depicted as containing

subsystems associated with the operator, the machine, and the environment. A human factors model adapted from Helander (1997) with associated subsystems is illustrated in Figure 8.2. A central focus of study in human factors is the human-machine system (Carayon, Alvarado, & Hundt, 2007). The human-machine system combines one or more humans and one or more physical components that interact to transform inputs into outputs. This interaction occurs as a result of specific task requirements and can be affected by social and organizational environments where tasks are performed. Human factors that affect performance within the human-machine system are related to human capabilities, human-machine interfaces, and the environment. Each of these components will be discussed.

HUMAN FACTORS SUBSYSTEMS

The Operator Subsystem

Within human-machine systems, humans assume the roles of operators and end users of machines and are

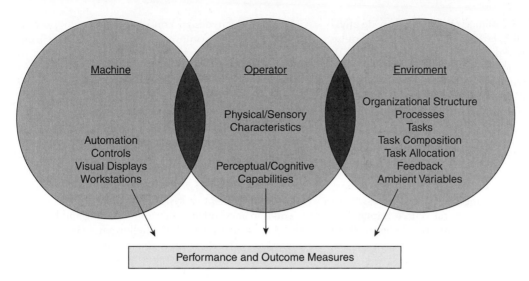

Machine

Automation
Controls
Visual Displays
Workstations

Operator

Physical/Sensory
Characteristics

Perceptual/Cognitive
Capabilities

Enviroment

Organizational Structure
Processes
Tasks
Task Composition
Task Allocation
Feedback
Ambient Variables

Performance and Outcome Measures

• **FIGURE 8.2.** Human factors subsystems.

situated at the core of the human factors subsystems. Human operators have distinct, individual, and identifiable personal attributes that characterize who they are, how they will interact with the system, and how they may perform. One goal of human factors is to optimize the total system by adopting indirect ways of accommodating people and their distinct traits within the system. This goal can be met by designing technology that fits 2 dimensions of human capabilities that are basic to human factors: physical and sensory characteristics and perceptual and cognitive abilities.

Physical and Sensory Characteristics. Human performance in work and other venues is a consequence of information processing, including some or all of the following human functions: attention, sensation, perception, coding and decoding, learning, memory, recall, reasoning, making judgments, making decisions, transmitting information, and executing physical responses. Depending on the functions that have to be performed, options exist in human-machine environments to allocate certain functions to humans or to physical (machine) components. Decisions to allocate certain functions to humans or machines are based on some preconceived notions of human-machine abilities and can affect performance within the system. For example, novice and expert nurses have different levels of experience; the use of clinical decision support, one component of a machine system, has been shown to be more important to less experienced nurses and less important

to expert nurses, especially in problem list identification. An advantage of this type of system is that all potentially relevant patient problems could be considered all at once for less experienced nurses or prioritized in subsets for nurses with greater clinical mastery. This part of the machine system can be used as a reminder to nurses who are sifting through volumes of data, and convenient for finding targeted data (Cho, Staggers, & Park, 2010).

The most basic physical and sensory capacities for humans include vision, hearing, smell, taste, manual dexterity, strength, and reach. *Ergonomics*, a term used interchangeably with human factors, attempts to define working conditions that enhance individual safety, comfort, and productivity by combining knowledge of human physical and sensory capacities with engineering principles (Hannah, Ball, & Edwards, 2006). With the advancement of smaller and smaller technologies, human factors engineers and clinicians must consider the obtrusiveness of ergonomic designs in the end user's environment during the technological development and implementation phases.

Examples of obtrusive designs are invasive types of technologies that adhere to the body, are worn by a person, can be carried by a person, or may be ingested, such as through inhalation of nanoparticles used in drug delivery systems (Staggers, McCasky, Brazelton, & Kennedy, 2008). In contrast, unobtrusive technologies, such as sensors, smart carpets, or cameras embedded in end users' environments, can provide remote monitoring of human activity levels within a residence or provide physiologic monitoring for restlessness, breathing, and pulse (Skubic, Alexander, Popescu, Rantz, & Keller, 2009). Each of these technologies provides a unique design and interface used to enhance patient care. These technologies will affect how data may be captured and used for patient assessments, will change how patients are monitored, change the nature of nursing work, and influence nurse, provider, and patient interactions. Within the Nurse-Patient Trajectory Framework (Figure 8.1) these changes are manifested within nurse and patient trajectories, which refer to the assembling, scheduling, monitoring, and coordinating of all steps necessary to complete patient care. It is imperative that human factors principles be incorporated into the design of these novel medical devices before they are widely used. This will require substantial collaborations between clinicians, patients, and engineers as these devices are developed from infancy.

Research in healthcare that has incorporated ergonomic considerations for an operator's human characteristics and physical senses into the design of technology is abundant in the literature. For example, as alarms have increased with the use of technology, to substitute for an operator's attention, ergonomic variables that have been considered include alarm outputs, design of alarm displays and control settings, alarm test procedures, and preparation of labeling and instructional materials. Researchers studying anesthetic errors and mishaps have found that complex jobs such as anesthesiology require maximum vigilance, a state of maximal physiologic and psychological readiness to react (Weinger & Englund, 1990). Applying human factors to complex jobs such as anesthesiology increases human reliability, reduces the probability of error, and improves performance. However, tasks associated with nurse anesthetists are distinct from anesthesiologists, and human factors evaluations within this community of nurses as well as other nursing disciplines are limited to date (Gorges & Staggers, 2008).

Experts in human factors also consider physiologic dimensions to be an important component of design. For instance, the dimensional ranges of female hands including length, breadth, and circumference can be used to improve medical device design. This is an important design consideration in nursing since many more females choose to become nurses than males. Improved designs will affect a female nurse's ability to apply force while moving heavy equipment (Hasler, 1996). For example, consider a situation where a busy staff nurse has to assist in the transport of an obese patient, lying on a heavy, specially designed air bed, to an emergent

procedure. Such design considerations could prevent physical harm and improve outcomes resulting from fewer lost work days due to injury, decreased time to patient intervention, and improved job satisfaction.

Perceptual and Cognitive Abilities. Perception provides humans with the capability to detect, identify, and recognize sensory input, while cognition refers to higher-level mental phenomena such as memory, information processing, use of rules or strategies, formulating hypotheses, problem solving, learning, and judgment (Wickens, Lee, Liu, & Gordon-Becker, 2004). The human perceptual system is responsible for general orientation and body equilibrium, listening and locating vibrations, touching, tasting, smelling, and visualization. Cognitive research is used to describe psychological processes associated with the acquisition, organization, and use of knowledge (Hollnagel, 2003).

Perceptual and cognitive processes in human-machine interactions are complex and involve continuous exchanges of information between operators and the machines they use, which is a type of shared cognition. For example, nurses and physicians work in tandem to deliver optimal care for each patient. The design of human-machine interfaces, such as nursing and physician interfaces, used for documentation and medical record review must consider the nature of interdisciplinary work. Unfortunately, studies typical of evaluating nursing workflow disruption have not been a focus in similar studies assessing physician workflow; for instance, investigating how nursing roles and activities are affected by physician orders when implementing a clinical information system would provide valuable design input for electronic medical record designs (Lee & McElmurry, 2010). Medical devices are also an important human-machine interface that are sometimes shared and need to be tested collaboratively by interdisciplinary healthcare teams, but these evaluations are limited. Evaluations including both nurses and pharmacists should provide important design considerations for computerized provider order entry for pharmacy and medication administration systems to ensure safe execution of orders and delivery of medications (Alexander & Staggers, 2009).

Perceptual and cognitive processes in human-machine systems involve the operator providing input to the machine, the machine acting on the input and displaying information back to the operator; the operator processing information through sensing mechanisms such as visual, auditory, somatosensory, and vestibular systems; and finally, the operator determining if the information from the machine is accurate, providing correct communication, deciding what actions to take, and providing new input to the machine (Proctor & Proctor, 2006). Attempts to understand and exploit human capabilities and strengths within the area of human perception and cognitive ability are critical to the safe design of technology. Safe design includes responses to human stress and is an important variable in human factors research. For example, the ability of a nurse to make timely and accurate decisions and to be vigilant of machine alarms during periods of sleep deprivation while working several 12-hour night shifts in a row is a common work scenario that is worthy of attention in human factors research. Furthermore, human factors experts in nursing have begun using mapping techniques, called *link analysis*, to map the cognitive processes of nursing work and to understand what stresses nurses encounter during work that contribute to cognitive delay. For example, nonlinearity of nursing work, which requires frequent shifts in the process of delivering care, results in interruptions and delays in care that contribute to unsafe environments (Potter et al., 2004). Understanding the perceptual and cognitive abilities of operators in the healthcare sector provides better understanding of the physical and operational structures that affect clinical decision making and clinical reasoning that may lead to potential system failures.

The Machine Subsystem

The machine subsystem, illustrated in Figure 8.2, is broadly conceptualized and may be represented by any artifact controlled by a human such as a knife, a pocket calculator, a toilet seat, or a computer. Features that make a machine unique, more user-friendly, and safer, such as an appropriately designed curvature of a toilet seat or bedpan to avoid cutting off circulation and numbness in lower extremities, can be aesthetically pleasing as well as functionally attractive. In machine systems, such as computers, design features including automation, controls, visual displays, and workstations have effects on the human operator's ability to perform work when interacting with the machine. These design features are discussed next.

Automation. Increasing attention to error in medicine and concern for patient safety have prompted general recommendations for the development of automated technologies to support clinical decision making to ensure that errors are caught, to promote data standards, and to develop systems that communicate with each other. *Automation* is defined as the execution by a machine of functions previously carried out by humans ranging from full manual control to full automation. Under conditions of full manual control particular functions are controlled by the human, whereas with full automation machines control all aspects of functioning, including monitoring (Parasuraman & Riley, 1997). Introducing automation can change the nature of cognitive demands and the responsibilities of system users, often in ways that were unintended or unanticipated by designers. Underscoring the importance of human factors design in systems evaluation, unintended consequences of technology have been highlighted as important sources of error in healthcare (Ash, Berg, & Coiera, 2004). For example, unintended consequences of the implementation of computerized clinical decision support systems resulted in problems related to content and presentation of information (Ash, Sittig, Campbell, Guappone, & Dykstra, 2007). Content problems were related to eliminating or shifting human roles; for instance, removing nurses from the medication-ordering loop required physicians to have knowledge of the quantities of IV solutions used and to manually calculate drip rates. Presentation alerts were related to alert fatigue when clinicians received too many alerts for drug-drug interactions. Similar implementation problems occurred when electronic health records implemented in nursing homes contained messaging systems which were not standardized, creating confusion and omission of necessary patient care tasks (Alexander, Rantz, Flesner, Diekemper, & Siem, 2007).

As technology evolves, research continues to be produced to better understand and improve how humans interact with automated systems. In safety-critical systems, human factors methods have been used to understand how automated systems improved hazard awareness, alerting mechanisms, identified conflicts, and reduced unnecessary communication in congested situations. Similarly, human factors methods are being used in healthcare. For example, clinical reminders and automated decision support systems used to take advantage of existing electronic patient information to alert providers of recommended actions have been used to improve compliance with established treatment guidelines and improve diagnoses (Patterson, Nguyen, Halloran, & Asch, 2004). Furthermore, research regarding the design of automated medical equipment has led to safer systems and improved patient outcomes (Vicente, Kada-Bekhaled, Hillel, Cassano, & Orser, 2003). However, there are many automated machine components that nurses and other professionals use in their daily work lives, which have had no human factors evaluations. The absence of an emphasis on using human factors to evaluate interactions between healthcare professionals and the automated machines they use before the machines are implemented could lead to unintended consequences that are harmful to patients, result in poorer outcomes of care, and reduce effectiveness of healthcare providers' care delivery.

Controls. Controls, used to facilitate human-machine interaction, are interface elements that allow humans to transfer mechanical energy into a technical system in order to perform automated control functions (Bullinger, Kern, & Braun, 1997). The dimensions of a control design include shape, size, material, surface, and control task. These dimensions must be compatible with anatomic, anthropometric, and physiologic conditions of the human or performance levels may suffer. Performance factors that are particularly influenced by task control design include resistance, accuracy, and speed and can be influenced by human stature, structure, and physical function. Controls that are not well designed may increase stress during human-machine interaction resulting in unsatisfying, frustrating, and threatening interactions that affect human performance.

In healthcare, the American National Standards Institute (ANSI) and Association for the Advancement of Medical Instrumentation (AAMI) recently issued a set of guidelines and preferred practices for the design of medical device controls (ANSI/ AAMI, 2009). In the guidelines, ANSI/AAMI has described design elements or features for medical devices to be considered human factored. Interface controls of patient-controlled analgesia (PCA) pumps have been studied to verify the redesign of PCA interfaces using human factors engineering processes. Use of human factors approaches improved patient safety by decreasing drug concentration errors and reducing task completion times for experienced users of the device; however, many devices, some which have not been studied extensively (e.g., intensive care unit ventilators, electronic health records) continue to place a significant cognitive burden on the end user, resulting in greater error during usage, and are not well integrated into existing systems (Alexander & Staggers, 2009).

Visual Displays. One of the current barriers to creating an effective healthcare information infrastructure is a lack of standard design for clinical information systems that influence user effectiveness, efficiency, and satisfaction. One of the problems associated with designing technology is that physical aspects of the human-computer domain can be touched and inspected, while the abstract functional aspects, including the concepts and relationships of underlying data elements defining the practitioners domain, must be understood by the end users. Human factors experts use cognitive ergonomics to overcome these barriers by explaining how humans think and use knowledge and by applying this to machine learning environments. A goal of cognitive ergonomics experts is to provide important clues for designing information systems that match how people think and perform. Cognitive ergonomists will design tasks within visual displays that enhance reliable, safe, and effective user performance (Wilson, Jackson, & Nichols, 2003). One method for designing effective and safe retrieval systems is to take advantage of established semantic and symbolic approaches to visual display and menu design by considering human expectancies and mental models (Staggers & Norcio, 1993).

Humans are habitual. Designers take advantage of these stereotypical behaviors in the general population, as well as established protocols and standards in the medical community to develop visual displays that are consistent with these behaviors. Building conceptual models and designs that match human expectancies allows users to predict the effects of their interactions with technology; without a good conceptual model, users operate blindly, are unable to function independently, and have little knowledge of what to expect from the system (Norman, 2002). Conceptual models that clash with human expectancies can lead to errors and system failures.

Conceptual models are part of an important concept in design called mental models. Difficulties in representing accurate mental models in computer systems arise from inequalities between what users think images mean and what they accomplish. When inequalities occur significant barriers to utilization result; for example, data entry may fail as a result of poorly designed content, fields that do not represent what the user expects, and poor usability design (Cimino, Patel, & Kushniruk, 2001). One illustration of this occurred during the evaluation of a novel sensor system interface used to monitor elderly people's activity levels in an assisted living facility (Alexander et al., 2008). One of the sensors used to monitor cooking activity also sensed the temperature of the stove in the resident's apartment. The visual display on the interface for the stove temperature was labeled "Temperature"; subsequently, during heuristic and usability studies on the interface, designers realized that nurses mistakenly thought this output represented a vital sign rather than a stove-top temperature. Other noted research in display design includes the effects of off-ward trend graphs on clinical decision making in a neonatal intensive care unit, use of different interface designs and their impact on the ability of novice nurses to learn to use computer simulation and performance in critical care environments, and finally, comparisons of response time, errors, and satisfaction between text-based versus graphical user interfaces in the process of completing nursing care (Alberdi et al., 2003; Staggers & Kobus, 2000; Effken & Doyle, 2001).

Workstations. Traditional workplace designs, depending on an employee's job responsibility, might consider such issues as posture, visual acuity, office structure including height of office furniture, or exposure to environmental factors like lighting, radiant temperature, and noise. The physical design of the workspace should include ergonomic dimensions associated with user height, weight, and strength. Furthermore, in analyzing the workspace, designers should consider what users should see, what they need to hear, what users manipulate or reach while performing work, space requirements, potential for disturbance or inactivation of controls, if the work environment is adequate for emergency situations, and what other systems or devices are in use (Alvarado, 2007).

With the "new frontiers" in remote healthcare delivery methods, such as telenursing, miniature, and wireless computing, the nature of the workstation is changing in healthcare environments. Healthcare providers who are implementing and using these tools should consider the benefits and challenges of remote computerization in healthcare. The benefits of remote computerization include greater efficiency of work processes, error reduction since data can be entered at the point of care, and inclusion of tailored outputs such as still and moving imagery to support decision making. The challenges of remote computerization include geographical considerations such as where dead zones occur, battery life, memory limitations, and its impact on the patient-clinician relationship (Fischer, Stewart, Mehta, Wax, & Lapinsky, 2003; Hebda & Czar, 2009). Additionally, as technology becomes more integrated into our daily lives individual person factors become an important variable to predict the implementation success of information technology. These differences in utilization of information resources may lead to different clinical decisions or judgments regarding treatments, potential outcomes, diagnoses, or utilization of healthcare resources. Age, for example, is an important variable. One study demonstrated that older Internet users tend more often to both know how to and use internet search mechanisms for information related to illnesses and medical conditions, doctors, nursing homes, home health agencies,

or other healthcare providers than older, non-Internet users. However, significantly larger numbers of these non-Internet users actually used information they found to treat an illness or condition or to change an exercise or nutritional plan when compared with the Internet users (Taha et al., 2009).

The Environmental Subsystem

The final subsystem component in the human factors model, shown in Figure 8.1, concerns the environment. Critical environmental issues that are important in human factors research include organizational structures and processes that address communication, responsibilities, training and relationships among co-workers; tasks, task composition, allocation of tasks, and feedback mechanisms in the system; and ambient variables in the environment (see Figure 8.1). Each of these attributes is discussed.

Organizational Structures and Processes. Our society is just beginning to understand the impact that the substantial growth of technology, such as social networking interactions on the internet (e.g.,. Web 2.0, Twitter, and Facebook), wikis, folksonomies, blogs, and hosts of other tools used to manage the collective intelligence of large groups of people (Thede & Sewell, 2010). Organizational survival will depend on the ability of leaders to communicate to stakeholders within the system how technology will fit within and affect organizational culture. Task and role changes, resulting from the adoption of new technologies, will result in task uncertainty and require greater coordination, feedback, and training within the organization to prevent system failures.

Tasks. Tasks involve interplay between physical and cognitive activities and may be considered to follow a continuum between nearly pure physical tasks, such as transporting a patient to an X-ray, to nearly pure cognitive tasks, such as assessing hemodynamic status. The terms *task* and *function* are often used interchangeably. Tasks tend to describe discrete, detailed behaviors needed to carry out functions, whereas functions tend to describe continuous, macrolevel behaviors, such as analyzing or detecting (Sharit, 1997). Task composition, allocation of tasks, and feedback mechanisms are important elements in designing task sequences and are discussed in the following section.

Task Composition. A task or action sequence starts with a goal. Then, steps are initiated based upon the user's intentions. This is followed by the sequence of actions to be performed or that are intended to be performed, and the steps in the execution of the task. After tasks are executed they are assessed based on user perception, interpretation, and evaluation of the interpretations of the actions. Task structures may be shallow, narrow, wide, and deep. Most everyday tasks, which occupy most of a human's time, are considered shallow, narrow structures that are opportunistic in nature, requiring little complexity in analysis and minimal conscious activity. In shallow and narrow structures, humans need only examine alternative actions and act; alternatively, wide and deep structures require a considerable amount of conscious planning and thought, and usually require deliberate trial and error functions (Norman, 2002).

Formal task load models have been used to determine appropriate levels and forms of human-machine interactions. Cognitive task analysis (CTA) used to evaluate task load has been used in healthcare settings. Examples of CTA in healthcare research include the following: identification of potential errors performed with computer-based infusion devices used for terbutaline administration in preterm labor; evaluation of cognitive and physical burdens during periods of high workload and stress while using computer-based physiologic monitoring systems in cardiac anesthesia; and gaining new perspectives in the work of nursing processes to understand how disruptions can contribute to nursing error in acute care environments (Obradovich & Woods, 1996; Potter, et al., 2004; Cook & Woods, 1996).

Task Allocation. Function allocation is used to assign the performance of each function or task to the elements, including humans, hardware, and software, that is best suited to perform it. Function allocation models using systems design methodologies have been proposed. These models use decision matrices to determine performance demands between human and automated functions in computers. Function allocation models can be used to ensure that design considerations: (1) promote the development and updating of adequate mental models, (2) ensure that appropriate levels of human involvement in tasks are maintained, (3) human capabilities are maximized, and (4) the negative consequences of human limitations are reduced (Sharit, 1997).

Feedback. Conditions that have been found to hinder feedback in healthcare environments include incomplete awareness that system failures have occurred, time and work pressures, delays in action or outcome sequences, case infrequence, deficient follow-up, failed communication, deficient reporting systems, case review biases, shift work, and handoffs (Croskerry, 2000). Feedback is an important element that may be derived from display information in human-computer interactions and is fed back to the environmental subsystem where it becomes important in the perception, implementation, and evaluation of tasks. Not all system feedback mechanisms are technical in nature; sometimes feedback mechanisms are created through human quality audits, peer reviews, and data mining. Emotional risks associated with the failure to provide feedback include loss of confidence, uncertainty about performance, and increased stress.

Feedback mechanisms have been recognized as important components in nurse-computer interactions. Improvements have been recognized in the visibility and standardization of coordination of care mechanisms in wireless computerized information systems in nursing home information systems. In these settings, improved feedback mechanisms positively affected staff documentation and communication patterns in automated wireless nursing home environments where personal digital assistants (PDAs) were used by nurse assistants to document activities of daily living as they occurred; simultaneously, nurses were able to see what care had been completed and outcomes related to the care. This seamless transition resulted in better quality and efficiency of patient care (Rantz et al., 2010). In other reports, evaluations of response times to critical laboratory results using automated feedback mechanisms resulted in decreased response times following an appropriate treatment order (Kuperman et al., 1999). Information technologies that facilitate transmission of important patient data can improve the quality of care.

Ambient Variables. Adaptation is a set of changes in an individual response that make it possible to deal with adverse conditions that may result in reduced stress levels and improved performance. Numerous ambient variables in the environment may create adverse conditions by creating acute, prolonged, or chronic stressors for human operators. External acute stressors, or those that affect learning, performance, and decision making, may include heat, cold, darkness, noise, vibration, or sleep loss and can result in eye strain, hearing loss, heatstroke, and frost bite. External and prolonged stressors include repeated motion and excessive climates, which can result in chronic degenerative conditions such as carpal tunnel syndrome or dehydration. Internal and prolonged acute stressors may be recognized as fear or anxiety and may include phobias; these conditions may result in inhibition, avoidance, withdrawal, depression, ulcers, and other somatic symptoms.

Performance and Outcome Measures in Human Factors

One goal of human factors is to design safe and healthy work systems, especially during human-machine interactions occurring between individual operators, while considering variable factors associated with the work system. The result is improved overall user performance and function. Performance measures include system output, input, and reliability measures. These measures are affected by performance capabilities and limitations, performance affordances, and performance requirements.

Performance Capabilities and Limitations. In safety-critical systems, such as healthcare, humans and machines may jointly be responsible for executing tasks, performing certain operations, and monitoring system safety. The probability that human error will occur during human-machine interactions is influenced by performance-shaping factors like the amount of training that an employee receives to understand human-machine interfaces, the amount and frequency of tasks to perform certain functions of a job, or environmental noise that interacts with the frequency of patient care alarms. Human performance measures are affected by the capability of a human to know what is going on around them, which is called situational awareness (SA) (Endsley, 2000).

Three fundamental levels of SA that are important in performance include the following: level 1, perception of important information or cues in order to form a correct perception of the situation; level 2, comprehension as measured by the ability to combine, interpret, store, and retain information and to determine the relevance of the information to goals; and level 3, projection, the highest level of SA or understanding, is the ability to project the future state of events and dynamics within the system. Important for understanding SA are temporal variables for operators, such as the ability to estimate how much time is available until an event occurs, when action needs to be taken, and the rate at which information changes. Determining situations where decision making is compromised, such as in congested surroundings and where outcomes may be affected, is critical in dynamic environments where situations are always changing. For example, in an ICU or emergency setting where large amounts of data are regularly processed during times when nursing workload is frequently high and the environment is often loud, unintended consequences could result, such as inadequate patient supervision, greater nurse fatigue, and higher burnout.

Performance-based measurement in SA is any measurement that infers an operator's awareness of the situation from observable actions or the effects of the actions on the system (Pritchett & Hansman, 2000). This type of system is often used in biosurveillance and public health informatics.

Performance Affordances. Performance affordances are the perceived and actual properties of an object that determine how it is to be used; affordances provide strong clues about the operations of things. At any point in the existence of an object it is said to exist in a certain state; states change, therefore objects exhibit an affordance for transformation that may lead to other changes in a system state (Dowell & Long, 1989). A good example of this phenomenon occurs when a data field that has a critical laboratory value in a patient care information system has a brighter highlighted text, or even the entire field is highlighted, to increase user awareness of the critical value to prompt action. Examples in other clinical information systems specifically used in nursing homes include the use of certified nursing aides and RN tasks lists, which turn pink when certain daily tasks have not been completed. These colored displays provide visual prompts and reminders for all staff so that important patient care tasks are not overlooked.

Affordances consider the relationship between properties of the environment and the operator's capability to act. Implications for system affordances are that operators with different capabilities may perceive the environment differently resulting in different action selections, and thus, possibly resulting in different outcomes. For instance, informatics nurses and other providers have been exploring response times, accuracy of clinical decision making, error rates, drug usage, and target ranges for specified treatments by using integrated graphical user interfaces to demonstrate their effectiveness, efficiency, and satisfaction in healthcare settings (Alexander & Staggers, 2009). Furthermore, these types of human-machine evaluations provide insights into how denser data displays may enhance patient care, save user time, and increase satisfaction.

Some of these enhanced interfaces promote a different type of interaction by enabling nurses to visualize multiple data outputs differently and assess hemodynamic responses to nurse interventions. It is important that these types of evaluations involve usability testing of actual medical devices in real settings by end users, rather than in mock laboratory settings where environmental influences might be different. If medical equipment is not properly tested in real environments unexpected things will happen.

Outcome Measures in Human Factors Research

Data is important for determining whether outcomes in human factors goals have been achieved. Potential contributors to outcomes have been discussed and include the individual tasks to be performed, tools and technology to accomplish the tasks, and the environments where tasks are performed. A study of the relationships between outcome measures and nursing work helps human factors researchers in the design process by identifying elements that need attention.

Nursing services are beginning to utilize human factors methods to capture relevant data about nursing services in the field. Papers about the creation of nursing human factors laboratories and investigations are beginning to appear, which describe methods for evaluating impressions of human-machine components and tasks associated with heparin and insulin infusion devices, for evaluating labeling of injectable drugs, to address display design related to clinical documentation, and organizational issues that contribute to patient risk by nurses (Despins, Scott-Cawiezell, Rouder, 2010; Momtahan, Burns, Jeon, Hyland, & Gabriele, 2008; Etchells et al., 2006; Boston-Fleischhauer, 2008a; Boston-Fleischhauer, 2008b). In other healthcare studies, human factors barriers in the use of clinical reminders in an information system were identified, including workload during patient visits, documenting clinical relevancy of reminders, inapplicability of the clinical reminders, limited training, perceived reduction of quality of provider-patient interactions, and the decision to use paper forms prior to order entry (Patterson, Nguyen, Halloran, & Asch, 2004). In these cases, reducing the human factors barriers could have increased the use of clinical reminders and improved the quality of care.

CONCLUSION

Human factors evaluations are increasingly important as the growth of technology continues to expand into healthcare settings. Informatics nurses are playing a significant role in understanding the complex interactions between human-machine systems as they are implemented. Specific systems components identified as being important in human factors research include the operator of the system, the machine, the interactions the operator has with the machine, environmental variables that impact the human-machine interaction, and feedback mechanisms affecting the work of individuals in the system, performance, and outcome measures. Understanding human factors enables nurses to understand how work is performed, to develop human-machine systems that support the work of the organization, and facilitate organizational and individual goal achievement. Greater knowledge of these human-machine interactions enables nurses to intercede before unintended consequences happen.

REFERENCES

Alberdi, E., Gilhooly, K., Hunter, J., Logie, R., Lyon, A., McIntosh, N. et al. (2003). Computerisation and decision making in neonatal intensive care: A cognitive engineering investigation. *Journal of Clinical Monitoring, 16,* 85–94.

Alexander G.L. (2007). The nurse-patient trajectory framework. In K. A. Kuhn, J. R. Warren, & T-Y. Leon (Eds.), Medinfo 2007 (pp. 910–914).

Alexander, G. L., Rantz, M. J., Flesner, M. K., Diekemper, M., & Siem, C. (2007). Clinical information systems in nursing homes: An evaluation of initial implementation strategies. *Computers, Informatics, Nursing, 25,* 189–197.

Alexander, G. L., Rantz, M. J., Skubic, M., Aud, M. A., Wakefield, B., Florea, E. et al. (2008). Sensor systems for monitoring functional status in assisted living residents. *Research in Gerontological Nursing, 1,* 238–244.

Alexander, G. L., & Staggers, N. (2009). A systematic review on the designs of clinical technology: Findings and recommendations for future research. *Advances in Nursing Science, 32,* 252–279.

Alexander, G. L. & Stone, T. T. (2000). System review: A method for investigating medical errors in healthcare settings. *Case Management, 5,* 202–213.

Alvarado, C. J. (2007). The physical environment in healthcare. In P. Carayon (Ed.), *Handbook of human factors and ergonomics in healthcare and patient safety* (pp. 287–307). Mahwah, NJ: Lawrence Erlbaum Assoc.

American National Standards Institute (ANSI)/ Association for the Advancement of Medical Instrumentation (AAMI). (2009). *Human factors engineering: Design of medical devices* (Rep. No. HE 75). Arlington, VA: ANSI/AAMI.

Ash, J. S., Berg, M., & Coiera, E. (2004). Some unintended consequences of information technology in healthcare: The nature of patient care information system-related errors. *Journal of the Americal Medical Informatics Association, 11,* 104–112.

Ash, J. S., Sittig, D. F., Campbell, E. M., Guappone, K. P., & Dykstra, R. H. (2007). Some unintended consequences of clinical decision support systems. In J. M. Teich, J. Suermondt, & G. Hripcsak (Eds.), Bethesda, MD: American Medical Informatics Association.

Berwick, D. M. (1991). Controlling variation in healthcare. *Medical Care, 29,* 1212–1225.

Boston-Fleischhauer, C. (2008a). Enhancing healthcare process design with human factors engineering and reliability science part 1. *Journal of Nursing Administration, 38,* 27–32.

Boston-Fleischhauer, C. (2008b). Enhancing healthcare process design with human factors engineering and reliability science, part 2: Applying the knowledge to clinical documentation systems. *Journal of Nursing Administration, 38,* 84–89.

Bullinger, H., Kern, P., & Braun, M. (1997). Controls. In Salvendy G (Ed.), *Handbook of Ergonomics and Human Factors* (2nd ed., pp. 697–727). New York: John Wiley & Sons, Inc.

Carayon, P., Alvarado, C. J., & Hundt, A. S. (2007). Work system design in healthcare. In P. Carayon (Ed.), *Handbook of Human Factors and Ergonomics in Healthcare and Patient Safety* (pp. 61–78). Mahwah, NJ: Lawrence Erlbaum Assoc.

Cho, I., Staggers, N., & Park, I. (2010). Nurses' responses to differing amounts and information content in a diagnostic computer-based decision support application. *Computers, Informatics, Nursing, 28,* 95–102.

Cimino, J. J., Patel, V. L., & Kushniruk, A. W. (2001). Studying the human-computer-terminology interface. *Journal of the American Medical Informatics Association, 8,* 163–173.

Cook, R. I., & Woods, D. D. (1996). Adapting to new technology in the operating room. *Human Factors, 38,* 593–613.

Croskerry, P. (2000). The feedback sanction. *Academic Emergency Medicine., 7,* 1232–1238.

Despins, L. A., Scott-Cawiezell, J., & Rouder, J. N. (2010). Detection of patient risk by nurses: a theoretical framework. *Journal of Advanced Nursing, 66,* 465–474.

Dowell, J., & Long, J. (1989). Towards a conception for an engineering discipline of human factors. *Ergonomics, 32,* 1513–1535.

Effken, E. (2003). An organizing framework for nursing informatics research. *Computers Informatics Nursing, 21,* 316–325.

Effken, J. A., & Doyle, M. (2001). Interface design and cognitive style in learning an instructional computer simulation. *Computers in Nursing, 19,* 164–171.

Endsley, M. R. (2000). Theoretical underpinnings of situation awareness: A critical review. In M.R. Endsley & D. J. Garland (Eds.), *Situation Awareness Analysis and Measurement* (pp. 3–32). Mahwah, New Jersey: Lawrence Erlbaum Associates.

Etchells, E., Bailey, C., Biason, R., DeSousa, S., Fowler, L., Johnson, K. et al. (2006). Human factors in action: Getting "pumped" at a nursing usability laboratory. *Healthcare Quarterly, 9,* 69–74.

Fischer, S., Stewart, T. E., Mehta, S., Wax, R., & Lapinsky, S. E. (2003). Handheld computing in medicine. *Journal of the American Medical Association, 10,* 139–149.

Gorges, M., & Staggers, N. (2008). Evaluations of physiological monitoring displays: A systematic review. *Journal of Clinical Monitoring and Computing, 22,* 45–66.

Graves, J. R., & Corcoran, S. (1989). The study of nursing informatics. *Image Journal of Nursing Scholarship, 21,* 227–231.

Hannah, K. J., Ball, M. J., & Edwards, M. J. A. (2006). Ergonomics. In *Introduction to Nursing Informatics* (3rd ed., pp. 234–242). New York: Springer.

Hasler, R. A. (1996). Human factors design: What is it and how can it affect you? *Journal of Intravenous Nursing, 19,* S5–S8.

Hebda, T., & Czar, P. (2009). Hardware, software, and the roles of support personnel. In *Handbook of informatics for nurses & healthcare professionals* (4th ed.), (pp. 49–77). Upper Saddle River, NJ: Pearson/Prentice Hall.

Helander, M. G. (1997). The human factors profession. In Salvendy G (Ed.), *Handbook of human factors and ergonomics* (pp. 3–16). New York: John Wiley & Sons, Inc.

Hollnagel, E. (2003). Prolegomenon to cognitive task design. In E.Hollnagel (Ed.), *Handbook of cognitive task design* (pp. 3–15). Mahwah, New Jersey: Lawrence Erlbaum Associates.

Johnson, J. K., & Barach, P. (2007). Clinical microsystems in healthcare: The role of human factors in shaping the microsystem. In P.Carayon (Ed.), *Handbook of human factors and ergonomics in healthcare and patient safety* (pp. 95–107). Mahwah, NJ: Lawrence Erlbaum Assoc.

Kuperman, G. J., Teich, J. M., Tanasijevic, M. J., Ma'Luf, N., Rittenberg, E., Jha, A. et al. (1999). Improving response to critical laboratory results with automation. *Journal of the American Medical Informatics Association, 6,* 512–522.

Lee, S., & McElmurry, B. (2010). Capturing nursing care workflow disruptions: Comparison between nursing and physician workflows. *Computers, Informatics, Nursing, 28,* 151–159.

Momtahan, K., Burns, C. M., Jeon, J., Hyland, S., & Gabriele, S. (2008). Using human factors methods to evaluate the labeling of injectable drugs. *Healthcare Quarterly, 11,* 122–128.

Nemeth, C. P. (2004). *Human factors methods for design: Making systems human centered.* Boca Raton: CRC Press.

Norman, D. A. (2002). *The design of everyday things.* New York: Double Day.

Obradovich, J. H., & Woods, D. D. (1996). Users as designers: How people cope with poor HCI design in computer-based medical devices. *Human Factors, 38,* 574–592.

Parasuraman, R., & Riley, V. (1997). Humans and automation: Use, misuse, disuse, abuse. *Human Factors, 39,* 230 253.

Patterson, E. S., Nguyen, A. D., Halloran, J. P., & Asch, S. M. (2004). Human factors barriers to the effective use of ten HIV clinical reminders. *Journal of the American Medical Informatics Association., 11,* 50–59.

Potter, P., Boxerman, S., Wolf, L., Marshall, J., Grayson, D., Sledge, J. et al. (2004). Mapping the nursing process: A new approach for understanding the work of nursing. *Journal of Nursing Administration, 34*, 101–109.

Pritchett, A. R., & Hansman, R. J. (2000). Use of testable responses for performance based measurement of situation awareness. In M. R. Endsley & D. J. Garland (Eds.), *Situation awareness analysis and measurement* (pp. 189–209). Mahwah, New Jersey: Lawrence Erlbaum Associates.

Proctor, R. W., & Proctor, J. D. (2006). Sensation and perception. In Gavriel Salvendy (Ed.), *Handbook of human factors and ergonomics* (3rd ed., pp. 53–88). Hoboken NJ: John Wiley and Sons, Inc..

Rantz, M. J., Hicks, L., Petroski, G. F., Madsen, R. W., Alexander, G. L., Galambos, C. et al. (2010). Cost, staffing, and quality impact of bedside electronic medical record (EMR) in nursing homes. *Journal of the American Medical Directors Association,* 11(7), 485–493.

Reason, J. (1990). *Human Error.* New York: Cambridge University Press.

Reason, J. (1995). Understanding adverse events: Human factors. *Quality in Healthcare, 4*, 80–89.

Schwirian, P. M. (1986). The NI pyramid: A model for research in nursing informatics. *Computers in Nursing, 4*, 134–136.

Sharit, J. (1997). Allocation of functions. In G. Salvendy (Ed.), *Handbook of Human Factors and Ergonomics* (2nd ed., pp. 302–337). New York: John Wiley & Sons, Inc.

Simmons, D., & Graves, K. (2008). Tubing misconnections—A systems failure with human factors: Lessons for nursing practice. *Urologic Nursing, 28*, 460–464.

Skubic, M., Alexander, G. L., Popescu, M., Rantz, M. J., & Keller, J. (2009). A smart home application to eldercare: Current status and lessons learned. *Technology and Healthcare, 17*, 183–201.

Staggers, N. (1991). Human factors: The missing element in computer technology. *Computers in Nursing, 9*, 47–49.

Staggers, N. (2002). Human-computer interaction. In S. Englebardt & R. Nelson (Eds.), *Information technology in healthcare: An interdisciplinary approach* (pp. 321–345). Philadelphia: Harcourt Health Science Company.

Staggers, N. (2003). Human factors: Imperative concepts for information systems in critical care. *AACN Clinical Issues, 14*, 310–319.

Staggers, N., & Kobus, D. (2000). Comparing response time, errors, and satisfaction between text-based and graphical user interfaces during nursing order tasks. *Journal of the American Medical Informatics Association, 7*, 164–176.

Staggers, N., McCasky, T., Brazelton, N., & Kennedy, R. (2008). Nanotechnology: Implications for patients, providers and informatics. *Nursing Outlook, 56*, 268–274.

Staggers, N., & Norcio, A. (1993). Mental models: Concepts for human-computer interaction research. *International Journal of Man-Machine Studies, 38*, 587–605.

Staggers, N., & Parks, P. L. (1993). Description and initial applications of the Staggers & Parks nurse-computer interaction framework. *Computers in Nursing, 11*, 282–290.

Taha, J., Sharit, J., & Czaja, S. J. (2009). Use of and satisfaction with sources of health information among older internet users and nonusers. *The Gerontologist, 49*, 663–673.

Thede, L. Q. & Sewell, J. P. (2010). Professional networking. In *Informatics and nursing: competencies and applications* (3rd ed., pp. 101–119). Philadelphia: Wolters Kluwer/Lippincott Williams & Wilkins.

Turley, J. (1996). Toward a model for nursing informatics. *Image Journal of Nursing Scholarship, 28*, 309–313.

Vicente, K. J., Kada-Bekhaled, K., Hillel, G., Cassano, A., & Orser, B. A. (2003). Programming errors contribute to death from patient-controlled analgesia: case report and estimate of probability. *Canadian Journal of Anaesthesia, 50*, 328–332.

Weinger, M., Pantiskas, C., Wiklund, M. E., & Carstensen, P. (1998). Incorporating human factors into the design of medical devices. *Journal of the American Medical Association., 280*, 1484.

Weinger, M. B., & Englund, C. E. (1990). Ergonomic and human factors affecting anesthetic vigilance and monitoring performance in the operating room environment. *Anesthesiology, 73*, 995–1021.

Werley, H. H., & Grier, M. R. (1981). *Nursing Information Systems.* New York: Springer Publishing.

Wickens, C. D., Lee, J. D., Liu, Y., & Gordon-Becker, S. E. (2004). *An introduction to human factors engineering.* (2nd ed.) Upper Saddle River, NJ: Pearson Prentice Hall.

Wilson, J. R., Jackson, S., & Nichols, S. (2003). Cognitive work investigation and design in practice: The influence of social context and social work artefacts. In E.Hollnagel (Ed.), *Handbook of cognitive work design* (pp. 83–97). Mahwah, New Jersey: Lawrence Erlbaum Associates.

Open Source and Free Software

Peter J. Murray / W. Scott Erdley

• OBJECTIVES

1. Describe the basic concepts of open source software (OSS) and free software (FS).
2. Describe the differences between open source and free software, and proprietary software, particularly in respect of licensing.
3. Discuss why an understanding of open source and free software is important in a healthcare context, in particular where a choice between proprietary and open source or free software is being considered.
4. Describe some of the open source and free software applications currently available, both healthcare-specific and for general office/productivity use.
5. Introduce some of the organizations and resources available to assist the nurse interested in exploring the potential of open source software.

• KEY WORDS

open source software
free software
Linux

INTRODUCTION

It is estimated that, worldwide, over 350 million people use open source software products and thousands of enterprises and organisations use open source code (Anderson & Dare, 2009); free and open source software are increasingly recognised as a reliable alternative to proprietary products. Most nurses use open source and free software (OSS/FS) (Table 9.1) on a daily basis, often without even realizing it. Everybody who sends an e-mail or uses the Web uses OSS/FS most of the time, as the majority of the hardware and software that allows the Internet to function (Web servers, file transmission protocol [FTP] servers, and mail systems) are OSS/FS. As Vint Cerf, Google's "Chief Internet Evangelist" who is seen by many as the "father of the Internet," has stated, the Internet "is fundamentally based on the existence of open, non-proprietary standards" (Openforum Europe, 2008). Many popular Web sites are hosted on Apache (OSS/FS) servers, and increasingly people are using OSS/FS Web browsers such as Firefox. While in the early days of computing software was often free, free software (as defined by the Free Software Foundation [FSF]; Table 9.1) has existed since the mid-1980s, the GNU is Not Unix Project (GNU)/Linux operating system (Table 9.1) has been developing since the early 1990s, and the open source initiative (OSI) (Table 9.2) definition of open source software has existed since the late 1990s. It is only more recently that widespread interest has begun to develop in the possibilities of OSS/FS within health, healthcare, and nursing, and within nursing informatics (NI) and health informatics.

TABLE 9.1	Some Common Acronyms and Terms

A number of acronyms are used to denote a combination of free software and open source software. OSS/FS is the term that is used for preference in this chapter; others include the following:

OSS: Open source software

OSS/FS: Open source software/free software

FOSS: Free and open source software

FLOSS: Free/libre/open source software

GNU: GNU is Not Unix Project (a recursive acronym); This is a project started by Richard Stallman, which turned into the Free Software Foundation (FSF, www.fsf.org), to develop and promote alternatives to proprietary Unix implementations.

GNU/Linux or Linux: The complete operating system including the Linux kernel, the GNU components, and many other programs. GNU/Linux is the more accurate term because it makes a distinction between the kernel—Linux—and much of the software that was developed by the GNU Project in association with the FSF.

In healthcare facilities in many countries, in both hospital and community settings, healthcare information technology (IT) initially evolved as a set of facility-centric tools to manage patient data. This was often primarily for administrative purposes, such that there now exists, in many facilities, a multitude of different, often disconnected, systems, with modern hospitals often using more than 100 different software applications. One of the major problems that nurses and all other health professionals currently face is that many of these applications and systems do not interface well for data and information exchange to benefit patient care. A major challenge in all countries is to move to a more patient-centric system, integrating facilities such as hospitals, physicians' offices, and community or home healthcare providers, so that they can easily share and exchange patient data and allow collaborative care around the patient. Supporters of OSS/FS approaches believe that only through openness, in respect to open standards and access to applications' source codes, is the user in control of the software and able to adapt the application to local needs, and prevent problems associated with vendor lock-in (Murray, Wright, Karopka, Betts, & Orel, 2009).

However, many nurses have only a vague understanding of what OSS/FS are and their possible applications and relevance to nursing and NI. This chapter aims to provide a basic understanding of the issues, as it is only through being fully informed about the relative merits, and potential limitations, of the range of proprietary software and OSS/FS, that can nurses make informed choices, whether they are selecting software for their own personal needs or involved in procurements for large healthcare organizations. This chapter will provide an overview of the background to OSS/FS, explaining the differences and similarities between open source and free software, and introducing some particular applications such as the GNU/Linux operating system. Licensing issues will be addressed, as they are one of the major issues that exercise the minds of those with responsibility for decision making, and issues such as the interface of OSS/FS and proprietary software, or use of OSS/FS components are not fully resolved. Some commonly available and healthcare–specific applications will be introduced, with a few examples being discussed. Some of the organizations working to explore the use of OSS/FS within healthcare and nursing, and some additional resources, will be introduced.

The chapter will conclude with a case study of what many consider the potential "mother of OSS/FS healthcare applications," Veterans Health Information System and Technology Architecture (VistA) (Tiemann, 2004), and recent moves to develop fully OSS/FS versions.

OSS/FS—THE THEORY

Background

While we use the term *open source* (and the acronym OSS/FS) in this chapter, we do so loosely (and, some would argue, incorrectly) to cover several concepts, including open source software, free software, and GNU/Linux. Each of these concepts and applications has its own definition and attributes (Table 9.2). While the 2 major philosophies in the OSS/FS world, i.e., the free software foundation (FSF) philosophy and the open source initiative (OSI) philosophy, are today often seen as separate movements with different views and goals, their adherents frequently work together on specific practical projects (FSF, 2010a).

The key commonality between FSF and OSI philosophies is that the source code is made available to the users by the programmer. Where FSF and OSI differ is in the restrictions placed on redistributed source code. FSF is committed to no restrictions, so that if you modify and redistribute free software, as a part or as a whole of aggregated software, you are not allowed to place any restrictions on the openness of the resultant source code (Wong & Sayo, 2004). The difference between the 2 movements

TABLE 9.2	Free Software and Open Source Definitions

Free Software

The term *free software* is defined as follows by the Free Software Foundation (FSF) (Version 1.92, 2010, http://www.gnu.org/philosophy/free-sw.html, emphasis added):

Free software is seen in terms of liberty, rather than price, and to understand the concept, you need to think of "free" as in free speech, not as in free beer. The differences are easier to understand in some languages other than English, where there is less ambiguity in the use of the word *free*. For example, in French, the use of the terms *libre* (freedom) software versus gratis (zero price) software. Free software is described in terms of the users' freedom to run, copy, distribute, study, change, and improve the software. More precisely, it refers to 4 kinds of freedom for the users of the software:

- The freedom to run the program for any purpose (freedom 0)
- The freedom to study how the program works, and change it to make it do what you wish (freedom 1). Access to the source code is a precondition for this.
- The freedom to redistribute copies so you can help your neighbor (freedom 2)
- The freedom to distribute copies of your modified versions to others (freedom 3). By doing this you can give the whole community a chance to benefit from your changes. Access to the source code is a precondition for this.

A program is free software if users have all of these freedoms.

Open Source Software

The term *open source* is defined exactly as follows by the open source initiative (OSI) (The Open Source Definition (OSD) Version 1.9, www.opensource.org/docs/osd):

Introduction

Open source doesn't just mean access to the source code. The distribution terms of open-source software must comply with the following criteria:

1. Free Redistribution
   The license shall not restrict any party from selling or giving away the software as a component of an aggregate software distribution containing programs from several different sources. The license shall not require a royalty or other fee for such sale.
   Rationale: By constraining the license to require free redistribution, we eliminate the temptation to throw away many long-term gains in order to make a few short-term sales dollars. If we didn't do this, there would be lots of pressure for cooperators to defect.

2. Source Code
   The program must include source code, and must allow distribution in source code as well as compiled form. Where some form of a product is not distributed with source code, there must be a well-publicized means of obtaining the source code for no more than a reasonable reproduction cost preferably, downloading via the Internet without charge. The source code must be the preferred form in which a programmer would modify the program. Deliberately obfuscated source code is not allowed. Intermediate forms such as the output of a preprocessor or translator are not allowed.
   Rationale: We require access to un-obfuscated source code because you can't evolve programs without modifying them. Since our purpose is to make evolution easy, we require that modification be made easy.

3. Derived Works
   The license must allow modifications and derived works, and must allow them to be distributed under the same terms as the license of the original software.
   Rationale: The mere ability to read source isn't enough to support independent peer review and rapid evolutionary selection. For rapid evolution to happen, people need to be able to experiment with and redistribute modifications.

4. Integrity of the Author's Source Code
   The license may restrict source-code from being distributed in modified form only if the license allows the distribution of "patch files" with the source code for the purpose of modifying the program at build time. The license must explicitly permit distribution of software built from modified source code. The license may require derived works to carry a different name or version number from the original software.

(continued)

TABLE 9.2	Free Software and Open Source Definitions *(continued)*

Open Source Software

Rationale: Encouraging lots of improvement is a good thing, but users have a right to know who is responsible for the software they are using. Authors and maintainers have reciprocal right to know what they're being asked to support and protect their reputations.

Accordingly, an open-source license must guarantee that source be readily available, but may require that it be distributed as pristine base sources plus patches. In this way, "unofficial" changes can be made available but readily distinguished from the base source.

5. No Discrimination Against Persons or Groups

The license must not discriminate against any person or group of persons.

Rationale: In order to get the maximum benefit from the process, the maximum diversity of persons and groups should be equally eligible to contribute to open sources. Therefore we forbid any open-source license from locking anybody out of the process.

Some countries, including the United States, have export restrictions for certain types of software. An OSD-conformant license may warn licensees of applicable restrictions and remind them that they are obliged to obey the law; however, it may not incorporate such restrictions itself.

6. No Discrimination Against Fields of Endeavor

The license must not restrict anyone from making use of the program in a specific field of endeavor. For example, it may not restrict the program from being used in a business, or from being used for genetic research.

Rationale: The major intention of this clause is to prohibit license traps that prevent open source from being used commercially. We want commercial users to join our community, not feel excluded from it.

7. Distribution of License

The rights attached to the program must apply to all to whom the program is redistributed without the need for execution of an additional license by those parties.

Rationale: This clause is intended to forbid closing up software by indirect means such as requiring a non-disclosure agreement.

8. License Must Not Be Specific to a Product

The rights attached to the program must not depend on the program's being part of a particular software distribution. If the program is extracted from that distribution and used or distributed within the terms of the program's license, all parties to whom the program is redistributed should have the same rights as those that are granted in conjunction with the original software distribution.

Rationale: This clause forecloses yet another class of license traps.

9. License Must Not Restrict Other Software

The license must not place restrictions on other software that is distributed along with the licensed software. For example, the license must not insist that all other programs distributed on the same medium must be open-source software.

Rationale: Distributors of open-source software have the right to make their own choices about their own software.

10. License Must Be Technology-Neutral

No provision of the license may be predicated on any individual technology or style of interface.

Rationale: This provision is aimed specifically at licenses which require an explicit gesture of assent in order to establish a contract between licensor and licensee. Provisions mandating so-called "click-wrap" may conflict with important methods of software distribution such as FTP download, CD-ROM anthologies, and web mirroring; such provisions may also hinder code re-use. Conformant licenses must allow for the possibility that (a) redistribution of the software will take place over non-Web channels that do not support click-wrapping of the download, and that (b) the covered code (or re-used portions of covered code) may run in a non-GUI environment that cannot support popup dialogues.

is said to be that the free software movement's fundamental issues are ethical and philosophical, while for the open source movement, the issues are more practical than ethical ones; thus, the FSF asserts that open source is a development methodology, while free software is a social movement (FSF, 2010a).

OSS/FS is contrasted with proprietary or commercial software, again the 2 terms often being conflated but strictly needing separating. Proprietary software is that on which an individual or company holds the exclusive copyright, at the same time restricting other people's access to the software's source code and/or the right to copy, modify, and study the software. (Sfakianakis, Chronaki, Chiarugi, Conforti, & Katehakis, 2007) Commercial software is software developed by businesses or individuals with the aim of making money from its licensing and use. Most commercial software is proprietary, but there is commercial free software, and there is noncommercial nonfree software.

OSS/FS should also not be confused with freeware or shareware. Freeware is software offered free of charge, but without the freedom to modify the source code and redistribute the changes, so it is not free software (as defined by the FSF). Shareware is another form of commercial software, which is offered on a "try before you buy" basis. If the customer continues to use the product after a short trial period, or wishes to use additional features, they are required to pay a specified, usually nominal, license fee.

Free Software Definition

Free software is defined by the FSF in terms of 4 freedoms for software users: to have the freedom to use, study, redistribute, and improve the software in any way they wish. A program is only free software, in terms of the FSF definition, if users have all of these freedoms (see Table 9.2). The FSF believes that users should be free to redistribute copies, either with or without modifications, either gratis or through charging a fee for distribution, to anyone, anywhere without a need to ask or pay for permission to do so (FSF, 2010a).

Confusion around the use and meaning of the term *free software* arises from the multiple meanings of the word *free* in the English language. In other languages, there is less of a problem, with different words being used for the "freedom" versus "no cost" meanings of *free*, for example the French terms *libre* (freedom) software versus *gratis* (zero price) software. The "free" of free software is defined in terms of liberty, not price, thus to understand the concept, the common distinction is in thinking of free as in free speech, not as in free beer (FSF, 2010b). Acronyms such as FLOSS (free/libre/OSS—a combination of the above 2 terms emphasizing the "libre" meaning of the word *free*) or OSS/FS are increasingly used, particularly in Europe, to overcome this issue (International Institute of Infonomics, 2005).

Open Source Software Definition

Open source software is any software satisfying the open software initiative's definition (OSI, n.d.). The open source concept is said to promote software reliability and quality by supporting independent peer review and rapid evolution of source code as well as making the source code of software freely available. In addition to providing free access to the programmer's instructions to the computer in the programming language in which they were written, many versions of open source licenses allow anyone to modify and redistribute the software.

The open source initiative (OSI) has created a certification mark, "OSI certified." In order to be OSI certified, the software must be distributed under a license that guarantees the right to read, redistribute, modify, and use the software freely (OSI, n.d). Not only must the source code be accessible to all, but also the distribution terms must comply with 10 criteria defined by the OSI (see Table 9.2 for full text and rationale).

OSS/FS Development Models and Systems

OSS/FS has existed as a model for developing computer applications and software since the 1950s (Waring & Maddocks, 2005); at that time, software was often provided free (gratis), and freely, when buying hardware (Murray et al., 2009). The freedoms embodied within OSS/FS were understood as routine until the early 1980s with the rise of proprietary software. However, it was only in the 1980s that the term free software (Stallman, 2002) and in the 1990's that the term open source software, as we recognise them today, came into existence to distinguish them from the proprietary models.

The development models of OSS/FS are said to contribute to their distinctions from proprietary software. Shaw et al. (2002) state that as OSS/FS is "developed and disseminated in an open forum," it "revolutionizes the way in which software has historically been developed and distributed." A similar description, in a United Kingdom government report, emphasizes the open publishing of source code and that development is often largely through voluntary efforts (Peeling & Satchell, 2001).

While OSS/FS is often described as being developed by voluntary efforts, this description may belie the professional skills and expertise of many of the developers. Many of those providing the volunteer efforts are highly skilled programmers who contribute time and efforts freely to the development of OSS/FS. In addition, many OSS/FS applications are coordinated through formal groups. For example, the Apache Software Foundation (www.apache.org) coordinates development of the Apache hypertext transfer protocol (HTTP) server and many other products.

OSS/FS draws much of its strength from the collaborative efforts of people who work to improve, modify, or customize programs, believing they must give back to the OSS/FS community so others can benefit from their work. The OSS/FS development model is unique, although it bears strong similarities to the openness of the scientific method, and is facilitated by the communication capabilities of the Internet that allow collaboration and rapid sharing of developments, such that new versions of software can often be made available on a daily basis.

The most well-known description of the distinction between OSS/FS and proprietary models of software development lies in Eric Raymond's famous essay, "The Cathedral and the Bazaar" (Raymond, 2001). Cathedrals, Raymond says, were built by small groups of skilled workers and craftsmen to carefully worked out designs. The work was often done in isolation, and with everything built in a single effort with little subsequent modification. Much software, in particular proprietary software, has traditionally been built in a similar fashion, with groups of programmers working to strictly-controlled planning and management, until their work was completed and the program released to the world. In contrast, OSS/FS development is likened to a bazaar, growing organically from an initial small group of traders or enthusiasts establishing their structures and beginning businesses. The bazaar grows in a seemingly chaotic fashion, from a minimally functional structure, with later additions or modifications as circumstances dictate. Likewise, most OSS/FS development starts off highly unstructured, with developers releasing early, minimally functional code and then modifying their programs based on feedback. Other developers may then join, and modify or build on the existing code; over time, an entire operating system and suite of applications develops, evolves, and improves continuously.

The bazaar method of development is said to have been proven over time to have several advantages, including the following:

- Reduced duplication of efforts through being able to examine the work of others and through the potential for large numbers of contributors to use their skills. As Moody (2001) describes it, there is no need to reinvent the wheel every time as there would be with commercial products whose codes cannot be used in these ways

- Building on the work of others, often by the use of open standards or components from other applications

- Better quality control; with many developers working on a project, code errors (bugs) are

uncovered quickly and may be fixed even more rapidly (often termed Linus' Law, "given enough eyeballs, all bugs are shallow" [Raymond, 2001])

- Reduction in maintenance costs; costs, as well as effort, can be shared among potentially thousands of developers (Wong & Sayo, 2004).

CHOOSING OSS/FS OR NOT

Proposed Benefits of OSS/FS

OSS/FS has been described as the electronic equivalent of generic drugs (Bruggink, 2003; Goetz, 2003; Surnam & Diceman, 2004). In the same way as the formulas for generic drugs are made public, so OSS/FS source code is accessible to the user. Any person can see how the software works and can make changes to the functionality. It is also suggested by many that there are significant similarities between the open source ethos and the traditional scientific method approach (supported by most scientists and philosophers of science), as this latter method is based on openness, free sharing of information, and improvement of the end result. As OSS/FS can be obtained royalty free, it is less expensive to acquire than proprietary alternatives. This means that OSS/FS can transform healthcare in developing countries just as the availability of generic drugs have.

This is only one of several benefits proposed for OSS/FS, with further benefits including lack of the proprietary lock-in that can often freeze out innovation, and with OSS/FS projects supporting open standards and providing a level playing field, expanding the market by giving software consumers greater choice (Dravis, 2003).

Besides the low cost of OSS/FS, there are many other reasons why public and private organizations are adopting OSS/FS, including security, reliability and stability, and developing local software capacity. Many of these proposed benefits have yet to be demonstrated or tested extensively, but there is growing evidence for many of them, and we will address some of them in the next section.

Issues in OSS/FS

There are many issues in the use of OSS/FS that we cannot address here in detail. However, by providing nurses who are exploring, using, or intending to use OSS/FS with a basic introduction and pointers to additional resources, we facilitate their awareness of the issues and support them in their decision making. The issues that we introduce include, not necessarily in any order of importance:

- Licensing
- Copyright and intellectual property
- Total cost of ownership (TCO)
- Support and migration
- Business models
- Security and stability

Licensing and copyright will be addressed in the next section, but the other issues will be covered briefly here, before concluding the section with a short description of one possible strategy for choosing OSS/FS (or other software, as the issues are pertinent to any properly-considered purchase and implementation strategy).

Total Cost of Ownership. TCO is the sum of all the expenses directly related to the ownership and use of a product over a given period of time. The popular myth surrounding OSS/FS is that it is always free as in free of charge. This is true to an extent, as most OSS/FS distributions (e.g., Ubuntu [www.ubuntu.com], Red Hat [www.redhat.com], SuSE [www.opensuse.org], Debian [www.debian.org]) can be obtained at no charge from the Internet; however, copies can also be sold.

No true OSS/FS application charges a licensing fee for usage, thus on a licensing cost basis OSS/FS applications are almost always cheaper than proprietary software. However, licensing costs are not the only costs of a software package or infrastructure. It is also necessary to consider personnel costs, hardware requirements, migration time, changes in staff efficiency, and training costs, among others. Without all of this information, it is impossible to really know which software solutions are going to be the most cost effective. There are still real costs with OSS/FS, specifically around configuration and support (examples are provided in Wheeler, 2007 and Wong & Sayo, 2004).

Wheeler (2007) lists the main reasons why OSS/FS comes out cheaper, including the following:

- OSS/FS costs less to initially acquire, because there are no license fees.
- Upgrade and maintenance costs are typically far less due to improved stability and security.
- OSS/FS can often use older hardware more efficiently than proprietary systems, yielding smaller hardware costs and sometimes eliminating the need for new hardware.

- Increasing numbers of case studies using OSS/FS show it to be especially cheaper in server environments.

Support and Migration. Making an organization-wide change from proprietary software can be costly, and sometimes the costs will outweigh the benefits. Some OSS/FS packages do not have the same level of documentation, training, and support resources as their common proprietary equivalents, and may not fully interface with other proprietary software being used by other organizations with which an organization may work (e.g., patient data exchange between different healthcare provider systems).

Migrating from one platform to another should be handled using a careful and phased approach. The European Commission has published a document entitled the "IDA Open Source Migration Guidelines" (European Communities, 2003) that provides detailed suggestions on how to approach migration. These include the need for a clear understanding of the reasons to migrate, ensuring that there is active support for the change from IT staff and users, building up expertise and relationships with the open source movement, starting with noncritical systems, and ensuring that each step in the migration is manageable.

Security and Stability. While there is no perfectly secure operating system or platform, factors such as development method, program architecture, and target market can greatly affect the security of a system and consequently make it easier or more difficult to breach. There are some indications that OSS/FS systems are superior to proprietary systems in this respect, and the security aspect has already encouraged many public organizations to switch or to consider switching to OSS/FS solutions. The French Customs and Indirect Taxation authority, for example, migrated to Red Hat Linux largely because of security concerns with proprietary software (International Institute of Infonomics, 2005).

Among reasons often cited for the better security record in OSS/FS is the availability of the source code (making it easier for vulnerabilities to be discovered and fixed). Many OSS/FS have a proactive security focus, so that before features are added, the security considerations are accounted for and a feature is added only if it is determined not to compromise system security. In addition, the strong security and permission structure inherent in OSS/FS applications that are based on the Unix model are designed to minimize the possibility of users being able to compromise systems (Wong & Sayo, 2004). OSS/FS systems are well known for their stability and reliability, and many anecdotal stories exist of OSS/FS servers functioning for years without requiring maintenance. However, quantitative studies are more difficult to come by (Wong & Sayo, 2004).

Security of information is vitally important in the health domain, particularly in relation to access, storage, and transmission of patient records. The advocates of OSS/FS suggest that it can provide increased security over proprietary software, and a report to the U.K. government saw no security disadvantage in the use of OSS/FS products (Peeling & Satchell, 2001). Even the U.S. government's National Security Agency (NSA), according to the same report, supports a number of OSS/FS security-related projects. Stanco (2001) considers that the reason the NSA thinks that free software can be more secure is that when anyone and everyone can inspect source code, hiding backdoors into the code can be very difficult.

In considering a migration to OSS/FS, whether it is for everyday office and productivity uses, or for health-specific applications, there are some commonly encountered challenges that one may face. These challenges have traditionally been seen as including the following:

- There is a relative lack of mature OSS/FS desktop applications.

- Many OSS/FS tools are not user-friendly and have a steep learning curve.

- File sharing between OSS/FS and proprietary applications can be difficult.

As OSS/FS applications have matured in recent years, and the user community grown, many of these challenges have been largely overcome, such that today, many OSS/FA applications are indistinguishable from proprietary equivalents for many users in terms of functionality, ease of use, and general user-freiendliness.

Choosing the Right Software: The 3-Step Method for OSS/FS Decision Making. Whether one is working with OSS/FS or commercial/proprietary tools, choosing the right software can be a difficult process, and a thorough review process is needed before making a choice. A simple 3-step method for OSS/FS decision making can guide organizations through the process and works well for all kinds of software, including server, desktop, and Web applications (Surman & Diceman, 2004).

Step 1. Define the needs and constraints. Needs must be clearly defined, including those of the organization and of individual users. Other specific issues to consider include range of features, languages, budget (e.g., for training or integration with other systems), the implementation time frame, compatibility with existing systems, and the skills existing within the organization.

Step 2. Identify the options. A short list of 3 to 5 software packages that are likely to meet the needs can be developed from comparing software packages with the needs and constraints listed in the previous phase. There are numerous sources of information on OSS/FS packages, including recommendations of existing users, reviews, and directories (e.g., OSDir.com and OpenSourceCMS.com.) and software package sites that contain promotional information, documentation, and often demonstration versions that will help with the review process.

Step 3. Undertake a detailed review. Once the options have been identified, the final step is to review and choose a software package from the short list. The aim here is to assess which of the possible options will be best for the organization. This assessment can be done by rating each package against a list of criteria, including quality, ease of use, ease of migration, software stability, compatibility with other systems being used, flexibility and customizability, user response, organizational buy-in, evidence of widespread use of the software, and the existence of support mechanisms for the software's use. Hands-on testing is key and each piece of software should be installed and tested for quality, stability, and compatibility, including by a group of key users so as to assess factors such as ease of use, ease of migration, and user response.

Making a Decision. Once the review has been completed, if 2 packages are close in score, intuition about the right package is probably more important than the actual numbers in reaching a final decision.

Examples of Adoption or Policy Regarding OSS/FS

OSS/FS has moved beyond the closed world of programmers and enthusiasts. Governments around the world have begun to take notice of OSS/FS and have launched initiatives to explore the proposed benefits. There is a significant trend toward incorporating OSS/FS into procurement and development policies, and there are increasing numbers of cases of OSS/FS recognition, explicit policy statements, and procurement decisions. Many countries, regions, and authorities now have existing or proposed laws mandating or encouraging the use of OSS/FS (Wong & Sayo, 2004).

A survey from The MITRE Corporation (2003) showed that the U.S. Department of Defense (DoD) at that time used over 100 different OSS/FS applications. The main conclusion of their study (The MITRE Corporation, 2003) was that OSS/FS software was used in critical roles, including infrastructure support, software development, research, and that the degree of dependence on OSS/FS for security was unexpected. In 2000, the (U.S.) President's Information Technology Advisory Committee (PITAC, 2000) recommended that the U.S. federal government should encourage OSS/FS use for software development for high-end computing. In 2002, the U.K. government published a policy (Office of the e-Envoy, 2002), since updated, that it would "consider OSS solutions alongside proprietary ones in IT procurements" (p. 4), "only use products for interoperability that support open standards and specifications in all future IT developments" (p. 4) and explore the possibility of using OSS/FS as the default exploitation route for government-funded research and development (R&D) software. Similar policies have been developed in Denmark, Sweden, and The Netherlands (Wong & Sayo, 2004).

European policy encouraging the exploration and use of OSS/FS has been consequent on the European Commission's *eEurope2005—An Information Society for All* initiative (European Communities, 2004) and its predecessors, such as the i2010 strategy (European Communities, 2005) with their associated action plans. These have encouraged the exchange of experiences and best practice examples so as to promote the use of OSS/FS in the public sector and e-government across the European Commission and member states of the European Union (EU). In addition, the EU has funded R&D on health-related OSS/FS applications as well as encouraged open standards and OSS/FS where appropriate in wider policy initiatives.

In other parts of world, Brazil and Peru are among countries whose governments are actively moving toward OSS/FS solutions, for a variety of reasons, including ensuring long-term access to data through the use of open standards (i.e., not being reliant on proprietary software that may not, in the future, be interoperable) and cost reduction. The South African government has a policy favoring OSS/FS, Japan is considering moving e-government projects to OSS/FS, and pro-OSS/FS initiatives are in operation or being seriously considered in Taiwan, Malaysia, South Korea, and other Asia Pacific countries.

OPEN SOURCE LICENSING

While OSS/FS is seen by many as a philosophy and a development model, it is also important to consider it as a licensing model (Leong, Kaiser, & Miksch, 2007; Sfakianakis et al., 2007). In this section, we can only briefly introduce some of the issues of software licensing as they apply to OSS/FS, and will include definitions of licensing, some of the types of licenses that exist, and how licenses are different from copyright. While we will cover some of the legal concepts, this section cannot take the place of proper legal counsel, which should be sought when reviewing the impact of licenses or contracts. Licensing plays a crucial role in the OSS/FS community, as it is "the operative tool to convey rights and redistribution conditions" (Anderson & Dare 2009, p. 101).

Licensing is defined by Merriam-Webster (2010) as giving the user of something permission to use it; in the case here, that something is software. Most software comes with some type of licensing, commonly known as the end-user licensing agreement (EULA). The license may have specific restrictions related to the use, modification, or duplication of the software. The Microsoft EULA, for example, specifically prohibits any kind of disassembly, inspection, or reverse engineering of software (Zymaris, 2003). Most licenses also have statements limiting the liability of the software manufacturer toward the user in case of possible problems arising in the use of the software.

From this working definition of licensing, and some examples of what can be found in a EULA, we can examine copyright. While licensing gives a person the right to use software, with restrictions in some cases, copyright is described as the exclusively granted or owned legal right to publish, reproduce, and/or sell a work (Merriam-Webster, 2010). The distinctions between ownership of the original work and rights to use it are important, and there are differences in the way these issues are approached for proprietary software and OSS/FS. For software, the *work* means the source code or statements made in a programming language. In general, the person who creates a work owns the copyright to it and has the right to allow others to copy it or deny that right. In some cases the copyright is owned by a company with software developers working for that company, usually having statements in their employment contracts that assign copyright of their works to the company. In the case of OSS/FS, contributors to a project will often assign copyright to the managers of the project.

While in the case of proprietary software, licensing is generally dealt with in terms of restrictions (i.e., what the user is not allowed to do, for OSS/FS, licensing is seen in terms of permissions, rights, and encouraging users to do things). Most software manufacturing companies hold the copyright for software created by their employees. In financial terms, these works are considered intellectual property, meaning that they have some value. For large software companies, such as Oracle or Microsoft, intellectual property may be a large part of their capital assets. The open source community values software differently, and OSS/FS licenses are designed to facilitate the sharing of software and to prevent an individual or organization from controlling ownership of the software. The individuals who participate in OSS/FS projects generally do realize the monetary value of what they create; however, they feel it is more valuable if the community at large has open access to it and is able to contribute back to the project.

A common misconception is that if a piece of software, or any other product, is made freely available and open to inspection and modification, then the intellectual property rights (IPR) of the originators cannot be protected, and the material cannot be subject to copyright. The open source community, and in particular the FSF, have adopted a number of conventions, some built into the licenses, to protect the IPR of authors and developers. One form of copyright, termed *copyleft* to distinguish it from commercial copyright terms, works by stating that the software is copyrighted and then adding distribution terms. These are a legal instrument giving everyone the rights to use, modify, and redistribute the program's code or any program derived from it but only if the distribution terms are unchanged. The

code and the freedoms become legally inseparable, and strengthen the rights of the originators and contributors (Cox, 1999; FSF, 2010c).

Types of OSS/FS Licenses

A large and growing number of OSS/FS licenses exists. Table 9.3 lists some of the more common ones, while fuller lists of various licenses and terms can be found in Wong and Sayo (2004). The OSI website currently lists over 60 (www.opensource.org/licenses), while the FSF website lists over 40 general public license (GPL)-compatible free software licenses (www.gnu.org/licenses/license-list.html). The 2 main licenses are the GNU GPL and the Berkeley system distribution (BSD)-style licenses. It is estimated that about 75% of OSS/FS products use the GNU GPL (Wheeler, 2010), and this license is designed to ensure that user freedoms under the license are protected in perpetuity, with users being allowed to do almost anything they want to a GPL program. The conditions of the license primarily affect the user when it is distributed to another user (Wong & Sayo, 2004). BSD-style licenses are so named because they are identical in spirit to the original license issued by the University of California, Berkeley. These are among the most permissive licenses possible, and essentially permit users to do anything they wish with the software, providing the original licensor is acknowledged by including the original copyright notice in source code files and no attempt is made to sue or hold the original licensor liable for damages (Wong & Sayo, 2004).

TABLE 9.3	Some Common OSS/FS Licenses

GNU GPL: A free software license and a copyleft license. Recommended by FSF for most software packages (www.gnu.org/licenses/gpl.html).

GNU Lesser General Public License (GNU LGPL): A free software license, but not a strong copyleft license, because it permits linking with nonfree modules (www.gnu.org/copyleft/lesser.html).

Modified BSD License: The original BSD license, modified by removal of the advertising clause. It is a simple, permissive noncopyleft free software license, compatible with the GNU GPL (www.oss-watch.ac.uk/resources/modbsd.xml).

W3C Software Notice and License: A free software license and is GPL compatible (www.w3.org/Consortium/Legal/2002/copyright-software-20021231).

MySQL Database License: (www.mysql.com/about/legal)

Apache License, Version 2.0: A simple, permissive noncopyleft free software license that is incompatible with the GNU GPL (www.apache.org/licenses/LICENSE-2.0).

GNU Free Documentation License: A license intended for use on copylefted free documentation. It is also suitable for textbooks and dictionaries, and its applicability is not limited to textual works (e.g., books) (www.gnu.org/copyleft/fdl.html).

Public domain: Being in the public domain is not a license, but means the material is not copyrighted and no license is needed. Public domain status is compatible with the GNU GPL.

Further information on licenses is available at www.gnu.org/licenses/licenses.html and www.opensource.org/licenses.

Here is an example from the GNU GPL that talks about limitations:

16. Limitation of Liability. In no event unless required by applicable law or agreed to in writing will any copyright holder, or any other party who may modify and/or redistribute the program as permitted above, be liable to you for damages, including any general, special, incidental, or consequential damages arising out of the use or inability to use the program (including but not limited to loss of data or data being rendered inaccurate or losses sustained by you or third parties or a failure of the program to operate with any other programs), even if such holder or other party has been advised of the possibility of such damages. (FSF, 2007, para. 16)

Like the Microsoft EULA, there are limitations relating to liability in the use of the software and damage that may be caused, but unlike the Microsoft EULA, the GPL makes it clear what you can do with the software. In general, you can copy and redistribute it, sell or modify it. The restriction is that you must comply with the parts of the license requiring the source code to be distributed as well. One of the primary motivations behind usage of the GPL in OSS/FS is to ensure that once a program is released as OSS/FS, it will remain so permanently. A commercial software company cannot legally modify a GPL program and then sell it under a different proprietary license (Wong & Sayo, 2004).

In relation to using OSS/FS within a healthcare environment, as with use of any software, legal counsel should be consulted to review any license agreement made; however, in general terms, when using OSS/FS there are no obligations that would not apply to using any copyrighted work. Someone cannot legally take a body of work, the source code, and claim it as their own. The licensing terms must be followed as with any other software.

Perhaps the most difficult issue comes when integrating OSS/FS components into a larger infrastructure, especially where it may have to interface with proprietary software. Much has been said about the "viral" nature of the open source license, which comes from the requirement of making source code available if the software is redistributed. Care must be taken that components utilized in creating proprietary software either utilize OSS/FS components in such a way as to facilitate distribution of the code or avoid their use. If the component cannot be made available without all of the source code being made available, then the developer has the choice of not using the component or making the entire application open source. Some projects

have created separate licensing schemes to maintain the OSS/FS license and provide those vendors that wish to integrate components without making their product open source. MySQL, a popular open source database server offers such an option (Table 9.3).

Licensing is a complex issue; we have only touched on some of the points, but in conclusion, the best advice is always to read the license agreement and understand it. In the case of a business decision on software purchase or use, one should always consult legal counsel; however, one should remember that OSS/FS licenses are more about providing freedom than about restricting use.

OSS/FS APPLICATIONS

Many OSS/FS alternatives exist to more commonly known applications. Not all can be covered here, but if one thinks of the common applications that most nurses use on a daily basis, these are likely to include the following:

- Operating system
- Web browser
- E-mail client
- Word processing or integrated office suite
- Presentation tools

For each of these, OSS/FS applications exist. Using OSS/FS does not require an all or nothing approach (Dravis, 2003) and much OSS/FS can be mixed with proprietary software and a gradual migration to OSS/FS is an option for many organizations or individuals. However, when using a mixture of OSS/FS and proprietary or commercial software, incompatibilities can be uncovered and cause problems whose severity must be assessed. Many OSS/FS applications have versions that will run on non-OSS/FS operating systems, so that a change of operating system, for example, to one of the many distributions of Linux, is not necessarily needed. Most OSS/FS operating systems now have graphical interfaces that look very similar to Windows or Apple interfaces.

Operating Systems: GNU/Linux

A GNU/Linux distribution (named in recognition of the GNU Project's significant contribution, but often just called Linux) contains the Linux kernel at its heart and all the OSS/FS components required to produce full operating system functionality. *GNU/Linux* is a term that is increasingly used by many people to cover

TABLE 9.4	Some Common Linux Distributions

Ubuntu: Ubuntu is a Linux-based operating system for desktop, server, netbook, and cloud computing environments. First released in 2004, it is loosely based on Debian OS. Ubuntu now releases updates on a 6-month cycle. There are increasing numbers of customised variants of Ubuntu, aimed at, for example, educational use (Edubuntu), professional video and audio editing (Ubuntu Studio), and server editions (www.ubuntu.com).

Debian: Debian GNU/Linux is a free distribution of the Linux-based operating system. It includes a large selection of prepackaged application software, plus advanced package management tools to allow for easy installation and maintenance on individual systems and workstation clusters (www.debian.org).

Mandriva (formerly Mandrakelinux): Available in multiple language versions (including English, Swedish, Spanish, Chinese, Japanese, French, German, Italian, and Russian). Mandrakelinux was first created in 1998 and is designed for ease of use on servers and on home and office systems (www2.mandriva.com).

Red Hat (Enterprise): Red Hat Enterprise Linux is a high-end Linux distribution geared toward businesses with mission-critical needs (www.redhat.com).

Fedora: The Fedora Project was created in late 2003, when Red Hat Linux was discontinued. Fedora is a community distribution (fedoraproject.org).

SuSE: SuSE, now a subsidiary of Novell, was first developed in 1992. It is a popular mainstream Linux distribution (www.novell.com/linux).

KNOPPIX: KNOPPIX is a bootable Live system on CD or DVD, consisting of a representative collection of GNU/Linux software, automatic hardware detection, and support for many graphics cards, sound cards, and peripheral devices. KNOPPIX can be used for the desktop, educational CD, as a rescue system, or adapted and used as a platform for commercial software product demos. As it is not necessary to install anything on a hard disk, but can be run entirely from CD-ROM or DVD, it is ideal for demonstrations of Linux (www.knoppix.com).

There are many Web sites and organisations that maintain lists of the most used Linux distributions, for example distrowatch. com/dwres.php?resource=major, en.wikipedia.org/wiki/Comparison_of_Linux_distributions, and www.linux.com/directory/ Distributions.

a distribution of operating systems and other associated software components. However, Linux was originally the name of the kernel created by Linus Torvalds, which has grown from a one-man operation to now having over 200 maintainers representing over 300 organizations.

A kernel is the critical center point of an operating system that controls central processing unit (CPU) usage, memory management, and hardware devices. It also mediates communication between the different programs running within the operating system. The kernel influences performance and the hardware platforms that the OSS/FS system can run on, and the Linux kernel has been ported to run on almost any hardware, from mainframes and supercomputers, through desktop, laptop, and tablet machines, to mobile phones and other mobile devices. The Linux kernel is OSS/FS, licensed under the GNU GPL.

Over time, individuals and companies began distributing Linux with their own choice of OSS/FS packages bound around the Linux kernel; the concept of the *distribution* was born, which contains much more than the kernel (usually only about 0.25% in binary file size of the distribution). There is no single Linux distribution, and many commercial distributions and freely available variants exist, with numerous customized distributions that are targeted to the unique needs of different users (Table 9.4). While all distributions contain the Linux kernel, some contain only OSS/FS materials, while others additionally contain non-OSS/FS components, and the mix of OSS/FS and other applications included and the configurations supported vary. The Debian GNU/Linux distribution is one of the few distributions that is committed to including only OSS/FS components (as defined by the open source initiative) in its core distribution.

Ubuntu, Linux Mint, and PCLinuxOS are generally viewed as the easiest distributions for new users who wish to simply test or gain a general familiarity with Linux. Slackware Linux, Gentoo Linux, and FreeBSD are distributions that require a degree of expertise and familiarity with Linux if they are to be used effectively and productively. openSUSE, Fedora, Debian GNU/Linux, and Mandriva Linux are mid-range distributions in terms of both complexity and ease of use. Recently, Google has released their version of an open source operating system called Android. It is suited for a wide range of devices from personal computer to mobile device. In particular, there is a smartphone now running Android. There are rumors of tablet computers running Android soon to come to market.

Web Browser and Server: Firefox and Apache

While for most people the focus may be on their client-end use of applications, many rely on other, server-side applications, to function. Web browsing is a prime example where both server and client-side applications are needed. Web servers, such as Apache, are responsible for receiving and fulfilling requests from Web browsers. An OSS/FS application, the Apache HTTP server, developed for Unix, Windows NT, and other platforms, is currently the top Web server with 55% of the market share (over twice that of its next-ranked competitor), and serving 67% of the million busiest Web sites. Apache has dominated the public Internet Web server market ever since it grew to become the number 1 Web server in 1996 (Wheeler, 2007; NetCraft Ltd., 2010). Apache began development in early 1995 and is an example of an OSS/FS project that is maintained by a formal structure, the Apache Software Foundation.

Firefox (technically Mozilla Firefox) is an OSS/FS graphical Web browser, designed for standards compliance, and with a large number of browser features. It derives from the Mozilla Application Suite, and aims to continue Netscape Communicator as an open project and is maintained by the Mozilla Organization and employees of several other companies, as well as contributors from the community. Firefox source code is OSS/FS, and is tri-licensed, under the Mozilla Public License (MPL), the GNU GPL, and the GNU Lesser General Public License (LGPL), which permit anyone to view, modify, and/or redistribute the source code, and several publicly released applications have been built on it. As of May 2010, Firefox had over 24% worldwide usage share of web browsers, making it the second most used browser, after Internet Explorer (Netmarketshare, 2010), although reports show higher market shares, up to 30%, in some European countries (AT Internet, 2010).

Word Processing or Integrated Office Suite: Open Office (Office Productivity Suite)

While OSS/FS products have been strong on the server side, OSS/FS desktop applications are relatively new and few. Open Office (strictly OpenOffice.org), which is based on the source code of the formerly proprietary StarOffice, is an OSS/FS equivalent of Microsoft Office, with most of its features. It supports the ISO/IEC standard OpenDocument Format (ODF) for data interchange as its default file format, as well as Microsoft Office formats among others. As of November 2009, Open Office supports over 110 languages. It includes a fully featured word processor, spreadsheet, and presentation software. One of the advantages for considering a shift from a Windows desktop environment to Open Office is that it reads most Microsoft Office documents without problems and will save documents to many formats, including Microsoft Word (but not vice versa). This makes the transition relatively painless and Open Office has been used in recent high profile switches from Windows to Linux. Open Office has versions that will run on Windows, Linux, and other operating systems. (Note that the text for this chapter was originally written using OpenOffice.org Writer, the word processing package within the OpenOffice.org suite.)

The word *PowerPoint* has become almost synonymous with software for making presentations, and is even commonly used as a teaching tool. The OpenOffice.org suite contains a presentation component, called Impress, which produces presentations very similar to PowerPoint; they can be saved and run in OpenOffice format on Windows or Linux desktop environments, or exported as PowerPoint versions.

Some Other OSS/FS Applications

BIND. The Berkeley Internet Name Domain (BIND) is a domain name system (DNS) server, or in other words, an Internet naming system. Internet addresses, such as www.google.com or www.openoffice.org, would not function without DNS. These servers take these human-friendly names and convert them into computer-friendly numeric Internet protocol (IP) addresses and vice versa. Without these servers, users would have to memorize numbers such as 74.125.19.104 in order to use a Web site, instead of simply typing www.google.com.

The BIND server is an OSS/FS program developed and distributed by the University of California at Berkeley. It is licensed under a BSD-style license by the Internet Software Consortium. It runs 95% of all DNS servers including most of the DNS root servers. These servers hold the master record of all domain names on the Internet.

Perl. Practical Extraction and Reporting Language (Perl) is a high-level programming language that is frequently used for creating CGI (common gateway interface) programs. Started in 1987, and now developed as an OSS/FS project, it was designed for processing text and derives from the C programming language and many other tools and languages. It was originally developed for Unix and is now available for many platforms. Perl modules and add-ons are available to do almost anything, leading some to call it the "Swiss Army chain-saw" of programming languages (Raymond, 2003).

PHP. PHP stands for PHP Hypertext Preprocessor. The name is an example of a recursive acronym (the first word of the acronym is also the acronym), a common practice in the OSS/FS community for naming applications. PHP is a server-side, HTML-embedded scripting language used to quickly create dynamically-generated Web pages. In an HTML document, PHP script (similar syntax to that of Perl or C) is enclosed within special PHP tags. PHP can perform any task any CGI program can, but its strength lies in its compatibility with many types of relational databases. PHP runs on every major operating system, including Unix, Linux, Windows, and Mac OS X and can interact with all major Web servers.

LAMP. The Linux, Apache, MySQL, PHP (LAMP) architecture has become very popular as a way of affordably deploying reliable, scalable, and secure Web applications (the "P" in LAMP can also stand for Perl or Python). MySQL is a multithreaded, multiuser, SQL (Structured Query Language) relational database server, using the GNU GPL. The PHP-MySQL combination is also a cross-platform (i.e., it will run on Windows as well as Linux servers) (Murray & Oyri, 2005).

Content Management Systems. Many OSS/FS applications, especially modern content management systems (CMS) that are the basis of many of today's interactive Web sites, use LAMP. A CMS has a flexible, modular framework that separates the content of a Web site (the text, images, and other content) from the framework of linking the pages together and controlling how the pages appear. In most cases, this is done to make a site easier to maintain than would be the case if it was built exclusively out of flat HTML pages. There are now over 200 OSS/FS FLOSS content management systems (see php.opensourcecms.com for an extensive list) designed for developing portals and Web sites with dynamic, fully searchable content. Drupal (drupal.org), for example, is one of the most well-known and widely used CMS and is currently used for the official site of the White House (www.whitehouse.gov), the United Nations World Food Programme (www.wfp.org), and the South African Government for their official 2010 FIFA World Cup website (www.sa2010.gov.za). MyOpenSourcematrix, a CMS designed for large organisations, has been used by the UK's Royal College of Nursing to provide a content and communications portal for its 400,000 members (Squiz UK, 2007).

A CMS can be easily administrated and moderated at several levels by members of an online community, which gives complete control of compliance with the organisation's policy for published material and provides for greater interactivity and sense of ownership by online community members. In addition, the workload relating to publication of material and overall maintenance of the Web site can be spread among many members, rather than having only one Web spinner. This secures frequent updates of content and reduces individual workloads, making the likelihood of member participation greater. The initial user registration and redistribution of passwords and access can be carried out automatically by user requests, while assignment to user groups is made manually by the site administrators or moderators.

FLOSS applications are gaining widespread use within education sectors, with one example of a widely used e-learning application being Moodle (www.moodle.org). Moodle is a complete e-learning course management system, or virtual learning environment (VLE), with a modular structure designed to help educators create high-quality, multimedia-based online courses. Moodle is translated into more than 30 languages, and handles thematic or topic-based classes and courses. As Moodle is based in social constructivist pedagogy (moodle.org/doc/?frame=philosophy.html), it also allows the construction of e-learning materials that are based around discussion and interaction, rather than static content. (Kaminski, 2005)

OSS/FS HEALTHCARE APPLICATIONS

It is suggested that in healthcare, as in many other areas, the development of OSS/FS may provide much-needed competition to the relatively closed market of commercial, proprietary software (Smith, 2002), and thus encourage innovation. This could lead to lower cost and higher quality systems that are more responsive to changing clinical needs. OSS/FS could also solve many of the problems health information systems currently face including lack of interoperability and vendor lock-in, cost, difficulty of record and system maintenance given the rate of change and size of the information needs of the health domain, and lack of support for security, privacy, and consent. This is because OSS/FS more closely conforms to standards and its source code open to inspection and adaptation. A significant motive for supporting the use of OSS/FS and open standards in healthcare is that interoperability of health information systems requires the consistent implementation of open standards (Sfakianakis et al., 2007). Open standards, as described by the International Telecommunications Union (ITU), are made available to the general public and developed, approved, and maintained via a collaborative and consensus-driven process (ITU, 2009, Sfakianakis et al., 2007) A key element of the process is that, by being open, there is less risk of being dominated by any single interest group.

Bowen et al. (2009) summarize a number of advantages that open source software offers when compared with proprietary software, including, but not limited to, the following: (1) ease of modification and or customization, (2) the large developer community and its benefits, (3) increased compliance with open standards, (4) enhanced security, (5) increased likelihood of source code availability in the event of the demise of the vendor or company, (6) easier to adapt for use by healthcare students, and (7) the flexibility of source code to adapt to research efforts. The cost effectiveness of open source software also lends well to communities or organizations requiring such an approach (e.g., long-term care facilities, assisted living communities, clinics (public health and educational venue clinics), and home care.

Yellowlees, Marks, Hogarth, & Turner (2008) are among those who suggest that many current EHR systems tend to be expensive, inflexible, difficult to maintain, and rarely interoperable across health systems; this is often due to their being proprietary systems. This makes clinicians reluctant to use them, as they are seen as no better than paper-based systems. OSS/FS has been very successful in other information-intensive industries, and so is seen as having potential to integrate functional EHR systems into, and across, wider health systems. They believe that interoperable open source EHR systems would have the potential to improve healthcare in the United States, and cite examples from other areas around the world.

Currently, there is much interest in interoperability testing of systems, not only between proprietary systems, but also among OSS/FS systems, and between OSS/FS systems and proprietary systems. Integrating the Healthcare Enterprise (IHE) has developed a range of open source interoperability testing tools, called MESA, KUDU, and its next generation tool GAZELLE, to test healthcare interoperability according to the standards profiled by the IHE in its technical frameworks. The Certification Commission for Health Information Technology (CCHIT) has developed an open source program called Laika to test EHR software for compliance with CCHIT interoperability standards.

There are, of course, potential limitations regarding open source EHRs. Technology staff may require education in order to be adept with understanding and supporting open source solutions. Open source efforts are more likely to be underfunded, which impacts not only the ability to upgrade but also support of the software.

Another limitation is the perception of open source solutions as the forgotten stepchild of certification (at least in the U.S.). Only recently (mid-2009) did the CCHIT modify requirements to allow for more than just proprietary EHRs to become certified. Additional barriers include limited interoperability, fuzzy ROI, slower uptake by users than proprietary software, personnel resistance to this change, and, as previously alluded, IT employees unfamiliar with open source software. Other barriers to use of OSS/FS for implementation of EHRs or health information systems (HISs) have been identified, including resistance to change among users and IT departments, lack of documentation associated with some OSS/FS projects, and language barriers in some countries, in particular due to the documentation around many OSS/FS developments being in English, without translation (Bagayoko, Dufour, Chaacho, Bouhaddou, & Fieschi, 2010).

In the case study, we will look at one project, probably the largest, most sophisticated, and furthest developed— VistA. Here we will provide a brief overview of examples of some of the other projects currently existing, some of which have been in development for over 15 years. Many share commonalities in trying to develop components of EHRs and several have online demonstration versions available for exploration. A useful summary of the known projects and products has been provided by the AMIA OSWG (Valdes, 2008), while a number of Web sites provide catalogues of known OSS/FS developments in health (e.g., www.medfloss.org).

Examples exist of OSS/FS electronic medical records (EMRs), hospital management systems, laboratory information systems, radiology information systems, telemedicine systems, picture archiving and communications systems, and practice management systems (Janamanchi, Katsamakas, Raghupathi, & Gao, 2009). A few examples indicate this range, and more extensive lists and descriptions are available at several Web portals, including www.medfloss.org.

ClearHealth

www.clear-health.com

ClearHealth is a Web-based, fully comprehensive medical suite offering a wide range of tools to practices of all sizes. It includes scheduling and registration features; EMR including alerts, patient dashboard, laboratory ordering and results, barcode generation and uses SNOMED; access via mobile devices; billing and reporting features; and specialist clinical modules (Goulde & Brown, 2006).

Indivo

indivohealth.org

Indivo is an OSS/FS personally controlled health record (PCHR) system, using open standards. A PCHR enables individuals to own and manage a complete, secure, digital copy of their health and wellness information. Indivo integrates health information across sites of care and over time, and is actively deployed in diverse settings, for example in the Children's Hospital Boston and the Dossia Consortium (Mandl, Simons, Crawford, & Abbett, 2007; Bourgeois, Mandl, Shaw, Flemming, & Nigrin, 2009).

GNUMed

wiki.gnumed.de/bin/view/Gnumed

The GNUmed project builds free, liberated open source EMR software in multiple languages to assist and improve longitudinal care (specifically in ambulatory settings, i.e., multiprofessional practices and clinics). It is made available at no charge and is capable of running on GNU/Linux, Windows, and Mac OS X. It is developed by a handful of medical doctors and programmers from all over the world.

OpenMRS

openmrs.org/wiki/OpenMRS

OpenMRS® is a community-developed, open source enterprise EMR system platform (Wolfe et al., 2006). Of particular interest to this project is supporting efforts to actively build and/or manage health systems in the developing world to address AIDS, tuberculosis, and malaria, which afflict the lives of millions. Their mission is to foster self-sustaining health IT implementations in these environments through peer mentorship, proactive collaboration, and a code base equaling or surpassing any proprietary equivalent. OpenMRS is a multi-institution, nonprofit collaborative led by Regenstrief Institute, Inc. (regenstrief.org) and Partners In Health (pih.org), and has been implemented in 20 countries throughout the world ranging from South Africa and Kenya to Haiti, India, and China as well as in the United States. This effort is supported in part by organizations such as the World Health Organization (WHO), the Centers for Disease Control (CDC), The Rockefeller Foundation, and the President's Emergency Plan for AIDS Relief (PEPFAR).

PatientOS

www.patientos.org

PatientOS (pronounced patient-oh-es, where O and S stand for open source) is designed to function as an HIS. The software architecture, design patterns, and framework is constructed to meet the complexities of an enterprise-wide information system. Internationalization and localization are expected, including translation into multibyte languages such as Japanese.

District Health Information System

sourceforge.net/projects/dhis/

The District Health Information System (DHIS) provides for data entry, report generation, and analysis. It is part of a larger initiative for healthcare data in developing countries, called the Health Information System Programme (HISP).

OpenEHR

www.openehr.org

The openEHR Foundation is an international, not-for-profit organization working toward the development of interoperable, lifelong EHRs. However, it is also looking to reconceptualize the problems of health records, not in narrow IT-implementation terms, but through an understanding of the social, clinical, and technical challenges of electronic records for healthcare in the information society. The openEHR Foundation was created to enable the development of open specifications, software, and knowledge resources for health information systems, in particular EHR systems. It publishes all its specifications and builds reference implementations as OSS/FS. It also develops archetypes and a terminology for use with EHRs.

Tolven

www.tolvenhealth.com

Tolven is developing a range of electronic personal and clinician health record applications, using open source software and health industry standards, including Unified Medical Language Systems and Health Level 7.

European Projects and Initiatives

The EU, specifically through research and development programmes funded by the European Commission has, over the past 15 years, funded a number of OSS/FS projects and initiatives designed to explore and promote the use of OSS/FS within EU member states and organisations within the EU. While many of the earlier initiatives were projects whose outputs were not further developed, or are no longer available, several of them laid the basis for current initiatives, such as the Open Source Observatory and Repository Portal (www.osor.eu). Among the early EU projects are the following:

- SMARTIE sought to offer a comprehensive collection, or suite, of selected medical software decision tools, ranging from clinical calculators (i.e., risk factor scoring) up to advanced medical decision support tools (i.e., acute abdominal pain diagnosis)
- openECG (www.openecg.net) sought to consolidate interoperability efforts in computerized electrocardiography at the European and international levels, encouraging the use of standards. The project aimed to promote the consistent use of format and communications standards for computerized ECGs and to pave the way toward developing similar standards for stress ECG, Holter ECG, and real-time monitoring. The openECG portal still provides information on interoperability in digital electrocardiography, and one of the project's outputs, the Standard Communications Protocol for Computer-Assisted Electrocardiography (SCP-ECG) was approved as an ISO standard, ISO/DIS 11073-91064
- Open source medical image analysis (OSMIA) (www.tina-vision.net/projects/osmia.php) was designed to provide an OSS/FS development environment for medical image analysis research in order to facilitate the free and open exchange of ideas and techniques
- PICNIC (www.minoru-development.com/) was designed to help regional healthcare providers to develop and implement the next generation of secure, user-friendly regional healthcare networks, to support new ways of providing health and social care;
- FOSS: Policy Support (FLOSSpols) (www.flosspols.org/) aim to work on 3 specific tracks: government policy toward OSS/FS; gender issues in open source; and the efficiency of open source as a system for collaborative problem solving; however, it should be noted that many of these are R&D projects only and not guaranteed to

have any lasting effect or uptake beyond the lifespan of the project.

The Open Source Observatory and Repository for European public administrations (www.osor.eu) is a major portal that supports and encourages the collaborative development and reuse of publicly-financed free, libre, and open source software (FLOSS) applications developments for use in European public administrations. It is a platform for exchanging information, experiences, and FLOSS-based code. It also promotes and links to the work of national repositories, encouraging the emergence of a pan-European federation of open source software repositories. OSOR.eu is financed by the European Commission through the initiative Interoperable Delivery of European eGovernment Services to Public Administrations, Businesses and Citizens (IDABC) and is supported by European governments at national, regional, and local levels.

OSOR.eu indexes and describes a number of health-related initiatives, some directly related to providing healthcare and others with lessons that might be applicable across a number of sectors, including healthcare. Among the health-specific initiatives listed are:

- Health Atlas Ireland (www.hse.ie/eng/about/Who/Population_Health/Health_Intelligence/): An OSS/FS application using geographical information systems (GIS), health related datasets, and statistical software. It received the Irish Prime Minister Public Service Excellence Award because of its capacity to innovate and to improve the quality and the efficiency health services. Health Atlas Ireland is an open source application developed to use a Web environment to add value to existing health data; it also enables controlled access to maps, data, and analyses for service planning and delivery, major incident response, epidemiology, and research to improve the health of patients and the population.
- Santé Libre CD-ROM (silibre.free.fr/spip/): A French nurse, Christophe Tavernier, at Centre Hospitalier in La Rochelle, central France compiled a CD-ROM of OSS/FS applications for use in health organisations. It is designed to encourage students and health workers to use open source applications.

Many hospitals and healthcare institutions in the EU are increasing their use of open source software (OSOR.eu, n.d.). The University Hospital of Clermont Ferrand began using OSS/FS to consolidate data from multiple computer systems in order to improve its invoicing. The Centre Hospitalier Universitaire Tivoli in Louvière, Belgium in 2006 estimated that about 25% of its software was OSS/FS, including enterprise resource planning (ERP) software, e-mail applications, VPN software openVPN, and the K-Pacs OSS/FS DICOM viewing software. Additionally, many hospitals are moving their Web sites and portals to OSS/FS content management systems, such as Drupal. The St. Antonius hospital in the cities of Utrecht and Nieuwegein (The Netherlands) are migrating to an almost completely OSS/FS IT environment, with 3,000 desktops running Ubuntu GNU/Linux, and using OpenOffice for office productivity tools. Growing numbers of examples of the use of OSS/FS for developing hospital and HISs exist, especially in developing countries.

ORGANIZATIONS AND RESOURCES

Over the past 10 years a number of organizations have sought to explore and, where appropriate, advocate the use of OSS/FS within health, healthcare, and nursing. While some of these are still active, others have struggled to maintain activity due to having to rely primarily on voluntary efforts, which can be difficult to sustain over long periods. As a result, current efforts in promoting and publicising OSS/FS seem to be based around looser collaborations and less formal groups, often working on developing and maintaining information resources. The American Medical Informatics Association (AMIA), International Medical Informatics Association (IMIA), and the European Federation for Medical Informatics (EFMI) all have working groups dealing with OSS/FS who develop position papers, contribute workshops and other activities to conferences, and undertake a variety of other promotional activities. Each of these groups have nurses actively involved.

National (in all countries) and international health informatics organizations seem to be late in realizing the need to consider the potential impact of OSS/FS. The IMIA established an Open Source Health Informatics Working Group in 2002. It aims to work both within IMIA and through encouraging joint work with other OSS/FS organizations to explore issues around the use of OSS/FS within healthcare and health informatics. The mission of the AMIA OSWG (www.amia.org/working-group/open-source) is to act as the primary conduit between AMIA and the wider open source community. Its specific activities include providing information regarding the benefits and pitfalls of OSS/FS to other AMIA working groups, identifying useful

open source projects, and identifying funding sources and providing grant application support to open source projects. The AMIA OSWG produced a White Paper in late 2008 that not only addressed and summarised many of the issues on definitions and licensing addressed in this chapter but also provided a list of the major OSS/FS electronic health and medical record systems in use, primarily in the U.S., at the time (Valdes, 2008). The AMIA OSWG identified 12 systems, in use in over 2,500 federal government and almost 900 non–federal government sites, which among them held over 32 million individual patient records (Samuel & Sujansky, 2008; Valdes, 2008).

The IMIA-OSWG, in collaboration with several other organisations, including the AMIA-OSWG, organized a series of think-tank meetings in 2004, in Winchester, U.K., and San Francisco, U.S. The main purpose of these events was to "identify key issues, opportunities, obstacles, areas of work and research that may be needed, and other relevant aspects, around the potential for using open source software, solutions and approaches within healthcare, and in particular within health informatics, in the UK and Europe" (Murray, 2004, p.4). Three-quarters of attendees at the first event (U.K., February 2004) described their ideal vision for the future use of software in healthcare as containing at least a significant percentage of OSS/FS with nearly one-third of the attendees wanting to see an "entirely open source" use of software in healthcare. Similar findings arose from the U.S. meeting of September 2004, which had broader international participation. The emergence of a situation wherein OSS/FS would interface with proprietary software within the healthcare domain was seen to be achievable and desirable. Such use was also likely if the right drivers were put in place and barriers addressed. Participants felt the strongest drivers included the following:

- Adoption and use of the right standards
- The development of a FLOSS "killer application"
- A political mandate toward the use of FLOSS
- Producing positive case studies comparing financial benefits of FLOSS budget reductions

Participants rated the most important issues why people might use or do use FLOSS within the health domain as quality, stability, and robustness of software and data as well as long-term availability of important health data because of not being "locked up" in proprietary systems that limit interoperability and data migration. They felt the 2 most important areas for FLOSS activity by IMIA OSWG and other FLOSS groups were political activity and efforts toward raising awareness among healthcare workers and the wider public. There was a feeling, especially from the U.S. meeting, that lack of interaction between OSS/FS groups was a barrier to adoption in healthcare.

Discussions at meetings in 2008 and 2009, and in particular at the Special Topic Conference of the European Federation for Medical Informatics (EFMI) held in London in September 2008, and at the Medical Informatics Europe (MIE) 2009 conference held in Sarajevo, Bosnia and Herzegovina, reflected back on progress made since 2004 (Murray et al., 2009). It was concluded that many of the issues identified in 2004 remained relevant, and while some progress had been made in raising awareness within health and nursing communities of the possibilities of OSS/FS, the same issues were still relevant.

To date, few nursing or NI organizations have sought to address the implications of OSS/FS from a nursing-focused perspective. The first nursing or NI organization to establish a group dealing with OSS/FS issues was the Special Interest Group in Nursing Informatics of IMIA (IMIA/NI-SIG). Established in June 2003, the IMIA-NI Open Source Nursing Informatics (OSNI) Working Group has many aims congruent with those of the IMIA OSWG, but with a focus on identifying and addressing nursing-specific issues and providing a nursing contribution within multiprofessional or multidisciplinary domains. However, it has been difficult to maintain specific nursing-focused activity and many members now work within other groups, to provide nursing input.

Among providers of resources (see Table 9.5), the Medical Free/Libre and Open Source Software Web site (www.medfloss.org) provides a comprehensive and structured overview of OSS/FS projects for the healthcare domain; it also offers an open content platform to foster the exchange of ideas, knowledge, and experiences about projects.

The International Open Source Network (IOSN, www.iosn.net), funded by the United Nations Development Programme (UNDP), is a center of excellence for OSS/FS in the Asia-Pacific region. It is tasked specifically with facilitating and networking OSS/FS advocates in the region, so developing countries in the region can achieve rapid and sustained economic and social development by using affordable, yet effective, OSS/FS solutions to bridge the digital divide. While its work and case studies have a focus on developing countries, and especially those of the Asia-Pacific region, the materials they produce are of wider value. In particular, they publish a series of FOSS primers, which serve as introductory documents to OSS/FS in general as well as covering particular topic areas in greater detail. Their purpose is to raise FLOSS awareness, particularly among policy makers, practitioners and educators. While there is not currently a health offering, the general lessons from the primers on education, open standards, OSS/FS licensing and the general introductory primer to OSS/FS are useful materials for anyone wishing to explore the issues in greater detail (IOSN, n.d.).

Open Health Tools (http://www.openhealthtools.org) is an open source community, with members including national health agencies from several countries, medical standards organizations, and software product and service companies. Its vision is of enabling a ubiquitous ecosystem where members of the health and informatics professions can collaborate to build interoperable systems.

SUMMARY

OSS/FS has been described as a disruptive paradigm, but one that has the potential to improve not only the delivery of care, but also healthcare outcomes (Bagayoko et al., 2010). This chapter provides a necessarily brief introduction to OSS/FS. While we have tried to explain the underlying philosophies of the 2 major camps, only an in-depth reading of the explanations emanating from each can help to clarify the differences.

Many of the issues we have addressed are in a state of flux, therefore we cannot give definitive answers or solutions to many of them, as debate and understanding will have moved on. As we have already indicated, detailed exploration of licensing issues is best addressed with the aid of legal counsel. Readers wishing to develop a further understanding of OSS/FS are recommended to read the International Open Source Network's (IOSN) Free and Open Source Software (FOSS) Primer (Wong & Sayo, 2004). Additional resources are identified in Table 9.5.

CASE STUDY: VISTA (VETERANS HEALTH INFORMATION SYSTEM AND TECHNOLOGY ARCHITECTURE)

This case study focuses on the long-standing HIS of the U.S. Department of Veterans Affairs (VA). As outlined above, VistA is an acronym for Veterans Health Information systems and Technology Architecture. Started in the early 1980's with efforts at electronic record keeping via the Decentralized Hospital Computer Program (DHCP) information system, the

TABLE 9.5	Selected Information and Resource Web Sites

Linux Medical News: The leading news resource for health and medical applications of OSS/FS. The site provides information on events, conferences and activities, software development, and any other issues that contributors feel are relevant to the use of OSS/FS in healthcare (www.linuxmednews.com).

Medical Free/Libre and Open Source Software: A comprehensive and structured overview of Free/Libre and Open Source Software (FLOSS) projects for the healthcare domain. The Web-based resource also offers an open content platform to foster the exchange of ideas, knowledge, and experiences about the projects (www.medfloss.org).

SourceForge: SourceForge is the largest repository and development site for open source software. Many healthcare applications and other OSS/FS applications use it as the official repository of their latest versions (sourceforge.net).

Free and Open Source Software (FOSS) for Health Web Portal: The FOSS for Health Web portal aims to be a dynamic, evolving repository and venue for interaction, sharing, and supporting those who are interested in using OSS/FS in health and e-Health. It is part of the Open Source and Standards PCTA (PANACeA Common Thematic Activities) of the PAN Asian Collaboration for Evidence-based eHealth Adoption and Application (PANACeA) (www.foss-for-health.org/portal).

FOSS Primers: The IOSN is producing a series of primers on FOSS. The primers serve as introductory documents to FOSS in general, as well as covering particular topic areas in greater detail. Their purpose is to raise FOSS awareness, particularly among policy makers, practitioners, and educators. The following Web site contains summaries of the primers that have been published or are currently being produced (www.iosn.net/publications/foss-primers).

OSS Watch: OSS Watch is an advisory service that provides unbiased advice and guidance on the use, development, and licensing of free and open source software. OSS Watch is funded by the JISC and its services are available free-of-charge for higher and further education within the U.K. (www.oss-watch.ac.uk).

The Open Source Observatory and Repository (OSOR): OSOR is a platform for exchanging information, experiences, and FLOSS-based code for use in public administrations (www.osor.eu).

FOSS Open Standards/Government National Open Standards Policies and Initiatives: Many governments all over the world have developed policies and/or initiatives that advocate and favour open source and open standards in order to bring about increased independence from specific vendors and technologies, and at the same time accommodate both FOSS and proprietary software (en.wikibooks.org/wiki/FOSS_Open_Standards/Government_National_Open_Standards_Policies_and_Initiatives.).

Free & Open Source Software Portal: A gateway to resources related to free software and the open source technology movement (UNESCO, www.unesco-ci.org/cgi-bin/portals/foss/page.cgi).

The Top 100 Open Source Software Tools for Medical Professionals: (www.ondd.org/the-top-100-open-source-software-tools-for-medical-professionals)

Open Source methods, tools, and applications; open source downloads: (www.openclinical.org/opensourceDLD.html)

25 Open Source Software Projects that Are Changing Healthcare: - (mastersinhealthintformatics.com/2009/25-open-source-software-projects-that-are-changing-healthcare)

Open Source Software for Public Health: - (www.ibiblio.org/pjones/wiki/index.php/Open_Source_Software_for_Public_Health)

Clearhealth: (www.clear-health.com/content/view/41/51 & www.clear-health.com/content/blogcategory/0/38)

VistA Resources

VistA Monograph: (www4.va.gov/VistA_MONOGRAPH/index.asp)

VistA Modernization Report: (www.actgov.org/knowledgebank/studies/Documents/VistA%20Modernization%20Report%20-%20 Legacy%20to%20Leadership,%20May%204,%202010.pdf)

VistA eHealth: (www.ehealth.va.gov/EHEALTH/index.asp)

VistA Documentation Library: (www.va.gov/vdl)

Latest version of OpenVistA: (sourceforge.net/projects/worldvista)

A description of the historical development of VistA: (worldvista.org/AboutVistA/VistA_History)

Veterans Health Administration disseminated this system country-wide by the early 1990s. The name *VistA* dates back to 1996, when the project previously known as the DHCP was renamed to VistA (VistA Monograph, www4.va.gov/VistA_MONOGRAPH/ index.asp, WorldVista, worldvista.org/AboutVistA/ VistA_History).

VistA is widely believed to be the largest integrated HIS in the world. Because VistA was originally developed and maintained by the U.S. Department of VA for use in veterans' hospitals it is public domain. Its development was based on the systems software architecture and implementation methodology developed by the U.S. Public Health Service jointly with the National Bureau of Standards. VistA is in production today at hundreds of healthcare facilities across the country, from small outpatient clinics to large medical centers. It is currently used by all VA facilities throughout countries where there is a U.S. military presence, as well as in non-military clinics with both military and civilian focuses.

VistA itself is not strictly open source or free software, but because of its origin was released to, and remains in, the public domain. Because of this free availability it has been promoted by many OSS/FS organizations and individuals with some suggesting it is the "mother of OSS/FS healthcare applications" (Tiemann, 2004).

Over the years VistA has demonstrated its flexibility by supporting a wide variety of clinical settings and medical delivery systems, inside and outside of facilities ranging from small outpatient-oriented clinics to large medical centers with significant inpatient populations and associated specialties, such as surgical care or dermatology. Hospitals and clinics in many countries depend on it to manage such things as patient records, prescriptions, laboratory results, and other medical information. It contains, among other components, integrated hospital management, patient records management, medication administration (via barcoding), and medical imaging systems.

There are many versions of the VistA system in use in the U.S. Department of Defense Military Health System, the U.S. Department of Interior's Indian Health Service, and internationally, including, for example, the Berlin Heart Institute of Germany (Deutsches Herzzentrum Berlin, Deutschland), and National Cancer Institute of Cairo University in Egypt.

The use of VistA helps demonstrate some of the proposed benefits of OSS/FS. The costs associated with the acquisition and support of an HIS can indirectly affect the quality of healthcare provided by limiting the availability of timely and accurate access to electronic patient records. One solution is to lower the cost of acquiring an HIS by using a software stack consisting of open source, free software (OSS/FS). Since VistA is in the public domain and available through the U.S. Freedom of Information Act (FOIA), software license fees are not an issue with regard to deployment.

Two projects associated with, and deriving from, VistA are WorldVistA (worldvista.org/) and OpenVistA (worldvista.sourceforge.net/openvista/index.html). WorldVistA was formed as a U.S.-based nonprofit organization committed to the continued development and deployment of VistA. It aims to develop and support the global VistA community, through helping to make healthcare IT more affordable and more widely available, both within the United States and internationally.

WorldVistA extends and improves VistA for use outside its original setting through such activities as developing packages for pediatrics, obstetrics, and other hospital services not used in veterans' hospitals. WorldVistA also helps those who choose to adopt VistA to learn, install, and maintain the software.

Historically, running VistA has required adopters to pay licensing fees for the systems on which it runs: the programming environment (Massachusetts General Hospital Utility Multi-Programming System [MUMPS]) and the operating system underneath (such as Microsoft Windows or VMS [Virtual Memory System]). OpenVistA will help its adopters eliminate these fees by allowing VistA to run on the GT.M programming environment and the Linux operating system, which are both open source and free. By reducing licensing costs, OpenVistA allows users to spend their money on medicine, medical professionals, and other resources more likely to directly improve patient care. The OpenVistA project effort also transfers knowledge and expertise and builds long-term relationships between adopters and the rest of the worldwide VistA community.

The complete OpenVistA package comprises the following:

- GNU/Linux operating system GT.M, an implementation of the Standard M programming system, (M = MUMPS)VistA

- EsiObjects, a standards-compliant, object-relational, database management, and interoperability system

- Information on VistA, OpenVistA, and WorldVistA and software downloads are available at a number of Web sites, including the following:
  - www.va.gov/vdl/—VistA Documentation Library
  - www1.va.gov/vista_monograph/—VistA Monograph
  - sourceforge.net/projects/worldvista/—latest versions of OpenVistA software

A description of the historical development of VistA is available at www.worldvista.org/vista/history/index.html. A demonstration of OpenVista as a Web-based application is also available to try out. It is an installable package for Windows OS computers found at www.ehealth.va.gov/EHEALTH/CPRS_demo.asp. Once installed, the application links to a demonstration server hosted by VA Information Services, thereby allowing the user to enter and retrieve data without risk.

Started in 2000, the sharing of veterans' health information between the U.S. Department of Defense (DoD) and the VA became fullly fledged in 2004. A Directorate (VA/DoD Health Information Sharing Directorate) administers this effort between both of the agencies regarding interoperability along with other initiatives related to IT, healthcare, and data sharing. Efforts coordinated and supported by this intermediary organization currently include bidirectional health information interoperability exchange (BHIE), clinical and health information repository efforts (Clinical Data Repository/ Health Data Repository [CHDR]) initiated in 2006, transition of active personnel to veteran status via the Federal Health Information Exchange (FHIE) initiative between the DoD and the VA, laboratory data sharing (Laboratory Data Sharing Interoperability [LDSI]) not only between the DoD and the VA but also among commercial laboratory vendors, and, increased quality of care for polytrauma patients due to data exchange. The Directorate also coordinates report generation for the VA, the DoD, and the Office of Management and Budget (OMB) (VA HealthIT Sharing, www1.va.gov/ vadodhealthitsharing).

The VA also provides Web access for its veterans through VistA. These include the HealtheVet project, which provides 24 × 7 Web-based access to VA health services and information; and the Compensation and Pension Records Interchange (CAPRI), which enables veterans service organizations (VSOs) to view-only a member's EHR if necessary to assist the individual with benefit claims and drug refills.

WebVista

An example of adapting to current technology is a third party Web-based version of Vista. ClearHealth adapted the VistA EMR system to Web 2.0 tools as WebVista. Users are able to utilize the capabilities of VistA via a standard Web browser (see earlier entry on ClearHealth).

Future Direction

Based on the VistA Modernization Report (see Table 9.5 for Web address), the software is to be updated with current technologies and more importantly the source code is to be replaced with current, and more modern, code language. Of greater import is the recommendation to shift completely to an open source, open standards environment along with development efforts to support and advance VistA 2.0.

REFERENCES

Anderson, H., & Dare, T. (2009). Passport without a visa: Open source software licensing and trademarks. *International Free and Open Source Software Law Review, 1*(2), 99–110. Retrieved from http://www. ifosslr.org/ifosslr/article/view/11.

AT Internet. (2010). Web visit distribution by browser family (graphic). Retrieved from http://www. atinternet-institute.com/en-us/browsers-barometer/ browser-barometer-march-2010/index-1-2-3-195.html.

Bagayoko, C-O., Dufour, J-C., Chaacho, S., Bouhaddou, O., & Fieschi, M. (2010). Open source challenges for hospital information system (HIS) in developing countries: A pilot project in Mali. *BMC Medical Informatics and Decision Making, 10*(22). doi:10.1186/1472-6947-10-22.

Bourgeois, F. C., Mandl, K. D., Shaw, D., Flemming, D., & Nigrin, D. J. (2009). Mychildren's: Integration of a personally controlled health record with a tethered patient portal for a pediatric and adolescent population. *AMIA Annual Symposium Proceedings*, 65–69. Retrieved from http://www.ncbi.nlm.nih.gov/ pmc/articles/PMC2815447.

Bowen, S., Valdes, I., Hoyt, R., Glenn, L., McCormick, D., & Gonzalez, X. (2009). Open-source electronic Health records: Policy implications. In *Open Source EHR public policy wiki*. Retrieved from http://www. openmedsoftware.org/wiki/Open_Source_EHR_ Public_Policy

Bruggink, M. (2003). *Open source in africa: Towards informed decision-making*. The Hague, The Netherlands: International Institute for Communication and Development (IICD). Retrieved from http://www.iicd. org/files/Brief7.pdf.

Certification Commission for Health Information Technology (CCHIT). (n.d.) *Project Laika*. Retrieved from http://www.cchit.org/laika.

Cox, A. (1999). *The risks of closed source computing*. Retrieved from http://www.ibiblio.org/oswg/oswg-nightly/oswg/en_US.ISO_8859-1/articles/alan-cox/ risks/risks-closed-source/index.html.

Dravis, P. (2003). *Open source software: Perspectives for development*. Washington, DC: Global Information and Communication Technologies Department, The World Bank. Retrieved from http://www.infodev.org/en/ Publication.21.html.

European Communities. (2003). *The IDA open source migration guidelines*. Morden, Surrey: Netproject Ltd. and Interchange of Data between Administrations, European Commission. Retrieved from http:// ec.europa.eu/idabc/en/document/2623/5585.

European Communities. (2004). *e-Europe Action Plan 2005*. Brussels: European Commission, Directorate-General Information Society. Retrieved from http:// europa.eu/legislation_summaries/information_society/ l24226_en.htm.

European Communities (2005). *i2010 – A European information society for growth and employment.* Brussels: European Commission, Directorate-General Information Society. Retrieved from http://www.epractice.eu/node/281014.

Free Software Foundation (FSF). (2007). *GNU General Public License. Version 3, 29 June 2007.* Retrieved from http://www.gnu.org/licenses/gpl.html.

Free Software Foundation (FSF). (2010a). *Why 'free software' is better than 'open source'.* Boston, MA: Free Software Foundation. Retrieved from http://www.gnu.org/philosophy/free-software-for-freedom.html.

Free Software Foundation (FSF). (2010b). *The free software definition. version 1.92.* Boston, MA: Free Software Foundation. Retrieved from http://www.gnu.org/philosophy/free-sw.html.

Free Software Foundation (FSF). (2010c). *What is copyleft?* Retrieved from http://www.gnu.org/copyleft/copyleft.html.

Goetz, T. (2003). Open source everywhere. *WIRED, 11*(11), 158–167, 208–211. Retrieved from http://www.wired.com/wired/archive/11.11/opensource.html.

Goulde, M., & Brown, E. (2006). *Open source software: A primer for healthcare leaders.* California Healthcare Foundation/Forrester Research. Retrieved from http://www.chcf.org/publications/2006/03/open-source-software-a-primer-for-health-care-leaders.

International Institute of Infonomics. (2005). *Free/libre and open source software: Survey and study: FLOSS final report.* University of Maastricht, The Netherlands: International Institute of Infonomics. Retrieved from http://flossproject.org/report/index.htm.

International Open Source Network (IOSN). (n.d.). *FOSS Primers.* Retrieved from http://www.iosn.net/publications/foss-primers

International Telecommunications Union (ITU). (2009). *Definition of "open standards."* Retrieved from http://www.itu.int/ITU-T/othergroups/ipr-adhoc/openstandards.html.

Janamanchi, B., Katsamakas, E., Raghupathi, W., & Gao, W. (2009). the state and profile of open source software projects in health and medical informatics. *International Journal of Medical Informatics, 78*(7), 457–472.

Kaminski, J. (2005). *Moodle: A user-friendly, open source course management system.* Retrieved from http://www.nursing-informatics.com/moodle_article.pdf.

Leong, T. Y., Kaiser, K., & Miksch, S. (2007). Free and open source enabling technologies for patient-centric, guideline-based clinical decision support: A survey. In A. Geissbuhler, R. Haux, & C. Kulikowski (Eds.), *IMIA yearbook of medical informatics 2007.* Retrieved from http://www.schattauer.de/de/magazine/uebersicht/zeitschriften-a-z/imia-yearbook/imia-yearbook-2007/issue/special/manuscript/8416/show.html.

Mandl, K. D., Simons, W. W., Crawford, W. C. R., & Abbett, J. M. (2007). Indivo: A personally controlled health record for health information exchange and communication. *BMC Medical Informatics and Decision Making, 7*(25). doi:10.1186/1472-6947-7-25.

Merriam-Webster (2010). *Merriam-Webster OnLine.* Retrieved from http://www.merriam-webster.com/netdict/license.

Moody, G. (2001). *Rebel code: Inside linux and the open source revolution.* Cambridge, MA: Perseus Publishing.

Murray, P. J. (2003). Open source and free software— What's in it for nurses? *Information Technology in Nursing, 15*(1), 15–20.

Murray, P. J. (2004). *Open steps, release 1.0. Report of a thinktankmMeeting on free/libre/open source software in the health and health informatics domains.* Retrieved from http://www.peter-murray.net/chiradinfo/marwell04/marwell%20release%201.0.pdf.

Murray, P. J. & Oyri, K. (2005). Developing online communities with LAMP (Linux, Apache, MySQL, PHP)—The IMIA OSNI and CHIRAD experiences. In R. Englebrecht, A. Geissbuhler, C. Lovis, & G. Mihalas (Eds.), *Connecting medical informatics and bio-informatics: Proceedings of MIE2005—The XIXth international congress of the european federation for medical informatics,* 361–366. Amsterdam: IOS Press.

Murray, P. J., Oyri, K., & Wright, G. (2005). Osni. info—Using open source tools to build an international community of nurse informaticians. *Revista Cubana de Informatica Medica, 2*(5). Retrieved from http://www.cecam.sld.cu/pages/rcim/revista_8/articulo_htm/osni_info.htm.

Murray, P., Shaw, N., & Wright, G. (2002). Open source and health informatics: Taking forward the discussions. *British Journal of Healthcare Computing and Information Management 19*(5), 14.

Murray P. J., Wright G., Karopka T., Betts H., & Orel A. (2009). Open source and healthcare in europe— Time to put leading edge ideas into practice. In K. P. Adlassnig, B. Blobel, J. Mantas, & I. Masic, (Eds.), *Medical informatics in a united and healthy europe, proceedings of MIE2009,* 963–967. Amsterdam: IOS Press. Retrieved from http://person.hst.aau.dk/ska/MIE2009/papers/MIE2009p0963.pdf.

Netcraft Ltd. (2010). *May 2010 web server survey.* Retrieved from http://news.netcraft.com/archives/2010/05/14/may_2010_web_server_survey.html.

Netmarketshare. (2010). *Browser market share.* Retrieved from http://marketshare.hitslink.com/browser-market-share.aspx?qprid=0&qptimeframe=M&qpsp=136&qpnp=2.

Office of the e-Envoy. (2002). *Open source software: Use within uk government, version 1.* London: Office of the e-Envoy, e-Government Unit. Retrieved from http://archive.cabinetoffice.gov.uk/e-envoy/frameworks-oss-policy/$file/oss-policy.pdf.

Openforum Europe Ltd. (2008). *The importance of open standards in interoperability (OFE onepage brief no.1 (31.10.08.))*. Retrieved from http://www. openforumeurope.org/library/onepage-briefs/ofe-open-standards-onepage-2008.pdf.

Open Source Initiative (OSI). (n.d.). *The open source definition, version 1.9*. Retrieved from http://www. opensource.org/docs/osd.

Oyri, K., & Murray, P. J. (2005). Osni.info—Using free/libre/open source software to build a virtual international community for open source nursing informatics. *International Journal of medical Informatics, 74*, 937–945.

Peeling, N., & Satchell, J. (2001). *Analysis of the impact of open source software*. Farnborough: QinetiQ Ltd. Retrieved from http://citeseerx.ist.psu.edu/viewdoc/download?doi=10.1.1.115.8510&rep=rep1&type=pdf.

President's Information Technology Advisory Panel (PITAC). (2000). *Developing open source software to advance high end computing*. Arlington, VA: National Coordination Office for Computing, Information, and Communications. Retrieved from http://www.itrd.gov/pubs/pitac/pres-oss-11sep00.pdf.

Raymond, E. S. (2001). *The cathedral and the bazaar: Musings on linux and open source by an accidental revolutionary* (Rev. ed.). Sebastopol, CA: O'Reilly and Associates.

Raymond, E. S. (2003). *The jargon file, version 4.4.7*. Retrieved from http://www.catb.org/~esr/jargon/html/S/Swiss-Army-chainsaw.html.

Samuel, F., & Sujansky, W. (2008). *Open-source EHR systems for ambulatory care: A market assessment*. California Healthcare Foundation. Retrieved from http://www.chcf.org/~/media/Files/PDF/O/OpenSourceEHRSystemsExecSummary.pdf.

Sfakianakis, S., Chronaki, C. E., Chiarugi, F., Conforti, F., & Katehakis, D. G. (2007). Reflections on the role of open source in health information system interoperability. In A. Geissbuhler, R. Haux, & C. Kulikowski (Eds.), *IMIA yearbook of medical informatics 2007*. Retrieved from http://www.schattauer.de/de/magazine/uebersicht/zeitschriften-a-z/imia-yearbook/imia-yearbook-2007/issue/special/manuscript/8412/download.html.

Shaw, N. T., Pepper, D. R., Cook, T., Houwink, P., Jain, N., & Bainbridge, M. (2002). Open source and international health informatics: Placebo or panacea? *Informatics in Primary Care 10*(1), 39–44.

Smith, C. (2002). *Open source software and the NHS: A white paper*. Leeds, U.K.: NHSIA.

Squiz UK Ltd. (2007). *Royal college of nursing case study*. Retrieved from http://www.squiz.co.uk/clients/case-studies/royal-college-of-nursing.

Stallman, R. M. (2002). *Free software free society: Selected essays of Richard M. Stallman*. Boston, MA: GNU Press/Free Software Foundation.

Stanco, T. (2001). *World bank: InfoDev presentation*. Retrieved from http://lwn.net/2002/0117/a/stanco-world-bank.php3.

Surman, M., & Diceman, J. (2004). *Choosing open source: A guide for civil society organizations*. Toronto, Canada: Commons Group. Retrieved from http://commons.ca/articles/fulltext.shtml?x=335.

The MITRE Corporation. (2003). *Use of free and open-source software (FOSS) in the U.S. Department of Defense, version 1.2.04*. Retrieved from http://www.microcross.com/dodfoss.pdf.

Tiemann, M. (2004). *Open source: The solution in many countries*. Presentation at HIMSS Annual Conference and Exhibition 2004, Orlando, FL.

U.S. Department of Veterans Affairs. (2008). *VistA monograph*. Retrieved from http://www4.va.gov/VistA_MONOGRAPH/index.asp.

U.S. Department of Veterans Affairs (2010). *VA HealthIT sharing*. Retrieved from http://www1.va.gov/vadodhealthitsharing.

Valdes, I. (2008). *Free and open source software in healthcare 1.0. American Medical Informatics Association open source working group white paper*. Retrieved from https://www.amia.org/files/Final-OS-WG%20White%20Paper_11_19_08.pdf.

Waring, T., & Maddocks, P. (2005). Open source software implementation in the UK public sector: Evidence from the field and implications for the future. *International Journal of Information Management, 25*(5), 411–442.

Wheeler, D. A. (2007). *Why open source software/free software (OSS/FS, FLOSS or FOSS)? Look at the numbers!* Retrieved from http://www.dwheeler.com/oss_fs_why.html.

Wheeler, D. A. (2010). *Make your open source software GPL-compatible. or else*. Retrieved from http://www.dwheeler.com/essays/gpl-compatible.html.

Williams, S. (2002). *Free as in freedom: Richard Stallman's crusade for free software*. Sebastopol, CA: O'Reilly and Associates.

Wolfe, B. A., Mamlin, B. W., Biondich, P. G., Fraser, H. S. F., Jazayeri, D., Allen, C., Miranda, J., & Tierney, W. M. (2006). The OpenMRS system: Collaborating toward an open source EMR for developing countries. *Proceedings of the AMIA Annual Symposium 2006*, 1146.

Wong, K., & Sayo, P. (2004). *Free/open source software: A general introduction*. Kuala Lumpur, Malaysia: International Open Source Network (IOSN). Retrieved from http://www.iosn.net/downloads/foss_primer_current.pdf.

WorldVista (n.d.). *VistA history*. Retrieved from http://worldvista.org/AboutVistA/VistA_History.

Yellowlees, P. M., Marks, S. L., Hogarth, M., & Turner, S. (2008). Standards-based, open-source electronic health record systems: A desirable future for the U.S. health industry. *Telemedicine and e-Health, 14*(3): 284–288. doi:10.1089/tmj.2007.0052.

Zymaris, C. (2003). *A comparison of the GPL and the Microsoft EULA*. Retrieved from http://www.cyber.com.au/cyber/about/comparing_the_gpl_to_eula.pdf.

Mobile Computing Platforms

Kathleen G. Charters / Thomasine D. Guberski

• OBJECTIVES

1. Describe utilization of a mobile computing platform in clinical care.
2. Apply principles of the Health Insurance Portability and Accountability Act of 1996 (HIPAA) to the utilization of a mobile computing platform in clinical practice.
3. Analyze the usefulness of specific clinical applications for a mobile computing platform using a structured critique format.
4. List 3 advantages and 3 disadvantages of utilizing a mobile computing platform in clinical practice.

• KEY WORDS

mobile computing
form factor
mobile healthcare system
mHealth
HIPAA
clinical applications

MOBILE COMPUTING PLATFORMS

Mobile computing is pervasive. Although some mobile devices do not provide wireless communication, the trend since 2000 (Turisco, 2000) has been an ever-expanding constellation of devices that provide wireless connectivity, are small in size and lightweight, consume little power, and have a full range of functionality with intuitive interactions. The public expectation is that people will be connected to the Internet at all times and in all places. This expectation has driven development of a robust infrastructure.

The explosion of consumer wireless technology has also triggered a rapid evolution of public expectations. The public no longer accepts having to use a separate device for each type of communication or activity. Public expectation is that a single device will perform multiple functions. This expectation has driven development of software applications that run on a variety of devices. Due to a limited display area on the smallest devices, interfaces have evolved to be simpler and more intuitive. This convergence of public expectation with technological infrastructure and innovation has produced a greater range of computer devices used in a greater range of environments and activities (Poslad, 2009).

Individual use of mobile information technology (IT) follows a continuum along several dimensions: the desired physical size and characteristics of the platform, the length of time a mobile device operates before requiring recharging, the way a device accesses a network, the availability of applications to support an individual's work, and the type and level of security.

157

When evaluating usefulness of a computing platform for an individual, all these factors are evaluated against the individual's workflow to determine what combination best supports their work. The question, "What works best for a nurse?" has no one right or wrong answer; however, it is possible to come up with a best fit to meet a given nurse's needs.

Mobile computing technologies have been widely applied to a variety of businesses (May, 2009). Many healthcare applications exist for individual mobile computing; for example, as of August 2010, the Apple iTunes store lists over 5,300 iPhone apps categorized as Health, 3,000 iPad apps categorized as Health, and over 1,300 iTunes University courses under the heading Health and Medicine. These applications are for healthcare team members and healthcare consumers. Applications for large-scale organizational mobile computing in healthcare delivery systems are under development (Hardy, 2009).

Use of mobile computing in a healthcare system depends on acceptance by healthcare professionals. Wu, Wang, and Lin (2007, p. 66) found "compatibility, perceived usefulness, and perceived ease of use significantly affected healthcare professional behavioral intent." Compatibility refers to the degree to which use is perceived to be consistent with values, experiences, and needs. Perceived usefulness is defined as the degree to which a healthcare professional believes use will enhance the professionals' performance. Perceived ease of use refers to the degree to which a healthcare professional believes use will be free of physical and mental effort. Behavioral intention to use refers to the degree to which a healthcare professional's motivation is to use a mobile healthcare system. Wu, Wang, and Lin found younger healthcare providers are more fluent with new technology, and that tablet computers are the major platform for mobile computing in healthcare systems. Although they found practice compatibility is the most significant antecedent for mobile healthcare system success, they suggested other factors influencing acceptance by healthcare professionals include privacy and security, system and information quality, and mobile device limitations. Lehmann, Prasad, and Scornavacca (2008) found that factors such as hardware and device selection, network coverage, immediacy of decision-making information and an information system governance structure that recognizes the specifics of mobile technology management are essential enhancements to the Information System Success Model for predicting the fate of mobile applications.

Mobility brings with it constraints. Mobile device limitations include screens and keyboards too small to use easily, health hazards (distraction leading to automobile or workplace accidents, medical device interference), security concerns (a multilayered approach is required, but few devices have any security), power consumption (long battery life should not significantly add to size or weight), connectivity quality (need ubiquitous, accurate signal reception), and bandwidth (high speed over a long range).

Appropriate strategies and workflows must be created to mitigate these limitations. Gebauer and Shaw (2004) found screen and keyboard size are the most significant factors for mobile application usage. This is synergistic with not needing to take a lot of time and effort to learn or reach familiarity with a mobile healthcare application and the perceived benefit. Selection of screen and keyboard size must take into account the intended use. To support extensive reading of text and a significant amount of typing, select the appropriate device sized to support that level of activity (e.g., a 7-inch screen with a landscape keyboard). Avoid texting or speaking on the phone while driving (The White House, 2009). Post restricted areas where mobile devices interfere with medical devices (e.g., the neonatal intensive care unit). Employ a multilayered approach to security to protect mobile devices from multiple threats. When securing data on wireless networks, the data at rest and the data in transit must be secured (Yasin, 2009). This may entail using a virtual private network (VPN), user authentication, network access control, encryption, and client-level security to protect mobile devices from "malicious code, hackers, data theft, and unauthorized access" (Mobile Defense Measures, 2009, p. 7). Select mobile devices with a battery life long enough to cover a typical workday before requiring recharging. Ensure the wireless network adequately covers the work area and facilitates timely responses.

MOBILE HEALTHCARE SYSTEMS

Early adopters of mobile technology are leading the way in adapting this platform for healthcare purposes. This adaptation is occurring at the individual level in the healthcare professional community and in the healthcare consumer community. Because of the expectations of the healthcare consumer community and the experiences of early adopters in the healthcare professional community, in the future healthcare organizations will offer mobile healthcare systems as an extension of existing healthcare delivery applications. User expectations and requirements are driving mobile healthcare application content. Relevant materials and functions are incorporated into both lifestyle and workflow.

When the practice of healthcare and public health is supported by mobile technology, this is referred to as mHealth (also known as mobile health). Using mobile communication devices to provide health services and healthcare information increases access to healthcare, improves the ability of the healthcare team to diagnose and track diseases, and expands healthcare team access to ongoing education and training. Mobile communication technologies enable communication in motion, allowing individuals to contact each other irrespective of time and place. This is especially useful in remote areas. Mobile technology integration in healthcare has the potential to promote healthy lifestyles, and improve decision making by healthcare professionals and their patients. Healthcare quality is enhanced through improved access to medical and health information and instantaneous communication. Increased use of mobile technology can help reduce healthcare costs by improving efficiencies in the healthcare system and promoting prevention through communication supporting behavior change. Mobile communication technologies can be leveraged to support existing workflows within the healthcare system and between the healthcare delivery system and the general public.

To be successful in making the transition to mobile healthcare systems, organizations need to provide healthcare professionals with education regarding the organizational goals that are met through the use of mobile computing and the advantages for the healthcare professional. The most common fear expressed by healthcare professionals is that mobile computing will add yet another layer of activities to an already overburdened healthcare delivery system. However, early adopters have discovered that mobile computing is not an addition to what they were doing, but rather a substitution for activities in which they were already engaged. The mobile platform gives healthcare professionals the advantage of not being tied to a specific location in order to complete their tasks. Mobile healthcare computing allows real-time access to information and resources at the point of care. The variety of sizes of devices allows individuals to select the form factor that best conforms to their needs. The intended use of the device drives selection of the size.

The smallest form factor may suffice if the primary need is to listen to a continuing education podcast (Kleinpell & Bruinsma, 2010; Kleinpell, Hravnak, Settles, & Melander, 2009). For example, the nurse is using an MP4 player to listen to a podcast about mobile telemedicine. If the primary need is to stay connected by voice and by real-time messages while having access to other sources of information, a smart phone with 2 different networking modalities may best meet that need (Spader, 2009). For example, the user selects an iPhone with G3 network access and both voice and data services. The user is able to receive phone calls, e-mail, and text messages, and can seamlessly look up information while they are engaged in a conversation (Gamble, 2009). For example, a patient calls and indicates he is suicidal. The healthcare professional needs to locate and activate the support system closest to where that patient is located while continuing to engage the patient.

If the primary need is to have access to text and images, a slightly larger mobile device such as a tablet with an e-reader application may be the best solution. For example, the provider is making rounds and wants to look up relevant medical reference material on a device that fits in a lab coat pocket, so the user selects an iPad. If the primary need is to share text, images, and multimedia with patients and collect patient-entered data, a notebook-sized device may best meet that need. For example, a provider wants to educate a patient about an institutional review board (IRB)-approved experimental procedure, so the provider uses a Macbook Air to show a short video and administer a Web-based quiz to check for understanding. The patient consents to complete a secure Web-based screening form, which is stored in a research database (Fetter, 2009a, 2009b).

The healthcare consumer community is engaging in parallel decision making about what form factor best fits their lifestyle (Godwin-Jones, 2008). For example, a healthy man wants to capture the number of steps taken during the day, so he selects an iPod nano and uses the fitness application. When he synchronizes his iPod nano, he uploads his data to the Nike application to see his progress toward the fitness goal he selected. A patient is taking a course on chronic disease management and uses an MP4 player to listen to deep relaxation exercises. A child with a chronic disease uses mobile technology to get health reminders and report her health activities. Using mobile technology, she records her readings and activities in real time wherever she happens to be. Mobile technology gives a diabetic teenager a degree of freedom that would otherwise not be possible. Using a smartphone does not set a teenager apart from other teenagers, because using a smartphone is common practice. For example, a juvenile-onset diabetic teenager uses a smartphone to get reminders about checking his blood glucose and taking insulin (Project HealthDesign, 2010). The teenager documents a blood sugar level that exceeds the limit set by his healthcare coordinator. When the measure recorded exceeds the set limit, an alert is sent. The healthcare coordinator gets a message on her smartphone that a patient safety alert is available. The healthcare coordinator uses her smartphone to logon and retrieve the alert, and then calls the patient to have a conversation about what is going on. Based on this real-time communication the healthcare coordinator can provide guidance about what steps to take.

Older Internet users are significantly more likely than younger generations to look online for health information. Health questions drive Internet users age 73 and older to the Internet just as frequently as they drive Generation Y users, outpacing teens by a significant margin. Researching health information is the third most popular online activity with the most senior age group, after e-mail and online search (Jones & Fox, 2009, p. 7). Generation X is the most likely group to look for health information online (p. 10).

Geriatric patients may use mobile technology to update their health information in their personal health record. For example, a geriatric patient in stage 3 renal failure cannot sit at the computer for long periods because her feet swell. She uses an iPad because she can sit in her recliner with her feet elevated while she updates her medication list in My HealtheVet (http://www.myhealth.va.gov) prior to her healthcare appointment. She wants to let her primary care provider know about the medication changes her nephrologist made. The patient selected the iPad because the screen is large enough to see easily and to type on comfortably. She has a concern that one of her new medications is causing a problem, because she has periods when her heart starts racing. From her recliner she looks up a drug-drug interaction checker, and discovers there is a known interaction between the new medication and a medication she routinely takes for her heart (Jonas & Burns, 2010; Perez, 2009). She then uses the iPad to securely message her primary care provider with the updated medication list and her concern about this new symptom, and asks if she can discuss this when she comes in for her appointment. Her provider receives an e-mail on his mobile device indicating there is a secure message, and logs on to read the message. This gives the provider an opportunity to assign the secure message to the clinical pharmacist for her input prior to the scheduled appointment.

As with any application of technology, there are advantages and disadvantages to using a mobile platform for healthcare. Setting realistic expectations about response times is essential for health and well-being. Being connected at all times in all places makes setting boundaries and managing expectations a survival skill.

CONTINUUM OF PLATFORMS FOR MOBILE COMPUTING

Mobile Device Physical Characteristics

The distinctions between different forms of personal computers used for mobile computing are relative according to characteristics such as weight, display size, and interface for data entry. In general, platforms used for mobile computing weigh less than 5 pounds, have screens 13 inches or smaller, and support wireless network access (see Table 10.1). A smartphone (a hybrid device combining wireless telephone, e-mail, Internet access, and device-optimized applications) is at the opposite end of the networking continuum. A smartphone represents a convergence between computing and communication. A smartphone fits in a shirt pocket, weighs ounces, has a 2-inch or slightly larger display, and can access a cellular network for both voice and data (see Table 10.1). In contrast, an ultralight MP4 handheld device is used without

TABLE 10.1	Continuum of Mobile Device Physical Characteristics				
Characteristic	Laptop	Netbook	Tablet	Smartphone	Ultralight MP4
Weight	4 lbs	2 lbs	<2 lbs	2–9 oz	1–2 oz
Screen size	10–13 in.	7–9 in.	4–7 in.	1.5–4 in.	1–2.5 in.
Wireless network access	WiFi WiMax	WiFi WiMax	WiFi G3	Cellular data network Bluetooth	None
Voice communication	VoIP	VoIP	VoIP	Cellular network	None

TABLE 10.2	Examples of Mobile Devices				
Characteristic	**Laptop**	**Netbook**	**Tablet**	**Smartphone**	**Ultralight MP4**
Device	MacBook	MacBook Air	iPad	iPhone 4	iPod nano
Weight	4.7 lbs	3.0 lbs	1.6 lbs	4.8 oz	1.28 oz
Screen size	13.3 in.	13.3 in.	9.7 in.	3.5 in.	2.2 in.
Wireless network access	Wi-Fi	Wi-Fi Bluetooth	Wi-Fi	Wi-Fi 3GS GSM	None
Camera	Front facing	Front facing	No	Front facing Rear facing With HD video	Yes with video
Input	Full-size keyboard and trackpad	Full-size keyboard and trackpad	Full-size multi-touch screen	Miniature multi-touch screen*	Click wheel
Battery life	10 hours for wireless Web browsing	5 hours for wireless Web browsing	10 hours using Wi-Fi 9 hours using 3G for wireless Web browsing	10 hours using Wi-Fi 7 hours using 3G for wireless Web browsing	24 hours for playing music

*A Bluetooth full-size external keyboard is supported

wireless network connectivity. It does provide mobile computing support, but it does not provide communication support.

Laptop Notebook Tablet Smartphone and MP4 Physical Characteristics

A laptop computer is light enough to hand carry, has a slightly larger display, and slightly more processing power and storage capacity than a notebook computer (see Table 10.2). It is possible to add external devices to a laptop or a notebook to enhance any shortcoming. The trade-off is that adding external devices increases the weight and decreases the mobility of the system. Laptop and notebook computers are designed to run on battery power. This greatly enhances the ability of the user to have a computer available when traveling. The next step in the progression of mobile computing devices is the tablet, a smaller lighter computer. The most important difference between a laptop or notebook and a tablet is the use of a touchcreen for input on a tablet.

An even more mobile form of computer is the smartphone. Weighing in at a half pound or less, it is small enough to fit in a shirt pocket (see Table 10.2). Features differentiating a tablet from a smartphone include the size of the keyboard and the technology used for voice communication. A smartphone comes with a

miniature keyboard. An MP3 has many characteristics in common with the smartphone, but tends to have a longer battery life since it does not support voice communication.

Mobile devices depend on batteries. The length of time a battery supports use of the device and the length of time it takes for the battery to recharge determine the usefulness of the device. Users are frustrated by limited battery life that does not support their workflow. Rechargeable batteries may be used under a reasonably wide temperature range; however, recharging batteries should only be done at room temperature. Moderate temperatures produce better results and a safer environment.

Mobile Device Form Factor Trade-Offs

The key to a mobile device is the nonbulky display. A computer that can be held in the palm of one hand and used with the other hand is a handheld device. For example, an iPod Touch is considered a handheld. The key to a handheld device is the miniature keyboard. Note the trade-off in functions. As size gets smaller, there are corresponding limitations on what a computer can do. The smallest mobile devices are also the most limited in screen size, memory, storage space, and ease of entering data (e.g., using a miniature keyboard).

A mobile computer may be used as a stand-alone device or as part of a network. (Smartphones, by definition, are part of a cellular network.) The Institute of Electrical and Electronics Engineers (IEEE) establishes the rules that govern how networks work. Greater bandwidth means a higher rate of data transmission.

An MP4 device is designed to work both as a stand-alone computer and as a device that communicates with a computer. The most common way for an MP4 device to communicate with a computer is through a Universal Serial Bus (USB) cable. The MP4 device is synchronized and recharged through the USB cable. The person doing the synchronization has control over what is shared (e.g., music, podcasts, videos).

Wireless Devices

For a computer to connect wirelessly to a network it must have special hardware meeting specific standards for wireless communication (see the IEEE 802.11 series). The most common standard used for this is IEEE 802.11 that governs how local area networks (LANs) connect wirelessly using wireless fidelity (Wi-Fi). Specific airwave GHz bands have specific communication standards (IEEE 802.11a, 802.11b, 802.11g, and 802.11i).

Laptop and notebook computers may come equipped to do both hardwired (Ethernet) and wireless (Wi-Fi or Bluetooth) connections. Mobile laptop and notebook computers are also wireless enabled, most commonly using Wi-Fi following IEEE 802.11 standards to connect to a wireless LAN (WLAN). Tablet computers typically are designed for both hardwire and 2 types of wireless connectivity. They often have an Ethernet port for cable connection to the LAN as well as both Wi-Fi (following IEEE 802.11 standards) and Bluetooth (an open wireless technology standard for exchanging data over short distances using short wavelength radio transmissions). Bluetooth creates personal area networks (PANs) with high levels of security. Smartphones use cellular telephone technology for voice communication and may use any of the other wireless communication protocols as well.

Why Use a Mobile Device?

In the clinical practice setting, time is a precious commodity. Practices that allow a nurse to manage and organize time effectively and efficiently are valuable. One strategy for better use of time is to organize data and information so that it is readily available when needed. Most nurses would like to eliminate sticky notes and other small paper reminders and the multiple small reference books that fill (and fall out of) lab-coat pockets. Nurses in the acute care setting would like to document data as they collect it, instead of writing data down one place and transcribing it into the health record at a later point in time. Nurses with the Visiting Nurses' Association gather information at the time of the visit and need to turn that information into an electronic version to support documentation requirements for billing and reimbursement (Barthold, 2009). In primary care, nurses complain about the lack of time to accurately bill for office visits and procedures. Other clinic nurses would like a method to track patients. Lack of time to look up pertinent clinical information is a complaint often voiced by nurses in clinical practices.

One potential solution to manage and organize time is a paper-based daily planner. That helps solve some time management issues, but a paper-based daily planner does not address several other issues, especially availability of clinical information at the point of care. What if one small device that fits easily into the palm of a hand, or more importantly, in a lab-coat pocket, could help nurses improve patient care by bringing information to the nurse at the point of care at the moment that information is most needed? That device is the mobile computer. Although mobile computers share basic functions such as an address book, calculator, date book, memo pad, to-do list, and security, the attractiveness for nurses and other healthcare providers lies in the ability to customize the mobile computer's usefulness with applications specifically developed to assist healthcare providers in the clinical setting. The usefulness of standard applications in clinical practice as well as categories of specific clinical application software categories follow.

Generic Functions and Their Application to Clinical Practice. The mobile computer evolved as an information technology to support personal information management. A mobile computer is a handheld device that allows the user to organize and manage personal information. A mobile computer provides an address book, a calculator, date book, memo pad (for typed input), notepad (for hand-written input), to-do lists, and a way to synchronize part or all of this information with another computer in order to help the user organize their time and tasks. Most mobile computers allow the user to access the Internet via a Wi-Fi connection. The focus of generic applications is to allow individuals to organize and manage their information, including their time, data, and money. Most mobile computers provide voice recognition, take photos, and play music.

The *address book* is an always-alphabetical list that has fields for name, address, phone number, organization, e-mail, and other data. The entries can be categorized, however, as the nurse likes. This allows multiple categories such as attending physicians, nursing units, clinics, and staff members to be created.

The *calculator* is a basic function calculator, capable of basic mathematical operations. Calculators for specific medical calculations are available.

The *date book* or calendar function allows nurses to keep track of their schedules, from a daily, weekly, or monthly perspective. Reminder alarms can be set to alert nurses to upcoming events for themselves or their patients. Reoccurring events can be entered once and repeated multiple times. Some systems will allow providers to download their patient schedule.

The *memo pad* provides a place to compose memos, which can be synchronized with another computer. One use is to produce and edit project outlines. Many people use this function to download their written personalized "peripheral brains."

The *to-do list* allows the nurse to create multiple lists and keep track of tasks to be done daily, weekly, or monthly. Components of the lists can be prioritized by level of importance and/or due date.

Standard mobile computer functions supporting personal information management can readily be adapted to assist in professional activities management. The advantages for healthcare providers using the standard functions include saving time through improved access to and management of information. Common examples include saving time and improving information management. Nurses save time looking up contact information when information for frequently contacted individuals is in one place, eliminating searching for beeper numbers and phone numbers in several sources. The ability to download a patient schedule into the date book saves time by enabling the provider to review test results prior to the patient encounter. The *notepad* feature is useful in keeping track of changes in patient orders during rounds.

Applications

Several very useful applications that facilitate professional time management are available for mobile devices. These applications may work as stand-alone programs with no need to connect to anything once they are loaded onto the mobile computer (e.g., a viewer for reading an e-book). Some applications require periodic asynchronous updating (e.g., a subscription with quarterly updates). Other applications are designed to connect to a WLAN each time they are launched (e.g., a wireless e-mail application), and still others can be downloaded directly to the device. Typically, an application is downloaded to a computer and then during synchronization the application is put on the mobile device. If the application requires periodic updating, it will prompt the user when it is time to load the update. If the application depends on connecting with a WLAN, it will seek out a WLAN when it is launched. When the mobile computer has wireless capability and access to a WLAN, e-mail can be accessed by, and responses sent directly from, the device in real time.

General Freeware, Shareware, and Commercial Applications

A mobile computer may be used for viewing information, or to perform office automation tasks (e.g., to create, view, and edit documents, spreadsheets, and databases), or to browse the Internet. There are 3 types of general applications: document and image viewers, office automation applications, and Web browsers.

Document viewers allow the user to download and read text files. Many publishers use special formats for their publications that require document viewers. Document viewers allow formatting, indexing of content, and special characters to be preserved when documents are downloaded. Some programs allow the viewer to bookmark sections of the document for quick reference. Most do not permit editing of a commercially purchased publication. Several document readers are available and many publishers specify which document reader must be used for their publication.

There is a mobile device version of Adobe Reader or Acrobat Reader available for free download. The application allows .pdf extension documents to be downloaded and read on a mobile device. Although documents not specially formatted for the device can be opened using this application, formatting may not be preserved, making the document difficult to read.

A *graphics viewer* for image viewing may be useful for individuals practicing in specialties where images are a basic requirement. Most mobile devices allow the user to take digital photos.

Office utilities allow the user to download, view, revise and upload documents to a computer. Database programs are available to read data files and can be used to create databases. A database is especially useful for remote data capture of research data that is aggregated in one central database.

Web browsers are another popular application. These applications may also function as offline HTML document readers. Content is provided, often free of charge, to the subscriber, through a wide variety of channels (specially formatted Web sites). The content is updated regularly and provides news about a particular area or topic selected by the user. The user can do an update as part of the synchronization process or using a wireless or Wi-Fi hot spot connection.

With these additional applications, a travel charger, and a portable keyboard, the mobile device may function as a mobile office. A user so equipped may leave the larger computer behind when traveling. All the information and equipment needed to do a presentation can be available in a handheld.

Clinical Applications by Functional Categories

Once users discovered the effectiveness of a handheld device for managing personal information, they envisioned the usefulness of a mobile device in supporting their workflow. Numerous applications that support healthcare professionals in their delivery of care are now available. There are applications that support clinical care (e.g., medications, treatments, documentation, clinical decision making), administrative functions (e.g., reporting), research (e.g., data collection), and education (e.g., presentations) (Health Sciences & Human Services Library, 2010). Available healthcare applications range from simple reference material (e.g., electronic books and journal articles), to interactive tracking databases (e.g., coding care delivery services for billing purposes), to highly sophisticated decision support systems (e.g., interactive clinical consultation applications).

Clinicians utilize their mobile devices to support their workflow by having ready access to relevant information at the point of care. Clinical applications are the reason information is readily available. Because of its mobility, a handheld provides information and decision support at the point of care. Mobile computing value to the clinician increases with wireless connectivity to clinical information sources at the point of care. The ability to quickly check on signs and symptoms that could indicate a medical emergency, review appropriate drug doses for a less familiar drug, check for drug interactions, review the latest evidence-based management guidelines for a particular problem, and utilize applications for differential diagnoses and clinical decision making including management, all contribute to improving patient care. Available applications generally fall into 1 of 3 categories: clinical references, patient tracking, and billing and coding.

Clinical Applications by Category

Categories of *clinical references* include journals, general and specialty references, pharmacologic references, medical calculators, and clinical decision support tools for treatment and/or clinical consultation. Mobile clinical references include applications that scan journals for specified topics, general and specialty practice electronic resources, pharmacology databases, medical calculators, and clinical decision-making applications. Clinical references account for most of the freeware and shareware healthcare applications.

The amount of new patient care information available in journals can be overwhelming and often providers do not have the luxury of setting aside time each day for reading. The ability to access the Internet to find comprehensive clinically relevant information related to patient care is extremely valuable. There is the ability to customize the selection of journals by area of interest. With some Web browsing services, MEDLINE and PubMed searches are possible. Other Web sites allow the user to order searches on a particular topic and then deliver appropriate journal abstracts and articles to the mobile device.

Most well-known healthcare references are commercially available in a special format that works well on a mobile device. Specialty information is available in the form of standard text references. For example, the National Institutes of Health Web site, through the National Heart, Lung, and Blood Institute (NHLBI), provides electronic guidelines and applications for the diagnosis and management of asthma, cholesterol, hypertension, and obesity. The Centers for Disease Control and Prevention provides screen reader device text-only versions of documents such as the Childhood Immunization Schedule, STD Treatment Guidelines, and Guidelines for Management of CommunityAcquired Pneumonia. Evidence-based clinical practice guidelines, which support provider decisions about appropriate healthcare, provide the recommended course of action in specific situations. Guidelines are available from government agencies and professional organizations. The National Guideline Clearing House has links to multiple practice guideline sites.

Other Web sites are sources of clinical practice information and are subscription based. PEPID has customized programs available through subscription. Subscribers have a variety of evidence-based information tools.

Pharmacology databases are probably the most frequently used application. Many applications are available, including both freeware (see eDruginfo.com) and subscription applications. All applications contain drug information for prescription drugs and some are bundled with additional applications that support clinical decision making.

Some applications allow the user to easily check for multiple drug-drug interactions.

Medical calculator applications are available to assist providers who use standard formulas for calculation of body mass index (BMI), creatinine clearance, and so forth. Many are available as free downloads and may be included as a module in other applications.

Several drug database programs to aid in the selection of antibiotics are available and function as *clinical decision support* tools. There are hyperlinks between the treatments suggested and detailed information about the specific antibiotic. Information about drug interactions, renal dosing, and other data are available.

Infectious disease applications contain information that providers need at the point of care. A clinical decision support tool is designed to assist providers in the area of differential diagnosis by chief complaint. Once the problem has been translated into a medical condition, the provider can seamlessly navigate to tests. Information available includes the advantages and disadvantages of the test, normal and abnormal results and their cause, and factors affecting the test. When the drugs and other therapies section is accessed, detailed information about the drug is available without having to access another application.

In summary, mobile devices can be optimized for clinical practice through the utilization of applications designed to support healthcare providers by providing ready access to journals and electronic resources, pharmacology databases, medical calculators, and clinical decision support tools. Bringing this information to the point of care should improve patient outcomes.

Patient tracking software is a handheld patient management tool that allows the provider to track a variety of patient information. Fields often included in the application include demographic information, physical examination findings, laboratory and other test results, clinical progress, and assessment notes. Entering data on each patient, especially in a busy office practice, can be time consuming. This is often a reason cited not to use patient tracking software. Some time can be saved with the use of pull-down menus available on several programs for demographic information, names of common laboratory and other tests, and

physical examination findings. An alternative to entering all data on the mobile device is to enter data on the desktop and synchronize it. Many programs can be integrated with a desktop computer system. The ability to share patient information is most helpful for on-call coverage. Several patient tracking programs are available as freeware or commercial products. One limiting factor with patient tracking software occurs when there is a lack of communication with other hospital information systems such as the laboratory or X-ray department. Another limiting factor is when the clinical information system does not support mobile device data sharing, so information cannot be downloaded to the mobile device from other departments and the information must be entered by hand. Many mobile computing users do not consider patient tracking valuable unless it is integrated with the hospital computer system.

Billing and coding applications are designed to document charges for patient visits, procedures, and medical diagnoses. The utilization of these applications may increase charges for practices. These applications allow coding of evaluation and management (E&M) charges, International Classification of Diseases (ICD) codes, and Current Procedural Terminology (CPT) codes.

HIPAA Implications

The HIPAA administrative simplification provisions include electronic transactions and code sets, security, unique identifiers, and privacy. If a computer has individually identifiable health information or protected health information stored on it, the person who maintains or transmits that information is responsible for reasonable and appropriate safeguards.

Asynchronous Communication

A reasonable level of security for a mobile device with individually identifiable health information is to have the device protected by having to enter an ID and password in order to use it. In case the device is lost or stolen, there should be an application that will wipe any information on the device in the event the user incorrectly enters an ID and password a set number of times. If the hardwire synchronization is between a protected device and a desktop computer that is secure (located in a locked room, protected by an ID and password to log on) that point-to-point transmission is secure. Users should be trained by the organization in their responsibility for maintaining privacy and security of the data.

Synchronous Communication and Wireless Devices

All the considerations for asynchronous communication remain, but in addition, when a device is wireless enabled, the individually identifiable health information that is transmitted must be protected during the process of transmission as well as when it resides on a mobile device. This is typically done through encryption. The data exchanged is encrypted when it leaves and is decrypted when it arrives at its destination. Encryption and decryption take time, so system performance will be slower than if the data were not encrypted.

Evaluation of Clinical Applications

There are hundreds of applications available to support healthcare providers. Some problems exist. The quality of all applications is not equal. Not all applications are peer reviewed. Information may not be updated quickly (e.g., the standard for updating drug information may be a minimum of quarterly), if the vendor only provides annual updates. This is a serious deviation from the standard of practice. Some freeware applications collect information about users and make the information available commercially. Most sites will allow the nurse to preview software prior to purchase. Some sites will allow the nurse to download a preview application or the entire application to use for a short time in order to evaluate usefulness before making a purchase. If the nurse should have a problem with the download or running the application, sites often provide technical support to assist in problem resolution.

A systematic approach to evaluating clinical applications starts with an understanding of the goal of the nurse selecting and using that software. Factors to consider include the amount of time and level of effort required to install and successfully run the application. There should be a way to install and back up the application. The human-computer interface should allow the user to comfortably view the information (it may be necessary to change the font size or color scheme to enhance the contrast). The user should be able to comfortably enter information (e.g., use a stylus and the keyboard for input). If the mobile device "hangs" the user should be able to do a soft reset and not lose data. The user should have control over the synchronization process. The battery life should accommodate the user's workflow. The user should be able to get the information desired out of the application in the

format desired. The benefit derived from using the application should offset the cost of the application.

CASE STUDY: INTEGRATION OF INFORMATION TECHNOLOGY INTO CLINICAL PRACTICE

You have downloaded your clinic schedule for today (Monday) onto your handheld computer. All the patients are familiar to you including Ms. Y who has rescheduled an appointment and has not been seen for several months. Ms. Y arrives for her appointment. You open your PatientKeeper application and update the following information during the visit: Ms. Y is a 55-year-old African American woman with a history of diabetes mellitus type 2 and hyperlipidemia. She was seen in the emergency room over the weekend for vomiting and diarrhea and was told she had dehydration and a urinary tract infection. She was given IV fluids and a prescription for Macrobid, which she was unable to fill. She takes Lipitor 40 mg orally every evening and Glucotrol XL 5 mgm daily. The diarrhea is gone and she has very little nausea today. She has no drug allergies. On physical examination, she has a temperature of 100°F oral, a pulse of 92, respirations of 16 per minute, a BP of 116/75, and her height is 65 inches. She weighs 146 pounds. The BP is within her normal range. Her random BS in the office was 103. She has some slight tenderness over the L flank. The rest of the physical examination is unremarkable.

The question is: What are the current treatment options for this patient? You access the TheraDoc application on your mobile handheld. When you enter the data, serum creatinine is requested. You access the ER labs and her creatinine at that time was 1.6. You review her previous labs and discover her previous creatinine was 1.2. You make a note to reorder a creatinine today. A urinalysis done in the office was negative for WBCs but a small amount of leukocyte esterase is present. The recommendations list several drugs, including ciprofloxacin, which you prefer to use. You access the Johns Hopkins Antibiotic Guide to review the evidence-based practice guideline information. The preferred antibiotic, by the Infectious Disease Society of America, is ciprofloxacin. Concerned about her increased creatinine, you access a medmath program and calculate her creatinine clearance which is 41. Using Epocrates Rx, you check to see if a dose adjustment of Cipro is necessary. It is not. You also run a drug interaction check. There is an interaction that can result in a slight risk of hypoglycemia. Since she does her own blood sugars at home you remind her about calling if her blood sugar drops below 70. You make a note to follow up on her creatinine, which was drawn today, and schedule her to return in a few days. You review the Electronic Preventive Services Selector (ePSS) U.S. Preventive Services Task Force (USPSTF) and remind her that you need to discuss her health maintenance at the next visit. At the end of the day, you synchronize your mobile device with your desktop, updating the databases.

REFERENCES

Barthold, M. (2009). Standardizing electronic nursing documentation. *Nursing Management, 40*(5), 15–17.

Fetter, M. (2009a). Interoperability: Making information systems work together. *Issues in Mental Health Nursing, 30*(7), 470–472.

Fetter, M. (2009b). The Internet: Backbone of the World Wide Web. *Issues in Mental Health Nursing, 30*(4), 281–282.

Gamble, K. (2009). Cutting the cord: CIOs are leveraging wireless technologies to help nurses deliver patient care safely and efficiently. *Healthcare Informatics, 26*(9), 30, 32–33.

Gebauer, J., & Shaw, M. (2004). Success factors and impacts of mobile business applications: Results for a mobile e-procurement study. *International Journal of Electronic Commerce, 8*(3), 19–41.

Godwin-Jones, R. (2008). Emerging technologies mobile-computing trends: Lighter, faster, smarter. *Language, Learning & Technology, 12*(3), 3–9.

Hardy, K. (2009). Mobile apps keep doctors on the go. *Healthcare IT News, 6*(9), 1, 21.

Health Sciences & Human Services Library. (2010). Mobile Apps (Smart Phones & PDAs). Retrieved August 17, 2010 from http://guides.hshsl.umaryland.edu/mobileapps

Jonas, D., & Burns, B. (2010). The transition to blended e-learning: Changing the focus of educational delivery in children's pain management. *Nurse Education in Practice, 10*(1), 1–7.

Jones, S., & Fox, S. (2009). Generations online in 2009. *Pew Internet & American life project.* Retrieved from http://pewinternet.org/Reports/2009/Generations-Online-in-2009.aspx.

Kleinpell, R., & Bruinsma, S. (2010). E-learning resources for acute care nurse practitioners. *The Nurse Practitioner, 35*(1), 12–13.

Kleinpell, R., Hravnak, M., Settles, J., & Melander, S. (2009). Making the Web work for acute care NP education. *The Nurse Practitioner, 34*(4), 8–10.

Lehmann, H., Prasad, M. & Scornavacca, E. (2008). Adapting the IS success model for mobile technology in health: A New Zealand example. *Proceedings of The 10th International Conference on Electronic Commerce,* article no. 22.

May, T. (2009). The three paths to mobile victory. *Computerworld, 43*(23), 44.

Mobile Defense Measures. (2009, August). *Federal Solutions,* (pp. 4–7).

Perez, E. (2009). E-Health: How to make the right choice. *Nursing Forum 44*(4), 277–282.

Polsad, S. (2009). Ubiquitous computing: Smart devices, environments and interactions. West Sussex, U.K.: John Wiley & Sons.

Project Health Design. (2010). Retrieved from http://www.projecthealthdesign.org/

Spader, C. (2009, August 10). Cool tools: Cutting-edge gadgets sharpen nurses' efficiency. *Nursing Spectrum,* (pp. 20–21).

Turisco, F. (2000). Mobile computing is next technology frontier for healthcare providers. *Healthcare financial management.* Retrieved from http://www.allbusiness.com/technology/telecommunications-cell-phones-phone-services/668879-1.html.

The White House. (2009). Executive order: Federal leadership on reducing text messaging while driving. Retrieved from http://www.whitehouse.gov/the_press_office/Executive-Order-Federal-Leadership-on-Reducing-Text-Messaging-while-Driving.

U.S. Department of Health & Human Services, Agency for Healthcare Research & Quality. (2010). U.S. Preventive Services Task Force. Retrieved August 17, 2010 from http://www.ahrq.gov/clinic/uspstfix.htm

Wu, J., Wang, S., & Lin, L. (2007). Mobile computing acceptance factors in the healthcare industry: A structural equation model. *International Journal of Medical Informatics, 76*, 66–77.

Yasin, R. (2009). Wireless lockdown. *Government Computer News, 28*(16), 20–23.

PART 3

Informatics Theory

Virginia K. Saba

11

The Practice Specialty of Nursing Informatics

Kathleen M. Hunter / Carol J. Bickford

- OBJECTIVES
    1. Discuss core concepts and the scope of practice of nursing informatics.
    2. Describe nursing informatics as a distinct specialty.
    3. Relate the functional areas of nursing informatics practice.
    4. Identify available organizational resources.

- KEY WORDS

    informatics
    competencies
    terminologies
    scope and standards of practice

ABSTRACT

Nursing informatics is an established and growing area of specialization in nursing. All nurses employ information technologies in their practice. Informatics nurses are key persons in the design, development, implementation, and evaluation of these technologies and in the development of the specialty's body of knowledge.

This chapter addresses pertinent concepts, definitions, and interrelationships of nursing and nursing informatics. The core concepts of nursing informatics are described and related to one another. The recognition of nursing informatics as a distinct nursing specialty, its scope of practice, and certification are discussed.

INTRODUCTION

Decision making is an integral part of daily life. Nurses regularly make frequent, critical, life-impacting decisions. These decisions often are made within very short time frames (McCauhan, 2002). Good decisions require accurate and accessible data as well as skill in processing information. At the heart of nursing informatics is the goal of providing nurses with the data, information, and support for information processing to make effective decisions. This decision making can encompass any and all of the following areas of nursing practice: client care, research, education, and administration.

Effective practice of nursing informatics—a recognized nursing specialty—requires understanding of foundational documents, concepts and practices, definitions, and the specialty's metastructures and core phenomena. The accompanying discussion of the scope of practice, informatics competencies, standards of practice and professional performance, and associated measurement criteria provide more detail for a better understanding of this specialty.

INFORMATICS NURSE/INFORMATICS NURSE SPECIALIST

An informatics nurse (IN) is a registered nurse who has experience in nursing informatics. Informatics nurse specialists (INS) are prepared at the graduate level (master's degree) with courses in nursing informatics. An INS functions as a graduate-level-prepared specialty nurse.

Foundational Documents Guide Nursing Informatics Practice

In 2001, the American Nurses Association (ANA) published the *Code of Ethics for Nurses with Interpretive Statements*, a complete revision of previous ethics provisions and interpretive statements that guide all nurses in practice, be it in the domains of direct patient care, education, administration, or research. Nurses working in the informatics specialty are professionally bound to follow these provisions. Terms such as decision making, comprehension, information, knowledge, shared goals, outcomes, privacy, confidentiality, disclosure, policies, protocols, evaluation, judgment, standards, and factual documentation abound throughout the explanatory language of the interpretive statements. Examine this guidance by reviewing

the entire document posted for public access at http://nursingworld.org/ethics/code/protected_nwcoe629.htm.

In 2003, a second foundational professional document, *Nursing's Social Policy Statement, 2nd Edition*, provided a new definition of nursing that was reaffirmed in the 2010 *Nursing's Social Policy Statement: The Essence of the Profession*:

> Nursing is the protection, promotion, and optimization of health and abilities, prevention of illness and injury, alleviation of suffering through the diagnosis and treatment of human response, and advocacy in the care of individuals, families, communities, and populations. (ANA, 2010b, p. 3)

Again, informatics nurses must be cognizant of the statements and direction provided by this document to the nursing profession, its practitioners, and the public.

The ANA's *Nursing: Scope and Standards of Practice, Second Edition* (2010) further reinforces the recognition of nursing as a cognitive profession. The exemplary competencies accompanying each of the 16 Standards of Professional Nursing Practice, comprised of Standards of Practice and Standards of Professional Performance, reflect the specific knowledge, skills, abilities, and judgment capabilities expected of registered nurses. The standards include data, information, and knowledge management activities as core work for all nurses. This cognitive work begins with the critical-thinking and decision-making components of the nursing process that occur before nursing action can begin (see Table 11.1).

The nursing process provides one delineated pathway and process for decision making. Assessment, or data collection and information processing, begins the

TABLE 11.1	Standards of Professional Nursing Practice (ANA, 2010a)		
	Standards of Practice		**Standards of Professional Performance**
1	Assessment	7	Ethics
2	Diagnosis	8	Education
3	Outcomes identification	9	Evidence-based practice and research
4	Planning	10	Quality of practice
5	Implementation	11	Communication
5A	Coordination of care	12	Leadership
5B	Health teaching and health promotion	13	Collaboration
5C	Consultation	14	Professional practice evaluation
5D	Prescriptive authority	15	Resource utilization
6	Evaluation	16	Environmental health

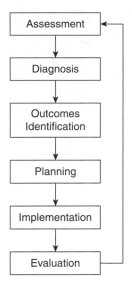

• **FIGURE 11.1.** The nursing process (ANA, 2010b).

nursing process. Diagnosis or problem definition, the second step, reflects the interpretation of the data and information gathered during assessment. Outcomes identification is the third step, followed by planning as the fourth step. Implementation of a plan is the fifth step. The final component of the nursing process is evaluation. Figure 11.1 shows how the nursing process is most often presented as a linear process with evaluation listed as the last step. However, the nursing process really is iterative, includes numerous feedback loops, and incorporates evaluation activites throughout the sequencing. For example, evaluation of a plan's implementation may prompt further assessment, a new diagnosis or problem definition, and decision making about new outcomes and related plans. Figure 11.2 demonstrates the interactivity of the nursing process and connects the standards of practice and professional performance to the appropriate nursing process steps.

The collection of data about a client or about a management, education, or research situation is guided by

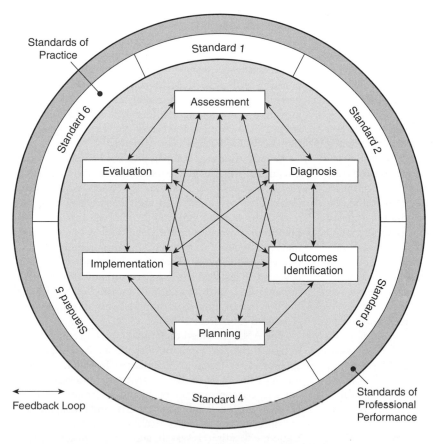

• **FIGURE 11.2.** The nursing process and standards (ANA, 2010b).

a nurse's knowledge base built on formal and informal educational preparation, evidence and research, and previous experiences. In healthcare, as in most areas of our lives, data, information, and knowledge are growing at astronomical rates and demand increasing reliance on computer and information systems for collection, storage, organization and management, analysis, and dissemination. For example, in clinical nursing practice, consider the significant expansion in the amount and types of data that *must* be collected for legal, regulatory, quality, and other reasons; the data, information, and knowledge, like genetic profiles, related to specific client health conditions; and the information and knowledge about the healthcare environment, such as that associated with billing and reimbursement, health plan, and available formulary options. Collecting data in a systematic, thoughtful way, organizing data for efficient and accurate transformation into information, and documenting thinking and actions are critical to successful nursing practice. Nursing informatics is the nursing specialty that endeavors to make the collection, management, and dissemination of data, information, and knowledge—to support decision making—easier for the practitioner, regardless of the domain and setting.

INFORMATICS AND HEALTHCARE INFORMATICS

Informatics is a science that combines a domain science, computer science, information science, and cognitive science. Thus, it is a multidisciplinary science drawing from varied theories and knowledge applications. Healthcare informatics may be defined as the integration of healthcare sciences, computer science, information science, and cognitive science to assist in the management of healthcare information. Healthcare informatics is a subset of informatics. Imagine a large umbrella named informatics and imagine many persons under this umbrella. Each person represents a different domain science, one of which is healthcare informatics.

Because healthcare informatics is a relatively young addition to the informatics umbrella, you may see other terms that seem to be synonyms for this same area, such as health informatics or medical informatics. Medical informatics, historically, was used in Europe and the United States as the preferred term for healthcare informatics. Now, medical informatics is more clearly realized as a subset of healthcare informatics, and health informatics may mean informatics used in educating healthcare clients and/or the general public.

As healthcare informatics evolves, so will the clarity in definition of terms and scopes of practice.

Healthcare informatics addresses the study and management of healthcare information. A model of overlapping discrete circles could depict the integrated content most often considered representative of the multiple and diverse aspects of healthcare informatics. Healthcare informatics would be the largest encompassing circle surrounding smaller intersecting circles. These aspects include specific content areas such as information retrieval, ethics, security, decision support, patient care, system life cycle, evaluation, human-computer interaction (HCI), standards, telehealth, healthcare information systems, imaging, knowledge representation, electronic health records (EHRs), education, and information retrieval.

Nursing Informatics

Nursing informatics (NI) is a subset of healthcare informatics. It shares common areas of science with other health professions and, therefore, easily supports interprofessional education, practice, and research focused on healthcare informatics. Nursing informatics also has unique areas that address the special information needs for the nursing profession. Nurses work both collaboratively with other healthcare professionals and independently when engaged in clinical and administrative nursing practice. Nursing informatics reflects this duality as well, moving in and out of integration and separation as situations and needs demand.

In 1985, Kathryn Hannah proposed a definition that nursing informatics is the use of information technologies in relation to any nursing functions and actions of nurses (Hannah, 1985). In their classic article on the science of nursing informatics, Graves and Corcoran presented a more complex definition of nursing informatics. Nursing informatics is a combination of computer science, information science, and nursing science designed to assist in the management and processing of nursing data, information, and knowledge to support the practice of nursing and the delivery of nursing care (Graves & Corcoran, 1989).

The ANA modified the Graves and Corcoran definition with the development of the first scope of practice statement for nursing informatics. The ANA defined nursing informatics as the specialty that integrates nursing science, computer science, and information science in identifying, collecting, processing, and managing data and information to support nursing practice, administration, education, research, and the expansion of nursing knowledge (ANA, 1994). The explanation of the accompanying standards of practice for nursing informatics followed in 1995 with ANA's publication of the *Standards of Nursing Informatics Practice*.

In 2000, the ANA convened an expert panel to review and revise the scope and standards of nursing informatics practice. That group's work included an extensive examination of the evolving healthcare and nursing environments and culminated in the publication of the *Scope and Standards of Nursing Informatics Practice* (2001b). This professional document includes an expanded definition of nursing informatics that was slightly revised in the 2008 *Nursing Informatics: Scope and Standards of Practice* to include wisdom:

> Nursing informatics (NI) is a specialty that integrates nursing science, computer science, and information science to manage and communicate data, information, knowledge, and wisdom in nursing practice. NI supports consumers, patients, nurses, and other providers in their decision-making in all roles and settings. This support is accomplished through the use of information structures, information processes, and information technology. (ANA, 2008, p. 1)

Further into the revised 2008 document, a slightly amended definition is provided:

> Nursing informatics is a specialty that integrates nursing science, computer science, and information science to manage and communicate data, information, knowledge, and wisdom in nursing practice. Nursing informatics facilitates the integration of data, information, knowledge, and wisdom to support patients, nurses, and other providers in their decision-making in all roles and settings. This support is accomplished through the use of information structures, information processes, and information technology. (ANA, 2008, p. 65)

The Nursing Informatics Special Interest Group of the International Medical Informatics Association (IMIA-NI) adopted the following definition in 2009:

> Nursing informatics science and practice integrates nursing, its information and knowledge and their management with information and communication technologies to promote the health of people, families, and communities world wide. (Nursing Informatics Special Interest Group of the International Medical Informatics Association, 2009)

These multiple definitions illustrate the dynamic, developing nature of this still-young nursing specialty.

Development of different definitions and a healthy debate on those definitions promotes validation of key elements and concepts. A willingness to continue exploring possible definitions can prevent premature conceptual closure, which may lead to errors in synthesis and knowledge development.

Nursing Informatics as a Specialty

Characteristics of a nursing specialty include: differentiated practice, a well-derived knowledge base, a defined research program, organizational representation, educational programs, and a credentialing mechanism.

In early 1992, the ANA recognized nursing informatics as a specialty in nursing with a distinct body of knowledge. Unique among the healthcare professions, this designation as a specialty provides official recognition that nursing informatics is indeed a part of nursing and that it has a distinct scope of practice.

The core phenomena of nursing are the nurse, person, health, and environment. Nursing informatics focuses on the information of nursing needed to address these core phenomena. Within this focus are the metastructures or overarching concepts of nursing informatics: data, information, knowledge, and wisdom. It is this special focus on the information of nursing that differentiates nursing informatics from other nursing specialties.

Research programs in NI are guided by the National Institute for Nursing Research's research priorities for NI. These priorities, first identified in 1993, are: using data, information, and knowledge to deliver and manage care; defining and describing data and information for patient care; acquiring and delivering knowledge from and for patient care; investigating new technologies to create tools for patient care; applying patient care ergonomics to the patient-nurse-machine interaction; integrating systems for better patient care; and evaluating the effects of nursing informatics solutions. Table 11.2 summarizes these research priorities.

Nursing informatics is represented in international, national, regional, and local organizations. For example, there is a nursing informatics working group in the American Medical Informatics Association (AMIA) and in the International Medical Informatics Association (IMIA). Nursing informatics is part of the clinical section of the Healthcare Information and Management Systems Society (HIMSS). The International Council of Nurses regularly addresses NI issues and NI use in nursing practice.

Increasingly, nursing school curricula include content, and sometimes complete courses, on information

TABLE 11.2	Summary of NI Research Priorities from NINR Expert Panel (1993) and Delphi Survey (1998)

Priority Research Areas

User needs
Identification of users' (nurses, patients, families) information needs
Nature and processes of clinical decision making and skill development
Match information technologies to nursing work patterns
Capture, representation, and storage of data, information, and knowledge
Develop, validate, and formalize nursing language terms, taxonomies, and classifications
Interdigitate nursing language schemes with larger standards initiatives
Design and management of nursing information databases for use in patient management, clinical records, and research
Develop and test clinical data storage schemes that optimize single-recording, multiple use in nursing
Develop alternative modes of conceptualizing, operationalizing, quantifying, and representing nursing information for
    incorporation into future information systems
Demonstrate connectivity architecture for capture and storage of patient care information across settings
Informatics support for nursing and healthcare practice
Technology development, including decision support systems to support nursing practice (integrates human-computer interaction)
Use of telecommunications technology for nursing practice
Professional practice issues (e.g., competencies, confidentiality)
Informatics support for patients/families/consumers
Patients' use of information technology
Consumer health informatics
Informatics support for practice-based knowledge generation
Develop systems to build clinical databases to generate and analyze knowledge linkages among resource consumption (structure),
    care processes (including nursing diagnoses and interventions), and outcomes to guide practice and policy
Design and evaluation methodologies
Develop evaluation methodologies for studying system use and impact on nursing decision making, nursing practice, and, if
    possible, patient outcomes
Systems modeling and evaluation

Adapted from: Bakken, S., Stone, P. W., & Larson, E. L. (2008). A nursing informatics research agenda for 2008-18: Contextual influences and key components. *Nursing Outlook, 56*(5), 206–214.e3.

technologies in healthcare and nursing. In 1989, the University of Maryland established the first graduate program in nursing informatics. The University of Utah followed in 1990. Now there are several in-person and online programs for graduate work in this specialty. Doctoral programs in nursing informatics have also been established.

Following the publication of the first nursing informatics scope of practice and standards documents, the American Nurses Credentialing Center (ANCC) established a certification process and examination in 1995 to recognize those nurses with basic informatics specialty competencies.

Scope of Nursing Informatics Practice

A scope of practice statement answers the who, what, when, where, why, and how questions related to practice and establishes the boundaries of a particular profession or specialization within a profession. Boundaries describe what is, and what is not, within the purview of an occupational group.

The scope of nursing informatics practice includes developing and evaluating applications, tools, processes, and strategies used for information handling. Information handling—the processes involved in managing data, information, and knowledge—includes naming, organizing, grouping, collecting, processing, analyzing, storing, retrieving, transforming, and communicating data and information. Nursing informatics makes use of a broad range of information technologies, not just computers.

As noted earlier in this chapter, nursing informatics is one component of the broader field of healthcare informatics. Nursing informatics intersects with other domains and disciplines concerned with the management of data,

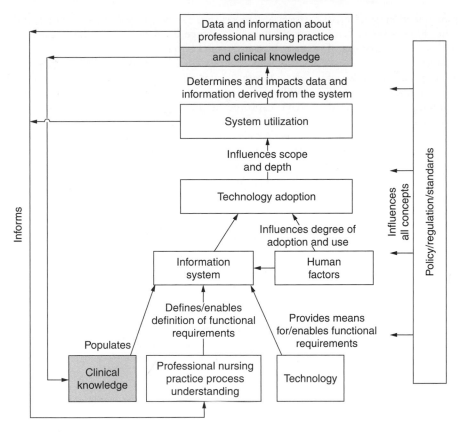

• **FIGURE 11.3.** The organizing framework for clinical information systems: Critical knowledge as the critical factor (Androwich et al., 2003).

information, and knowledge. The boundaries and intersections are flexible and allow for the inevitable changes and growth that evolve over time.

Models for Nursing Informatics

Models are representations of some aspect of the real world. Models show particular perspectives of a selected aspect and may illustrate relationships. Models evolve as knowledge about the selected aspect changes and are dependent on the "worldview" of those developing the model. It is important to remember that different models reflect different viewpoints and are not necessarily competitive; that is, there is no one "right" model.

A clinical information system (CIS) model (Fig. 11.3) shows how modeling can be used to organize different concepts into a logical whole. The purpose of this model is to depict system components, influencing

factors, and relationships that need to be considered when attempting to capture the complexities of professional nursing practice.

Different scholars in nursing informatics have proposed different models. Some of these models are presented here to provide further perspectives on nursing informatics, to demonstrate how differently scholars and practitioners may view what seems to be the same thing, and to show that nursing informatics is an evolutionary, theoretical, and practical science. Again, remember that there is no one right model nor are any of the models presented here exhaustive of the possible perspectives of nursing informatics.

Graves and Corcoran's seminal work included a model of nursing informatics. Their model placed data, information, and knowledge in sequential boxes with one-way arrows pointing from data to information to knowledge. The management processing box is directly above, with arrows pointing in one direction from management processing to each of the three boxes (Graves & Corcoran, 1989). The model is a direct depiction of their definition of nursing informatics.

In 1986, Patricia Schwirian proposed a model of nursing informatics intended to stimulate and guide systematic research in this discipline. Her concern at that time was over the sparse volume of research literature in nursing informatics. The model provides a framework for identifying significant information needs, which in turn can foster research. There are four primary elements arranged in a pyramid with a triangular base. The four elements are the raw material (nursing-related information), the technology (a computing system comprised of hardware and software), the users surrounded by context (nurses, students), and the goal (or objective) toward which the preceding elements are directed. Bidirectional arrows connect the three base components of raw material, user, and computer system to form the pyramid's triangular base. The goal element is placed at the apex of the pyramid to show its importance. Similarly, all interactions between the three base elements and the goal are represented by bidirectional arrows (Schwirian, 1986).

Turley, writing in 1996, proposed another model in which the core components of informatics (cognitive science, information science, and computer science) are depicted as intersecting circles. Nursing science is a larger circle that completely encompasses the intersecting circles. Nursing informatics is the intersection between the discipline-specific science (nursing) and the area of informatics (Turley, 1996).

Data, Information, Knowledge, and Wisdom

Data, information, knowledge, and wisdom are the current metastructures or overarching concepts for nursing informatics with specific definitions in the *Nursing Informatics: Scope and Standards of Practice* (ANA, 2008). Data are discrete entities that are described objectively without interpretation and would include some value assigned to a variable. Another term that might be used for a datum is fact. For example, a systolic blood pressure is a variable, and the number measured for that blood pressure is the value. Another datum may be a nursing intervention, a patient problem, or an outcome. A single datum, in isolation, lacks meaning. A systolic blood pressure of 150 mm Hg is a fact or datum. What this fact means for the patient and for the nurse requires more data—a data set. Other parameters—diastolic blood pressure, pulse, weight, age, medications, activity at time of measuring the blood pressure and so on—

form a data set that can be processed for meaning and decision making. Once the data set is available, the data may be transformed into information.

A concept related to data is that of atomic-level data. Atomic level data are raw, uninterpreted facts with values and cannot be further subdivided. These data, captured at the source in the course of nursing practice, are very useful in tracking the effectiveness of nursing decisions and are amenable to inclusion in electronic information systems as well as multiple forms of manipulation (Graves & Corcoran, 1989; Zielstorff et al., 1993). Analysis, combination, aggregation, and summarization are ways in which an information system can transform atomic level data to information.

Information reflects interpretation, organization, or structuring of data. Information is the result of processing data. As well, information is required to process data. Context is part of the information applied to a set of data to transform that set. Context enables a nurse to place the data set into the current client or patient situation—to apply the uniqueness of that client or patient. Knowledge is also required to transform data into information. A nurse applies knowledge from academic learning, information sources (e.g., guidelines and protocols) and practice experience. Data processing or transformation occurs when raw facts are transformed through the application of context to give those facts meaning or via the organization of data into a structure that connotes meaning (Graves & Corcoran, 1989).

Knowledge emerges from the transformation of information. "Knowledge is information that is synthesized so that relationships are identified and formalized" (ANA, 2008, p. 92). Consider the continuity, the overlap reflected in the intersections, and the somewhat linear process with numerous bidirectional feedback loops in Figure 11.4 (ANA, 2008, p. 5). Knowledge is the understanding of patterns from many experiences with specific data and information transformation. Understanding of patterns provides the practitioner with greater ability to predict what will happen in specific client or patient situations. Knowledge derived from transforming information over many client experiences may be integrated into a nurse's experiential knowledge base. Publications that share such experiential knowledge make these synthesized insights more widely available and may generate research. Research formally transforms data and information into evidence-based knowledge. Note, however, that processing of information does not always result in the development of knowledge. Further, knowledge itself may be processed to generate decisions and new knowledge (Graves & Corcoran, 1989).

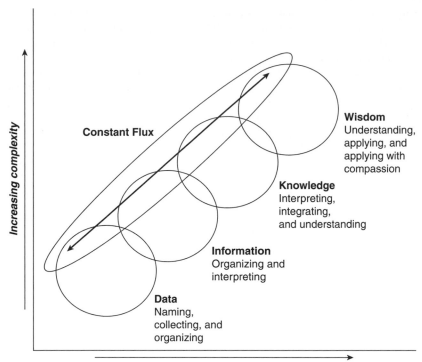

Increasing complexity

Constant Flux

Wisdom
Understanding,
applying, and
applying with
compassion

Knowledge
Interpreting,
integrating,
and understanding

Information
Organizing and
interpreting

Data
Naming,
collecting, and
organizing

Increasing Interactions and Inter-relationships

• **FIGURE 11.4.** The relationship of data, information, knowledge, and wisdom (ANA, 2008).

Wisdom became incorporated as part of the nursing informatics model in the 2008 NI scope of practice statement. Wisdom is defined as the appropriate use of knowledge to manage and solve human problems, including when and how to apply knowledge. Wisdom implies that decisions and judgements are sensible, that the outcomes of these decisions and judgements are optimal, and a sense of truth or rightness is involved. Haggerty and Grace (2008) conceptualize three key elements of wisdom: (1) providing for the common good as well as the good of one another, (2) using both intellect and affect in problem solving, and (3) using experience-based tacit knowing to address problems. Current evidence-based practice and outcomes research efforts are attempts to operationalize the application of wisdom into practice.

FUNCTIONAL AREAS OF PRACTICE

Informatics nurses are found in many diverse places, in direct healthcare settings, in supporting healthcare industries, government, professional organizations, medical device vendors, software companies, and elsewhere. The various role and position names attached to the individuals in these settings are as varied as the places where informatics nurses are found.

Because of this variety, and the often confusing terms describing roles and positions, a better approach for looking at the work of informatics nurses is to examine functional areas of practice. Functional areas in nursing informatics are: administration, leadership, and management; analysis, compliance and integrity management; consultation; coordination, facilitation and integration; development; educational and professional development; policy development and advocacy; and research and evaluation. Areas of integrated functions—intersections of clinical practice and informatics—include telecommunications for healthcare delivery (telehealth). Detailed descriptions of these functional areas are found in *Nursing Informatics: Scope and Standards of Practice* (ANA, 2008).

The administration, leadership, and management functional area can encompass activities such as scheduling, staffing, communication improvement, budget assistance, quality management, outcomes management, issue tracking, and case management. Informatics nurse specialists may be found in mid-level and senior-level leadership positions, including chief information officer (CIO) and chief nursing officer (CNO). Mid-level leadership roles include director of an informatics-related department, project officer, and program manager.

Analysis may be defined as the study of relevant information to develop a solution to a problem. The analyst must evaluate available options, determine cost and feasibility for each solution, and select the best resolution. An analyst (often known as a systems analyst) will convert user specifications into functional specifications, working closely with the users to ensure the conversion meets user needs. Workflow analysis is an important skill. Analysts may design databases or help data administrators design those resources. Compliance involves development, implementation, and monitoring of processes for meeting internal and external performance expectations. External performance expectations include the requirements associated with the Health Insurance Portability and Accountability Act (HIPAA) of 1996, national and international standards related to information technology, and The American Recovery and Reinvestment Act of 2009 (ARRA), which provides Medicare and Medicaid incentive payments to providers and hospitals for the "Meaningful Use" of certified health information technology products. Integrity management, in nursing informatics, focuses on data integrity—ensuring the data captured in an information system retains its validity. Participation in policy development related to assignment and use of passwords and access authority is an example of data integrity management.

The consultant function in nursing informatics is very fluid. Consultants do many different things in many different arenas, and most do a lot of travel. But, the focus of consultant work might be categorized as follows: system design, system selection, system implementation, analysis of work flow and system impact, knowledge management, and assisting clients with informatics issues. Consultants may work for a large organization that only does consulting, for a vendor who provides consulting services for customers, or independently.

Coordination is undertaken to synchronize the work of many into a unified effort. This function may focus on sharing information among many different units responsible for deploying and maintaining an information technology (IT) infrastructure. Coordination is needed in nursing informatics work because decisions may be made in one unit without sufficient consideration of problems or issues impacting other units. Unilateral decisions can lead to misunderstanding and wasted effort.

When working with group processes, facilitation involves designing and overseeing successful experiences or meetings for others who have come together for a common purpose. This common purpose may be to enable decision making, problem solving, or the exchange of ideas. A facilitator does not lead, distract, or entertain.

Integration, at first consideration, is similar to facilitation as it brings together two or more entities with the goal of having those disparate entities work effectively as a whole. The entities may be components, systems, and/or people. Data integration involves extraction, transformation, and loading (ETL) of data (a component) from different systems into one entity (a data warehouse or data mart) in order to manipulate and evaluate the data. Information integration focuses on bringing together data from multiple systems and representing these data in a unified, accurate, and consistent manner that supports viewing, manipulation, analysis, and decision making. Information integration facilitates the work of end users required to deal with multiple systems.

On a large scale, information integration may be known as enterprise information integration (EII). EII has its own unique requirements and constraints. The data must be available in real time—meaning the disparate systems are accessed directly (for example, laboratory data would be accessed directly from the laboratory information system). Data semantics (the meanings assigned to each data element) must be the same (consistent) across systems. Each system may have data represented by different labels and/or formats to support relevancy for each system's primary users; the sense of the data element, however, must be the same. The people side of integration may focus on bringing those people together with computers to foster effective use of this information technology. Technology integration can help people overcome fear, explore a system's capabilities, and build competencies.

Educational development functions can involve designing, producing, and teaching in formal, academic programs about informatics. Informatics content may be provided at the undergraduate, graduate, post-graduate, and doctoral level. Activities within the professional development sector relate to offering opportunities to learners for developing and maintaining knowledge, skills, and abilities in nursing and health informatics. Learners may be students in healthcare professions, informatics nurses, informatics nurse specialists, and clients. Specific activities are online course management, tracking, grade management, computer-assisted instruction (CAI), course delivery, management of remote information sources, distance conferencing, and presentation support.

Examples of systematic inquiry in nursing informatics include searching bibliographic systems, analyzing aggregate data for trends, formally evaluating different ways of presenting information on a monitor screen, and experiments aimed at testing theories or conceptual frameworks. Nursing informatics research focuses on the metastructures of data, information, and knowledge—their acquisition, storage, manipulation, and presentation to support decision making.

In 1993, the National Institute for Nursing Research (NINR) published a report entitled *Nursing Informatics: Enhancing Patient Care*. This report encouraged innovative research on using nursing informatics to improve clinical care and established a prioritized agenda for nursing informatics research. A Delphi study published in 1998 confirmed the relevancy of this research agenda (Brennan, Zielstorff, Ozbolt, & Strombom, 1998). Writing in 2008, Bakken, Stone, and Larson noted the continued relevance of these research priorities. They recommended expanding the users of this agenda to interdisciplinary researchers. Bakken and colleagues suggested research addressing genomic and environmental data, nursing-practice reengineering, empowering collaborative knowledge development by patients and caregivers, supporting complex data manipulation through development of user-configurable software, development of middle-range nursing informatics theories, and evaluation methods related to human-computer-interface factors.

Policy is a course of action or inaction chosen by authorities to manage a problem or a group of problems. Policy can be proactive or reactive. Policies are developed for a variety of reasons, including regulatory and legal requirements, guiding professional and personal behavior, enhancing communication, obtaining feedback on situations not met by existing policy, identifying new, improved ways of working, and reflecting operational, management, or technical directives. Thus, policies can be regulatory, advisory, or informative.

Policy advocacy occurs when individuals or groups wish to influence the development of specific policy, including that addressing consumer health. Informatics nurse specialists can influence internal and public policy development through sharing expertise on data and information needs, structure, management, and availability. Serving on task forces, lobbying, writing letters, and publishing opinion pieces are some methods of policy advocacy.

Telehealth is an example of a functional area where nursing informatics is tightly integrated with the delivery of healthcare. Telehealth is the delivery of healthcare, health-related education, public health services, and administrative functions over distance. Typically, electronic communication technologies are involved in telehealth. As with health informatics, there are numerous subdomains associated with telehealth: telenursing, telemedicine, teledentistry, etc. Nursing informatics specialists do not, usually, provide direct telenursing services. Instead, they serve a support role. The American Nurses Association and the International Council of Nurses have published standards, principles, and competencies on telenursing.

STANDARDS OF PRACTICE

The NI standards of practice are divided into two parts: standards of practice and standards of professional performance. Three overarching principles apply to all nursing informatics practice and should be considered by informatics nurses and informatics nurse specialists when addressing the application of the standards of practice. Briefly, these overarching principles advise that an informatics nurse incorporates theories, principles, and concepts from sciences into informatics practice; integrates ergonomics and human-computer-interaction (HCI) principles; and systematically determines the social, legal, regulatory, and ethical impact of an informatics solution (ANA, 2008).

There are six practice standards organized around a problem-solving process framework: assessment, identify the issue or problem, identify outcomes, develop a plan, implement the plan, and evaluation. This set of standards addresses the practice of nursing informatics by both informatics nurses and informatics nurse specialists. It is similar in structure to the nursing practice standards in the ANA publication, *Nursing: Scope and Standards of Practice* (ANA, 2004). Each standard provides accompanying measurement criteria.

The standards of professional performance consist of ten standards addressing the professional behavior of the informatics nurse and informatics nurse specialist. Again, measurement criteria are provided with each standard. These standards focus on education, quality of nursing informatics practice, professional practice evaluation, collegiality, ethics, collaboration, research, resource utilization, advocacy, and leadership.

COMPETENCIES

Benner's (1982) work, built on the Dreyfus model of skill acquisition that describes the evolution of novice to expert, merits discussion for nursing informatics. This desired change in skills involves the evolution from a novice level to advanced beginner to competent to proficient to, finally, an expert level. Every nurse must continually exhibit the capability to acquire and then demonstrate specific skills, beginning with the very first student experience. As students, most individuals can be described as novices having no experience with the situations and related content in those situations where they are expected to begin developing competencies by performing tasks that refine their skills. The advanced beginner can marginally demonstrate acceptable performance, having built on lessons learned in an expanding experience base. Individuals at these levels often need oversight by teachers or experienced colleagues to help structure the learning experience and support appropriate and successful workplace decision making and action.

Increased proficiency over time results in enhanced competencies reflecting mastery and the ability to cope with and manage many contingencies. Continued practice, combined with additional professional experience and knowledge, allows the nurse to evolve to the proficient level of appreciating the rules and maxims of practice and the nuances that are reflected in the absence of the normal picture. The expert has developed the capacity to intuitively understand the situation and immediately target the problem with minimal effort or problem solving.

Staggers, Gassert, and Curran are most often cited as the first published information about their research identifying the informatics competencies necessary for all nurses (Staggers, Gassert, & Curran, 2001). Their conceptual framework guiding the research included computer skills, informatics knowledge, and informatics skills as the informatics competencies (Staggers, Gassert, & Curran, 2002, p. 385). Their research, however, only identified informatics competencies for four levels of nurses: beginning nurse, experienced nurse, informatics specialist, and informatics innovator (Staggers, Gassert, & Curran, 2001). The comprehensive list of 304 competencies posed a significant challenge for professional development and academic faculties wishing to address each of the competencies when preparing curricula and then teaching educational programs for all skill levels. Further competencies definition work was completed by the workgroup that developed the current NI scope and standards document. Their review of the literature culminated in a 2-page matrix that included delineation by computer and information literacy (ANA, 2008, pp. 38–39).

The Technology Informatics Guiding Educational Reform (TIGER) initiative moved from an invitational conference to volunteer task forces, also known as collaboratives, to systematically develop key content related to discrete topics, including nursing informatics competencies. See Chapter 42 for further discussion on *The Tiger Initiative* and http://tigersummit.com/Competencies_New_B949.html for the final informatics competencies report.

The American Nurses Credentialing Center (ANCC) has used the competencies work and its own role delineation studies to develop and maintain the nursing informatics certification examination. The ANCC designated NI content expert panel has oversight responsibility for the content of this examination and considers the current informatics environment and research when defining the test content outline. Currently, the content outline topics address: human factors, system life cycle (system planning, analysis, design, implementation and testing, evaluation, maintenance, and support), information technology (hardware, software, communications, data representation, and security), information management and knowledge generation (data, information, knowledge), professional practice, trends, and issues (roles, trends and issues, ethics), and models and theories, and management and leadership. The detailed test content outline is available at http://www.nursecredentialing.org/Documents/Certification/TestContentOutlines/InformaticsNurseTCO.aspx.

The Healthcare Information and Management Systems Society (HIMSS) has established a CPHIMS (Certified Professional in Healthcare Information & Management Systems) certification program that may be of interest to informatics nurses. The content outline for the examination and other administrative and application details are available at the HIMSS Web site at http://www.himss.org/ASP/certification_cphims.asp.

TERMINOLOGIES

Why are informatics nurses and nurse scholars so interested in terminologies? Nursing terminologies focus on the patient and care process, not reimbursement or mortality, and are increasingly important as EHRs become an integral component of healthcare services delivery. These terminologies are used to capture, store, and manipulate data in EHRs. Nursing is both blessed and challenged by the wealth of terminologies available for describing nursing practice and nurses' contributions to healthcare. This diversity offers practitioners choices in how to best describe their patient population and practice.

To convey important data and information to others, the communication must be understood by the listener and be interpreted as having meaning. This is best accomplished by using standard communication formats and terminologies and recognized conventions for describing the concepts being presented. Concept representation involves the set of terms and relationships that describe the phenomena, processes, and practices of a discipline, such as nursing. Data elements, classifications, nomenclatures, vocabularies, and languages are some of the ways in which nursing concepts may be represented. Data elements are terms for which data are collected and for which values are assigned. A specific, purposeful group of data elements, representing a subset of concepts within a discipline, is a data set.

The Nursing Minimum Data Set (NMDS), developed through Dr. Harriet Werley's research, is considered the foundational work for nursing languages and represents the first attempt to standardize the collection of essential nursing data. This data set contains 16 data elements divided into patient, service, and nursing care elements, and fosters the comparison of nursing data across time, settings, and populations (Werley & Lang, 1988). The 4 nursing care elements include nursing diagnosis, nursing intervention, nursing outcome, and intensity of nursing care. Patient or client demographic elements address personal identification, date of birth, gender, race, and residence. The 7 service elements include unique facility or service agency number, unique health record number of patient or client, unique number of principal registered nurse provider, episode admission or encounter data, discharge or termination date, disposition of patient or client, and expected payer.

Most of these data elements, except for the nursing care elements and the unique identifier for the primary registered nurse, have long been captured in healthcare information systems. Werley and her colleagues envisioned collecting these data from everywhere nursing care is delivered, aggregating and storing these data in large databases, and using these data for policy analysis, evaluation of care, strategic planning, and nursing research. There are other data sets that contain nursing data elements, such as the Minimum Data Set (MDS) developed for long-term care facilities (http://www.cms.gov/home/medicaid.asp) and outcome and assessment information set (OASIS), the home health data set that is used by home health agencies (http://www.cms.gov/OASIS/).

Much of the early nursing terminologies research that helps describe nursing practice received initial federal funding support from the National Library of Medicine. The ANA further highlighted these efforts through establishment of a standardized recognition program for terminologies and data sets, based on defined review criteria. The ANA program for recognition of terminologies that support nursing has evolved, in concert with the advancements in the research and terminology development efforts, to include new recognition criteria. The Committee for Nursing Practice Information Infrastructure (CNPII) provides oversight to this ANA program.

ANA-RECOGNIZED TERMINOLOGIES

This section provides a brief description of the current 12 ANA-recognized terminologies. A detailed presentation of each terminology recognized by the ANA as of 2010 is outside the scope of this chapter. Interested readers are referred to the Websites or custodians presented in Table 11.3 for more details. What is important to remember is that each of the ANA-recognized terminologies was developed for specific purposes and does not yet provide the language to describe every segment of the nursing process.

Nursing Minimum Data Set (NMDS) is the minimum set of items of information with uniform definitions and categories concerning the specific dimension of professional nursing that meets the information needs of multiple data users in the healthcare system.

Nursing Management Minimum Data Set (NMMDS) contains data variables, categorized into environment, nurse resources, and financial resources, that are needed to inform the decision-making process of nurse executives related to leading and managing nursing-services delivery and care coordination.

Clinical Care Classification (CCC) System is a research-based, empirically developed terminology that identifies the discrete data elements of nursing practice. The CCC System includes a holistic framework and coding structure of diagnoses, interventions, and outcomes for assessing, documenting, and classifying care in all healthcare settings. It is used to track and measure patient/client care holistically over time, across settings, population groups, and geographic locations. More details are available in Chapter 14: Overview of CCC System and at www.sabacare.com.

International Classification for Nursing Practice® **(ICNP)** is a combinatorial terminology for nursing practice that facilitates cross-mapping of local terms and

TABLE 11.3	Current ANA-Recognized Terminologies and Data Sets		
Category		**Setting**	**Content**
Data Element Sets			
1. NMDS Nursing Minimum Data Set http://www.nursing.umn.edu/ICNP/USANMDS/home.html		All nursing	Clinical data elements
2. NMMDS Nursing Management Minimum Data Set http://www.nursing.umn.edu/ICNP/USANMMDS/home.html		All settings	Nursing administrative data elements
Interface Terminologies			
3. CCC System Clinical Care Classification (CCC) System www.sabacare.com and www.clinicalcareclassification.com		All settings	Diagnoses, interventions, and outcomes
4. ICNP® International Classification of Nursing Practice www.icn.ch/pillarsprograms/international-classification-for-nursing-practicer/		All Nursing	Diagnoses, interventions, and outcomes
5. NANDA NANDA International www.nanda.org		All nursing	Diagnoses

6. NIC
Nursing Intervention Classification
    www.nursing.uiowa.edu/excellence/nursing_knowledge/clinical_effectiveness/
    index.htm
		All nursing	Interventions

7. NOC
Nursing Outcome Classification
    www.nursing.uiowa.edu/excellence/nursing_knowledge/clinical_effectiveness/
    index.htm
		All nursing	Outcomes

8. Omaha System Omaha System www.omahasystem.org		Home care, public health, and community	Diagnoses, interventions, and outcomes
9. PNDS Perioperative Nursing Data Set www.aorn.org/PracticeResources/PNDSAndStandardizedPerioperativeRecord/		Perioperative	Diagnoses, interventions and outcomes
Multidisciplinary Terminologies			
10. ABCCodes ABC Codes www.abccodes.com		Nursing and Other	Interventions
11. LOINC Logical Observation Identifiers Names and Codes www.loinc.org		Nursing and other	Outcome and assessments
12. SNOMED CT Systematic Nomenclature of Medicine-Clinical Terms www.ihtsdo.org/snomed-ct/		Nursing and other	Diagnoses, interventions, and outcomes

existing vocabularies and classifications. ICNP includes nursing phenomena (nursing diagnoses), nursing actions, and nursing outcomes.

NANDA International (Nursing Diagnoses, Definitions, and Classification) (NANDA) is a nursing diagnoses classification developed to describe the important judgments nurses make in providing nursing care for individuals, families, groups, and communities. These judgments, or diagnoses, are the basis for selection of nursing outcomes and interventions. The terminology is updated every 2 years.

Nursing Interventions Classification (NIC) is a comprehensive, research-based, standardized classification of interventions that nurses perform and use for clinical documentation, communication of care across settings, integration of data across systems and settings, effectiveness research, productivity measurement, competency evaluation, reimbursement, and curricular design. In NIC, an intervention is defined as "any treatment, based upon clinical judgment and knowledge that a nurse performs to enhance patient/client outcomes." (http://www.nursing.uiowa.edu/excellence/nursing_knowledge/clinical_effectiveness/nicoverview.htm) NIC includes interventions that nurses do on behalf of patients, both independent and collaborative interventions, both direct and indirect care.

Nursing Outcomes Classification (NOC) provides a comprehensive, standardized classification of patient/client outcomes developed to evaluate the effects of nursing interventions. For NOC, an outcome is a measurable individual, family, or community state, behavior, or perception that is measured along a continuum and is responsive to nursing interventions.

Omaha System is a comprehensive practice and documentation tool used by multidisciplinary healthcare practitioners in any setting, from the time of client admission to discharge. Omaha System includes an assessment component (Problem Classification Scheme), an intervention component (Intervention Scheme), and an outcomes component (Problem Rating Scale for Outcomes).

Perioperative Nursing Data Set (PNDS) describes perioperative nursing practice with a subset of terms that specifically describe perioperative nursing diagnoses, nursing interventions, and patient outcomes in surgical settings from preadmission until discharge.

Alternative Billing Codes (ABC) contains terminologies describing alternative medicine, nursing, and other integrative healthcare interventions. These codes include the type of provider and the recognized level of licensed practitioner by state.

Logical Observation Identifiers Names and Codes (LOINC) is a set of universal names and ID codes for identifying laboratory and clinical test results; these codes can be used to describe laboratory and clinical results when stored in electronic databases or transmitted in electronic messages. The clinical portion of the LOINC database includes entries for vital signs, hemodynamics, intake/output, electrocardiogram, obstetric ultrasound, cardiac echo, urologic imaging, gastroendoscopic procedures, pulmonary ventilator management, selected survey instruments, and other clinical observation.

Systematic Nomenclature of Medicine Clinical Terms (SNOMED CT) is a core terminology providing a common language that enables a consistent way of capturing, sharing, and aggregating health data across specialties and sites of care.

ORGANIZATIONS AS RESOURCES

Many organizations have emerged to provide information resources and value-added membership benefits that support those individuals interested in healthcare and nursing informatics. Clinical specialty and other professional organizations have also appreciated the evolving healthcare information management focus and have established organizational structures such as informatics sections, divisions, workgroups, or special interest groups. Some have incorporated informatics and information system technology initiatives in strategic plans with dedicated staffing and ongoing financial support. In many instances, informal networking groups have evolved into international organizations with hundreds of members connected via the Web.

The nature, purposes, and activities of the multiple informatics organizations have sufficient differences that there is bound to be at least one organization, if not more, for everyone interested in nursing informatics. Information about a few of these organizations is provided here. Only national or international informatics-related organizations with nursing groups are included. All of the groups presented here are accessible to individual nurses for more information and/or participation. This content is in no way an exhaustive presentation. To learn more about these organizations and others, consult the Internet, informatics colleagues, and the literature.

American Nurses Association and Specialty Nursing Organizations

The ANA and its affiliates and several nursing specialty organizations have informatics committees and government affairs offices addressing information technology, EHRs, standards, and other informatics issues. Membership and active participation in such professional organizations demonstrate compliance with Provisions 8 and 9 of the *Code of Ethics for Nurses with Interpretive Statements* (ANA, 2001a) and Standard 16. Leadership described in *Nursing Informatics: Scope and*

Standards of Practice (ANA, 2008). Within the ANA, the CNPII provides the major policy generation and management for informatics-related topics and issues.

AMIA Nursing Informatics Working Group (NIWG)

AMIA is a nonprofit membership organization of individuals, institutions, and corporations dedicated to developing and using information technologies to improve healthcare. The NIWG within AMIA aims to promote and advance nursing informatics within the larger context of health informatics.

The NIWG pursues this mission in many areas, such as professional practice, education, research, governmental and other service, professional organizations, and industry. Member services, outreach functions, official representation to Nursing Informatics Special Interest Group of the International Medical Informatics Association (IMIA-NI) and liaison activities to other national and international groups are some of the activities of this working group.

One NIWG project of great interest is the Nursing Informatics History Project. The purpose of this project is documentation and preservation of the history of nursing informatics. Three main activities are set up to accomplish this purpose:

- Preservation of materials from nursing informatics pioneers and nursing informatics organizations in an archive at the National Library of Medicine started by Dr. Virginia K. Saba in 1997

- Videotaping of the stories of nursing informatics pioneers (available on the AMIA Website)

- Documentation of the evolution of informatics as a specialty in nursing

NIWG has established three awards that recognize excellence in nursing informatics: the Student Award, the Harriet Werley Award, and the Virginia K. Saba Informatics Award. Explore the rich resources at the NIWG Website at https://www.amia.org/working-group/nursing-informatics.

ANIA-CARING

In January 2010, two nursing informatics organizations (American Nursing Informatics Association and CARING) merged to form ANIA-CARING. The combined organization, with a 3000-plus membership in 50 states and 34 countries, is one of the largest associations of its kind in the United States. The organization is dedicated to advancing the field of nursing informatics through communications, education, research, and professional activities. Annual spring conferences are scheduled through 2012. A newsletter is published quarterly and is indexed in CINAHL and Thompson. ANIA-CARING runs a very active e-mail list and has provided public access to a large job bank, listing over 800 employer-paid positions. The ANIA-CARING web presence and membership application can be accessed at www.ania-caring.org.

British Computer Society (BCS) Nursing Specialist Group (NSG)

The BCS promotes wider social and economic progress through the advancement of information technology science and practice. The NSG is the leading United Kingdom organization for nurses and therapists interested in the management and use of information to improve care, the development of learning programmes for all staff, enabling better response to patient inquiry, and improved direction to nursing and therapy specialities for clinical information and education. NSG members are eligible for the annual prestigious Dame Phyllis Friend Award. The executive committee provides coordination and liaison with a range of national and international bodies in the field of health informatics and holds a significant body of knowledge in this emerging domain. Further details are available at http://www.bcs.org/server.php?show=nav.10013.

HIMSS Nursing Informatics Community

The Healthcare Information and Management Systems Society (HIMSS) provides leadership for the management of healthcare-related technology, information, and change through publications, educational opportunities, and member services. Founded in 2003, the HIMSS Nursing Informatics Community reflects the increased recognition of the role of the informatics nurse professional in healthcare information and management systems. This community speaks in a unified voice for the HIMSS members who practice in the nursing informatics community and provides nursing informatics expertise, leadership, and guidance internally to HIMSS and externally with the global nursing informatics community. The HIMSS Nursing Informatics Committee serves as the leadership for this community. The Nursing Informatics Community has a membership of more than 2000 nurses, representing nearly 10% of HIMSS members.

One unique feature of the Nursing Informatics Community is its online collection of initiatives and resources to promote and support the field of nursing informatics, including:

- The role of the nurse informaticist
- Educational presentations on nursing informatics as a driver of quality
- Professional and career links to stimulate career development
- Best practice tools for project management
- Information on education reform and workforce solutions from the TIGER Initiative
- A unified voice for all nursing informatics organizations—the Alliance for Nursing Informatics
- Current industry news

Access this content at http://www.himss.org/ASP/topics_nursingInformatics.asp.

Educational Technology and Information Management Advisory Council (ETIMAC)

The mission of the National League for Nursing (NLN) is to advance quality nursing education that prepares the nursing workforce to meet the needs of diverse populations in an ever-changing healthcare environment. The ETIMAC was established to promote the effective use of technology in nursing education, both as a teaching tool and as an outcome for student and faculty learning, and to advance the integration of information management into educational practices and program outcomes. See http://www.nln.org/getinvolved/AdvisoryCouncils_TaskGroups/etimac.htm.

Nursing Informatics Australia (NIA)

The NIA is a special interest group of the Health Informatics Society of Australia (HISA) and is the preeminent group of nursing informaticians in Australia. The NIA sees the priorities for nursing informatics in Australia as use of appropriate language, education, and ongoing research. It aims to encourage nurses to embrace information and communication technologies and to establish strong foundations for taking these developments forward. The NIA works to ensure nursing has the data and resources to continue providing evidence-based, quality, cost-effective, and outcome-driven care for patients and clients into the future. The NIA holds an annual conference on nursing informatics. See http://www.hisa.org.au/nursing/.

Nursing Informatics Special Interest Group of the International Medical Informatics Association (IMIA/NI-SIG)

This special interest group was originally established by IMIA in 1983 as Working Group 8 of IMIA, dedicated to serving the specific needs of nurses in the field of nursing informatics. IMIA-NI is focused on fostering collaboration among nurses and others who are interested in nursing informatics; exploring the scope of nursing informatics and its implication for information handling activities associated with nursing care delivery, nursing administration, nursing research, and nursing education, and the various relationships with other healthcare information systems; supporting the development of nursing informatics in the member countries; providing appropriate informatics meetings, conferences, and post-conferences that provide opportunities to share knowledge and research that facilitates communication of developments in the field; encouraging the publication and dissemination of research and development materials in the field of nursing informatics; and developing recommendations, guidelines, and courses related to nursing informatics.

IMIA-NI holds a triennial conference, has an annual General Assembly meeting, and pursues other activities through its Working Groups. A Working Group consists of experts selected and assigned, without consideration of nationality, to work in a specified area. The Chairperson of a WG is elected by the General Assembly upon recommendation of the Executive Committee. Current Working Groups are NI-Consumer/Client Health Informatics, NI-Education, NI-Evidence Based Practice, NI-Management, and NI-Health Informatics Standards

More details are available at http://www.imiani.org/index.php.

Alliance for Nursing Informatics (ANI)

The ANI is a collaboration of organizations, representing a unified voice for nursing informatics. NI brings together over 25 nursing informatics groups mainly in the United States that function separately at local, regional, national, and international levels. Each of these organizations has their own established programs, publications, and organizational structures for their members.

The ANI aims to foster further development of a united voice for nursing informatics through providing a single point of connection between nursing informatics individuals and groups and the broader nursing and healthcare community. The ANI is a mechanism for transforming care and developing resources, guidelines and standards for nursing informatics practice, education, scope of practice, research, certification, public policy, terminology, best practice guidelines, mentoring, advocacy, networking, and career services. See www.allianceni.org.

TIGER (Technology Informatics Guiding Education Reform)

The TIGER initiative seeks to better prepare practicing nurses and nursing students to use technology and informatics to improve the delivery of patient care. Phase one of TIGER engaged stakeholders to create a common vision of ideal EHR-enabled nursing practice. In 2007, ANI became the enabling organization for the TIGER Initiative Phase II Activities by facilitating collaboration among participating organizations to achieve the vision. Phase III of the TIGER Initiative is a call to action to leaders, organizations, and informatics and other nurses. All stakeholders are charged with ACTION in the following crucial areas: standards and interoperability, national health IT agenda, informatics competencies, education and faculty development, staff development, usability and clinical application design, virtual demonstration center, leadership development, consumer empowerment and personal health records. Individuals as well as organizations can participate in and contribute to this initiative. More details are available in Chapter 42 The Tiger Initiative and at www.tigersummit.com.

Canadian Nursing Informatics Association (CNIA)

The CNIA's mission is to be the voice for nursing informatics in Canada. Recognizing the importance of the work the CNIA is undertaking, the Canadian Nurses Association has granted associate group status to the CNIA. The CNIA is also affiliated with COACH, Canada's National Health Informatics Association. Through this strategic alliance, CNIA is the Canadian nursing nominee to the International Medical Informatics Association–Special Interest Group in Nursing Informatics (IMIA-NI). The *Canadian Journal of Nursing Informatics* began publishing in the Spring of 2006. Four issues are published each year. See http://cnia.ca.

American Academy of Nursing (AAN)

The American Academy of Nursing and its invited membership of fellows create and execute knowledge-driven and policy-related initiatives to drive reform of America's healthcare system through work of its committees, panels, and the workforce commission. The recent Technology Drill Down (TD2) effort provided an opportunity to develop an improved process for identifying technological solutions to medical/surgical-unit-workflow inefficiencies. See www.aannet.org.

Sigma Theta Tau International (STTI)

Sigma Theta Tau International, another invited member organization, has a mission to support the learning, knowledge, and professional development of nurses committed to making a difference in health worldwide. It has established the Virginia K. Saba Informatics Award given to an informatics expert whose contributions have the capacity and scope to enhance quality, safety, outcomes, and decision making in health and nursing care from a national or an international perspective. The Ruth Lilly Nursing Informatics Scholar is a 2-year award to an individual to contribute to the vision and plan for the Virginia Henderson International Nursing Library's continued contributions to nursing knowledge. See www.nursingsociety.org.

SUMMARY

Concepts of informatics, healthcare informatics, and nursing informatics were explained and their relationships to each other were discussed. The core concepts of nursing informatics were presented and described. The establishment of the specialty of nursing informatics was explained. Functional areas, scope of practice, and standards of practice of nursing informatics were explored. A brief discussion of terminologies supporting nursing practice placed core concepts into the context of nursing informatics. Competency work related to the practice of nursing informatics was presented. International and national resources for informatics nurses were provided.

REFERENCES

Androwich, I. M., Bickford, C. J., Button, P. S., Hunter, K. M., Murphy, J., & Sensmeier, J. (2003). *Clinical information systems: A framework for reaching the vision.* Washington, DC: American Nurses Publishing.

American Nurses Association. (1994). *The scope of practice for nursing informatics.* Washington, DC: American Nurses Publishing.

American Nurses Association. (1995). *Standards of nursing informatics practice.* Washington, DC: American Nurses Publishing.

American Nurses Association. (2001a). *Code of ethics for nurses with interpretive statements*. Washington, DC: American Nurses Publishing.

American Nurses Association. (2001b). *Scope and standards of nursing informatics practice*. Washington, DC: American Nurses Publishing.

American Nurses Association. (2003). *Nursing's social policy statement*. 2nd ed. Washington, DC: nursesbooks.org.

American Nurses Association. (2004). *Nursing: Scope and standards of practice*. Washington, DC: nursesbooks.org.

American Nurses Association. (2008). *Nursing informatics: Scope and standards of practice*. Silver Spring, MD: nursesbooks.org.

American Nurses Association. (2010a). *Nursing: Scope and standards of practice, 2nd edition*. Silver Spring, MD: nursesbooks.org.

American Nurses Association. (2010b). *Nursing's social policy statement: The essence of the profession*. Silver Spring, MD: nursesbooks.org.

Bakken, S., Stone, P. W., & Larson, E. L. (2008). A nursing informatics research agenda for 2008-18: contextual influences and key components. *Nursing Outlook, 56*(5), 206–214.e3.

Benner, P. (1982). From novice to expert. *American Journal of Nursing, 82*(3), 402–407.

Brennan, P. F., Zielstorff, R. D., Ozbolt, J. G., & Strombom, I. (1998). Setting a national research agenda in nursing informatics. *Medinfo, 9,* 1188–1191.

Graves, J. R., & Corcoran, S. (1989). The study of nursing informatics. *IMAGE: Journal of Nursing Scholarship, 21*(4), 227–231.

Haggerty, L. A., & Grace, P. (2008). Clinical wisdom: the essential foundation of "good" nursing care. *Journal of Professional Nursing, 24*(4), 235–240.

Hannah, K. (1985). Current trends in nursing informatics: Implications for curriculum planning. In K. Hannah, E. J. Guillemin, & D. N. Conklin (Eds.), *Nursing uses of computer and information science*. Amsterdam: North-Holland.

McCauhan, D. (2002). What decisions do nurses make? In C. Thompson, & D. Dowding, *Clinical Decision Making and Judgement in Nursing (pp.95–108)*. London: Churchill Livingston.

NINR Priority Expert Panel on Nursing Informatics. (1993). *Nursing informatics: Enhancing patient care*. Bethesda, MD: U.S. Department of Health and Human Services, U.S. Public Health Service, National Institutes of Health.

Nursing Informatics Special Interest Group of the International Medical Informatics Association (2009). IMIA-NI General Assembly 2009 Meeting Minutes. Helsinki: Finland. Retrieved July 17, 2010 from http://www.imiani.org/index.php?option=com_docman&task=cat_view&gid=15&Itemid=30

Schwirian, P. M. (1986). The NI Pyramid-A model for research in nursing informatics. *Computers in Nursing, 4*(3), 134–136.

Staggers, N., Gassert, C. A., & Curran, C. (2001). Informatics competencies for nurses at four levels of practice. *Journal of Nursing Education, 40*(7), 303–316.

Staggers, N., Gassert, C. A., & Curran, C. (2002). A Delphi study to determine informatics competencies for nurses at four levels of practice. *Nursing Research, 51*(6), 383–390.

Turley, J. (1996). Toward a model for nursing informatics. *IMAGE: Journal of Nursing Scholarship, 28*(4), 309–313.

Werley, H. & Lang, N. (Eds.). (1988). *Identification of the Nursing Minimum Data Set*. New York: Springer.

Zielstorff, R., Hudgings, C., & Grobe, S. (1993). *Next-generation nursing information systems: Essential characteristics for professional practice*. Washington, DC: American Nurses Publishing.

12

Advanced Terminological Approaches in Nursing

Nicholas R. Hardiker / Suzanne Bakken / Tae Youn Kim

- OBJECTIVES
    1. Describe the need for advanced terminology systems.
    2. Identify the components of advanced terminology systems.
    3. Compare and contrast two approaches for representing nursing concepts within an advanced terminology system.

- KEY WORDS

    concept representation
    terminology
    vocabulary
    standardized nursing language

INTRODUCTION

The failure to achieve a single, integrated terminology with broad coverage of the healthcare domain has been characterized as the "vocabulary problem." Evolving criteria for healthcare terminologies for implementation in computer-based systems suggest that concept-oriented approaches are needed to support the data needs of today's complex, knowledge-driven healthcare and health management environment. This chapter focuses on providing the background necessary to understand recent approaches to solving the vocabulary problem. It also includes several illustrative examples of these approaches from the nursing domain.

BACKGROUND AND DEFINITIONS

The primary motivation for standardized terms in nursing is the need for valid, comparable data that can be used across information system applications to support clinical decision making and the evaluation of processes and outcomes of care. Secondary uses of the data for purposes such as clinical, translational, and comparative effectiveness research, development of practice-based nursing knowledge, and generation of healthcare policy are dependent on the initial collection and representation of the data. Given the importance of standardized terminology, one might ask, "Why, despite the extensive work to date, is the vocabulary problem not yet solved?"

The Vocabulary Problem

Several reasons for the vocabulary problem have been posited in health and nursing informatics literature. First, the development of multiple, specialized terminologies has resulted in areas of overlapping content, areas for which no content exists, and large numbers of codes and terms (Chute, Cohn, & Campbell, 1998; Cimino, 1998a). Second, existing terminologies are most often developed to provide sets of terms and

TABLE 12.1	Evaluation Criteria Related to Concept-oriented Approaches

Atomic-based—concepts must be separable into constituent components (Chute et al., 1998)

Compositionality—ability to combine simple concepts into composed concepts, eg, "pain" *and* "acute" = "acute pain" (Chute et al., 1998)

Concept permanence—once a concept is defined it should not be deleted from a terminology (Cimino, 1998b)

Language independence—support for multiple linguistic expressions (Chute et al., 1998)

Multiple hierarchy—accessibility of concepts through all reasonable hierarchical paths with consistency of views (Chute et al., 1998; Cimino, 1998b; Cimino et al., 1989)

Nonambiguity—explicit definition for each term, eg, "patient teaching related to medication adherence" defined as an *action* of "teaching", *recipient* of "patient", and *target* of "medication adherence" (Chute et al., 1998; Cimino, 1998b; Cimino et al., 1989)

Nonredundancy—one preferred way of representing a concept or idea (Chute et al., 1998; Cimino, 1998b; Cimino et al., 1989)

Synonymy—support for synonyms and consistent mapping of synonyms within and among terminologies (Chute et al., 1998; Cimino, 1998b; Cimino et al., 1989)

definitions of concepts for human interpretation, with computer interpretation as only a secondary goal (Rossi Mori, Consorti, & Galeazzi, 1998). The latter is particularly true for nursing terminologies that have been designed for direct use by nurses in the course of clinical care (Association of Operating Room Nurses [AORN], 2007; Johnson et al., 2006; Martin, 2005; Saba, 2006). Unfortunately, knowledge that is eminently understandable to humans is often confusing, ambiguous, or opaque to computers, and, consequently, current efforts have often resulted in terminologies that are inadequate in meeting the data needs of today's healthcare systems. This chapter focuses on providing the background necessary to understand recent concept-oriented approaches to solving the vocabulary problem. It also includes illustrative examples of these approaches from the nursing domain. Note that the word "terminology" is used throughout this chapter to refer to the set of terms representing a system of concepts.

Concept Orientation

An appreciation of the approaches discussed in this chapter has as a prerequisite an understanding of what it means for a terminology to be concept oriented. Previous published reports provide an evolving framework that enumerates the criteria (Table 12.1) that render healthcare terminologies suitable for implementation in computer-based systems. In particular, it is clear that such terminologies must be concept oriented (with explicit semantics), rather than based on surface linguistics (Chute et al., 1998; Cimino, 1998b; Cimino, Hripcsak, Johnson, & Clayton, 1989). Several previous studies have reported that many existing

nursing terminologies do not meet the criteria related to concept orientation (Henry & Mead, 1997; Henry, Warren, Lange, & Button, 1998).

In order to appreciate the significance of concept-oriented approaches, it is important to first understand the definitions of and relationships among things in the world (objects), our thoughts about things in the world (concepts), and the labels we use to represent and communicate our thoughts about things in the world (terms). These relationships are depicted by a model commonly called the semiotic triangle (Fig. 12.1) (Ogden & Richards, 1923). The International Organization

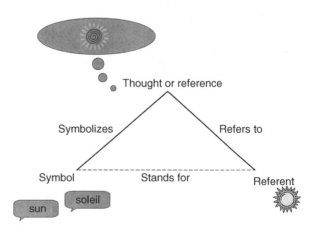

• **FIGURE 12.1.** The semiotic triangle depicts the relationships among objects in the perceivable or conceivable world (referent), thoughts about things in the world, and the labels (symbols or terms) used to represent thoughts about things in the world.

for Standardization (ISO) international standard ISO 1087-1:2000 provides definitions for elements that correspond to each vertex of the triangle:

Concept (ie, thought or reference): Unit of knowledge created by a unique combination of characteristics—a characteristic is an abstraction of a property of an object or of a set of objects.

Object (ie, referent): Anything perceivable or conceivable.

Term (ie, symbol): Verbal designation of a general concept in a specific subject field—a general concept corresponds to two or more objects which form a group by reason of common properties (International Organization for Standardization [ISO], 1990).

As specified by the criteria in Table 12.1 and illustrated in Figure 12.1, a single concept may be associated with multiple terms (synonymy); however, a term should represent only one concept.

COMPONENTS OF ADVANCED TERMINOLOGY SYSTEMS

Within the context of the high-level information model provided by the Nursing Minimum Data Set (NMDS) (Werley & Lang, 1988), there has been extensive development and refinement of terminologies for describing patient problems, nursing interventions, and nursing-sensitive patient outcomes (AORN, 2007; Moorhead, Johnson, & Maas, 2004; Martin, 2005; Dochterman & Bulechek, 2004; North American Nursing Diagnosis Association [NANDA], 2008; Ozbolt, 1998; Saba, 2006), including the development of the International Classification for Nursing Practice (ICNP) (Coenen, 2003; International Council of Nurses [ICN], 2009). These terminologies are described elsewhere in this text. The main component of more advanced terminology systems, however, is a concept-oriented terminology model or ontology representing a set of concepts and their interrelationships. The model is constructed using an ontology language that may be implemented using description logic within a software system or by a suite of software tools.

Terminology Model

A terminology model is a concept-based representation of a collection of domain-specific terms that is optimized for the management of terminological definitions. It encompasses both schemata and type definitions (Campbell, Cohn, Chute, Shortliffe, & Rennels, 1998; Sowa, 1984).

Schemata incorporate domain-specific knowledge about the typical constellations of entities, attributes, and events in the real world and, as such, reflect plausible combinations of concepts, eg, "dyspnea" may be combined with "severe" to make "severe dyspnea." Schemata may be supported by either formal or informal composition rules (ie, grammar).

Type definitions are obligatory conditions that state only the essential properties of a concept (Sowa, 1984), eg, a nursing activity must have a *recipient*, an *action*, and a *target*.

There have been several published reports related to terminology models for nursing (Bakken, Cashen, & O'Brien, 1999; Hardiker & Rector, 1998; ICN, 2001), which contributed to the development of an international standard for a reference terminology model for nursing (ISO, 2003).

Representation Language

Terminology models may be formulated and elucidated in an ontology language such as Knowledge Representation Specification Syntax (KRSS) (Campbell et al., 1998) or Web Ontology Language (OWL) (Rector, 2004). Ontology languages represent classes (also referred to as concepts, categories, or types) and their properties (also referred to as relations, slots, roles, or attributes). In this way, ontology languages are able to support, through explicit semantics, the formal definition of concepts in terms of their relationships with other concepts (Fig. 12.2); they also facilitate reasoning about those concepts, eg, whether two concepts are equivalent or whether one concept, such as "pain", subsumes (is a generalization of) another, such as "acute pain."

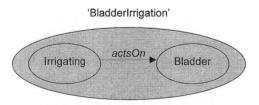

• **FIGURE 12.2.** A simple graphical example of a formal representation of the nursing activity concept "Bladder Irrigation."

Computer-based Tools

A representation language may be implemented using description logic within a software system or by a suite of software tools. The functionality of these tools varies but may include among other things management and internal organization of the model, and reasoning on the model, such as automatic classification of composed concepts based on their formal definition, eg, "teaching medication regime" is a kind of "teaching."

In addition, the software may facilitate transformation of concept representations into canonical form (eg, "cardiomegaly of the heart" is transformed to "cardiomegaly" since the location of the pathology is inherent in the concept itself), or support a set of sanctions (ie, constraints) that test whether a proposed composed concept is sensible (eg, "decubitus ulcer of the heart" and "impaired normal cognition" are not coherent terms). Other software support may be provided for knowledge engineering, operations management, and conflict detection and resolution.

The extent to which a terminology may be suitable for computer processing has previously been characterized in terms of "generations" (Rossi Mori et al., 1998). *First-generation terminology systems* consist of a list of enumerated terms, possibly arranged as a single hierarchy. They serve a single purpose or a group of closely related purposes and allow minimal computer processing. *Second-generation systems* include an abstract terminology model or terminology model schema that describes the organization of the main categories used in a particular terminology or set of terminologies. The abstract terminology model is complemented by a thesaurus of elementary descriptors (ie, terms) and templates or rules (ie, grammar) for defining how categories may be combined. For example, "pain" and "severe" may be combined into "severe pain." Second-generation systems can be used for a range of purposes, but they allow only limited computer processing, eg, automatic classification of composed concepts is not possible. *Third-generation systems* support sufficient formalisms to enable computer-based processing, ie, they include a grammar that defines the rules for automated generation and classification of new concepts. Third-generation language systems have also been referred to as formal concept representation systems (Ingenerf, 1995) or reference terminologies (Spackman, Campbell, & Cote, 1997).

Because they were designed primarily for direct manual use by nurses in the process of care or for classification purposes, the majority of existing nursing terminologies [eg, NANDA, Nursing Interventions Classification (NIC)] can be characterized as first-generation systems. The beta 2 version of the ICNP provided an example of a second-generation system (ICN, 2001)—this has

subsequently been superseded. Advanced terminology systems, ie, third-generation terminology systems are the focus of the remainder of this chapter.

ADVANTAGES OF ADVANCED TERMINOLOGY SYSTEMS

Computer-based systems that support clinical applications such as electronic health records and decision support require more granular (ie, less abstract) data than that typically contained in terminologies designed primarily for manual use or for the purpose of classification (Campbell, Carpenter, Sneiderman, Cohn, Chute, & Warren, 1997; Chute, Cohn, Campbell, Oliver, & Campbell, 1996; Cimino, 1998b; Cimino et al., 1989). Advanced concept-oriented terminology systems allow much greater granularity through controlled composition while avoiding a combinatorial explosion of pre-coordinated terms, thereby enhancing the ability of computer-based systems to process clinical data for meaningful use.

In addition, as described previously in this chapter, advanced terminology systems facilitate two important facets of knowledge representation for computer-based systems that support clinical care: (a) describing concepts and (b) manipulating and reasoning about those concepts using computer-based tools. Advantages resulting from the first facet include (1) nonambiguous representation of concepts, (2) facilitation of data abstraction or de-abstraction without loss of original data (ie, "lossless" data transformation), (3) nonambiguous mapping among terminologies, (4) data reuse in different contexts, and (5) data exchange across settings. These advantages are particularly important for clinical uses of the terminology. Advantages gained from the second facet include auditing the terminology system, automated classification of new concepts, and an ability to support multiple inheritance of defining characteristics (eg, "acute postoperative pain" is both a "pain" and a "postoperative symptom"). Both facets are vital to the maintenance of the terminology itself as well as to the ability to subsequently support the clinical utility of the terminology (Campbell et al., 1998; Rector, Bechhofer, Goble, Horrocks, Nowlan, & Solomon ,1997).

ADVANCED TERMINOLOGICAL APPROACHES IN NURSING

Over recent years, there have been a number of initiatives that support the development of advanced concept-oriented terminology systems for the nursing domain. Following a brief description of approaches underpinning three of these initiatives (terminology models within ISO 18104:2003, modified KRSS underpinning the original development of SNOMED RT (Systematized Nomenclature of Medicine Reference Terminology), and the OWL representation of ICNP), a nursing term is represented under ICNP and SNOMED CT (Clinical Terms) approaches in order to illustrate similarities and differences between representations. A further illustrative example demonstrates one of the potential functions of an advanced terminology system for nursing, ie, cross-mapping between existing terminologies.

Terminology Models—ISO 18104:2003

An international standard (ISO 18104:2003) covering reference terminology models for nursing diagnoses (Fig. 12.3) and nursing actions (Fig. 12.4) was approved in 2003 (ISO, 2003). The standard was developed by a group of experts within ISO Technical Committee 215 (Health Informatics) Working Group 3 (Semantic Content) under the collaborative lead-

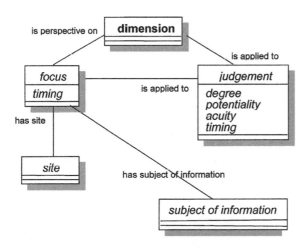

• **FIGURE 12.3.** Reference terminology model for nursing diagnoses. (The terms and definitions taken from ISO 18104:2003 Health Informatics—Integration of a reference terminology for nursing, Figures 1 and 2 [corresponding to Figs. 12.3 and 12.4 in this text] are reproduced with the permission of the International Organization for Standardization [ISO]. The standard can be obtained from any ISO member and from the Website of the ISO Central Secretariat at www.iso.org. Copyright remains with ISO.)

ership of the International Medical Informatics Association–Nursing Special Interest Group (IMIA-NI) and the International Council of Nurses (ICN). The model built on work originating within the European Committee for Standardization (European Committee for Standardization, 2000).

The development of ISO 18104:2003 was motivated in part by a desire to harmonize the plethora of nursing terminologies in use around the world (Hardiker, 2004). Another major incentive was to integrate with other evolving terminology and information model standards—the development of ISO 18104:2003 was intended to be "consistent with the goals and objectives of other specific health terminology models in order to provide a more unified reference health model" (ISO, 2003, p. 1). Potential uses identified for the terminology models include to (1) facilitate the representation of nursing diagnosis and nursing action concepts and their relationships in a manner suitable for computer processing, (2) provide a framework for the generation of compositional expressions from atomic concepts within a reference terminology, (3) facilitate the mapping among nursing diagnosis and nursing action concepts from various terminologies, (4) enable the systematic evaluation of terminologies and associated terminology models for purposes of harmonization, and (5) provide a language to describe the structure of nursing diagnosis and nursing action concepts in order to enable appropriate integration with information models (ISO, 2003). The standard is not intended to be of direct benefit to practicing nurses. It is intended to be of use to those who develop coding systems, terminologies, terminology models for other domains, health information models, information systems, software for natural langue processing, and markup standards for representation of healthcare documents.

ISO 18104:2003 has undergone substantial bench testing, both during its development and through independent research (Hwang, Cimino, & Bakken, 2003; Moss, Coenen, & Mills, 2003). The standard was under review at the time of writing for consideration of revisions.

Modified KRSS—SNOMED RT/CT

A concept-oriented approach was developed, through collaboration between the College of American Pathologists and Kaiser Permanente, based on SNOMED International. SNOMED Reference Terminology (RT) was a reference terminology optimized for clinical data retrieval and analysis (Spackman et al., 1997) that, along with UK Clinical Terms, SNOMED RT has

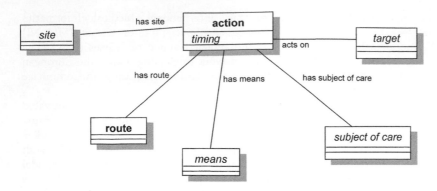

• **FIGURE 12.4.** Reference terminology model for nursing actions. (The terms and definitions taken from ISO 18104:2003 Health Informatics—Integration of a reference terminology for nursing, figures 1 and 2 [corresponding to Figs. 12.3 and 12.4 in this text] are reproduced with the permission of the International Organization for Standardization [ISO]. The standard can be obtained from any ISO member and from the Website of the ISO Central Secretariat at www.iso.org. Copyright remains with ISO.)

been used as a foundation for a new terminology system, SNOMED Clinical Terms (CT). Concepts and relationships in SNOMED RT were represented using modified KRSS (Campbell et al., 1998). Concept definition and manipulation were supported through a set of tools with functionality such as (1) acronym resolution, word completion, term completion, spelling correction, display of the authoritative form of the term entered by the user, and decomposition of unrecognized input (Metaphrase) (Tuttle, Keck, Cole et al., 1998), (2) automated classification (Ontylog), and (3) conflict management, detection, and resolution (Galapagos) (Campbell et al., 1998). Table 12.2 illustrates the representation, using generic description logic representation and modified KRSS, of a single nursing activity. SNOMED CT was developed collaboratively by the College of American Pathologists and the UK National Health Service (Wang, Sable, & Spackman, 2002). SNOMED CT possesses both reference terminology properties and user interface terms. SNOMED CT is considered to be the most comprehensive, multilingual clinical healthcare terminology in the world and integrates, through external mappings, concepts from multiple nursing terminologies and classification systems, including the Clinical Care Classification (CCC) System (see Chapter 14: Overview of CCC System or www.sabacare.com), the International Classification for Nursing Practice, the North American Nursing Diagnosis Association Taxonomy, the Nursing Interventions Classification, the Nursing Outcomes Classification, the Omaha System, and the Perioperative

TABLE 12.2	Possible Representations of the Nursing Activity Concept "Bladder Irrigation," Using Generic Description Logic Representation and Modified KRSS
Generic Description Logic Representation (with corresponding OWL constructors)	BladderIrrigation $\equiv$ Irrigating $\sqcap$ $\exists$ actsOn.Bladder
	Key
	$\equiv$ equivalentClass
	$\sqcap$ intersectionOf
	$\exists$ someValuesFrom
Modified KRSS Representation	(Define-concept BladderIrrigation (and Irrigating) (actsOn Bladder))

TABLE 12.3	Possible OWL Representation (in XML) of the Nursing Activity Concept "Bladder Irrigation"

```
<owl:Class rdf:ID="BladderIrrigation">
  <owl:equivalentClass>
    <owl:Class>
      <owl:intersectionOf rdf:parseType="Collection">
        <owl:Class rdf:about="#Irrigating"/>
        <owl:Restriction>
          <owl:onProperty>
            <owl:FunctionalProperty rdf:about="#actsOn"/>
          </owl:onProperty>
          <owl:someValuesFrom>
            <owl:Class rdf:about="#Bladder"/>
          </owl:someValuesFrom>
        </owl:Restriction>
      </owl:intersectionOf>
    </owl:Class>
  </owl:equivalentClass>
</owl:Class>
```

Nursing Data Set. SNOMED CT is distributed through the International Health Terminology Standards Development Organisation (IHTSDO). IHTSDO is an international nonprofit organization based in Denmark whose purpose is to develop, maintain, promote, and enable adoption and correct use of its terminology products such as SNOMED CT.

OWL–ICNP

Outside the health domain, work in relation to the Semantic Web has resulted in an emerging "standard" (ie, a W3C recommendation) ontology language, OWL (McGuiness & van Harmelen, 2004). OWL is intended for use where applications, rather than humans, are to process information. As such, it should be able to meet the requirements of advanced terminology systems that support contemporary healthcare. OWL builds on existing recommendations such as eXtensible Markup Language (XML) (surface syntax for structured documents), Resource Description Framework (RDF) (a data model for resources), and RDF Schema (a vocabulary for describing the properties and classes of resources) by providing additional vocabulary and a formal semantics. Software, both proprietary and open source, is available for (a) managing terminology models or ontologies developed in OWL (eg, Protégé (Protégé, 2010) and (b) reasoning on the model (eg, FaCT++) (Tsarkov, 2009). Work within nursing is maturing. For

example, ICNP is maintained in OWL—it is a compositional standards-based terminology for nursing practice (Hardiker & Coenen, 2007). The compositionality of ICNP further facilitates the development of and the cross-mapping among local terminologies and existing classification systems (ICN, 2009).

An OWL representation (in XML) of the nursing activity concept "Bladder Irrigation" is provided in Table 12.3 for comparison with the KRSS representations in Table 12.2.

ADVANCED TERMINOLOGY SYSTEMS IN PRACTICE

Figure 12.5 displays a potential mapping (to the right of the figure) between the NIC concept "Bladder Irrigation" (Dochterman & Bulechek, 2004) and the pre-coordinated Omaha System concept "Treatments and Procedures: Bladder Care" (Martin, 2005). A computer-based reasoner can use the formal definitions of the corresponding composed concepts to infer a hierarchical relationship. The asserted properties for both concepts (in the center of the figure) are identical. The existing hierarchy (to the left of the figure) asserts that "Performing" subsumes "Irrigating." Thus, "BladderCare," which maps to the Omaha System concept "Treatments and Procedures: Bladder Care," is a generalization of "BladderIrrigation," which maps to the NIC concept

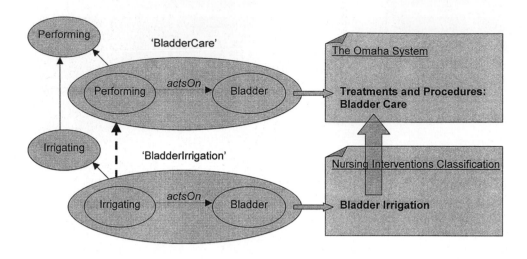

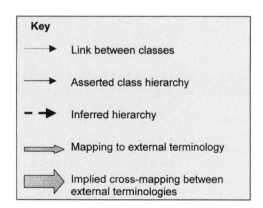

• **FIGURE 12.5.** An illustration of a potential mapping using an advanced terminology system between nursing activity concepts from two existing terminology systems.

"Bladder Irrigation." Hence, the NIC concept "Bladder Irrigation" potentially maps onto the Omaha System concept "Treatments and Procedures: Bladder Care" (but *not* vice versa).

SUMMARY AND IMPLICATIONS FOR NURSING

Previous studies have supported the need for advanced concept-oriented terminology systems that (a) provide for nonambiguous concept definitions, (b) facilitate composition of complex concepts from more primitive concepts, and (c) support mapping among terminolo-

gies (Campbell et al., 1997; Cimino, Clayton, Hripcsak, Johnson,1994; Chute et al., 1996; Henry, Holzemer, Reilly, Campbell, 1994). Because of the magnitude of resources and collaboration required, the development of advanced concept-oriented terminology systems is a fairly recent phenomenon. However, a number of benefits have been proposed: (1) facilitation of evidence-based practice (eg, linking of clinical practice guidelines to appropriate patients during the patient-provider encounter); (2) matching of potential research subjects to research protocols for which they are potentially eligible; (3) detection of and prevention of potential adverse drug effects; (4) linking online information resources; (5) increased reliability and validity of data for quality evaluation; and (6) data mining for purposes such as clinical research, health services research, or knowledge discovery.

The developers of nursing and healthcare terminologies and informatics scientists have made significant progress. From decades of nursing language research, there exists an extensive set of terms describing patient problems, nursing interventions and activities, and nursing-sensitive patient outcomes (AORN, 2007; ICN, 2009; Dochterman & Bulechek, 2004; Martin, 2005; Moorhead et al., 2004; NANDA, 2008; Ozbolt, 1998; Saba, 2006). Through the efforts of nursing professionals, new terms have been integrated into large healthcare terminologies as demonstrated by nursing informatics research, which are useful for representing nursing-relevant concepts (Bakken, Cimino, Haskell, et al., 2000; Bakken, Warren, Lundberg, et al., 2002; Henry et al., 1994; Lange, 1996; Matney, Bakken, & Huff, 2003). Ontology languages supported by suites of software tools have been developed within the context of terminologies with broad coverage of the healthcare domain (Campbell et al., 1998). Applicability of these tools to the nursing domain has been demonstrated (Hardiker & Rector, 1998; Zingo, 1997). A major remaining challenge is the development of content. However, there is significant progress in that area as well; existing standardized nursing terminologies have shown themselves to be an excellent source.

A number of efforts within nursing (eg, ICNP) and the larger healthcare arena (eg, SNOMED CT) are aimed toward the achievement of advanced terminology systems that support semantic interoperability across healthcare information systems. In addition, other research has focused on examining how terminology models and advanced terminology systems relate to other types of models that support semantic interoperability, such as a domain model for nursing, the Health Level 7 Reference Information Model (RIM) (Goossen et al., 2004), open EHR Archetypes (Beale, 2003), Detailed Clinical Models (Goossen, 2008), and an ontology for document naming (Hyun, Shapiro, Melton, et al., 2009). Such interoperability is a prerequisite to meeting the information demands of today's complex healthcare and health management environment.

REFERENCES

Association of Operating Room Nurses (2007). *PNDS – Perioperative Nursing Data Set* (2nd ed., rev.). Denver, CO: AORN Inc.

Bakken, S., Cashen, M., & O'Brien, A. (1999). Evaluation of a type definition for representing nursing activities within a concept-based terminologic system. In N. Lorenzi (Ed.), *1999 American Medical Informatics Association Fall Symposium* (pp. 17–21). Philadelphia, PA: Hanley & Belfus Inc.

Bakken, S., Cimino, J. J., Haskell, R., Kukafka, R., Matsumoto, C., Chan, G. K., & Huff, S. M. (2000). Evaluation of the clinical LOINC (Logical Observation Identifiers, Names, and Codes) semantic structure as a terminology model for standardized assessment measures. *Journal of the American Medical Informatics Association, 7*(6), 529–538.

Bakken, S., Warren, J. J., Lundberg, C., Casey, A., Correia, C., Konicek, D., & Zingo, C. (2002). An evaluation of the usefulness of two terminology models for integrating nursing diagnosis concepts into SNOMED clinical terms. *International Journal of Medical Informatics, 68*(1–3), 71–77.

Beale, T. (2003). Archetypes and the EHR. *Studies in Health Technology and Informatics, 96*, 238–244.

Campbell, J., Carpenter, P., Sneiderman, C., Cohn, S., Chute, C., & Warren, J. (1997). Phase II evaluation of clinical coding schemes: Completeness, taxonomy, mapping, definitions, and clarity. *Journal of the American Medical Informatics Association, 4*(3), 238–251.

Campbell, K., Cohn, S., Chute, C., Shortliffe, E., & Rennels, G. (1998). Scalable methodologies for distributed development of logic-based convergent medical terminology. *Methods of Information in Medicine, 37*(4–5), 426–439.

Chute, C., Cohn, S., & Campbell, J. (1998). A framework for comprehensive terminology systems in the United States: Development guidelines, criteria for selection, and public policy implications. ANSI Healthcare Informatics Standards Board Vocabulary Working Group and the Computer-based Patient Records Institute Working Group on Codes and Structures. *Journal of the American Medical Informatics Association, 5*(6), 503–510.

Chute, C. G., Cohn, S. P., Campbell, K. E., Oliver, D. E., & Campbell, J. R. (1996). The content coverage of clinical classifications. *Journal of the American Medical Informatics Association, 3*(3), 224–233.

Cimino, J. (1998a). The concepts of language and the language of concepts. *Methods of Information in Medicine, 37*(4–5), 311.

Cimino, J. (1998b). Desiderata for controlled medical vocabularies in the twenty-first century. *Methods of Information in Medicine, 37*(4–5), 394–403.

Cimino, J., Hripcsak, G., Johnson, S., & Clayton, P. (1989). Designing an introspective, multi-purpose, controlled medical vocabulary. In L. C. Kingsland, III (Ed.), *Symposium on Computer Applications in Medical Care* (pp. 513–518). Washington, DC: IEEE Computer Society Press.

Cimino, J. J., Clayton, P. D., Hripcsak, G., & Johnson, S. B. (1994). Knowledge-based approaches to the maintenance of a large controlled medical terminology. *Journal of the American Medical Informatics Association, 1*(1), 35–50.

Coenen, A. (2003). Building a unified nursing language: The ICNP. *International Nursing Review, 50*(2), 65–66.

Dochterman, J. & Bulechek, G. M. (2004). *Nursing interventions classification* (4th ed.). St. Louis, MO: C. V. Mosby.

European Committee for Standardization. (2000). *CEN ENV health informatics—Systems of concepts to support nursing*. Brussels, Belgium: CEN.

Goossen, W., Ozbolt, J., Coenen, A., Park, H., Mead, C., Ehnfors, M., & Marin, H. (2004). Development of a provisional domain model for the nursing process for use within the Health Level 7 reference information model. *Journal of the American Medical Informatics Association, 11*(3), 186–194.

Goossen, W. T. F. (2008). Using detailed clinical models to bridge the gap between clinicians and HIT (pp. 3–10). In E. de Clercq et al. (Eds.), *Collaborative patient centred ehealth*. Brussels, Belgium: IOS Press.

Hardiker, N. (2004). An international standard for nursing terminologies. In J. Bryant (Ed.), *Current perspectives in healthcare computing* (pp. 212–219). Swindon, UK: Health Informatics Committee of the British Computer Society.

Hardiker, N. & Rector, A. (1998). Modeling nursing terminology using the GRAIL representation language. *Journal of the American Medical Informatics Association, 5*(1), 120–128.

Hardiker, N. R. & Coenen, A. (2007). Interpretation of an international terminology standard in the development of a logic-based compositional terminology. *International Journal of Medical Informatics, 76S2*, S274–S280.

Henry, S. B., Holzemer, W. L., Reilly, C. A., & Campbell, K. E. (1994). Terms used by nurses to describe patient problems: Can SNOMED III represent nursing concepts in the patient record? *Journal of the American Medical Informatics Association, 1*(1), 61–74.

Henry, S. B. & Mead, C. N. (1997). Nursing classification systems: Necessary but not sufficient for representing "what nurses do" for inclusion in computer-based patient record systems. *Journal of the American Medical Informatics Association, 4*(3), 222–232.

Henry, S. B., Warren, J. J., Lange, L., & Button, P. (1998). A review of major nursing vocabularies and the extent to which they have the characteristics required for implementation in computer-based systems. *Journal of the American Medical Informatics Association, 5*(4), 321–328.

Hwang, J. I., Cimino, J. J., & Bakken, S. (2003). Integrating nursing diagnostic concepts into the medical entities dictionary using the ISO Reference Terminology Model for Nursing Diagnosis. *Journal of the American Medical Informatics Association, 10*(4), 382–388.

Ingenerf, J. (1995). Taxonomic vocabularies in medicine: The intention of usage determines different established

structures (pp. 136–139). In R. A. Greenes, H. E. Peterson, & D. J. Protti (Eds.), *MedInfo 95*. Vancouver, BC: HealthCare Computing and Communications, Canada.

International Council of Nurses. (2001). *International Classification for Nursing Practice* (beta 2 version). Geneva, Switzerland: International Council of Nurses.

International Council of Nurses (2009). *International Classification for Nursing Practice* (version 2). International Council of Nurses. Retrieved July 27, 2010 from www.icn.ch/pillarsprograms/international-classification-for-nursing-practicer/

International Organization for Standardization. (1990). *International Standard ISO 1087 1:2000 Terminology—Vocabulary—Part 1: Theory and application*. Geneva, Switzerland: International Organization for Standardization.

International Organization for Standardization. (2003). *International Standard ISO 18104:2003 Health Informatics—Integration of a reference terminology model for nursing*. Geneva, Switzerland: International Organization for Standardization.

Johnson, M., Bulechek, G., Butcher, H., Dochterman, J. M., Maas, M., Moorhead, S., & Swanson, E. (2006). *NANDA, NOC, and NIC Linkages: Nursing diagnoses, outcomes, & interventions*. St. Louis, MO: Mosby.

Lange, L. (1996). Representation of everyday clinical nursing language in UMLS and SNOMED. In J. Cimino (Ed.), *1996 American Medical Informatics Association Fall Symposium* (pp. 140–144). Philadelphia, PA: Hanley & Belfus, Inc.

Martin, K. S. (2005). *The Omaha System: A key to practice, documentation, and information management*. St. Louis, MO: Elsevier.

Matney, S., Bakken, S., & Huff, S. M. (2003). Representing nursing assessments in clinical information systems using the logical observation identifiers, names, and codes database. *Journal of Biomedical Informatics, 36*(4–5), 287–293.

McGuiness, D. L. & van Harmelen. F. (eds.) (2004). *OWL Web Ontology Language Overview*. World Wide Web Consortium. Retrieved July 27, 2010 from www.w3.org/TR/owl-features/.

Moorhead S., M. Johnson M. & Maas M. (Eds.) (2004). *Nursing outcomes classification* (3rd ed.). St. Louis, MO: C. V. Mosby.

Moss, J., Coenen, A., & Mills, M. (2003). Evaluation of the draft international standard for a reference terminology model for nursing actions. *Journal of Biomedical Informatics, 36*(4–5), 271–278.

North American Nursing Diagnosis Association. (2008). *NANDA nursing diagnoses 2009–20011: Definitions and classification 2009–2011*. Philadelphia, PA: North American Nursing Diagnosis Association.

Ogden, C. & Richards, I. (1923). *The meaning of meaning*. New York: Harcourt, Brace & World.

Ozbolt, J. G. (1998). *Ozbolt's patient care data set* (version 4.0). Nashville, TN: Vanderbilt University.

Protégé (2010). *What is Protégé-OWL?* Retrieved July 27, 2010 from http://protege.stanford.edu/overview/protege-owl.html

Rector, A. L. (2004). Defaults, context, and knowledge: Alternatives for OWL-indexed knowledge bases (pp. 226–237). *Pacific Symposium on Biocomputing.* January 6–10, 2004; Hawaii.

Rector, A. L., Bechhofer, S., Goble, C. A., Horrocks, I., Nowlan, W. A., & Solomon, W. D. (1997). The GRAIL concept modelling language for medical terminology. *Artificial Intelligence in Medicine, 9,* 139–171.

Rossi Mori, A., Consorti, F., & Galeazzi, E. (1998). Standards to support development of terminological systems for healthcare telematics. *Methods of Information in Medicine, 37*(4–5), 551–563.

Saba, V. (2006). Clinical Care Classification System. Retrieved July 27, 2010 from www.sabacare.com.

Sowa, J. (1984). Conceptual structures. Reading, MA: Addison-Wesley.

Spackman, K. A., Campbell, K. E., & Cote, R. A. (1997). SNOMED RT: A reference terminology for healthcare. In D. Masys (Ed.), 1997 American Medical Informatics Association Annual Fall Symposium (pp. 640–644). Philadelphia, PA: Hanley & Belfus, Inc.

Tsarkov, D. (2009). factplusplus. Retrieved July 27, 2010 from http://code.google.com/p/factplusplus/

Tuttle, M., Keck, K. D., Cole, W. G., Erlbaum, M. S., Sherertz, D. D., Chute, C. G., Elkin, P. L., Atkin, G. E., Kahoi, B. H., Safran, C., Rind, D., & Law, V. (1998). Metaphrase: An aid to the clinical conceptualization and formalization of patient problems in healthcare enterprises. Methods of Information in Medicine, 37(4–5), 373–383.

Wang, A., Sable, J. H., & Spackman, K. (2002). The SNOMED clinical terms development process: Refinement and analysis of content. In I. Kohane (Ed.), 2002 American Medical Informatics Association Fall Symposium (pp. 845–849). Philadelphia, PA: Hanley & Belfus, Inc.

Werley, H. H. & Lang, N. M. (Eds.) (1988). Identification of the Nursing Minimum Data Set. New York: Springer.

Zingo, C. A. (1997). Strategies and tools for creating a common nursing terminology within a large health maintenance organization. In U. Gerdin, M. Tallberg, & P. Wainwright. (Eds.), NI97 (pp. 27–31). Stockholm, Sweden: IOS Press.

13

Nursing Minimum Data Set Systems

Connie White Delaney / Bonnie Westra

- OBJECTIVES
  1. Define the concept Nursing Minimum Data Set (NMDS).
  2. Compare and contrast national NMDSs.
  3. Analyze which of the defined/published NMDSs support the International Nursing Minimum Data Set (i-NMDS).
  4. Apply the concept of "context" to the definition and use of NMDSs.

- KEY WORDS

  Minimum Data Set
  Nursing
  Nursing Minimum Data Set (NMDS)
  Nursing Minimum Management Data Set (NMMDS)

INTRODUCTION—CLINICAL NURSING VISIBILITY FROM NATIONAL TO INTERNATIONAL CONTEXTS

The impetus for access to and use of nursing data and information has never been stronger. Recognition of this growing need for nursing data has been powered by forces both internal and external to nursing (Institute of Medicine, 2000, 2001, 2004, 2010; Brooten, Youngblut, Kutcher, & Bobo, 2004; Maas &Delaney, 2004; American Nurses Credentialing Center [ANCC], 2008; Centers for Medicare and Medicaid Services, 2008; U.S. Department of Health and Human Services [U.S.-DHHS], n.d.; Dunton & Montalvo, 2009). Moreover, this growing need has been fuelled by international as well as national factors. The identification of the Nursing Minimum Data Set (NMDS), visionary work begun in the United States in 1980s by Werley and Lang (1988), has indeed spurred activity extending to national efforts to develop similar data sets around the world. Moreover, these national

efforts have supported an initiative to develop an international i-NMDS. This chapter provides a synthesis of historical, current, and future NMDS systems which can increase nursing data and information capacity to drive knowledge building for the discipline and profession and contribute to the standards supportive of the electronic health record (EHR).

NMDS HISTORICAL SUMMARY

The NMDS identifies essential, common, and core data elements to be collected for all patients/clients receiving nursing care. The NMDS is a standardized approach that facilitates the abstraction of these minimum, common, essential core data elements to describe nursing practice (Werley & Lang, 1988) from both paper and electronic records. It is intended for use in all settings where nurses provide care, spanning, for example, acute care, ambulatory centers, home healthcare, community practices, occupational health, and school health.

The NMDS was conceptualized through a small group work at the nursing information systems (NISs) conference held in 1977 at the University of Illinois College of Nursing. Werley and colleagues took the NMDS forward at the NMDS conference in 1985, held at the University of Wisconsin-Milwaukee School of Nursing. It was during this invitational conference that the NMDS was developed consensually through the efforts of 64 conference participants and formalized (Werley & Lang, 1988).

The NMDS includes 3 broad categories of elements: (a) nursing care, (b) patient or client demographics, and (c) service elements (see Table 13.1). Many of the NMDS elements are consistently collected in the majority of patient/client records across healthcare settings in the United States, especially the patient and service elements. The aim of the NMDS is not to be redundant of other data sets, but rather to identify what are the minimal data needed to be collected from records of patients receiving nursing care.

The NMDS was developed by building on the foundation established by the U.S. Uniform Hospital Discharge Data Set (UHDDS). The number of new items—mainly the nursing care items—is relatively less. The nursing care elements of the NMDS (nursing diagnosis, nursing interventions, nursing outcome, and intensity of nursing care) were derived from the nursing process. Additionally an item was added for an unique number of principle registered nurse provider (Table13.1).

Eight benefits of the NMDS, when adopted and implemented nationally or internationally with a system of ongoing data collection, were identified:

1. Access to comparable, minimum nursing care, and resources data on local, regional, national, and international levels
2. Enhanced documentation of nursing care provided
3. Identification of trends related to patient or client problems and nursing care provided
4. Impetus to improved costing of nursing services
5. Improved data for quality assurance evaluation
6. Impetus to further development and refinement of NISs
7. Comparative research on nursing care, including research on nursing diagnoses, nursing interventions, nursing outcomes, intensity of nursing care, and referral for further nursing services
8. Contributions toward advancing nursing as a research-based discipline

TABLE 13.1	The U.S. NMDS Data Elements

Nursing Care Elements
Nursing diagnosis
Nursing intervention
Nursing outcome
Intensity of nursing care

Patient or Client Demographic Elements
Personal identification[a]
Date of birth[a]
Sex[a]
Race and ethnicity[a]
Residence[a]

Service Elements
Unique facility or service agency number[a]
Unique health record number of patient or client[a]
Unique number of principle registered nurse provider
Episode admission or encounter date[a]
Discharge or termination date[a]
Disposition of patient or client[a]
Expected payer for most of this bill (anticipated financial guarantor for services)[a]

[a]Elements of the Uniform Hospital Discharge Data Set (UHDS).

STANDARDS AND RESEARCH ERA—21st CENTURY

Although the full benefits of the NMDS are still being realized, the NMDS work has influenced a number of advances. The NMDS influenced the work of the professional nurses association. In 1991, the American Nurses Association (ANA) recognized the NMDS as the minimum data elements to be included in any data set or patient record. The ANA consequently established the American Nurses' Association Steering Committee on Data Bases to Support Clinical Nursing Practice (since renamed the Committee on Nursing Practice Information Infrastructure). This committee launched a recognition process for standardized nursing vocabularies needed to capture the NMDS data elements for nursing diagnoses, interventions, and outcomes in a patient record. To date 10 languages have been recognized by ANA (2010); in addition, two data sets have been recognized by ANA: the NMDS and the Nursing Management Minimum Data Set (NMMDS) to complement the clinically oriented NMDS (ANA, 2010) as shown in Table 13.2.

TABLE 13.2	American Nurses Association Recognized Languages and Data Sets Supporting Nursing Practice (April 2009)
Languages	**Data Sets**
ABC codes	Nursing Minimum Data Set (NMDS)
Clinical Care Classification (CCC) System (formerly HHCC)	Nursing Management Minimum Data Set (NMMDS)
International Classification for Nursing Practice (ICNP)	
Logical Observations Identifiers Names and Codes (LOINC)	
NANDA—nursing diagnoses, definitions, and classification	
Nursing Outcomes Classification (NOC)	
Nursing Interventions Classification (NIC) system	
Omaha System	
Patient Care Data Set (PCDS)	
Perioperative Nursing Data Set (PNDS)	
Systematized Nomenclature of Medicine, Clinical Terminology (SNOMED CT)	

The NMDS served as a key component of the standards developed by the Nursing Information & Data Set Evaluation Center (NIDSEC) (American Nurses Association, 1997). The advancement of the NMDS has supported nurses' participation in developing computerized health information systems (HISs) (Androwich, Bickford, Button, Hunter, Murphy, & Sensmeier, 2003), utilization of data and information to support evidence-based practice (Pierce, 2000; Pravikoff, Pierce, & Tanner, 2003; Tanner, 2000), and inclusion of information management as an essential component of the discipline. The American Association of Colleges of Nursing (AACN) White Paper on the Clinical Nurse Leader (AACN, 2003), the position papers on the Baccalaureate Essentials (AACN, 2008), and the Doctorate of Nursing Practice

(AACN, 2004) are examples of the recognition of the essential core function of informatics expertise within practice. The NMDS is a principal driver in determining the research agenda for informatics (McCormick, Delaney, Brennan, et al., 2007). The NMDS has been core to advancing the science of understanding the complexity of nursing practice within complex systems through methods based on cutting edge intelligent systems (Clancy, Delaney, Morrison, & Gunn, 2006).

Moreover, the NMDS has triggered extensive attention, study, and deliberations related to nursing staffing and care quality and safety (Aiken, Clarke, Cheung, Sloane, & Silber, 2003; U.S.-DHHS, n.d.; Welton, Zone-Smith, & Fischer, 2006; Welton, Unruh, & Halloran, 2006; Welton, 2007; Welton & Dismuke, 2008; Welton, Zone-Smith, & Bandyopadhyay, 2009; Unruh 2008). The national Health Information Technology initiative under the oversight of the Office of the National Coordinator (2010) and healthcare reform (HealthCare Reform, 2010) provide timely opportunities for the advancement of the NMDS to address quality, safety, and cost.

Tools and Methods

Tools and methods to facilitate comparability of nursing data continue to evolve, including the International Classification for Nursing Practice (ICNP) and the International Standards Organization Reference Terminology Model for Nursing. Mapping of many of the recognized ANA languages into SNOMED CT (http://www.snomed/snomedct/), development of a validation method for this mapping (Lu, Eichmann, Konicek, Kanak, & Delaney, 2007; Park, Lu, Ucharattana, Konicek, & Delaney, 2007; Park, Lu, Konicek, & Delaney, 2007; Westra, Bauman, Delaney, Lundberg, & Peterson, 2008), and inclusion of the NMDS elements in SNOMED CT recognized nursing's contribution to healthcare as well. The NMDS has likewise been recognized by Health Level 7 (HL7) and validation of the inclusion of the NMDS elements within the HL7 information model has been completed (www.hl7.org).

NATIONAL NURSING MINIMUM DATA SETS

Established NMDSs

The early NMDS work in the United States spurred the development of NMDSs in numerous other countries. To date 7 countries have identified NMDS systems, including Australia, Canada, Belgium, Iceland, The

Netherlands, Switzerland, and Thailand (see Table 13.3). A perusal of these data sets reveals a definite consensus on the importance of the nursing care elements across all countries with identified NMDSs. There is variability as to the level of granularity in the specification of these data sets. Some are very granular in specifying specific patient problems and specific interventions of interest, while other data sets maintain a high conceptual focus and emphasize empowering nursing to establish NMDSs that can address all nursing problems/interventions/outcomes per encounter. There is also support for collection of key characteristics related to the patient/client and the service. There is variation as to applicability of the data sets to settings other than acute care.

Emergent NMDSs

Several countries across most continents beyond North America are exploring development of NMDS systems. For example, in Europe, the World Health Organization (Ryan & Delaney, 1995) has been concerned with variables including nursing care, personal data, medical diagnosis, and service data. Many of these elements are similar to the U.S. NMDS. Work is ongoing in the United Kingdom, eg, Scotland, to identify NMDSs to be congruent with the initiatives of the National Health Service. The Nordic countries likewise have much ongoing activity to identify NMDSs, eg, Finland (Turtiainen, Kinnunen, Sermeus, & Nyberg, 2000), Denmark, and Sweden (Hansebo, Kihlgren, & Ljunggren, 1999). France is pursing identification of a NMDS.

Moreover, Brazil is leading efforts in South America to identify a NMDS. South Korea and Japan are focusing on development efforts as well. New Zealand has focused efforts on a diabetes-specific data set to date. In summary, it is clear that there is major work being accomplished across the globe to ensure that nursing essential data will be more comprehensively available in the future. There is varying capacity to capture variables related to the context of care. NMDS research has begun at an international level (Goossen, Delaney, Coenen, et al., 2006).

Call for Standardized Contextual Data

Ample studies have demonstrated the significance of nurse staffing, patient/staff ratios, professional autonomy and control, organizational characteristics, unit internal environment, work delivery patterns, work group characteristics, external environment, staff work satisfaction, education of staff, multidisciplinary coordination/collaboration, and educational level on the quality and outcomes of patient care. For example, Aiken et al. (2003); Aiken et al. (2002); and Aiken, Smith, and Lake (1994) have maintained extensive research programs focused on examining the significance of these factors for quality of care. These studies have influenced the identification and use of NMDSs elements. Table 13.3 clearly indicates that several countries with established NMDSs have included some contextual data in the NMDSs. For example, Belgium calls for data related to number of beds and number of nurses available; Switzerland includes specific workload data related to each nursing intervention. The U.S. NMDS addresses "intensity"; however, no current NMDS addresses the essential breadth of contextual variables.

The development within the United States of the NMMDS addresses this void. The 18 NMMDS elements are organized into 3 categories: environment, nursing care resources, and financial resources (see Table 13.4). The NMMDS is the minimum set of items of information with uniform definitions and categories concerning the specific dimension of the context of patient/client care delivery. It represents the essential data used to support the management and administration of nursing care delivery across all types of settings. The NMMDS most appropriately focuses on the nursing delivery unit/service/center of excellence level across these settings. The NMMDS supports numerous constructed variables as well as aggregation of data, eg, unit level, institution, network, system. This minimum data set provides the structure for the collection of uniform information that influences quality of patient care, directly and indirectly. These data, in combination with actual patient data identified in the NMDS, support clinical decision making; management decisions regarding the quantity, quality, and satisfaction of personnel; costs of patient care; clinical outcomes; and internal and external benchmarking.

As previously indicated, the ANA, noting the importance of available standardized research-based nurse relevant data sets that encompass both the clinical and contextual data, has recognized two nursing datasets: the NMDS and the NMMDS. The NMMDS has been integral to several national quality initiatives, including the *National Database of Nursing Quality Indicators®* *(NDNQI)*, Magnet Status recognition and the management quality indicators in the National Quality Forum (NQF) nurse-sensitive quality indicators (Montalvo, 2007; ANCC, 2008; Kurtzman, & Kizer, 2005). Adoption of the NMMDS beyond the United States is

TABLE 13.3	National NMDS

Australia (Community Nursing Minimum Data Set [CNMDSA])[a]	Canada (Health Information: Nursing Components Data Set (HI: NC Data Set)[a]
Community Nursing	**National Scope Across All Settings[b]**
Purpose: compare performance of institutions, allocate resources, monitor and compare health status of the population, and deliver information	Purpose: deliver information about nursing care, and to demonstrate unique contribution of nurses to the public
NANDA	**NANDA**
Goals of nursing care	Nursing Interventions Classification (NIC)
Nursing interventions	Omaha System
Client dependency	Clinical Care Classification (CCC)
Nursing diagnosis	Nursing outcomes
Nursing resource utilization	
Patient Demographics	**Patient Demographics**
Birth date of client	Racial/ethnic
Sex of client	Unique geographical location
Ethnicity—country of birth	Unique lifetime identifier
Ethnicity—language spoken at home	Language
Location of client	Occupation
	Living arrangement
	Home environment, including physical structure
	Responsible caregiver on discharge
	Functional health status
	Burden on care provider
	Education level
	Literacy level
	Work environment
	Lifestyle data
	Income level
Medical diagnoses	Medical diagnoses
	Medical procedures
Resource utilization	Unique nurse identifier
Episode	Principal nurse provider
Agency/provider service	Mortality
Agency identifier	Physician, nurses, and consultant identifiers
Client identifier	Admit/discharge dates
Admission date	Length of stay
Referral source	
Discharge date	
Discharge destination (also a nursing element)	
Other support service	

(continued)

TABLE 13.3	National NMDS *(continued)*
NMDS Belgium Minimate Verpleegkundige Gegevens (MVG)/Resume Infirmier Minimum (RIM), Minimale Psychiatricsche Gegevens (MPG)[a–d]	**NMDS in Iceland**[e]
Use in general hospitals throughout the country, including psychiatric hospitals	Use across all healthcare settings
	Nursing diagnoses (NANDA)
	Nursing interventions (NIC)
Main diagnosis	Main medical diagnosis
Complications	Additional medical procedures and operation
Medical procedure and operations	Date of operation
	Responsible doctor for operation
Activities of daily living: (1) hygiene, (2) mobility, (3) elimination, (4) feeding assistance, (5) tube feeding, (6) mouth care, (7) dressing, (8) prevention of pressure sore, (9) intubation, (10) assessment, (11) training of activities of daily living, (12) crisis intervention, (13) reality orientation, (14) isolation, (15) taking vital signs, (16) physical parameters, (17) cast care, (18) taking blood samples, (19) medication management, (20) infusion care, and (21) wound care	Personal identifier
	Sex
	Residence
	Marital status
	Nationality
	Primary care doctor/district
Patient number	Principal nurse provider number
Year of birth	Provider nurse
Sex	Facility-agency
	Admission date
	Admission time
	Admission way
	Admission circumstance
	Admission reason
	Admit from
	Remitted by
	Discharge date
	Discharge time
	Discharge to
	Discharge destination
	Disposition of patienty
	Date of ended effective medical treatment
	Date of arrival outpatients
	Days on day-unit
	Control after discharge
	Readmission
Code of the hospital	
Code of the department	
Code of the nursing unit	

TABLE 13.3	National NMDS *(continued)*

NMDS Belgium Minimate Verpleegkundige Gegevens (MVG)/Resume Infirmier Minimum (RIM), Minimale Psychiatricsche Gegevens (MPG)[a–d]	NMDS in Iceland[e]
Day of admission	
Day of stay	
Day of discharge	
Nursing hours available on the nursing unit	
Number of nurses available	
Number of beds	
Nurse qualification mix	

The Netherlands (NMDSN)[f,g]	Switzerland (the Swiss Nursing Maximum Data Set)[h]
Aim for NMDSN: budget parameter for nursing	
Ten nursing processes: (1) assessment, (2) patient problems, (3) goals, (4) interventions, (5) daily reports, (6) flow chart, (7) forms to ascertain continuity of care, (8) risk for bedsore, (9) problems in vital signs, and (10) risk for falls	
Twenty-four nursing diagnoses/patient problems/nursing phenomena:	
(1) problematic communication; (2) need for information, knowledge; (3) fear; (4) uncertainty about the future; (5) problems in contact with family; (6) insufficient insight in the health situation; (7) difficulty managing therapy; (8) lack of motivation to co-operate in treatment and care; (9) behavioral problems; (10) disorientation in time, place; (11) memory problem; (12) restlessness; (13) pain; (14) problems with rest/sleep; (15) difficulty with stressful situations; (16) pressure ulcer; (17) impairment in elimination; (18) fever; (19) breathing; (20) problems with food and fluids; (21) self-care limitation; (22) functional problem with activities of daily living; (23) high risk; and (24) impairment in vital functions	
Thirty-two nursing interventions/actions	
Four outcomes/results of nursing care: (1) patient falls, (2) satisfaction with care, (3) satisfaction with information, and (4) satisfaction with pain management	
Three complexity of care: (1) calculation of nursing intensity, (2) visual analogue scale on which nurses score the complexity of care, and (3) visual analogue scale on which nurses score the appropriateness of the amount of care that could be given	
Patient characteristics:	Semistandard languages: LEP, PRN, PLAISIR, RAI
Sex	
Year of birth	(Considering NANDA, NIC, NOC)
Admission date	Health status: nursing phenomena and results

(continued)

TABLE 13.3	National NMDS (continued)
The Netherlands (NMDSN)[f,g]	**Switzerland (the Swiss Nursing Maximum Data Set)[h]**
Discharge date Unique patient code Age	Interventions: treatment and nursing care, principal intervention, secondary interventions, frequency, contribution of social network, care times, individualized required care time, individualized given care time Action modalities: frequency, duration, presence/absence of activity, volume, number of contributors, constant presence, nurture of assistance, contribution of social network
Seven items described medical conditions: (1) admission medical diagnoses, (2) additional medical diagnoses, (3) complications, (4) predictability of the health situation (5) stability of the health situation, (6) life-threatening situations, and (7) the derived item multiple health problems	Name Date of birth Sex Town/city of residence nationally Civil status Professional status on admission Language used during care Interpreter Religion Type of insurance Payment of basic care Other source of payment Homecare and assistance Type of dwelling Persons living at the same address Neonate: weight at birth, length, congenital deformity, and length of pregnancy
Healthcare settings: Hospital Ward Specialty Type of nursing delivery system Date of data collection	Nonnursing care and treatment: surgical operation, examinations, domiciliary assistance, other intra/extrainstitutional treatments or services, medication, pharmacotherapy
	Place: nature of location, services offered by each unit Unit infrastructure: number of beds per unit Institution: identification Status Type of institution Professionals: Care personnel number/sex/ Swiss or non-Swiss; professional training: number, diploma level
Thailand[i,j]	
Nursing care elements: Nursing problems Nursing interventions Nursing outcomes Patient elements: Patient first name and last name	

TABLE 13.3	National NMDS *(continued)*
Thailand[i,j]	
Sex	
Medical diagnosis	
Health history of patient and family allergy	
Address and phone number of patients	
Referral	
Laboratory tests	
Patient's condition and medical instruments use before discharge	
Discharge plan	
Service elements:	
Hospital number	
Admission umber	
Date of admission	
Date of discharge/expiry	
Health insurance	

[a]Ryan & Delaney (1995); [f]Goossen et al. (1998); [g]Goossen et al. (2001); [h]Berthou & Junger (2000); iKunaviktikul et al. (2001); [j]Volrathongchai, Delaney & Phuphaibul (2003).
Incomplete information data sets: [b]Based on U.S. NMDS and Belgium data set; [d]Evers (2000); [e]Haraldsdottir (2001); [c]Sermeus (1992).

also occurring. Nurses in Iceland have taken the lead in translating and testing the NMMDS for an entire nation. G. A. Hardardottir's dissertation research focuses on translation and validation of the NMMDS in Iceland (e-mail communication, March 7, 2011). M. Ólafsdóttir Thorlacius' thesis focused on validating the NMMDS-ICE (Icelandic version) across pediatric units in Icelandic hospitals and testing whether the NMMDS-ICE survey includes information needed to support daily nurse decision making in these settings (e-mail communication, February 2, 2011).

Last major advances are occurring to support the integration and open source availability of the NMMDS. To be useful in computerized healthcare systems, the datasets and other recognized terminologies must be structured in a format that can support electronic exchange of data. In an effort to support interoperable use and to meet ANA recommendations, the NMMDS is currently undergoing a major revision to align the data elements, definitions, and codes with other national standards. The revision process requires harmonization of the NMMDS data elements with comparable research, national requirements for nursing management data, and other national terminology standards. The

TABLE 13.4	Nursing Management Minimum Data Set (NMMDS) Data Elements
Environment	
Facility unique identifiers	
Nursing delivery unit or service	
Patient/client population	
Volume	
Method of care delivery	
Patient/client accessibility	
Clinical decision making complexity	
Environmental complexity	
Autonomy	
Accreditation	
Nursing Care	
Management demographic profile	
Staff demographic profile	
Staffing	
Staff satisfaction	
Financial Resources	
Payer type	
Reimbursement	
Budget	
Expense	

Federal Consolidated Health Informatics (CHI) initiative, now subsumed by the public-private Health Information Technology Standards Panel (HITSP) organization, recommends terminology standards for use in electronic health records within the United States (Healthcare Information Technology Standards Panel, 2010). The Logical Observations Identifiers Names and Codes (LOINC) is one of the federally recognized terminologies. Moreover, LOINC has been officially designated by the ANA as an ANA-recognized nomenclature because it represents and captures observations or assessments important for nursing. Given the above, in 2007 the NMMDS research team approached the LOINC committee with a proposal for a collaborative effort to include the revised version of the NMMDS in the LOINC database. The goals of this combined work were to ensure that the NMMDS codes are harmonized with an existing federally recognized standard and to provide a mechanism for NMMDS public distribution through LOINC (Westra, Matney, Subramanian, Hart, & Delaney, 2010; Westra, Subramanian, Hart, et al., 2010).

NMDSs RELATIONSHIP TO INTERNATIONAL NURSING MINIMUM DATA SET (i-NMDS)

Evolution of Concept

The i-NMDS includes the core, internationally relevant, essential, minimum data elements to be collected in the course for providing nursing care (Clark & Delaney, 2000). These data can provide information to describe, compare, and examine nursing practice around the globe. Work toward the i-NMDS is intended to build on the efforts already underway in individual countries. It is imperative that the national healthcare infrastructure supports the collection and reuse of nursing data. Consequently, partner countries participating in the development of the i-NMDS are encouraged to establish triads composed of (a) representative(s) of the National Nurses Association (preferably International Council of Nurses [ICN] member), (b) International Medical Informatics Association Nursing Informatics Special Interest Group (IMIA NI-SIG) representative, and (c) informatics expert(s). Project teams provide coordination and communication of project work in each country.

The i-NMDS project is intended to build on and support data set work already underway in individual countries, as well as the work with another ICN initiative, the ICNP. Data collected in the i-NMDS pilot project will be cross-mapped and normalized to the ICNP. This i-NMDS work will assist in testing the i-NMDS and also advancing the ICNP as a unifying framework. Overall, the i-NMDS project focuses on coordinating ongoing international data collection and analyses of the i-NMDS to support the description, study, and improvement of nursing practice (Goossen, Delaney, Semeus, et al., 2004).

Cosponsorship

The i-NMDS Research Center (http://www.nursing.umn.edu/ICMP.html) is lead by a steering committee of international representatives of countries with existing and emerging NMDSs as well as professional cosponsorship and areas of informatics expertise (www.inmds.org). The project is cosponsored by the ICN and the IMIA NI-SIG. Project work is also coordinated with international standards organizations and other stakeholders to assure harmonization of these efforts.

Purposes

The contribution of nursing care and nurses is essential to healthcare globally. The i-NMDS as a key data set will support:

- Describing the human phenomena, nursing interventions, care outcomes, and resource consumption related to nursing services
- Improving the performance of healthcare systems and the nurses working within these systems worldwide
- Enhancing the capacity of nursing and midwifery services
- Addressing the nursing shortage, inadequate working conditions, poor distribution and inappropriate utilization of nursing personnel, and the challenges as well as opportunities of global technological innovations
- Testing evidence-based practice improvements
- Empowering the public internationally

Data Elements

The i-NMDS elements are organized into 3 categories: setting, subjects of care, and nursing elements (Delaney, Goossen, Park, et al., 2003). Setting variables include country characteristics as well as descriptors of the location of care, whether the setting is acute, ambulatory, home, and so on. Measures include care personnel characteristics, including numbers, full-time equivalents, education, gender, and so on. Subjects of care can include individuals, families, groups, or communities. Demographics of the subject (individuals, families, groups, and communities) are included, eg, country of residence, disposition, age, gender, medical diagnosis are described. Last, nursing care elements include nursing diagnosis/subject of care problems, interventions, and outcomes. A measure of intensity of resource consumption will be developed. Nursing care data may be collected using standardized languages, eg, Clinical Care Classification (CCC) System, Omaha System, NANDA, NIC, NOC. Some nursing care data will be normalized using the ICNP.

Issues

Continuing attention needs to focus on consistency with the i-NMDS as well as supporting development of NMDSs across all countries. Consensus has been established to support the development and adoption of NMDSs that support all core nursing data collection in information systems across all settings. However, congruent with the state-of-adoption, specific studies addressing critical areas of international import will be designed to support the inclusion of countries with the capacity to collect the data which is the focus of specific studies. Normalization of data definitions must occur. Normalization of data collection time periods is a difficult issue.

FUTURE DIRECTIONS

The power of NMDSs to describe nursing practice from an international perspective is daunting (Delaney, 1996; Delaney &Moorhead, 1995; Delaney, Ruiz, Clarke, & Srinivasan, 2000; Delaney, Mehmert, Prophet, & Crossley, 1998; Junger, Berthou, & Delaney, 2004; Karpiuk, Delaney, & Ryan, 1997; Maas & Delaney, 2004; Mehmert & Delaney, 1991; Park & Delaney, 2003; Rios-Iturrine, Delaney, Mehmert, Kruckeberg, & Chung, 1991; Saba, 1997, 2007). Knowing the human phenomena served by nursing, the interventions given and the outcomes realized are essential to improving outcomes, assuring patient/client safety, and providing wise stewardship of all resources, from human to financial. Information and knowledge are key to supporting an essential knowledge-driven professional service and improving healthcare through effective policy changes.

Addressing the nursing shortage, inadequate working conditions, personnel satisfaction, all factors that research shows affect the quality of care, is dependent on nursing administration access to contextual as well as clinical data captured in the i-NMDS.

Access to the large data sets populated by the i-NMDS empowers nursing to capitalize on the emerging technologies of knowledge discovery, decision support, and advanced clinical information systems (Delaney, Reed, & Clarke, 2000; Delaney, Herr, Mass, & Specht, 2000; Irwin & Saba, 2003). Hypotheses generation as well as pattern discoveries will revolutionize many aspects of nursing research. Moreover, these data and valid and reliable knowledge generation likewise can revolutionize education and educating knowledge workers.

CASE SCENARIO

There is a need to determine quality and outcomes of care for pain management in elders with fractured hip diagnoses both across settings of care within one healthcare system and within and across national healthcare system boundaries. The National Health Service in collaboration with the World Health Organization wishes to establish benchmarks for care. You are asked to file a report addressing the following:

1. What is the relationship between and among the number, education, certification, and experience of healthcare workers and the vacancy rate?

2. What is the relationship between and among the number, education, certification, and experience of healthcare workers and turnover rates?

3. What is the relationship between and among the number, education, certification, and experience of healthcare workers and the following outcomes:

   (a) Nosocomial infections

   (b) Discharge effectiveness (teaching/planning)

   (c) Patient/family satisfaction with care received

   (d) Length of stay appropriate to diagnosis

   (e) Morbidity/mortality

   (f) Nurse satisfaction

REFERENCES

Aiken, L. H., Clarke, S. P., Cheung, R. B., Sloane, D. M., & Silber, J. H. (2002). Hospital nurse staffing and patient mortality, nurse burnout and job dissatisfaction. *Journal of the American Medical Association, 288*(16), 1987–1993.

Aiken, L. H., Clarke, S.P., Cheung, R. B., Sloane, D. M., & Silber, J. H. (2003). Educational levels of hospital nurses and surgical patient mortality. *Journal of the American Medical Association, 290*(12), 1617–1623.

Aiken, L. H., Smith, H. L., & Lake, E. T. (1994). Lower Medicare mortality among a set of hospitals known for good nursing care. *Medical Care, 32*(8), 771–787.

American Association of Colleges of Nursing. (2003). White paper on the clinical nurse leader. Washington, DC: AACN.

American Association of Colleges of Nursing. (2004). *Position statement on the practice doctorate in nursing.* Retrieved August 13, 2010 from http://www.aacn. nche.edu/DNP/DNPPositionStatement.htm

American Association of Colleges of Nursing. (2008). *The essentials of baccalaureate education for professional nursing practice.* Retrieved August 13, 2010 from http:// www.aacn.nche.edu/Education/pdf/BaccEssentials08. pdf

American Nurses Association. (1997). *Nursing Information & Data Set Evaluation Center (NIDSECSM).* Washington, DC: ANA.

American Nurses Association. (2010). Retrieved March 8, 2011 from http://journals/lww.com/ cinjournal/Abstract/2007/09000/Use_of_NIDSEC_ Compliant_CIS_in_community_based.11.aspx.

American Nurses Credentialing Center (ANCC). (2008). *Application manual: Magnet recognition program.* Silver Spring, MD: American Nurses Credentialing Center.

Androwich, I., Bickford, C., Button, P., Hunter, K., Murphy, J., & Sensmeier, J. (2003). *Clinical information systems: A framework for reaching the vision.* Washington, DC: American Nurses Association.

Berthou, A. & Junger, A. (2000). *Nursing data: Final report short version 1998–2000 period.* Retrieved April 1, 2002 from http://www.hospvd.ch/public/ise/nursingdata

Brooten, D., Youngblut, J. M., Kutcher, J., & Bobo, C. (2004). Quality and the nursing workforce: APNs, patient outcomes, and healthcare costs. *Nursing Outlook, 52,* 45–52.

Clancy, T., Delaney, C., Morrison, B., & Gunn, J. (2006). The benefits of standardized nursing languages in complex adaptive systems such as hospitals. *Journal of Nursing Administration, 36*(79), 426–434.

Clark, J. & Delaney, C. (2000). Conceptualization and feasibility of an international nursing minimum data set (i-NMDS) [abstract] (p. 865). In V. Saba, R. Carr, W. Sermeus, & P. Rocha (Eds.), *One step beyond: The evolution of technology & nursing, Proceedings of the 7th Congress on Nursing Informatics.* Auckland, New Zealand: Adis International.

Centers for Medicare and Medicaid Services. (2008). Retrieved August 18, 2010 from www.cms.gov

Delaney, C. (1996). Use of nursing informatics in advanced nursing practice roles for building healthier populations (clinical innovations). *Journal for Advanced Nursing Quarterly, 1*(4), 48–53.

Delaney, C., Goossen, W., Park, H., Junger, A., Oyri, K., Saba, V., & Coenen, A. (2003). Seeking international consensus on elements of the international nursing minimum data set (iNMDS) [abstract] (pp. 74–75). In H. Marin, E. Marques., E. Hovenga, and W. Goossen (Eds.), *Proceedings of the 8th International Congress in Nursing Informatics.* Rio de Janeiro, Brazil: Brazil E-Papers Ltd.

Delaney, C., Herr, K., Maas, M., & Specht, J. (2000). Reliability of nursing diagnoses documented in a computerized nursing information system. *Nursing Diagnosis, 11*(3), 121–134.

Delaney, C., Mehmert, P., Prophet, C., & Crossley, J. (1998). Establishment of the research value of nursing minimum data sets [reprint]. In V. Saba (Ed.), *Nursing and computers: An anthology, 1987–1996.* New York: Springer.

Delaney, C., & Moorhead, S. (1995). The nursing minimum data set, standardized language & healthcare quality. *Journal of Nursing Care Quality, 10*(1), 16–30.

Delaney, C., Reed, D., & Clarke, M. (2000). Describing patient problems & nursing treatment patterns using nursing minimum data sets (NMDS & NMMDS) and UHDDS repositories [paper] (pp. 176–179). In J. M. Overhage (Ed.), *AMIA 2000 converging information, technology, & healthcare.* Philadelphia, PA: Hanely & Belfus Inc.

Delaney, C., Ruiz, M., Clarke, M., & Srinivasan, P. (2000). Knowledge discovery in databases: Data mining the NMDS [paper] (pp. 61–65). In V. Saba, R. Carr, W. Sermeus, & P. Rocha (Eds.), *One step beyond: The evolution of technology & nursing, Proceedings of the 7th Nursing Informatics Congress.* Auckland, New Zealand: Adis International.

Dunton, N. & Montalvo, I. (Eds.). (2009). *Sustained improvement in nursing quality: Hospital performance on NDNQI indicators, 2007–2008.* Silver Spring, MD: American Nurses Association.

Goossen, W., Delaney, C., Coenen, A., Saba, V., Park, H., Casey, A., & Oyri, K. (2006). Towards the International Nursing Minimum Data Set. In C.Weaver, C. Delaney, P.Weber, & R.Carr, (Eds.), *Nursing and informatics for the 21st Century: An international look at cases, practice, and the future.* Chicago, IL: Healthcare Information and Management Systems Society.

Goossen, W., Delaney, C., Semeus, W., Junger, A., Saba, V., Oyri, K., & Coenen, A. (2004). Preliminary results of a pilot of the international nursing minimum data set (i-NMDS) [abstract] (p. S103). In *Proceedings of MedInfo 11th World Congress on Medical Informatics of the International Medical Informatics Association.* Amsterdam, The Netherlands: IOS Press.

Goossen, W. T. F., Epping, P. M. M., Feuth, T., Dassen, T. W. N., & Hasman, A. (1998). A comparison of nursing minimum data sets. *Journal of the American Medical Informatics Association, 5*(2), 152–163.

Goossen, W. T. F., Epping, P. J. M. M., Feuth, T., van den Heuvel, W. J. A., Hasman, A., & Dassen, T. W. N. (2001). Using the nursing minimum data set for the Netherlands (NMDSN) to illustrate differences in patient populations and variations in nursing activities. *International Journal of Nursing Studies, 38,* 243–257.

Hansebo, G., Kihlgren, M., & Ljunggren, G. (1999). Review of nursing documentation in nursing wards-changes after intervention for individualized care. *Journal of Advanced Nursing, 29*(6), 1462–1473.

Healthcare Reform. Retrieved August 13, 2010 from www.healthcare.gov/

Healthcare Information Technology Standards Panel. Retrieved August 13 2010 from http://www.hitsp.org/

Institute of Medicine Committee on Quality of Healthcare in America. (2000). *To err is human.* Washington, DC: National Academy Press.

Institute of Medicine Committee on Quality of Healthcare in America. (2001). *Crossing the quality chasm: A new health system for the 21st century.* Washington, DC: National Academy Press.

Institute of Medicine Committee on the Work Environment for Nurses & Patient Safety. (2004). *Keeping patients safe.* Washington, DC: National Academy Press.

Irwin, R. G. & Saba, V. (2003). An electronic 3 care tracking system. In e-Health for all: Designing nursing agenda for the future. In H. Marin, E. Marques, E. Hovenga, & W. Goossen (Eds.), *Proceedings of the 8th International Congress in Nursing Informatics.* Rio-de-Janeiro, Brazil: Brazil E-Papers Ltd.

Junger, A., Berthou, A., & Delaney, C. (2004). Modeling, the essential step to consolidate and integrate a national NMDS [paper]. MEDINFO-2004:*World Congress on Medical Informatics.* International Medical Informatics Association (IMIA) in San Francisco: CA. Amsterdam, The Netherlands: IOS Press.

Karpiuk, K., Delaney, C., & Ryan, P. (1997). South Dakota statewide nursing minimum data set project. *Journal of Professional Nursing, 13*(2), 76–83.

Kunaviktikul, W., Anders, R. L., Srisuphan, W., Chontawan, R., Nuntasupawat, R., & Pumparporn, O. (2001). Development of quality of nursing care in Thailand. *Journal of Advanced Nursing, 36*(6), 776–784.

Kurtzman, E. T., & Kizer, K. W. (2005). Evaluating the performance and contribution of nurses to achieve an environment of safety. *Nursing Administration Quarterly, 29,* 14–23.

Lu, D. F., Eichmann, D., Konicek, D., Kanak, M., & Delaney, C. (2007). SNOMED CT & Post–mapping Validation Methodology for Nursing Vocabularies. *Computers, Informatics, & Nursing.*

Maas, M. & Delaney, C. (2004). Nursing process outcome linkage: An assessment of literature & issues. *Medical Care, 42*(2)(Suppl.), II-40-II-48.

McCormick, K., Delaney, C., Brennan, P., Effken, J., Kendrick, K., Murphy, J., Skiba, D., Warren, J., Weaver, C., Weiner, B., & Westra, B. (2007). Guideposts to the future – An agenda for nursing informatics. *Journal of the American Medical Informatics Association, 14*(1), 19–24.

Mehmert, P. & Delaney, C. (1991). Validating impaired physical immobility. *Nursing Diagnosis, 2*(4), 143–154.

Montalvo, I. (2007). The national database of nursing quality indicators (NDNQI). *Online Journal of Issues in Nursing,16*(1), 12–13.

Office of the National Coordinator for Health Information Technology. Retrieved August 13, 2010 from http://healthit.hhs.gov/portal/server.pt?open=512&objID=1200&mode=2

Park, H., Lu, D., Konicek, D., & Delaney, C. (2007) Nursing interventions classification in systematized nomenclature of medicine clinical terms: A cross-mapping validation. *Computers, Informatics & Nursing, 25*(4), 198–208.

Park, M., & Delaney, C. (2003). Enhanced nursing care profile of older patients with dementia using nursing minimum data set (NMDS) & uniform hospital discharge data set (UHDDS) in an acute care setting [paper] (pp. 490–494). In H. Marin, E. Marques., E. Hovenga, & W. Goossen (Eds.), *Proceedings of the 8th International Congress in Nursing Informatics.* Rio-de-Janeiro, Brazil: Brazil E-Papers, Ltd.

Park, H.,Lu, D. F., Ucharattana, P., Konicek, D., & Delaney, C. (2007). Nursing Intervention Classification in the Systematized Nomenclature of Medicine Clinical Terms: A Cross-Mapping Validation. *Computers, Informatics, & Nursing, 25*(4), 198–208.

Pierce, S. (2000). Readiness for evidencebased practice: Information literacy needs of nursing faculty and students in a southern U.S. state. *Dissertation Abstracts International, 62*(12B), 5645. UMI No. 3035514.

Pravikoff, D., Pierce, S., & Tanner, A. (2003). Are nurses ready for evidence-based practice? *American Journal of Nursing, 103*(5), 95–96.

Rios-Iturrine, H., Delaney, C., Mehmert, P., Kruckeberg, T., & Chung, Y. (1991). Validation of defining characteristics of four nursing diagnoses using a computerized database. *Journal of Professional Nursing, 7*(5), 293–299.

Ryan, P., & Delaney, C. (1995). The nursing minimum data set: Research findings and future directions. *Annual Review of Nursing Research, 13,* 169–194.

Saba, V. K. (1997). Why the Home Healthcare Classification is a recognized nomenclature. *Computers in Nursing, 15*(20), S67–S73.

Saba, V. K. (2007). *Clinical Care Classification (CCC) System: A guide to nursing documentation.* New York: Springer Publishing.

Tanner, A. (2000). Readiness for evidence-based practice: Information literacy needs of nursing faculty and students in a southern U.S. state. *Dissertation Abstracts International, 62*(12B), 5647. UMI No. 3035515.

Turtiainen, A. M., Kinnunen, J., Sermeus, W., & Nyberg, T. (2000). The cross-cultural adaptation of Belgium Nursing Minimum Data Set to Finnish Nursing. *Journal of Nursing Management, 8*, 281–290.

Unruh, L. (2008). Nurse staffing, and patient, nurse, and financial outcomes. *American Journal of Nursing, 108*(1), 62–71.

U.S. Department of Health and Human Services (DHHS). *Hospital compare, A quality tool provided by Medicare.* Retrieved August 2010 from http://hospitalcompare.hhs.gov/

Volrathongchai, K., Delaney, C., & Phuphaibul, R. (2003). The development of NMDSs in Thailand. *Journal of Advanced Nursing, 43*(6), 1–7.

Welton, J. M. (2007). Mandatory hospital nurse to patient staffing ratios: Time to take a different approach. *Online Journal of Issues in Nursing, 12.* Retrieved from www.nursingworld.org/MainMenuCategories/ANAMarketplace/ANAPeriodicals/OJIN/TableofContents/Volume122007/No3Sept07/MandatoryNursetoPatientRatios.aspx

Welton, J. M. & Dismuke, C. E. (2008). Testing an inpatient nursing intensity billing model. *Policy, Politics, & Nursing Practice, 9*, 103–111.

Welton, J. M., Unruh, L., & Halloran, E. J. (2006). Nurse staffing, nursing intensity, staff mix, and direct nursing care costs across Massachusetts hospitals. *Journal of Nursing Administration, 36*, 416–425.

Welton, J. M., Zone-Smith, L., & Bandyopadhyay, D. (2009). Estimating nursing intensity and direct cost using the nurse-patient assignment. *Journal of Nursing Administration, 39*, 276–284.

Welton, J. M., Zone-Smith, L., & Fischer, M. H. (2006). Adjustment of inpatient care reimbursement for nursing intensity. *Policy, Politics, & Nursing Practice, 7*, 270–280.

Werley, H., & Lang, N. (Eds.). (1988). *Identification of the Nursing Minimum Data Set (NMDS).* New York: Springer.

Westra, B., Bauman, R., Delaney, C., Lundberg, C., & Peterson, C. (2008). Validation of the PNDS (Perioperative Nursing Data Set) and Systematized Nomenclature Medicine Clinical Terms (SNOMED CT). Concept Mapping. *AORN Journal, 87*(6), 1217–1229.

Westra, B., Matney, S., Subramanian, A., Hart, C., Delaney, C. (2010). Update of the NMMDS and Mapping to LOINC. In C. Weaver, C. Delaney, P. Weber, & R. Carr (Eds.), *Nursing and informatics for the 21st century: An international look at cases, practice, and the future* (2nd ed.). Chicago, IL: Healthcare Information and Management Systems Society.

Westra, B. L., Subramanian, A., Hart, C. M., Matney, S. A., Wilson, P. S., Huff, S. M., Huber, D. L., & Delaney, C. W. (2010) Achieving "Meaningful Use" of electronic health records through the integration of the Nursing Management Minimum Data Set. *Journal of Nursing Administration, 40*(7/8), 336–343.

Overview of the Clinical Care Classification System: A National Nursing Standard Coded Terminology

Virginia K. Saba / Jacqueline Moss / Luann Whittenburg

- **• OBJECTIVES**
  1. Provide an overview of the Clinical Care Classification (CCC) System.
  2. Identify why a coded nursing terminology is required to document nursing plans of care.
  3. Describe how the CCC System can be used to cost nursing care.

- **• KEY WORDS**

  electronic health record
  nursing documentation
  clinical information system
  CCC System
  nursing care costs
  nursing terminology
  national standard

"In attempting to arrive at the truth, I have applied everywhere for information, but in scarcely an instance have I been able to obtain hospital records fit for any purpose of comparison...if wisely used, these improved statistics would tell us more of the relative value of particular operations and modes of treatment than we have any means of obtaining at present."
—Florence Nightingale, 1863

As Florence Nightingale observed, the lack of standardized clinical information in healthcare records is a deterrent to our ability to track and measure patient responses to care interventions. And, the standardization of nursing information has changed little with the implementation of electronic healthcare records. The lack of progress in this area is a serious deficiency that undermines nursing's ability to determine the effectiveness of patient healthcare services and threats to public health. The lack of standardized nursing data collection also increases healthcare costs by constraining the ability of nurses to share data efficiently, resulting in patient safety concerns, increased administrative costs due to replication of data collection, and lack of efficient data transfer between healthcare professionals.

CURRENT TRENDS

In the United States, the federal government has made the use of electronic health record (EHR) technology a national priority and has mandated that every person must have an EHR by 2015. In 2004, the Office of the

TABLE 14.1	Major Characteristics of the Clinical Care Classification System

- Free with permission
- Atomic-level concepts
- Open architecture: PC, Mac, tablets, PDA mobile computing
- Designed for all computer-based systems: electronic health records (EHRs), electronic medical records (EMRs), personal health records (PHRs), health information technology (HIT), clinical information systems (CISs), etc.
- Tested as applicable in all healthcare settings
- Interoperable with Health Level Seven (HL7)
- Integrated in SNOMED-CT and National Library of Medicine's Unified Medical Language System (UMLS)
- Conforms to Cimino criteria for a standardized terminology for EHRs
- Coding structure is based on ICD-10 for information exchange, promoting interoperability
- Recognized Nursing Terminology by American Nurses Association
- Conforms to ISO Reference Terminology Model for Nursing (ISO-18104)
- Developed empirically from research of live patient care data records
- Designed for determining care costs, workload, and productivity
- Electronically links nursing diagnoses to interventions and outcomes
- Coded standardized and unified framework for electronic documentation, processing, retrieval, and analysis following the nursing process

National Coordinator (ONC) for Health Information Technology (HIT) and the position of National Coordinator were established in the Department of Health and Human Services (HHS). The ONC's mission is to promote the development of a nationwide health information and technology infrastructure that allows for the electronic use and exchange of information. The National Coordinator's role is to provide the leadership to develop the information standards and infrastructure necessary to harness the use of technology to improve patient care and reduce healthcare costs. The National Coordinator also leads the health information and technology implementation of the American Recovery and Reinvestment Act (ARRA) of 2009, including a portion of the bill called the Health Information Technology for Economic and Clinical Health (HITECH) Act of 2009.

For this initiative, incentives will be offered to healthcare providers who use EHR technology in a manner that is deemed 'meaningful use' by the federal government. The first stage of this initiative mandates that providers capture health information in a coded format and uses the coded data to track clinical conditions and to communicate information for care coordination and the reporting of clinical outcomes (Centers for Medicare & Medicaid Services, 2009). Data describing the contributions of nurses to healthcare and patient outcomes are not collected in a coded format that meets the federal requirements for "meaningful use" of EHR technology and therefore are not included in the national or regional healthcare information record data repositories

for healthcare data sharing, making nursing's contribution to patient care invisible.

The Clinical Care Classification (CCC) System is the first national nursing standard selected as a coded, standardized, and interoperable terminology to document nursing practice, making nursing data visible in the EHR. In 2007, the CCC System was named the 1st National Nursing Terminology Standard recommended by the Healthcare Information Technology Standards Panel (HITSP) to meet the interoperability specifications for EHRs. The HITSP recommendation was accepted by the U.S. HHS Secretary in 2008. The CCC system was initially proposed for the exchange of the encounter message component of clinical data, chief complaints, and nurses' triage notes. The CCC was adopted for EHR interoperability because of the major characteristics that are listed in Table 14.1.

OVERVIEW

This chapter will provide an overview of the CCC System and how the incorporation of the CCC system into EHRs can meet nursing's data collection and sharing needs. The CCC System provides a unique framework and coding structure for capturing the "essence of nursing care" electronically by nurses and allied health professionals in all healthcare settings. The CCC enables the ongoing analysis of patient data for the generation of evidence-based and clinical practice guidelines. The CCC facilitates the collection of coded data to describe nursing practice that enhances nursing care planning, nursing documentation, the analyses of nurse-sensitive outcomes, and aids in determining workload measures, resources, and costs of nursing care.

CCC SYSTEM DEVELOPMENT

The CCC System was originally created to document nursing care in home health and ambulatory care settings, but research has shown that the CCC also applies to nursing care in acute care settings (Holzemer, Dawson, Sousa, Bain, & Hsieh, 1997; Moss, Dangrongsak, Gallichio, 2005) and in all types of healthcare facilities. The CCC System was developed empirically from a federally (Healthcare Financing Administration) funded research study conducted by Dr. Virginia K. Saba and her research staff at Georgetown University, School of Nursing to develop a computerized methodology for assessing and classifying Medicare patients to predict nursing resource needs and to measure outcomes of care. To accomplish this goal, data on actual resource use were collected from 8,900 patient records, which included approximately 40,000 textual phrases representing nursing diagnoses and patient problems and 72,000 phrases depicting patient care services and/or actions (Saba & Taylor, 2007). Using "keyword sorts" and research analyses the data revealed that the content of the textual phrases could be organized hierarchically into 2 interrelated classification systems, describing nursing diagnoses and nursing interventions and actions, and resulted in the development of CCC Version 1.0 (originally known as the Home Healthcare Classification [HHCC]), which was published in 1991.

In the development of the CCC System, a determination was made using the live empirical research data to code terms and phrases at all levels of the terminology hierarchy, allowing a high level of specificity when documenting nursing care. As a result, the CCC System, consisting of 2 interrelated terminologies, forms a single system specifically designed for computer-based clinical information systems to facilitate nursing documentation at the point-of-care.

CCC SYSTEM

The current version of the CCC System, Version 2.1, consists of 2 interrelated terminologies: the CCC Nursing Diagnoses and Outcomes, and the CCC Nursing Interventions/Actions. Together, they form a single system classified by 21 Care Components and organized by 4 Healthcare Patterns. The CCC is used to document the process of nursing care by linking nursing diagnoses, interventions, and outcomes together and from the CCC System to other terminologies (e.g., reference terminologies such as SNOMED-CT).

CCC SYSTEM STRUCTURE

The standardized framework of the CCC System consists of 4 levels designed to allow the data to flow between the lowest level upward to the highest level or the highest level downward to the lowest level. The CCC System framework allows nursing data to be coded at multiple levels of abstraction, providing the ability to analyze nursing data at multiple levels of granularity. This standardized information framework provides the format for the documentation of nursing practice and supports the linkages between the 2 interrelated terminologies—(1) CCC of Nursing Diagnoses and Outcomes and (2) CCC of Nursing Interventions/Actions—to enable the analyses of outcome measures, workload, resources, and cost.

CCC HEALTHCARE PATTERNS

At the highest level of the CCC System Famework are 4 healthcare patterns: (1) Health Behavioral, (2) Functional, (3) Physiological, and (4) Psychological. Each represents a different set of Care Components. The healthcare patterns serve to organize the 2 CCC terminologies—nursing diagnoses and nursing interventions—and describe the domain of nursing in relationship to the 6 standards of the nursing process. Figure 14.1 illustrates the CCC System standardized framework.

CCC CARE COMPONENTS

At a second level of the CCC terminology hierarchy are 21 Care Components that serve to further classify the CCC System's 2 terminologies—nursing diagnoses and nursing interventions. The Care Components also provide the coding framework to facilitate electronic processing. A *Care Component* (CC) is defined as follows (Saba, 2007):

> "A cluster of elements that depicts the four healthcare patterns: Functional, Health Behavioral, Physiological, and Psychological representing a holistic approach to patient care." (p.158)

The Care Components are used to code and classify the 6 standards of the nursing process: assessment, diagnosis, outcome identification, planning, implementation,

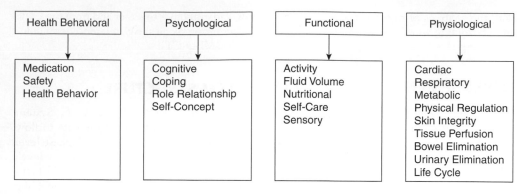

• **FIGURE 14.1.** CCC System framework.

and evaluation (ANA, 2003). The Care Components are also used to link, map, and track the care process for an episode of illness, facilitate computer processing, and statistical analyses as well as used to track and measure patient care holistically over time and across settings, population groups, and geographic locations. A complete listing of the CCC System Care Components can be found in Figure14.1.

The 21 Care Components were found to be clinically relevant nursing assessment classes, the best predictors of healthcare resources, and the most appropriate standardized framework for coding and classifying nursing diagnoses, interventions, and outcomes (Holzemer et al., 1997). Holzemer indicated that the 21 Care Component method of classification was 99% compliant for coding disease conditions in a variety of healthcare settings. See Figure 14.1 for the organizational structure of the 21 Care Components by the 4 Healthcare Patterns.

CCC OF NURSING DIAGNO\SES

The CCC Nursing Diagnoses terminology consists of 182 nursing diagnostic concepts (58 major diagnostic concepts representing concrete patient problems and 123 subcategories providing precise, granular-related concepts describing the specific variations of the major diagnostic problems). The CCC Nursing Diagnoses depicts patient conditions requiring clinical care by nurses and allied health providers. These diagnoses were derived from the over 40,000 phrases depicting patient problems and/or nursing diagnoses that required nursing services and that also included the outcomes of care processes or patient outcomes on discharge from an episode of illness. Some of the concepts originally

collected include North American Nursing Diagnosis Association (NANDA) terms that were adapted and converted from verb phrases to noun clauses for the CCC System (Saba, 2007).

The CCC System's definition for nursing diagnoses is based on a nursing diagnosis definition approved by the North American Nursing Diagnoses Association at the ninth conference in 1990 (NANDA, 1992).

> "Nursing Diagnosis is a clinical judgment about individual, family, or community responses to actual and potential health problems/life processes. A nursing diagnosis provides the basis for selection of nursing interventions to achieve outcomes for which the nurse is accountable. (p. 5)."

Examples of Core Nursing Diagnoses with their 3 or 4 alphanumeric codes:

- Activity Alteration (A01)
- Dying Process (E10)
- Polypharmacy (H21.1)
- Alcohol Abuse (N58.2)

A complete listing of the CCC Nursing Diagnoses can be found in Appendix A.

CCC OF NURSING OUTCOMES

Each of the CCC System Nursing Diagnoses can be paired with 1 of 3 qualifiers (i.e., Improve, Stabilize, or Deteriorate) depicting the expected outcome of care or 1 of 3 qualifiers depicting the actual outcome of care. In pairing the 182 Nursing Diagnoses with the 3 outcome qualifiers results in 549 Expected Nursing Outcomes and 549 Actual Nursing Outcomes for the documentation of nursing process data. The Expected Outcome Qualifiers are used in nursing documentation based on the plan of care when a patient's nursing diagnosis, problem, or particular condition is anticipated.

1. *Improve*: Patient's diagnosis or problem will change and/or improve and will not require any further care.
2. *Stabilize*: Patient's diagnosis or problem will stabilize and/or not change and will not require further care.
3. *Deteriorate*: Patient's diagnosis or problem will deteriorate or worsen and/or the patient may die.

Whereas when the nursing interventions are completed at a particular point in time or on discharge, the 3 Actual Outcome Qualifiers are used to document the nursing care results and/or status of the identified nursing diagnoses. The CCC System's Actual Outcome Qualifiers are:

1. *Improved*: Patient's diagnosis or problem improved and/or resolved.
2. *Stabilized*: Patient's diagnosis or problem did not change and/or remained the same.
3. *Deteriorated*: Patient's diagnosis or problem worsened and/or patient died.

Examples of Expected and Actual Outcomes:
- Substance Abuse : Will Improve or has Improved (N40.0.**1**).
- Substance Abuse: Will Stabilize or has Stabilized (N40.0.**2**).
- Substance Abuse: Will Deteriorate or has Deteriorated (N40.0.**3**).

CCC OF NURSING INTERVENTIONS

The CCC of Nursing Interventions consists of 792 Nursing Interventions/Actions (198 Nursing Interventions [72 major and 126 subcategories]) with 4 Action Types. The interventions are used to document the essence of care provided by the nurse treating the assessed diagnosis, problem, or condition. The 72 major interventions represent major intervention concepts and the 126 subcategories represent precise nursing interventions or specific intervention concepts. The nursing interventions were derived from approximately 72,000 research phrases depicting nursing interventions, actions, treatments,

procedures, activities, or services provided by nurses and other allied health providers during episodes of illness.

In the CCC System a *nursing intervention* is defined as follows (Saba, 2007):

"A single nursing action, designed to achieve an outcome for a nursing or medical diagnoses for which the nurse is accountable." (p. 328)

Examples of the Core Nursing Interventions with their 3 or 4 alphanumeric codes are listed as follows:
- Bowel Care (B06.0)
- Medication Care (H24.0)
- Cast Care (A02.1)
- Dying/Death Measures (E14.2)

A complete listing of the CCC Nursing Interventions can be found in Appendix A.

Intervention Action Types

The nursing care and service phrases used to develop the CCC terminology were found to contain 2 parts: (1) a core nursing intervention or service, and (2) an action type that expanded the scope of the intervention or service. Thus, both nursing interventions and action types are considered essential nursing care processes and coded separately in the terminology. Therefore, each of the nursing interventions was further expanded by combining it with 1 of 4 action type qualifiers: (1) Assess or Monitor; (2) Perform or Direct Care; (3) Teach or Educate, and (4) Manage or Refer.

The 4 Action Types depict 4 distinct 'essence of nursing care' and are defined as follows:

1. *Assess or Monitor:* Collect and analyze data on the health status.
2. *Perform or Direct Care:* Provide a therapeutic action.
3. *Teach or Educate:* Provide information, knowledge, or skill.
4. *Manage or Refer:* Administer, coordinate, or manage care or services.

These 4 qualifiers define the action dimension to modify each nursing intervention or service and are reflected in the coding process, making it easier to code, process, retrieve, and analyze the intervention data. For example, the nurse requires more time and expertise to *Assess Wound Care* than to *Teach Wound Care*. The more precise coding provides better predictions of care outcome measures, resources, workload,

TABLE 14.2	Example of Skin Integrity Alteration with Each of 4 Nursing Intervention Actions to Achieve Each of 3 Actual Outcomes	
Nursing Diagnosis	**Nursing Intervention**	**Nursing Outcome**
Skin Integrity Alteration (R46)	Assess Skin Care (R54.0.**1**)	Skin Integrity Stabilized (R46.0.**2**)
Skin Integrity Alteration (R46)	Perform Skin Care (R54.0.**2**)	Skin Integrity Improved (R46.0.**1**)
Skin Integrity Alteration (R46)	Teach Skin Care (R54.0.**3**)	Skin Integrity Deteriorated (R46.0.**3**)
Skin Integrity Alteration (R46)	Manage Skin Care (R54.0.**4**)	Skin Integrity Improved (R46.0.**1**)

and/or costs. Each Core Nursing Intervention must include 1 of the 4 action types. Here are some examples using the Core Nursing Intervention of Cast Care (B02.1) with an Action Type code inserted as the last, or fifth, digit:

Assess Cast Care (A02.1.1)

Perform Cast Care (A02.1.2)

Teach Cast Care (A02.1.3)

Manage Cast Care (A02.1.4)

Documentation using the CCC System enables linkage between nursing diagnoses, interventions, and outcomes to provide a complete picture of how the nursing process influences patient outcomes. For example, the diagnosis Skin Integrity Alteration could be combined with each of the 4 action types and outcome labels to describe very different patient scenarios, as illustrated in Table 14.2. An example of Skin Integrity Alteration is used for each of the 4 Nursing Intervention Action Types to achieve each of the 3 Nursing Outcomes.

CODING STRUCTURE

The CCC System data are coded based on a 5-level structure similar to the coded structure of the International Classification of Diseases and Health Related Problems: Tenth Revision (ICD-10) (WHO, 1992). Each concept in the CCC System is assigned a unique code comprising 5 alphanumeric characters:

First character: An alpha character that represents a Care Component class

Second and third digits: Numeric digits that represent a Major Category.

Fourth digit: Numeric digit that represents a Subcategory

Fifth digit: Last numeric digit that represents a Qualifier

One of 3 Outcome Qualifiers describes the Expected and/or Actual Outcomes of care.

One of 4 Action Type Qualifiers modifies and expands the description of the Nursing Intervention(s).

See Table 14.3 for examples of the CCC System Nursing Diagnosis with Outcomes and Nursing Interventions with Actions Coding Structures.

CCC SYSTEM TERMINOLOGY SCOPE

The CCC System Terminology classified by 21 Care Components consists of the following:

182 Nursing Diagnoses

546 Nursing Outcomes (182 Nursing Diagnoses plus 3 Expected or Actual Outcomes)

792 Nursing Interventions (198 Core Nursing Interventions plus 4 Action Types)

Information Model

The CCC System follows the CCC Information Model shown in Figure 14.2 for the documentation of patient care by nursing and allied health providers. The Information Model illustrates the interactive continuous feedback of care data and the interrelationships between the CCC Nursing Diagnoses and Outcomes and the CCC Nursing Interventions and Actions.

CCC Care Plan Example

The CCC System is used for the documentation of a nursing plan of care based on the nursing process. A

TABLE 14.3	Example of Clinical Care Classification System—Nursing Diagnosis with Expected and Actual Outcomes and Nursing Intervention with Action Coding Structures
Nursing Diagnosis	**Blood Pressure Alteration (C06.1)**
Class	Cardiac Care Component: **C**
Major concept	Cardiovascular Alteration: **Co6.0**
Minor/subcategory concept	Blood Pressure Alteration: **C06.1**
Expected outcome:	Blood Pressure Alteration *Will Improve*: C06.1.**1**
Nursing Intervention	**Perform Cardiac Rehabilitation (C08.1.2)**
Class	Cardiac Care Component: **C**
Major concept	Cardiac Care: **C08.0**
Minor/subcategory concept	Cardiac Rehabilitation: **C08.1**
Action type qualifier	Perform Cardiac Rehabilitation: C08.1.**2**
Actual outcome:	Blood Pressure Alteration *Stabilized*: C06.1.**2**

care plan, as outlined in the CCC Information Model (Figure 14.3), is initiated with the signs and symptoms identified from the admission and/or follow-up assessment, from which a Care Component is selected and used to map the appropriate CCC Nursing Diagnoses with the Expected Outcomes/Goals for the Nursing Diagnosis. Each Nursing Diagnosis is then mapped to the CCC Nursing Interventions and Action Types (nursing orders) to develop and provide a plan of care. Once the goals of the CCC Nursing Diagnoses are met (the nursing interventions resolved), then the

Actual Outcomes are recorded and the care plan is completed. The care evidence is based on the number and frequency of nursing interventions and action types.

The plan of care guides the continuity of care and assists in the evaluation of nursing care outcomes. The example in Figure 14.3 is displayed as a clinical pathway. The plan focuses on the acute pain, as assessed, and is mapped to the nursing care orders. Once the goal for the acute pain is met, the nursing orders are discontinued and the plan ends.

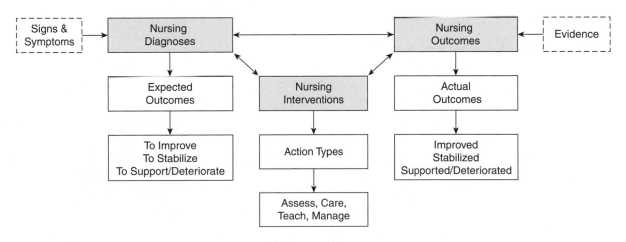

• **FIGURE 14.2.** Clinical Care Classification Information Model.

Care Component/ Nursing Dx Signs & Symptoms	Care Component/ Nursing Dx Expected Outcome	Encounter/Day 1 Nursing Interventions Action Types	Encounter Day 2 Nursing Interventions Action Types	Care Component/ Nursing Dx Actual Outcome
Q 45.1 Acute Pain Alteration * Pain when coughing or deep breathing	Q 451.1.1 Improve Acute Pain	Q47.1.1 Assess Acute Pain Control * Determine location and intensity of pain	>>>>>>>>>>>>>>>>	Q45.1.1 Acute Pain Alteration Improved/Goal Met
		Q47.1.3 Teach Acute Pain Control * Splint with pillow when coughing	>>>>>>>>>>>>>>>>	* Patient does complain of pain & does not Cough
		H24.3.2 Perform Medication Treatment * Give pain medication PRN	>>>>>>>>>>>>>>>>	* No Pain Mediation required

• **FIGURE 14.3.** Sample Nursing Care Plan for Acute Pain Alteration..

CCC—NURSING PRACTICE

Numerous home healthcare agencies have implemented the CCC System, which has been incorporated into agency database dictionaries and used for the documentation of nursing care in many formats. With the introduction of Version 2.0 numerous national and international healthcare organizations have successfully implemented the CCC System. In Finland, the CCC is being implemented throughout the entire country as an integral part of the patient healthcare record, such as the Orthon Hospital in Helsinki and the Kupio Hospital in Kupio. Siemens Medical Solutions, a vendor of hospital information technology (HIT) systems, has integrated the CCC System into the latest version of its HIT system, called Sorian, which has been distributed in all the hospitals using the Siemens HIT around the world as of August 2009. Nationally, the CCC System can be found in numerous hospitals that have completed or are in the process of implementing a Plan of Care Application, regardless of vendor, such as the Southcoast Hospitals Group, Fall River, MA; Claxton-Hepburn Medical Center, Ogdensburg, NY; Hospital Corporation of American (HCA) for its approximately 163 hospitals around the country; Rush Hospital, Chicago, IL, Vanderbilt Medical Center, Nashville, TN, and so on.

The Southcoast Hospitals Group, Fall River, MA, has implemented and coded their care planning system using the CCC System. A sample screen is shown in Figure 14.4. Their nurses assess the patient on admission, from which the patient's nursing diagnoses, or problem list, is generated. However, for each shift the nurse selects only the 2 or 3 nursing diagnoses that will be treated during that time period.

Safety Component	
.... Name/Discipline	COTTER, SUSAN L RN
.... To Stabilize	Injury Risk
.... Assess/Monitor	Equipment Safety Environmental Safety
.... Care/Perform	Equipment Safety Environmental Safety
.... Teach/Instruct	Equipment Safety Environmental Safety
.... Safety Plan	Assist with ADLs Bed-low locked position Bed exit alarm Brakes-wc, stretcher & bed Patient Checks PRN Encourage call light use Notify MD of Changes Orient Pt to Environment Ruby Slipper Program Side rails up

• **FIGURE 14.4.** Sample Screen from the Southcoast Hospitals Group, Fall River, MA.

CCC—NURSING RESEARCH

More than 17 studies have been conducted using the CCC System and its predecessor, the HHCC, to evaluate the ability of the classification to represent and support nursing care in electronic information systems. In research studies, the CCC has been shown to be successful in adequately documenting nursing care in patients with AIDS (Holzemer et al., 1997), depressive disorder (Parlocha & Henry, 1998), and coronary artery bypass grafts (Moss, Dangrongsak, Gallichio, 2005). The CCC has also been used successfully in the design of decision support to aid nurses in tailoring and evaluating interventions to enhance adherence to treatment regimens for HIV and AIDS patients (Bakken et al., 2005). In this study, nurses evaluated a patient's propensity for medication adherence through the use of an evaluation tool, the Client Adherence Profiling-Intervention Tailoring (CAP-IT) program. CAP-IT is used to assign patients a score reflecting their individual reasons for potentially not taking medication as prescribed. Each individualized profile was matched with a set of CCC System Interventions to be delivered to that specific patient (Bakken et al., 2005). Using this approach, the researchers were able to track what interventions were delivered to each patient, how long nurses spent delivering those interventions, and how intervention plans were adjusted over time.

The CCC System has been used to show practice patterns through analysis of nursing data entered during the course of patient documentation in electronic information systems (Bakken et al., 2005; Holzemer et al., 1997; & Moss et al., 2005). In a recent study of medication counselling in Finland (Saranto, Moss, & Jylha, 2010), the CCC was found to be useful in documenting the occurrence and type of medication counselling nurses used in an acute care setting. Through examining nurses' documentation regarding medication counselling in both the standardized portion and narrative portion of the record, the researchers were able to determine deficiencies in the amount, type, and the timing of counselling. The researchers found in this study that nurses were not documenting many occurrences of medication counselling, that nurses were not verifying that patients understood the implications of their medications, and that medication counselling often was not offered at the optimum time (i.e., immediately prior) before discharge (Saranto et al., 2010). Understanding nurses' documentation allows for the design of targeted strategies to improve the approach to provide nursing care in a more effective manner.

CCC—NURSING EDUCATION

For educational purposes, the CCC System has been incorporated into the creation of a simulated clinical information system, allowing students to learn the electronic documentation process prior to entering the actual clinical environment. In 2002, Bakken, at Columbia University School of Nursing, designed a system for advanced practice nurse (APN) students to enter clinical encounter data in a customized software program on a personal digital assistant (PDA) using the standardized nursing terminology of the CCC System. The overarching framework for the application was the nursing process, depicting its 6 steps using the concepts from the CCC System.

Dr. Veronica Feeg and colleagues designed a simulated system using a personal computer and the software Microsoft Access. The purpose of the simulation system project was to integrate and evaluate a stand-alone, free, electronic documentation application for nursing students in their clinical laboratories. The project staff compared the ability of nursing students to prepare a plan of care using the electronic application of the CCC System and a laptop PC with their ability to prepare a plan of care in narrative text using word processing software. The project staff wanted to conduct research to evaluate the effectiveness of the electronic system in teaching students the nursing process in an electronic environment (Feeg & Saba, 2008). The researchers found that students using the simulated electronic information system to document their plans of care using the CCC System terminology enhanced their learning of the nursing process, nursing diagnoses, and interventions. Feeg and colleagues have expanded and tested the research in another setting and found that the students also endorsed the electronic application for documenting their plans of care (Molloy College, 2010).

CCC—ANALYSES

The analysis of the data generated from nursing documentation utilizing the CCC System can provide nursing directors, managers, and nursing staff with a great deal of information. Because the CCC System provides a standardized framework that is coded, patient care data can be processed and retrieved to provide evidence of nursing care. The following are examples of possible analyses:

1. Number and categories of nursing diagnoses can be totaled to establish standardized plans of care for specific medical conditions.

2. Nursing diagnoses can be related to the nursing intervention services, which will lead to establishing best practices evidence-based outcomes.

3. Actual outcomes can be compared with the expected outcomes, linking performed nursing interventions to actual changes in each patient's condition.

4. Number and type of nursing interventions by care component can be related to medical conditions, establishing pathways for standardized care. They can also be related to the care provider's clinical performance.

5. Nursing intervention action types (if timed) can provide staff workload, resource needs, and care costs.

COSTING CARE

While government efforts to improve healthcare quality through the introduction of pay-for-performance initiatives for physicians has gained considerable traction over the past several years (e.g., the physician quality reporting initiative [PQRI]), broad reaching efforts to include nursing care are beginning to emerge. One factor driving interest in including nursing in pay-for-performace programs is the recognition that nurses are central to improving the quality and safety of care. Since October 2008, the Centers for Medicare and Medicaid Services (CMS) has decreased hospital reimbursement for the treatment of complications arising from inadequate care. Four of these conditions are related to deficiencies in nursing care: (1) falls, (2) pressure ulcers, (3) catheter-associated urinary tract infections, and (4) central-line-associated infections (Robert Wood Johnson Foundation, 2009). While these outcomes can be documented and measured, data related to the nursing processes leading to the occurrence and the cost of nursing delivery is lacking in healthcare and hospital information systems.

Nurses provide the majority of care patients receive when admitted to hospitals. However, nursing care is not directly billed to the insurance company, federal government, or patient; hospitals' bills are based on a fixed daily room rate and the cost of nursing service is included within the per diem charge (Welton & Harris, 2007). Currently, there is no reliable method to determine the actual cost of nursing care to hospitals because the per diem rates do not differentiate between the direct care expenses associated with nursing-specific tasks, such as medication administration and other patient care activities (Dejohn, 2008). Thus, nursing costs are included in overall financial summaries—departmental and organizational—but are not itemized by professional nursing service. This method of billing for nursing care significantly contributes to the invisibility of the critically important role of the nurse in the delivery of direct and indirect patient care.

To determine the full cost of nursing services and overcome the invisibility of nursing care services, we must overcome the lack of knowledge regarding what nurses actually do and the lack of documentation of nursing process in a standardized manner. The continuation and resistance to directly costing and charging for nursing services as a reimbursable line item has led to the development of nursing documentation systems that contain mostly patient physiological and medication administration data and little nursing process data (Moss, Andison, & Sobko, 2007). Renewed interest in how nurses impact patient care quality and safety provides an opportunity for a renewed focus on the design of nursing documentation systems that contain nursing interventional data. The nursing data can then be used both for estimating nursing costs and estimating the impact nursing interventions have on patient care outcomes.

Using a standardized intervention terminology with associated costs will enable the costs of nursing care to be calculated as an end-product of documentation in an electronic record and eliminate the need for additional data collection. Due to the ability of the CCC System to code individual interventions at a level of abstraction that describe individual nursing activities, the CCC System has been used successfully to cost nursing care.

CLINICAL CARE CLASSIFICATION SYSTEM COSTING METHOD

The CCC System can be used to study workload as well as nursing costs using the Clinical Care Classification System Costing Method (CCC-CM). The CCC-CM uses the CCC System Nursing Intervention and Action Types combined with Relative Value Units developed by Relative Value Studies Inc. (RVS Inc.) to determine a relative value for each coded intervention.

The RVUs were selected as one of very few measures available that have been developed and tested by RVS Inc. to determine the actual cost of patient care for Pay for Performance for Medicaid physician services. Originally, RVUs were developed through an agreement with Alternative Link Systems, Inc. and were being used for the reimbursement of selected allied healthcare

TABLE 14.4	Mean Costs of Clinical Care Classification Nursing Interventions with Actions	
Intervention	**Mean Duration**	**Mean Cost**
Nursing Care Coordination Manage/Refer (15.6%)	2 min 6 sec	$2.42
Nursing Status Report Assess/Monitor (12%)	4 min 20sec	$4.22
Medication Treatment Perform/Direct (11.6%)	3 min 9 sec	$6.33
Physical Exam Assess/Monitor (10.2%)	3 min 40 sec	$3.20
Universal Precautions Perform/Direct (9.3%)	57.52 sec	$1.96

professionals. The RVU manual designed for clinicians included selected nursing interventions, coded listings of integrative healthcare services, interventions, or procedures with unit values to indicate the relative effort of each service provided to patients (Relative Value Studies, 2006; ABC Coding Solutions, 2006).

The RVUs for the 4 Action Types used in the CCC-CM were developed by RVS Inc. using data from ABC codes that were developed for the reimbursement of selected allied healthcare professionals. Each value that was used was developed through a survey of providers asking for a value for each action based on time, skill, risk to the patient, risk to the provider, and severity of illness.

To test the CCC-CM's ability to cost nursing interventions in practice, Moss and Saba conducted a pilot study to cost 21 commonly executed CCC System core intervention codes combined with 1 of the 4 action types to describe 84 specific nursing interventions. Ten registered nurses were observed over the course of approximately 22 hours and the nursing interventions were recorded on the electronic data collection tool. A total of 251 interventions were observed, coded, and entered into the database representing the intervention's CCC code and duration. The electronic forms–based data collection tool was created in a Microsoft Access database using a tablet personal computer (PC). The pilot data collectors followed nurses during the course of patient care, and each time a nurse performed an Action Type with a Core Nursing Intervention, the pilot data collectors entered the corresponding Action Type and Core Nursing Intervention codes. The tool automatically calculated the duration (length of time) of the intervention through the use of a built-in stopwatch-type device.

During the study nurses performed 37 unique interventions and a total of 224 interventions during the course of patient care. The 5 most frequently performed interventions were (1) Nursing Care Coordination/Manage-Refer (15.6%), (2) Nursing Status Report/Assess-Monitor (12%), (3) Medication Treatment/Perform-Direct (11.6%), (4) Physical Exam/Assess-Monitor (10.2%), and (5) Universal Precautions/Perform-Direct (9.3%). After applying the appropriate calculation to each intervention, a cost for the intervention could be calculated. Table 14.4 describes the duration and calculated cost of these most frequently performed interventions.

Dykes conducted a pilot study with similar results (2010, unpublished data).

The Dykes pilot was designed to provide an initial evaluation of RVS Inc.'s RVUs for estimating cost of care based on the actual time that medical unit nurse participants at Brigham and Women's Hospital (BWH), a teaching affiliate of Harvard Medical School, Boston, MA, took to provide a single Action Type with a single Core Nursing Intervention to a patient. A sample of 270 observations of the 4 Action Types using only 21 Core CCC Nursing Interventions was collected through workflow observations of 2 medical units at BWH.

Based on the sample of observations, the cost of care was logically estimated. The findings suggest that the CCC System holds promise as a standard to support data capture for measuring nursing workload based on interventions and action types performed and the cost of care.

CCC—AVAILABILITY

As noted, the CCC System establishes an ICD-like and a Common Procedural Terminology (CPT)-like, coded terminologies for nursing care. Each concept is coded, defined, and never duplicated. The CCC System is a dynamic classification for nursing that is continually updated based on the needs of the nurses and allied health professionals addressing the changes in nursing practice or incorporating research study results. The CCC Scientific Advisory Board meets annually and reviews requests from CCC System stakeholders to modify, add, or retire nursing diagnoses and interventions and/or revise codes and definitions in the terminology. The CCC System is available for use under 'Copyright with Permission' without cost. A permission Form is available and has been designed to be compatible with EHRs, regardless of vendor system, for those who want to implement the CCC System in their healthcare facility. The Permission Form provides a user with a password to obtain the software files (data dictionaries) ready for computer uploading from its web site. The CCC System Version 2.0 has been translated into many different languages including German, Finnish, Portuguese, Korean, Dutch, Spanish, Norwegian, and Chinese and is currently being translated into other languages.

A complete guide to the system as well as codes for Nursing Diagnoses, Nursing Interventions, and Nursing Outcomes can be found in the *Clinical Care Classification (CCC) System Manual: A Guide to Nursing Documentation* (Saba, 2007) or on the Internet at www.sabacare.com or www.clinicalcareclassification.com.

CONCLUSION

The collection and analysis of data are a critical thrust of current health services research. Data analysis is aimed at cost, quality, and effectiveness outcomes. Collecting data that describes the processes and outcomes of nursing care electronically has the potential to provide evidence for care protocols and delivery models. Nurses collect and document enormous amounts of data during the course of caring for each patient that could contribute to furthering the science of nursing care. Although process and outcomes are used to inform the delivery of practice with evidence, data used to develop practice-based evidence (PBE) and evidence-based practice (EBP) are derived from different sources. Deriving evidence for informing practice from research is termed EBP, informing practice from the analysis of patient data collected during the delivery of care is termed PBE (DeJong, 2007). The contribution of these sources of data to nursing practice and science rest with logically structuring the research input, providing adequate processing and memory, and assuring valid and reliable

output. Clear definition, valid linkage between datasets, and the clear coding of input are essential in securing meaningful output for practical application at the point-of-care. The aggregation of information over time and how the aggregation affects the quality of information is especially important to uniform datasets. Using PBE requires the compilation of clinical data into a *clinical data repository*. This compilation may also be called an *information warehouse* or simply a *data repository* where data are stored longitudinally over multiple episodes of care. The data can then be accessed to provide continuity of care to the individual patient, to measure care effectiveness and productivity, to provide evidence for care delivery, or to inform public policy.

The CCC System is a coded national nursing terminology standard proven useful and consistent for nursing documentation including nursing plans of care. The implementation of the CCC System in the EHR will allow the contribution of nursing practice to become visible and strengthen the viability of the nursing profession. With the accumulation of nursing data for populations over time, more in-depth analysis can be performed and the comparison of outcomes across healthcare facilities will be possible. The availability of accurately coded essence-of-nursing-care data will validate nursing's contribution to patient care outcomes and contribute to advancing nursing science.

REFERENCES

ABC Solutions. (2006). *Relative values for integrative healthcare using ABC codes*. Albuquerque, NM: ABC Coding Solutions—Alternative Link Inc.

American Nurses Association (2003). *Nursing: Scope & Standards of Practice*. Sliver Spring: ANA.

Bakken, S., Holzemer, W., Portillo, C. J., Grimes, R., Welch, J., & Wantland, D. (2005). Utility of a standardized nursing terminology to evaluate dosage and tailoring of an HIV/AIDS adherence intervention. *Journal of Nursing Scholarship, 37*, 251–257.

Centers for Medicare and Medicaid Services. (2009). CMS proposes definition of meaningful use of certified electronic health records technology, *Fact Sheets*. Baltimore, MD: Department of Health and Human Services.

Dejohn, P. (2008). What comes after value analysis? *OR Manager, 24*(5), 15–18.

DeJong, G. (2007). *Setting the Stage: The Case for Another Paradigm*. Paper presented at the Council for the Advancement of Nursing Science Special Topics Conference, Washington, DC.

Feeg, V., & Saba V.K. (2008). Testing a bedside personal computer clinical care classification system for nursing students using Microsoft Access. *Computers Informatics Nursing, 26*(6), 339–349.

Holzemer, W. L., Henry, S. B., Dawson, C., Sousa, K., Bain, C., & Hsieh, S. F. (1997). An evaluation of the utility of the home healthcare classification for categorizing patient problems and nursing interventions from the hospital setting. In T. U. Gerdin & M. Wainwright (Ed.), *NI-99: Nursing informatics: The impact of nursing knowledge on healthcare informatics* (pp. 21–26). Stockholm: IOS Press.

Moss, J., Andison, M., & Sobko, H. (2007). *An Analysis of Narrative Nursing Documentation in an Otherwise Structured Intensive Care Clinical Information System.* Paper presented at the Proceedings of the American Medical Informatics Association Annual Symposium, Chicago.

Moss, J., Dangrongsak, M, & Gallichio, K. (2005). *Representing critical care data using the clinical care classification.* Paper presented at the Proceedings of the American Medical Association Annual Symposium, Washington, DC.

Nightingale, F., (1863). *Notes on hospitals.* London: Longman, Green, Roberts, Longman, & Green.

North American Nursing Diagnoses Association. (1992). *Nanda nursing diagnoses: Definitions and classifications.* St. Louis, MO: North American Nursing Diagnoses Association.

Parlocha, P. K., & Henry. S. B. (1998). The usefulness of the Georgetown home healthcare classification system for coding patient problems and nursing interventions in psychiatric home care. *Computers Informatics Nursing, 16,* 45–52.

Relative Value Studies, Inc. (2006). *Relative value for integrative healthcare using ABC codes.* Broomfield, CO: Relative Value Studies, Inc.

Robert Wood Johnson Foundation. (2009). *Perspectives on pay for performance in nursing: Key considerations in shaping payment systems to drive better patient care outcomes.* Pittsburgh, PA: Robert Wood Johnson Foundation.

Saba, V. K. (2007). *Clinical care classification (CCC) system manual: A guide to nursing documentation.* New York, NY: Springer.

Saba, V. K., & Taylor, S. L. (2007). Moving past theory: Use of a standardized coded nursing terminology to enhance nursing visibility. *Computers in Nursing, 25*(6), 324–331.

Sarento, K. M, Moss, J., & Jylha, V (2010). Medication counseling: Analysis of electronic documentation using the Clinical Care Classification System. Proceedings of the 13th World Congress on Medical and Health Informatics, MEDINFO-13. (pp.284-288) Cape Town, South Africa: IOS Press.

Welton, J. M, & Harris, K. (2007). Hospital billing and reimbursement. *JONA, 37*(4), 164–166.

PART 4

Current Issues in Informatics

Kathleen A. McCormick

15

Health Data Standards: Development, Harmonization, and Interoperability

Joyce Sensmeier

- OBJECTIVES

    1. Discuss the need for health data standards.
    2. Describe the standards development process and related organizations.
    3. Delineate the importance of standards harmonization and interoperability.
    4. Describe current health data standards initiatives.
    5. Explore the business value of health data standards.

- KEY WORDS

    standards
    health information exchange
    knowledge representation
    interoperability
    Nationwide Health Information Network
    terminology

Standards are foundational to the development, implementation, and exchange of electronic health records (EHRs). The effectiveness of healthcare delivery is dependent on the ability of clinicians to access health information when and where it is needed. The ability to exchange health information across organizational and system boundaries, whether between multiple departments within a single institution or among a varied cast of providers, payers, regulators, and others, is essential. A harmonized set of rules and definitions, both at the level of data meaning as well as at the technical level of data exchange, is needed to make this possible. In addition, there must be a sociopolitical structure in place that recognizes the benefits of shared information and incentivizes the adoption and implementation of such standards.

This chapter examines health data standards in terms of the following topic areas:

- Need for health data standards
- Standards development process, organizations, and categories
- Knowledge representation
- Standards coordination and harmonization
- Standards and interoperability
- Health data standards initiatives
- Business value of health data standards

INTRODUCTION TO HEALTH DATA STANDARDS

The ability to communicate in a way that ensures the message is received and the content is understood is dependent on standards. Data standards are intended to reduce ambiguity in communication so that the actions taken based on data are consistent with the actual meaning of that data. The Health Information Technology for Economic and Clinical Health (HITECH) Act is driving U.S. efforts to transform healthcare through the meaningful use of health data. This goal will be advanced through a phased-in series of improved clinical data capture processes that support more rigorous quality measures and improvements. This transformation requires data capture and sharing and advanced clinical processes, which will enable improved outcomes. The ultimate end state can only be achieved through the organized structuring and effective use of information to support better decision making and more effective care processes, thus improving health outcomes and reducing cost growth.

While current information technology (IT) is able to move and manipulate large amounts of data, it is not as proficient in dealing with ambiguity in the structure and semantic content of that data. The term *data standards* is generally used to describe those standards having to do with the structure and content of health information. However, it may be useful to differentiate data from information and knowledge. Data are the fundamental building blocks on which healthcare decisions are based. Data are collections of unstructured, discrete entities (facts) that exist outside of any particular context. When data are interpreted within a given context and given meaningful structure within that context, they become information. When information from various contexts is aggregated following a defined set of rules, it becomes knowledge and provides the basis for informed action (Nelson, 2006). Data standards represent both data and their transformation into information. Data analysis generates knowledge, which is the foundation of professional practice standards.

Standards are created by several methods (Hammond, 2005): (1) A group of interested parties comes together and agrees upon a standard; (2) The government sanctions a process for standards to be developed; (3) Marketplace competition and technology adoption introduces a de facto standard; (4) A formal consensus process is used by a standards development organization (SDO). The standards development process typically begins with a use case or business need that describes a system's behavior as it responds to a request that originates from outside of that system. Technical experts then consider what methods, protocols, terminologies, or specifications are needed to address the requirements of the use case. An open acceptance or balloting process is desirable to ensure that the developed standards have representative stakeholder input, which minimizes bias and encourages marketplace adoption and implementation.

Legislated, government-developed standards are able to gain widespread acceptance by virtue of their being required by either regulation or in order to participate in large, government-funded programs, such as Medicare. Because government-developed standards are in the public domain, they are available at little or no cost and can be incorporated into any information system; however, they are often developed to support particular government initiatives and may not be as suitable for general, private sector use. Also, given the amount of bureaucratic overhead attached to legislative and regulatory process, it is likely that they will lag behind changes in technology and the general business environment.

Standards developed by SDOs are typically consensus-based and reflect the perspectives of a wide variety of interested stakeholders. They are generally not tied to specific systems. For this reason, they tend to be robust and adaptable across a range of implementations; however, most SDOs are nonprofit organizations that rely on the commitment of dedicated volunteers to develop and maintain standards. This often limits the amount of work that can be undertaken. In addition, the consensus process can be time consuming and result in a slow development process, which does not always keep pace with technologic change. Perhaps the most problematic aspect of consensus-based standards is that there is no mechanism to ensure that they are adopted by the industry, since there is usually little infrastructure in place to actively and aggressively market them. This has resulted in the development of many technically competent standards that are never implemented. The U.S. Standards Strategy (ANSI, 2005) states that, "The goal of all international standards forums should be to achieve globally relevant and internationally recognized and accepted standards that support trade and commerce while protecting the environment, health, safety, and security."

There are a number of drivers in the current standards landscape that are working to accelerate health data standards adoption and implementation through innovative efforts and incentives to address this charge.

STANDARDS CATEGORIES

Four broad areas are identified to categorize health data standards (Department of Health and Human Services, 2010). Transport standards are used to establish a common, predictable, secure communication protocol between systems. Vocabulary standards consist of standardized nomenclatures and code sets used to describe clinical problems and procedures, medications, and allergies. Content exchange standards and value sets are used to share clinical information such as clinical summaries, prescriptions, and structured electronic documents. Security standards include standards used for authentication, access control, and transmission of health data.

Transport Standards

Transport standards primarily address the format of messages that are exchanged between computer systems, document architecture, clinical templates, the user interface, and patient data linkage (Committee on Data Standards for Patient Safety, 2004). To achieve data compatibility between systems, it is necessary to have prior agreement on the syntax of the messages to be exchanged. The receiving system must be able to divide the incoming message into discrete data elements that reflect what the sending system wishes to communicate. The following section describes some of the major SDOs involved in the development of transport standards.

Accredited Standards Committee X12N/Insurance. Accredited Standards Committee (ASC) X12N has developed a broad range of electronic data interchange (EDI) standards to facilitate electronic business transactions. In the healthcare arena, X12N standards have been adopted as national standards for such administrative transactions as claims, enrollment, and eligibility in health plans, and first report of injury under the requirements of the Health Insurance Portability and Accountability Act (HIPAA). Due to the uniqueness of health insurance and the varying policies for protection of personal health information from country to country, these standards are primarily used in the U.S. HIPAA directed the Secretary of the Department of Health and Human Services (HHS) to adopt standards for transactions to enable health information to be exchanged electronically, and the Administrative Simplification Act (ASA), one of the HIPAA provisions, requires standard formats to be used for electronically submitted healthcare transactions. The American National Standards Institute (ANSI) developed these, and the ANSI X12N 837 Implementation Guide has been established as the standard of compliance for claims transactions.

Institute of Electrical and Electronic Engineers. The Institute of Electrical and Electronic Engineers (IEEE) has developed a series of standards known collectively

as P1073 Medical Information Bus (MIB), which support real-time, continuous, and comprehensive capture and communication of data from bedside medical devices such as those found in intensive care units, operating rooms, and emergency departments. These data include physiologic parameter measurements and device settings. These standards are used internationally. IEEE standards for IT focus on telecommunications and information exchange between systems including local and metropolitan area networks. Current activities include efforts to develop standards that support wireless technology. The IEEE 802.xx suite of wireless networking standards, supporting local and metropolitan area networks, has advanced developments in the communications market. The most widely known standard, 802.11, commonly referred to as Wi-Fi, allows anyone with a "smart" mobile device or a computer with either a plug-in card or built-in circuitry to connect to the Internet wirelessly through myriad access points installed in offices, hotels, airports, coffeehouses, convention centers, and even parks, among other locations. Many healthcare organizations are evaluating and implementing wireless solutions that support point-of-care technology.

National Electrical Manufacturers Association. The National Electrical Manufacturers Association (NEMA), in collaboration with the American College of Radiologists (ACR) and others, formed DICOM (Digital Imaging and Communications in Medicine) to develop a generic digital format and a transfer protocol for biomedical images and image-related information. DICOM enables the transfer of medical images in a multi-vendor environment and facilitates the development and expansion of picture archiving and communication systems (PACS). The specification is usable on any type of computer system and supports transfer over the Internet. The DICOM standard is the dominant international data interchange message format in biomedical imaging. The Joint NEMA/The European Coordination Committee of the Radiological and Electromedical Industry/Japan Industries Association of Radiological Systems (COCIR/JIRA) Security and Privacy Committee (SPC) issued a white paper that provides a guide for vendors and users on how to protect medical information systems against viruses, Trojan horses, denial of service attacks, Internet worms, and related forms of so-called malicious software.

World Wide Web Consortium. The World Wide Web Consortium (W3C) is the main international standards organization for development of the World Wide Web (abbreviated WWW or W3). W3C also publishes XML (Extensible Markup Language), which is a set of rules for encoding documents in machine-readable format. XML is most commonly used in exchanging data over the Internet. It is defined in the XML 1.0 Specification produced by the W3C and several other related specifications, all of which are available in the public domain. XML's design goals emphasize simplicity, generality, and usability over the Internet, which also makes it desirable for use in cross-enterprise health information exchange. It is a textual data format, with strong support for the languages of the world. Although XML's design focuses on documents, it is widely used for the representation of arbitrary data structures such as Web Services. Web Services use XML messages that follow the Simple Object Access Protocol (SOAP) standard and have been popular with traditional enterprise. Other transport protocols include the Representational State Transfer (REST) architectural style, which was developed in parallel with the Hypertext Transfer Protocol (HTTP) used in Web browsers. The largest known implementation of a system conforming to the REST architectural style is the World Wide Web.

Vocabulary Standards

A fundamental requirement for effective communication is the ability to represent concepts in an unambiguous fashion between both the sender and receiver of the message. Natural human languages are incredibly rich in their ability to communicate subtle differences in the semantic content, or meaning, of messages. While there have been great advances in the ability of computers to process natural language, most communication between health information systems relies on the use of structured vocabularies, terminologies, code sets, and classification systems to represent healthcare concepts. Standardized terminologies enable data collection at the point of care, and enable retrieval of data, information, and knowledge in support of clinical practice. The following examples describe several of the major systems.

Current Procedural Terminology. The Current Procedural Terminology (CPT) code set, maintained by the American Medical Association (AMA), accurately describes medical, surgical, and diagnostic services. It is designed to communicate uniform information about medical services and procedures among physicians, coders, patients, accreditation organizations, and payers for administrative, financial, and analytical purposes. The current version is the CPT 2010. In addition to descriptive terms and codes, it contains modifiers, notes, and

guidelines to facilitate correct usage. While primarily used in the U.S. for reimbursement purposes, it has also been adopted for other data purposes.

International Statistical Classification of Diseases and Related Health Problems: Ninth Revision and Clinical Modifications. The International Statistical Classification of Diseases and Related Health Problems: Ninth Revision and Clinical Modifications (ICD-9-CM) (World Health Organization, 1980) is a version of a mortality and morbidity classification used since 1979 for reporting in the U.S. It is widely accepted and used in the healthcare industry and has been adopted for a number of purposes including data collection, quality-of-care analysis, resource utilization, and statistical reporting. It is the basis for the diagnostic-related groups (DRGs) developed for Medicare, which are used extensively in the U.S. for hospital reimbursement as part of the prospective payment system. While ICD-9 procedure codes are the acceptable HIPAA code set for inpatient claims, Healthcare Common Procedure Coding System/Current Procedural Terminology (HCPCS/CPT) codes are the valid set for outpatient claims.

International Statistical Classification of Diseases and Related Health Problems: Tenth Revision. The International Statistical Classification of Diseases and Related Health Problems: Tenth Revision (ICD-10) is the most recent revision of the ICD classification system for mortality and morbidity, which is used worldwide. In addition to diagnostic labels, the ICD-10 also encompasses nomenclature structures. The U.S. version, ICD-10-CM, has yet to be broadly implemented in part due to its complexity; however, the transition to ICD-10-CM and ICD-10 Procedural Coding System (ICD-10-PCS) is anticipated to improve the capture of healthcare information and bring the U.S. in step with coding systems worldwide. For those who prepare appropriately, leveraging the ICD-10 investment will allow organizations to move beyond compliance to achieve competitive advantage (Bowman, 2008). Moving to the new code sets will also improve efficiencies and lower administrative costs due to replacement of a dysfunctional classification system.

Nursing and Other Domain-Specific Terminologies. The American Nurses Association (ANA) has spearheaded efforts to coordinate the various minimum data sets and standardized nursing terminologies. The ANA Committee for Nursing Practice Information Infrastructure (CNPII) evaluates minimum data sets and standardized terminologies to determine if they meet specific criteria. The ANA has recognized the following nursing terminologies that support nursing practice: ABC Codes, Clinical Care Classification, International Classification of Nursing Practice, Logical Observation Identifiers Names and Codes (LOINC), North American Nursing Diagnosis Association, Nursing Interventions Classification (NIC), Nursing Outcome Classification (NOC), Nursing Management Minimum Data Set, Nursing Minimum Data Set, Omaha System, Patient Care Data Set (retired), Perioperative Nursing Data Set, and SNOMED-CT (Rutherford, 2008). These standard terminologies enable knowledge representation of nursing content. Nurses use assessment data and nursing judgment to determine nursing diagnoses, interventions, and outcomes. These elements can be linked together using standards to represent nursing knowledge.

RxNorm. RxNorm is a standardized nomenclature for clinical drugs and drug delivery devices produced by the National Library of Medicine (NLM). Because every drug information system follows somewhat different naming conventions, a standardized nomenclature is needed for the consistent exchange of information, not only between organizations but even within the same organization. For example, a hospital may use one system for ordering and another for inventory management. Still another system might be used to record dose adjustments or to check drug interactions. The goal of RxNorm is to allow various systems using different drug nomenclatures to share data efficiently at the appropriate level of abstraction. RxNorm contains the names of prescription and many nonprescription formulations that exist in the U.S., including the devices that administer the medications.

Unified Medical Language System. Currently, the Unified Medical Language System (UMLS) consists of a metathesaurus of terms and concepts from dozens of vocabularies, a semantic network of relationships among the concepts recognized in the metathesaurus, and an information sources map of the various biomedical databases referenced. There are specialized vocabularies, code sets, and classification systems for almost every practice domain in healthcare. Most of these are not compatible with one another, and much work needs to be done to achieve usable mapping and linkages between them. There have been a number of efforts to develop mapping and linkages among various code sets, classification systems, and vocabularies. One of the most successful is the UMLS project undertaken by the NLM.

The NLM supports the development, enhancement, and distribution of clinically specific vocabularies to facilitate the exchange of clinical data to improve retrieval of health information. In 1986, the NLM began an ambitious long-term project to map and link a large number of vocabularies from a number of knowledge sources to allow retrieval and integration of relevant machine-readable information. The NLM is the central coordinating body for clinical terminology standards within HHS (National Library of Medicine, 2010). The NLM works closely with the Office of the National Coordinator for Health Information Technology (ONC) to ensure NLM's efforts are aligned with the goal of the President and HHS Secretary to achieve nationwide implementation of an interoperable health IT infrastructure to improve the quality and efficiency of healthcare.

Other domain-specific terminologies include Current Dental Terminology (CDT), International Medical Terminology (IMT), and Diagnostic and Statistical Manual of Mental Disorders (DSM-IV-TR) to name just a few.

Content Standards

Content Standards are related to the data content within information exchanges. Information content standards define the structure and content organization of the electronic message's or document's information content. They can also define a "package" of content standards (messages or documents). In addition to standardizing the format of health data messages and the lexicons and value sets used in those messages, there is widespread interest in defining common sets of data for specific message types. The concept of a *minimum data set* is defined as "a minimum set of items with uniform definitions and categories concerning a specific aspect or dimension of the healthcare system which meets the essential needs of multiple users" (Health Information Policy Council, 1983).

A related concept is that of a *core data element*. It has been defined as "a standard data element with a uniform definition and coding convention to collect data on persons and on events or encounters" (National Committee on Vital and Health Statistics, 1996). Core data elements are seen as serving as the building blocks for well-formed minimum data sets and may appear in several minimum data sets. The following are some examples of minimum, or core, data sets currently in use. As with code sets, professional specialty groups are often the best source for current information on minimum data set–development efforts. A number of SDOs, which develop messaging format standards such as HL7 and ASC X12N, have been increasingly interested in incorporating domain-specific data sets into their messaging standards.

American Society for Testing and Materials. The American Society for Testing and Materials (ASTM) is one of the largest SDOs in the world and publishes standards covering all sectors in the economy. The ASTM Committee E31 on Healthcare Informatics has developed a wide range of standards supporting the electronic management of health information. One of these standards, the Continuity of Care Record (CCR), was developed in collaboration with the Massachusetts Medical Society, HIMSS, the American Academy of Family Physicians, and the American Academy of Pediatrics. The CCR is a core data set of the most relevant and timely facts about a patient's healthcare. It is prepared by a practitioner at the conclusion of a healthcare encounter in order to enable the next practitioner to readily access such information. It includes a summary of the patient's health status (e.g., problems, medications, allergies) and basic information about insurance, advance directives, care documentation, and care plan recommendations. The primary use for the CCR is to provide a snapshot in time containing the pertinent clinical, demographic, and administrative data for a specific patient.

Clinical Data Interchange Standards Consortium. The Clinical Data Interchange Standards Consortium (CDISC) is a global, multidisciplinary consortium that has established standards to support the acquisition, exchange, submission, and archive of clinical research data and metadata. CDISC develops and supports global, platform-independent data standards that enable information system interoperability to improve medical research and related areas of healthcare. One example is the Biomedical Research Integrated Domain Group (BRIDG) Model, which is a domain analysis model representing protocol-driven biomedical and clinical research. The BRIDG model emerged from an unprecedented collaborative effort among clinical trial experts from CDISC, the National Institutes of Health (NIH)/National Cancer Institute (NCI), the Food and Drug Administration (FDA), HL7, and other volunteers. This structured information model is being used to support development of data interchange standards and technology solutions that will enable harmonization between the biomedical and clinical research and healthcare arenas.

Health Level Seven. Health Level Seven (HL7) is an SDO that develops standards in multiple categories including transport and content. HL7 standards focus on facilitating the exchange of data to support clinical practice both within and across institutions. HL7 standards cover a broad spectrum of areas for information exchange including medical orders, clinical observations, test results, admission/transfer/discharge, document architecture, clinical templates, user interface, EHR, and charge and billing information. A primary example of an HL7 standard is the HL7 Clinical Document Architecture (CDA) Release 2, Continuity of Care Document (CCD), which is an implementation guide for sharing Continuity of Care Record (CCR) patient summary data using the HL7 CDA document exchange model for clinical documents.

The HL7 EHR System Functional Model and Standard defines key functions of electronic health record systems (EHR-S) to enable consistent expression of system functionality (HL7, 2007). The function list is described from a user perspective with the intent to enable consistent expression of system functionality. This EHR-S Functional Model, through the creation of functional profiles for care settings and realms, enables a standardized description and common understanding of functions sought or available in a given setting (e.g., intensive care, oncology, cardiology, office practice in one country, or primary care in another country). HL7 standards are widely implemented by healthcare provider organizations worldwide, many of which have adapted the basic standards for use in their particular settings.

International Health Terminology Standards Development Organisation. The International Health Terminology Standards Development Organisation (IHTSDO) is a not-for-profit association in Denmark that develops and promotes use of SNOMED-CT to support safe and effective health information exchange. It was formed in 2006 with the purpose of developing and maintaining international health terminology systems. SNOMED-CT is a comprehensive clinical terminology, originally created by the College of American Pathologists (CAP) and, as of April 2007, owned, maintained, and distributed by the IHTSDO. The CAP continues to support SNOMED-CT operations under contract to the IHTSDO and provides SNOMED-related products and services as a licensee of the terminology. The NLM is the U.S. member of the IHTSDO and, as such, distributes SNOMED-CT at no cost in accordance with the member rights and responsibilities outlined in the IHTSDO's Articles of Association. SNOMED-CT is one of a suite of designated standards for use in U.S. federal government systems for the electronic exchange of clinical health information.

National Council for Prescription Drug Programs. The National Council for Prescription Drug Programs (NCPDP) develops both content and transport standards for information processing in the pharmacy services sector of the healthcare industry. This is a very successful example of how standards can enable significant improvements in service delivery. Since the introduction of this standard in 1992, the retail pharmacy industry has moved to 100% electronic claims processing in real time. NCPDP standards are forming the basis for electronic prescription transactions. Electronic prescription transactions are defined as EDI messages flowing between healthcare providers (i.e., pharmacy software systems and prescriber software systems) that are concerned with prescription orders. NCPDP's Telecommunication Standard Version 5.1 was named the official standard for pharmacy claims within HIPAA, and NCPDP is also named in other U.S. federal legislation titled the Medicare Prescription Drug, Improvement, and Modernization Act. Other NCPDP standards include the SCRIPT Standard for Electronic Prescribing, and the Manufacturers Rebate Standard.

National Uniform Claim Committee Recommended Data Set for a Noninstitutional Claim. Organized in 1995, the scope of the National Uniform Claim Committee (NUCC) was to develop, promote, and maintain a standard data set for use in noninstitutional claims and encounter information. The committee is chaired by the AMA, and its member organizations represent a number of the major public and private sector payers. The NUCC was formally named in the administrative simplification section of HIPAA as one of the organizations to be consulted by ANSI-accredited SDOs and the Secretary of HHS as they develop, adopt, or modify national standards for healthcare transactions. As such, the NUCC has authoritative voice regarding national standard content and data definitions for noninstitutional healthcare claims in the U.S.

Security Standards

HIPAA Security Standards for the Protection of Electronic Health Information at 45 CFR Part 160 and Part 164, Subparts A and C. The HIPAA Security Rule was developed to protect electronic health information and implement reasonable and appropriate administrative safeguards that establish the foundation for a covered entity's security program (CMS, 2007). Prior to HIPAA, no generally accepted set of security standards or general requirements for protecting health information existed in the healthcare industry. Congress passed the Administrative Simplification provisions of HIPAA to protect the privacy and security of certain health information, and promote efficiency in the healthcare industry through the use of standardized electronic transactions.

ISO IEC 27002:2005 Standard. The ISO IEC 27002:2005 Standard consists of recommended information security practices. It establishes guidelines and general principles for initiating, implementing, maintaining, and improving information security management in an organization. The objectives outlined provide general guidance on the commonly accepted goals and best practices for control objectives and controls for information security management. ISO/IEC 27002:2005 is intended as a common basis and practical guideline for developing organizational security standards and effective security management practices, and to help build confidence in interorganizational activities.

STANDARDS COORDINATION AND HARMONIZATION

It has become clear to both public and private sector standards development efforts that no one entity has the resources to create an exhaustive set of health data standards that will meet all needs. New emphasis is being placed on leveraging and harmonizing existing standards to eliminate the redundant and siloed efforts that have contributed to a complex, difficult to navigate health data standards environment. Advances are being made in the area of standards harmonization through the coming together of industry groups to accelerate and streamline the standards development and adoption process.

In addition to the various SDOs described above, the following organizations are working at international, national, and regional levels to create synergistic relationships between and across organizations. These emerging organizations are involved in standards development, coordination, and harmonization in all sectors of the economy. Since many of the health data standards issues, such as security, are not unique to the healthcare sector, this breadth of scope offers the potential for technology transfer and advancement across multiple sectors. The following is a brief description of some of the major international, national, and regional organizations involved in broad-based standards development, harmonization, and coordination.

American National Standards Institute

The American National Standards Institute (ANSI) serves as the U.S. coordinating body for voluntary standards activity. Standards are submitted to ANSI by member SDOs and are approved as American National Standards through a consensus methodology developed by ANSI. ANSI is the U.S. representative to the International Organization of Standardization (ISO), and as such, is responsible for bringing forward U.S. standards to that organization.

European Technical Committee for Standardization

In 1990, TC 251 on medical informatics was established by the European Committee for Standardization (CEN). CEN/TC 251 works to develop a wide variety of standards in the area of healthcare data management and interchange. CEN standards are adopted by its member countries in Europe and are also submitted for harmonization with ISO standards.

Health IT Standards Committee

The American Recovery and Reinvestment Act (ARRA) provided for the creation of the Health IT Standards Committee under the auspices of the Federal Advisory Committee Act (FACA). The Committee is charged with making recommendations to the U.S. National Coordinator for Health IT on standards, implementation specifications, and certification criteria for the electronic exchange and use of health information. In developing, harmonizing, or recognizing standards and implementation specifications, the Committee also provides for the testing of the same by the National Institute for Standards and Technology (NIST). The Committee has formed several workgroups to further the work of the FACA. These workgroups are comprised of stakeholder representatives and subject matter experts focused on the following topic areas: Clinical Operations, Clinical Quality, Privacy and Security, and Implementation.

Healthcare Information Technology Standards Panel

ONC has as its mission to enhance healthcare quality and contain costs for widespread adoption of interoperable EHRs by 2014. In the fall of 2005, ONC awarded multiple contracts to advance this goal. ANSI, in cooperation with strategic partners HIMSS, Booz Allen Hamilton, and Advanced Technology Institute, was awarded a contract for creating processes to harmonize standards. This standards harmonization collaborative established the Healthcare Information Technology Standards Panel (HITSP) through an an open, inclusive, and consensus-based process with broad stakeholder representation of more than 900 organizational members from the private and public sector.

Objectives

- To serve and establish a cooperative partnership between the public and private sectors to achieve a widely accepted and useful set of standards that will enable and support widespread interoperability among healthcare software applications in a nationwide health information network for the U.S.

- To harmonize relevant standards in the healthcare industry to enable and advance interoperability of healthcare applications, and the interchange of healthcare data, to assure accurate use, access, privacy and security, both for supporting the delivery of care and public health.

- To facilitate the efforts of SDOs to maintain, revise, or develop new standards as required to support the HITSP specifications.

Impact. As of January 2010, HITSP has published over 165 interoperability specifications and related constructs, the majority of which were recognized and accepted by the HHS Secretary. While ANSI's contract with HHS concluded on April 30, 2010, this body of work will significantly advance our nation's efforts toward enabling the secure and reliable exchange of electronic health information nationwide to enhance the quality and efficiency of care delivery. Most recently, an HITSP specification, HITSP/C32 Summary Documents Using HL7 CCD, was adopted by HHS in the Final Rules identifying the criteria for hospitals and eligible providers to become meaningful users of health IT, and the certification criteria and standards for achieving meaningful use in order to qualify for incentive payments under the ARRA.

Integrating the Healthcare Enterprise

Standards, while a necessary part of the interoperability solution, are not sufficient alone to fulfill the needs. Simply using a standard does not necessarily guarantee health information exchange within and across organizations and systems. Standards can be implemented in several ways, so implementation specifications or guides are critical to make interoperability a reality (Sensmeier, 2010). Standard-implementation specifications are designed to provide specific configuration instructions or constraints for implementation of a particular standard or set of standards.

Integrating the Healthcare Eneterprise (IHE) is an international organization that provides a detailed framework for implementing standards, filling the gaps between standards and their implementations. While IHE is not a standards body and does not create standards, it offers a common framework, available in the public domain, to understand and address critical integration needs. Vendors publish IHE integration statements to document the IHE integration profiles supported by their products that were successfully tested at an IHE Connectathon. Users can reference the appropriate integration profiles in requests for proposals, thus simplifying the systems acquisition process.

IHE has published a large body of detailed specifications that are being implemented globally today by healthcare providers and regional entities to enable standards-based, safe, secure and efficient health information exchange.

International Organization for Standardization

The International Organization for Standardization (ISO) develops, harmonizes, and publishes standards internationally. ISO standards are developed, in large part, from standards brought forth by member countries and through liaison activities with other SDOs. Often, these standards are further broadened to reflect the greater diversity of the international community. In 1998, the ISO Technical Committee (TC) 215 on Health Informatics was formed to coordinate the development of international health information standards, including data standards. Consensus on these standards influences health informatics standards adopted in the U. S. and the interoperability of national and international HIE. This Committee published the first international standard for nursing content titled *Integration of a Reference Terminology Model for Nursing*. This standard includes the development of reference terminology models for nursing diagnoses and nursing actions with relevant terminology and definitions for implementation.

Object Management Group

While the organizations described thus far are made up of volunteer-based SDOs, the Object Management Group (OMG) is representative of a different approach to standards development. OMG is an international consortium of primarily for-profit vendors of information systems technology who are interested in the development of standards based on object-oriented technologies. While its standards are developed by private organizations, it has developed a process to lessen the potential problems noted previously with proprietary standards. Standards developed in OMG are required to be implemented in a commercially available product by their developers within one year of the standard being accepted; however, the specifications for the standard are made publicly available. The OMG CORBAMed working group is responsible for development of object-based standards in the health information arena.

Public Health Data Standards Consortium

The Public Health Data Standards Consortium (PHDSC) is a national nonprofit membership-based organization of federal, state, and local health agencies; professional associations and academia; public and private sector organizations; international members; and individuals. Its goal is to empower the healthcare and public health communities with health IT standards that improve individual and community health. PHDSC represents a common voice from the public health community about the national effort toward standardization of health information for healthcare and population health by identifying priorities for new standards, promoting integration of health data systems, and educating the public health community about health data standards.

It is increasingly recognized that combining the strengths of these efforts and their approaches tends to minimize individual weaknesses and can lead to significant gains for the healthcare sector as a whole. As we have discussed, this melding of approaches is being achieved both at the organizational and international levels by the development of coordinating bodies and consortia, as well as through national, government-directed laws, regulations, committees, and initiatives.

STANDARDS AND INTEROPERABILITY

ONC Standards and Interoperability Framework

At the March 24, 2010 Health IT Standards Committee, Doug Fridsma, MD, PhD, Acting Director, ONC Office of Interoperability and Standards, announced several projects intended to support the national Standards and Interoperability Framework and Nationwide Health Information Network (NHIN) (Fridsma, 2010). In February 2010, the ONC released more than 10 contracts that provided funding to support activities designed to develop the standards, tools, interoperability framework, and technical infrastructure to support the overall U.S. goals of improving adoption of health IT.

Use Case Development and Functional Requirements

A foundational component of the ONC Standards and Interoperability Framework is use case development and functional requirements for interoperability. ONC will leverage the National Information Exchange Model (NIEM) framework and apply it to healthcare as a best practice for use case development and data integration. The NIEM framework, developed by the U.S. Department of Justice and the Department of Homeland Security, enables information sharing, focusing on information exchanged among organizations as part of their current or intended business practices. Working in collaboration with a wide community including consumers, providers, government organizations, and other stakeholders, this process will identify real-world needs, prioritize them, and create explicit documentation of the use cases, functional requirements, and technical specifications for interoperability.

Harmonization of Core Concepts

ONC will also leverage the NIEM framework to support data exchange harmonization. This harmonization process will merge related core data concepts, add new concepts, and map concepts from use case to another. The framework delineates 3 parts to harmonization: (1) the standards (the data that is exchanged), (2) the services (the functions that will be supported in the exchange), and (3) the policy (the trust, business rules, etc.). In order to address the needs of the use cases and increased use of health IT, there may be a need to modify or extend the existing standards or develop new standards. The ONC will work with SDOs and research organizations to extend existing or develop new standards as necessary.

Implementation Specifications

In order to test and implement the standards in real-life settings, they must be specified to a higher degree of detail. An implementation specification becomes an explicit description of the standards, services, and policies that then conform to the adopted standards and have sufficient detail to be implemented. These implementation specifications will be packaged together to support individual use cases. New implementation specifications will be created where they don't currently exist.

Reference Implementations

A reference implementation is a software solution that is analyzed to be compliant with the standards and serves as a "reference" to other software developers of what an interoperable solution looks like. Reference implementations will be accessible as a public resource with compiled code, source code, and supporting documentation. They can then be used by others to guide their own implementation or to identify problems with the specification that will be communicated as feedback to the ONC.

Testing and Certification

To accelerate the development, use, maintenance, and adoption of interoperability standards across the industry, and to spur innovation, the ONC will develop tools to facilitate the entire standards lifecycle and maximize reuse of concepts and components, including tools and repositories for browsing, selecting, and implementing appropriate standards. The ONC will work with NIST to provide testing tools to validate that a particular implementation conforms to a set of standards and implementation specifications. The ONC will also support the development of an integration testing "harness" that will test how a particular component that has satisfied conformance testing requirements integrates into the reference implementation.

A certification process is also being established so that organizations can be approved as certifying entities to which vendors may submit their EHR systems for review and certification. The Health Information Technology: Initial Set of Standards, Implementation Specifications, and Certification Criteria for Electronic Health Record Technology (45 CFR Part 170) Final Rule, published in 2010 by HHS, identifies the technical standards that must be met in the certification process, and coordinates those requirements with the meaningful use objectives.

CURRENT INITIATIVES

Regional Health Information Exchange

Formal entities are now emerging to provide both the structure and the function for health information exchange efforts, both at independent and governmental or regional/state levels. These organizations, called Regional health information exchanges (HIEs), are geographically-defined entities that develop and manage a set of contractual conventions and terms, and arrange for the governance and means of electronic exchange of information.

The HITECH Act authorized the establishment of the State Health Information Exchange Cooperative Agreement Program in the U.S. to advance appropriate and secure health information exchange across the healthcare system. The purpose of this program is to continuously improve and expand these services to reach all healthcare providers in an effort to improve the quality and efficiency of healthcare. Cooperative agreement recipients have been funded, and are now advancing the necessary governance, policies, technical services, business operations, and financing mechanisms for HIE over a 4-year performance period. This program builds from existing efforts to advance regional and state-level HIEs, while moving toward nationwide interoperability.

Nationwide Health Information Network

The Nationwide Health Information Network (NHIN) is a set of standards, services, and policies that enable secure health information exchange over the Internet. (Fridsma, 2010). The U.S. intent for the NHIN is to provide a foundation for the exchange of health IT across diverse entities, within communities and across the country, to achieve the goals of the HITECH Act. This component of the national health IT agenda will enable health information to follow the consumer, be available for clinical decision making, and support appropriate use of health information beyond direct patient care so as to improve population health. The NHIN architecture is a specific network architecture that realizes health information implementation specifications based on open standards. The ONC recognizes a broad range of exchange needs for the NHIN including simple, local applications and more robust exchanges with federal agencies or large nationwide entities. Work is currently underway to establish minimum requirements for local applications through the NHIN Direct project.

THE BUSINESS VALUE OF HEALTH DATA STANDARDS

The importance of data standards to enhancing the quality and efficiency of healthcare delivery is being recognized by national and international leadership. Reviewing the business value of defining and using data standards is critical for driving the implementation of these standards into applications and systems. Having data standards for data exchange and information modeling will provide a mechanism against which deployed systems can be validated (Loshin, 2004). Reducing manual intervention will increase worker productivity and streamline operations. Defining information exchange requirements will enhance the ability to automate interaction with external partners, which in turn will decrease costs.

A standardized nursing language is necessary so that nursing knowledge can be represented and communicated consistently among nurses and other healthcare providers. Identifying key data elements, defining them consistently, and capturing them in a database will build a library of evidenced-based care that can be measured and validated (Rutherford, 2008). Enhanced data collection will contribute to greater adherence to standards of care, assessment of nursing competencies, and evaluation of nursing outcomes, thus increasing the visibility of nursing interventions and improving patient care.

By using data standards to develop their emergency department data collection system, New York State demonstrated that it is good business practice (Davis, 2004). Their project was completed on time without additional resources and generated a positive return on investment. The use of standards provided the basis for consensus between the hospital industry and the state, a robust pool of information that satisfied the users, and the structure necessary to create unambiguous data requirements and specifications.

Other economic stakeholders for health IT include software vendors or suppliers, software implementers who install the software to support end-user requirements, and the users who must use the software to do their work. The balance of interests among these stakeholders is necessary to promote standardization to achieve economic and organizational benefits (Marshall, 2009). Defining clear business measures will help motivate the advancement and adoption of interoperable health IT systems, thus ensuring the desired outcomes can be achieved. Considering the value proposition for incorporating data standards into products, applications, and systems should be a part of every organization's IT strategy.

SUMMARY

This chapter introduces health data standards, the organizations that develop, coordinate, and harmonize them, the process by which they are developed, examples of current standards initiatives, and a discussion of the business value of health data standards. Four broad areas are described to categorize health data standards. Transport standards are used to establish communication protocols between systems. Vocabulary standards are used to describe clinical problems and procedures, medications, and allergies. Content exchange standards and value sets are used to share clinical information such as clinical summaries, prescriptions, and structured electronic documents. And security standards are those used for authentication, access control, and transmission of health data. Organizations involved in the development, harmonization, and coordination of health data standards are profiled.

A discussion of the standards development process highlights the international and sociopolitical context in which standards are developed and the potential impact they have on the availability and currency of standards. The increasingly significant role of the federal government in influencing the development and adoption of health data standards is discussed. Several key initiatives, including the ONC Standards and Interoperability Framework, Regional HIEs, and the NHIN are described, and their potential impacts are highlighted. Finally, the business value and importance of health data standards to improving the quality and efficiency of healthcare delivery and the role their adoption plays in improving patient outcomes are emphasized.

REFERENCES

ANSI. (2005). *The United States Standards Strategy*. New York: American National Standards Institute.

Bowman, S. (2008). Why ICD-10 is worth the trouble. *Journal of AHIMA, 79*(3), 24–29.

Centers for Medicare and Medicaid Services (CMS). (2007). *HIPAA security series: Security 101 for covered entities.* (Vol. 2, paper 1, pp. 1–11). Washington, DC: Centers for Medicare and Medicaid Services.

Committee on Data Standards for Patient Safety. (2004). *Patient safety: Achieving a new standard for care.* Washington, DC: Institute of Medicine.

Davis, B. (2004). Return-on-investment for using data standards: A case study of New York State's data system. *Public Health Data Standards Consortium*. Retrieved from http://www.phdsc.org/standards/pdfs/ROI4UDS.pdf.

Department of Health and Human Services. (2010). *Health information technology: Initial set of standards, implementation specifications, and certification criteria for electronic health record technology.* (45 CFR Part 170). Washington, D. C.: Office of the Secretary.

Fridsma, D. (2010). *Interoperability framework overview.* Presentation to the HIT Standards Committee, March 24, 2010. Washington, DC.

Hammond, W. E. (2005). The making and adoption of health data standards. *Health Affairs, 23*(5), 1205–1213.

Health Information Policy Council. (1983). *Background Paper: Uniform minimum health data sets.* Washington, DC: Department of Health and Human Services.

Health Level Seven (HL7) EHR Technial Committee. (2007 February). Electronic health record—System functional model, release 1. Ann Arbor, MI: Health Level Seven.

Loshin, D. (2004). The business value of data standards. *DM Review. 14*(6), 20.

Marshall, G. (2009). The standards value chain. *Journal of AHIMA, 10*, 58–65.

National Committee on Vital and Health Statistics. (1996). *Report of the National Committee on Vital and Health Statistics: Core health data elements.* Washington, DC: Government Printing Office.

National Library of Medicine. (2010). Health information technology and health data standards at NLM. Retrieved from http://www.nlm.nih.gov/healthit.html.

Nelson, R. (2006). Data processing. In V. K. Saba & K. A. McCormick (Eds.), *Essentials of Nursing Informatics* (4th ed.). New York, NY: McGraw-Hill.

Rutherford, M. A. (2008). Standardized nursing language: What does it mean for nursing practice? *The Online Journal of Issues in Nursing, 13*(1).

Sensmeier, J. (2010). The impact of standards and certification on EHR Systems. *Foundations of Nursing Informatics*. Atlanta, GA: HIMSS10.

WEB SITES

The field of data standards is a very dynamic one with existing standards undergoing revision and new standards being developed. The best way to learn about specific standards activities is to get involved in the process. All of the organizations discussed in this chapter provide opportunities to be involved with activities that support standards development, coordination, and implementation. Listed below are the World Wide Web addresses for each organization. Most sites describe current activities and publications available, and many have links to other related sites.

Accredited Standards Committee (ASC) X12. *www.wpc-edi.com*

American Medical Association (AMA). *www.ama-assn.org*

American National Standards Institute (ANSI). *www.ansi.org*

American Nurses Association (ANA). *www.nursingworld.org*

American Society for Testing and Materials (ASTM). *www.astm.org*

Clinical Data Interchange Standards Consortium (CDISC). *www.cdisc.org*

Digital Imaging Communication in Medicine Standards Committee (DICOM). *www.nema.org*

European Committee for Standardization Technical Committee 251Health Informatics (CEN/TC 251). *www.cen.eu/cen*

Health Level Seven (HL7). *www.hl7.org*

Healthcare Information Technology Standards Panel (HITSP). *www.hitsp.org*

Institute of Electrical and Electronic Engineers (IEEE). *www.ieee.org*

Integrating the Healthcare Enterprise (IHE). *www.iheusa.org*

International Health Terminology Standards Development Organisation (IHTSDO). *www.ihtsdo.org*

International Organization for Standardization (ISO). *www.iso.org*

International Statistical Classification of Diseases and Related Health Problems (ICD-9, ICD-9CM, ICD-10). *www.cdc.gov/nchswww*

Logical Observation Identifiers Names and Codes (LOINC). *loinc.org*

National Committee on Vital and Health Statistics (NCVHS). *aspe.os.dhhs.gov/ncvhs*

National Council for Prescription Drug Programs (NCPDP). *www.ncpdp.org*

National Electrical Manufacturers Association (NEMA). *www.nema.org*

National Library of Medicine (NLM).*www.nlm.nih.gov/healthit.html*

National Uniform Claims Committee (NUCC). *www.nucc.org*

Object Management Group (OMG). *www.omg.org*

Office of the National Coordinator for Health Information Technology (ONC). *www.hhs.gov/healthit*

Public Health Data Standards Consortium (PHDSC). *www.phdsc.org*

RxNorm. *www.nlm.nih.gov/research/umls/rxnorm*

Unified Medical Language System (UMLS). *www.nlm.nih.gov/research/umls*

World Wide Web Consortium (W3C). *www.w3.org*

16

Nursing Informatics and Healthcare Policy

Judy Murphy / Elizabeth Johnson

• OBJECTIVES

1. Discuss the significant impact of federal legislation from 2009 and 2010 on the use of health information technology.
2. Describe the creation of the office of the National Coordinator for Health Information Technology and summarize the major role it plays in the implementation of health information technology.
3. Discuss the implications of policy on nursing informatics as a specialty.
4. Identify the impact that national trends and events focused on information and information technology have on nursing informatics practice.

• KEY WORDS

informatics
health information technology
public policy
health policy

On March 23, 2010, President Barack Obama signed into law the landmark Patient Protection and Affordable Care Act (PPACA), a federal statute that represents the most recent legislation in a sweeping healthcare reform agenda passed into law by the 111th Congress and the Obama administration. The new law is dedicated to replacing a broken system with one that ensures all Americans have access to healthcare that is both affordable and driven by quality standards. It includes broad provisions for the improvement of healthcare delivery that will take effect between March 23, 2010 and January 1, 2018 (Patient Protection and Affordable Care Act, Wikipedia).

For the new administration, the hard-fought legislative success of PPACA turns the spotlight on the growing recognition that advanced healthcare information technology (HIT) is and will be essential to support the massive amounts of electronic information exchange foundational to reform. In fact, the universal agreement that meaningful healthcare reform cannot be separated from the national—and arguably global—integration of HIT based on accepted, standardized, and interoperable methods of data exchange provided the linchpin for other critically important legislation that created the glide path for PPACA.

It was such consensus that resulted in the broad support and passage into law of the American Recovery and Reinvestment Act (ARRA) of 2009 and its key Health Information Technology (HITECH) Act provision in the early weeks of President Obama's presidency. Backed with an allocation of $19.2 billion, this legislation authorized the Centers for Medicare & Medicaid

Services (CMS) to provide reimbursement incentives for eligible professionals and hospitals that take steps to become "meaningful users" of certified electronic health record (EHR) technology to improve care quality and better manage care costs (American Recovery and Reinvestment Act, Wikipedia).

At the core of the new reform initiatives, the incentivized adoption of EHRs will improve care quality and better manage care costs, meeting clinical and business needs by capturing, storing, and displaying clinical information when and where it is needed to improve individual patient care and to provide aggregated, cross-patient data analysis.

EHRs will manage healthcare data and information in ways that are patient-centered and information-rich. Improved information access and availability will increasingly enable both the provider and the patient to better manage each patient's health by using capabilities provided by enhanced clinical decision support and customized educational materials.

In this massive transformation from disconnected, inefficient, paper-based "islands" of care delivery to a nationwide, interconnected, and interoperable system driven by EHRs and advancing HIT innovation, the importance of nurses and nursing informatics (NI) will be difficult to overstate. For decades, nurses have proactively contributed resources to the development, use, and evaluation of information systems. Today, they constitute the largest single group of healthcare professionals, including experts who serve on national committees and participate in interoperability initiatives focused on policy, standards and terminology development, standards harmonization, and EHR adoption. In their frontline roles, nurses will continue to have a profound impact on the quality and cost of healthcare and are emerging as leaders in the effective use of HIT to improve the safety, quality, and efficiency of healthcare services. (Alliance for Nursing Informatics (ANI), 2009).

Informatics nurses are key contributors to a working knowledge about how evidence-based practices designed in information systems can support and enhance clinical processes and decision making to improve patient safety and outcomes. With the responsibilities of care coordination and promotion of wellness, nurses are the "glue" of acute care delivery settings and often the patient's primary contact—and last defensive line—in care delivery, where medical errors or other unintended actions can be caught and corrected. In addition, as drivers in organizational planning and process reengineering to improve the healthcare delivery system, informatics nurses are increasingly sought out by nurses and nurse managers for leadership as their profession works to

bring IT applications into the mainstream healthcare environment (ANI, 2009).

Therefore, it is increasingly essential to the success of today's healthcare reform movement that nurses are involved in every aspect of selecting, designing, testing, implementing, and developing health information systems. Further, the growing adoption of EHRs must incorporate nursing's unique body of knowledge with the nursing process at its core.

CHAPTER OVERVIEW

Given the importance of today's healthcare transformation to the nursing profession, and the pivotal involvement of nurses in the reform process, it is important to understand the key components driving change in the industry: the primary influencers, organizations, programs, and processes that have shaped or defined polices for the integration of HIT that will affect all segments of healthcare, especially nursing. Therefore, the purpose of this chapter is to identify and define the historic and present roles of such influencers, including sections on the following topics:

- Forces of change in today's national healthcare system
- Mandate for reform: ARRA and its HITECH Act provision
- State and regional HIT programs
- HIT federal advisory committees and agencies
- Nursing informatics and healthcare reform
- The future

FORCES OF CHANGE IN TODAY'S NATIONAL HEALTHCARE SYSTEM

The long journey to the passage of PPACA, ARRA, and HITECH Act goes back several decades. In 1991, the Institute of Medicine (IOM) concluded that computerization can help to improve patient records and information management leading to higher quality of care in its landmark report, *The Computer-Based Patient Record: An Essential Technology for Healthcare* (Dick, 1997). That was followed nearly a decade later with other groundbreaking reports calling for the use of HIT to improve the efficiency, safety, and quality of the U.S. healthcare system: *To Err Is Human in 1999* (Kohn, 1999) and *Crossing the Quality Chasm in 2001* (Institute of Medicine, 2001). These reports were calls for a paradigm shift in managing patient care—from reliance on paper and verbal communication to a new era where nurses' clinical decision making is supported by technology.

In looking back at other significant forces of change, one of the earliest and most influential was The President's Information Technology Advisory Committee (PITAC).

The President's Information Technology Committee: The Winds of Change

In 1997, an Executive Order of President Clinton established the visionary, 24-member President's Information Technology Advisory Committee (PITAC), which was comprised of both corporate and academic leaders from across the United States. Since its inception, the committee has provided the President, Congress, and those Federal agencies involved in networking and information technology (IT) research and development with expert, independent advice on maintaining American preeminence in advanced IT. These technologies include critical elements of the national IT infrastructure such as high-performance computing, large-scale networking, cyber security, and high-assurance software and systems design (National Coordination Office for Networking and Information Technology Research and Development, n.d.).

In 1999, as part of its seminal work to define how IT could drive progress in the 21st Century, PITAC established a panel to provide guidance on how IT could be leveraged to transform healthcare and increase access to care for all citizens. Driving the panel's work was the firm conviction that the federal government's role in leading the way to healthcare reform through technology was both critical and, at the time, sorely lacking (Computing Research Association, 1999).

A few years later, in a report entitled, *Transforming Healthcare through Information Technology*, PITAC found that "at present, the U.S. lacks a broadly disseminated and accepted national vision for information technology in healthcare" (President's Information Technology Advisory Committee (PITAC), 2001, p. 4). To rectify the situation, the panel strongly recommended that the Department of Health and Human Services (HHS) define a clear vision for how IT could improve the U.S. healthcare system, follow up with resources sufficient to accomplish its objectives, and appoint a senior IT person to provide strategic leadership.

President Bush's Executive Order and the Birth of the Office of the National Coordinator

On January 20, 2004, President George W. Bush said in his State of the Union address, "… an electronic health record for every American by the year 2014 … by computerizing health records, we can avoid dangerous medical mistakes, reduce costs, and improve care." He went on to issue the executive order, "Incentives for the Use of Health Information Technology and Establishing the Position of the National Health Information Technology Coordinator", that has impacted every healthcare entity, provider, and informatics nurse professional in the United States (Bush, 2004).

Components of the order are as follows: (1) establish a national health information technology coordinator position; (2) develop a nationwide interoperable health IT infrastructure; and (3) develop, maintain, and direct implementation of a strategic plan to guide implementation of interoperable health IT in both public and private sectors. Interoperable health IT was seen as a means to reduce medical errors, improve quality, and produce greater value for healthcare expenditures. That same year, Dr. David Brailer was appointed by then Secretary of the Department of Health and Human Services (HHS) Tommy Thompson as the first National Health Information Technology Coordinator.

The Office of the National Coordinator for Health Information Technology (referred to as the ONC) remains today as the principal federal entity charged with coordination of nationwide efforts to implement and use the most advanced HIT and the electronic exchange of health information. The ONC is a key player in the execution of the provisions in ARRA and the HITECH Act. The current coordinator is Dr. David Blumenthal.

On the road to healthcare reform, many other organizations and initiatives provided the vision, leadership, and processes that paved the way toward the legislative action seen in ARRA, the HITECH Act, and PPACA. Ensuring the translation mandated by the legislation, other groups such as the ONC's HIT Policy and Standards Committees are defining and shaping the healthcare agenda on an ongoing basis.

HIT Training Programs: An Essential Element of Reform

PITAC's 2001 recommendations to President George W. Bush included a call for trained professionals who could apply HIT to healthcare reform, noting that it would be necessary to "establish programs to increase the pool of biomedical research and healthcare professionals with training at the intersection of health and information technology" (PITAC, 2001, p. 12.). In its findings, the report warned that the pool of professionals at the time was "remarkably small."

Today, the urgent need for HIT experts is challenged by a shortage of the very professionals who are best positioned to carry transformation forward. The dilemma is nowhere more relevant than in nursing. In the face of insufficient numbers of nurses to meet future demands, the importance of HIT training programs designed to infuse new efficiencies into the work nurses perform has gained paramount importance (Gassert, 2006).

With consensus around the essential requirement for advanced HIT and the mounting pressures of shortages in nursing and other medical professions, HHS has enlisted the talent and resources of some of the nation's leading universities, community colleges, and major research centers to advance the widespread adoption and meaningful use of HIT. These schools are offering a wide variety of training programs that are helping to build the depth and breadth of the health informatics workforce as a critical component in the transformation of American healthcare delivery. Both on-campus and online programs in HIT are available at the certificate, associate, bachelors, and masters degree levels. Certificate programs typically consist of between 15 and 30 credit hours and are often designed for working professionals (Education-Portal.com, n.d.). The American Medical Informatics Association (AMIA) created the revolutionary 10×10 Program in 2005, with the goal of training 10,000 healthcare professionals in applied health informatics by 2010, and became a model for certificate-based programs (American Medical Informatics Association, n.d.[b]).

Through ARRA, federal awards and grants totaling some $84 million to 16 universities and junior colleges are providing incentives for HIT education to speed the growth of a new pool of HIT professionals. These programs are now supporting the training and development of more than 50,000 new HIT professionals (Health Information Technology Grants). For more information, see the section on Workforce Training under Mandate for Reform: ARRA and Its HITECH Act Provision.

The Health Insurance Portability and Accountability Act: Privacy and Security

The Health Insurance Portability and Accountability Act (HIPAA), which passed in 1996, required HHS to develop regulations protecting the privacy and security of electronic health information as well as facilitate its efficient transmission (Health Insurance Portability and Accountability Act of 1996). HIPAA's goals are to allow the flow of health information needed to provide and promote high quality healthcare while protecting the public's health and well being. Prior to HIPAA, no generally accepted set of standards or requirements for protecting health information existed in the health-care industry. At the same time, new technologies were evolving to move the healthcare industry away from paper-based processes and toward increasing reliance on electronic information systems to conduct a host of administrative and clinically-based functions, such as providing health information, paying claims, and answering eligibility questions (Gassert, 2006).

To comply with the requirements of the HIPAA, HHS published what are commonly known as the HIPAA Privacy Rule and the HIPAA Security Rule. The rules apply to all health plans, healthcare clearinghouses, and to any healthcare provider that transmits health information in electronic form (Health Insurance Portability and Accountability Act, Wikipedia; Health Insurance Portability and Accountability Act of 1996).

The HIPAA Privacy Rule. The HIPAA Privacy Rule, which took effect on April 14, 2003, established national standards for the protection of individually identifiable health information. As such, the rule regulates the use and disclosure of an individual's health information, referred to as protected health information, and sets forth standards for individuals' privacy rights to understand and control how their health information is used. The rule applies to those organizations identified as "covered entities," including healthcare clearinghouses, employer-sponsored health plans, health insurers, and other medical service providers that engage in the transfer of protected health information. Protected health information is defined broadly and includes any part of an individual's medical record or payment history (Department of Health & Human Services, 2003).

The HIPAA Security Rule. The HIPAA Security Rule took effect on April 21, 2003 with a compliance date of April 21, 2005 for most covered entities. The Security Rule complements the Privacy Rule; while the Privacy Rule pertains to all protected health information including both paper and electronic records, the Security Rule deals specifically with electronic protected health information. Still, a major goal of the Security Rule is to protect the privacy of individuals' protected health information while allowing covered entities to adopt new technologies to improve the quality and efficiency of patient care. Given the diversity of the healthcare marketplace, the Security Rule is designed to be flexible and scalable so that a covered entity can implement policies, procedures, and technologies that are appropriate for the entity's particular size, organizational structure, and risks to consumers' electronic protected health information (Department of Health & Human Services, n.d.[a]).

In the years following its passage and implementation, HIPAA regulations have had a significant impact on health informatics, including nursing informatics. For example, under HIPAA, patients must be permitted to review and amend their medical records. Healthcare providers have expressed concern that patients who choose to access their records could experience increased anxiety. However, studies have determined that counter-benefits already include enhanced doctor-patient communications and associate only minimal risk with increasing patients' access to their records.

Most recently, the passage of ARRA has expanded HIPAA's mandate to impose new privacy and security requirements. (For details, see Mandate for Reform: ARRA and Its HITECH Act Provision later in this chapter.)

EHR Certification and the Changing Role of CCHIT

With the passage of ARRA and the HITECH Act, the ONC has become the driving force behind the definition of meaningful use of EHRs and the certification of EHR systems. This new reality has changed the operating environment for the Certification Commission for Healthcare Information Technology (CCHIT), which until recently had been the sole agency designated to certify EHR systems.

CCHIT was founded in 2004 (Certification Commission for Health Information Technology, 2010) with support from 3 industry associations in healthcare information management and technology: the American Health Information Management Association (AHIMA), the Healthcare Information and Management Systems Society (HIMSS), and the National Alliance for Health Information Technology (NAHIT). In September 2005, HHS awarded CCHIT a contract to develop the certification criteria and inspection process for EHRs and the networks through which they interoperate. Since then, in its work to certify EHRs, CCHIT established the first comprehensive, practical definition of the capabilities that were required in such systems. The certification criteria were developed through a voluntary, consensus-based process engaging diverse stakeholders. Many informatics nurses were involved in this process, helping to define the certification criteria for the hospital and ambulatory environments as well as to outline the testing processes used by CCHIT (Certification Commission for Health Information Technology, Wikipedia).

However, in the months following the 2009 passage of ARRA, questions surfaced about CCHIT's future role. On March 2, 2010, the ONC confirmed the merits of this debate when it issued a new Notice of Proposed Rulemaking (NPRM) (Notice of Proposed Rulemaking, Wikipedia), which would establish 2 certification programs for the purposes of testing and certifying EHRs—a temporary program and a permanent program. These new programs were not limited to CCHIT. On June 24, 2010, the ONC published its Final Rule on the Temporary Certification Program for EHRs.

Under the temporary program, the ONC will authorize approved organizations, called ONC-Authorized Testing and Certification Bodies (ONC-ATCBs), to both test and certify EHRs and EHR modules, thereby assuring the availability of certified EHR technology prior to the beginning of the reporting period defined under ARRA. The permanent certification program will replace the temporary program after the first year and will separate the responsibilities for performing testing and certification. In addition to EHR and EHR modules certification, the permanent program will include the certification of other types of HIT, such as personal health records (PHRs) and health information exchange (HIE) networks (Premier, Inc., 2010).

Standards and the National Health Information Network

In late 2005, the U.S. Department of Health and Human Services commissioned the Healthcare Information Technology Standards Panel (HITSP) to assist in developing a National Health Information Network (NHIN), which would create a nationwide, interoperable, private, and secure exchange of heath information between EHRs (Health Information Technology Standards Panel, n.d.).

As envisioned then and now, NHIN is intended to provide a set of standards that regulate the connections among providers, consumers, and others involved in supporting health and healthcare. The purpose of these standards is to enable normalized health information to follow the consumer; making health records, laboratory results, medication information, and related medical data readily available and accessible to providers, pharmacists, and even consumers over the Internet, thereby helping to achieve the goals of the HITECH Act today. At the same time, NHIN is also dedicated to ensuring that consumers' health information remains secure and confidential in the electronic environment.

Interoperability

Interoperability is the ability of health information systems to work together within and across organizational boundaries to advance the effective delivery of healthcare for individuals and communities by sharing data between EHRs. To facilitate interoperability, standards for data transport, content exchange, and vocabulary management are necessary. This is why standards development is so important: it enables the interoperability needed for regional and national health data exchange and is essential to the development of the NHIN.

Debate exists about how interoperability should develop with regard to the timing of EHR adoption. On the one hand, many industry leaders believe that interoperability should precede EHR use. They are convinced that the ability to share information should be designed into EHRs and that the infrastructure and industry capacity for securely networking this information should exist up front. On the other hand, others argue that interoperability will follow widespread EHR adoption. This side of the debate believes that once health information becomes electronic and everyone is using EHRs, interoperability will naturally follow since it will be easier and cheaper than manual data sharing (Barr, 2008; Connor, 2007).

Integrating the Healthcare Enterprise. Integrating the Healthcare Enterprise (IHE) is a global initiative, now in its tenth year, to create the framework for passing vital health information seamlessly from application to application, system to system, and setting to setting across multiple healthcare enterprises. IHE brings together HIT stakeholders to demonstrate the implementation of standards for communicating patient information efficiently throughout and among healthcare enterprises by developing a framework of interoperability. Because of its proven process of collaboration, demonstration, and real-world implementation of interoperable solutions, IHE is in a unique position to significantly accelerate the process for defining, testing, and implementing standards-based interoperability among EHR systems (Integrating the Healthcare Enterprise, n.d.). Additional details on healthcare data standards development, harmonization, and interoperability can be found in Chapter 15.

Nonprofit Organizations Driving Reform: AMIA and HIMSS

Among the many nonprofit organizations advancing HIT and health informatics today, few have had such positive impact on the industry as the AMIA and the HIMSS. Both organizations have significant numbers of nurse members as well as committees, task forces, and working groups for the nursing community.

AMIA. The AMIA is dedicated to promoting the effective organization, analysis, management, and use of information in healthcare to support patient care, public health, teaching, research, administration, and related policy. For over thirty years, the members of AMIA and its honorific college, the American College of Medical Informatics (ACMI), have sponsored meetings, education, policy, and research programs. The federal government frequently calls upon AMIA as a source of informed, unbiased opinions on policy issues relating to the national health information infrastructure, uses and protection of personal health information, and public health considerations, among others (AMIA, n.d.[a]).

With an overall mission of advancing the informatics profession relating to health and disease, AMIA champions the use of health information and communications technology in clinical care and research, personal health management, public health/population, and transactional science with the ultimate objective of improving health. The association is also dedicated to expanding the size and strengthening the competency of the U.S. health informatics workforce and supporting the continued development of the health informatics profession.

HIMSS. The HIMSS was founded in 1961 and is a comprehensive healthcare–stakeholder membership organization exclusively focused on providing leadership for the optimal use of IT and management systems for the betterment of healthcare. The HIMSS is a global organization that represents over 23,000 members, 73% of whom work in patient care delivery settings, and has offices in Chicago, Washington, D.C., Brussels, and Singapore. The HIMSS also includes corporate members and not-for-profit organizations that share its mission to transform healthcare through the effective use of IT and management systems (Healthcare Information and Management Systems Society, 2009).

The society was founded on the premise that an organized exchange of experience among members could promote a better understanding of the principles underlying healthcare systems and improve the skills of those who direct HIT programs and the practitioners who analyze, design, or evaluate HIT systems. In today's environment of rapid reform and transformation, HIMSS frames and leads healthcare public policy and industry practices through its educational, professional development, and advocacy initiatives designed to promote information and management systems' contributions to ensuring quality patient care (HIMSS Legacy Workgroup, 2007).

MANDATE FOR REFORM: ARRA AND ITS HITECH ACT PROVISION

ARRA and its important HITECH Act provision were passed into law on February 17, 2009. Commonly referred to as "The Stimulus Bill" or "The Recovery Act," the landmark legislation allocated $787 billion to stimulate the economy, including $147 billion to rescue and reform the nation's seriously ailing healthcare industry. Of these funds, $19 billion in financial incentives were earmarked for the relatively short period of 5 years to drive reform through the use of advanced HIT and the adoption of EHRs. The incentives were intended to help healthcare providers purchase and implement HIT and EHR systems, and the HITECH Act also stipulated that clear penalties would be imposed beyond 2015 for both hospitals and physician providers who failed to adopt use of EHRs in a meaningful way. This section describes some of the key components of ARRA and the HITECH Act (American Recovery and Reinvestment Act, Wikipedia).

HITECH Incentives for Meaningful Use of EHRs

The majority of funding from the HITECH Act will be used to reward hospitals and eligible providers for "meaningful use" of certified EHRs by "meaningful users" with increased Medicare and Medicaid payments. Both programs have start dates of fiscal year 2011 (October 1, 2010) for hospitals and calendar year 2011 (January 1, 2011) for eligible providers. On December 31, 2009, the Centers for Medicare and Medicaid Services (CMS), with input from the ONC and the HIT Policy and Standards Committees, published the Proposed Rule on Meaningful Use of EHRs and began a 60-day public comment period. After reviewing more than 2,000 comments, HHS issued the final rule on July 13, 2010. The final criteria for meeting meaningful use are divided into 5 initiatives (Blumenthal, 2010):

1. Improve quality, safety, efficiency, and reduce health disparities.

2. Engage patients and families.

3. Improve care coordination.

4. Improve population and public health.

5. Ensure adequate privacy and security protections for personal health information.

Specific objectives were written to demonstrate that EHR use has a "meaningful" impact on 1 of the 5 initiatives. Under the final rule, there are 14 core objectives that require compliance for hospitals, and 15 for providers. Additionally, both hospitals and providers must choose 5 additional objectives from a "menu set." If the objectives are met during the specified year and the hospital or provider submits the appropriate measurements, then the hospitals or providers will receive the incentive payment. The hospital incentive amount is based on the Medicare and Medicaid patient volumes; the provider incentives are fixed per provider. The incentives are paid over 5 years, and the hospital or provider must submit measurement results annually during each of the years to continue to qualify. The objectives will mature every other year, with new criteria and standards being published in 2011, 2013, and 2015 (Goedert, 2010).

Quality Measures

One of the meaningful use criteria for both hospitals and providers is the requirement to report quality measures to either CMS (for Medicare) or to the state (for Medicaid). For providers, the final rule lists 44 measures, with a requirement to comply with 6. For hospitals, the rule lists 15 measures and requires compliance with all of them (Goedert, 2010).

Because HHS will not be ready to electronically accept quality measure reporting in 2011, the Proposed Rule specifies that hospitals and eligible providers will submit summary information on clinical quality measures to CMS through attestation in 2011. HHS expects to be ready to electronically accept quality measure reporting in 2012.

Quality measurement is considered one of the most important components of the incentive program under ARRA and the HITECH Act, since the purpose of the HIT incentives is to promote reform in the delivery, cost, and quality of healthcare in the U.S. Dr. David Blumenthal, current National Coordinator of HIT, emphasized this point when he said that "HIT is the means, but not the end. Getting an EHR up and running in healthcare is not the main objective behind the incentives provided by the federal government under ARRA. Improving health is. Promoting healthcare reform is" (Blumenthal, 2009).

The ONC and Establishment of the HIT Policy and Standards Committees

To drive the rapid, HIT-based reform under such an aggressive plan, the HITECH legislation re-energized the ONC with specific accountabilities and significant funding, and created 2 new Federal Advisory Committees under its control: the HIT Policy Committee and the HIT Standards Committee. These 2 committees are comprised of public and private stakeholders (including physicians and nurses) tasked to provide recommendations on the HIT policy framework, standards, implementation specifications, and certification criteria for electronic exchange and use of health information (AMA, 2009). Also see HIT Federal Advisory Committees and Agencies later in this chapter.

Standards and Interoperability

ARRA and the HITECH Act recognized that a key element of the widespread adoption and use of HIT would be the development of uniform electronic standards that would allow various HIT systems to communicate with each other, thereby interconnecting the industry. ARRA placed a deadline of December 31, 2009 on the development of such standards.

The ONC and its HIT Standards and Policy Committees have made considerable progress to address concerns over interoperability implementation through their work on a new ONC Interoperability Framework, NHIN, and standards development. The NHIN Work Group is developing recommendations for extending the secure exchange of health information using NHIN standards, services, and policies to the broadest audience possible. Further, a group of federal agencies; local-, regional-, and state-level health information exchange (HIE) organizations; and integrated delivery networks, formerly known as the NHIN Cooperative, has been helping to develop the NHIN standards, services, and policies and demonstrate live health information exchange through the NHIN Exchange (Department of Health and Human Services, n.d.[c]).

The NHIN Direct Project, a new initiative based on initial recommendations from the NHIN Work Group, is being launched to explore the NHIN standards and services required to enable secure health information exchange at a more local and less complex level, such as a primary care provider sending a referral or care summary to a local specialist electronically.

Privacy and Security

The HITECH Act significantly expanded federal privacy and security laws under HIPAA as follows (American Medical Association, 2009):

- HIPAA privacy and security laws now apply directly to business associates of covered entities.
- The law defines actions that constitute a breach of patient health information (including inadvertent disclosures) and requires notification to patients if breaches occur.
- Patients are allowed to pay out of pocket for a healthcare item or service in full and to request that the claim not be submitted to the health plan.

- Physicians are required to provide patients, upon request, an accounting of disclosures of health information made through the use of an EHR.
- The sale of a patient's health information without the patient's written authorization is prohibited, except in limited circumstances involving research or public health activities.
- Covered entities are prohibited from being paid to use patients' health information for marketing purposes without patient authorization, except limited communication to a patient about a drug currently prescribed for that patient.
- PHR vendors must notify individuals of a breach of patient health information.
- Noncovered HIPAA entities such as HIEs, regional health information organizations, e-prescribing gateways, and PHR vendors are required to have business associate agreements with covered entities for the electronic exchange of patient health information.
- HIPAA can now authorize increased civil monetary penalties for HIPAA violations.
- HIPAA authorizes increased authority for state attorneys general to enforce HIPAA.

For additional information on privacy and security, see Chapter 17.

Comparative Effectiveness Research

ARRA and the HITECH Act increased funding by more than $1 billion for comparative effectiveness research (CER) and established the Federal Coordinating Council for Comparative Effectiveness Research (FCC-CER). This group is an advisory board comprised of clinical experts responsible for reducing duplication of efforts and encouraging coordination and complementary use of resources, coordinating related health services research, and making recommendations to the President and Congress on CER infrastructure needs. As part of this legislation, the Agency for Healthcare Research and Quality (AHRQ) will receive additional funding for CER, nearly half of which must be shared with the National Institutes of Health (NIH) to conduct or support CER (American Medical Association, 2009).

Workforce Training

ARRA funding has also been designated to educate the workforce required to modernize the healthcare system by promoting and expanding the adoption of HIT by 2014

(Department of Health and Human Services, n.d.[d]). There are 4 grant programs set up to support the training and development necessary for a skilled workforce (Department of Health and Human Services, n.d.[d]):

- $32 million to establish 9 university-based certificate and advanced degree HIT training programs, including a program sponsored by the University of Colorado-Denver School of Nursing
- $360 million to create 5 regional Community College Consortia of more than 80 member community colleges in all 50 states to help address the demand for skilled HIT specialists
- $10 million to support HIT education curriculum development
- $6 million to develop an HIT competency examination program.

National Institutes of Health and National Library of Medicine Grants to Support HIT Research

The passage of ARRA and the HITECH Act provision earmarked substantial funding in support of HIT research, in addition to programs supporting HIT training. For its part, the NIH received an infusion of funds for 2009 and 2010 as part of ARRA. Presently, the NIH has designated over $200 million, to be used throughout 2009 and 2010, for a new initiative called the NIH Challenge Grants in Health and Science Research. This program supports research on topics that address specific scientific and health research challenges in biomedical and behavioral research that would benefit from significant, 2-year jump-start funds. NIH anticipates funding 200 or more grants, each up to $1 million, depending on the number and quality of applications (National Center for Research Resources, n.d.).

In addition, the National Library of Medicine (NLM) offers Applied Informatics grants to health-related and scientific organizations that wish to optimize use of clinical and research information. These grants help organizations exploit the capabilities of HIT to bring usable, useful biomedical knowledge to end users by translating the findings of informatics and information science research into practice through novel or enhanced systems, incorporating them into real-life systems and service settings (Department of Health & Human Services, 2010).

SHARP Research Grants

Alongside the NIH and NLM focus on incentivizing research, the ONC also made $60 million available to support the development of Strategic Health IT Advanced Research Projects (SHARP). The SHARP program funds research focused on the following achievements: (1) breakthrough advances that address well-documented problems impeding HIT adoption, and (2) accelerating progress toward achieving nationwide meaningful use of HIT in support of a high-performing, continuously-learning healthcare system. The ONC awarded 4 cooperative agreements of $15 million, with each awardee implementing a research program addressing a specific research focus area: HIT security, patient-centered cognitive support, healthcare application and network architectures, and secondary use of HIT data (Department of Health & Human Services, 2010).

Beacon Communities

Also funded by the HITECH Act, the Beacon Community Program includes $250 million in grants to build and strengthen the HIT infrastructure and HIE capabilities within 17 communities. These communities will demonstrate the vision of a future where hospitals, clinicians, and patients are meaningful users of HIT, and together the community achieves measurable improvements in healthcare quality, safety, efficiency, and population health. The program awarded funding to communities at the cutting edge of EHR adoption and health information exchange, enabling them to reach a new level of sustainable healthcare quality and efficiency. The program is anticipated to demonstrate how HIT can help providers and consumers develop innovative ways of delivering care, leading to measurable health and efficiency improvements. Additionally, the program will generate lessons learned that other communities can use to achieve similar HIT goals (Monegain, 2010).

STATE AND REGIONAL HIT PROGRAMS

With recognition that the regional electronic exchange of health information is essential to the successful implementation of the NHIN and to the success of national healthcare reform in general; the HITECH Act authorized and funded a State HIE Cooperative Program and a Regional HIT Extension Program. Taken together, these grant programs offer much needed local and regional assistance and technical support to providers, while enabling coordination and alignment within and among states. Ultimately, this will allow information to follow patients anywhere they go within the U.S. healthcare system (Department of Health & Human Services n.d.[b]).

State Health Information Exchange Cooperative Agreement Program

This grant program awarded funding to 56 states, eligible territories, and qualified state-designated entities (SDEs) to establish HIE capacity among healthcare providers and hospitals in their jurisdictions. These efforts are expected to rapidly build capacity for exchanging health information across the healthcare system, both within and across states. Awardees are responsible for increasing connectivity and enabling patient-centric information flow to improve the quality and efficiency of care. Key to this goal is the continual evolution and advancement of necessary governance, policies, technical services, business operations, and financing mechanisms for HIE over each state, territory, and SDE's 4-year performance period. This program builds on existing efforts to advance regional and state HIE while moving toward nationwide interoperability via the NHIN.

HIT Extension Program

The HIT Extension Program consists of Regional Extension Centers (RECs) and a national Health Information Technology Research Center (HITRC). The program is designed to support the training and consulting needs of the many healthcare providers seeking to adopt EHRs and achieve meaningful use by offering education, outreach, and technical assistance. RECs will help providers in their geographic service areas select, successfully implement, and meaningfully use certified EHR technology to improve the quality and value of healthcare. The ONC has funded 60 RECs in virtually every geographic region of the United States to ensure adequate support to healthcare providers in communities across the country. The HITRC promotes communication and learning among the RECs and collaborates with them by offering technical assistance, guidance, and information on best practices to support and accelerate healthcare providers' efforts to become meaningful users of EHRs. They are especially helpful to small provider practices that have limited resources for the selection, implementation, and evaluation of EHRs.

HIT FEDERAL ADVISORY COMMITTEES AND AGENCIES

In 1972, decades before ARRA, the HITECH Act, and PPACA, the Federal Advisory Committee Act became law and is still the legal foundation defining how Federal Advisory Committees and Agencies (FACAs) should operate. As then prescribed, characteristics of such groups included openness and inclusiveness, specific authorization by either the President or the head of the overseeing agency, transparency, and clearly defined timelines for operation, termination, and renewal. In 2009, as mandated by ARRA and the HITECH Act, the ONC created 2 new Federal Advisory Committees: the HIT Policy Committee and the HIT Standards Committee, in order to gain broad input on the use of HIT to support healthcare reform.

The HIT Policy Committee. The HIT Policy Committee is charged with making recommendations to the ONC on a policy framework for the development and adoption of a nationwide health information infrastructure, including standards for the exchange of patient medical information. Serving the Committee are 7 workgroups to address and make recommendations to the full committee on key reform issues such as meaningful use of EHRs, certification and adoption of EHRs, information exchange, NHIN, the strategic plan framework, privacy and security policy, and enrollment in federal and state health and human services programs. Connie Delaney, a nurse and coauthor of a chapter in this book, sits on this 25-member committee.

The HIT Standards Committee. The HIT Standards Committee is charged with making recommendations to the ONC on standards, implementation specifications, and certification criteria for the electronic exchange and use of health information. In harmonizing or recognizing standards and implementation specifications, the HIT Standards Committee is also tasked with providing for all associated testing by the National Institute of Standards and Technology (NIST). Serving the Committee are 4 workgroups addressing clinical operations, clinical quality, privacy and security requirements, and implementation strategies that accelerate the adoption of proposed standards. There are 3 nurses that participate on this 25-member committee, including Judy Murphy and Elizabeth Johnson who are the coauthors of this chapter.

In addition to the HIT Policy and Standards Committees, 2 other key agencies involved in the national healthcare reform movement include the National Committee on Vital and Health Statistics and the National Quality Forum.

The National Committee on Vital and Health Statistics. The National Committee on Vital and Health Statistics (NCVHS) was originally established more than 50 years ago by Congress to serve as an advisory body to the HHS on health data, statistics, and national health information policy. It fulfills important review and advisory functions relative to health data and statistical problems of national and international interest, stimulates or conducts studies of such problems, and makes proposals for improvement of U.S. health statistics and information systems. In 1996, the NCVHS was restructured to meet expanded responsibilities under HIPAA. In 2009, the committee was the first to hear testimony and make recommendations to the ONC regarding meaningful use criteria to measure effective EHR use (The National Committee on Vital and Health Statistics, n.d.).

The National Quality Forum. The National Quality Forum (NQF) is a nonprofit organization that aims to improve the quality of healthcare for all Americans through fulfillment of its 3-part mission: to set national priorities and goals for performance improvement; to endorse national consensus standards for measuring and publicly reporting on performance; and to promote the attainment of national goals through education and outreach programs. The NQF has taken the lead in defining quality measures to qualify for the meaningful use incentives under the HITECH Act (National Quality Forum, n.d.).

NURSING INFORMATICS AND HEALTHCARE REFORM

In 2009, a survey sponsored by the HIMSS Nursing Informatics community, entitled *Informatics Nurse Impact Survey*, concluded that the passage of ARRA and its provision of incentives to promote the meaningful use of EHRs created new opportunities for informatics nurses "to apply their ability not only to understand all sides of the IT process, but to act as a translator between those who understand the language of the technology and the language and needs of clinicians and patients" (HIMSS, 2009, p. 2).

For years, informatics nurses have contributed to the work of healthcare reform implementation teams, creating increasingly stronger positions from which to help put the new national healthcare infrastructure in place. Given the aggressive timeframes written into the new healthcare reform legislation, however, collaboration between public and private healthcare entities has never been more important. This call to action in the transformation of the healthcare industry has raised the visibility of a number of respected nursing and nursing informatics professional organizations, whose missions seek to advance the practice of informatics nurses and strengthen the profession's collective voice and impact.

The proceeding section highlights some of the involvement that nurses have had in the work of HIT and healthcare reform.

Nursing Informatics Organizations

Of the professional nursing informatics organizations active in helping to define and drive policies in the process of implementing ARRA and the HITECH Act, the following are among the most influential.

Alliance for Nursing Informatics. The Alliance for Nursing Informatics (ANI) is dedicated to furthering the development of a united voice for nursing informatics, providing a single point of connection between individual informatics nurses, nursing informatics groups, and the broader nursing and healthcare community. The ANI is a collaborative representing thousands of nurses and more than 40 NI groups in the United States that function separately at local, regional, national, and international levels. The ANI works to provide a mechanism for transforming care and developing resources, guidelines, and standards for NI practice, education, scope of practice, research, certification, public policy, terminology, best practice guidelines, mentoring, advocacy, networking, and career services. It supports individual membership in affiliated NI groups and organizations. Formed in 2004, a key goal remains its constant engagement and leadership in issues of national importance in HIT (Alliance for Nursing Informatics, 2009).

American Medical Informatics Association—Nursing Informatics Working Group Policy Committee. The American Medical Informatics Association—Nursing Informatics Working Group Policy Committee (AMIA-NIWG) was founded in 1990 to promote the practice of NI within the larger interdisciplinary context of health informatics. The members pursue this goal in many arenas: professional practice, education, research, governmental and other service, professional organizations, and industry. The AMIA-NIWG is the official representative to IMIA-NI and liaises to other national and international groups. They are the sponsors of the Nursing Informatics History Project, which documents and preserves the history of nursing informatics (American Medical Informatics Association, n.d.[a]).

International Medical Informatics Association Special Interest Group for Nursing Informatics. The International Medical Informatics Association Special Interest Group for Nursing Informatics (IMIA/NI-SIG) was formed in 1982 to foster collaboration among nurses and others interested in nursing informatics to facilitate development in the field. Its purpose is to share knowledge, experience, and ideas with nurses and healthcare providers worldwide about the practice of nursing informatics and the benefits of enhanced information management (International Medical Informatics Association, n.d.).

HIMSS Nursing Informatics Community. The HIMSS Nursing Informatics Community was formed in 2003 in response to increased recognition of the roles of informatics nurses, with a mission to advance NI practice, education, and research by articulating a cohesive voice for the HIMSS NI Community and to provide strategic guidance and tactical support for the programs and activities for NI within the HIMSS. The group articulates a cohesive voice for the HIMSS informatics nurses and provides domain expertise, leadership, and guidance to HIMSS activities, initiatives, and collaborations within the global NI community (HIMSS, 2009).

Nursing Organizations

Professional nursing organizations with the ability to influence and inform policy activities through government agencies, decision makers, and the public include the following.

The American Nurses Association. The American Nurses Association (ANA) is the core professional organization representing the interests of the nation's more than 3 million nurses. The ANA advances the nursing profession by fostering high standards of nursing practice, promoting the rights of nurses in the workplace, projecting a positive and realistic view of nursing, and lobbying the Congress and regulatory agencies on healthcare issues affecting nurses and the public (American Nurses Association, n.d.).

The American Association of Critical-Care Nurses. The American Association of Critical-Care Nurses (AACN) was established to help educate nurses working in newly developed intensive care units. Today, it is the world's largest specialty nursing organization, representing the interests of more than 500,000 nurses responsible for the care of acute and critically ill patients (American Association of Critical-Care Nurses, n.d.).

American Organization of Nurse Executives. The American Organization of Nurse Executives (AONE) is the voice of nursing leadership in healthcare. The organization provides leadership, professional development,

advocacy, and research to advance nursing practice and patient care, promotes nursing leadership excellence, and shapes public policy for healthcare (American Organization of Nurse Executives, n.d.).

American Academy of Nursing Informatics and Technology Expert Panel. The American Academy of Nursing Informatics and Technology Expert Panel (AAN) serves the public and the nursing profession by advancing health policy and practice through the generation, synthesis, and dissemination of nursing knowledge. The AAN's 1,500 elected-to-fellowship members are among nursing's most accomplished leaders in education, management, practice, and research. In order to advance health policy and assist in driving healthcare reform, the AAN works through a system of expert panels. Each expert panel generates, synthesizes, and disseminates nursing knowledge in a specific area that is important to the AAN and society as a whole. There are 17 expert panels, including one for informatics and technology. This panel provides informatics and technology leadership through communication, education, publication, and policy appointment recommendations (American Academy of Nursing Informatics and Technology Expert Panel, n.d.).

The TIGER Initiative. The Technology Informatics Guiding Education Reform (TIGER) initiative aims to identify information and knowledge-management best practices and effective technology capabilities for nurses. TIGER's goal is to create and disseminate action plans that can be duplicated within nursing and other multidisciplinary healthcare training and workplace settings (Technology Informatics Guiding Education Reform Initiative, n.d.).

The TIGER Initiative is working to catalyze a dynamic, sustainable, and productive relationship between the ANI, with its 20 NI professional societies, and major nursing organizations including the ANA, the AONE, the AACN, and others which collectively represent over 2 million nurses. It is important to acknowledge the involvement of nurses and nursing organizations in this initiative that are not informatics nurse specialists. Having their collective voice at the table with informatics nurses strengthens the value of nursing's role and position on HIT issues.

During the first and second phases of TIGER's operations, the group worked to create a common vision for an ideal EHR-enabled nursing practice and then facilitated collaboration among participating organizations to achieve this vision. Now in its third phase, TIGER is working with leaders and other organizations in the healthcare reform movement in 9 critical areas: standards and interoperability, the national HIT agenda, informatics competencies, education and faculty development, staff development, usability and clinical application design, a virtual demonstration center, leadership development, and consumer empowerment and personal health records. For more information on the TIGER Initiative see Chapter 42.

Nursing Informatics Competencies

Today's informatics nurse combines clinical knowledge with IT to improve the ways nurses diagnose, treat, care for, and manage patients. Essentially, informatics nurses support, change, expand, and transform nursing practice through the design and implementation of IT. The ANI defines nursing practice as "a specialty that integrates nursing science, computer science, and information science to manage and communicate data, information, knowledge, and wisdom in nursing practice" (RNDegrees.net, n.d.).

In the transforming healthcare environment, informatics nurses help to design the automated tools that help clinicians, nurse educators, nursing students, nurse researches, policymakers, and consumers as they increasingly seek to manage their own health. Therefore, it is essential that a nursing culture that promotes the acceptance and use of IT is sustained and advanced by establishing informatics nurse competencies and the educational processes that help nurses achieve them.

Many in the profession emphasize the need for every nurse, whether employed in a practice or educational setting, to develop a minimum or "user" level of computer literacy and informatics theory. A second tier includes the intermediate level of literacy, which includes nurses who may work part time on teams to design, modify, or evaluate HIT systems. The third level of competency is the advanced, or innovator, level where a nurse is considered to specialize. A more complete discussion of competencies and competency development for nurses is provided in Chapter 44.

Again, it is important to note that the informatics competencies described here are for nurses and nurse leaders, not informatics nurses. Practicing nurses' understanding of the role HIT plays to drive quality care and healthcare reform directly impacts their adoption of HIT and their definition of best practice use of HIT.

The Intersection of HIT Policy and Nursing Informatics

Informatics nurses are poised to play pivotal leadership roles in defining new policies that help to make the goals of ARRA and the HITECH Act a reality over the coming years. To make such a profound difference in today's constantly changing healthcare environment, informatics professionals must be aware of existing and proposed healthcare policy on an ongoing basis. Policy is defined as a course of action that guides present and future decisions, is based on given conditions, and is selected from identified alternatives. Healthcare policy is established on local, state, and national levels to guide the implementations of solutions for the population's health needs. Both existing conditions and emerging trends in the healthcare industry influence policy decisions. Policy decisions often establish the direction for future trends that impact informatics. Informatics nurse professionals, therefore, must become more cognizant of events and the healthcare policies that will affect their practices (Gassert, 2006).

As aptly summarized by one of nursing's most active and respected organizations, the ANI, "…'meaningful use' of HIT, when combined with best practice and evidence-based care delivery, will improve healthcare for all Americans. This is an essential foundation for the future of nursing, and informatics nurses must be engaged as leaders in the effective use of information technology to impact the quality and efficiency of healthcare service" (Alliance for Nursing Informatics (ANI), 2009, p. 9).

Influencing HIT Transformation through Testimony and Comment

This chapter has discussed the need for HIT competencies, awareness of how HIT is changing the way we diagnose, treat, care for, and manage patients, as well as healthcare policies that affect healthcare practices and the global healthcare landscape. In addition, informatics nurses should never underestimate the power of communication to bring about meaningful change in our nation's healthcare delivery system.

In 2005, the World Health Organization's Commission on the Social Determinants of Health asked, "What narrative will capture the imaginations, feelings, intellect and will of political decision-makers and the broader public and inspire them to action?" (World Health Organization, 2005, p. 44). Years later, the question is more important than ever to the nursing profession and to informatics nurses who stand in an unprecedented position to effect change. Public comment through a growing number of media outlets—supported by the emergence of the Internet and social media—translates theory and knowledge into meaningful activity that can drive and define local, state, and federal policy, addressing key health and social issues and improving the lives of patients affected by them (Kaminski, 2007).

Outlets for communication that can reach pivotal segments of society and the ears of key influencers in healthcare reform include not only traditional media (newspapers, magazines, books) but also new mass media formats like Web-based video and blogs, Twitter, and other social media sites. Whether commenting over these outlets from organizations like the HIMSS, the ANI, and the AMIA or as an individuals active in healthcare transformation, such communication can change public perceptions of current issues and help form and influence public attitudes and decisions.

For example, through the ANI's efforts and those of its members, nursing informatics experts are tapped as valued resources for providing expert testimony and serving on national committees and initiatives focused on HIT policy, standards harmonization, and EHR adoption and certification. Many times over the past 5 years, nurses have provided testimony on NI- and HIT-related topics for the AMIA, the HIMSS, the CCHIT, the NCVHS, and others.

THE FUTURE

Leaders in both healthcare and nursing agree that the future of nursing depends on a profession that will continue to innovate using HIT and informatics to play an instrumental role in patient safety, change management, and quality improvement, as evidenced by quality outcomes, enhanced workflow, and user acceptance. These areas highlight the value of informatics nurses as knowledge workers and their roles in the adoption of HIT to deliver higher quality clinical applications across healthcare organizations.

That value can only increase as new directions and priorities emerge in healthcare. In an environment where the roles of all healthcare providers are diversifying, informatics nurses must prepare to guide the profession appropriately from their positions as project managers, consultants, educators, researchers, product developers, decision support and outcomes managers, chief clinical information officers, chief information officers, advocates, policy developers, entrepreneurs, and business owners. This is especially true where informatics nurses can contribute leadership in the effective design and use of EHR systems. To achieve our nation's healthcare reform goals, the healthcare community must leverage the sources of patient care technologies and information management competence that informatics nurses provide to ensure that the national investment in HIT and EHRs is implemented properly and effectively over the coming years.

In fact, in its October 2009 recommendations to the Robert Wood Johnson Foundation (RWJF) on the future of nursing, the ANI argued that nurses will be integral to achieving a vision that will require a nationwide effort to adopt and implement EHR systems in a meaningful way: "This is an incredible opportunity to build upon our understanding of effectiveness research, evidence-based practice, innovation and technology to optimize patient care and health outcomes. The future of nursing will rely on this transformation, as well as on the important role of nurses in enabling this digital revolution"[emphasis added] (ANI, 2009, p. 9).

For no professional group does the future hold more excitement and promise from so many productive perspectives than it does for informatics nurses.

SUMMARY

The passage of landmark healthcare reform legislation, including ARRA and the HITECH Act in 2009 and the PPACA in 2010, have changed the landscape of the U.S. healthcare Industry forever, perhaps more than any expert envisioned just scant years ago. The Obama administration's hard-fought legislative success is testimony to the growing recognition that advanced HIT is essential to support the enormous amounts of electronic information that will be collected and exchanged and will be foundational to industry transformation and healthcare reform. As the nation undergoes a massive transformation from disconnected, inefficient, paper-based "islands" of care delivery to a nationwide, interconnected, and interoperable system driven by EHRs and HIT innovation, the importance of nurses and NI will become increasingly evident. For decades, nurses have proactively contributed resources to the development, use, and evaluation of information systems. Today, they constitute the largest single group of healthcare professionals, and include experts who serve on national committees and initiatives focused on HIT policy, standards and terminology development, standards harmonization, and EHR adoption. Performing their frontline roles, nurses will continue to have a profound impact on the quality and effectiveness of healthcare and are emerging as leaders in the effective use of HIT to improve the quality and efficiency of healthcare services.

REFERENCES

Alliance for Nursing Informatics (ANI). (2009). *Statement to the Robert Wood Johnson Foundation Initiative— Future of nursing: Acute care.* Retrieved from http:// www.himss.org/handouts/ANIResponsetoRWJ_ IOMonTheFutureofNursing.pdf.

Alliance for Nursing Informatics (ANI). (n.d.). *Welcome to the new Alliance for Nursing Informatics Web site.* Retrieved from http://www.allianceni.org/.

American Academy of Nursing Informatics and Technology Expert Panel (AAN). (n.d.). *About AAN.* Retrieved from http://www.aannet.org/i4a/pages/index.cfm?pageid=3284.

American Association of Critical Care Nurses (AACN). (n.d.). Retrieved from http://www.aacn.org.

American Association of Nurse Executives (AONE). (n.d.). Retrieved from http://www.aone.org.

American Medical Association (AMA). (n.d.). *American Recovery And Reinvestment Act of 2009 (ARRA).* Retrieved from http://www.ama-assn.org/ama/pub/advocacy/current-topics-advocacy/hr1-stimulus-summary.shtml.

American Medical Informatics Association (AMIA). (n.d.[a]). Retrieved from https://www.amia.org

American Medical Informatics Association. (n.d.[b]). *AMIA 10 × 10 Program.* Retrieved from http://www.amia.org/10x10/students.asp.

American Nurses Association (ANA). (n.d.). Retrieved from http://www.nursingworld.org/.

American Recovery and Reinvestment Act (ARRA),. (n.d.). In *Wikipedia.* Retrieved May 10, 2010 from http://en.wikipedia.org/wiki/American_Recovery_and_Reinvestment_Act_of_2009.

Barr, F. (2008, November 6). Healthcare interoperability: The big debate. *e-Health Insider,* Retrieved from http://www.e-health-insider.com/comment_and_analysis/359/healthcare_interoperability:_the_big_debate.

Blumenthal, D. (2009, September 16). National HIPAA Summit in Washington, D.C.

Blumenthal, D. (2010, July 13). The "meaningful use" regulation for electronic health records. *The New England Journal of Medicine.* Retrieved from http://healthcarereform.nejm.org/?p=3732.

Bush, G. W. (2004, January 20). *State of the union address.* Retrieved from http://www.americanrhetoric.com/speeches/stateoftheunion2004.htm.

Bush, G. W. (2004). *Executive order, incentives for the use of health information technology and establishing the position of the national health information technology coordinator.* Retrieved from http://edocket.access.gpo.gov/cfr_2005/janqtr/pdf/3CFR13335.pdf.

Certification Commission for Health Information Technology (CCHIT). (2010). *About the Certification Commission for Health Information Technology.* Retrieved from http://www.cchit.org/about.

Certification Commission for Healthcare Information Technology (CCHIT). (n.d.). In *Wikipedia.* Retrieved May 9, 2010 from http://en.wikipedia.org/wiki/Certification_Commission_for_Healthcare_Information_Technology.

Computing Research Association. (1999). *President's information technology advisory committee (PITAC) final report: Fact sheet.* Retrieved from http://www.cra.org/govaffairs/advocacy/pitac_fs.pdf.

Connor, D. (2007). Healthcare pros debate interoperability standards. *Network World.* Retrieved from http://www.networkworld.com/news/2007/022707-healthcare-pros.html.

Department of Health & Human Services. (2003, May, rev.). *Summary of the HIPAA privacy rule, HIPAA compliance assistance.* Retrieved from http://www.hhs.gov/ocr/privacy/hipaa/understanding/summary/privacysummary.pdf.

Department of Health & Human Services. (2010). *NLM applied informatics grants.* Retrieved from http://www.grants.nih.gov/grants/guide/rfa-files/RFA-LM-09-001.html.

Department of Health & Human Services. (2010, April 2). *News release: HHS awards $144 million in Recovery Act funds to institutions of higher education and research to address critical needs for the widespread adoption and meaningful use of health information technology.* Retrieved from http://www.hhs.gov/news/press/2010pres/04/20100402a.html.

Department of Health & Human Services. (n.d.[a]). *Health information privacy: Summary of the HIPAA security rule.* Retrieved from http://www.hhs.gov/ocr/privacy/hipaa/understanding/srsummary.html.

Department of Health & Human Services. (n.d.[b]). *HITECH priority grants program: Health IT workforce development program, facts at a glance.* Retrieved from http://healthit.hhs.gov/portal/server.pt?open=512&objID=1432&mode=2.

Department of Health and Human Services. (n.d.[c]). *Nationwide health information network: Overview.* Retrieved from http://healthit.hhs.gov/portal/server.pt?open=512&mode=2&cached=true&objID=1142.

Department of Health and Human Services. (n.d.[d]). *Recovery act-funded programs.* Retrieved from http://www.hhs.gov/recovery/programs/index.html#Health.

Dick, R., & Steen, E. (1997). *The computer-based patient record: An essential technology for healthcare.* Institute of Medicine, Committee on Improving the Patient Record. Washington, DC: National Academy Press.

Education-Portal.com. (n.d.). *Online education programs in health information technology with training info.* Retrieved from http://education-portal.com/online_education_programs_in_health_information_technology.html.

Gassert, C. A. (2006). Nursing informatics and healthcare policy. In V. Saba & K. McCormick (Eds.), *Essentials of Nursing Informatics* (pp. 183–194). New York, NY: McGraw-Hill.

Geodert, J. (2010, July 13). A first look at final MU criteria. *Health Data Management.* Retrieved from http://content.nejm.org/cgi/reprint/NEJMp1006114.pdf?ssource=hcrc.

Healthcare Information and Management Systems Society (HIMSS). (2009, April 2). *HIMSS*

2009 informatics nurse impact survey: Sponsored by McKesson. Executive summary. Retrieved from http://www.himss.org/content/files/HIMSS2009InformaticsNurseImpactSurvey.pdf.

Health Information Management and Systems Society (HIMSS). (n.d.). Retrieved from http://www.himss.org.

Health Information Technology Standards Panel (HITSP) & American National Standards Institute (ANSI). (n.d.). *Enabling healthcare interoperability.* Retrieved from http://www.hitsp.org/government.aspx

Health Insurance Portability and Accountability Act of 1996. Public law 104-191, 104th Congress. Retrieved from https://www.cms.gov/HIPAAGenInfo/Downloads/HIPAALaw.pdf.

Health Insurance Portability and Accountability Act. (n.d.) In *Wikipedia.* Retrieved May 9, 2010 from http://en.wikipedia.org/wiki/Health_Insurance_Portability_and_Accountability_Act.

HIMSS Legacy Workgroup. (2007). *The history of HIMSS.* Retrieved from http://www.himss.org/content/files/HIMSS_HISTORY.pdf.

HIPAA Survival Guide. (n.d.). *HIPAA security rule.* Retrieved from http://www.hipaasurvivalguide.com/hipaa-survival-guide-16.php.

Integrating the Healthcare Enterprise (IHE). (n.d.). *Changing the way healthcare connects.* Retrieved from http://www.ihe.net/

Institute of Medicine, Committee on Quality of Healthcare in America. (2001). *Crossing the quality chasm: A new health system for the 21st Century.* Washington, DC: National Academy Press. Retrieved from http://www.nap.edu/catalog.php?record_id=10027.

International Medical Informatics Association (IMIA). (n.d.). Retrieved from http://www.imia.org.

Kaminski, J. (2007). Activism in education focus: Using communicative and creative technologies to weave social justice and change theory into the tapestry of nursing curriculum. *EcoNurse.* Retrieved from http://econurse.org/EthelJohns.html.

Kohn, L., Corrigan, J., & Donaldson, M. (Eds.) (1999). *Institute of Medicine, To Err is Human: Building a Safer Health System.* Washington, DC: National Academy Press. Retrieved from http://www.nap.edu/openbook.php?isbn=0309068371.

Monegain, B. (2010, May 4). Health IT 'Beacon Communities' awarded $220 million. *Healthcare IT News.* Retrieved from http://www.healthcareitnews.com/news/health-it-beacon-communities-awarded-220-million.

National Center for Research Resources. (n.d.). *NIH challenge grants in health and science research—NCRR topics.* Retrieved from http://www.ncrr.nih.gov/the_american_recovery_and_reinvestment_act/challenge_grant_initiative.

National Committee on Vital and Health Statistics (NCVHS). (n.d.). Retrieved from http://www.ncvhs.hhs.gov/intro.htm.

National Coordination Office for Networking and Information Technology Research and Development. (n.d.). *President's information technology advisory committee (PITAC) - Archive.* Retrieved from http://www.nitrd.gov/Pitac/index.html.

National Quality Forum (NQF). (n.d.). Retrieved from http://www.qualityforum.org/About_NQF/About_NQF.aspx.

Notice of Proposed Rulemaking. In *Wikipedia.* Retrieved May 10, 2010 from http://en.wikipedia.org/wiki/Notice_of_proposed_rulemaking.

Patient Protection and Affordable Care Act. In *Wikipedia.* Retrieved May 6, 2010 from http://en.wikipedia.org/wiki/Patient_Protection_and_Affordable_Care_Act.

Premier, Inc. (2010, March 9). *Summary of proposed rule certification programs for health information technology.* Retrieved from http://www.premierinc.com/about/advocacy/issues/10/hit/Premier-Summary-ONC-NPRM-EHR-Certification.pdf.

President's Information Technology Advisory Committee (PITAC). (2001, February). *Panel on transforming healthcare, transforming healthcare through information technology, report to the President.* Retrieved from http://www.internet2.edu/health/files/pitac-hc-9feb01.pdf.

RNDegrees.net. (n.d.). *Nursing Informatics Degree Programs.* Retrieved from http://rndegrees.net/nursing-informatics-degree-programs.html.

Technology Informatics Guiding Education Reform (TIGER) Initiative. (n.d.). Retrieved from http://www.tigersummit.com.

World Health Organization Secretariat of the Commission on Social Determinants of Health. (2005). *Action on the social determinants of health: Learning from previous experiences, background report,* (p. 44).

OTHER RESOURCES

American College of Physicians. (2006, November 20). *American College of Physicians to offer health information technology training course.* (Press release). Retrieved from http://www.medicalnewstoday.com/articles/57084.php.

American Nursing Informatics Association (ANIA). (n.d.). Retrieved from http://www.ania.org.

Blumenthal, D. (2010, April 27). Promoting use of health IT: Why be a meaningful user. *Health IT Buzz Blog.* Retrieved from http://healthit.hhs.gov/blog/onc/index.php/2010/04/27/promoting-use-of-health-it-why-be-a-meaningful-user.

Department of Health & Human Services. (2010). *Proposed establishment of certification programs for health information technology notice of proposed rulemaking.* Retrieved from http://www.aamc.org/members/gir/onc_hit_certrule_presentation_hitpc.ppt.

Fischetti, L., & Deering, M. J. (2006). Electronic health record systems: U.S. federal initiatives and public/

private partnerships. In V. Saba & K. McCormick (Eds.), *Essentials of Nursing Informatics* (pp. 229–237). New York, NY: McGraw-Hill.

Fortner P. (2009, December 15). Nurses claim their seat at the health IT decision-making table. *iHealthBeat*. Retrieved from http://www.ihealthbeat.org/features/2009/nurses-claim-their-seat-at-the-health-it-decisionmaking-table.aspx.

WorldwideLearn. (n.d.). *Guide to college majors in health information technology*. Retrieved from http://www.worldwidelearn.com/online-education-guide/health-medical/health-information-technology-major.htm.

Halamka, J. (2010, March 30). The ONC interoperability framework. *Healthcare IT News*. Retrieved from http://www.e-health-insider.com/comment_and_analysis/359/healthcare_interoperability.

Halamka, J. (2010, March 30). The ONC interoperability framework. *Life as a Healthcare CIO Blog*. Retrieved from http:/geekdoctor.blogspot.com/2010/03/onc-interoperability-framework.html.

HITECH Priority Grants Program. *Health information technology extension program facts-at-a-glance*. Retrieved from http://www.hhs.gov/recovery/programs/hitech/factsheet.html.

Integrating the Healthcare Enterprise (IHE). (n.d.). Retrieved from http://www.himss.org/ASP/topics_ihe.asp.

Murphy, J. (2009, Fall). Meaningful use for nursing: Six themes regarding the definition for meaningful use, nursing informatics commentary. *Journal of Healthcare Information Management*, 23(4), 9–11.

Murphy, J. (2010, Winter). This is our time: How ARRA changed the face of health IT," nursing informatics commentary. *Journal of Healthcare Information Management*, 24(1), 8–9.

Nursing Informatics History Project. (n.d.). Retrieved from https://www.amia.org/niwg-history-page.

Patient Protection and Affordable Care Act. Retrieved from http://docs.house.gov/energycommerce/ppaca.pdf

Ray, A. (2010, May 5). Understanding certification: Evaluating certified EHR technology. AHQA 2010 Annual Meeting. Retrieved from http://www.ahqa.org/uploads/A1CCHIT.pdf.

National Alliance for Health Information Technology. (2010, April 28). *Report to the Office of the National Coordinator for Health Information Technology on defining key health information technology terms*. Retrieved from http://healthit.hhs.gov/portal/server.pt/gateway/PTARGS_0_10741_848133_0_0_18/10_2_hit_terms.pdf.

Rogers, R. F. (2008, October 7-8). *Addressing pending health information technology worker shortages*. South Dakota health IT summit, Sioux Falls, SD. Retrieved from http://freedownloadbooks.net/index.php?keyword=The+Health+Information+Technology+Workforce%3A+Addressing+Pending+HIT+Worker+Shortages&filetype=ppt&page=results.

Rowley, R. (2010, March 4). Rules for designating EHR certification bodies now defined. EHR Bloggers. *Practice Fusion*. Retrieved from http://www.ehrbloggers.com/2010/03/rules-for-designating-ehr-certification.html.

Sensmeier, J. (2009, September-October). Don't overlook the role of nurses in the digital revolution. *GHIT*. Retrieved from http://www.allianceni.org/docs/GHIT_JSensmeier.pdf.

17

Trustworthy Systems for Safe and Private Healthcare

Dixie B. Baker

- OBJECTIVES
    1. To explain the critical role that "trustworthiness" plays in health information technology (HIT) adoption, and healthcare quality and safety.
    2. To introduce and describe a trust framework comprising 7 layers of protection essential for establishing and maintaining trust.
    3. To identify, where applicable, how regulatory provisions relate to this framework – and what is left up to the enterprise to address.

- KEY WORDS
    healthcare
    privacy
    security
    patient safety
    trustworthy systems

INTRODUCTION

The healthcare industry is undergoing a dramatic transformation from today's inefficient, costly, manually intensive, crisis-driven model of care delivery to a more efficient, consumer-centric, science-based model that proactively focuses on health management and quality measurement. This transformation is driven by several major factors including the skyrocketing cost of healthcare delivery, the exposure of patient safety problems, and an aging, socially networked population that recognizes the potential for using health information technology (HIT) to dramatically reduce the cost and improve the quality of care, while enabling consumers to play a more active role in their own health.

The U.S. Health Information Technology for Economic and Clinical Health (HITECH) Act, enacted in 2009 as part of the American Recovery and Reinvestment Act (USC, 2009), provided major structural changes; funding for research, technical support, and training; and financial incentives all designed to significantly expedite and accelerate this transformation. The HITECH Act codified the Office of National Coordinator (ONC) for HIT and assigned it responsibility for developing a nationwide infrastructure that would facilitate the use and exchange of electronic health information, including policy, standards, implementation specifications, and certification criteria. In enacting the HITECH Act, Congress recognized that the meaningful use and exchange of electronic health records (EHRs) were key to improving the quality, safety, and efficiency of the U.S. healthcare system.

At the same time, the HITECH Act recognized that as more health information was recorded and exchanged electronically to coordinate care, monitor quality, measure outcomes, and report public health threats, the risk to personal privacy and patient safety would be heightened. This recognition is reflected in that 4 of the 8 areas identified in the HITECH Act as priorities for the ONC specifically address risks to individual privacy and information security:

1. Technologies that *protect the privacy* of health information and *promote security* in a qualified EHR, including for the *segmentation and protection from disclosure* of specific and sensitive individually identifiable health information, with the goal of minimizing the reluctance of patients to seek care (or disclose information about a condition) because of privacy concerns, in accordance with applicable law, and for the use and disclosure of *limited data sets* of such information.

2. A nationwide HIT infrastructure that allows for the electronic use and *accurate exchange* of health information.

3. Technologies that, as part of a qualified EHR, allow for an *accounting of disclosures* made by a covered entity (as defined by the Health Insurance Portability and Accountability Act of 1996) for purposes of treatment, payment, and healthcare operations.

4. Technologies that allow individually identifiable health information to be *rendered unusable, unreadable, or indecipherable to unauthorized individuals* when such information is transmitted in the nationwide health information network or physically transported outside the secured, physical perimeter of a healthcare provider, health plan, or healthcare clearinghouse.

As noted by National Coordinator David Blumenthal, MD, MPP, "Information is the lifeblood of modern medicine. Health information technology is destined to be its circulatory system. Without that system, neither individual physicians nor healthcare institutions can perform at their best or deliver the highest-quality care" (Blumenthal, 2009). To carry Dr. Blumenthal's analogy one step further, at the heart of modern medicine lies trust. Caregivers must trust that the technology and information they require will be available when needed at the point of care. They must trust that the information in a patient's EHR is accurate and complete and that it has not been accidentally or intentionally corrupted, modified, or destroyed. Consumers must trust that their caregivers will keep their most private health information confidential and will disclose and use it only to the extent necessary and in ways that are legal,

ethical, and authorized as consistent with their personal expectations and preferences. Above all else, consumers must trust that their caregivers and the technology they use will "do no harm."

The nursing field is firmly grounded in a tradition of ethics, patient advocacy, care quality, and human safety. The registered nurse is well indoctrinated on clinical practice that respects personal privacy and protects confidential information and life-critical information services. The American Nurses Association's (ANA's) *Code of Ethics for Nurses with Interpretive Statements* includes a commitment to "promote, advocate for, and strive to protect the health, safety, and rights of the patient" (ANA, 2001). The International Council of Nurses (ICN) Code of Ethics for Nurses affirms that the nurse "holds in confidence personal information" and "ensures that use of technology…[is] compatible with the safety, dignity, and rights of people" (ICN, 2000). Fulfilling these ethical obligations is the individual responsibility of each nurse, who must trust that the information technology she relies upon will help her ensure that personal information will be protected and that the technology is safe.

Recording, storing, and exchanging information electronically does indeed introduce new risks. As anyone who has used a personal computer knows, it takes only a few keystrokes to instantaneously send information to millions of people throughout the world. Try doing that with a paper record and a fax machine! We also know that nefarious spyware, viruses, and Trojan horses skulk around the Internet and insert themselves below our keyboards, eager to capture our passwords, identities, and credit card numbers. At the same time, the capability to receive laboratory results within seconds after a test is performed; to continuously monitor a patient's condition remotely, without requiring him to leave his home; or to be given expert guidance and decision support specifically applicable to a patient's condition and history, all are enabled through HIT.

As HIT assumes a greater role in the provision of care and in healthcare decision making, the nurse increasingly must trust HIT to provide timely access to accurate and complete health information and to use that information to offer personalized clinical decision support, while assuring that individual privacy is continuously protected. Legal and ethical obligations, as well as consumer expectations, drive requirements for assurance that data and applications will be available when they are needed; that private and confidential information will be protected; that data will not be modified or destroyed other than as authorized; that systems will be responsive and usable; and that systems designed to

TABLE 17.1	The Nationwide Privacy and Security Framework Defines 8 Privacy Principles
Principle	**Description**
Individual access	Individuals should be provided simple and timely means to access and obtain their individually identifiable health information in a readable form and format.
Correction	Individuals should be provided a timely means to dispute the accuracy or integrity of their individually identifiable health information and to have erroneous information corrected or the dispute documented.
Openness and transparency	Policies, procedures, and technologies that directly affect individuals and their individually identifiable health information should be open and transparent.
Individual choice	Individuals should be provided a reasonable opportunity and capability to make informed decisions about the collection, use, and disclosure of their individually identifiable health information.
Collection and use	Individually identifiable health information should be collected, used, and/or disclosed only to the extent necessary to accomplish a specified purpose(s) and never to discriminate inappropriately.
Data quality and integrity	People and entities should take reasonable steps to ensure that individually identifiable health information is complete, accurate, and up-to-date to the extent necessary for intended purposes and that it has not been altered or destroyed in an unauthorized manner.
Safeguards	Individually identifiable health information should be protected with reasonable administrative, technical, and physical safeguards to ensure its confidentiality, integrity, and availability and to prevent unauthorized or inappropriate access, use, or disclosure.
Accountability	These principles should be implemented, and adherence assured, through appropriate monitoring and other means, and methods should be in place to report and mitigate nonadherence and breaches.

perform health-critical functions will do so safely. These are the attributes of trustworthy HIT—technology that is worthy of our trust. The Markle Foundation's Connecting for Health identified privacy and security as a technology principle fundamental to trust: "All health information exchange, including in support of the delivery of care and the conduct of research and public health reporting, must be conducted in an *environment of trust*, based on conformance with appropriate requirements for patient privacy, security, confidentiality, integrity, audit, and informed consent" (Markle, 2006).

Many people think of *security* and *privacy* as synonymous. Indeed, these concepts are related in that security mechanisms can help protect personal privacy by ensuring that confidential personal information is accessible only by authorized individuals and entities. However, privacy is more than security, and security is more than privacy. Healthcare privacy principles were first articulated in the United States Department of Health, Education, and Welfare's 1973 report entitled *Records, Computers, and the Rights of Citizens* as "fair information practice principles" (DHEW, 1973). The Markle Foundation's Connecting for Health updated these principles to incorporate new risks created by a networked environment in which health information is routinely electronically captured, used, and exchanged

(Markle, 2006). Based on these works, as well as other national and international privacy and security principles focusing on individually identifiable information in an electronic environment (including but not limited to health), the ONC developed a *Nationwide Privacy and Security Framework for Electronic Exchange of Individually Identifiable Health Information* that identified 8 principles intended to guide the actions of all people and entities that participate in networked, electronic exchange of individually identifiable health information (ONC, 2008). These principles, described in Table 17.1, essentially articulate the rights of individuals to openness, transparency, fairness, and choice in the collection and use of their health information.

Where privacy relates to individual rights, security deals with protection. Security mechanisms and assurance methods are used to protect the confidentiality and authenticity of information, the integrity of data, and the availability of information and services, and to provide an accurate record of activities and accesses to information. While these mechanisms and methods are critical to protecting personal privacy, they are also essential in protecting patient safety and care quality and in engendering trust in electronic systems and information. For example, if laboratory results are corrupted during transmission, or historical data in an EHR are overwritten, the nurse is likely to lose confidence that the HIT can be trusted to help her provide quality care. If a sensor system designed to track wandering Alzheimer patients shuts down without alarming those depending upon it, patients' lives are put at risk.

Trustworthiness is an attribute of each system component and of integrated enterprise systems as a whole, including those components that may exist in "clouds." Trustworthiness is difficult to retrofit, as it must be designed and built into the system from the outset and conscientiously preserved as the system evolves. Discovering that an operational system cannot be trusted generally indicates that extensive—and expensive—changes to the system are needed. In this chapter, we introduce a framework for achieving and maintaining trustworthiness in HIT.

WHEN THINGS GO WRONG

Although we would like to be able to assume that computers, networks, and software are as trustworthy as our toasters and refrigerators, unfortunately that is not the case. One of the more dramatic examples became the cover story for the February 2003 issue of CIO, which relates in detail the occurrence and recovery from "one of the worst healthcare IT crises in history"—a catastrophic failure in the network infrastructure that supported CareGroup, one of the most prestigious healthcare organizations in the United States. The source of the problem was ultimately traced to network switches that directed network traffic over a highly overburdened and fragile network, which was further taxed when a researcher uploaded a multigigabyte file into the picture archiving and communication system (PACS). The failure resulted in a 4-hour closure of the emergency room, a complete shutdown of the network, and 2 days of paper-based clinical operations—a true "retro" experience for many of the physicians who had never practiced without computers. Network services were not fully recovered until 6 days after the onset of the disaster (Berinato, 2003), and CareGroup learned a valuable lesson about network sizing and scalability.

Between May 2005 and June 2006, an employee with access to electronic patient information at the Cleveland Clinic's office in Weston, Florida, downloaded the personal identification information of approximately 1,500 patients. The medical identity information stolen included patients' names, dates of birth, Social Security numbers, Medicare numbers, and home addresses. The Medicare numbers and patient identity information were ultimately used by medical services providers in Miami Dade County to fraudulently bill Medicare for approximately $8 million for medical services that had not been delivered and medical equipment that had not been supplied (USA-FL, 2008).

Identity theft can imperil individuals' lives as well. In 2006, a 27-year-old mother of 4 children in Salt Lake City received a phone call from a Utah social worker notifying her that her newborn had tested positive for methamphetamines and that the state planned to remove all of her children from her home. The young mother had not been pregnant in more than 2 years, but her stolen driver's license had ended up in the hands of a meth user who gave birth using the stolen identity. After a few tense days of urgent phone calls with child services, the victim was allowed to keep her children, and she hired an attorney to sort out the damages to her legal and medical records. Months later, when she needed treatment for a kidney infection, she carefully avoided the hospital where her stolen identity had been used. But her caution did no good because her electronic record, with the identity thief's medical information intermingled, had circulated to hospitals throughout the community. The hospital worked with the victim to correct her charts to avoid making life-critical decisions based on erroneous information. The data corruption damage could have been far worse had the thief's baby not tested positive for methamphetamines, bringing the theft to the victim's attention (Rys, 2008).

In July 2009, after noting several instances of computer viruses affecting the United Kingdom's National Health Service (NHS) hospitals, a British news broadcasting station conducted a survey of the NHS trusts throughout England to determine how many of their systems had been infected by computer viruses. Seventy-five percent replied, reporting that over 8,000 viruses had penetrated their security systems, with 12 incidents affecting clinical departments, putting patient care at risk, and exposing personal information. One Scottish trust was attacked by the Conficker virus, which shut down computers for 2 days. Some attacks were used to steal personal information, and at a cancer center, 51 appointments and radiotherapy sessions had to be rescheduled (Cohen, 2009). The survey seemed to have little effect on reducing the threat—less than a year later, NHS systems were victimized by the Qakbot data-stealing worm, which infected over a thousand computers and stole massive amounts of information (Goodin, 2010).

Even antivirus software may not be as trustworthy as one would hope. In April 2010, computers throughout the U.S. began rebooting themselves when a software update caused an antivirus program to identify a normal Microsoft Windows file as a virus. The problem forced about one-third of the hospitals in Rhode Island to postpone elective surgeries and stop treating non-trauma, emergency-room patients (Tobin, 2010).

The HITECH Act introduced a federal requirement for covered entities to notify individuals whose unsecured protected health information may have been exposed due to a security breach. It further required that breaches affecting 500 or more individuals be immediately reported to the secretary of the Department of Health and Human Services (HHS), who must post a list of the reported breaches to a public Web site. Between September 22, 2009, and June 11, 2010, a total of 92 breaches, from 27 states and the District of Columbia, were reported on the HHS Web site—affecting nearly 2.5 million individuals (HHS, 2010). Fifty-seven of the breaches were attributed to theft or loss of computer equipment, portable devices, and electronic media—the most visible and easily detected types of breaches. Thus one might surmise that this accounting may be just the tip of the iceberg of electronic breaches of health information.

The bottom line is that systems, networks, and software applications, as well as the enterprises within which they are used, are highly complex, and the only safe assumption is that "things will go wrong." Trustworthiness is an essential attribute for the systems, software, services, processes, and people used to manage individuals' health information and to help provide safe, high-quality healthcare.

HIT TRUST FRAMEWORK

Trustworthiness can never be achieved by implementing a few policies and procedures, and some security technology. Protecting sensitive and safety-critical health information and ensuring that the systems, services, and information nurses rely upon to deliver quality care are available when they are needed, require a complete HIT trust framework that starts with an objective assessment of risk and is conscientiously applied throughout the development and implementation of policies, operational procedures, and security safeguards built on a solid system architecture. This trust framework is depicted in Figure 17.1 and comprises 7 layers of protection, each of which is dependent upon the layers below it (indicated by the arrows in the figure), and all of which must work together to provide a trustworthy HIT environment for healthcare delivery.

Layer 1: Risk Management

Risk management is the foundation of the HIT trust framework. Objective risk assessment informs decision making and positions the organization to correct those physical, operational, and technical deficiencies that pose the highest risk to the information assets within the enterprise and to put into place protections that will enable the organization to manage the residual risk and liability. Patient safety, individual privacy, and information security all relate to *risk*, which is simply the probability that some bad thing will happen. Risk is always with respect to a given context comprising relevant threats, vulnerabilities, and valued assets. Threats can be natural occurrences (e.g., earthquake, hurricane), accidents, or malicious people and software programs. Vulnerabilities are present in facilities, hardware, software, communication systems, business processes, workforces, and electronic data. Valued assets can be anything from reputation to business infrastructure to information to human lives.

A security risk is the probability that a threat will exploit a vulnerability to expose confidential information, corrupt or destroy data, or interrupt or deny essential information services. If that risk could result in the unauthorized disclosure of an individual's private health information or the compromise of an individual's identity, it also represents a privacy risk. If the risk could result in the corruption of clinical data or an interruption in the availability of a safety-critical system, causing human harm or the loss of life, it is a safety risk as well.

Information security is widely viewed as the protection of information confidentiality, data integrity, and service availability. Indeed, these are the 3 areas of safeguards directly addressed by the technical safeguards discussed in the Health Insurance Portability and Accountability Act (HIPAA) Security Rule (HHS, 2003). Generally, safety is most closely associated with protective measures for data integrity and the availability of life-critical information and services, while privacy is more often linked to confidentiality. However, the unauthorized exposure of private health information, or corruption of one's personal electronic health record as a result of an identity theft, can put an individual's health and safety at risk.

Risk management is an ongoing, individualized discipline wherein each individual or each organization examines its own threats, vulnerabilities, and valued assets and decides for itself how to deal with identified risks: to reduce or eliminate them, counter them with protective measures, or tolerate them and prepare for the consequences. Risks to personal privacy, patient

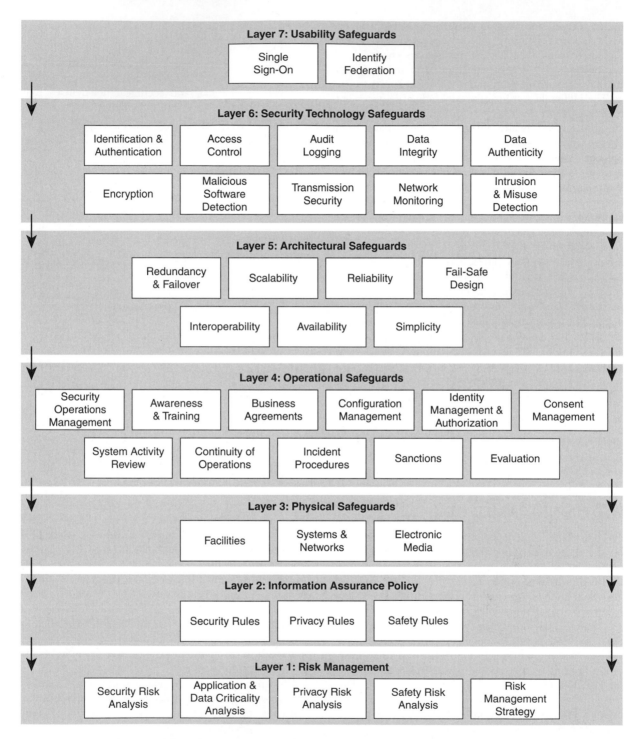

• **FIGURE 17.1.** A framework for achieving and maintaining trustworthiness in health information technology comprises multiple layers of trust, beginning with objective risk assessment that serves as the foundation for information assurance policy, and operational, architectural, and technological safeguards.

safety, care quality, financial stability, and public trust all must be considered in developing an overall strategy for managing risks, both internal and external, to an organization. Resource virtualization, from Internet transmissions to "cloud" computing, present particular challenges because the computing and networking resources used may be outside the physical and operational control of the subscriber.

Layer 2: Information Assurance Policy

The risk management strategy will identify what risks need to be addressed through an information assurance policy governing operations, information technology, and sanctions. The information assurance policy defines rules that guide organizational decision making, define behavioral expectations, and govern individual actions. The policy should define rules for protecting individuals' private information and for providing choice and transparency with respect to how their health information is used and shared. It should include rules that protect human beings, including patients, employees, family members, and visitors, from physical harm that could result from data corruption or service interruption. Overall, the information assurance policy should define the rules needed to protect the organization's valued information assets from identified risks to confidentiality, data integrity, and availability.

Some policy rules will be mandated by applicable state and federal laws and regulations. For example, the HIPAA Security Rule requires compliance with a set of administrative, physical, and technical standards, and the HIPAA Privacy Rule (HHS, 2002) sets forth privacy policies to be implemented. The HITECH Act's privacy and security provisions strengthened and built upon the HIPAA standards. In addition, state and local privacy and security laws will need to be translated into organizational policy rules.

The policy that codifies the nurse's obligation to protect patients' privacy and safety is embodied in the ICN Code of Ethics for Nurses (ICN, 2000):

- The nurse holds in confidence personal information and uses judgment in sharing this information.

- The nurse takes appropriate action to safeguard individuals when their care is endangered by a co-worker or any other person.

The HIT information assurance policy provides the foundation for the development and implementation of physical, operational, architectural, and security technology safeguards. Nursing professionals can provide valuable insights, recommendations, and advocacy in the formulation of information assurance policies within the organizations where they practice, as well as within their professional organizations and for state and federal governments.

Layer 3: Physical Safeguards

Physically safeguarding health information, and the information technology used to collect, store, retrieve, analyze, and exchange that information is essential to ensuring that information needed at the point and time of care is available, trustworthy, and usable in providing quality healthcare. Although the electronic signals that represent health information are not themselves "physical," the facilities within which data are generated, stored, displayed, and used; the media on which data are recorded; the information system hardware used to process, access, and display the data; and the communications equipment used to transmit and route the data are. So are the people who generate, access, and use the information the data represent. Physical safeguards are essential to protecting these assets in accordance with the information assurance policy.

The HIPAA Security Rule prescribes 4 standards for physically safeguarding electronic health information protected under HIPAA: facility access controls, workstation use policies and procedures, workstation security measures, and device and media controls. Physically safeguarding the lives and well-being of patients is central to the roles and responsibilities of nurses. Protecting patients requires the physical protection of the media on which their health data are recorded, as well as the devices, systems, networks, and facilities involved in data collection, use, storage, and disposal.

Layer 4: Operational Safeguards

Operational safeguards are processes, procedures, and practices that govern the creation, handling, usage, and sharing of health information in accordance with the information assurance policy. The HIT trust framework shown in Figure 17.1 includes the following operational safeguards.

Security Operations Management. HIPAA regulations require that each healthcare organization designate a security official and a privacy official to be responsible for developing and implementing security and privacy policies and procedures. The management of services relating to the protection of health information and patient privacy touches every function within a healthcare organization.

Awareness and Training. One of the most valuable actions a healthcare organization can take to maintain public trust is to inculcate a culture of safety, privacy, and security. If every person employed by, or associated with, an organization feels individually responsible for protecting the confidentiality, integrity, and availability of health information, and the privacy and safety of patients, the risk for that organization will be vastly reduced! Recognition of the value of workforce training is reflected in the fact that the HIPAA Security and Privacy Rules require training in security and privacy, respectively, for all members of the workforce. Formal privacy and security training should be required to be completed at least annually, augmented by simple reminders.

Business Agreements. Business agreements help manage risk and bound liability, clarify responsibilities and expectations, and define processes for addressing disputes among parties. The HIPAA Privacy and Security Rules require that each person or organization that provides to a covered entity services involving individually identifiable health information must sign a "business associate" contract obligating the service provider to comply with HIPAA requirements, subject to the same enforcement and sanctions as covered entities. The HIPAA Privacy Rule also requires data use agreements defining how limited data sets will be used. Organizations wishing to exchange health information as part of the Nationwide Health Information Network (NWHIN) Exchange must sign a Data Use and Reciprocal Support Agreement (DURSA) in which they agree to exchange and use message content only in accordance with the agreed upon provisions (NHIN, 2009). Agreements are only as trustworthy as the entities that sign them. Organizations should exercise due diligence in deciding with whom they will enter into business agreements.

Configuration Management. Configuration management refers to processes and procedures for maintaining an accurate and consistent accounting of the physical and functional attributes of a system throughout its life cycle. From an information assurance perspective, configuration management is the process of controlling and documenting modifications to the hardware, firmware, software, and documentation involved in the protection of information assets.

Identity Management and Authorization. Identity management involves the establishment and validation of the identity of each individual or entity with access to system resources; the authorization and assignment of roles, capabilities, and privileges to that identity; the control of accesses related to those entitlements, including the authentication of asserted identity; the termination of identities and authorizations; and the maintenance of the governance processes that support this life cycle. In a healthcare environment, identity management extends to assuring that patients are whom they claim to be—a serious data integrity and patient safety issue. As noted in the previous section, medical identity theft has become a significant risk that identity management processes and procedures must address.

Consent Management. Both federal and state laws, including the HIPAA Privacy Rule, set forth requirements for obtaining an individual's permission before collecting, retaining, or exchanging his personal health information. Certain types of information, such as psychiatric notes and substance abuse records, have special restrictions and authorization requirements. In addition, medical ethics require that providers obtain a patient's informed consent before administering treatment or retaining biological specimens. Managing these permissions, and ensuring that the consumer's privacy preferences are consistently adhered to, is a complex process essential to protecting personal privacy. Today, consent management is primarily a manual process, though standards for electronically representing, exchanging, and enforcing consumer consent directives are emerging.

System Activity Review. One of the most effective means of detecting potential misuse and abuse of privileges is by regularly reviewing records of information system activity, such as audit logs, facility access reports, and security incident tracking reports. Although automated audit review tools exist, they are not widely used in healthcare. Most healthcare organizations rely on either manual review or auto-assisted review (HIMSS, 2009). As EHR systems and exchanges become more prevalent, the volume of audit data that will be generated will rapidly exceed the capacity for human review. Further, the HITECH Act's requirements for maintaining an accounting of disclosures between organizations, and for notifying individuals affected by breaches, will necessitate the use of automated review.

Continuity of Operations. Unexpected events, both natural and human-produced, do happen, and when they do, it is important that critical health services can continue to be provided. As healthcare organizations become increasingly dependent on electronic health information and information systems, the need to plan for unexpected events, and for operational procedures to enable the organization to continue to function, become more urgent. The HIPAA Security Rule requires that organizations establish and implement policies and procedures for responding to an emergency. The first step in planning for contingencies is to identify those software applications and data that are essential for enabling operations to continue under emergency conditions and for returning to full operations. These business-critical systems are those to which architectural safeguards such as fail-safe design, redundancy and failover, and availability engineering should be applied.

Incident Procedures. Awareness and training should include a clear explanation of what an individual should do if she suspects a security incident, such as a malicious code infiltration or denial-of-service attack or a breach of confidential information. Organizations need to plan their response for when an incident is reported, including procedures for investigating and resolving the incident, notifying individuals whose health information may have been exposed as a result of the incident, and penalizing parties responsible for the incident. As noted above, the HITECH Act requires notification of individuals whose information may have been exposed as a result of a breach.

Sanctions. The HIPAA law (USC, 1996) and the HITECH Act prescribe severe civil and criminal penalties for sanctioning entities that fail to comply with the privacy and security provisions. Organizations must implement appropriate sanctions to penalize workforce members who fail to comply with privacy and security policies and procedures.

Evaluation. Periodic, objective evaluation of the operational and technical safeguards in place helps measure the outcomes of the security management program. A formal evaluation should be conducted at least annually and should involve independent participants who are not responsible for the program. Independent evaluators can be from within or from outside an organization, so long as they can be objective. In addition to the annual programmed evaluation, security technology safeguards should be evaluated whenever changes in circumstances or events occur that affect the risk profile of the organization.

Layer 5: Architectural Safeguards

A system's architecture comprises its individual hardware and software components, their relationships among each other and with the environment, and the principles that govern the system's design and evolution

over time. As shown in Figure 17.1, specific architectural design principles, and the hardware and software components that support those principles, establish the technical foundation for security technology safeguards. These design principles are discussed below.

Redundancy and Failover. Security- and safety-critical system components should be integrated such that no single point of failure exists. If a given component fails, the system should engage a second, backup component with no breach of sensitive information or corruption of data.

Scalability. As more health information is recorded, stored, used, and exchanged electronically, systems and networks must be able to deal with that growth. The catastrophic failure at CareGroup, discussed earlier, resulted from the network's inability to scale to the capacity required. The latest stage in the evolution of the Internet specifically addresses the scalability issue by virtualizing computing resources into services, including software as a service (SaaS), platforms as a service (PaaS), and infrastructure as a service (IaaS); these are collectively referred to as *cloud* services. Indeed, the Internet itself was created on the same principle as cloud computing—the creation of a virtual, ubiquitous, continuously expanding network through the sharing of resources (servers) owned by different entities. Whenever one sends information over the Internet, the information is broken into small packets that are then sent from source to destination via a series of "hops" between servers, some or all of which probably belong to someone other than the sender or the receiver. Cloud computing, a model for providing on-demand computing services accessible over the Internet, pushes virtualization to a new level through the sharing of applications, storage, and computing power, to offer scalability beyond what would be economically possible otherwise.

Reliability. Reliability is the ability of a system or component to perform its specified functions consistently, over a specified period of time—an essential attribute of trustworthiness.

Fail-Safe Design. Safety-critical components, software, and systems should be designed such that if they fail, the failure will not cause people to be physically harmed. Note that fail-safe design may indicate that, under certain circumstances, a component should be shut down, or forced to violate its functional specification, to avoid harming someone. So the interrelationships among redundancy and failover, reliability, and fail-safe design are complex, yet critical to patient safety. The "break-the-glass" feature that enables an unauthorized user to gain access to patient information in an emergency situation is an example of fail-safe design. If, in an emergency, an EHR system fails to provide a nurse access to the clinical information he needs to deliver care, the break-the-glass feature will enable the system to "fail" safely and provide the access required. Fail-safe methods are particularly important in research where new treatment protocols and devices are being tested for safety.

Interoperability. Interoperability is the ability of systems and system components to work together. To effectively exchange health information requires that healthcare systems interoperate not only at the technical level, but also at the syntactic and semantic levels. The Internet and its protocols, which have been adopted for use within enterprises as well, transmit data (packets of electronic bits) over a network such that they arrive at their destination the same as when they were sent. But then, the receiving system must be able to decrypt encrypted data, open electronic messages, extract content, and translate the bits into health information that its applications and users will understand. Open standards, including encryption and messaging standards, and standard vocabulary for coding and exchanging security attributes and permissions (e.g., Security Assertion Markup Language [SAML], eXtensible Access Control Markup Language [XACML]), are fundamental to implementing interoperable healthcare systems.

Availability. Required services and information must be available and usable when they are needed. Availability is measured as the proportion of time a system is in a functioning condition. A reciprocal dependency exists between security technology safeguards and high-availability design: security safeguards depend upon the availability of systems, networks, and information to enable those safeguards to protect enterprise assets against threats to availability, such as denial-of-service attacks. Resource virtualization and cloud computing are important technologies for helping ensure availability.

Simplicity. Safe, secure architectures are designed to minimize complexity. The simplest design and integration strategy will be the easiest to understand, to maintain, and to recover in the case of a failure or disaster.

Layer 6: Security Technology Safeguards

Security technology safeguards are software and hardware services specifically designed to perform security-related functions. All of the security services depicted in Figure 17.1 are technical safeguards required by the HIPAA Security Rule. Table 17.2 identifies a number of open standards that are used to implement these functions

Identification and Authentication. The identity of all entities, whether people or software applications, must be clearly established before they are allowed to access protected systems, applications, and data. Identity management and authorization processes are used to validate identities and to assign them system rights and privileges. Then, whenever the person or application requires access, it asserts an identity and authenticates that identity by providing some proof in the form of something it has (e.g., smartcard), something it knows (e.g., password, private encryption key), or something it is (e.g., fingerprint). While only people can authenticate themselves using biometrics, both people and software applications can authenticate themselves using public-private key exchanges.

Access Control. Access control services help ensure that people, computer systems, and software applications are able to use all of and only those resources (e.g., computers, networks, applications, services, data files, information) that they are authorized to use and only within the constraints of the authorization. Access controls protect against unauthorized use, disclosure, modification, and destruction of resources and unauthorized execution of system functions. Access-control rules are based on federal and state laws and regulations, the enterprise's information assurance policy, as well as consumer-elected preferences. These rules may be based on the user's identity, the user's role, the context of the request (e.g., location, time of day), and/or a combination of the sensitivity attributes of the data and the user's authorizations.

Audit Logging. Security auditing is the process of collecting and recording information about security-relevant events. Audit logs are generated by multiple software components within a system, including operating systems, servers, firewalls, applications, and database management systems. Many healthcare organizations rely heavily on audit log reviews to detect potential intrusions and misuse.

Data Integrity. Data integrity services provide assurance that electronic data have not been modified or destroyed except as authorized. Cryptographic hash functions are commonly used for this purpose. A cryptographic hash

TABLE 17.2	Many Open Standards Address Security Technology Safeguards	
Safeguard	**Standard**	**Description**
Identification and authentication	ITU-T X.509: Information Technology— Open Systems Interconnection—The Directory: Public-key and attribute certificate frameworks	Standard for public key infrastructure (PKI), single sign-on, and privilege management infrastructure; includes standard formats for public-key certificates, certificate revocation lists, attribute certificates, and a certification path-validation algorithm
	OASIS Security Assertion Markup Language (SAML)	XML-based protocol for exchanging authentication and authorization data (assertions) between an identity provider and a service provider; used to enable single sign-on
Access control	ANSI/INCITS 359-2004: Information Technology – Role Based Access Control (RBAC)	Specifies RBAC elements (users, roles, permissions, operations, objects) and features required by an RBAC system
	HL7 Version 3 Confidentiality Code System 2.16.840.1.113883.5.25	HL7 V3 value set for coding confidentiality attributes
	HL7 V3 Version 3 Role Based Access Control (RBAC) Healthcare Permission Catalog	Permission vocabulary to support RBAC, consistent with OASIS XACML and ANSI INCITS RBAC standards
	OASIS eXtensible Access Control Markup Language (XACML)	XML-based language for expressing information technology security policy
Audit logging	ASTM E-2147-01: Standard Specification for Audit and Disclosure Logs for Use in Health Information Systems	Specifies how to design audit logs to record accesses within a computer system, and disclosure logs to document disclosures to external users
Data integrity	FIPS PUB 180-3 Secure Hash Standard (SHS).	Specifies 5 hash algorithms that can be used to generate message digests used to detect whether messages have been changed since the digests were generated
Data authenticity (nonrepudiation)	ASTM E-1762-95(2003): Standard Guide for Electronic Authentication of Healthcare Information	Standard on the design, implementation, and use of electronic signatures to authenticate healthcare data
	ETSI TS 101 903: XML Advanced Electronic Signatures (XadES)	Defines XML formats for advanced electronic signatures, based on the use of public key cryptography supported by public key certificates
Encryption (confidentiality)	FIPS 197, Advanced Encryption Standard, Nov 2001	Specifies a symmetric cryptographic algorithm that can be used to protect electronic data
Transmission security	IETF Transport Layer Security (TLS) Protocol: RFC 2246, RFC 3546	Standard for establishing secured channel at layer 4 (transport) of the Open Systems Interconnection model; includes authentication of sender and receiver, and encryption and integrity protection of the communication channel
	IETF IP Security Protocol (ipsec): RFCs listed at datatracker.ietf.org/wg/ipsec	Standard for establishing virtual private network (VPN) at layer 3 (network) of the OSI model; includes authentication of sender and receiver, and encryption and integrity protection of the communication channel
	IETF Secure/Multipurpose Internet Mail Extensions (S/MIME): RFC 2633	Internet mail protocol for providing authentication, message integrity and nonrepudiation of origin (digital signatures), and confidentiality protection (encryption)

(continued)

TABLE 17.2	Many Open Standards Address Security Technology Safeguards. *(continued)*	
Safeguard	**Standard**	**Description**
	OASIS WS-Security (WSS)	Extension to the Simple Object Access Protocol (SOAP) transport protocol used to access Web services; includes encryption and digital signing of messages, and exchange of security tokens, including SAML assertions

ANSI, American National Standards Institute; ASTM, ASTM International (originally American Society for Testing and Materials); ETSI, European Telecommunications Standards Institute; FIPS, National Institute of Standards and Technology (NIST) Federal Information Processing Standard; HL7, Health Level Seven; IETF, Internet Engineering Task Force; INCITS, InterNational Committee for Information Technology Standards; ITU-T, International Telecommunication Union—Telecommunication Standardization Sector; OASIS, Organization for the Advancement of Structured Information Standards

function is a mathematical algorithm that uses a block of data as input to generate a "hash value" such that any change to the data will change the hash value that represents it.

Data Authenticity. Sometimes the need arises to ensure not only that data have not been modified inappropriately, but that the data are in fact from an authentic source. This need, sometimes referred to as *nonrepudiation*, can be met through the use of digital signatures. Digital signatures use public-key (assymetric) encryption (see Encryption later in this section) to encrypt a block of data using the signer's private key. To authenticate that the data block was signed by the entity claimed, one only needs to try decrypting the data using the signer's public key; if the data block decrypts successfully, its authenticity is assured.

Encryption. Encryption is simply the process of obfuscating information by running the data representing it through an algorithm (sometimes called a *cipher*), such that the information is unreadable until the data are decrypted by someone possessing the proper encryption key. *Symmetric* encryption uses the same key to both encrypt and decrypt data, while *asymmetric* encryption (also known as *public-key encryption*) uses two keys that are mathematically related such that one key is used for encryption and the other for decryption. One key is called a private key and is held secret; the other is called a public key and is openly published. Which key is used for encryption and which for decryption depends upon the assurance objective. For example, secure e-mail encrypts the message contents using the recipient's public key (so that only the recipient can decrypt and view it) and then digitally signs the message using the sender's own private key (so that if the sender's public

key will decrypt it, the recipient will be assured that the sender actually sent it).

Malicious Software Protection. Malicious software, also called *malware*, is any software program designed to infiltrate a system without the user's permission, with the intent to damage or disrupt operations, or to use resources to which the developer is not authorized. Malicious software includes programs commonly called viruses, worms, Trojan Horses, and spyware. Protecting against malicious software requires not only technical solutions to prevent, detect, and remove these intruders, but also policies and procedures for reporting suspected attacks.

Transmission Security. Sensitive and safety-critical electronic data that are transmitted over vulnerable networks must be protected against unauthorized disclosure and modification. For example, the Internet protocol provides no protection against the disclosure or modification of any transmissions, and no assurance of the identity of any transmitters or receivers (or eavesdroppers). Protecting network transmissions between two entities (people, organizations, or software programs) requires that the communicating entities authenticate themselves to each other, confirm data integrity using something like a cryptographic hash function, and encrypt the channel over which data are to be exchanged.

Both the Transport Layer Security (TLS) protocol (IETF, 2008) and Internet Protocol security (IPsec) protocol suite (IETF, 1998) support these functions, except at different layers in the Open System Interconnection model (ISO, 1996). TLS establishes protected channels at the Open System Interconnection transport layer (layer 4), allowing software applications to exchange information securely. For example, TLS might be used to establish a secure link between a user's browser and a merchant's "check out" application on the Web. IPsec establishes protected channels at the Open System Interconnection network layer (layer 3), allowing Internet gateways to exchange information securely. For example, IPsec might be used to establish a virtual private network (VPN) that allows all hospitals within an integrated delivery system to openly exchange information securely. Because IPsec is implemented at the network layer, it is less vulnerable to malicious software applications than TLS and also less visible to users (for example, IPsec does not display an icon in a browser).

Network Monitoring. Network monitoring tools continuously monitor computer networks to detect slow or failing components, or bottlenecks in the network, that could indicate an impending or actual service outage. Network monitoring tools can detect problems caused by overloaded or crashed servers, network connections, or other devices connected to the network, and can alert system administrators when they need to take action.

Intrusion and Misuse Detection. Intrusion and misuse detection tools use information from network monitoring logs, system audit logs, application audit logs, and database audit logs to detect undesirable behavior. The principal difference between the two is that intrusion-detection tools attempt to detect intrusions originating from outside the enterprise, and misuse detection tools target undesirable behavior within an organization. While intruders are almost always unauthorized to access the resources they are attempting to obtain, misusers may be "authorized" users who are inappropriately using their authorizations.

Layer 7: Usability Features

The top layer of the trust framework includes services that make life easier for users. *Single sign-on* often is referred to as a security service when in fact it is a usability service that makes authentication services more palatable. Both single sign-on and identity federation enable a user to authenticate herself once and then to access multiple applications, multiple databases, and even multiple enterprises for which she is authorized, without having to reauthenticate herself. Single sign-on enables a user to navigate among authorized applications and resources within a single organization. Identity federation enables a user to navigate between services managed by different organizations. Both single sign-on and identity federation require the exchange of *security assertions*. Once the user has logged into a system, that system can pass the user's identity, along with other attributes, such as role, method of authentication, and time of login, to another entity using a security assertion. The receiving entity then enforces its own access control rules, based on the identity passed to it.

Neither single sign-on nor identity federation actually adds security protections other than to reduce the need for users to post their passwords to their computer monitors. In fact, if the original authentication method is weak, the risk associated with that weakness will be propagated to any other entities to which the identity is passed. Therefore, whenever single sign-on or federated identity is implemented, a key consideration is the strength of the method used to authenticate the individual whose identity will be passed on to others.

SUMMARY AND CONCLUSIONS

Healthcare is in the midst of a dramatic and exciting transformation that will enable individual health information to be captured, used, and exchanged electronically using interoperable HIT. The potential impacts on individuals' health and on the health of entire populations are dramatic. Outcomes-based decision support will help improve the safety and quality of healthcare. The availability of huge quantities of de-identified health information will help scientists discover the underlying genetic bases for diseases, leading to earlier and more accurate detection and diagnoses, more targeted and effective treatments, and ultimately personalized medicine.

In this chapter we have explained the critical role that trustworthiness plays in HIT adoption and in providing safe, private, high-quality care. We have introduced and described a trust framework comprising 7 layers of protection essential for establishing and maintaining trust in a healthcare enterprise. Many of the safeguards included in the trust framework have been codified in HIPAA standards and implementation specifications. Building trustworthiness in HIT always begins with objective risk assessment, a continuous process that serves as the basis for developing and implementing a sound information assurance policy and physical, operational, architectural, and technological safeguards to mitigate and manage risks to patient safety, individual privacy, care quality, financial stability, and public trust.

REFERENCES

American Nurses Association (ANA). (2001). *Code of Ethics for Nurses with Interpretive Statements*. Silver Spring, MD: Nursesbooks.org.

Berinato, S. (2003). All systems down. *CIO* (pp. 46–53).

Blumenthal, D. (2009). Launching HITECH. *The New England Journal of Medicine*. December 31, 2009.

Cohen, B (2009). NHS hit by a different sort of virus. Channel 4 News. July 9, 2009. Retrieved from http://www.channel4.com/news/articles/science_technology/nhs+hit+by+a+different+sort+of+virus/3256957.

Department of Health and Human Services (HHS). (2002). Health insurance reform: Standards for privacy of individually identifiable health information: final rule. 45 CFR Parts 160 and 164. *Federal Register*, December 28, 2000; amended August 14, 2002.

Department of Health and Human Services (HHS). (2003). Health insurance reform: Security standards, final rule. 45 CFR Parts 160, 162, and 164. *Federal Register*. February 20, 2003.

Department of Health and Human Services (HHS). (2010). Health information privacy: Breaches affecting 500 or more individuals. Retrieved from http://www.hhs.gov/ocr/privacy/hipaa/administrative/breachnotificationrule/postedbreaches.html.

Department of Health, Education, and Welfare (DHEW). (1973, July). Records, computers and the rights of citizens: Report of the Secretary's Advisory Committee on Automated Personal Data Systems. Retrieved from http://aspe.hhs.gov/DATACNCL/1973privacy/tocprefacemembers.htm.

Goodin, D. (2010, April 23). NHS computers hit by voracious, data-stealing worm. *The Register*. Retrieved from http://www.theregister.co.uk/2010/04/23/nhs_worm_infection.

Healthcare Information and Management Systems Society (HIMSS). (2009, November 3). 2009 HIMSS Security Survey.

International Council of Nurses (ICN). (2000). *The ICN Code of Ethics for Nurses*. Geneva: International Council of Nurses.

International Organization for Standardization (ISO). (1996). Information technology – open systems interconnection – basic reference model: The basic model. ISO/IEC 7498-1. Second Edition, 1994-11-15. Corrected and reprinted, 1996-06-15. Retrieved from http://standards.iso.org/ittf/licence.html.

Internet Engineering Task Force (IETF). (1998). Security architecture for the internet protocol. RFC 2401. November, 1998. Retrieved from http://www.ietf.org/rfc/rfc2401.txt.

Internet Engineering Task Force (IETF). (2008). The transport layer security (TLS) protocol. Version 1.2. RFC 5246. August, 2008. Retrieved from http://tools.ietf.org/html/rfc5246.

Markle Foundation Connecting for Health (Markle). (2006). *The Common Framework: Overview and Principles*. New York: The Markle Foundation.

NHIN Cooperative DURSA Team (NHIN). (2009, November 18). Nationwide Health Information Network (NHIN) Data Use and Reciprocal Support Agreement (DURSA). Retrieved from http://healthit.hhs.gov/portal/server.pt/document/910070/dursa_2009_versionforproductionpilots_20091123_pdf.

Office of the National Coordinator for Health Information Technology, U.S. Department of Health and Human Services (ONC). (2008, December 15). *Nationwide Privacy and Security Framework for Electronic Exchange of Individually Identifiable Health Information*. Retrieved from http://healthit.hhs.gov/portal/server.pt/gateway/PTARGS_0_10731_848088_0_0_18/NationwidePS_Framework-5.pdf.

Rys, R. (2008, March 13). The imposter in the ER: medical identity theft can leave you with hazardous errors in health records. msnbc.com. Retrieved from http://www.msnbc.msn.com/id/23392229/ns/health-health_care

Tobin, D. (2010, April 21). University Hospital computers plagued by anti-virus glitch. *The Post Standard*. Retrieved from http://www.syracuse.com/news/index.ssf/2010/04/university_hospital_plagued_by.html.

United States Attorney's Office, Southern District of Florida (USA-FL). (2008, April 1) Miami-Dade DME and clinic owners indicted for using stolen patient information in multi-million dollar medicare fraud scheme. (Press Release). Retrieved from http://miami.fbi.gov/dojpressrel/pressrel08/mm20080401.htm.

United States Congress, 104th Session (USC). (1996, August 21). Health Insurance Portability and Accountability Act of 1996. Public Law 104-191.

United States Congress (USC). (2009, February 17). American Recovery and Reinvestment Act of 2009 (ARRA). H.R. 1. Retrieved from http://frwebgate.access.gpo.gov/cgi-bin/getdoc.cgi?dbname=111_cong_bills&docid=f:h1enr.pdf.

18

Shaping Nursing Informatics Through the Public Policy Process

Amy M. Walker

• OBJECTIVES

1. Examine the critical pathways to public healthcare policy, public health policy, and healthcare and nursing informatics policy.
2. Define the policy process.
3. Analyze the skills informaticists must possess in order to effectively communicate with policy makers and those in positions to sway policy makers.
4. Explores how nursing informaticists at all levels can and do impact public healthcare policy, public health policy, and informatics policy.
5. Explain how education for nurses is changing to focus more on technology.
6. Encourage the profession to coordinate, educate, and consolidate roles in policy formulation to support our roles in quality, safety and patient advocacy.

• KEY WORDS

nursing informatics
public healthcare policy
public health policy
healthcare and nursing informatics policy
politics in healthcare

INTRODUCTION

Public healthcare policy helps determine standards of care, data metrics, as well as care and documentation processes. As such, public healthcare policy also guides equipment features, functionality, and systems selection. Although nursing informatics (NI) has had a role in shaping public informatics policy, it has not played a large enough part in shaping public healthcare policy and public health policy. In this era of the U.S. Health Information Technology for Economic and Clinical Health (HITECH) Act, it is especially critical for the NI community to understand public healthcare policy drivers and how to deliver a unified message to those who create public healthcare policy. This will not happen by chance; carefully crafted strategy and collaboration needs to occur now. Those who will lead the efforts to ensure that NI public policy issues are heard need education, advisement, competencies, and support. This paper examines the critical pathways to public healthcare policy, public health policy, and NI policy including an analysis of the skills informaticists must possess in order to effectively communicate with policy makers and those in positions to sway policy makers.

This paper explores how nursing informaticists at all levels can and do impact public policy. It provides an overview explaining how education for nurses is changing to focus more on technology, and a case is made for expanding this focus to the skills required for the NI community to educate, advocate, and collaborate with those outside of nursing—even those outside the care environment—to ensure technologies and processes advance with both the patient and the nurse in mind. In this chapter, 3 domains of policy will be described: public healthcare policy, public health policy, and healthcare and NI policy. Public healthcare policy will be described from the perspective of those national organizations and structures that work on the healthcare reform bills, Medicare and Medicaid reimbursement, provider shortages, and professional education. Public health policy will be described from the organizations that support the growth and staffing to conduct epidemiology and prevention in public health. Healthcare and NI policy will be developed from the perspectives of the organizations and missions supporting healthcare informatics policy.

CRITICAL PATHWAYS TO PUBLIC HEALTHCARE POLICY

Collaboration at the public healthcare policy level impacts the future of nursing and care delivery while setting expectations for standards of care that nurses are responsible for advancing at the most salient level. With over 3.1 million nurses in the United States alone, nurses are the apparatus for implementation of public healthcare policy (HRSA, 2010).

The extent to which nurses contributed to the Patient Protection and Affordable Care Act (PPACA) is nearly impossible to comprehend. The American Nurses Association (ANA) created *Healthcare Reform: Key Provisions Related to Nursing* and the American Association of Colleges of Nursing (AACN) created *Healthcare Reform Review: Nursing Education and Practice Provisions*, each of which is a chart outlining how the law supports continued nurse education and all sectors of the nursing workforce (American Nurses Association, 2010; American Association of Colleges of Nurses, 2010). These charts also explain how PPACA addresses the nursing shortage (especially as related to skilled nursing), quality improvement, best practices, and public health initiatives (Center to Champion Nursing in America, 2010). You can be sure that nurses and organizations such as the ANA and the AACN contributed at a high level to bring about these provisions. While impressive,

nursing's participation to engineer these changes is only one aspect of the role played in creating PPACA. Nurses are involved in numerous other initiatives related to improving the quality and delivery of care.

Policy changes can occur on the micro or macro levels. On the micro level, changes transpire within an organization (operational or process) or within the construct of a clinical information system. Public healthcare policy occurs on the macro level, where there is greater diversification among stakeholders and where policies have far greater range and impact. During the Institute of Medicine's (IOM's) Forum on the Future of Nursing, Selecky noted, "Public health cannot be separated from politics…as demonstrated by the term 'public'" (Institute of Medicine, 2010, p. 10). The New Jersey Collaborating Center for Nursing appears to agree. While noting the nursing profession's "long history of shaping public and health policy", the organization provides the best, most succinct definition of health policy and public policy that is available (New Jersey Collaborating Center for Nursing, n.d.):

> …health policy is a course of action that influences healthcare decisions (www.aacn.org). Public policy refers to policy that is generated by governmental agencies and enacted through legislation. Public policy is made on behalf of the public and is influenced by factors such as economics, social issues, research, and technology. Health policy influences decisions about the health of a society. Similar to public policy, health policy is also influenced by factors such as health status of the citizenry, research, and economics.

While PPACA is just beginning to take effect in some areas, most of the law's provisions will continue to change the course of healthcare for at least the next 5 to 10 years. The overall impact of the changes set forth in PPACA will undoubtedly alter the way care is delivered and received, as well as the ways in which nurses are educated, retained, and supported in perpetuity.

CRITICAL PATHWAYS TO HEALTHCARE AND NURSING INFORMATICS POLICY

Nurses have led several initiatives throughout the United States and beyond that are widely recognized as unquestionable successes. These initiatives include vaccination campaigns (Institute of Medicine, 2010, p. 7), AIDS prevention and awareness, infection control, and disaster response mobilization (Robert Wood Johnson Foundation, 2008).

The increasingly important role of nurses in the creation and execution of public health policy cannot be overlooked. Summarizing nursing's role in the development of public policy as discussed by Mary Selecky at the 2009 Forum on the Future of Nursing, the IOM writes, "Nurses need to understand their role in the development and implementation of public policies that impact health. They also need to inform public policy with science and evidence-based facts and be ethical, professional and collaborative" (Institute of Medicine, 2010, p. 11). The most important insight resulting from this forum is quite possibly that "[p]ublic health leaders and nurses need to provide *a buffer* and *a bridge* between the political world and the health world" [emphasis added] (Institute of Medicine, 2010, p. 11).

Providing that NI leaders have successfully convinced counterparts in the socioeconomic-political realm to align with their cause, collaboration with these entities often becomes crucial. This political strategizing requires more than just ensuring that clinical information systems adequately support documentation and knowledge sharing, both of which require collaboration for design and implementation. It also includes ensuring that the right people have the right knowledge when it comes to policy formation on federal, state, and local levels. The Robert Wood Johnson Foundation explains (Robert Wood Johnson Foundation, 2008):

> As the public health mandate expands in the face of 21st-century challenges, the visibility of nurse policymakers will likely increase. Their expertise in prevention and health promotion and their experience in delivering care have become valued assets, positioning them to play major roles in developing effective policies for assuring the public's health. (p. 2)

Additionally, and separately from the funding noted above, section 5314 of PPACA authorizes the Secretary to (Public Health Institute, 2010):

> Expand existing CDC public health training fellowships in epidemiology, laboratory science and *informatics*, the Epidemic Intelligence Service (EIS), and other related training programs. For each of fiscal years 2010 through 2013, $24.5 million is authorized for EIS fellowships and $5 million each for epidemiology, laboratory and informatics fellowships *[emphasis added]*. (p. 4)

To be clear, PPACA takes no action to expressly support or fund NI; however, achieving the goals of the Healthcare Reform Bill that relate to health information technology (HIT) would be difficult, or even impossible, if NI is not included as part of the equation.

Opportunities for improving awareness of informatics, enhancing HIT skill levels, and better positioning NI within healthcare policy will increase simply by virtue of the "follow-the-money" principle.

As one might anticipate, nursing is also widely influential within state and local policy initiatives. The Robert Wood Johnson Foundation does a wonderful job characterizing "policies that can transform patient care" in its *Chartering Nursing's Future* publication. Their studies include topics such as the contribution of nursing to HIT (March 2009), and an analysis of executive positions in public health nursing with a discussion of the policies that support public health nursing (September 2008). There are also case studies examining specific, state-by-state health policies and outcomes. Where, but through health informatics, would the data to support claims-related public health come from?

THE IMPACT OF NURSING INFORMATICISTS ON HEALTHCARE INFORMATICS AND NURSING INFORMATICS POLICY

Nursing informatics is defined by the ANA (2010) as an applied science that:

> ...integrates nursing science, computer science, and informatics science to manage and communicate data, information and knowledge in nursing practice. Nursing informatics facilitates the integration of data, information, knowledge, and wisdom to support patients, nurses, and other providers in their decision-making in all roles, and setting. This support is accomplished through the use of information structures, information processes, and information technology. (p17)

The promotion of standardization and knowledge sharing through NI has played a critical role in the establishment of public healthcare policy, healthcare and NI policy, and the creation of healthcare delivery standards (Ozbolt & Saba, 2008). Over the last decade, the NI community has made healthcare reform a necessary and obtainable goal, utilizing the same framework for interdisciplinary collaboration, standards development, and migration success that has fostered significant achievements in other nursing-related competencies. At the core of these achievements is the informatics nurse's ability to recognize opportunities for improvement; communicate need in actionable terms to various stakeholders; and collaborate with others, both internally and externally, to produce favorable outcomes.

It is in these areas that informatics nurses play an exceedingly crucial role. All nurses are, by definition, concerned with patient health and information related to patient health; however, informatics nurses, with their unique ability for using technology to enhance communication, documentation and reporting, have carved out a special niche in healthcare. Kaminski (2007) notes that "Nursing informatics is advanced by exploring the ways that nurses are shaping and contributing to the virtual environment—as professionals, peers, disseminators of health information and client education, researchers, advocates and activists." With these unique skills come indisputable responsibilities, such as advocating, leadership, engaging stakeholders, and collaborating with others, including those outside the discipline of nursing, to develop and implement practical solutions.

The leading organizations impacting healthcare informatics and NI policy are The Alliance for Nursing Informatics (ANI) in coordination with the American Medical Informatics Association (AMIA) and the Healthcare Information and Management Systems Society (HIMSS).

In many cases, professional organizations like the AMIA can legitimize claims made by those in NI leadership positions by accepting their recommendations. These organizations network with other professional organizations, as well as professional lobbyists, to promote the causes of nursing informatics and effective care delivery. Some of these organizations, like the AMIA, are lobbyists themselves (American Medical Informatics Association, n.d.):

> AMIA is committed to building a greater awareness and federal government investment in biomedical and health informatics education, practice, and research...Informatics is key to achieving these objective[s]. Through education of policy-makers, legislative action and grassroots activity, we know it is possible to strengthen and expand recognition and funding for biomedical and health informatics education, practice, and research.

The AMIA also details many of the avenues they, along with others, use to promote policy change. These approaches include creating panels and committees, with or without the cooperation of other organizations, to discuss policies and creating white papers expounding how informatics can effectively resolve certain healthcare delivery issues. These professional organizations also provide experts to educate and make recommendations to policy makers and testify to the impact of certain policies on healthcare (American Medical Informatics Association, n.d.). At

the very least, the goal is to keep moving the issue higher and higher up the chain of command until it gets the attention required for action and a solution is implemented.

The HIMSS has a national advocacy office. In addition to a nursing section, the association is also engaged with the AMIA and other organizations in coordinating nursing organizations focused on advocacy in informatics. The ANI is a collaboration of organizations that enables a unified voice for the NI community to engage in issues in the public healthcare policy process; information technology standards; information systems design, implementation and evaluation; and shared communication and networking opportunities (McCormick, Sensmeier, Delaney, & Bickford, 2010). It includes over 25 nursing organizations across academia, practice, vendor industries, and nursing specialties. HIMSS Analytics, a subsidiary of the HIMSS, conducts surveys on the numbers of nurses and the impact of nurses in informatics.

The HIMSS 2009 Informatics Nurse Impact Survey revealed that though "informatics nurses are involved in a wide variety of job responsibilities relating to IT," informatics nurses enjoy distinction in 3 specific clinical areas: patient safety, workflow analysis, and user education and acceptance (HIMSS Nursing Informatics, 2009). The survey also indicated that organizations rely on informatics nurses for input on medical device integration, patient medication administration, and clinical and quality reporting. Further, this survey confirms that informatics nurses have roles outside the patient care environment; many vendors employ informatics nurses to aid system integration, workflow analysis, end-user education, and overall system buy-in.

Beyond the clinical setting, nurses impact public healthcare policy creation and execution. Though nursing's contribution to PPACA has already been addressed, there are a number of examples of NI's influence on the Healthcare Reform Bill that have not yet been discussed. This includes standardization among healthcare reporting and documentation methods to support Medicare payments and reimbursement (Raths, 2010, p. 36). Informaticists will be directly responsible for implementing many of the provisions of the HITECH Act, even without direct guidelines, protocols, or available systems. This will require process and data knowledge as well as innovation.

In an online article of *The New England Journal of Medicine*, National Coordinator for Health IT, David Blumenthal, MD (2010), described the provisions of the HITECH Act. While not explicitly

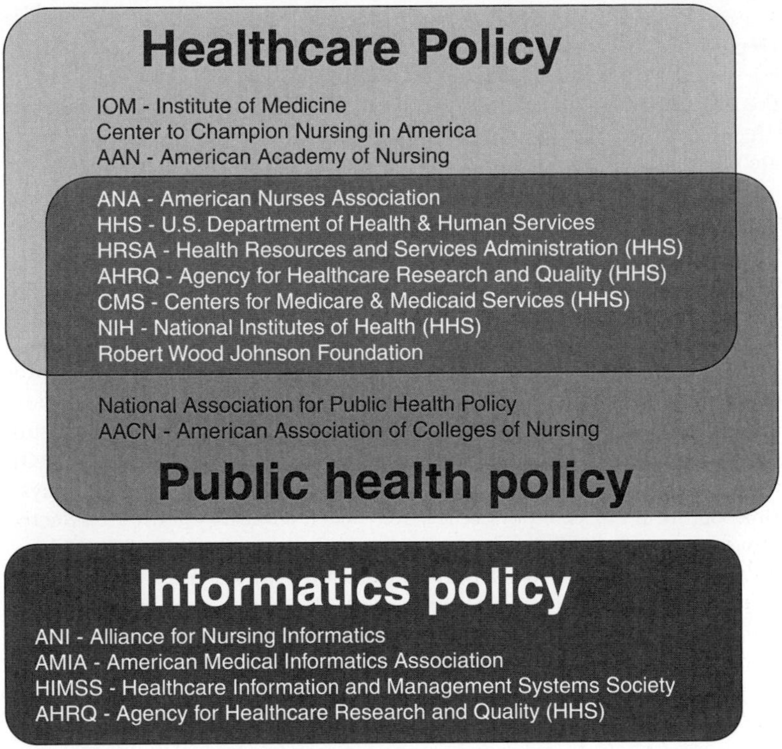

Healthcare Policy

IOM - Institute of Medicine
Center to Champion Nursing in America
AAN - American Academy of Nursing

ANA - American Nurses Association
HHS - U.S. Department of Health & Human Services
HRSA - Health Resources and Services Administration (HHS)
AHRQ - Agency for Healthcare Research and Quality (HHS)
CMS - Centers for Medicare & Medicaid Services (HHS)
NIH - National Institutes of Health (HHS)
Robert Wood Johnson Foundation

National Association for Public Health Policy
AACN - American Association of Colleges of Nursing

Public health policy

Informatics policy

ANI - Alliance for Nursing Informatics
AMIA - American Medical Informatics Association
HIMSS - Healthcare Information and Management Systems Society
AHRQ - Agency for Healthcare Research and Quality (HHS)

• **FIGURE 18.1.** Organizations that influence healthcare, public health, and informatics policy.

stated, each of the new regulations—meaningful use, certification, and regulation of certification and criteria standard—required input from informaticists. Going forward, informaticists will be responsible for supporting these provisions on the ground and providing the data to support meaningful use and certification criteria. Of the 8 new programs created by the HITECH Act (U.S. Department of Health & Human Services, 2010), 7 clearly fall in the NI realm for proper execution and/or support of the program's objectives. These include the following: regional extension centers, health information exchange, workforce training programs, strategic HIT advanced research pprojects (SHARP), the Nationwide Health Information Network (NHIN), the Beacon Community Program, and standards and certification.

To assuage any doubt about the expanding influence of NI in the healthcare arena, Blumenthal (2010) estimates that implementing the provisions of the HITECH Act will require 50,000 new, highly-skilled employees (Dombrowski & Kaye, 2010). Recognizing

that healthcare already suffers from a nursing shortage exacerbated by a lack of qualified faculty (Institute of Medicine, 2010, p. 8), the Obama administration is set to infuse $124 million from the Office of the National Coordinator (ONC) into training programs for HIT (Dombrowski & Kaye, 2010). Funds allotted from other governmental entities also focus on nursing education initiatives. The National Institutes of Health (NIH), for example, recently awarded 2 grants totaling just under $4 million to the Duke Center for Health Informatics (Bonnett, 2010), which combines Duke's Schools of Medicine and Nursing, the Pratt School of Engineering, and the Fuqua School of Business to "train the next generation of doctors, nurses and healthcare administrators in implementing and managing electronic medical record systems to improve patient care." The grants fund 2 programs: Curriculum Development Centers, and Consortia for University-Based Training of Health IT Professionals in Healthcare. Figure 18.1 describes the organizations that influence healthcare, public health, and informatics policy.

THE PUBLIC HEALTHCARE POLICY DEVELOPMENT PROCESS

So how do the ideas that originated at the grassroots, clinical practice level become laws? While the exact process varies from state to state and from state to national levels, if the right people and organizations have been engaged, the nursing informaticist's recommended best practices are sponsored by a legislator and introduced in a bill. From here, the bill goes to committee and experts from various groups that the committee anticipates will be impacted by the bill are asked to provide their reasons for supporting or opposing the bill. The committee may also seek recommendations for modification. Eventually, this bill goes to the floor where the House will vote on whether to approve it. If the bill isn't passed, it will either be dropped, sent back to the committee for modification, or sit for a time before it is reintroduced. If and when the bill is passed in one House, the bill is sent to the other House where this process is repeated. This is why it is ideal to have both chambers introduce the same bill, known as a companion bill. When both Houses agree on a bill, it is sent to the highest-ranking official in the state (i.e., Governor or President). The President or Governor then either signs the bill into law or employs veto power to prohibit passage of the bill. If the bill is vetoed, it needs to be reintroduced in one of the Houses before any lawmaking activities resume.

While this process may read easily on paper, there are many factors that impact the bill's viability in Congress, such as the number of Congressional co-sponsors supporting the bill, the level of support from constituents and national organizations, and the current political agenda. On average, it can take 7 to 8 years for legislation to pass if it is not on the national agenda. Although there are no guarantees; some bills based on the national agenda are never even reported out of committee. For these reasons, it is important that nurses understand the politics and policy of the issues they are working with to create change. They must work closely with experts in the field, in addition to political strategy and advocacy experts, to move an issue forward.

Skills Informaticists Need to Communicate with Policy Makers

It seems that advocating on behalf of others would be self-explanatory and intuitive for nurses; after all, nurses are patient advocates. However, as it relates to informatics, advocating is a far more complex responsibility that requires in-depth knowledge of both clinical processes and clinical systems. The informatics nurse is advocating not only on behalf of patients, but also on behalf of all nurses and caregivers, as well as known and anticipated technological capabilities. The informatics nurse must recognize inconsistencies in the care plan and the terminology available to electronically document care. The informatics nurse is also the first to recognize quality improvement opportunities as they relate to patient documentation (e.g., Is the desired patient data available, standard, and easily retrieved?). In addition to maintaining awareness about operations and clinical systems, the informatics nurse must constantly monitor clinical systems and assess their usefulness for a variety of users and uses. Informatics nurses also must ensure that nursing considerations are evaluated equally with other considerations (e.g., costs, interoperability, physician preference, etc.) when clinical systems are selected and implemented.

To advocate, informatics nurses must be (1) strategists, (2) leaders, and (3) great communicators; they must (4) engage stakeholders across multiple spectrums to ensure patient, nursing, and technological needs are understood and met. This includes creating buy-in from managers, administrators, and IT within the organization, as well as consultants, developers, and implementation specialists. It further includes those who may be outside the clinical setting, like investors and policy makers, whose decisions can have a huge impact on clinical systems and processes. According to Suzanne Begeny, Director of Government Affairs at the American Association of the Colleges of Nursing, "In order to effectively shape public policy, nurses need to realize that it takes a significant financial investment to compete on the national level. In addition to money, nurses must act as the impetus for the message, orchestrate support, and prepare our leaders for the political stage." In this way, nursing informatics issues will gain the recognition necessary to be taken seriously as healthcare reform progresses.

In a study on nursing leadership, Antrobus and Kitson (1999) observed that:

> Nursing leadership has both an internal and external focus. This dual perspective seems integral to understanding nursing leadership. Internally within nursing it is the relationship which leaders develop between the political, academic, management and clinical domains which enables access to and explication of nursing knowledge. Externally, it is the relationship leaders create between nursing and the socio-political context which enables leaders to position nursing to acquire power and influence. (p. 749)

Antrobus and Kitson (1999) go on to explain that nurse leaders must develop mastery over the languages used in each domain in order to "translate" and engage respective stakeholders in a meaningful exchange that moves nursing from the "invisible to the visible" (p. 750). The informatics nurse's success as a leader is likely the ability to draw on practical nursing experience and relate to other users within the environment. To explain the nurse's natural progression to leadership within the clinical environment and policy development, Antrobus and Kitson (1999) explain that "it was nursing knowledge from nursing practice which gave them legitimacy for their leadership influence" (p. 749). This knowledge is based on a philosophical understanding of nursing ethics and care ideologies.

The informatics nurse's role is akin to being a politician or salesperson. Nursing informaticists must be able to convey their concerns about data, and its availability for reporting and dissemination, in terms that are easily understood within the context of the recipient's own constitutional paragon. In other words, nursing informaticists must engage key stakeholders at the intersection of the stakeholder's ability and willingness to influence change. There are many ways to ascertain this understanding: participation in task forces, summits, conferences; creation of white papers; lobbying and support of lobbying efforts; membership in relevant organizations; acting as an expert witness; leading selection committees; and so on. With so many options, it is also necessary that NI leaders are strategic when determining who to engage and with whom to collaborate. They must learn to read others' willingness to assume a shared responsibility for quality informatics, and speak to them in a manner that causes these key players to want to take up the cause. Finally, NI leaders must learn to recognize appropriate engagements, and terms of engagement—even when it comes to their own involvement in promoting a particular cause.

In creating awareness about informatics, processes, and technological capabilities, it is possible to make too many lateral moves. Clearly, at the grassroots level, omnidirectional communication is an important and necessary action to uncover all facets of the informatics practices employed and ideas about how to improve data gathering and knowledge sharing. However, at a certain point, an NI leader must collect this information and move it beyond the realm of her core competencies to connect with others who can help resolve the issue or promote the cause. One method for doing so involves campaigning with phone calls and letters until someone within the clinical, professional, or political organization addresses the concern. When a professional organization, such as the AMIA or the AAN, expresses interest in the campaign, these grassroots efforts must still continue. Although, the most visible efforts may no longer be conducted by the NI leader(s) who initially brought the informatics issue to the forefront. In fact, it's very likely that by the time any policy recommendations make it in front of state or federal legislators, professional lobbyists will have become involved.

TAKING STOCK: NURSING INFORMATICS REPORT CARD— A CALL TO COLLABORATION

The need for skilled informatics nurses is not going away; it's growing stronger. Our education programs and healthcare institutions must be prepared to accommodate the demand for nurses experienced in patient care and readily able to tackle technology-related problems. This means more than just being comfortable with the technologies or attending a lunch-and-learn session to acclimate to new products and procedures. The 2009 Forum on the Future of Nursing recognized technology as a potential stumbling block for nurses who are not prepared to do more than "tweet" (Institute of Medicine, 2010):

> Nurses need to be fluent in *technology*. That means much more than following someone on Twitter or being competent with a BlackBerry or a computer. It involves such tasks as retrieving data, sharing information and mining health charts for information about both patients and the community. Programs that educate nurses need to emphasize technology and how to use it not only to communicate but also to plan, provide, and evaluate care. (p. 9)

We must not only prepare nurses for the technologies they're sure to encounter, we must assess their ability and willingness to adapt. Adequate training is an important aspect to successful adoption of any policy or procedure. Since nurses are critical, logical thinkers, educating them about the reasons for proposed changes and expected outcomes is integral. Change for the sake of change, especially among more seasoned nurses, is typically denigrated.

However, technological readiness isn't the only critical juncture. Inevitably, nursing informaticists will foray into policy on some level. This may be internal to the healthcare organization (e.g., how-to's, do's, don'ts, data for process improvement, fixes, etc.), where nursing informaticists perform a number of functions to ensure colleagues operate equipment and clinical information systems correctly and effectively, and ensure that process and patient data are available to managers and administrators. Nursing informatics will often be required to navigate hospital and public policy, as well. Informaticists will be responsible for ensuring that data is available for public reporting metrics and will be expected to communicate policy requirements to vendors and nursing colleagues. Nursing informatics education must include communication; relationship building; and an understanding of shared values, judgment, collaboration, leadership, and strategic thinking (Institute of Medicine, 2010, pp. 10–11). Curiously, these are the same skills required for nursing informaticists to advocate, engage, and collaborate on the public healthcare policy level.

SUMMARY

Nurses have always been patient advocates; it's our duty to care for the patient. We are attentive, loving, skilled, and patient—masters of the patient care domain. But we're stretched thin! And as the ratio of nurses to patients grows smaller, we grow older, the scope of practice evolves, treatments become more complex, and documentation grows both more necessary and more cumbersome, technology can and does help alleviate some of the strain on nursing. We must be willing to recognize this, and advocate for advancements in technology and processes that will not only promote patient care, but also make our lives easier. We must take leadership seats at the decision-making table. We must strategically collaborate and plan to have a voice; we must not give away our advocacy voice!

The formation of good public health policy relies on quality, unbiased, substantial data as well as the expertise of those who provide care within the healthcare environment. We need to lead the charge and engage leadership on every necessary level to ensure that public policy supports NI initiatives. No one is better positioned to collaborate with system vendors and politicians to ensure that healthcare technologies and public policies promote patient care at the extraordinary level we have always ascribed to in nursing.

REFERENCES

American Association of Colleges of Nurses. (2010, April 14). *Government Affairs*. Retrieved from http://www.aacn.nche.edu/Government/pdf/HCRreview.pdf.

American Medical Informatics Association. (n.d.). *AMIA Public Policy*. Retrieved from https://www.amia.org/public_policy.

American Nurses Association. (2010). *Health System Reform*. Retrieved from http://www.nursingworld.org/MainMenuCategories/HealthcareandPolicyIssues/HealthSystemReform.

Antrobus, S., & Kitson, A. (1999). Nursing leadership: influencing and shaping health policy and nursing practice. *Journal of Advanced Nursing, 29*(3), 746–753.

Bonnett, C. (2010, May 7). *The next frontier in healthcare reform*. Retrieved from https://www.dchi.duke.edu/publications/dchi-in-the-news/the-next-frontier-in-health-care-reform.

Blumenthal, D, Office of the National Coordinator for Health Information Technology. (2010, February 4). Launching HITECH. *New England Journal of Medicine, 362*(5), 382–385.

CENTER to Champion Nursing in America. (2010, April 21). *Nursing related provisions in healthcare reform legislation: A chart*. Retrieved from http://championnursing.org/resources/nursing-related-provisions-health-care-reform-legislation-chart.

Dombrowski, P., & Kaye, R. (2010, February). *Putting people to work in health IT – fast*. (HIMSS, Producer). Retrieved from http://www.himss.org/CI_Insights/CI_Insights_20100208.htm#1.

HIMSS Nursing Informatics. (2009, April 2). *HIMSS 2009 informatics nurse impact survey*. Retrieved from http://www.himss.org/ASP/topics_FocusDynamic.asp?faid=243.

HRSA. (2010, March 17). *HRSA study finds nursing workforce is growing and more diverse*. Retrieved from http://www.hrsa.gov

Institute of Medicine. (2010). A summary of the December 2009 forum on the future of nursing: Care in the community. Washington, D.C.: The National Academies Press.

Kaminski, J. (2007, Spring). Virtual nursing practice and culture: Shaping our place in cyberspace. *Nursing Informatics News, 4*(2). Retrieved from http://www.nursing-informatics.com/ninewsv4n2a.html. Page 1–2.

McCormick, KA, Sensmeier, J, Delaney, C, Bickford, C. Introduction to informatics and nursing in the new healthcare environment. In J. Bronzino (Ed.), *BME Handbook* (4th ed.). CRC Press/Taylor & Francis Group, LLC, NewYork. In Press 2012.

New Jersey Collaborating Center for Nursing. (n.d.). *Nursing in public and health policy*. Retrieved from http://www.njccn.org/public_policy.asp.

Ozbolt, J., & Saba, V. (2008, September/October). A brief history of nursing informatics in the United States of America. *Nursing Outlook, 56*, 199–205.

Public Health Institute. (2010, May). *Health reform and local health departments: Opportunities for the centers for disease control and prevention, Section VII — Attachments*. Bill Summary.

Raths, D. (2010, May). Healthcare reform and IT. *Healthcare Informatics, 27*(5), 36–37.

Robert Wood Johnson Foundation. (2008, October). Strengthening public health nursing part II: how nurse leaders in policymaking positions are

transforming public health. *Charting Nursing's Future*.

U.S. Department of Health & Human Services. (2010). *HITECH Programs*. Retrieved from http://healthit.hhs.gov.

Home Health: The Missing Ingredient in Healthcare Reform

Charlotte A. Weaver / Jennifer V. Moore

• OBJECTIVES

1. Home Health's potential role in the transformation of care delivery
2. Impact of Home Health's exclusion from Meaningful Use exclusion for incenting EHR adoption
3. Relationship of Affordable Care Act and opportunities to expand role of Home Health as primary care provider to elderly
4. Current state for EHR and information communication technologies use in Home Health

• KEY WORDS

EHR use in Home Health
Mobile devices, Telehealth, Remote monitoring
Home Health and Health Reform
Primary Care in the Home
Elderly and Care Transitions

INTRODUCTION

Home health has historically played a backstage role in healthcare delivery strategies in the United States. This has been due in part to health policy, but also to the "cottage industry" nature of the home health market. Altogether, there are about 11,000 home health agencies in operation as of 2010. About 1,600 of these agencies belong to the 4 publically traded companies that, based on revenues, are the largest providers in the industry but still only represent 5% of the market share. In terms of market dominance and volume of services delivered, the various state and metropolitan Visiting Nurse Associations and Services along the Eastern seaboard are large providers with average revenues of $25 million to $40 million, with the exception of the Visiting Nursing Service of New York, which consistently runs about $200 million per year. Chesney (personal communication, 2010, July 26), a health market analyst, reports that in 2008 there were only 744 agencies out of 9,432 that had revenues of $5 million or more. That means 93% of agencies have annual revenues of less that $5 million per year. While an accurate count of home health organizations by number of branch agencies is not available, industry analysts agree that more than 50% are single-site providers and 75% have 10 or fewer site locations.

Since Medicare's inception, reimbursement schemas have covered the spectrum of payment methods—from fee-for-service to those based on visits, episodes, cost, capitation, illness and functional severity levels, and combinations thereof. Each decade has seen new reimbursement schemas introduced, with the Centers for Medicaid and Medicare Services (CMS) making as many as 3 changes in a single decade (Randall, 2008). Up until the health reform legislation of 2009 and 2010, health policy for home health has focused primarily on cost containment reimbursement schemas meant to limit utilization and contain costs.

REIMBURSEMENT SCHEMAS AND THEIR DELETERIOUS AFFECTS

The iterations of reimbursement rate schemas over the last 30 years have played out like a dance between the industry and health policy makers (Bishop, 1996; MedPAC, 2010; Murtaugh, 2003; Randall, 2010). Containment efforts have been reactionary, sometimes with deleterious effects as when the 1997 Balanced Budget Act introduced the interim payment system (IPS). The IPS was a direct response to home health costs that had grown an average of 33% per year between 1990 and 1995 under fee-for service reimbursement (Bishop, 1996). The IPS introduced capitation by imposing per visit and beneficiary limits. While it affected an immediate drop in costs and utilization, in just a 3-year period, fully one-third of home health agencies closed or were acquired (Chesney, personal communication, 2010, July 26). As a correction factor, CMS introduced the prospective payment system (PPS) in 2000, and Medicare's spending on home health increased from 8% in 2001 to 18.3% in 2009, mirroring a doubling of expenditures for all postacute care expenditures in this same period.

Unfortunately, over the decades, CMS's reimbursement policies have tended to incentivize a business and operations focus within home health agencies. This focus has tended to encourage care delivery structured according to the latest reimbursement schema, rather than guided by the knowledge of clinically appropriate care and rewarded based on quality and care delivery metrics. Mary Naylor, in her research on transitional care innovations, notes that despite a compelling body of evidence, transitional care practices have not been adopted by home healthcare agencies or other providers primarily because Medicare reimbursement does not cover these services (Naylor, 2006). Rather than moving toward an integrated and coordinated approach focused on rehabilitative, independent function and self-management, Randall (2010) makes the further observation that the reimbursement schemas in the federal Medicare program have been inflexibly committed to an "acute homecare model", and that the industry's response to reimbursement changes since the late 90s has been fewer services

to homecare patients, shorter lengths of stay, and a much more "acute" Medicare benefit than prior to the 1997 capitated IPS schema. Randall states, "This repositioning of home health back to an acute care model was one of the CMS aims during the 2001-8 Bush administration, and it has succeeded" (p. 9).

The reimbursement rate changes enacted in the 2010 Patient Protection and Affordable Care Act (PPACA) will introduce a 3-year series of rate cuts capped by a market basket reevaluation in 2014. CMS expects these reductions to effect a significant constriction of Home Health providers in the marketplace and address the 3.4% growth rate that has occurred year-over-year from 2001 to 2009 (Medpac, 2010). This growth rate equates to about 500 new agencies entering the market every year and is viewed as an indicator of possible exploitation and Medicare fraud. This growth trend has been viewed with alarm by home health professional organizations as well. Organizations such as the National Association of Home Care (NACH) and the Alliance for Home Health Quality and Innovation (Alliance) have actively lobbied for approaches and measures for CMS to use to target the fraudulent new entries.

The need for spending CMS funds to obtain maximum health value for every dollar spent is a very real challenge for the United States, made even more pressing by the looming threat of Medicare's insolvency projected by the Congressional Budget Office for 2017 (Medpac, 2010, p. 13). The critique that we offer here is that a health policy that focuses solely on reimbursement and regulations is misdirected. The innovation being pushed in PPACA still misses integrating maximum use of home health and community services for prevention and population health in the at-risk populations by its failure to incentivize electronic medical record adoption in these healthcare sectors. While health spending constraints are a reality, our health policy in regards to home health's role in health reform needs new thinking. We would argue that home health needs to be incentivizeded under the Health Information Technology for Economic and Clinical Health (HITECH) Act's meaningful use eligibility for electronic health record (EHR) adoption, if we hope to use these capabilities and health information exchange across the care continuum (HITECH, 2010). To continue this exclusive focus on acute care and physician practices is at odds with the policies and practices of the major industrialized countries who spend considerably less on healthcare with higher health indices than the United States (Anderson, 2008).

In this chapter we compare U.S. health policy in home health and use of technology with other industrialized countries. We review how the historical relationship between the Department of Health and Human Services (HHS) and its administrative arm, CMS, is reflected in the current state of care delivery services, health information technology (HIT) adoption levels, and workforce challenges; and end with a future-focused perspective on the potential for innovative change. Future opportunity and hope rest with the 2010 PPACA legislation mandates and new regulations that push for more coordinated, patient-centered, multidisciplinary team care for the chronically ill and elderly populations. We are also optimistic that a current HHS study examining the inclusion of providers other than hospitals and physicians in the 2009 American Recovery and Reform Act's (ARRA) meaningful use incentive will allow both advance practice registered nurses (APRN) and home health organizations to be included as eligible providers in the near future.

US POLICY TOWARD HOME HEALTH COMPARED WITH OTHER COUNTRIES

Reimbursement Denial for Technology in Home Health

A constant throughout recent decades, and even maintained in the 2009 and 2010 health reform legislation, has been CMS's denial to reimburse for the use of technology in home care delivery, specifically telemonitoring using medical devices for blood pressure, weight, and glucometer readings. Nor are physicians or nurse practitioners reimbursed for telehealth home visits. This denial continues in spite of a body of evidence indicating that telemonitoring and telehealth for unstable, high-risk patients within the home reduces hospitalizations. Home health provider organizations that use telemonitoring and telehealth in their care delivery protocols and strategies do so at their own cost burden. Considering the extent to which the current and past administrations have pushed and incentivized EHR adoption in acute care and physicians' practices, it is mindboggling that this obstructive stance to the use of HIT in home health has not been overturned and aligned with approaches in other healthcare delivery sectors.

To understand how out of sync US home health policy is when compared with other countries that employ single-payer, government healthcare systems, it's helpful to look at the United Kingdom. The U.K.'s National Health Service (NHS) has a strong emphasis on restorative care, health maintenance, and supporting functional independence in their chronically ill and elderly populations. The U.K.'s NHS is actively targeting the health maintenance

needs of its aging population through its Whole System Demonstrator program that extends telemonitoring services and telehealth to elderly individuals living at home. This demonstration project funded at 81 million British pounds is just one of numerous projects aimed at defining effective use of technology in the home and new care delivery strategies for better and cost effective ways of caring for their large elderly population. Similarly, other countries like Scotland, Ireland, Germany, and Finland are actively working on developing strategies for using telehealth, medical monitoring and technology devices in homehealthcare for their growing elderly populations (Cleland et al., 2005; Koch et al., 2009; SAINI, 2008; SITRA, 2009 Bott & Haux, 2007; Vimarlund, 2008). The literature clearly shows that to maintain the chronically ill and elderly in their homes, full use of available communication and information technology is crucial. Internet-connected phones, medical device monitoring, and health data exchange between providers and patients or caregivers are all key enablers to care coordination and cost effective, quality care. While this body of literature speaks clearly at a common-sense level to clinicians; health economists caution that the studies lack clear economic evaluation that allows for like comparisons to determine "value for money" (Whitten, 2002). Within the U.S., however, informatics thought leaders like David Bates are calling for the extended use of EHR technologies to support more effective primary care delivery to the elderly and chronically ill in their homes and communities (Bates, 2010).

Hospital-at-Home Care Delivery Models

U.S. health policy has kept home health marginalized from mainstream healthcare delivery strategies by not looking to develop home healthcare as an integral component to cost-efficient, equitable, person-centered, quality healthcare for the elderly, disabled, and chronically ill. Countries, such as the United Kingdom, Australia, Canada, Finland, and Germany have a long history of aggressively using community and home healthcare programs for preventive, restorative, and palliative care in vulnerable populations. In addition, there is an acute care model, termed *hospital at home*, in which hospital-level care is delivered in the home to avoid the hazards of an acute hospital admission for the elderly with common acute medical conditions. Different variations of this model have been in practice throughout Europe, Australia, and the United Kingdom for over a decade (Ram, 2004; Nicholson, 2001; Aimonino, 2004, 2005). Despite differences in care models, the body of evidence points to avoidance of the iatrogenic illness, functional decline, and other adverse events that accompany the risk of acute hospitalization in the elderly (Leape, 1991; Baker, 2004). Lower healthcare costs, fewer complications, shorter lengths of stay, higher patient satisfaction, and better quality of life for the patient are some of the notable benefits (Aimonino, 2004, 2005, 2008; Ram, 2004; Leff, 2005, 2006; Montalto, 2002).

U.S. Hospital-at-Home Demonstration Projects

In the U.S., Leff and colleagues tested the hospital-at-home approach within elderly patient populations having 4 common conditions: community-acquired pneumonia, congestive heart failure, chronic obstructive pulmonary disease, and cellulitis. Leff's physician-led model worked closely with community-based laboratories and home health agencies to provide the same level of care as delivered in hospitals, including intravenous antibiotics, respiratory treatments, radiology, and lab diagnostic exams. Similar to the model used by Aimonino and colleagues in Italy, there was close coordination between the hospital and emergency room and the hospital-at-home program physicians. Upon discharge, there was a coordinated handoff to the primary care provider. Leff and colleagues found no difference between the hospitalized population and the at-home intervention group in mortality rates, functional levels, or readmission rates after an 8-week follow-up. However, the at-home treated patients had statistically significant differences for the following: higher satisfaction with all dimensions of their care, shorter lengths of stay, fewer complications, less care utilization, and cost differences greater than $2 thousand to $8 thousand per patient. Leff and colleagues conclude, "our study shows that an innovative substitutive hospital-at-home model for selected older patients with common acute medical conditions is feasible and efficacious in selected healthcare systems" (Leff, 2005, p. 807).

Nurse Practitioner–Led Hospital-at-Home Project

Importantly, the major tenets of the model used by the Leff and Aimonino teams are also reflected in a United Kingdom study testing Nurse Practicitioners' ability to act in the medical oversight role for an elderly population with chronic obstructive pulmonary disease (COPD). Ansari, Shamssain, Farrow, and Keaney (2009), from the University of Sunderland, conducted a case-controlled study using a nurse practitioner as the team lead for the hospital-at-home program, partnering with home health agencies for the nursing and care team services. The authors reported similar results of positive outcomes, no difference in hospital readmission rates post discharge,

less cost and resource expenditures, and higher patient satisfaction as compared with the hospitalized cohort. The hospital-at-home body of evidence speaks to the efficacy and quality of care potential for elder care in the U.S. healthcare system by partnering with home health to develop new care modalities and new health policy directions.

CLINICAL INFORMATION SYSTEMS IN HOME HEALTH—CURRENT STATE

OASIS Clinical Documentation

In October 2000, CMS introduced the Outcome and Assessment Information Set (OASIS) and required its use as a condition of participation for healthcare providers. The initial version of OASIS contained 79 data elements, all of which have been sustained through 2010. The OASIS tool is to be used at admission, readmission after an emergent care or hospitalization, and at discharge in order to compare functional levels. The difference in functional levels between admission and discharge serve as the quality indicators that are publically reported by CMS. The initial start-of-care assessment drives both a baseline functioning score and a derived payment amount based on the case mix score, termed the Home Health Resource Group (HHRG) score. Thus, with the introduction of OASIS, clinical documentation became directly linked to an agency's CMS reimbursement. There have been 3 versions of OASIS released since 2000, with the most recent being OASIS C, introduced on January 1, 2010. OASIS C changes target risk assessments, coordination of care, timeliness of communications with physician, and patient teaching for self-management skills. These changes represent a coordinated effort between CMS and the National Quality Forum to bring best practices into home health and are directed toward clinical practice behaviors.

Evolution of Clinical Information Systems in Home Health

The complexity of the OASIS documentation and the workflow involved to get the data back to the office for entry and transmission to enable reimbursement created a compelling need for clinical information systems. In anticipation of the 2000 OASIS introduction, agencies started looking to their legacy billing and admission, transfer, and discharge (ATD) system vendors to provide OASIS documentation capture. Vendors quickly responded by developing documentation systems that would allow clinicians to capture the OASIS data and pass it directly into the back-end system, eliminating the need for office staff to re-enter the OASIS documentation. In 2000, few legacy systems offered a clinical solution to capture even the routine visit notes in the home. Patient records and clinical documentation were collected on paper, and agencies' medical records were paper-based. Billing and ADT system vendors adopted a "bolt-on" approach to capture OASIS documentation. Consequently, the structure of the clinical documentation was based on a task concept that organized the patient record by visit-note type in chronologic order, with each discipline having their separate documentation tasks. A decade later, the remnants of this developmental approach are evident in the system offerings in the marketplace today. Current state still has limited workflow support functionality, and lacks integrated patient record views, multidisciplinary team workflow and patient care data views, clinical decision support, structured terminologies, and/or flexible quality reporting capabilities.

Antiquated Architectures and Limited R&D Budgets

The regulatory documentation burden for clinicians in home health is certainly the heaviest of any venue of care, with the average start-of-care admission, re-evaluations, and discharges each taking 1 to 2 hours on average. Through the required OASIS documentation, CMS aims to structure best practices, effect standardization, and provide quantitative quality measures; the result, however, for clinicians has been an onerous documentation burden. To manage this documentation load, clinicians need robust clinical documentation systems that facilitate workflow through clinical decision supports, clinician-specific views of patient care data, and reminders that support efficient and clinically sound documentation. Unfortunately, the HIT software suppliers for the home health industry reflect the cottage industry nature of home health itself. There are a myriad of small vendors who supply their local markets with systems developed to cover the basic front office and billing functions with added functionality to capture OASIS documentation. These basic systems require minimal capital outlay, making them affordable for the thousands of small-sized agencies that make up the bulk of the home health industry. However, that segment of the market with bigger buying power— the larger home health agencies and organizations, and the hospital-based agencies—began looking for more comprehensive clinical systems with advanced functionality to integrate with their referral sources and hospital information systems.

In response to the OASIS-driven market demand, HIS vendors began acquiring existing systems with the largest home health market shares and interfacing them to their legacy systems or selling them as stand-alone solutions. However, these HIS vendors have not been able to keep their promise of integrating multiple service line functionality, providing information exchange and seamless integration, standard terminology, and matching electronic medical record (EMR) functionality available in acute and ambulatory care systems. Nor have the vendors been able to invest to update these acquisitions from their 20-year-old architectures. Most of the major vendors' systems in the market today remain on their original technical platform architectures.

While the HIS vendors have matured their products to deliver point-of-care clinical documentation, the systems still have a strong focus on driving the reimbursement process rather than supporting clinical workflow and decision support. Lack of structured clinical data still characterizes the industry today, and has long challenged the ability of home health organizations to provide meaningful clinical outcome measures. The most evolved products offer the ability to maximize reimbursement by managing the number of patient visits and identifying patients at risk of rehospitalization; clinician views are still task and note based, siloed by discipline.

Given the limited buying power within the home health industry as compared with the acute care sector, vendors' research and development dollars will often go to hospital and physician solutions in their product lines. The ARRA stimulus and meaningful use incentives for acute care and physicians adds to this imbalance. The home health market is not large enough or lucrative enough to warrant vendors' investment to re-engineer the product line's technical platform and data model. For these reasons, the home health industry faces the prospect of entering into the next decade's health reform imperatives at a distinct disadvantage.

EHR ADOPTION AND MEANINGFUL USE: HEALTH POLICY

The 2000 National Home and Hospice Care Survey (NHHCS) conducted the first national survey on EMR use within the industry. The results showed that 32% of the agencies surveyed reported use of a computerized medical records system and an additional 22% indicated that they had plans to implement an electronic records system within the next year. Missing from this important benchmark, however, is specific functionality that is basic to EMR standards today: clinical decision support; flexibility of views of patient care information; point-of-care support for clinical documentation; telemedicine; and standardized, structured terminologies.

Without a doubt, there has been significant change in the adoption of EMR technologies within home health and hospice care providers since the NHHCS' 2000 survey. A 2007 to 2008 national survey conducted by the American Association of Homes and Services for the Aging reports a 43% current use of EMRs, with an additional 31% of agencies in the process of or planning to implement an EMR over the following year. These 2007 numbers represent a 33% increase over the 2000 national survey results. Resnick and Alwan (2010), the authors of the 2007 survey study, also looked at the functionality used in EMR systems. The following list includes some of their findings:

- Patient demographics   95%
- Clinical notes   34%
- Clinical decision support   23%
- Physician orders   50%

Telemedicine was used in about 38% of the surveyed agencies, but this represented telephone downloads of vital sign device monitoring to more sophisticated wireless transmissions to a centralized entity doing 24-hour surveillance. Only 29% of survey respondents reported using point of care for clinical documentation (PoCD). However, in the agencies using PoCD about 95% used this technology for OASIS documentation capture. Sharing of health information data with other providers was almost negligible, stemming from the lack of this functionality in the EMR systems in use.

Health information exchange capabilities require interoperability between the organizations sharing their EMR data. Until the standard setting initiatives mandated within ARRA are in place, true interoperability will remain out of reach, and EMR vendors and provider organizations will be limited in their abilities to engage in health information exchange. Resnick and Alwan (2010) also observe that the goal for state-level health information exchange with the ability of record sharing functionality for health providers would be greatly helped if long-term and postacute care settings were included in national ARRA-funded initiatives. The authors go on to note that it is hopeful that the ARRA includes a mandate to HHS to conduct a study to determine if HIT adoption incentive payments should be offered to providers other than hospitals and physicians.

DISCUSSION AND LOOKING TO THE FUTURE

The Demographic Imperative for New Health Policy: Future Focus

The goal of containing healthcare costs may be better served by broadening our thinking on how to use home healthcare more extensively and in coordinated partnership with the acute care and ambulatory care providers. Looking forward, the challenge in health policy is in determining how best to include the ethical and social perspectives of equity in access to care in the face of unsupportable growth in Medicare and Medicaid expenditures.

Both the ARRA of 2009 and the PPACA of 2010 are transformative pieces of health legislation that aim to stimulate EHR adoption throughout the acute care and physician practice sectors for greater efficiency, patient safety, and improved quality with better coordination of care across providers, venues, and geographies. New clinical care delivery strategies and programs are called for that will address the fragmentation and waste in our siloed healthcare systems. These new models and initiatives must also allow for an expanded resource capacity to accommodate the healthcare needs that will be coming from the rapid growth in our elderly population.

Health Workforce Challenges

In 2008, the IOM, under the auspices of the National Academies, released an urgent press release entitled, *Healthcare Work Force Too Small, Unprepared For Aging Baby Boomers; Higher Pay, More Training, And Changes In Care Delivery Needed To Avert Crisis*. In this release, the IOM noted that as the first of the U.S.'s 78 million baby boomers begin reaching age 65 in 2011, the U.S. will face a healthcare work force that is too small and woefully unprepared to meet their specific health needs. The IOM's subsequent 2008 report, *Retooling for an Aging America: Building the Healthcare Workforce*, called for bold initiatives to immediately start training all healthcare providers in the basics of geriatric care and to prepare family members and other informal caregivers, who currently receive little or no training in how to tend to their aging loved ones. The IOM set a target date of 2030 for the necessary reforms to take place—

the year by which all baby boomers will have turned 65 or older.

Today, the professional healthcare workforce, including nursing, receives insufficient geriatric education and clinical training in geriatric settings. And yet caring for the aged requires specialty knowledge of the pathophysiology of aging and geriatric syndromes that encompass such conditions as fall risks, cognitive impairments, depression, and malnutrition in conjunction with underlying chronic illnesses. Normal aging carries increasing degrees of loss of independence and personal health challenges even for healthy seniors. For the population over 65 years of age in 2008, 75% are estimated to have at least one chronic illness that requires ongoing medical management, but even more sobering is that about 20% of Medicare beneficiaries have 5 or more chronic conditions (IOM, 2008). Caring for the aged requires a highly skilled team of health professionals trained in geriatrics. Consequently, the burden of training falls largely on the shoulders of the home healthcare provider organization. While the NLN and the ACCN have mandated the inclusion of geriatrics within nursing curricula, curriculum content is not sufficient for the medical complexity presented by the geriatric populations, and clinical practicums in home health or community placements are scarce. Additionally, effective and efficient home healthcare requires the expertise of multiple domains—speech pathologists, occupational therapists, physical therapists, medical social workers, and nursing—delivered as highly coordinated teams with a patient-centered focus. Health professional educational centers are still not able to prepare new graduates to work within a multidisciplinary, team context. So in the authors' experience, the challenge of preparing the home healthcare professional workforce to have the clinical competencies, knowledge, and skills needed to optimally deliver effective and person-centered care to our geriatric population rests hugely on the provider organizations. For the lead author's organization, which is 3% of the home health industry, this educational investment averages close to $23 million per year for a clinical workforce of 10,250 individuals.

Recognizing Home Health's Potential

In order to see home health achieve its appropriate role in U.S. healthcare delivery strategies for the elderly, disabled, and chronically ill, confronting its status as the "orphan child" is crucial. All too often, when stakeholders and health professionals do think of home health, they have a perception that the clinical services delivered are of a low clinical skills task level, of questionable value, and the work environment is decidedly low tech in comparison to high-tech, acute care environments. Contributing to that less than glamorous image is the aged and chronically ill populations that largely comprise the home health patient population. Clinicians who choose home healthcare for their careers commonly describe having to counter perceptions like, "Home health is where those who couldn't make it in acute care go," or similarly, "Home health is where clinicians go to retire."

The Gentiva Story

At Gentiva Health Services, to counter the historical and policy disincentives, we have introduced a number of clinical programs and initiatives. We have used specialty programs developed and implemented over the past decade to introduce new product lines, care delivery modalities, the latest clinical science and best practices, as well as telemonitoring technologies. We have also defined geriatrics as our practice specialty. Mandatory for every clinician is the completion of 4 courses in basic geriatrics and an integrated comprehensive exam. About 20 hours of course study and practicum labs are required for a clinician to be certified in a given specialty program. To reward and incentivize this degree of continuing education and professionalism, we introduced a 6-stage clinical ladder that allows direct care clinicians to advance from entry level to a Vice President, equivalent in role and salary.

Each specialty program's clinical content, assessment, and interventions are based on the latest science and best practices. Some specialty programs are disease specific, as in Neurorehabilitation (strokes, MS, and Parkinson) and Cardiopulmonary (CHF, hypertension, and COPD). The Orthopedic Rehabilitation program focuses on joint surgery, and is protocol-driven by specific procedures. The Safe Strides and Senior Health programs target the geriatric syndromes of falls prevention and cognitive impairment. The Cardiopulmonary program uses telemonitoring and is supported by a 24-hour telemonitoring center based in Tampa. Gentiva absorbs the overhead expense for telemonitoring since CMS denies reimbursement for this expense.

Gentiva is able to leverage its size to fund infrastructure investment in its clinical workforce and point-of-care technologies. To enable this level of educational investment in its clinical workforce, Gentiva invests in a team of over 20 advanced-level clinical specialists, in addition to educational designers, software for interactive online courses, and a learning management system for tracking. Gentiva has also made the commitment to do extensive in-house development of a vendor's product to put a state-of-the-art, point-of-care system in the hands of its clinicians. This approach was adopted only after doing comprehensive market reviews at 2 different intervals 5 years apart, which found antiquated architecture that was unable to scale and had limited EMR functionalities.

Gentiva Health Services is fortunate to be positioned to make these workforce and technology investments. However, all home health providers have these same needs for a highly trained workforce and EMR-level technologies, but the reality of small business size and poor margins between reimbursement and costs severely limit the industry's capacity for these essential investments. As mentioned previously, the PPACA carries another round of reimbursement cuts for the home health industry. CMS estimates that the impact of all of the PPACA policies will lower home health agency reimbursement by 4.63% beginning January 1, 2011. Additive rate cuts will continue for 2012 and 2013, with a ray of hope offered by the rebasing discussions scheduled for 2014. There is hope and optimism that in these 2014 rebasing discussions, CMS and the ONC will validate technology costs such as telemonitoring, EHR technologies, and clinical information systems in home health and hospice to be necessary costs for quality and efficiencies needed for meaningful health reform. It is crucial that nurse leaders understand this key pivot point and support the extension of incentive payments for IT in home health if we are to realize the full potential of the healthcare reforms envisioned in the new legislation.

OPPORTUNITIES IN HEALTH REFORM LEGISLATION

The healthcare reform environment driven by the ARRA and the PPACA legislation is beginning to close the gap between current care practices and research-based best practices. Foremost amongst these best practices are the medical home, hospital-at-home, and care transitions models. Quality improvement initiatives are embedded in the PPACA act, such as bundling payments to hospitals to partner with primary care providers and encouraging community and home healthcare agencies to provide integrated, across-sectors care for the highly vulnerable populations in their local markets who are at risk for high readmission rates. Other mandates in the PPACA that open up new opportunities for the best

care delivery practices to be adopted broadly in home health are the Accountable Organization and 24-hour Primary Care Visit requirements. These initiatives have the potential to encompass the core tenants of the care transitions model and the reinvention of primary care practice embodied in the medical home model. The care transitions model has over a decade of research findings that show the human and economic advantages for using coaches and facilitators to coordinate services and do follow-up for patient teaching in self-management and personal health record use. Naylor and colleagues (2004) have demonstrated a highly effective model using nurse practitioners to bridge between hospital and home for high-risk populations, such as those with heart failure. Additionally, Coleman and his University of Colorado team (2004) have developed a broader model that uses a hospital-based coach who crosses from the hospital into the home to teach self-management and ensure that the patient is connected to primary care and follow-up services as needed.

But as Naylor points out, we have the capacity and structure in home health today to accommodate this care transitions model of care delivery without adding new layers, roles, or programs (Naylor, 2006):

> More than any other segment of healthcare services, home healthcare practitioners are uniquely poised to address the challenges and capitalize on the opportunities to ensure that these patients and their caregivers do not fall through the cracks. Home healthcare is the component of the healthcare industry best positioned to bridge gaps in care between hospitals and home, especially for high-risk groups such as older adults coping with multiple health problems (p. 48).

For broad adoption of the transition care model in home healthcare to be possible, the payment and reimbursement structures incentives will need to be extended to all stakeholders with equal opportunity and risk—hospitals, home health agencies, and primary care providers.

There are a plethora of quality improvement demonstration projects, initiatives, and directives outlined in the PPACA to incentivize new care delivery modalities based on best practice research evidence and workforce development. The breadth of the reform initiatives encompassed in the entirety of PPACA are unprecedented, and if put into practice, would address the limitations covered in this critique. We encourage all to spend time reading this body of work because the comprehensiveness of its reach means that it touches every sector and every role. As thought leaders we will want to be knowledgeable, informed, and engaged in the opportunities that touch our respective worlds. The full text of PPACA can be retrieved from the following Web site:finance.senate.gov/legislation/details/?id=61f4fb98-a3d0-d85c-d33f-f2c598e1d138

Key Reform Initiatives

We offer here a condensed summary of key initiatives in the PPACA that involve geriatrics and workforce development for nursing, opportunities for home healthcare, as well as those that target integrating care delivery with care transitions principles and extended primary care. Common in these demonstration pilot specifications are the abilities to collect and report the designated quality and economic measures and use of EHRs. This HIT requirement should serve as advance notice to home healthcare providers and others that we are moving to a "new day" in the U. S. healthcare industry, and current levels of EMR use in most home health organizations today will be insufficient to meet those laid out in the PPACA.

1. **Center for Medicare and Medicaid Innovation** (section3021): This program launched in November 2010, is to test innovative payment and services delivery models, including community-based health teams for medical homes led by primary care physicians; patient-centered medical home models; utilizing geriatric assessments and comprehensive care plans to coordinate the care of applicable individuals with multiple chronic conditions; funding home health providers who offer chronic care management services to applicable individuals in cooperation with interdisciplinary teams; improving postacute care through continuing care hospitals that offer inpatient rehabilitation, long term care hospitals, and home health or skilled nursing care; establishing community-based health teams to support small-practice medical homes be assisting primary care practitioners in chronic care management, including patient self-management; supporting care coordination for chronically-ill applicable individuals at high risk of hospitalization through an HIT-enabled provider network that includes care coordinators, a chronic disease registry, and home telehealth technology; and developing, documenting, and disseminating best practices and proven care models.

2. **Accountable Care Organizations** (section 3022): Groups of providers and suppliers manage and coordinate care for a given Medicare population, and those that meet quality performance standards receive payment for the shared savings. Home health providers that can accommodate this care delivery model and electronic information exchange functionality are ideally positioned to take advantage of this opportunity.

3. **Bundling Payments** (section 3023): The bundling pilot program will include all postacute care providers and is to focus on between 1 and 10 patient conditions. An *episode of care* is defined as 3 days prior to the admission of the beneficiary to a hospital for the identified condition and through 30 days following discharge from the hospital. Quality measures will be developed in consultation with the Agency for Healthcare Research and Quality. Of particular interest is a focus on areas such as care coordination, medication reconciliation, discharge planning, transitional care services, and other patient-centered activities.

4. **Independence at Home** (section 3024): This is a payment and service-delivery model using home-based primary care teams directed by physicians and nurse practitioners. The teams are accountable for providing comprehensive, coordinated, continuous, and accessible care to high-need populations at home and coordinating healthcare across all treatment settings. It reflects tenets of the medical home, hospital-at-home, and care transitions models. The care teams may be led by nurse practitioners and are multidisciplinary, have skills in providing home-based primary care; are available 24 × 7; and "use electronic health information systems, remote monitoring, and mobile diagnostic technology" (p. 755). Participants are eligible for incentive payments if they demonstrate delivery of services at lower costs than the predefined estimates for their patient population (minimum of 200 patients).

5. **Hospital Readmission Reduction** (section 3025): This regulation reduces payment for patients with excessive readmission rates for designated diagnoses, primarily elderly with heart failure, chronic obstructive pulmonary disease, or pneumonia. Presents opportunity for care transition programs and integration of home health in transition care delivery.

6. **Face-to-face encounter with PCP Prior to Home Health Referral** (section 6407): This regulation requires that Medicare beneficiary's primary care physician who would be overseeing the patient's

care while admitted to home health, would have to have seen the patient 6 months prior to the home health referral in order to qualify for Medicare payment. Telehealth visits are allowed to meet this regulation and it is also anticipated that advanced practice registered nurses and physician assistants will be used to do the face-to-face visit with the elderly, home-bound patients to ensure that their access to care is not denied. This small regulation change will potentially create a huge impetus for advanced practice registered nurses to be integrated in large numbers into primary care practices. This would also allow the regulatory obstacles regarding reimbursement for telehealth visits to be overcome. These are major changes in the care delivery modalities for primary care in the home.

The PPACA act also addresses the workforce shortage issues, the need to expand the number of physicians and APRNs in primary care, and support more geriatrics curriculum content through faculty development. Under Title V section 5001-5605 of PPACA, there are expanded funds for nursing and allied health student loans with friendlier repayment terms; APRN education grants; specific geriatrics education and training centers for faculty development from all the health sciences, as well as for direct care providers and family caregivers; nursing education grants; nursing faculty development loans; and grants for APRN-led community clinics with the added stipulation that at least one APRN must hold an executive management position within the organizational structure.

SUMMARY

It is the aim of this chapter to provide readers with a window to view into the world of home health, its current state of technology adoption and use, and the context for its untapped potential as a player in healthcare reform. With the enactment of PPACA, dramatic health policy changes are now in play that will fundamentally rewrite the structure, function, and role of home healthcare in the broad U.S. healthcare system. In addition, the PPACA provides bold, first-time opportunities for APRNs in the form of primary care–led practices, nurse-managed clinics, and transitional care and medical home programs. Now it is up to us to take full advantage of these opportunities to be fully engaged partners and participants in these future-shaping initiatives for a better healthcare delivery system in the United States.

REFERENCES

Aimonino, R. N., Tibaldi, V., Marinello, R., Bo, M., Isaia, G., Scarafiotti C., et al. (2005). Acute ischemic stroke in elderly patients treated in hospital at home: A cost minimization analysis. *J Am Geriatr Soc, 53*, 1442–1443.

Aimonino, R. N., Bo M., Molaschi, M., Massaia, M., Salerno, D., Amati, D., et al. (2004). Home hospitalization service for acute uncomplicated first ischemic stroke in elderly patients: A randomized trial. *J Am Geriatr Soc, 52*, 278–283.

Aimonino, R. N., Tibaldi, V., Leff, B., Scarafiotti, C., Marinello, R., Zanocchi, M., et al. (2008). Substitutive "Hospital at Home" versus inpatient care for elderly patients with exacerbations of chronic obstructive pulmonary disease: A prospective randomized, controlled trial. *J Am Geriatr Soc, 56*(3):493–500.

American Recovery and Reinvestment Act. (2009). Retrievd from http://frwebgate.access.gpo.gov/cgi-bin/getdoc.cgi?dbname=111_cong_bills&docid=f:h1enr.pdf.

Anderson, G. F., & Frogner, B. K. (2008). Health spending in OECD countries: Obtaining value per dollar. *Hlt Aff, 27*(6), 1718–1727.

Ansari, K., Shamssain, M., Farrow, M., & Keaney, N. P. (2009). Hospital-at-home care for exacerbations of chronic obstructive pulmonary disease: an observational cohort study of patients managed in hospital or by nurse practitioners in the community. *Chron Respir Dis 6*(2), 69–74.

Baker, D. I., Gottschalk, M., Eng, C., Weber, S., & Tinetti, M. E. (2001). The design and implementation of a restorative care model for home care. *Gerontologist, 41*, 257–263.

Baker, G. R. (2004). Commentary: Harvard medical practice study. *Qual Saf Healthcare, 13*(2), 151–152.

Bates, D. W., & Bitton, A. (2010).The future of health information technology in the patient-centered medical home. *Hlt Aff, 29*(4), 614–621.

Bishop, C. E., Brown, R. S., Phillips, B., Ritter G., Skwara, K. C.(1996). The home health visit: An appropriate unit for medicare payment. *Hlt Aff, 15*(4), 145–155.

Blumenthal, D., & Tavenner, M. (2010, July 13). The "Meaningful Use" regulation for electronic health records. *New England Journal of Medicine.* Retrieved from http://healthcarereform.nejm.org/?p=3732&query=home.

Bos, J. T., Frijters, D. H., Wagner, C., Carpenter, G. I., Finne-Soveri, H., et al. (2007). Variations in quality of Home Care between sites across Europe, as measured by Home Care Quality Indicators. *Aging Clin Exp Res, 19*(4), 323–329.

Bott, O. J., Marschollek, M., Wolf, K. H., & Haux, R. (2007). Towards new scopes: Sensor-enhanced regional health information systems. Part 1 architectural challenges. *Medthods Inf Med, 4,* 476–483.

Brennan, T. A., Leape, L. L., Laird, N. M., Hebert, L., Localio, A. R., et al. (1991). Incidence of adverse events and negligence in hospitalized patients: Results of the Harvard Medical Practice Study I. *New England Journal of Medicine, 34,* 370–376.

Canada Health Infoway. (2009). Making health information work better for Canadians. Corporate Business Plan 2009/2010. Retrieved from http://www2.infoway-inforoute.ca/Documents/bp/Business_Plan_2009-2010_en.pdf.

Cleland, J. G., Louis, A. A., Rigby, A. S., Jansens, U., & Balk, A. H. (2005) Noninvasive home telemonitoring for patients with heart failure at high risk of recurrent admission and death: the Trans-European Network-Home Care Management System (TENHMS) study. *J Am Coll Cardiol, 45*(10), 1654–1664.

Coleman, E. A., Smith, J. D., Frank, J. C., Min, S. J., Parry, C., et al. (2004). Preparing patient and caregivers to participate in care delivered across settings: The Care Transitions intervention. *J Am Geria Soc, 52*(11), 1817–1825.

Department of Health. (2009, January). The NHS Constitution for England. Retrieved from http://www.dh.gov.uk/en/Publicationsandstatistics/Publications/PublicationsPolicyAndGuidance/DH_093419.

Department of Health and Ageing. Australian Government. (2009, June). A healthier future for all Australians – final report. Retrieved from http://www.health.gov.au/internet/main/publishing.nsf/Content/nhhrc-report.

Doty, P. (2000). Cost effectiveness of home and community-based long-term care services. Retrieved from http://aspe.hhs.gov/daltcp/reports/costeff.htm.

Foust, J. B., Naylor, M. D., Boling, P. A., & Cappuzzo, K. A. (2005). Opportunities for improving post-hospital home medication management among older adults. *Home Healthcare Services Quarterly, 24*(1/2), 101–22.

Freudenheim, M. (2010, June 28). Preparing more care of elderly. *New York Times.* Retrieved from http://www.nytimes.com/2010/06/29/health/29geri.html?_r=l&src=me&pagewanted=print.

Gilje, F., Lacey, L., & Moore, C. (2007). Gerontology and geriatric issues and trends in U.S. nursing programs: a national survey. *J Prof Nurs, 23*(1), 21–29.

Hernadez, C., Casaa, A., & Escarrabill, J. (2003). The CHRONIC Project. Home hospitalization of exacerbated chronic obstructive pulmonary disease patients. *Eur Respir J, 21,* 58–67.

HITECH Act. (2010). Retrieved from http://www.hhs.gov/ocr/privacy/hipaa/administrative/enforcementrule/hitechenforcementifr.html.

Koch et al. (2009). Institute of Medicine. Retooling for an aging america. Building the healthcare workforce. Washington DC: The National Academies Press

Latimer, D. G., & Thornlow, D. K. (2006). Incorporating geriatrics into baccalaureate nursing curricula: Laying the groundwork with faculty development. *J Prof Nurs, 22*(2), 79–83.

Leff, B., & Montalto, M. (2004). Home hospital – toward a tighter definition. *J Am Geriatr Soc, 52,* 2141.

Leff, B., Burton, L., Mader, S., Naughton, B., Burl, J., et al. (2006). Satisfaction with Hospital-at-Home care. *J Am Geriatric Soc, 54*(9), 1355–1363.

Leff, B., Burton, L., Mader, S. L., Naughton, B., Burl, J., Inouye, S. K., et al. (2005). Hospital at Home: Feasibility and outcomes of a program to provide hospital-level care at home for acutely ill older patients. *Ann Inter Med, 143*(11), 798–808.

Medicare Payment Advisory Commission (Medpac). (2010, June). *A data book: Healthcare spending and the Medicare program.* Retrieved from http://www.medpac.gov/documents/Jun10DataBookEntireReport.pdf.

Institute of Medicine. (2008a). *Healthcare work force too small, unprepared for aging baby boomers; higher pay, more training, and changes in care delivery needed to avert crisis. (Press release).* Washington, DC: National Academies Press. Retrieved from http://www8.nationalacademies.org/onpinews/newsitem.aspx?RecordID=12089.

Institute of Medicine (IOM) (2008b). *Retooling for an Aging America: Building the Healthcare Workforce.* Washington, DC: The National Academies Press.

Murtaugh, C. M., McCall, N., Moore, S., & Meadow, A. (2003). Trends in Medicare home healthcare use: 1997–2001. *Hlt Aff, 22*(5), 146–156.

National Council on Disability. (2006). *Consumer directed health: How well does it work? Report to the President of the United States by the National Council on Disability (NCD).* Retrieved from http://www.ncd.gov/newroom/publications/pdf/consumerdirected.pdf.

National Health Services (NHS). (2010). *Connecting for health. Assistive technology: Helping patients to monitor vital signs at home.* Retrieved from http://www.connectingforhealth.nhs.uk/factsandfiction/patientcases/telehealth/?searchterm=home%20health.

National Health Services. (2009). *NHS choices: Your health, your choices.* Retrieved from http://www.nhs.uk/choiceintheNHS/Yourchoices/Pages/Yourchoices.aspx.

Naylor, M. D. (2006). Transitional care: A critical dimension of the home healthcare quality agenda. *Journal for Healthcare Quality, 28*(1), 48–54.

Naylor, M. D., Brooten, D. A., Campbell, R. L., Maislin, G. M., McCauley, K. M., & Schwartz, J. S. (2004). Transitional care of older adults hospitalized with heart failure: A randomized clinical trial. *Journal of the American Geriatrics Society, 52*(5), 675–684.

Nicholson, C., Bowler, S., Jackson, C. et al. (2001). Cost comparison of hospital-and home-based treatment models for acute chronic obstructive pulmonary disease. *Aust Health Rev; 24*, 181–187.

NNS Scotland. (2009). *Patient focus and public involvement*. Retrieved from www.scotland.gov.uk/Resource/Doc/158744/0043087.pdf.

Pearson, W. S., & Bercovitz, A. R. (2006). Use of computerized medical records in home health and hospice agencies: United States. *Vital Health Stat, 13*, 1–14.

Polisena, J., Coyle, D., Coyle, K., & McGill, S. (2009). Home telehealth for chronic disease management: A systematic review and an analysis of economic evaluations. *Int J Technol Assess Healthcare, 25*(3), 339–349.

Ram, F. S., Wedzicha, J. A., Wright, J., et al. (2004). Hospital at home for patients with acute exacerbations of chronic obstructive pulmonary disease: Systematic review of evidence. *BMJ, 329*, 315–319.

Randall, D. A. (2010). Legal and reimbursement issues for home telehealth. *Remington Report, 18*(2), 8–10,12.

Resnick, H. E., & Alwan, M. (2010). Use of health information technology in home health and hospice agencies: United States, 2007. *J Am Med Infor Assoc, 17*(4), 389–395.

Ricauda, N. A., Tibaldi, V., Leff, B., Scarafiotti, C., Marinello, R., Zanocci, M., & Molaschi, M. (2008). Substitutive "Hospital at home" versus inpatient care for elderly patients with exacerbations of chronic obstructive pulmonary disease: A prospective randomized, controlled trial. *J Am Geriatr Soc, 56*(3), 493–500.

SAINI. (2008). *Electronic Healthcare Services Concept Road Map for implementation in Finland*. Retrieved from http://www.sitra.fi/fi/Julkaisut/OhjelmienJulkaisut/teho/terveydenhuolto.htm.

Shaughness, P. W., Crisler, K. S., Schlenker, R. E., & Arnold, A. G. (1997). Outcomes across the care continuum: home healthcare. *Med Care, 35*, 1225–1226.

SITRA. (2009). The Finnish healthcare system: A value-based perspective. Retrieved from http://www.sitra.fi/fi/Julkaisut/OhjelmienJulkaisut/teho/terveydenhuolto.htm.

Southern California Evidence-Based Practice Center. (2010). Costs and benefits of health information technology. AHRQ Publication No. 06-E006, April, 2006. Retrieved from http://www.ahrq.gov/downloads/pub/evidence/pdf/hitsyscosts/hitsys.pdf.

Tinetti, M. E., Baker, D., Gallo, W. T., Nanda, A., Charpentier, P, & O'Leary, J. (2002). Evaluation of restorative care vs usual care for older adults receiving an acute episode of home care. *JAMA, 287*(16), 2098–2105.

US Census. 2005. Retrieved from http://www.census.gov/population/www/projections/projectionssagesex.html.

Vimarlund, V., Olve, N. G., Scandurra, I., & Koch, S. (2008). Organizational effects of information and communication technology (ICT) in elderly homecare: a case study. *Hlt Informatics J, 14*(3), 195–210.

Whitten, P., & Mickus, M. (2007). Home telecare for COPD/CHF patients: Outcomes and perceptions. *J Telemed Telecare, 13*(2), 69–73.

Whitten, P. S., Mair, F. S., Haycox, A., May, C. R., Williams, T. L., & Hellmich, S. (2002). Systematic review of cost effectiveness studies of telemedicine interventions. *BMJ, 324*(7351), 1434–1437.

Wilson, L. D. (2010). The American Association of Colleges of Nursing's Geriatric Nursing Education Consortium. *J Gerontol Nurs, 36*(7), 14–17. doi: 10.3928/00989134-20100528-01.

Continuum of Care Information Technology Systems

Gail E. Latimer

20

Computerized Provider Order Entry

Emily B. Barey

- OBJECTIVES
  1. The reader will be able to state two reasons why CPOE is different from other healthcare information technology implementations.
  2. The reader will be able to state at least five strategies to ensure a successful CPOE implementation and end-user adoption.
  3. The reader will be able to state at least one future possible direction of CPOE.
  4. The reader will be able to state three core competencies required of the nurse informatician working with CPOE.

- KEY WORDS
  CPOE
  ARRA
  meaningful use
  change management

COMPUTERIZED PROVIDER ORDER ENTRY

Much of the attention paid to computerized provider order entry (CPOE) has historically been associated with early adopters at academic medical centers, such as Brigham and Women's Hospital, and leading community sites, such as El Camino Hospital, reporting on their experiences with clinical information systems in the 1980s and 1990s. Then, in 2000 and 2001, through the publications of the Institute of Medicine's (IOM's) *To Err is Human* (Institute of Medicine [IOM], 2000) and *Crossing the Quality Chasm* (IOM, 2001), and the subsequent focus of The Agency for Healthcare Research and Quality on preventing medical errors this past decade, CPOE received renewed attention as a patient safety tool. The private sector, through employer organizations such

as the Leapfrog Group for Patient Safety, has also pursued a similar agenda (The Leapfrog Group, 2010). Each consistently recommends the use of CPOE to improve healthcare quality. The frequently highlighted benefits range from the simple (e.g., physician order legibility) to the more complex (e.g., decision support related to allergy and drug interaction checking, medication dosing guidance), and in some cases result in an overall decrease in patient mortality and significant financial return on investment (Kaushal et al., 2006; Longhurst et al., 2010; Poissant, Pereira, Tamblyn, & Kawasumi, 2005).

Recently, however, the call for CPOE implementation has taken on a new dimension with the passage of The Health Information Technology for Economic and Clinical Health (HITECH) Act of 2009. As part of the American Recovery and Reinvestment Act (ARRA) of 2009, the aim of the HITECH Act is to promote the adoption and meaningful use of health information technology (HIT). Included in the HITECH Act are financial incentives to physicians and healthcare organizations that utilize electronic health records (EHRs), including CPOE. These incentives will come in the form of increased reimbursement rates from the Centers for Medicaid and Medicare Services (CMS), but ultimately will result in a penalty if adoption and meaningful use of the EHR are not met. The final rule was published by the Department of Health and Human Services (DHHS) in July 2010 for the first phase of implementation, and more details are expected in 2011 and 2012 for the second and third phases (Department of Health and Human Services [DHHS], 2010).

According to the KLAS 2010 CPOE report, only 14% of all U.S. hospitals have achieved the expected 10% CPOE level required for the initial stage of meaningful use (Hess, 2010). And, although there are many reports and articles citing the benefits of CPOE, a review of the literature also reinforces the wide range of barriers and challenges to a successful CPOE adoption, including physician resistance, system cost, product immaturity, unintended errors, and unexpected increases in patient mortality subsequent to CPOE implementation (Ash et al., 2007; Han et al., 2005; Poon et al., 2004).

This chapter discusses a brief history of CPOE and its recently renewed significance on a national level with the passage of ARRA. Benefits of CPOE have been long established; however, ARRA offers new incentives to promote widespread adoption more rapidly. This chapter provides a review of successful CPOE implementation strategies, with special attention devoted to strategies and tactics that address the most common barriers to CPOE success noted in the literature including organization readiness and change management. The implementation methods described are based on best practices and case studies from the literature, along with the author's experience. The methods do not represent a specific, exhaustive implementation plan, but, rather, are a collection of recommendations to guide any CPOE implementation. Finally, the chapter sets the stage for the future of CPOE, including the required core competencies of the nurse informaticist for leading this type of implementation now and into the future.

The significance of CPOE cannot be underestimated. Although CPOE implies a physician- or provider-centric tool, the workflow and subsequent management of those patient care orders involves the entire interdisciplinary team, with the nurse at the center as patient care coordinator. CPOE is also often the foundation for standardizing care delivery and best practices, along with being an important component of advanced decision support.

As such, in addition to the broader backdrop of patient safety, quality, and now financial incentives, it is essential to recognize the impact of CPOE on the work of the nurse and the significance of the nursing informaticist in obtaining a core competency in CPOE.

DEFINITION OF CPOE

CPOE is often used as an abbreviation to represent how an EHR system requires a clinician to electronically enter patient care orders. There have been electronic order communication tools available in the past that allowed for the transmission of lab, radiology, medication, and other types of orders to downstream ancillary systems; however, they relied largely on the transcription of a handwritten physician note by a department secretary, nurse, or pharmacist and offered limited rules checking capacity.

The *P* in CPOE has most commonly stood for provider, but will also appear as physician or prescriber. This is what makes CPOE different from basic electronic order submission. The transcription step is removed, and the provider places the order directly into the system. By using *provider* it is also implied that the user placing the order is authorized to give or sign that order and leaves room for other disciplines in addition to physicians who have a scope of practice that supports CPOE, such as advanced practice nurses and physician assistants. CPOE is also different in that it is inherently tied to a clinical decision support system that enables the checking and presentation of patient safety rules during ordering, such as drug-drug interaction checking, duplicate checking, corollary orders, and dose calculations (Tyler, 2009).

CPOE standards are evolving. Organizations such as the National Quality Forum (NQF) and the Leapfrog Group wrote early proposals for required features and functions of CPOE as a way to promote and evaluate hospitals utilizing the tool to support safe medication practices. Leapfrog has maintained its CPOE standards since 2001, and they include CPOE that is linked to error prevention software and the ability to acknowledge with a reason any overrides of alerts or warnings presented to the provider (The Leapfrog Group, 2010). The NQF also requires the ability to document the reason for any override of an error prevention notice and includes the ability for the provider to see pertinent clinical information about the patient, such as allergies, at the time of ordering (National Quality Forum, 2003).

In 2005, Dr. Michael McCoy proposed three types of CPOE: basic, intermediate, and advanced (McCoy, 2005).

Basic CPOE incorporates order entry with simple decision support features such as allergy or drug-drug interaction checking. Intermediate level CPOE includes the display of additional relevant results at the time of ordering and the ability for providers to save their order preferences. Dr. McCoy considered advanced CPOE to represent advanced clinical order management, and it is here that more sophisticated decision support in the form of "guided ordering" or "mentored ordering" would be available (McCoy, 2005, p. 11).

The Certification Commission for Healthcare Information Technology (CCHIT) was founded in 2004 as a nonprofit organization with a mission to accelerate healthcare information technology adoption (Certification Commission on Health Information Technology [CCHIT], 2010). CCHIT is recognized as a certifying body by the federal government and has been accrediting EHR products since 2006 (CCHIT, 2010). The certification process requires that an EHR meet a comprehensive set of standards, including the essential features and functions of CPOE. The standards are established through voluntary work groups with representatives from across healthcare and information technology, and are revised annually. The CCHIT certification enables healthcare organizations to evaluate systems more effectively as they embark on selecting and implementing CPOE and other healthcare information technologies. Building consumer confidence in EHRs was an important precursor to the widespread adoption of EHRs and CPOE, and certification plays an important role in that. Perhaps more importantly, ARRA is now also explicit that the EHR technology used must be certified and that certification should be consistent with the current CCHIT approach (Blumenthal, 2009). Currently, the DHHS has granted EHR certification authority to both CCHIT and the Drummond Group.

The definition chosen for CPOE is important to clarify, as it will impact the scope of the CPOE implementation and the related design, build, testing, and training requirements. Will it be basic or advanced? Will it include physicians only or, more broadly, providers? The definition and standards used will also be significant moving forward as the government determines a final ruling on metrics to measure meaningful use of EHRs and CPOE and the corresponding incentive payment scales by CMS.

IMPLEMENTATION

Implementing CPOE, in many ways, is not unlike other health information technology (HIT) projects. It requires a project plan, with appropriate time to complete workflow analysis, system build, testing, and training. Like other HIT projects, the most successful implementations have a good change management plan that facilitates end-user adoption of the new technology. CPOE, however, is unlike other HIT projects in that it often impacts the healthcare organization on a much broader and deeper scale than, for example, activating a clinical data repository, picture archiving and communication system (PACS), or a clinical notes dictation system. CPOE is at the heart of patient care and cannot be done in isolation to one department or discipline, as it ultimately demands not only a new medium in which providers will work—the electronic health record—but also a new way in which to work.

A number of studies and reports have been written about successful implementation strategies for CPOE. Factors consistently cited include executive leadership, physician involvement, a multidisciplinary approach to implementation, good EHR system response time, and flexible training strategies (Drazen, Kilbridge, Metzger, & Turisco, 2000). This next section will build on these recommendations by reviewing the steps required to implement CPOE and then expanding on the practical how-to strategies to be successful.

There are five steps to implement CPOE. The first step is planning, including identifying sponsors of the project, a brief current state analysis, system selection, and ultimately developing an implementation plan. The second step is the design and build of the system, followed by testing. Design and build of the system requires careful workflow analysis and deep application-level knowledge to be successful. Testing is more than technical validation of interfaces and order transmittal. It is also an important step to identify any unintended consequences of the implementation and may also be used as a change management activity. The fourth step is training, which will be discussed not only as a formal phase, but as an activity that persists long after go live. The fifth step is go live and post live. It is critical that post live be included in the project plan and ultimately addressed as a perpetually active state.

Change management and communication activities are part of each implementation phase; as project milestones, they build on each other toward unifying end users and solidifying their readiness for a new way of working. The requirement of a comprehensive change management plan is reinforced by Studer (2005), who completed an extensive literature review of effectiveness of EHR implementations and concluded that organizational factors must be considered before, during, and after the implementation in order to promote successful adoption. Lapointe and

Rivard (2005) further suggested that change management must be addressed at the individual, group, and organizational levels. With this in mind, the implementation section of this chapter pays close attention to strategies that address both technical and organizational readiness for CPOE, with particular emphasis on the planning phase, as an early investment in this type of strategy will influence all subsequent phases and increase chances of implementation success.

The nurse informaticist has a role in every phase, but broadly represents integrating the experience of the patient, the end user, and the healthcare organization in order to ensure success for all stakeholders with CPOE. His or her skills in application knowledge, workflow analysis, and change management will be important contributions to the project.

PROJECT PLANNING

Choosing the best sponsors of the CPOE implementation is arguably the first milestone of the project and one that must be gotten right in the planning phase. Executive sponsorship and establishing a steering committee is the initial signal to all stakeholders that this project is not simply another isolated information technology (IT) project or one that will be completed by the IT department alone. There are 3 roles that are consistently present and recommended for success: clinical and administrative executives, practicing providers and clinicians, and IT.

The chief executive officer (CEO) or the chief operations officer (COO), chief nursing officer (CNO), and chief medical officer (CMO) represent the triad that will help set the tone of the implementation and remove any barriers to success. More and more, it is common to see this triad delegate its roles to a chief information officer (CIO), chief nursing information officer (CNIO), and chief medical information officer (CMIO), but it is important to distinguish delegating executive sponsorship from leadership in executive operations. There is no doubt that CIOs, CNIOs, and CMIOs have important roles to play in the execution of the CPOE project and its success, but because CPOE will be a fundamental change in the way the entire organization works those that are ultimately responsible for the organization should be its sponsors, while the others are core members of the steering committee.

Other members of the steering committee include practicing providers and clinicians, often referred to as *champions*. Their role is to be the bridge between leadership and those clinicians and providers who will actually be making the change to CPOE in their day-to-day practice. The most common members include representatives from nursing, physician, and pharmacy management and staff. Depending on the type and scope of the organization, it may also be important to consider the source of the physician representation. For example, if there is a large population of community physicians who refer patients to the hospital or will be affiliate users in their offices and clinics, then plan to include a doctor from that population. If it is an academic institution, then be careful to choose a physician who remains active in practice and will be an end user of the system, not simply a department chair.

In addition, the CIO and the project director will be critical members of the steering committee since they are the technical partners to the providers and executives and are responsible for ensuring the integrity of all existing systems, along with implementing the new CPOE successfully. The CNIO and CMIO should also be included here, as they are also key advisors on aligning the clinical, technical, and operational goals of the organization. Some organizations may also have a chief technology officer (CTO), and if so, they would also be included as an IT representative on the steering committee.

Benefit may also be found in representation by a patient or family member, a board member, and a member of a union, if appropriate. An articulate patient or family member who is familiar with the organization can be a symbolic reminder to the steering committee of the broader CPOE mission: to improve safety and quality. Some organizations also choose to include a board member, given the large capital investment that CPOE implementation often represents. If the organization is heavily unionized, the implementation may also be a good opportunity for labor partnership, and involvement at the highest level facilitates cooperation and ensures transparency in all communication early.

Once the executive sponsors and steering committee are identified, there is a wide variety of ways to handle the organization of the people and processes that will be the building blocks of the CPOE implementation beneath them. There are a few guiding principles that can help establish a functional project structure.

The first is to think of the CPOE project organization chart as ultimately evolving into permanent processes, rather than a structure created simply for the sake of getting to system go live. This is often one of the hardest shifts for an organization to make, because it demands a level of clarity and standardization in decision making that is typically not present from the outset. It also demands that those decision-making processes move quickly to avoid delays in the project that could cost both money and goodwill capital with stakeholders.

The second is to avoid creating parallel organizational structures. In the same spirit of the project evolving into permanent processes, so too should the structure be integrated into existing work groups, committees, and communication channels, if possible. This clearly sets the stage for anticipating that CPOE will be permanent, and it will be everyone's job to ensure CPOE is successful—not just the physicians or the IT department. To underscore this further, any aspect of an EHR implementation, including pharmacy, medication administration, and clinical notes, should be integrated this way into the organization's day-to-day operations to promote meaningful use of these systems. Using existing structures also lends itself as a familiar way to think about the needs of the individual, group, and organization for change management.

One exception to this may be the establishment of a new physician or provider advisory council, if one does not already exist, to support the steering committee and IT project team. An advisory council is typically led by the physician champion along with the CMIO. Although physicians are usually well represented by the physician champion and CMIO, the council is an important body to help engage a broader physician stakcholder group in decision making. It is often the group that also facilitates communication about the CPOE project at a local or department level within the organization.

With the physician advisory council in mind, there is an important final guiding principle in organizing the structure of the CPOE project, which is to spend as much effort on executive sponsorship as grassroots engagement. The most effective implementations of CPOE have created deliberate communication and decision-making channels between the bedside and the steering committee. This is often accomplished through the combination of an existing shared governance structure and appointing a local-level physician, nurse, and pharmacy champion or deputy champions that mimic the executive sponsorship team. Not to be confused with the concept of super users, this triad's role is to ensure all decisions being made related to the CPOE implementation can be localized successfully, if not to bring forward questions or concerns for resolution.

One of the first tasks that local-level stakeholders or advisory councils can assist with in the planning phase is a brief current state review of existing workflows and clinical care processes in their departments. It is tempting to do an exhaustive review, but it is more effective to orient the review to core clinical workflows and cap-

ture both future state needs and vision. This work serves three purposes: (1) it will generate the data and ideas for establishing metrics of success related to CPOE that are meaningful at a local level, (2) it will provide an early test of the communication and decision-making processes established by the steering committee to facilitate individual, group, and organizational dialogue, and (3) it will ready the organization for CPOE selection process. This is a good example of where the nursing informaticist can provide helpful guidance to local-level stakeholders to complete the needs assessment process, and align the outputs into a cohesive set of organization-wide metrics.

The selection process of CPOE does not need to be protracted, but it does need to engage as many providers as possible and establish confidence at all levels that the system selected is a good fit for the organization. Common activities include watching product demonstrations and utilizing the future state documentation noted previously to guide system review and follow-up questions, attending site visits to other organizations using the system, and reading the literature about CPOE in order to informally benchmark the organization's readiness to work toward a successful implementation. The other prerequisite to system selection will be that the product meets CCHIT certification or appropriate requirements per the final specifications in ARRA and the HITECH Act.

Despite the emphasis here on physician and end-user engagement, it is essential that both the informatics and IT groups also complete a thorough due diligence of their ability to implement and support the system on behalf of their provider counterparts. A system recommendation should reflect the best thinking of both clinical and technical stakeholders.

DESIGN AND BUILD

The thoughtful planning in identifying CPOE project leadership, stakeholder groups, and decision-making processes, along with completing the current state review, helps set the stage for an effective system design and build phase. This is the second step of the implementation process and is concentrated on two primary activities: validating that the CPOE-related workflows in the EHR system will support the organization's clinical care processes and standards, and reviewing the clinical content, such as order sets, to use in those workflows. If neither is complete nor appropriate, then it is necessary to complete the system build changes or identify an alternative workflow support.

Selected by the steering committee and key stakeholder groups, the organization's end users and subject matter experts will review the CPOE-related workflows and clinical processes to ensure the system will meet their needs. Guiding principles, as well as technical change control processes will need to be established to enable the group to work effectively and consistently across disciplines and departments reviewing CPOE processes. These standards and the ability to track changes related to design and build decisions should not be overlooked, as they will serve as a blueprint for future system testing and maintenance. Individual flow diagrams may be used to help capture the process, along with related decisions. This will also serve as a way to do high-level conflict checking and resolve any integration issues within the process or its related technical build. It is also often an opportunity to look for process improvement opportunities for the organization that may be leveraged by using an EHR and CPOE.

As an extension, if the organization does not already have a clinical content management approach in place, now is the time to determine one. Here, instead of flow diagrams to capture a workflow or clinical process, the goal is to track the source and date of creation of standards of care, namely, order sets, clinical protocols, decision support rules, and preference lists, that will be the content utilized in the CPOE system during the order entry process. Accurately building this content in a user-friendly way is a confidence builder for the providers who will be using it in CPOE, as it is one of the main ways the system reflects that it was designed by providers like them in their specialty, and not generic primary care. The documentation and tracking of the content build is also especially important if the organization has made a commitment to utilizing evidence-based practices, as this type of content demands regular review to ensure it is up-to-date. It is also a simple way to avoid content duplication and to promote basic standardization in clinical care.

With this infrastructure in place, one of the first design questions that will need to be addressed is regarding the level of standardization. There are 2 types of standardization that need to be determined: workflow process and clinical content. Standardization is helpful to reduce IT maintenance, ensure consistent training and use of the system, and enable common reporting tools, but it is critical not to standardize at the expense of system usability. A good rule of thumb is to let the organization's current policy and procedures drive standardization of clinical content to promote best patient care practices, but to allow for some localization of display of that content, as well as minor workflow modifications to support ease of adoption. This is assuming, of course, that the organization's existing clinical practices are consistent and well documented in order to be used as a primary source.

For example, the pneumonia order set should be standardized at the organization level, but common defaults within that order set may be determined either by the department or an individual end user recognizing that the critical care unit and an intensivist may have slightly different needs and preferences than the primary care provider admitting a patient with pneumonia to the general medical-surgical unit. This approach allows each to remain consistent within current best practice recommendations but still have appropriate choices for their patients. Similarly, the workflow related to medication management within the pneumonia order set may be different in the critical care unit, where a clinical pharmacist could be staffed locally for real-time consultation and verification. On a medical-surgical unit, this happens in a decentralized, asynchronous way. Both the content and workflows presented here are acceptable, but both require an organization-wide agreement on level of standardization, because if the goal was to use the exact same order set defaults and workflow in both departments, then the implication would be that each department was staffed the same and taking care of similar patients, which is clearly not the case, nor feasible. This example also highlights that careful workflow analysis is required to ensure that from a technical build perspective, the CPOE order set and order transmittal functions can accommodate this simultaneous variation in clinical operations.

In addition to careful CPOE workflow analysis within the EHR system, it is imperative to complete careful workflow analysis across clinical information systems such as operating room, lab, radiology, dietary, and any other ancillary systems that will need to receive order messages, or that the CPOE system will need to receive messages from. This demands not only CPOE application knowledge, but also a close partnership with those who have ancillary system application and workflow knowledge to ensure there are no interruptions to the CPOE workflow and subsequent patient care delivery. These integration points will be highlighted in the workflow diagrams, but establishing a proactive forum to address the points is recommended during the design and build phase. Waiting until the testing phase, where integration conflicts or shortfalls often become more obvious, is too late to adequately address either a change in process or a change in system build.

During this phase, it is easy to be very focused on the technical aspects of CPOE and lose sight of the broader impact of CPOE changes on the day-to-day work of the providers and other end users. In order to better anticipate the communication and training needs related to these changes, it can be helpful to use a survey tool during workflow validation to ask participating end users and subject matter experts what changes will impact them most, what they believe will be positive and negative about the change, and any outstanding questions they might have about the change. Another strategy for eliciting this feedback is to incorporate an element of hands-on use of the system by the end users and subject matter experts. Typically, this type of activity is reserved for the testing phase, but done on a small scale here it can provide an enormous amount of early feedback on the integrity of the decisions made thus far, as well as an initial sense of system usability. Finally, engaging providers in order set and content review can again be a way of assuring them that this is a clinical project and every effort is being made to meet their given specialty's needs. This may be done through the physician advisory council or representatives they choose.

TESTING

Testing is very important before going live with any system. Before going live with a CPOE system, it is vital to do many different kinds of testing, since there is often a large, complex infrastructure of hardware and software involved. Important types of testing are: functional, integration, and regression. It goes without saying that these will be completed by creating the appropriate test plans and tracking and resolving any issues identified. The intent of this section is not to provide an exhaustive testing plan, but to focus on some of the nuances of testing CPOE that may also serve as change management activities or help promote provider adoption, including usability testing, response time, hardware and printing testing, and dress rehearsal activities. The secondary goal is to build a bridge between the design and build phase to the training phase. Much of the output of testing will lead not only to technical changes but also training curriculum points, and the teams responsible for this work will need to have a good communication plan.

Testing is the first opportunity to involve a larger group of providers and end users beyond the original stakeholders and subject matter experts who validated the CPOE workflows in the design and build phase. This group is often referred to as *super users*, but here the role is expanded. Selecting them early and engaging them through a specific training and orientation process will enable them to be a better support mechanism at the local level to the implementation team, the clinical champions, and training team. Using them to help with testing activities is a good way for them to gain system exposure and build relationships both with the implementation team and the local end users they represent.

Usability testing is an area that loans itself to the fresh perspective of a super user, who, until now, has most likely not been engaged with the implementation. Usability is a quality attribute that assesses how easy user interfaces are to use (Nielsen, 2003). There are many quality attributes that represent usability, and for the purposes of CPOE usability, those to focus on include learnability, efficiency, errors, satisfaction, and utility (Nielsen, 2003). Usability expert Jakob Nielsen stresses that it is better to run several small tests in an iterative approach, where five end users are typically enough to identify the most important usability problems (2003). With this in mind, there are three types of testing activities that will promote system usability and build exposure to the new system in a constructive way for the purposes of identifying additional change management needs.

The first activity is simply to have each super user pull an existing patient chart and try to replicate it in the new system utilizing a provider type of login for that specialty. For example, a labor and delivery nurse, unit secretary, or obstetrician super user would try to enter all of the orders in the patient chart into the new system and keep a log of what they could find, what they couldn't find, what default settings seemed incorrect, and the like. This feedback is then combined with others from different specialties to identify any repetitive themes that warrant reworking in system design or other more minor interventions, such as build changes or follow-up training points.

The second activity is to pair the super user with an implementation team member to shadow a provider on rounds and try to simultaneously complete the work in the new system while the provider uses the old system. Ideally, this is done across a majority of specialties at different times of day to achieve a reasonable spectrum in your sample. Keep in mind, however, that five times should identify the majority of issues worthy of following up proactively.

The third activity is for the super user to identify three to five others from the department to participate in a simulation activity, where the provider representative may place a set of orders, while the nurse, pharmacist, and unit secretary ensure that all the necessary order transmittal and management steps flow to the correct output for implementation of those orders.

System response time, hardware configuration, and printing are also particularly sensitive during CPOE adoption and should also be well tested, engaging super users and other provider representation for feedback. These may be incorporated as aspects of the usability testing activities outlined above, and may have specific testing plans as well for a complete review.

Other strategies that reinforce testing, change management, and provide a bridge between design and build and training include completing presentations of integrated CPOE workflows to larger audiences, dress rehearsal activities across departments to simulate patient admission, transfer and discharge workflows, and additional small-scale, hands-on activities such as piloting training modules and materials.

Wherever possible, the goal with these activities is for the local-level champions, along with the super users and local level leadership, to come together to take accountability for resolving any issues they may identify and to present regular updates and communication to those they represent. The emphasis should also be placed on testing both the most common workflows as well as the known higher-risk workflows, such as transfers and changes in level of care, or where multiple systems or modules may overlap and integration or interfaces are essential. In this way, usability testing can serve both technical and change management purposes.

TRAINING

Training for CPOE should not be underestimated; however, it does not need to all be didactic and classroom-based prior to go live to be effective. In fact, a combination of methods coordinated prior to, during, and post live will promote not only competency in the new system, but also instill confidence in the new way of working and delivering patient care with CPOE. While it is necessary to train a wide variety of end users in addition to the providers placing the orders using CPOE, it is also important to balance a standardized curriculum for consistency with tailoring approaches to address specific needs of different groups of end users. This flexibility will remove any barriers to training and ensure a successful go live. There are five guiding principles that will help facilitate the training plan.

The first guiding principle is to plan for training to take place before, during, and after go live. Most organizations only plan and budget for pre live, and yet almost all of them end up implementing some sort of follow-up or refresher training thirty to sixty days post live, because they underestimated the impact that CPOE would have on the clinical operations of the organiza-

tion. Likewise, most end users are more ready to learn on the job, when they need the knowledge immediately. While it is not recommended to save all training for the go-live date, it is recommended to again plan and budget for the necessary support during go live to assess competency with the new system and reinforce teaching points where necessary.

The second guiding principle is to consider mixed mediums for the delivery of training. Classroom-based has its advantages but is better leveraged as a place to reinforce and expand on introductory e-learning modules that an end user could complete independently as a prerequisite to the classroom. In addition, the classroom is a place to focus on provider specialty–specific examples and real-time question and answer periods. For example, pre live a provider may complete a series of 10- to 15-minute e-learning topics on finding patients in the system, medication reconciliation, placing orders, and managing orders during daily rounds and discharges. The provider would then come to class to have these principles reinforced, along with an opportunity to be introduced to more complex topics, such as creating his or her own preference list of orders, or how to manage a clinical decision support alert. During go live, at-the-elbow support is available to reinforce teaching points and answer questions ad hoc, but providing drop-in access in a provider lounge or a conference room for other end users to access for specific follow-up questions during go live is also a good way to promote additional learning in a lower stress environment than at the patient bedside.

The curriculum should be workflow-based. Too often, clinical information system training focuses on simple how-to functions rather than exposing providers and other end users to the full clinical process and their role in it using CPOE. This is important for two reasons: it highlights that their day-to-day work is going to change with CPOE, and, as such, is an opportunity to provide them with anticipatory guidance about the impact of CPOE at go live. It also reminds end users why it is essential that they utilize the tool as it is being trained to achieve the expected outcome for the order they are placing or managing in order to avoid any delay in patient care.

Workflow-based curriculum can seem daunting and time consuming at first. To address this, plan to begin socializing providers and end users to what a workflow is prior to training through brief department meeting agenda items, bulletin board examples, or e-learning. Every workflow of the organization does not need to be explicitly taught. Emphasis should be placed on those with highest risk, such as patients with changes in their levels of care, where the technical and clinical handoff must be correct, and on high-volume examples for each department to utilize in their training exercises and competencies. For example, an obstetrician must know how to order and manage pitocin effectively, whereas an orthopedic surgeon must understand the patient-controlled analgesia and packed red blood cell workflows, as does the care team who will implement those orders on behalf of the provider.

The fourth guiding principle is to train both order entry and order management to providers, nurses, pharmacists, unit clerks, and other ancillary users downstream, such as lab, radiology, and operating room. This is to ensure that patient care is not interrupted, but also to build in additional provider support if an issue needs to be resolved. There may be multiple clinical information systems in play here along with CPOE, and end users who may not directly use CPOE still need exposure to the upstream workflow and the output they should expect either within other modules of the EHR or within their ancillary system via an interface. Exposing providers to order management also reinforces that CPOE is a new way of working relative to sharing active orders lists with all providers on the care team and reconciling those orders daily for conflicts, duplicates, and the broader planning of patient care. Historically, order management was done largely through interpretation by downstream staff, such as nurses and pharmacists. With CPOE that responsibility returns to the originating provider and the level of specificity required by the provider now about his or her orders is often an enormous change that must be clearly addressed through early exposure to the concept and training.

The fifth guiding principle is to plan and promote training early. As outlined here, training is clearly more than a pre-live activity in the days leading up to a go live. It is also an important component of the change management plan and has a number of integration points to be addressed if it is truly to be workflow-based. Promoting training early is also essential for the organization to prepare to backfill staff as needed or change provider schedules, to set expectations about compliance with the required training plan, and to engage executive sponsors to address any points of resistance early. Temporary supplemental trainers will also need to be identified to address concurrent training classes and needs that the core training team will not be able to cover alone. Planning and promoting early training must also be carefully coordinated with the CPOE build team and IT department to be sure that appropriate access to system environments is available to support developing, testing, and deploying the training curriculum.

As noted previously in the testing recommendations, the role of super users may be expanded here as well to formalize their roles as extensions of the training team at a local level. The key is not only to engage them early, but to deliberately assign a manager to the group who can be the liaison to the training team and hold the super users accountable for specific deliverables, such as ensuring that all providers and end users in their department are registered for training, and utilizing a competency check list during go live to assess the department's end users, or to round with the clinical champions and IT team members to be sure everything is working as expected at go live.

GO LIVE

The best CPOE go lives are as close to a non-event as possible. In other words, all the investment of time and effort prior to golive preparing for CPOE and subsequent changes associated with it pays the organization back in dividends with no interruptions in patient care, providers and end users confidently working through the learning curve of CPOE and order management, and good system reliability and response time at go live. To accomplish this, some of the final preparations to note for a smooth activation include a thorough cutover plan, appropriate levels of at-the-elbow support, and an issue response system in place that allows quick follow-up communication and resolution to any problems reported with the system.

A cutover plan represents the preparations to transition from one order entry system to the new CPOE system. In most cases, this is a fairly complex process, given the number of systems involved other than the EHR and CPOE, and the number of end users expected to be impacted. It is also a high-risk process because a provider's orders represent a significant part of the patient's plan of care and should not be interrupted or delayed due to the system change. A reliable cutover plan is integrated across systems and disciplines, well rehearsed, and visible to providers and other end users at the point of care. This last point is often overlooked. Cutover is the first milestone of the go-live phase and has an enormous potential to make a positive impression on the organization if it is managed well. It is most common for existing patient care orders to be transitioned from one system to the new CPOE system behind the scenes by providers, pharmacists, and nurses. This remains the recommendation; however, it is worth considering a rolling or phased cutover strategy that would allow for a project team expert and the clinical champions for the department to be available in person while end users are verifying that the orders were transitioned correctly and resolve any issues in real time, avoiding end-user frustration and anxiety with early phone calls to a go-live command center. This is particularly helpful in higher-acuity or risk areas, such as critical care, labor and delivery, and oncology.

Appropriate levels of at-the-elbow support during a CPOE go live is often debated based on resource constraints of the organization; however, there is no consistent ratio noted in the literature that reliably states a minimum number of people or hours available to support providers and end users during the go-live transition. To be sure, educated estimates can and should be made, including consideration for the percentage of compliance of providers with the training plan, the number of super users and local level champions who have been engaged with the project, and the depth of completion of the change management plan. In other words, how close is the organization to CPOE adoption prior to go live? Other considerations include the acuity and complexity of a department or patient population, past history of that department with any large-scale change, and scope of the implementation—how many other systems are going live simultaneously with CPOE that may also demand support?

At a minimum, the organization should plan on some level of support 24 hours a day for two weeks, both in a centralized command center and decentralized on each patient care unit or department. It is also important to be sensitive to the fact that, during those two weeks it may be required to shift resources based on business patterns. For example, it is not unusual to go live on a weekend with relative calm, but as Monday morning begins and several other departments come online, such as hospital outpatient areas and day surgery, support needs will begin to peak. It can also be helpful to look proactively at the planned surgery admissions or to watch the emergency department track board closely for admissions and deploy support to address the high-intensity needs of a new admission workflow using CPOE. Although the bulk of your support efforts should be spent addressing the needs of the majority, there may be key opinion leaders within the provider group or clinical leadership that are worth assigning a concierge, one-on-one type of support to during their initial rounds with CPOE. This can obviously be an expensive approach, but the goodwill effort may also help the morale of the entire group.

In the end, like most things, it is more a matter of quality than quantity of support, and, ultimately, it is not the support that will determine if the go live is successful, but the processes and communication to handle any issues. There are two ways to handle issues that may arise: proactively and reactively. Proactively, members of the implementation team, clinical champions, and super users should round frequently to the departments to identify issues by interacting with providers and end users, and resolving any concerns as they go. During this time, it can be very powerful if a member of the executive team of the organization also attends these rounds, not only to acknowledge concerns and communicate efforts to resolve them, but to provide positive reinforcement for the effort being made by providers and other end users during the transition. Other proactive strategies include having leadership and steering committee members host daily town hall meetings for providers and end users to attend to receive updates and listen to any issues from the field. A daily blog by the chief medical or nursing officer that invites comments can also be a successful medium. The key is to have real problem solvers visible as much as possible to the organization, and for those leaders to be supported by an issue resolution process that is fast and reliable.

The issue resolution process is by nature reactive, as only what is known can be resolved, so both the proactive and reactive components are necessary. The issue resolution process is best represented in a workflow diagram so it is clear to all members of the go-live team—including executives, steering committee members, clinical champions, and super users—how issues will be tracked and managed. The basis of this blueprint should already be reflected in existing implementation technical or system change control documentation. The primary adjustment to make to the process during the go-live phase is the response time to issue resolution. Metrics should be set for a response back to the reporter of the issue, based on the priority level of that issue. Categorization of priority levels should be clear and actionable, including a specific path for any issue described as patient safety–related. The key is that the process allows as many issues to be resolved in real time, and that even the minor issues have a response back to the reporter within 24 hours. The issues list should also have frequent clinical review, particularly if those documenting issues are nonclinical by background, and be reported at least daily to the executive sponsorship team. It can be helpful to start using this go-live process in the weeks leading up to go live, or as early as a pilot during the testing phase, to dress-rehearse it well and better anticipate any changes that may need to be made to support it. This further reinforces the change management aspect of the project plan by initiating activities early and committing to adjusting as needed for the best possible outcome.

Although this has not been an exhaustive review of all go-live activities, these three along with the previously noted training recommendation to deliberately assess competency with the new system during go live will serve as a solid foundation for adoption of CPOE during the go-live phase, and help identify key considerations for the transition to the post live and optimization phase.

POST LIVE AND OPTIMIZATION

Transitioning to post live typically begins two to four weeks after go live. It is, however, helpful to remain in the spirit of implementation or as go live–oriented as you can to ensure that issue resolution continues, morale remains high, and communication about the new CPOE system does not diminish. In other words, the processes that have been utilized thus far should continue despite the fact that at-the-elbow support has been rolled back and the centralized command center may have closed with CPOE operations now returning to the IT department location.

The first step of the post-live phase is to evaluate the initial feedback from the go live and use of the CPOE system. This may be accomplished through end-user survey tools, CPOE system reports to provide initial statistics on use and compliance, and a review of outstanding issues. This review should help set the priorities for post-live training, as well as identify areas that require a more thorough process review before adjusting system design or build. This latter point can be a difficult aspect of the transition from go live to post live, as it is now necessary to balance the need for continuing to quickly resolve low-level system build issues while tackling some of the more persistent underlying operations, clinical practice, or workflow issues that may have surfaced during the go live and ultimately be the root cause of several issues. In order to prioritize this work, it can be helpful to go back to the basics with a mock Joint Commission survey, patient safety review, completing a series of chart reviews and tracers, or identifying significant changes to revenue or patient satisfaction to facilitate unified agreement on what should be worked on next by the implementation team. CPOE vendor partnership is a given throughout the implementation. It is particularly critical at this time to provide any assistance needed to resolve outstanding issues.

The second step comes soon after the initial review, or is concurrent with it to celebrate the organization's accomplishment in reaching the CPOE goal. The majority of healthcare organizations in the United States still do not have CPOE in place so any group that accomplishes this should feel very proud of their work. This provides a natural progression to the third step, which is to share your experience with others through the writing of papers, presentations at conferences, and being a site visit and resource to others implementing CPOE.

Although the terms *post live* and *optimization* are nebulous with regard to how long this phase should last, the working assumption should be forever. The issue review process will become a permanent, iterative one, along with maintaining the CPOE content and adding to it. CPOE is a new way of working and delivering patient care, the full benefits of which will not be realized without daily attention to making the system better, utilizing new features as they become available, and incorporating it as a tool in every discussion about process improvement at the organization. Although there are a number of other HIT and broader clinical operations priorities competing for the resources applied to the CPOE implementation, now is the time to take careful stock of those resources and processes to be sure they are aligned well and embedded within the rest of the organization to reinforce the sense of permanence in using this tool. The initial investment is too great to consider go live or post live the end, when in fact it is just barely the beginning to leveraging HIT, and the ARRA meaningful use standard should only be the organization's minimum.

THE FUTURE OF CPOE

There is no doubt that CPOE will be an important feature and function of EHRs for the foreseeable future. As noted previously, recent, renewed attention to the adoption of CPOE at a national level with the passage of ARRA has solidified CPOE's position as significant to the delivery of healthcare in the future. The increased number of providers using CPOE alone will change the course of future development in this area, not to mention advances in software, hardware, and interoperability standards.

The culture of adoption of CPOE today is still largely one of resistance. As CPOE becomes the norm, healthcare organizations and providers alike will begin to have different expectations of the tool and its application to practice. The focus of CPOE software development has been oriented to improving basic usability and addressing specific workflow concerns, such as medication reconciliation. In the future, the focus will be on making CPOE smarter and able to better anticipate the provider's next action based on past patterns of use. In addition, clinical decision support will continue to become more robust and patient-specific, but with it will be a more elegant management of alerting, to avoid alert fatigue.

The implementation of CPOE will also shift in the future. As CPOE becomes the norm, it will bring an increased confidence in implementation models and adoption strategies. The emphasis will shift from designing and building systems locally for each organization to accepting standard workflows and content that reflect collective best practices. This in turn will allow for more rapid deployment of advanced clinical decision support features and patient safety benefits realization.

Hardware platforms for personal computing are another exciting area to watch for the future of CPOE. Providers will be able to choose from a wide range of devices in size and portability that will be increasingly enabled for touch screen and tailored to the unique information needs of a care area, such as intensive care, surgery, or oncology. There will be continued improvement of integration between telecommunication systems and EHR software that will facilitate increased remote alerting, monitoring, and access capabilities.

As interoperability standards between EHR systems improve, it is quite possible that resurgence in a "best-of-breed" vendor approach to EHR software modules could occur. It would require a significant expansion of data exchange standards beyond medication, allergy, and problem lists, but it is not unfathomable, considering the leaps in HIT standardization in the past five years alone.

Research related to the impact of CPOE adoption on this new scale will be critical to guiding its future, and the nurse informaticist has as much to contribute to shaping that future as leaders of CPOE implementations.

CORE COMPETENCIES OF THE NURSE EXPERT IN CPOE

Sensmeier summarized the demand for nursing informatics professionals in 2006 and quoted the American Medical Informatics Association (AMIA) Chair, Charles Safran, MD as stating that "every hospital and care setting needs one [nurse informatician]" in order to meet the government's vision for EHRs (2006, p.169). This is further reinforced in the 20th Annual HIMSS Leadership Survey where "half of healthcare IT professionals indicated that a focus on clinical systems will be their organizations' top IT priority in the next year, with a specific focus on EMR and CPOE technology" (Health Information Management Systems Society [HIMSS], 2009, p. 7). A significant barrier identified by the survey was a lack of IT staffing, particularly in application-

level support and process or workflow design (HIMSS, 2009), 2 of the core competencies required for the nurse expert in CPOE and highlighted by this chapter as essential elements of successful CPOE implementations. Two additional competencies required for the nurse expert in CPOE would include the ability to prepare and lead a large-scale change management plan, and comfort in navigating the national healthcare policy waters currently driving many of the clinical information system implementations.

Application-level knowledge represents the ability to assemble the building blocks of a clinical information system in the most effective way to meet the needs of the end user. In the case of CPOE, this will require not only technical competency for the purposes of designing and building the workflows to deliver patient care orders into the application, but also content management knowledge to standardize those orders and reinforce them with evidenced-based practice. More broadly, application-level knowledge also includes the ability to assess the integration points and impact of a particular application like CPOE with other applications like a results interface or pharmacy information system.

Workflow and clinical process knowledge is essential for successfully translating and aligning the needs of the end user, the patient, and the healthcare organization into the application, and leveraging its features and functions to meet those needs. As no single nurse informaticist can know everything about all of an organization's processes, workflow analysis skills draw on the nurse's underlying ability to interview clients for their history, complete an assessment, and collaborate across disciplines to meet a common goal. These are skills that would have been learned in nursing school for the purpose of patient care, and here scale for the purpose of ensuring the best outcomes for the organization utilizing the CPOE being implemented. For example, a nurse would never implement a plan of care for a patient simply based on diagnosis alone. So too a nurse informaticist would never implement CPOE simply based on one provider or one department.

Basic change management skills are also learned by nurses early in their clinical careers, as they relate to providing patients with education about their plan of care. This may include anticipatory guidance for changes large and small to a patient's lifestyle, daily routine, relationships, and perception of themselves. The nurse's ability to establish a healthy, trusting relationship with the client is at the core of successful patient education. Preparing an organization for the changes related to CPOE is, at its core, fundamentally not that different; however, the scale is significantly bigger and broader as the learning styles, motivations, and metrics of success for the CPOE implementation will vary widely across providers, patients, the interdisciplinary team, and the organization itself. Subsequent "coping mechanisms" for the CPOE changes will also vary by organization based on culture, infrastructure, available resources, and the ability to apply those resources. The expert nurse in CPOE is competent in understanding and anticipating these needs, and proactively leads through them in a positive, constructive way.

National healthcare policy review has often been reserved for the scope of practice of nurse leaders in management or academia. The expert nurse in CPOE, however, can no longer isolate him or herself from the of work of government on healthcare information technology. As stated previously, the implications of healthcare reform and ARRA are now more than ever tightly intertwined with the daily care of patients and the clinical information systems that support that care delivery. While an advanced degree in healthcare policy is not necessary, the competent nurse informaticist should understand the regulatory and compliance landscape, and its impact on clinical processes and applications, as this will always be an influence on his or her future work.

CONCLUSION

CPOE is one of the most challenging areas within healthcare IT today, and yet it has the promise of significant benefits to both patient and provider. CPOE systems have improved over the years and will only continue to become more user-friendly and sophisticated in their clinical decision support capabilities as the demand increases from broader adoption. Cultural barriers to CPOE implementation will also shift as adoption becomes required to demonstrate meaningful use of an EHR. With core competencies of systems knowledge, workflow analysis, change management, and healthcare policy, the nurse informaticist will be well positioned to support CPOE implementations today and shape the systems of tomorrow.

REFERENCES

Ash, J. S., Sittig, D. F., Poon, E. G., Guappone, K., Campbell, E., & Dykstra, R. H. (2007). The extent and importance of unintended consequences related to computerized provider order entry. *Journal of the American Medical Informatics Association, 14*(5): 415–423.

Blumenthal, D. (2009). Stimulating the adoption of health information technology. *New England Journal of Medicine, 360*(15): 1477–1479.

Certification Commission for Health Information Technology. (2010). *About the certification commission for health technology.* Retrieved from http://www.cchit.org/about.

Department of Health and Human Services. (2010). *Medicare and medicaid programs; electronic health record incentive program.* Retrieved from http://www.ofr.gov/OFRUpload/OFRData/2010-17207_PI.pdf.

Drazen, E., Kilbridge, P., Metzger, J., & Turisco, F. (2000). *A primer on physician order entry.* Oakland, CA: California HealthCare Foundation.

Han, Y. Y., Carcillo, J. A., Venkataraman, S. T., Clark, R. S. B., Watson, R. S., Nguyen, T. C., . . . Orr, R. A. (2005). Unexpected increased mortality after implementation of a commercially sold computerized physician order entry system. *Pediatrics, 116*(6): 1506–1512.

Health Information Management Systems Society. (2009). 20th annual HIMSS leadership survey. Chicago, IL: Health Information Management Systems Society. Retrieved from http://www.himss.org/2010Survey/healthcareCIO_final.asp.

Hess, J. (2010). *CPOE Digest 2010: Traffic Jams on the Road to Meaningful Use.* Orem, UT: KLAS Research.

Institute of Medicine. (2000). *To Err is Human: Building a Safer Health System.* Washington, DC: National Academies Press.

Institute of Medicine. (2001). *Crossing the Quality Chasm: A New Health System for the 21st Century.* Washington, DC: National Academies Press.

Kaushal, R., Jha, A. K., Franz, C., Glaser, J., Shetty, K.D., Jaggi, T., . . . Bates, D. W. (2006). Return on investment for a computerized physician order entry system. *Journal of the American Medical Informatics Association, 13*(3), 261–266.

Lapointe, L., & Rivard, S. (2005). Clinical information systems: understanding and preventing their premature demise. *Electronic Healthcare 3*(4): 92–100.

The Leapfrog Group. (2010). *Factsheet: computerized physician order entry.* Washington, D.C.: The Leapfrog Group. Retrieved from http://www.leapfroggroup.org/media/file/FactSheet_CPOE.pdf.

Longhurst, C. A., Parast, L., Sandborg, C. I., Widen, E., Sullivan, J., Hahn, J. S., . . . Sharek, P. J. (2010). Decrease in hospital-wide mortality rate after implementation of a commercially sold computerized physician order entry system. *Pediatrics, 126*(1), e1–e8. Retrieved from http://www.pediatrics.org.

McCoy, M. J. (2005). Advanced clinician order management – a superset of CPOE. *Journal of Healthcare Information Management, 19*(4): 11–13.

National Quality Forum. (2003). *Safe practices for better healthcare: a consensus report.* Washington, DC: National Quality Forum.

Nielsen, J. (2003). *Usability 101: Introduction to usability.* Fremont, CA: Author. Retrieved from http://www.useit.com/alertbox/20030825.html.

Poissant, L., Pereira, J., Tamblyn, R., & Kawasumi, Y. (2005). The impact of electronic health records on time efficiency of physicians and nurses: a systemic review. *Journal of the American Medical Informatics Association, 12*(5), 505–516.

Poon, E. G., Blumenthal, D., Jaggi, T., Honour, M. M., Bates, D. W., & Kaushal, R. (2004). Overcoming barriers to adopting and implementing computerized physician order entry systems in U.S. hospitals. *Health Affairs, 23*(4), 184–190.

Sensmeier, J. (2006). Every organization needs them: nurse informaticians. In C.A. Weaver, C.W. Delaney, P. Weber, & R.L. Carr (Eds.), *Nursing and Informatics for the 21st Century* (pp. 169–178). Chicago, IL: Healthcare Information and Management Systems Society.

Studer, M. (2005). The effect of organizational factors on the effectiveness of EHR system implementation - what have we learned?" *Electronic Healthcare, 4*(2): 92–98.

Tyler, D. (2009). Administrative and clinical health information systems. In D. McGonigle & K.G. Mastrian (Eds.), *Nursing Informatics and the Foundation of Knowledge* (pp. 205–218). Sudbury, MA: Jones and Bartlett Publishers.

21

Electronic Health Record Vendor Applications

Ann Patricia Farrell / Sheryl L. Taylor

• OBJECTIVES

1. Focus attention on key trends, issues, opportunities, and risks facing the nursing profession with regard to electronic health records (EHRs).
2. Describe key new and emerging technologies that respond to nursing requirements and demands for improved information systems.
3. Describe the impact of federal intervention on the commercial EHR market and the challenges and opportunities related to achieving "meaningful use."
4. Provide a patient-centric, interdisciplinary, workflow-driven model—the CareFlow Diagram—as a conceptual framework for communicating with diverse stakeholders regarding EHR nursing components and processes.
5. Relay highlights of lead enterprise EHR vendors' nursing philosophies, product differentiations, future visions, and clinical content and terminology solutions.

• KEY WORDS

American Recovery and Reinvestment Act (ARRA)
Clinical content
Electronic Health Record (EHR)
Health Information Technology for Economic and Clinical Health (HITECH) Act
Medical device integration
Multidisciplinary
Nursing philosophy
Nursing terminology
Unified communication systems
Vendor
Wireless

CURRENT TRENDS TOWARD PATIENT-CENTRIC, INTEROPERABLE EHRS: THE FEDERAL GOVERNMENT INTERVENES

Landmark patient safety–related reports from the Institute of Medicine (IOM, 2000, 2001) and National Priorities and Goals established by the National Quality Forum (NQF, 2008) planted ideas that came to life in the Patient Protection and Affordability Act (PPACA) of 2010 as well as the Health Information Technology for Economic and Clinical Health (HITECH) portion of the American Recovery and Reinvestment Act (ARRA) of 2009. The HITECH Act provides hospitals strong financial incentives for adoption of electric health records (EHRs). In this historic legislation, the U.S. government clearly states its firm belief in the significant benefits of EHRs and its readiness to invest extensive federal resources to proliferate their "meaningful use" (HITECH, 2009).

The Commonwealth Fund, a private U.S. foundation that aims to improve healthcare performance, recently reported that while the U.S. spends the most on healthcare—$7,290 per person per year—it ranks dead last in healthcare quality when compared with six other industrialized nations (Commonwealth Fund, 2010). Ten years after groundbreaking IOM reports, the industry has made little progress in achieving the goals and embracing the principles set forth for a 21st-Century health system, with EHRs playing an essential role in the delivery of safe, efficient, patient-centered, timely, efficient, and equitable care envisioned by the IOM.

With no sense of urgency or inclination to change until now, hospitals have largely failed to heed dire patient safety warnings and calls to action for EHRs and quality reporting by diverse public and private sector groups, including the IOM, NQF, Physician Quality Reporting Initiative (PQRI), and others. The HITECH act, which calls for initial financial rewards for meaningful use (and later penalties for non-use) of EHRs, has galvanized the U.S market and aligned hospitals' and health information technology (HIT) vendors' focus and priorities relative to EHR adoption. The majority of U.S. hospitals report intend to qualify for EHR meaningful use payment. Thus, this groundbreaking law appears to be the long-awaited spark needed to ignite widespread EHR adoption.

Excitement regarding growing EHR momentum is tempered with legitimate concerns relative to challenges in automating complex clinical workflows, gaining physician acceptance, and delivering patient-centric, interoperable solutions. Although pioneers led the way

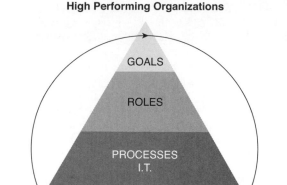

• **FIGURE 21.1.** High-Performing Organizations.

4 decades ago, electronic records failed to achieve envisioned industry adoption rates and wide-scale benefits.

When systems are poorly designed and/or implemented, errors have been introduced (The Joint Commission, 2008). Mistakes of the past could be amplified if EHR solutions fail to support clinician workflows or if rapid, poorly sequenced rollouts ignore change management, human factors, and process (re) design efforts proven critical for success.

Substantial capital and human investments are required to achieve EHR meaningful use objectives nationwide. It will be important to ascertain whether solutions and implementation methods support mission-critical business and clinical goals, as well as adhere to planned budgets and timelines—traditional HIT performance metrics. HIT vendors and hospital chief information officers (CIOs) have not historically been measured based on achievement of EHR goals and benefits. Meaningful use has, fortunately, refocused the industry on end users and outcomes, not merely buying, installing, and maintaining IT (see Figure 21.1).

HIT INDUSTRY STRUGGLES WITH AUTOMATING NURSING PROCESSES

Several well regarded, pioneering, hospital-centric EHR systems reflected a strong grasp of nursing roles and inextricable physician and interdisciplinary processes and data that must be well integrated. Vendors that lack a sound EHR design and nursing framework replicate paper models resulting in labor intensive, task-oriented, fragmented, and, at times, error-prone systems. In particular, the medication management process is broken, frequently supported with disjointed IT. With inefficient tools and increasingly onerous administrative and patient data collection requirements, some question if we are nursing the computer, rather than the patient.

Vendors and CIOs often fail to recognize the extreme complexity of nursing processes, nurse's often-chaotic work conditions, and the converging technologies nurses are asked to integrate at the point of care. And, nursing struggles to clearly explain these intricacies. Research by Joseph Ketcherside, MD, former Chief Medical Informatics Officer at Methodist Le Bonheur Healthcare, Memphis, TN, and Paul Cornell, PhD, Center for Healthcare and Technology, University of Memphis, Memphis, TN, (Cornell & Herrin, 2010) provide compelling, in-depth analyses of nursing activities, workflow, and computer use based in part on data farming, a technique originally used by the Marine Warfighting Laboratory in Quantico, Va to improve understanding of modern combat situations Not to be confused with data mining, data farming "grows" data by running thousands of simulations on imaginary patients and scenarios to evaluate options for providing care. Dr. Ketcherside concluded, "I thought what doctors did was hard, it turns out what nurses do in a day is 10 times more complicated in terms of workflow than what anyone else does in a day" (Manos, 2008). Michael B. Rothberg, MD, as Associate Medical Director for Quality at Baystate Medical Center, Springfield, MA, led research demonstrating how improving nurse-to-patient ratios can be a cost-effective patient safety intervention (Rothberg, 2005).

The IT journey to the point of care—nursing's domain—has clearly been daunting; it represents the next frontier. Although nursing has led EHR adoption, the industry struggles to deliver highly useful and useable seamless tools for nurses. Although a variety of portable, handheld and wearable mobile devices have been introduced, Workstations on Wheels (WOWs) remain the dominant nursing device form factor. While touted as point-of-care technology, WOWS are reported in Spyglass Consulting research by 76% of nurses to be used in the hallway as a stationary or mobile satellite nursing station due to myriad space, technical, cultural, ergonomic, and workflow factors (Malkary, 2007).

Rather than enter data in near real time at the point of care, nurses typically jot down values on scraps of paper, and later, at times *much* later, enter the data in the EHR. Recent research reveals an approximately 25%

error rate (one or more errors), whether vital sign data are transcribed onto paper records or entered into EHRs using a WOW (Wager, 2010). Critical care flowsheets often remain on paper long after the EHR is implemented, with resulting dual system problems.

While manual entry of vital signs into the EHR meets the HITECH Act's meaningful use criteria, it is a highly inefficient and error-prone process. Added risks are incurred if physicians (some remote) use aged or inaccurate data for decision support. A variety of technologies including barcode medication administration (BCMA), medical device integration (MDI), and computer-based provider order entry (CPOE) are propelling nursing toward a more real-time, point-of-care documentation model.

NURSING'S ROLE IN SUCCESSFUL EHR ADOPTION AND MEANINGFUL USE

Nursing assessment and care remain the primary reasons for hospitalization. Nurses play a pivotal role in every venue of care across the community. While use of EHRs can streamline nursing processes and improve patient outcomes, no technology can replace direct nurse observation and critical thinking. It is uncertain how well the HITECH Act's meaningful use criteria will address core nursing processes over time, and how taxpayer and hospital IT dollars invested in EHRs will pay off for nurses. Care team coordination and patient education and engagement, key goals in the HITECH Act, are nursing core competencies poised to be more fully exploited and well-automated (see Figure 21.2).

Although nursing represents the largest healthcare provider and EHR user group, government, IT vendor, and provider communities have traditionally underestimated the importance of and return on investment (ROI) in quality nursing services and enabling technologies. With nursing labor costs representing the largest line item in a hospital expense budget, nursing executives are under continual pressure to improve productivity and to justify staffing levels except where nurse-to-patient ratios are legislated.

Emerging payment schemes (e.g., Accountable Care Organizations, medical homes, etc.) and the HITECH Act reward eligible hospitals and providers for quality outcomes and increasingly penalize unsafe and poor-quality care. While physicians and CPOE play a central role in the HITECH Act, a 21st century health system and EHRs are patient-centric and depend on high-performing teams working in harmony. The

CARE MANAGEMENT TARGETS

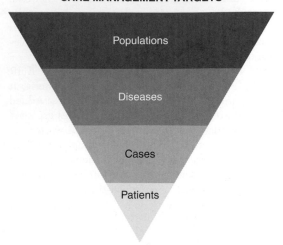

• **FIGURE 21.2.** Care management targets.

contributions of nursing and allied professionals are crucial to achieving the goals outlined in the HITECH Act, successfully implementing EHRs, and realizing high-quality patient outcomes.

While robust, hospital-wide EHR adoption is limited nationwide, successful organizations—from pioneers in the early 1970s to today—cite nursing's essential role in physician and clinician adoption and overall EHR benefits realization. With the rate of EHR adoption increasing rapidly, hopefully all stakeholders will become more enlightened regarding the essential role of nursing to a 21st century health system and the largely untapped potential power of nursing IT. Nursing processes are ripe for continued EHR vendor and hospital investment and IT innovation.

NEW TECHNOLOGIES

Nursing and interdisciplinary EHR applications have evolved and are maturing at varying rates related primarily to the level of vendor focus and investment. Evidence-based medicine (EBM), referred to in the HITECH Act as *comparative effectiveness*, is a fundamental element of EHR meaningful use and longer-term, sustained quality-of-care improvements and cost savings. Clinical content, including evidenced-based physician order sets and interdisciplinary plans of care, is a growing hospital requirement and EHR vendor priority.

Increasingly, third party content will be acquired by the hospital or health system, customized as needed to local practices, and approved by local clinician governance groups. Physicians and nurses personalize standard orders and plans of care based on the specific patient encounter and findings. Order sets and plans of care are increasingly embedded in EHRs, not just accessed via electronic links. EHR and clinical content vendors are creating and enhancing automated tools that enable more efficient integration of content into EHR workflows.

Although benefits of EBM have been well documented, resistance remains strong among some physicians who fear loss of autonomy and consumers voicing concerns regarding rationing of care (Carman, 2010). Nurses are well positioned to employ standards-based practices, if empowered by hospitals and EHR vendors with evidence-based, process-driven, not task-oriented, information systems.

While the technical framework established by Integrating the Healthcare Enterprise (IHE) begins to address standards harmonization, the current lack of a single, widely deployed nursing nomenclature has harmed the profession and hampered interoperability of nursing data. It impedes reporting and business intelligence analysis that could better tie nursing interventions to clinical, financial, service, and satisfaction outcomes and, thus, elevate the visibility and status of the Nursing profession (see Figure 21.3).

Clinicians are embracing wireless technologies. The strong demand for mobile, point-of-care EHR solutions has spawned unparalleled growth in spending

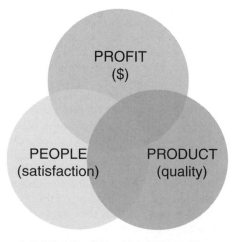

• **FIGURE 21.3.** Key performance indicators.

on wireless applications, clinical devices, and network infrastructure in spite of the recent U.S. economic downturn. Nurses are key beneficiaries of many wireless IT innovations. If well integrated in RN workflows and supported with reliable infrastructure, these technologies can significantly streamline and enhance care delivery and management and care team communication processes.

Emerging wireless unified communication systems offer sophisticated message and alert routing, along with escalation and management capabilities supported by diverse smartphone, badge-based and "purpose built" handheld and wearable devices. Information received from patients, other caregivers, computers, monitors and medical devices is delivered promptly to clinicians and administrators as data, voice, text, or alarms.

Effective communications and rapid response to critical information can have dramatic impacts on patient safety, clinician productivity, patient satisfaction, and organization performance. The most effective communication systems bring together and manage all message types and are tightly integrated with the EHR and other critical information systems and medical devices.

Lack of timely communication and prompt escalation of critical messages to appropriate clinicians can lead to patient deterioration without timely assessment and intervention. While enhanced communications can add value, communication overload and disjointed alarm systems pose key patient safety risks that can contribute to failure-to-rescue patient mortality rates. While some EHR alerts are helpful, many interrupt clinician workflow with annoying pop-up boxes and audible or visual alarms considered a nuisance that can create "alert fatigue," which can introduce rather than mitigate risk (HDM, 2009).

In addition to innovations in integrated communication systems, integrating monitor and device data with the EHR has generated dramatic improvements in nursing productivity. Medical device integration (MDI) recaptures hours of nursing time per day by eliminating unproductive, error-prone transcription of data. Once reviewed and validated by RN, medical device data are filed in the EHR. MDI enables access to more timely and accurate critical patient data by local and remote clinicians and care managers for more real-time patient assessment and clinical and financial decision making. Emerging payment schemes and tens of millions of additional citizens with healthcare coverage will create unprecedented demands for improved patient flow within the hospital and across the community.

MDI technology is becoming more prevalent, extending beyond continuous and spot-check bedside device interfaces to include vendor-agnostic, device-agnostic enterprise solutions. A handful of organizations have integrated smart pumps with the EHR. Use of smart pump technology and streamlining capture and validation of data acquired from bedside devices is intended to free up nursing for more direct care at the bedside, while providing additional accurate, real-time patient data in the EHR. Nursing culture must evolve to embrace a more real-time documentation mindset, with a new awareness of how point-of-care data are used with EHRs and CPOE.

Next-generation patient rooms, known as *smart rooms*, are equipped with a range of wireless technologies including computer screens that can display vital signs, medications, and helpful patient information and reminders. Healthcare professionals entering the room can be identified via advanced security systems, with names of all care providers listed for the patient and family.

Smart beds are being introduced with alarms and other features to maximize safety and reduce complications, such as pressure ulcers, associated with long-term bed rest. These beds are capable of assessing a patient's temperature, pulse and respiration rates, blood pressure, weight, sleep quality, and other metrics without the need to explicitly wire the patient. The patient can wear a vest with woven-in electrodes to provide a full EKG reading. Early adopters of smart room and smart bed technologies expect that as these innovations are proven successful and are cost effective, they will be more broadly adopted by hospitals throughout the nation.

Newer technologies that support remote patient monitoring include body area networks (sensors attached to patients to transmit vital sign information) and Telehealth, Telepresence, and Patient Infotainment (technologies that can support cross-continuum patient assessment and care management).

With a highly mobile clinician workforce and life-critical medical devices and systems relying on wireless technologies, a medical-grade network is becoming the backbone of the EHR. ABI Research reports that the strong WiFi adoption rates indicate the industry has overcome initial concerns about complexity and reliability of wireless IT within healthcare (Collins, 2010). Nurses are less sanguine with 71% of hospital-based nurses reporting in a prominent Spyglass Consulting study that the wireless network was not adequate to support communications at the point of care (Malkary, 2009).

Nurses can't be expected to be hardware, telecommunications, or biomed experts. They can set expectations and guidelines for IT regarding network coverage, reliability, quality of service and support, as well as enabling device requirements as part of EHR planning and budgeting efforts. If nurses lack access to sufficient numbers of useable clinical devices or the network performs poorly, the EHR will be underused, or abandoned, leading to diminished benefits and ROI.

THE RELATIONSHIP BETWEEN CPOE AND NURSING-COLLECTED POINT-OF-CARE DATA: NEW TECHNOLOGIES SUPPORT MEANINGFUL USE OF EHRS

Care delivery organizations are strongly encouraged to prioritize corporate goals, carefully consider interdisciplinary workflows, and deploy best practices in sequencing EHR rollouts. The HITECH Act's meaningful use guidelines are not a comprehensive set of requirements or implementation strategy and plan.

The HITECH Act has focused hospitals and IT vendors on physician use of EHRs, yet key CPOE adoption success strategies are not supported. The relationship between CPOE and nursing documentation is important but not always self-evident. Both the industry and the HITECH Act currently fail to recognize the importance of nursing-collected data, including vital signs, as the *primary* clinical decision support (CDS) information universally valued by physicians in determining treatment plans. CPOE is the culmination of a patient evaluation and complex decision-making process that requires access to relevant, timely, and accurate patient data and, at times, reference materials. CPOE is not simply a clerical (i.e., order entry) task that generates ancillary department requisitions. Use of scribes and other intermediaries greatly reduces potential CDS benefits of the EHR and CPOE.

In clinical decision making, physicians almost universally consider a common subset of patient data that includes laboratory and imaging results and patient assessment and medication administration data. Assessment data (e.g., allergies, height and weight, vital signs, intake and output, nurse-collected bedside lab values, etc.) are used in patient evaluation and treatment decisions by local and remote physicians. To provide up-to-date information to all care providers, nurses should document patient assessment data in near real time at the point of care.

For safe practice, in addition to patient assessment data, providers need online access to the current status of medications administered, not just ordered, for determining medication regimens and treatment protocols. Medication errors are the most frequent cause of adverse medical events and represent a decade-long area of industry concern.

Beyond providing key CDS information, an electronic medication administration record (eMar) along with barcode-enabled medication administration (BCMA) have a greater potential to decrease medication errors than CPOE. While physicians and nurses introduce similar numbers of errors, approximately 50% of physician errors are intercepted downstream while only 2% of administration errors are caught prior to reaching the patient (JAMA, 1995).

Physicians' heavy reliance on allergy, vital sign, and height and weight data is reflected by their inclusion in the HITECH Act's meaningful use criteria. Regrettably, other critical CDS data, in particular an eMar, are not part of the meaningful use criteria. However, to qualify for meaningful use 30% of patients on one or more medications must have at least one medication ordered via CPOE. Best practices indicate that key CDS data should be online prior to or concurrent with CPOE, and to remain up-to-date these data have to be documented by nurses in near real time at the point of care.

Clinical decision support data must be accurate and current. Ideally, critical information is "pushed" to clinicians in the EHR as part of ordering and care planning processes. Monitor and device data are increasingly integrated in the EHR with positive provider, patient, medication, and medical device identification and associations enabled with barcode and radio-frequency identification (RFID) technologies.

EHRS: REAL AND POTENTIAL IMPACTS ON MEDICAL ERRORS

While the Joint Commission had published a number of prior alerts related to specific IT, a Sentinel Alert was issued in 2008 targeting risks associated with "converging technologies" (e.g., the interrelationship between medical devices and HIT). Ronald A. Paulus, MD, Technology and Innovation Officer at Geisinger Health System, Danville, PA, aptly warned that "the science of the interplay between technology and humans or "human factors," is important and often gets short shrift" (The Joint Commission, 2008). This notification highlights the need for well-designed, workflow-driven human-computer interfaces and safe handoffs among clinicians and diverse information systems. The HIT industry has failed to allocate sufficient resources and focus attention on IT usability, resulting in significant inefficiencies and user frustrations that have negatively impacted the pace of EHR adoption and clinician satisfaction.

The U.S. Pharmacopeia MEDMARX database included 176,409 medication error records for 2006; 1.25% of these errors resulted in harm, of which approximately 25% involved some aspect of computer technology as at least one cause of the error. A 2007 survey conducted by the Institute for Safe Medication Practices (ISMP) showed that safety improvements with Automated Dispensing Cabinets (ADC) had not kept up with the growing popularity of the technology (The Joint Commission, 2008). Integrating EHRs and clinical devices with ADCs remains an ongoing workflow and IT challenge.

Kathleen Sebelius, secretary of the Department of Health and Human Services, which oversees the Agency for Healthcare Research and Quality (AHRQ), Medicare, and the Food and Drug Administration, recently reported that "there has not been a significant reduction in the number of medical errors, and what are getting worse are hospital-based infections that are preventable" (Crowley, 2009). Without a mandatory reporting system (which the Obama administration doesn't support), it is difficult to accurately estimate the scale or root causes of the problems. The lack of mandatory tracking cuts both ways—masking the degree of prevalence of errors on one hand, while enabling detractors to exaggerate the role of EHRs as a cause of errors on the other. A new committee was convened by IOM to study how HIT affects the safety of patient care. The 15-month project sponsored by the U.S. Department of Health & Human Services which plans to release its final report in 2012.

BUILDING ON HISTORY AND MOVING AHEAD

Transforming Care at the Bedside (TCAB), a highly publicized national program of the Robert Wood Johnson Foundation and the Institute for Healthcare Improvement (IHI) begun in 2003 and concluding in 2008, responded to the IOM report's findings and challenges in delivering quality care in medical surgical units. TCAB engaged a broad base of hospital and nursing leaders in an effort to identify ways to improve the quality and safety of patient care, increase the vitality and retention of nurses, enhance patients' and family members' care experience, and improve the effectiveness of the overall team—all key to U.S. healthcare goals. Efforts fostered by TCAB are reflected in emerging EHR and IT solutions and continue in many forms.

Nurses fear the routinization and "dumbing down" of the profession motivated by profit-driven medicine,

enabled by HIT. Nursing leadership is challenged to implement best practices for a 21st-Century Healthcare system, balancing the needs for evidence-based practice (structured data collection) and personalized patient care leveraging the power of IT—integrating and balancing high-tech and high-touch approaches. Success would move the national healthcare and HIT agendas forward and better the profession, patient outcomes, clinicians' experience, and the performance of healthcare organizations.

An uptick in involvement of Nursing and Nursing Informatics leadership in the design, selection, and implementation of EHRs is being reported. Though still insufficient, this engagement will hopefully grow and result in more workflow-enabling, nursing-friendly solutions. On the national scene, nursing influence appears to be growing, although the profession is woefully underrepresented and at times still invisible. Nurses lack a single compelling voice that speaks clearly to government, business, academia, clinical and IT leaders and stakeholders.

THE CAREFLOW DIAGRAM

An EHR has no walls but needs a foundation.

For this section, readers should refer to the CareFlow Diagram (Figure 21.4) for a graphical representation of the concepts presented.

The CareFlow Diagram provides a conceptual model including a framework for an inpatient-oriented EHR. It represents an ideal system, one that is patient-centric, interdisciplinary, workflow- and data-driven, evidence-based, and interoperable. While hospital-oriented, most of the concepts apply in other venues of care.

The original version of the CareFlow Diagram has been updated to include key emerging processes, such as medication reconciliation, and technoloprocesses, such as medication reconciliation, and technologies, such as the Continuity of Care Document standard. Electronic health records are expected to help break down the walls of individual organizations and silos of patient data, enabling the flow of key information to all authorized caregivers and the patient. The Careflow Diagram is agnostic regarding reimbursement and care models. It ties core clinical processes to EHR components, showing the interrelationships among physicians and the interdisciplinary care team processes and data.

Enterprise EHR vendors have traditionally focused largely on more episodic approaches to patient care. The market is demanding a patient-centric, holistic, interdisciplinary model with a long-term patient view supported by a single, longitudinal record and data sharing

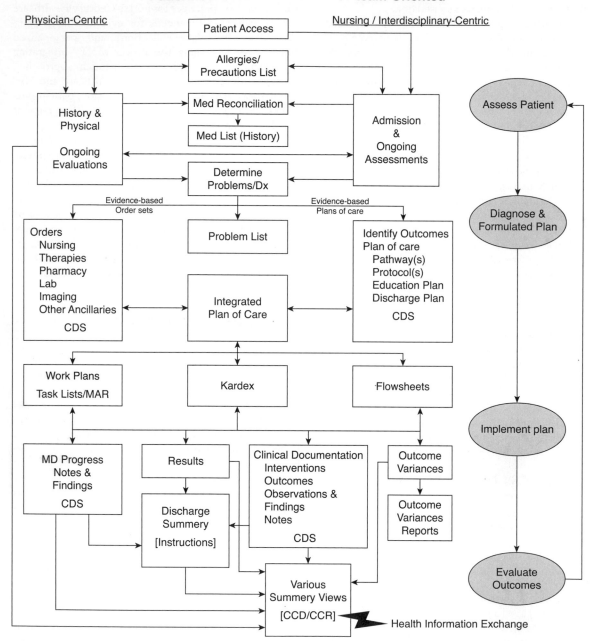

Patient Care Flow - Acute Care / team-Oriented

• **FIGURE 21.4.** The CareFlow diagram.

within the hospital and across the community. This will require a change in culture, roles, business models, processes, EHRs, and enabling technologies. Interoperability will require resolution of long-time issues with lack of standard data definitions and exchange mechanisms.

Though each vendor's solution is unique, the CareFlow diagram is intended as a conceptual model for collective use in communication and education, a framework for product design and evaluation, and a benchmark tool for EHR comparisons.

KEY CLINICAL SYSTEM NURSING AND INTERDISCIPLINARY CARE COMPONENTS

Patient Access

The patient record is initiated in the admission, discharge, and transfer (ADT) system or administrative portion of the EHR. The collection of initial registration and admission data establishes a patient record and begins the clinical and financial encounter with the provider organization. Patients may also be registered and preadmitted prior to arrival with increasing numbers of consumers expected to share targeted information via patient portals.

As part of the scheduling and admitting processes, select patient data are collected, stored, and available for retrieval by all authorized care providers. In organizations where data collected throughout each patient encounter are never archived, a birth-to-death patient record is available online. In a fully interoperable EHR environment, nurses can access patient records for all encounters and track patient progress versus goals and health status across multiple episodes of care throughout the community.

Every care process begins with a user sign-on to the information system. Due to increasingly frequent interactions with the EHR, single sign-on, biometric, and other advanced security technologies are being implemented to ease the burden of lengthy and multiple sign-on process. Frequent system access is especially burdensome to nursing, with RNs reportedly signing on to EHRs as many as 80 times a shift (Malkary, 2007). Patient lists are designed to support individual clinician permissions and are usually customized based on individual and group accountabilities and preferences.

While many patients enter the hospital via scheduled admissions, transfers from other facilities, referrals, walk ins, and other sources, an average of 55% of hospital admissions originate in the emergency department (Owens, 2003) along with 20% of hospital net profits (The Camden Group, 2003). The emergency department (ED) is the "gateway to the community." As a high-risk, high-impact, and increasingly high-volume department, the ED is under intense scrutiny by hospital chief executives and financial officers.

The ED continues to shed its former image as an IT "step child," with more sophisticated and better integrated ED departmental systems and enhanced EHR vendor ED modules. While there is a desire to have a single integrated electronic record that spans the ED visit and entire inpatient stay, ED requirements are challenging and unique. Thus many ED leaders continue to demand targeted niche solutions, particularly if the EHR vendor's ED application is immature or poorly designed and integrated.

Admission Assessments

Physicians perform history and physicals on patient admission and continually evaluate the patient's status during their stay. Similarly, nurses and clinicians (e.g., therapists) perform initial and ongoing patient assessments and therapeutic intakes. While a physician evaluation may focus on a specialty or body system, nurses' assessments are "head to toe" and holistic. EHR vendors' nursing documentation modules have historically automated narrative notes by creating body systems–based forms, with items typically selected from lists of predefined data. Systems that simply replicate the paper record online offer little value with no data analysis capability.

The amount and type of information collected on the nursing admission assessment has grown exponentially with a mounting number of accreditation, legislative, and compliance reporting rules and data collection by nurses. At the same time, the amount of pertinent clinical information nurses collect is rising with more complex, higher acuity and increasingly comorbid patients.

Research confirms that the admission assessment process is one of the most time consuming of all nursing processes (Cornell & Herrin, 2009). Newer technologies offer multiple input and documentation options, including handwriting, dictation, speech recognition, and free-text typing, with everything stored in digital format. Failure of a clinical device or wireless network during lengthy patient assessments where data are lost is noted by many nurses as the primary reason for device abandonment.

Assessment data should be entered once and shared across the EHR. With paper-based models, the same data are entered multiple times in different places and are not well integrated. Well-designed applications offer more streamlined data entry, eliminate duplicate data entry, and promote data sharing among providers (e.g., nursing assessment data populating the physician history and physical). Tablets are increasingly the device of choice for structured, template-driven, body systems–based clinical documentation.

Entry of nursing assessment data may prompt a system recommendation or trigger a plan of care, protocol (e.g., Fall Risk), and/or referral. For example, charting of out-of-range height and weight values may generate a recommended diet regimen and request to a dietician for nutrition counselling in the EHR.

Allergy and Precaution List

Patient precautions are a unique and often undervalued group of data and an essential component of the EHR. Patient precautions include medication allergies, difficult airway precautions, infection control precautions, and advance directives. A property of precautions is that the relevant aspects may be brought to the EHR user's attention at the time decisions must be made. This class of data is an important element of the patient record that makes it more valuable than the paper chart (Sands, 1995).

Medication Reconciliation Including Medication List (History)

Preventable adverse drug events are associated with 1 out of 5 injuries or deaths. Estimates reveal that 46% of medication errors occur on admission or discharge from a clinical unit or hospital when patient orders are written (Provost, 2003).

The Joint Commission defines *medication reconciliation* as follows:

[T]he process of comparing a patient's medication orders to all of the medications that the patient has been taking. This reconciliation is done to avoid medication errors such as omissions, duplications, dosing errors, or drug interactions. It should be done at every transition of care in which new medications are ordered or existing orders are rewritten. Transitions in care include changes in setting, service, practitioner or level of care.

The 5 steps comprising The Joint Commission's medication reconciliation process are:

1. Develop a list of current medications (medication history);
2. Develop a list of medications to be prescribed;
3. Compare the medications on the two lists
4. Make clinical decisions based on the comparison
5. Communicate the new list to appropriate caregivers and to the patient.

The Joint Commission established medication reconciliation as National Patient Safety Goal 8 in 2005. Since that time, many organizations have struggled to develop and implement efficient and effective processes to meet the intent of this goal. EHR vendors have been challenged to deliver fully automated, usable solutions for this process.

While the initial plan was to have The Joint Commission survey evaluate the medication reconcilia-

tion process beginning January 1, 2009, the Accreditation Committee agreed that expectations for accredited organizations should be refined. While this evaluation is being conducted, survey findings will not be factored into the accreditation decision, however organizations are expected to actively address this process.

Discussions with all stakeholders are expected to result in the crafting of a new guideline that both supports quality and safety of care and can be more readily implemented in the field in January 2011 (Joint Commission, March 2010). A medication reconciliation requirement with 50% threshold is included in the HITECH Act's Stage 1 meaningful use menu options, with reported intent to initially focus on admission and discharge transitions of care.

Diagnosis or Problem

"Medical diagnosis refers both to the process of attempting to determine the identity of a possible disease or disorder and to the opinion reached by this process." (Wikipedia, 2010a). Diagnostic criteria designate the combination of signs, symptoms, and test results that the clinician uses to attempt to determine the correct diagnosis. Primary and secondary medical diagnoses drive patient treatment plans and, increasingly, evidence-based order sets introduced with CPOE.

A nursing diagnosis is a clinical judgment about individual, family, or community experiences and responses to actual or potential health problems and life processes used to determine the appropriate plan of care for the patient. The nursing diagnosis drives interventions and patient outcomes, enabling the nurse to develop the patient plan of care.

Problem List (Interdisciplinary)

"A problem list is a list of a patient's problems that serves as an index to his or her record. Each problem, the date when it was first noted, the treatment, and the desired outcome are added to the list as each becomes known." (Wikipedia, 2010b). This list provides an ongoing guide for reviewing the health status and planning the care of the patient.

Medical diagnoses have been the major focus of problem lists. Traditionally, nursing problems have primarily appeared in the form of a plan of care (Henry, 1995). In a patient-centric EHR, an interdisciplinary problem list ensures that all views and needs of the patient are communicated.

Several long-identified themes continue to plague organizations seeking to implement interdisciplinary problem lists (Henry, 1995). Among these are ownership and responsibility for maintaining the problem list and development and maintenance of standardized codified lexicons that serve the needs of each discipline to reveal their specific contribution to patient care (Warren, 1997).

Enterprise EHR vendors provide varying degrees of support for problem lists, with advanced solutions providing a common list of all patient diagnoses and problems able to be sorted and filtered based on specific user and use and patient need. The HITECH Act's Stage 1 meaningful use criteria require more than 80% of patients to have an up-to-date problem list of current and active diagnoses with at least one entry recorded as structured data.

Plans of Care (Interdisciplinary)

Nursing plans of care are formed using the nursing process. First the nurse collects subjective and objective data, then organizes the data into a systematic pattern, such as Marjory Gordon's Functional health Status, which helps identify the areas in which the client needs nursing care. Based on this, the nurse makes a nursing diagnosis.

After determining the nursing diagnosis, the nurse must state the expected outcomes, or goals, for the plan individualized to the patient and situation. A common method of formulating the expected outcomes is to reverse the nursing diagnosis, stating what evidence should be present in the absence of the problem. The expected outcomes must also contain a goal date along with specific appropriate nursing interventions.

Progress toward the goals is continually monitored. An evaluation, with evidence, is provided at scheduled intervals to determine whether outcomes were met and if the plan is to be continued, discontinued, or modified. If the plan of care is problem-based and the client has recovered, the plan would be discontinued. If certain interventions are not helping or others are added, the care plan is modified and continued. If the client has not recovered, or if the plan was written for a chronic illness or ongoing problem, it may be continued and tracked in the EHR (Wikipedia, 2010c)

In early nursing applications, nurses built care plans "on the fly" by selecting appropriate interventions and expected outcomes from predefined checklists based on diagnoses and the individual patient's course of treatment. Even when automated, this process is labor intensive and repetitive. Hospitals are increasingly implementing evidence-based standards that include plans of care for nurses and allied health professionals.

Clinical pathways, also known as *care maps*, are interdisciplinary tools used to manage quality of care and streamline the care process. Their implementation reduces variability in clinical practice. Clinical pathways are based on evidence-based practices and have been proven to optimize outcomes in acute and home care settings.

Integrated pathways apply process management thinking to the improvement of patient healthcare. A key aim is to re-center the focus on the patient's overall journey, rather than the contribution of each specialty or caring function independently. Instead, all disciplines are emphasised as working together as a cross-functional team. (Wikipedia, 2010d)

Integrated Plans of Care

An integrated plan of care incorporates a comprehensive, patient-centric point of view. It includes all services to be provided for a patient, including physician orders and nursing and interdisciplinary plans of care.

Kardex

A Kardex is a patient management tool used by nurses to collect, organize, and display summary patient information in one place. Typically, a Kardex includes the patient name, medical record number, admission date, diagnosis, service, attending physician, primary nurse, patient age and date of birth, special needs and/or requests (e.g., prosthetics), allergies, medical alerts, and all currently active orders.

In an automated environment, the Kardex is more than just an online view of summary patient data. An electronic Kardex automatically gathers appropriate data already in the system via previously entered orders, plans of care, and clinical documentation. The Kardex can ideally be tailored to the needs and preferences of the individual organization, department, and work center.

In advanced nursing systems, direct entry of data into the Kardex will update associated parts of the electronic record; conversely, charting updates automatically populate the Kardex. A Kardex is not a legal document and, therefore, it is not saved in the permanent patient record.

Work Plans and Task lists

EHRs support generation of work plans, also known as task lists, as an automatic by-product of orders and plans of care. These task lists help nurses organize, document, and manage patient care activities and interventions for individual patients or groups of patients. Nurses can access task lists for an entire shift or view them in the system as needed for a particular period of time. Completion of an activity or set of activities can be charted directly on the task list. EHRs with paper-based models often promote task-oriented processes, failing to embed interventions within overall care and documentation processes.

Two types of activities are presented on task lists: (1) treatments and/or interventions and (2) medications. Some organizations integrate these activities into a single, chronologic list of assigned medications and non-medication related tasks. Most departments prefer a task list for treatments and interventions and a separate medication ("meds due") list including IVs, known as an electronic medication administration record (eMAR). Some vendors offer a separate IV administration record known as an IVAR.

The eMAR should contain all medication orders including one-time, scheduled, unscheduled, and PRN medications, IV additives, topical solutions, and any other pharmaceutical or homeopathic therapy. As soon as a medication order is entered and verified, it automatically appears on the eMAR and is accessible by authorized local and remote physicians, nurses, therapists, and pharmacists. An eMar offers clinicians a picture of the entire medication history, typically with 7-day views of data.

Nurses chart medications on the eMAR as *given* or *not given*, and adjust schedules, as authorized, to accommodate held or missed doses. If a medication is not charted within a predefined time frame, the nurse can be alerted electronically in the EHR via visual cues and, if desired, audible alerts sent to a device or other communication system.

Documentation of medications on the eMAR can prompt the nurse for specific charting actions (e.g., pain assessment) 30 minutes after administration of PRN pain medication per The Joint Commission requirements. Charting a medication as *given* can automatically send a charge to the revenue cycle management system and decrement the pharmacy inventory system or ADC.

Current patient safety initiatives have prompted the adoption of barcode technology for positive provider, patient, and medication identification to support the "5 rights" of mediation administration: the right patient, drug, dose, route, and schedule. BCMA requires access to the EHR at the point of care and charting via wall-mounted bedside terminals or mobile devices. One of the most daunting challenges for hospital and HIT vendors has been to design and implement efficient and effective BCMA and eMAR processes with seamlessly integrated applications, supporting devices and enabling technologies.

Results

Laboratory, imaging, and other ancillary department tests ordered by physicians, once completed, have results filed in the EHR database that are accessible to all authorized care providers. Lab values, radiology reports, and, in some cases, images from picture archiving systems (PACS) can be retrieved as needed during the care and, increasingly, the patient education processes.

In more advanced systems, key lab values and patient data are displayed automatically during the ordering process (e.g., a digitalis order automatically displays the last pulse rate and potassium level). Most systems can prompt users for orders of complementary tests or procedures where medically recommended.

In an EHR, results data can be viewed over time in tabular formats and graphed for display of trends. In advanced EHR systems, multiple data types including nursing interventions can be displayed on the same graph (e.g., digitalis administration, potassium values, and pulse rates).

Clinical Documentation

Physicians and the entire care team document observations and findings in progress notes and ongoing electronic charting. A confluence of factors, including patient-centric care models, is driving current heightened interest in interdisciplinary care and documentation.

Nurses document in the EHR in a number of online formats, including structured notes, checklists and interactive flowsheets. Narrative notes are minimized in EHRs, particularly if data cannot be extracted for later analysis.

Clinical documentation is the major method by which diverse care providers collaborate across multiple points of service. When attempts are made to implement more structured documentation models, nurses can resist, believing these approaches "depersonalize" care and mask the patient as an individual. Standardized charting is more readily adopted if RNs can add patient-specific observations and comments where needed. Certainly EHR user interfaces could be better designed and formatted to display and highlight findings that personalize the patient story.

Given the enormous amount of time nurses spend in documenting care, 30% to 50% in some organizations, speed and efficiency of data entry is a top priority. While most hospitals aim to minimize nursing charting time, patient care documentation must be legally defensible, regulatory-compliant, and clinically sound.

With a growing number of critical care beds and monitored patients throughout the hospital, integration of medical device and EHR data will increasingly proliferate.

The process to manually enter electronic data collected by patient monitors and devices (e.g., cardiac monitors, ventilators, IV pumps) into an EHR is error-prone, labor-intensive, and nonproductive. Where a monitor or device integration exists, data values captured are displayed and verified by the nurse prior to entry into the EMR data base.

Outcomes Variance Tracking and Reports

Virtually all care delivery organizations are focused on improving patient safety and quality of care. For organizations to thrive, clinicians must be committed to continual performance improvement including comparison of expected versus actual outcomes. In electronic systems, as a by-product of patient care documentation, data are collected that continually measure key clinical processes and progress against plans. Data analyses can pinpoint "lags" in process substeps, support root cause analysis of problems, and target process improvement efforts.

As evidence-based care and clinical pathways are more rapidly adopted and data are codified, more rigorous examination of care patterns can occur. Unexplained variances tracked by the system are available for clinician response and management reporting.

Outcomes variance reports can be used to identify outliers, compare performance across providers, and when appropriate, update pathways to reflect more effective practices. High-performing hospitals increasingly monitor processes and outcomes in real time. They continually benchmark performance against their prior outcomes, performance of peers, and best practices in healthcare and other industries for nonclinical services such as parking and food service.

Discharge Summary and Instructions

A discharge summary is a clinical report prepared by a physician or other health professional at the conclusion of a hospital stay or series of treatments. It outlines the patient's chief complaint, the diagnostic findings, the therapy administered, and the patient's response to it, along with recommendations upon discharge. A medication reconciliation is also performed on discharge.

The six components mandated by The Joint Commission for a hospital discharge summary include:

1. Reason for hospitalization
2. Significant findings
3. Procedures and treatments provided
4. Patient's discharge condition
5. Patient and family instructions (as appropriate)
6. Attending physician's signature

The discharge summary is an increasingly important component of care with inpatient stays shortening and postdischarge care often provided by multiple physician specialists and clinician providers. Discharge summaries support continuity of care goals by providing the key patient data needed for transfer of care to the family and other facilities and providers in the community, such as the patient's primary care physician.

The discharge summary includes patient instructions with follow-up information and recommended education forms or programs specific to the patient's condition. In an integrated EHR, discharge summary data are collected and updated throughout the patient stay and are available for final review and completion prior to patient discharge or transfer to another facility or home. The requirement to offer condition-specific educational resources to 10% of patients was reintroduced in the menu set of objectives for the HITECH Act's Stage 1 meaningful use criteria.

Summary Views

With the growing amount and density of patient data, key information is often difficult to extract and synthesize. EHRs offer a variety of data snapshots that provide customized views that facilitate rapid and timely evaluation of critical patient data and trends. Patient summaries are targeted for specific use and designed to meet the needs and preferences of an enterprise, medical specialty, or individual caregiver. Patient summaries can support rounding, initial patient evaluation by consulting physicians, end-of-shift or transition-of-care reporting by nurses and care teams, and other diverse patient care, care management, and care team communication activities. Providing a summary of care record for 50% or more of patient transfers or referrals is part of the optional meaningful use criteria in the HITECH Act.

THE CONTINUITY OF CARE DOCUMENT AND THE CONTINUITY OF CARE RECORD: HEALTH INFORMATION EXCHANGE

Both the Health Level Seven (HL7) Clinical Document Architecture (CDA) and the American Society for Testing and Materials (ASTM) International Continuity of Care Record (CCR) strive to facilitate the interchange of healthcare data among care providers. The Continuity of Care Document (CCD) specification is an XML-based mark-up standard intended to specify the encoding, structure, and semantics of a patient summary clinical document for health information exchange. The CCD specification is a constraint on the HL7 CDA standard.

The CDA specifies and mandates a textual part (which ensures human interpretation of the document contents) and optional structured parts (for software processing) of the patient summary. The structured part is based on the HL7 Reference Information Model (RIM) and provides a framework for referring to concepts from coding systems such as from systematized nomenclature of medicine (SNOMED CT®) and LOINC (Wikipedia, 2010e).

The patient summary contains a core data set of the most relevant administrative, demographic, and clinical information facts about a patient's healthcare, covering one or more healthcare encounters. It provides a means for healthcare practitioners, systems, and settings to aggregate and share pertinent data about a patient to support the continuity of care. Its primary use is to provide a snapshot in time.

The CCR standard is a patient health summary standard. It is a way to create flexible documents that contain the most relevant and timely core health information about a patient, and to send these electronically from one care giver to another. It contains various sections such as patient demographics, insurance information, diagnosis and problem list, medications, allergies, and plan of care. These represent a snapshot of a patient's health data that can be useful or possibly lifesaving, if available at the time of clinical encounter. The CCR standard is designed to permit easy creation by a physician using an EHR system at the end of an encounter.

The CCD and CCR are often seen as competing standards (Wikipedia, 2010f). While there is a growing belief that the CCD will become the dominant standard in the future, the HITECH Act's meaningful use criteria allow either a CCD or CCR, with the expectation that these standards will be harmonized later.

Vendor Responses

Table 21.1 represents targeted lead EHR vendors' self-reported nursing philosophies, product differentiations, and visions for the future.

STANDARD TERMINOLOGY PROVIDED WITH CLINICAL APPLICATIONS

Market Expectation

Despite the lack of a national consensus regarding one standard nursing terminology or data set, healthcare organizations (HCOs) expect their EHR vendor to deliver a standards-based set of nursing content for charting and planning care. Implementation of an EHR system is usually a lengthy project; but the cost, time, and effort required can be decreased if a set of valid content is included with the software and organizations can modify this set where necessary to meet their specific requirements. Without a "starter set" of clinical content encoded with a standard terminology, the nursing and information systems departments must devote significant time and resources to developing their own "from scratch" and configuring it into the tables and dictionaries of their EHR system.

Now that the federal government has recognized SNOMED CT® (systematized nomenclature of medicine) as the standard reference terminology, the expectation of HCOs has risen; they want the starter set of terminology provided with the EHR software to be one that maps to SNOMED CT®. SNOMED CT® facilitates sharing and aggregating healthcare information within and among HCOs. Facilities using terminologies that map to SNOMED CT® are able to take advantage of these capabilities and ultimately participate in national and potentially international healthcare initiatives.

As most HCOs have adopted a multidisciplinary or even interdisciplinary approach to delivery of care, their expectation for predefined content extends beyond meeting the needs of nursing. Content to support clinical documentation for therapists, social services, and other members of the care team is being requested and increasingly provided as part of clinical content.

Current Status

Responding to this market demand, most of the major HIT vendors now deliver at least a basic starter set of terminology. An increasing number of these vendors

TABLE 21.1	Vendors' Nursing Philosophies, Product Differentiations, and Visions for Future

Cerner Corporation[a]

Philosophy for nursing

Cerner's nursing philosophy recognizes professional nursing as both a science and an art. More than 400 nurses strong, Cerner is committed to enhancing the science of nursing by embedding evidence-based nursing practice in the workflow, providing the right information at the right time for the right person. The focus on individual clients/patients allows the nurse to meet patient or client unique needs, including physical, psychological, social, and spiritual needs. Cerner's clinical intelligence system uses technological innovations and data analysis to support nurses and patients in diverse settings. This approach enables critical thinking and clinical reasoning for actions by the practicing professional nurse.

Key differentiators

Cerner's patient-centric architecture strengthens care with knowledge, providing a single source of truth for patient information that is leveraged across the care continuum for all caregivers to communicate, document, evaluate, and coordinate each patient's progress.

Closed loop medication process: All caregivers manage a real-time view of the patients' medication profile, history, and medication adherence.

Integrating Devices with the Electronic Health Record (EHR): Cerner is leading the industry device suppliers to a plug-and-play workflow.

Evidenced-based interdisciplinary care planning: Cerner Knowledge Solutions place the latest clinical evidence, empirical data, and optimal practices at the clinician's fingertips at the appropriate time and place within the care process.

Vision of the future

Cerner's vision goes beyond the traditional EHR by including the devices attached to or in proximity to the patient, such as IV pumps, ventilators, and beds. These devices capture patient care data that are viewable currently only via the individual physical devices. The clinician must look at the data from multiple sources to see the complete picture of the patient's status. With advances in technology, these devices can stream data seamlessly into the EHR, enabling nurses to be knowledge workers rather than technology integrators, and allowing them to apply their skills toward a positive impact on patient outcomes (Karp & Gehrt, in press 2010).

Epic Systems Corporation[b]

Philosophy for nursing

Epic designs software with the diverse requirements of the novice and the expert nurse in mind, and their connections to the interdisciplinary team. Workflows provide access to information with few clicks. Upgrades are not released unless they are "as fast or faster" than the version they replace. Documentation is automated in many areas and multiple entry options are provided to match individual preferences. Our real-time patient summary timeline tells a patient's admission story visually, facilitating safe handoffs. Real-time and retrospective dashboards support broader clinical process improvement. Our customers are our partners in implementation and development—working closely with us to prioritize improvements and to optimize the practical benefits of implementation.

Key differentiators

Epic offers highly rated clinical ambulatory and inpatient systems built in-house on the same underlying database, one lifetime record accessible across the continuum of care. Creating a fast and user-friendly system that clinical staff can learn quickly and incorporate easily into day-to-day workflows has always been the focus of our development.

Our employee ratio reflects our focus on clients and products. Our client base includes 190 of the most prestigious organizations in the U.S., and over 40 clients have achieved Magnet Recognition. Our staff-to-client ratio is nearly 20:1, compared with an industry average of less than 2:1.

Vision of the future

Epic's vision is that nurses have the information they need, whether it comes from within their walls, from an affiliated practice, from an outside organization (with Care Everywhere), or directly from the patient (with MyChart or Lucy).

Epic is enhancing device integration. Rather than manual data entry, interfaced device data automatically populates patient records.

Epic is simplifying reporting for clinical quality and effectiveness, allowing users to meet regulatory requirements such as meaningful use, Joint Commission audits, and CMS core measures.

Epic has created EpicEarth, a network that will harness the diverse knowledge of Epic users, improving patient care, streamlining go lives, and expanding clinical knowledge.

(continued)

TABLE 21.1	Vendors' Nursing Philosophies, Product Differentiations, and Visions for Future *(continued)*

Eclipsys Corporation[c] (acquired by Allscripts)

Philosophy for nursing

Eclipsys recognizes that nurses have always been at the center of patient care, from performing clinical assessments and administering complex treatment plans to counselling and educating patients and their families. With our advanced clinical solutions, Eclipsys supports nurses as care coordinators, providing evidence-based content to support decision making at the point of care. With our one-patient, one-record approach, Eclipsys provides the nurse with relevant information from across the enterprise to support safe, effective care and optimal clinical outcomes. Eclipsys solutions help make healthcare safer for patients—and safer for nurses.

Key differentiators

Eclipsys uses a one-patient, one-record approach in delivering advanced clinical solutions, which facilitates workflow and helps all members of the healthcare team deliver safer, more effective patient care while optimizing clinical outcomes. When all healthcare team members have access to evidence-based practices, they can collectively work toward a common goal in partnership with the patient and the patient's family. Our solutions offer evidence-based clinical content that is interdisciplinary in design and consensually validated by thousands of practicing clinicians. Our clinical solutions put the right knowledge into the hands of the right person at the right place and time.

Vision of the future

The Eclipsys vision is to continue to be the leader in delivering advanced healthcare IT solutions that make a tangible difference in quality, safety, and cost effectiveness. Our solutions embed the latest best practices and workflows, evidence-based clinical content, and integrated technologies to promote excellent performance and superior care. In addition, Eclipsys' vision is to be a trusted value partner in a healthcare organization's pursuit of superior clinical, financial, and operational outcomes. Eclipsys strives to help nurses—and all healthcare professionals—reach their full potential.

GE Healthcare[d]

Philosophy for nursing

Nurses are key stakeholders in the delivery of healthcare with nursing practice spanning all settings and spectrums of healthcare delivery. Supporting these complex workflows means giving nurses the tools they need to work more efficiently and collaborate more effectively. Nursing will continue to lead and have a pivotal role in transforming healthcare in the United States. Nurses are boundaryless in their reach, engagement, and impact. As nursing continues to redefine models of care delivery and transform the culture of how care is delivered, GE Healthcare (GEHC) continues to innovate and develop the necessary technologies to support transformation and nursing practice.

Key differentiators

GE's key differentiators include the implementation of "Smart" intelligent functionality across the continuum of care to optimize patient safety and outcomes, clinician productivity, and cost effectiveness. Key differentiators facilitate interdisciplinary care collaboration integrating real-time and population-based health functionality for:

- Smart visualization
- Smart documentation
- Smart analytics and business intelligence

Vision of the future

The GE Healthymagination vision for the future is focused on reducing costs, increasing access, and improving quality as GE continuously develops innovations. Healthymagination is transforming the way nurses and other clinicians serve patients through increased focus on IT and the power of information. Through Healthymagination innovation and groundbreaking technology, GE is making IT solutions and real-time clinical decision support more accessible, giving caregivers access to increasingly valuable information insights. The vision of Healthymagination is to provide better health for more people. GE is committed to making health IT faster and more productive, enabling nurses to interact even more effectively with patients and their family members and other clinical staff.

(continued)

TABLE 21.1	Vendors' Nursing Philosophies, Product Differentiations, and Visions for Future *(continued)*

McKesson Information Solutions[e]

Philosophy for nursing

The challenges facing nursing today are tremendous: numerous regulatory and administrative requirements, labor and delivery requirements, and a lack of adequate nursing staff to facilitate care planning. First and foremost, however, nursing is always looking for ways to improve patient care and patient safety.

McKesson's nursing and nursing documentation solutions focus on meeting the needs of the frontline nurse through to the chief nursing officer, addressing the many challenges and requirements facing the nursing profession today.

Key differentiators

- Patient safety
  - First to market with barcode medication administration (BCMA)
  - Greatest breadth and depth of experience with BCMA
- Clinical performance
  - Comprehensive decision support from the point of ordering through documentation
  - Clinical analytics reporting packages and scorecards
  - Prescriptive content starter sets
  - Flexible tools to adjust as regulatory and quality initiatives evolve
- Care team efficiency
  - Interdisciplinary care planning and worklists to enhance care team communication
  - Tools that support the whole care team with a single record and source of truth
  - Interoperability strategies to support the continuum of care

Vision of the future

The economic incentives (and penalties) tied to meaningful use of electronic health records are rapidly accelerating the adoption of HIT. As the largest group of healthcare professionals, nurses will play a critical role in the impact this acceleration has on quality, efficiency, patient satisfaction, staff satisfaction, and the bottom line. If done right, we will see not incremental but transformational positive change. Therefore McKesson is focused on the near-term future—ensuring our customers achieve wide-scale adoption of systems that support optimal workflow, handle mandatory reporting requirements as a by-product of patient care, and give nurses more time to care.

QuadraMed Corporation[f]

Philosophy for nursing

QuadraMed CPR (QCPR) supports an interdisciplinary, holistic approach that encourages individualized patient-centered care. The strength of our philosophy is to promote complete, accurate, and timely documentation by adhering to a professional nursing best-practice model, avoiding a task-driven workflow in order to enhance the quality of nursing practice at the bedside.

Key differentiators

QCPR barcode medication administration supports 11 rights expanding the verification of the following:

1. Patient
2. Time
3. Drug
4. Dose
5. Route
6. Reason or diagnosis
7. Documentation
8. Form
9. Diluents
10. Concentration
11. Admixture

In addition, the QCPR workflow engine combined with clinical decision support and smart templates reduces inappropriate or unnecessary clerical tasks, and improves documentation in the areas of completeness, compliance, and accuracy.

(continued)

TABLE 21.1	Vendors' Nursing Philosophies, Product Differentiations, and Visions for Future *(continued)*

Vision of the future

QCPR will be able to deliver evidence-based order sets personalized to an individual patient, so that clinicians only interact with the pertinent information in a guideline or protocol. This revolutionary solution will help to minimize time spent at the computer, reduce unnecessary tests, and improve patient outcomes.

QuadraMed is focused on streamlining the use of the electronic health record and providing tools that will improve clinician, patient, and patient-family communication and education. The Interactive Whiteboard Engine will enable the development of site-specific HIPAA-compliant displays that can be used throughout the hospital.

Siemens Healthcare[g]

Philosophy for nursing

A myriad of challenges are face healthcare today with one constant—the need to provide safe, high-quality patient care supported by evidence-based practices implemented with greater efficiency.

Siemens Healthcare's solutions bring knowledge to the point of care as nurses look to evidence-based practices and sophisticated workflow technologies to assist them in meeting care delivery needs. Siemens Healthcare brings breadth and depth of clinical solutions designed to support healthcare's increasingly complex work environment.

Siemens Healthcare believes that being on the forefront of developing IT solutions to support clinical practice is a sound investment in the future. These solutions will help promote nursing professional practice as we enter a new world of healthcare.

Key differentiators

Siemens Healthcare is a fully integrated diagnostics company, bringing together imaging and lab diagnostics, therapy, and healthcare information technology to deliver solutions across the entire continuum of care. Solutions support clinical practice by leveraging Healthcare Process Management, which provides workflow technologies to manage care processes from admission to discharge, synchronize and allocate handoffs, and escalate notifications to care providers when appropriate. Coupled with embedded reporting analytics, organizations can effectively monitor care delivery processes and clinical outcomes from start to finish. With the assistance of these advanced IT tools, nurses are able to deliver safe, high-quality care to their patients with confidence.

Vision of the future

Siemens Healthcare strives to provide global breakthough innovations in healthcare to support the delivery of unsurpassed clinical excellence. Through the combination of information technology and imaging and diagnostics solutions, Siemens Healthcare focuses on addressing the entire healthcare continuum from prevention, early detection, and diagnosis to therapy and care. Providing integrated technologies that facilitate seamless access and offer workflow technologies to synchronize and monitor care delivery will support the transformation of clinical practice in the new decade. As the healthcare environment continues to evolve, Siemens Healthcare remains committed to leveraging IT to support and enhance the role of nursing by developing solutions that foster new clinical knowledge founded on research, innovation, and vision.

[a]Obtained from and published with permission of Cerner Corporation.
[b]Obtained from and published with permission of Epic Systems Corporation.
[c]Obtained from and published with permission of Eclipsys Corporation.
[d]Obtained from and published with permission of GE Healthcare.
[e]Obtained from and published with permission of McKesson Information Solutions.
[f]Obtained from and published with permission of QuadraMed Corporation.
[g]Obtained from and published with permission of Siemens Healthcare.

include standards-based terminology with their clinical documentation application, as well as evidence-based standards of care with their care planning and clinical pathways applications, and some are using standard terminologies that map to SNOMED CT®.

Table 21.2 contains a survey of the targeted leading vendors that offer enterprise EHR solutions, provides information about their current status regarding the terminologies they deliver, and the clinical applications in which they are deployed.

TABLE 21.2	Vendors' Evidence-Based Clinical Content and Standardized Terminology

Cerner Corporation[a]

Source of content for evidence-based plans of care

Cerner believes the changes needed in healthcare must be built on an integrated platform of academic, healthcare delivery, and corporate health information technology organizations. Cerner has formalized a unique partnership to develop evidence-based plans of care with the goal of transforming the practice and science of nursing (Lundeen, Harper, Kerfoot, 2009). These endeavors highlight Cerner's Millennium Lighthouse, a suite of solutions and services that promote rapid implementation and adoption of evidence-based practice, while simplifying the capture of data for CMS and Magnet indicators through configuring relevant, real-time data collection into the workflow, and producing real-time dashboards and various reports.

Standard vocabulary and terminology solutions utilized

Cerner supports the practice of nursing research through standardized coded data elements in SNOMED-CT®. Cerner has long defined concepts that are intuitive and meaningful for the clinician end user while maintaining the structure, integrity, and hierarchy of this reference terminology. The terminology core is necessary for decision support, variance studies, outcomes reporting, and general use and reuse of information for quality, safety, and efficiency. The coded terms provide the interoperability framework for reporting on operational, quality, and financial outcomes. Cerner identifies its major contribution to the science by philanthropic efforts by funding the ANCC/Cerner Magnet Prize.

Current partnerships with clinical content vendors

Cerner continues to develop content while partnering with the following content vendors:

- 3M for Medical Necessity content
- American Medical Association for CPT codes
- Rehabilitation Institute of Chicago for rehabilitation workflows
- British Medical Journal and Zynx for order sets
- Elsevier for First Consult and MD Consult
- Krames and ExitCare for patient education materials
- HLI for Cerner Controlled Medical Terminology
- IMO for linkages to and data from the National Library of Medicine's MeSH database and other services
- Lexi-Comp for drug interaction
- King Guide for IV compatibility data used with Multum

Epic Systems Corporation[b]

Source of content for evidence-based plans of care

Clients have the option of using evidence-based CPMRC Point of Care Integrated Solutions or Zynx Health ZynxCare content for their plans of care.

Standard vocabulary and terminology solutions utilized

Epic provides an open structure that allows organizations to incorporate their preferred standardized nursing languages into Epic workflows. Examples of vocabularies that can be used with Epic's system include:

- Clinical Care Classification System
- International Dietetics and Nutrition Terminology
- North American Nursing Diagnosis Association
- Nursing Interventions Classification
- Nursing Outcomes Classification
- Omaha
- Perioperative Nursing Data Set

Our Model System makes use of SNOMED CT® terms and can use SNOMED CT®'s hierarchical structure to create diagnosis or concept groupers that simplify decision support setup and reporting. Epic's enterprise EMR provides mapping to SNOMED CT® terms for selected fields and can use mapping imported from other terminology sets.

Current partnerships with clinical content vendors

Not applicable

(continued)

TABLE 21.2	Vendors' Evidence-Based Clinical Content and Standardized Terminology *(continued)*

Eclipsys Corporation[c] (acquired by AllScripts)

Source of content for evidence-based plans of care

Eclipsys partners with the Clinical Practice Model Resource Center (CPMRC), a subsidiary of Elsevier, to provide robust, interdisciplinary, evidence-based clinical content. Eclipsys' trademarked Knowledge Based Charting™ provides more than 200 evidence-based, interdisciplinary clinical practice guidelines (CPGs). Knowledge-Based Charting enhances safety and quality while enabling improved clinical outcomes by standardizing evidence-based care and providing knowledge at the point of care. CPGs drive the patient's plan of care, allowing the nurse to establish and monitor patient progress toward identified clinical goals.

Standard vocabulary and terminology solutions utilized

Eclipsys utilizes SNOMED-CT® as our primary source of standardized vocabulary and terminology.

Current partnerships with clinical content vendors

Eclipsys currently partners with Wolters Kluwer Health and Zynx Health for physician content and physician order sets. Eclipsys currently partners with the Clinical Practice Model Resource Center, a subsidiary of Elsevier, for evidence-based nursing and interdisciplinary clinical content and clinical practice guidelines.

GE Healthcare[d]

Source of content for evidence-based plans of care

Allowing customer preference of evidence-based interdisciplinary plans of care, GEHC retains an agnostic position to evidence-based sources. GEHC supports and emphasizes principles of sound and primary research for evidence and demonstrated best practices. Our current source for evidence-based plans of care is Zynx but we continue to explore the landscape for other partnership opportunities.

Standard vocabulary and terminology solutions utilized

GEHC has established partnerships with renowned healthcare delivery systems, which have deep integration of terminology and standards. Various Centricity solutions utilize the University of Nebraska Lexicon, ICD-9, ACOG, and AWHONN vocabulary and terminology. GE continues to evaluate additional opportunities to partner with industry thought leaders as well as continued enhancements to our products as standards evolve.

Current partnerships with clinical content vendors

Through its IT portfolio, GE Healthcare actively evaluates market-based opportunities to integrate leading-edge clinical content within its core clinical information systems. Current vendor-based alliances and partnerships include Zynx for care plans and order sets; First DataBank, Thompson Reuters, and Lexicomp for drug interaction, allergy, and dosing guidelines; and The Nebraska Medical Center for problem list lexicon. Future vendor relationships will be forthcoming.

McKesson Information Solutions[e]

Source of content for evidence-based plans of care

Current healthcare regulations and accreditation requirements, guidelines, quality improvement initiatives, and best practices are researched, reviewed, and evaluated for inclusion in McKesson's Knowledge Center Content for Horizon Expert Plan. The content leverages standard nomenclature from NANDA International, Nursing Interventions Classification and Nursing Outcomes Classification, International Dietetics and Nutrition Terminology, as well as SNOMED-CT®. Customers may supplement this content by purchasing care plans from Wolters Kluwer and Zynx.

Standard vocabulary and terminology solutions utilized

Horizon Clinicals uses terminologies required by Stage 1 of the Interim Final Rule issued by CMS. We use a large set of standardized terminologies, including:

- SNOMED CT® to document patient problems, facilitate rapid documentation, and generate meaningful clinical alerts
- ICD-9-CM for patient billing and reporting
- CPT for charge capture
- RxNorm to transmit medication information within continuity of care documents
- CVX to document and report immunizations

Standard and custom relationships between terminologies are used to facilitate efficient billing based on charting. A central terminology repository collects and distributes terminologies using preconfigured loading scripts.

(continued)

TABLE 21.2	Vendors' Evidence-Based Clinical Content and Standardized Terminology *(continued)*

Current partnerships with clinical content vendors

McKesson has partnerships with various third-party vendors for clinical content:

- Wolters Kluwer and Zynx for evidenced-based content for care plans and order sets
- Health Language for various types of structured and codified content such as ICD-9, SNOMED CT®, CVX, etc., and mappings among the various content sets
- First Data Bank for medication and allergy lists

QuadraMed Corporation[f]

Source of content for evidence

QuadraMed partners with CPMRC, an Elsevier company, to provide evidence-based plans of care. In addition, our partnership enables the offering of Practice Transformation services to assist organizations with clinical practice advancement, cultural changes, and improved processes.

Standard vocabulary and terminology solutions utilized

The Controlled Medical Vocabulary (CMV) enables the definition and management of clinical concepts to support the sharing of clinical information between clinicians, clinical disciplines and care settings. More importantly, the use of a CMV facilitates critical thinking and decision making at the point of care, and also provides a mechanism to extract and aggregate data to support analysis and improve the quality of patient safety and care. Embedding a CMV within QCPR provides the ability to support an unlimited number of code sets and provides organizations the capability to use their own terminologies.

Current partnerships with clinical content vendors

QuadraMed has partnered with CPMRC, an Elsevier company, to include their standardized, interdisciplinary, evidence-based clinical content in QCPR. Embedding CPMRC content provides clinical recommendations for interventions based on best practices to help organizations improve outcomes and meet quality and safety and compliance objectives. Links to articles, references, and abstracts supporting the value of the recommended approach are readily available to clinicians at the point of care.

Siemens Healthcare[g]

Source of content for evidence

Siemens Healthcare stays on the forefront of the healthcare industry to identify timely, research-based content and sources of content that our customers can leverage to help guide them in their care delivery decisions. Siemens Healthcare partners with ZynxHealth to help ensure our customers have access to rigorously reviewed research and performance measures. This evidence-based content can be used as the basis for developing and maintaining the patient plan of care. However, our solutions provide the flexibility to support our customers' clinical content initiatives whether obtained from content vendors or developed and validated internally.

Standard vocabulary and terminology solutions utilized

As the industry moves to adopting standard terminology to support national initiatives and address interoperability, Siemens Healthcare recognizes the need to adopt a consistent and standard vocabulary and terminology as part of our infrastructure.

Siemens Healthcare currently supports the ability to reference third-party terminologies such as Clinical Care Classification (CCC), LOINC, International Classification for Nursing Practice (ICNP), SNOMED CT®, and NIC/NOC/NANDA. So as to not limit our customers to any one vocabulary, our solutions allow for any terms to be used.

Current partnerships with clinical content vendors

Siemens Healthcare partners with industry providers of clinical knowledge that our customers can access to complement our starter content. Through our partnership with ZynxHealth, our customers leverage evidence-based orders sets and interdisciplinary plans of care which can serve as the basis of the care delivery process.

In addition, Siemens Healthcare utilizes First Databanks DAM to support clinical checking as part of the medication management process. The First Databanks monographs are also used in Siemens solutions to support patient education.

Vendor Information Sources

Cerner Corporation. (May 2010). Roy Simpson, Vice President, Nursing

Epic Systems Corporation. (May 2010). Emily Barry. Director of Nursing Informatics

Eclipsys Corporation. (May 2010), Jim Cato, Vice President, Chief Nursing Officer

McKesson Information Solutions. (May 2010) Billie Whitehurst, Vice President and Chief Nursing Officer

(continued)

TABLE 21.2	Vendors' Evidence-Based Clinical Content and Standardized Terminology *(continued)*

Vendor Information Sources *(continued)*

GE Healthcare IT Solutions A. (May 2010). Dana Andrews, Chief Nursing Officer

QuadraMed Corporation. (May 2010). Annette Edmonds, Enterprise Solution Architect Clinical Advisor

Siemens Healthcare. (May 2010). Gail Latimer, Vice President and Chief Nursing Officer

[a]Obtained from and published with permission of Cerner Corporation.
[b]Obtained from and published with permission of Epic Systems Corporation.
[c]Obtained from and published with permission of Eclipsys Corporation.
[d]Obtained from and published with permission of GE Healthcare.
[e]Obtained from and published with permission of McKesson Information Solutions.
[f]Obtained from and published with permission of QuadraMed Corporation.
[g]Obtained from and published with permission of Siemens Healthcare.

REFERENCES

The Camden Group. (2003). *Hospital Emergency Departments in Crisis: Aggressive Planning is Needed* (Vol. VII, No. 1).

Carman, K. L., et al. (2010). *Evidence that consumers are skeptical about evidence-based healthcare*. Washington, D. C.: American Institutes for Research.

CCDProblem List. (n.d.). In *Wikipedia*. Retrieved , June 1, 2011, from http://wikipedia.org/wiki

CCR. (n.d.). In *Wikipedia*. Retrieved , June 1, 2011, from http://wikipedia.org/wiki

CDA. (n.d.). In *Wikipedia*. Retrieved , June 1, 2011, from http://wikipedia.org/wiki

Clinical pathways. (n.d.). In *Wikipedia*. Retrieved , June 1, 2011, from http://wikipedia.org/wiki

Commonwealth Fund. (2010, June). Mirror mirror on the wall: How the performance of the U.S. healthcare system compares internationally.

Cornell, Paul PhD; Herrin-Griffith, Donna MSN (September 2010). Transforming Nursing Workflow, Part 1: The Chaotic Nature of Nurse Activities, Journal of Nursing Administration: 40(9) pp 366–373.

Crowley, C, F., & Nalder, E. (2009, August 10). Within healthcare hides massive, avoidable death toll. *Hearst Newspapers.*

(2009, October 1). Avoiding 'Alert Fatigue'. *Health Data Management Magazine.* Retrieved from http://www. healthdatamanagement.com/issues/2009_71/-39039-1. html

Henry, S. B. (1995). A comparison of problem lists generated by physicians, nurses and patients. Proc Annu Symp Comput Appl Med Care. 1995: 382–386 AMIA

U.S. Health Insurance Technology for Economic and Clinical Health Act. (2009). Pub. L. No. 115-5, Division A Title XIII (pp. 112–65) and Division B Title IV (pp. 353–398).

Horowitz, B. T. (2010, June). WiFi use grows strongly in healthcare industry: Report. Retrieved from http:// www.eweek.com/c/a/Health-Care-IT/WiFi-Use-Grows-Strongly-in-Health-Care-Industry-Report-785636.

Institute for Healthcare Improvement & Robert Wood Johnson Foundation. (n.d.). *Transforming Care at the Bedside.* Retrieved from http:// www.ihi.org/IHI/Programs/StrategicInitiatives/ TransformingCareAtTheBedside.htm.

Institute of Medicine. (2000). Kohn, L. T., Janet M. Corrigan, J. M., & Molla S. Donaldson, M. S. (Eds.). *To err is human: Building a safer health system.* Washington, D. C.: National Academy Press.

Institute of Medicine Report. (2001). Crossing the quality chasm: A new health system for the 21st century. Washington, D. C.: National Academy Press.

Joint Commission. (2008, December). Safely Implementing Health Information and Converging Technologies. *Joint Commission Sentinel Alert*, Issue 42.

Joint Commission. (2010, March 5). Medication reconciliation. National Patient Safety Goal to be Reviewed, Refined. Retrieved from http://www.ncbi. nlm.nih.gov/pmc/articles/PMC3041362/

Karp, E., & Gehrt, L. (in press). Health information technology: Acquisition, adoption, and transformation. M. A. Gullatte (Ed.), In *Nursing management: Principles and practice* (2nd ed.). Philadelphia, PA: Springer Publishing.

Leape, L. L., Bates, D. W., Cullen, D. J., et al. (1995). ADE Prevention Group. Systems Analysis of Adverse Drug Events. *JAMA, 274,* 35–43.

Lundeen, S., Harper, E., & Kerfoot, K. (2009). Translating nursing knowledge into practice: An uncommon partnership. *Nursing Outlook, 57*(3).

Malkary, G. (2007). Healthcare without bounds: Point of care computing for nursing. Location: Spyglass Consulting Group, Menlo Park, California.

Malkary, G. (2009, November). Healthcare without bounds: Point of care communications for nursing. Location; Spyglass Consulting Group, Menlo Park, California.

Manos, D. (2008, January 15). Data Farming Helps Hospital Keep Nurses at Bedside. *HealthIT News*. Retrieved from http://www.healthcareitnews.com/news/data-farming-helps-hospital-keep-nurses-bedside.

Medical Diagnosis. (n.d.). In *Wikipedia*. Retrieved June 1, 2011//wikipedia.org/wiki/

NANDA. (1992). *Nursing Diagnosis Frequently Asked Questions*. Retrieved from http://www.nanda.org/NursingDiagnosisFAQ.aspx.

National Priorities Partnership. (2008). National priorities and goals: Aligning our efforts to transform America's healthcare. Washington, DC: National Quality Forum.

Owens, P., et al. February 2006. Hospital admissions that began in the emergency department , 2003. AHRQ health cost and utilization project, AHRQ Statistical Brief #1. Retrieved from http://www.hcup-us.ahrq.gov/reports/statbriefs/sb1.pdf.

Plans of Care. (n.d.). In *Wikipedia*. Retrieved June 1, 2011//wikipedia.org/wiki/

Problem List. (n.d.). In *Wikipedia*. Retrieved , June 1, 2011, from http://wikipedia.org/wiki

Provonost, P., et al. (2003). A practical tool to reduce the risk of medication errors. *Journal of Critical Care Medication Reconciliation*: 18(4), pp (201-205)

Rothberg, M. B., et al. (2005, August). Improving nurse-to-patient staffing ratios as a cost-effective safety intervention. *Medical Care, 43*(8).

Sands, D. Z., et al. (1995). Patient precautions: A forgotten piece of the electronic patient record. Boston: Beth Israel Hospital and Harvard Medical School.

Wager, K. A., et al. (in press 2010). Comparison of Quality and Timeliness of Vital Signs Data during a multi-phase EHR implementation. *Computers in Nursing*. Intel Motion 2009, CIN Sept. 2010.

Warren, J. (1997). Organization and functional features of a multi-disciplinary problem list in an enterprise-wide computer-based patient record. Retrieved from AMIA http://www.ncbi.nlm.nih.gov/pmc/articles/PMC2233332/pdf/procamiaafs00001-0930.pdf. pp 897.

The Role of Technology in the Medication-Use Process

Matthew C. Grissinger / Michelle Mandrack

- OBJECTIVES
  1. Describe factors that will influence the adoption of technology in healthcare.
  2. Describe the challenges and rewards related to implementing a computerized prescriber order entry system (CPOE).
  3. Recognize the benefits and limitations of barcode-enabled point-of-care (BPOC) technology as it relates to overall efforts to reduce medication errors, including errors using these systems.
  4. Define the benefits and limitations of automated dispensing cabinets (ADC) in healthcare and its application to the medication-use process.
  5. Describe the benefits and limitations of smart infusion pump technology.
  6. Recognize the value of and a methodology for assessing an organization's readiness for implementing technology.

- KEY WORDS
  automated dispensing cabinet
  barcode-enabled point-of-care technology
  computer prescriber order entry
  failure mode and effects analysis
  high-alert medications
  medication error
  smart infusion pump delivery systems

INTRODUCTION

Due to the numerous steps required in the care of patients, the healthcare industry is an inherently error-prone process that is fraught with opportunities for mistakes to occur. This concept was confirmed in the oft-quoted 1999 Institute of Medicine (IOM) report, *To Err Is Human: Building a Safer Health System*, where the authors extrapolated that between 44,000 and 98,000 patients die each year in the United States from preventable medical error. These deaths were the results of practitioner interactions with "bad systems" (Kohn, Corrigan, & Donaldson, 1999). The authors emphatically state that the healthcare industry must place safety as the number 1 national priority and work diligently toward this goal. One explicit recommendation emanating from the first of a series of IOM reports on healthcare is to improve the safety design

341

of systems as is presently being employed in other high error-prone industries such as the aerospace and nuclear industries. These industries not only acknowledge and accept the notion that individuals will make errors from normal mental slips and lapses in memory, but recognize that enhancing safety system design through the use of technology is an invaluable tool in the prevention of potentially life-threatening mistakes. More recent estimates on the financial impact of adverse drug events (ADEs) attribute $2 billion of increased hospitalization costs to preventable ADEs (Adachi & Lodolce, 2005). The 2006 IOM report, *Preventing Medication Errors*, noted that to deliver safe drug care, healthcare organizations should make effective use of well-designed technologies, which will vary by setting. Although the evidence for this assertion is strongest in the inpatient setting, the use of technology will undoubtedly lead to major improvements in all settings (Aspden, Wolcott, Bootman, & Cronenwett, 2006).

TECHNOLOGY AND HEALTHCARE

Until recently, the majority of technology acquisitions have consisted of basic stand-alone computer systems, which were primarily used for data input to increase each department's efficiency with financial accountability measures. These computers were generally installed in the pharmacy, radiology, and laboratory departments, and could also be found in the administration and business offices. Each department was allowed to evaluate and purchase their own unique computer system, preventing any integration of data or dissemination of critical patient information, which is indispensable in providing safe care (Leape, Bates, Cullen, et al., 1995). But even as improving technologies have emerged allowing for seamless integration of information to occur, most organizations have shown little interest or incentive to incur the huge costs associated with replacing their present nonintegrated computer systems. According to an American Society of Health-System Pharmacists (ASHP) survey in 2007, nearly half of the responding hospitals stated that they have components of an electronic medical record (EMR), but a complete digital hospital with a fully implemented EMR is far in the future, with only 5.9% of hospitals being fully digital (without paper records). An estimated 12% of hospitals were using computerized prescriber order entry systems (CPOE) with decision support, 24.1% use barcode medication administration, and 44% were using intelligent infusion devices (smart pumps) (Pedersen & Gumpper, 2007).

INFLUENCES ON THE ADOPTION OF TECHNOLOGY

Consumers have become increasingly concerned that hospitals are less than safe following the numerous mass media reporting of medical mistakes, which have resulted in patient harm and deaths. In 1995, there were television and newspaper accounts that reported the tragic death of a patient from a preventable ADE due to an inadvertent administration of a massive overdose of a chemotherapy agent over 4 days. This particular error became a watershed event for patients, practitioners, and healthcare organizations alike, not only because it occurred at the world renowned Dana Farber Cancer Institute, but also because it happened to the prestigious *Boston Globe* healthcare reporter, Betsy Lehman. How could a mistake of this proportion occur in a leading healthcare facility where each practitioner is specifically educated in the care and treatment of cancer patients? A root cause analysis of the error revealed that there was no malpractice or egregious behavior, but that excellent, conscientious, and caring pharmacists and nurses simply interpreted an ambiguous handwritten chemotherapy order incorrectly. In retrospect, if technology had been available, the physician could have entered the medication order into a CPOE system and this heartbreaking error may not have happened.

Unfortunately, this example is by far not an isolated case. According to a 1994 American Medical Association report, medication errors related to the misinterpretation of physicians' prescriptions were the second most prevalent and expensive claim listed on malpractice cases filed over a 7-year period on 90,000 malpractice claims between 1985 and 1992 (Cabral, 1997). Also, it has been estimated in the outpatient setting that indecipherable or unclear orders resulted in more than 150 million telephone calls from pharmacists and nurses to prescribers requiring clarification, which not only is time-consuming for practitioners, but estimated to cost healthcare systems billions of dollars each year. Thus, the availability of critical clinical information needed at point-of-care (during prescribing, dispensing, and administering) can not only improve time management and contribute to cost-savings through improved utilization of medications, staff and patient satisfaction, but most importantly, reduce the incidence of error.

The first organized attempt to move acute care organizations toward improving patient safety through technology began from an initiative by The Leapfrog Group. Composed of more than 150 private and public organizations providing healthcare benefits, this group felt that they had a significant financial investment in preventing errors for their employees, thus increasing productivity by contracting only with those organizations that had hospital-wide adoption of CPOE technology. Yet, a survey by Leapfrog completed in 2003 showed that not only did this financial incentive result in no increase from the 2002 survey in the number of hospitals that had implemented CPOE, but there was also a drop of 17% in hospitals now fully committed to CPOE implementation before 2005 (Stefanacci, 2004). According to Leapfrog, 26% of the 1244 hospitals that completed their survey in 2009 report having a CPOE system in at least one inpatient department (Leapfrog, 2010). Even if an organization implements CPOE, this does not mean that the system will catch incorrect medication orders entered into the system. Another report from Leapfrog, based on a study between June 2008 and January 2010 of 214 hospitals from across the United States who completed Leapfrog's CPOE evaluation tool, revealed that these systems potentially missed half of the routine medication orders and one-third of potentially fatal medication orders (Leapfrog, 2010). Because little research is available on the effectiveness of CPOE on medication error prevention, other organizations such as the Joint Commission, a nonprofit organization that is the nation's leading standards-setting and accrediting body in healthcare, and the National Quality Forum (NQF) are presently refraining from uniformly requiring its adoption.

Probably the most important development to promote the implementation of technology is the announcement by the Centers for Medicare & Medicaid Services (CMS) of a proposed rule to implement provisions of the American Recovery and Reinvestment Act of 2009 (Recovery Act) that provide incentive payments for the meaningful use of certified electronic health records (EHR) technology. The Medicare EHR incentive program will provide incentive payments to eligible professionals, eligible hospitals, and critical access hospitals that are meaningful users of certified EHR technology. The Medicaid EHR incentive program will provide incentive payments to eligible professionals and hospitals for efforts to adopt, implement, or upgrade certified EHR technology or for meaningful use in the first year of their participation in the program and for demonstrating meaningful use during each of 5 subsequent years (CMS, 2010).

Interest in the use of barcoding technology increased due to the Food and Drug Administration's (FDA) February 25, 2004 ruling, which required medications to have machine-readable barcodes. In an optimally acute care, barcoded environment, a nurse would scan his or her barcode identification badge at the beginning of each medication administration time, the patient's barcode identification band, and the intended drug's barcoded label with a barcode scanner. A mismatch between the patient, the drug packaging applied during manufacturing or repackaging, an incorrect time, dose, route, and the patient's medication record would trigger a warning, prompting the nurse to investigate the discrepancy before administering the medication. One of the first healthcare facilities to adopt barcode technology was due to the inspiration of a nurse at the Department of Veterans Affairs (VA) in Topeka, Kansas. Her insight resulted in a 74% improvement in errors caused by the wrong medications being administered, a 57% improvement in errors caused by incorrect doses being administered, a 91% improvement in wrong patient errors, and almost a 92% improvement in wrong time errors between 1993 and 1999. Additional examples of evolving technology used to prevent medication errors include automated dispensing cabinets (ADCs) and smart infusion pumps. As more technology systems are introduced into healthcare, it is important that nurses understand their benefits and problems, and how technology will affect their practice. As noted by the IOM report, *Keeping Patients Safe: Transforming the Work Environment of Nurses*, despite its potential, patient safety experts caution that technology by itself is not a panacea. While able to remedy some problems, technology may also generate new forms of error and failure (IOM, 2004).

Computerized Prescriber Order Entry (CPOE)

To a large degree, healthcare practitioners still communicate information in the "old-fashioned way." According to the aforementioned ASHP technology survey, 17.8% of U.S. hospitals had a CPOE system in 2007. Clinical decision-support systems (CDSSs) are important components of CPOE, directing prescribers toward evidence-based drug therapy. Of those hospitals with CPOE, 67.2% had CDSSs in use to improve prescribing. Nearly one-third of hospitals with CPOE systems did not have a CDSS. In these facilities, clinicians entered orders into electronic systems that did not have rules that integrated order information, patient information, and clinical practice guidelines into computer system logic to provide feedback to prescribers. Therefore, it is estimated that only 12% of U.S. hospitals at the end of 2007 had CPOE with a CDSS (Pedersen, 2007).

Many factors demonstrate the need for a shift from a traditional paper-based system that relies on the practitioners' vigilance to automated order entry, record keeping, and clinical care. These factors include accessing patient information spread across multiple organizations that may be unavailable, especially in large organizations and, therefore, medical care would be provided without pertinent patient information. The structure of the patient's record often makes it difficult to locate valuable information as well as illegible handwritten entries by healthcare practitioners, and for those patients with chronic or complex conditions, the records can increase to multiple volumes over many years. These problems result in a variety of communication breakdowns when providing healthcare to patients from the duplication of services, delays in treatment, increased length of stay, and increased risk of medical errors. Additionally, human memory-based medicine can be inaccurate or not recalled.

Currently, practitioners rely heavily on the unaided mind, which has been proven to be unreliable, to recall a great amount of detailed information. Actually, only a portion of medical knowledge is ever loaded into the prescribers' minds and not all of this knowledge is retained. Also, much of the retained learned knowledge in healthcare quickly becomes obsolete with no assurance that they will acquire any new knowledge. Even if new knowledge is learned and retained, it is impossible for practitioners to integrate all knowledge with an infinite amount of patient data in a short period of time. Faced with knowledge overload, prescribers and other practitioners tend to fall back on clinical judgment rather than organized knowledge.

There are also many barriers that lead to ineffective communication of medication orders that include issues with illegible handwriting, use of dangerous abbreviations and dose designations, and verbal and faxed orders. Studies have shown that as a result of poor handwriting, 50% of all written physician orders require extra time to interpret. Sixteen percent of physicians have illegible handwriting (Cohen, 2007). Illegible handwriting on medication orders has been shown to be a common cause of prescribing errors and patient injury and death have actually resulted from such errors (Brodell, 1997; Cabral, 1997; ASHP, 1993). In a study at a large teaching hospital, published in 2005, 1 in 3 house physicians and medical students who believed their orders were always legible had been asked to clarify them because of poor legibility (Garbutt, Highstein, Jeffe, et al., 2005). Illegible orders may also lead to delays in the administration of medications. To clarify these illegible orders, the healthcare practitioner's workflow is typically interrupted (Cohen, 1999).

The use of a CPOE system has the potential to alleviate many of these problems. CPOE systems allow physicians to electronically order medications, tests, and consultations. They also provide advice on best practices and alerts to the possible adverse consequences of a therapy, such as an allergy or a harmful combination of drugs (American Hospital Association [AHA], 2007). But there are many other potential enhancements that even a basic CPOE system could offer to further enhance safe medication ordering practices, including features unique to the acute care setting, ambulatory care setting or both; allow for prescribers to access records and enter orders from their office or home; prescriber selectable, standardized single orders or order sets; implementation of organization-specific standing orders based on specific situations such as before or after procedures; menu-driven, organization-specific lists of medications on formulary; and passive feedback systems that present patient-specific data in an organized fashion, such as test results, charges, reference materials, and progress notes, or active feedback systems to provide clinical decision-making tools by providing specific assessments or recommendations through alerts and reminders or even therapeutic suggestions at the time the order is entered.

CPOE systems offer many other advantages over the traditional paper-based system. They can improve quality, patient outcomes, and safety by a variety of factors such as increasing preventive health guideline compliance by exposing prescribers to reminder messages to provide preventive care by encouraging compliance with recommended guidelines, identifying patients needing updated immunizations or vaccinations, and suggesting cancer screening and diagnosis reminders and prompts. Other advantages include reductions in the variation in care to improve disease management by improving follow-up of newly diagnosed conditions, reminder systems to improve patient management, automating evidence-based protocols, adhering to clinical guidelines, or providing screening instruments to help diagnosis disorders. Order entry systems can improve drug prescribing and administration by driving formulary usage, improving antibiotic usage, suggesting whether certain antibiotics or their dosages are appropriate for use. Medication refill compliance can be increased using reminder systems to increase adherence to therapies. Drug dosing could be improved, especially for those medications whose dosing is based on laboratory results, such as heparin or warfarin, to maintain adequate anticoagulation control.

Many studies have demonstrated a reduction in ADEs with the use of CPOE. For example, Bates and colleagues showed that serious medication errors were reduced by 55% and preventable ADEs were reduced by 17% (Bates, Leape, Cullen, et al., 1998). Another study has shown that non–missed-dose medication errors fell from 142/1000 patient-days to 26.6/1000 patient-days (Bates, Teich, Lee, et al., 1999). The same study showed a reduction of nonintercepted serious medication errors from 7.6/1000 patient-days to 1.1/1000 patient-days. A study of a pediatric critical care unit found a 41% reduction in potentially dangerous errors after implementation of CPOE (Potts, Barr, Gregory, et al., 2004). A recent evaluation of the potential benefit of CPOE over pharmacist review for ordering errors demonstrated that CPOE could reduce potentially dangerous prescribing errors but would have no effect on administration errors, which have a high risk of patient injury (Wang, Herzog, Kaushal, et al., 2007). In a meta-analysis of 12 original investigations that compared rates of prescribing medication errors with handwritten and computerized physician orders, 80% of those studies reported a significant reduction in total prescribing errors, 43% in dosing errors, and 37.5% in ADEs (Shamliyan, Duval, Du, et al., 2008). Errors of omissions would be reduced, such as failure to act on results or carry out indicated tests. Handwriting and interpretation issues would be eliminated. There would be fewer handoffs if the CPOE system was linked to information systems in ancillary departments which would eliminate the need for staff members to manually transport orders to the pharmacy, radiology department, and laboratory, resulting in fewer lost or misplaced orders and faster delivery time. The system has also eliminated the need for staff members in those departments to manually enter the orders into their information systems, reducing the potential for transcription errors (Healthcare Information and Management Systems Society, 2002). Medical data capture and display would be improved, enabling a more comprehensive and accurate documentation by prescribers and nurses. Access to pertinent literature and clinical information from knowledge bases and literature sources would enable ready access to updated drug information. These obvious improvements to patient care would not only improve patient safety but also increase efficiency, productivity, and cost-effectiveness.

Currently, the cost of providing healthcare is rising while reimbursement for services is declining. Total spending on healthcare in the economy has doubled over the past 30 years to a current level of about 16% of gross domestic product (GDP). The Congressional Budget Office estimates that this percentage will double again over the next 25 years to 31% of GDP (Bartlett, 2009). CPOE systems offer a variety of solutions to help reduce the cost in providing healthcare and making more appropriate utilization of services. In the outpatient setting, reductions in hospitalizations and decreased lengths of stay can be obtained from automated scheduling of follow-up appointments to reducing unnecessary diagnostic tests. Better use of formulary and generic drugs can be achieved by providing feedback of prescribing charges and patterns to encourage prescribers to substitute generic medications for more expensive branded medications. Properly designed systems can show an improvement in workflow and time-saving measures for prescribers, if the program makes sense to the prescriber and follows a rational process while performing order entry, by improving the availability and responses to information regarding diagnosis and treatment. Savings related to the storage of paper medical records could be substantial, compared with the cost of storing computerized backup storage devices. Entering medication and diagnostic orders into a computer system would allow for instantaneous capturing of charges, therefore enhancing revenue. Costs associated with the use of transcription notes would be eliminated as well by using an electronic patient record system. Lastly, there is patient and user satisfaction. For example, the admission process for patients from the outpatient setting into an acute care organization can be a cumbersome and time-consuming process. Electronic systems would improve communication, if connected to an outpatient clinical referral system, by decreasing the amount of time needed to complete the referral process in addition to providing important patient information such as patient allergies and diagnosis. The time spent searching for or organizing paper-based information would be substantially reduced, thus improving prescriber and nurse satisfaction as well.

Despite the many documented benefits of using a computerized system, many roadblocks and safety issues exist. One primary area of concern revolves around the costs of implementation. Investing in a CPOE system is not analogous to purchasing software off the store shelf, and it involves far more resources than spending money on a software package. Hospitals will need a minimum infrastructure to support its use, such as a fiber optic backbone network; time, space, and manpower to provide adequate staff education and development; and workstations and high-speed Internet access. The process of selecting the vendor is a costly and difficult process, especially if a vendor cannot address the organization's specific needs. In addition, staff resources will be needed to develop and program organization-specific rules, guidelines, or protocols and to implement the system, plus provide ongoing support for any needed enhancements or changes to the system. It is also difficult to prove or demonstrate any quantifiable benefits or returns on investment because it is hard to accurately measure the actual costs of using paper-based records. Benefits such as provider convenience, patient satisfaction, and service efficiency are not easily captured on the bottom line in terms of increase in revenue, decrease in expense, or avoidance of expense. Add on top of these competing priorities, including other forms of automation to enhance medication safety, such point-of-care barcoding systems and smart infusion pumps that are currently on the market. Another challenge involves the integration of "legacy" systems, those that have been in institutions for many years, which already exist in healthcare organizations. Many organizations are risk averse, waiting to let others be the clinical pioneers before they invest in these systems. Finally, despite the prospects of enhanced workflow and reduction in medication errors, there are real and potential problems with even the best CPOE systems.

As previously mentioned, CPOE systems have demonstrated a reduction in ADEs. Unfortunately, unsafe prescribing practices and medication errors are still possible with these systems. Some organizations, in fear of alienating prescribers, have an active CPOE system but the clinical order screening capability of warnings and alerts have been turned off. The capability to build rule-based safety enhancements, or clinical decision support (CDS), is often available in the software but the actual rules, such as prompts for prescribers to order potassium replacement for patients with lab results reporting below normal potassium levels, are not provided by the vendor nor are they typically programmed for use by organizations. CDS is a method for delivering clinical knowledge and intelligently filtered patient information to clinicians and/or patients for the purpose of improving healthcare processes and outcomes. CDS includes knowledge-delivery interventions, such as targeted documentation forms and templates, relevant data presentation, order and prescription creation facilitators, protocol and pathway support, reference information and guidance, and alerts and reminders (Osheroff, 2009).

A study by Nebeker and colleagues (2005) showed that high rates of ADEs may continue after CPOE implementation if the system lacks CDS for drug selection, dosing, and monitoring. Studies have shown those prescribers, using only the basic CPOE system alone, order appropriate medication doses for patients 54% of the time. By comparison, prescribers using the CPOE system with decision support tools prescribed appropriate doses 67% of the time. The addition of the decision support tools also increased the percentage of prescriptions considered ordered at appropriate intervals to 59%, from 35% with the basic CPOE system (Kaushal, Bates, Landrigan, et al., 2001). A national sample of 62 hospitals voluntarily used a simulation tool designed to assess how well safety decision support worked when applied to medication orders in computerized order entry. This simulation detected only 53% of the medication orders that would have resulted in fatalities and 10% to 82% of the test orders that would have caused serious adverse drug events (Metzger, Welebob, Bates, et al., 2010)

Complex and time-consuming order entry processes can often lead to practitioner frustration as evidenced by potential increases in the use of verbal orders, another error-prone process in communicating medication orders. Computer issues such as error messages, frozen screens, slow access to information, and other issues lead to problems of accessing critical patient or drug information as well as adding to prescriber frustration. It is important to have the ability to access past patient histories, particularly previous ADEs and comorbid conditions, yet some systems are unable to access prior patient care encounters. Problems may arise if drug information updates are not performed on a timely basis or if this information is difficult to access. One key error reduction strategy is the ability to install user-defined warnings (eg, "look-alike/sound-alike" drug name alert), yet some systems do not allow for this type of customization.

New types of medication errors can occur with the use of CPOE such as wrong patient errors, when the wrong patient is selected from a menu list of similar patient names; wrong drug errors, when the wrong medication is selected from a list due to look-alike similarity in either the brand or generic name; or orders intended for laboratory levels that are filled as medications.

Even though CPOE systems are intended for use by prescribers, their presence in organizations will affect nursing and other personnel as well. CPOE systems will affect or even change the work of nurses in many ways, both negative and positive (AHA, 2000). First, like prescribers, these systems will require nurses to possess basic computer skills. Depending on the design of the system, nurses may find it difficult to know when new orders have been entered into the system, a special concern with respect to "STAT" or other new orders. Nurses sometimes see off-site entry of orders by prescribers as detrimental, because it reduces the opportunity to communicate information or ask questions face-to-face with prescribers with regard to the care of patients. In some situations, prescribers are reluctant to enter orders and use verbal orders as a way of "getting around" entering orders into the CPOE system and, in fact, nurses may end up entering verbal orders from prescribers.

But there are many beneficial aspects of these systems for nurses. Providing the capability for computerized physician order entry and making patient education material available electronically to nurses also have been identified as strategies to facilitate communication. With computerized physician order entry, nurses do not have to engage in transcription or verification of orders. Electronic patient education materials, unlike printed materials, are easily modifiable to meet clinician and patient needs; it is also possible to track which materials were given and by whom, assess follow-up and comprehension, and link education activities and documentation (Case, Mowry, Welebob, 2002). Nurses may have more time with patients due to enhanced productivity due to a reduced frequency in contacting prescribers to clarify orders. Additionally, there would be reductions in time wasted in transcribing duplicate orders for the same medication or test; greater standardization of orders, lessening the need to understand and adhere to diverse regimens and schedules; improved efficiency when ordering tests or procedures, thus reducing time devoted to carrying out redundant orders; and less need to enter voice orders into the system as prescribers gain access to the system from other units and remote locations. Finally, orders would be usually executed faster, medications would be available more quickly and patients receive care more promptly. It is important for healthcare administration and nurses to understand that for a CPOE system to work as intended, it must be fully utilized by prescribers.

Barcode-enabled Point-of-Care (BPOC) Technology

Nurses play a vital role in the medication-use process, ranging from their involvement in the communication of medication orders to the administration of medications. As nurses know well, the administration of medications can be a labor intensive and error-prone process. One study showed that 38% of medication errors occur during the drug administration process (Leape et al., 1995). While about half of the ordering, transcribing, and dispensing errors were intercepted by the nurse before the medication error reached the patient, almost none of the errors at the medication administration stage were caught. In another study of medication administration errors in 36 healthcare facilities, Barker et al. found that some type of medication administration error occurred in almost 20% of medication doses administered (Barker, Flynn, Pepper, et al., 2002). In addition, nurses are burdened with larger patient loads and are caring for patients with higher degrees of acuity then ever before. To make

matters worse, the number of medications that have reached the market has grown 500% over the past 10 years to more than 17,000 trademarked and generic drugs in North America (Institute for Safe Medication Practices [ISMP], 2000). Rapid advances in technology have helped to make this process more efficient and safe. One form of technology that will have a great impact on medication safety during the administration process is barcode-enabled point-of-care (BPOC) technology.

For more than 20 years, barcode technology has clearly demonstrated its power to greatly improve productivity and accuracy in the identification of products in a variety of business settings, such as supermarkets and department stores. Proven to be an effective technology, it quickly spread to virtually all other industries. Yet, relatively few organizations in the healthcare industry have embraced this valuable technology as a method to enhance patient safety.

The American Society of Health-System Pharmacists National Survey reported that approximately 24.1% of hospitals stated using barcode technology (Pedersen et al., 2007). This survey showed that all Veterans Affairs hospitals used BPOC, and general and children's medical–surgical hospitals with 100 to 399 beds were more likely to have BPOC to verify the accuracy of medication administration at the point-of-care. The reasons for these few numbers are varied and may include the cost of implementation, challenges integrating with current informatics systems, and prioritization among other information technology projects. The survey also revealed that larger hospitals (400 or more staff beds) had adopted CPOE before starting to adopt BPOC.

For the healthcare industry, the potential effect of implementing barcode technology to improve the safe administration of medications is enormous. As previously stated, the VA Healthcare System, a pioneer in the use of barcode technology, looked at their medication error rate based on the number of incident reports related to medication errors before and after implementation of the BPOC system. The study showed that following the introduction of the BPOC, reported medication error rates declined from 0.02% per dose administered to 0.0025%. This is almost a 10-fold reduction in errors over 8 years (Johnson, Carlson, Tucker, & Willette, 2002). In a study that used the direct-observation methodology to monitor medication administration before and after the deployment of the electronic medication administration records (eMAR) and barcoded medication administration (BCMA) systems showed a 54% reduction of medication administration errors (Paoletti, Suess, Lesko, et al.,

2007). In another study that assessed rates of errors in order transcription and medication administration on units before and after implementation of the barcode eMAR, observers noted an 11.5% error rate in medication administration on units that did not use the barcode eMAR versus a 6.8% error rate on units that did use it—a 41.4% relative reduction in errors. The rate of potential adverse drug events (other than those associated with timing errors) fell from 3.1% without the use of the barcode eMAR to 1.6% with its use, representing a 50.8% relative reduction (Goon, Keohane, Yoon, et al., 2010).

BPOC can improve medication safety through several levels of functionality. At the most basic level, the system helps to verify that the right drug is being administered to the right patient at the right dose by the right route and at the right time. On admission, patients are issued an individualized barcode wristband that uniquely identifies their identity. When a patient is to receive a medication, the nurse scans their barcoded employee identifier and the patient's barcode wristband to confirm their identity. The Joint Commission has stated that a barcode with two unique, patient-specific identifiers will provide healthcare organizations a system that complies with the 2010 National Patient Safety Goal requirement of obtaining two or more patient identifiers before medication administration (Joint Commission, 2010). Prior to medication administration, each bar-coded package of medication to be administered at the bedside is scanned. The system can then verify the dispensing authority of the nurse, confirm the patient's identity, match the drug identity with their medication profile in the pharmacy information system, and electronically record the administration of the medication in an eMAR system.

The use of an eMAR is likely to be more accurate than traditional handwritten MARs. One study showed that by using BPOC, the medication-verification component greatly facilitates the documentation process for nurses and may be an important factor for its acceptance (Poon, Keohane, Bane, et al., 2008). In a survey of nurses who worked in a variety of clinical settings, the nurses believed that using barcoding and eMARs at the bedside was more time consuming, but they acknowledged that the extra time was worth it to assure verification. Saving time on transcribing orders or trying to read handwritten, paper-based medication sheets was seen by many to be a significant positive change (Hurley, Bane, Fotakis, et al., 2007). Furthermore, the barcode scanner can enable nurses to have greater accuracy in recording the timing of medication administration, as the computer generates an actual "real-time" log of medication administration.

Additional levels of functionality can include some of the following features:

- Up-to-date drug reference information from online medication references. This could include pictures of tablets or capsules, usual dosages, contraindications, adverse reactions and other safety warnings, pregnancy risk factors, and administration details.

- Customizable comments or alerts (eg, look-alike/sound-alike drug names, special dosing instructions [eg, 2 tablets = 10 mg]) and reminders of important clinical actions that need to be taken when administering certain medications (eg, do not crush, respiratory intubation is required for neuromuscular blockers).

- Monitoring the pharmacy and the nurse's response to predetermined rules such as alerts or reminders. This includes allergies, duplicate dosing, over/under dosing, checking for cumulative dosing for medications with established maximum doses such as acetaminophen.

- Reconciliation for pending or STAT orders (ie, a prescriber order not yet verified by a pharmacist). The ability of the nurse to enter a STAT order into the system on administration that is linked directly to the pharmacy profile and prevents the duplicate administration of the same medication.

- Capturing data for the purpose of retrospective analysis of aggregate data to monitor trends (eg, percentage of doses administered late, alerts that were overridden). However, this analysis should *not* be used to assess employee performance, especially if it could lead to punitive action.

- Verifying blood transfusion and laboratory specimen collection identification.

- Increased accountability and capture of charges for items such as unit stock medications.

It is important to understand that the successful implementation of an effective BPOC system "forces" nurses to accept and change some of their long-held practices when administering medications to achieve a higher level of medication safety. When BPOC technology is used correctly, it drives compliance with the proper identification of patients, it documents real-time administration, and acts as a double-check. It is also vitally important to its success that affected staff members, and specifically frontline nurses, are involved in all the decisions related to the purchase, education, and implementation of barcode technology. Before embarking on a BPOC implementation, it is critical to anticipate potential failures and develop contingency plans for unexpected results. Of course, a stringent testing phase should also be built into the system rollout phase using a technique such as failure mode and effects analysis (FMEA) to proactively address potential sources of breakdowns, workarounds, or new sources of medication errors.

One study noted significant changes to workflow that occurred during the implementation of a BPOC system at VA hospitals that might lead to the use of workarounds (Patterson, Cook, & Render, 2002). Negative effects and corresponding workarounds include the following:

- Nurses were sometimes caught "off guard" by the programmed automated actions taken by the BPOC software. For example, the BPOC would remove medications from a patient's drug profile list 4 hours after the scheduled administration time, even if the medication were never administered.

- Inhibited coordination of patient information between nurses and physicians. Before the BPOC was implemented, the prescriber could quickly review the handwritten MAR at the patient's bedside or in the unit's medication room.

- Nurses found it more difficult to deviate from the routine medication administration sequence with the BPOC system. For example, if a patient refused a medication, the nurses had to manually document the change since the medication had already been documented as given when it was originally scanned.

- Nurses felt that their main priority was the timeliness of medication administration because BPOC required nurses to type in an explanation when medications were given even a few minutes late. Particularly in long-term care settings, some nurses were observed to scan and prepour medications for unavailable patients so that they would appear "on time" in the computer record, thereby relying on memory to administer unlabeled medications when the patient returned to the unit.

- Nurses used strategies to increase efficiency that circumvented the intended use of BPOC. For example, some nurses routinely entered a patient's social security number by typing the numbers rather than scanning the patient's barcode wristband, because typing seemed to

be quicker. This was especially true if the nurse experienced difficulty in scanning the patient's barcode arm band (ie, curvature of barcode on patient's wrist band on patients with small wrists, or damaged barcodes) (Patterson et al., 2002).

The interaction between nurses and technology at the bedside is important and must be continually evaluated for safety. As previously mentioned, nurses tend to develop workarounds for ineffective or inefficiently designed systems. Koppel, Wetterneck, Telles, and Karsh (2008) sought to identify reasons for workarounds and found three categories that capture this phenomenon: (a) omission of process steps, (b) steps performed out of sequence, and (c) unauthorized process steps. The authors identified 15 types of workarounds, including, for example, affixing patient identification barcodes to computer carts, scanners, doorjambs, or nurses' belt rings; carrying several patients' pre-scanned medications on carts. The authors identified 31 types of causes of workarounds, such as unreadable medication barcodes (crinkled, smudged, torn, missing, covered by another label); malfunctioning scanners; unreadable or missing patient identification wristbands (chewed, soaked, missing); non-barcoded medications; failing batteries; uncertain wireless connectivity; emergencies. The authors found nurses overrode BCMA alerts for 4.2% of patients charted and for 10.3% of medications charted. The possible consequences of the workaround include wrong administration of medications, wrong doses, wrong times, and wrong formulations. Shortcomings in the BCMAs' design, implementation, and workflow integration encouraged workarounds.

One medication error reported to ISMP caused by a workarounds (overriding an alert), involved a mix-up with an order for digoxin elixir (used for congestive heart failure), which was stocked on the unit as a 0.05 mg/mL, 60 mL multidose bottle (usual dose is 0.125–0.25 mg [2.5–5 mL]). The nurse not only misinterpreted the dose of digoxin elixir as 60 mL, but accidentally retrieved a bottle of doxepin (used for depression), which was available as 10 mg/mL (usual dose is 75–150 mg per day [7.5–15 mL]) from unit stock and attempted to administer what she thought was digoxin elixir. This error occurred because she scanned the barcode on the bottle, which generated an error window on the laptop computer screen stating "drug not on profile" and did not investigate the error. The system allowed the nurse to manually enter the wrong medication's national drug code (NDC) number (a medical code set that identifies prescription drugs and some over-the-counter products), ignoring the correct drug NDC number that had been entered by the pharmacy which appeared on the laptop screen and administered 60 mL of doxepin elixir. This allowed the nurse a method to bypass the check system and simply type in numbers and administer a drug, whether it was the right or wrong ordered medication.

Alerts that are generated by BCMA systems often may not be noticeable. For example, a system may generate a visual display of the alert but not provide a distinct auditory alert. If a nurse does not look at the screen for any alerts after scanning a patient's wristband and/or barcoded medications, errors will ensue. Additionally, the alerts are not hard-stops, meaning that the system does not physically stop a practitioner from proceeding with scanning or administering a medication (Patient Safety Authority [PSA], 2008). Problems have also occurred when other processes surrounding medication administration have broken down. Although the steps directly involved with the scanning of the medication and patient may be completed, errors can be introduced if distractions occur or medications are laid down after the scanning process.

One major issue that initially hindered the widespread implementation of BPOC systems was with the pharmaceutical industry's unwillingness to adopt a universal barcode standard and apply a barcode consistently to the container of all medications, including unit-dose packages. But in February 2004, the FDA established a new rule that requires a barcode on most products in a linear format that meets the Uniform Code Council (UCC) or Health Industry Business Communications Council (HIBCC) standards. This barcode must contain the product's NDC number, but the expiration date and lot numbers are optional (ISMP, 2004).

Further complicating the issue is the unavailability of unit-dose packaging for some medications. At this point, if hospital pharmacies that employ barcode technology cannot purchase medications that are packaged in a unit-dose system, they must repackage these medications and relabel each with a barcode. This can only be done at considerable cost in manpower and/or automated repackaging equipment. In addition, the chance of a medication error occurring is increased because doses must be taken from their original container and then repackaged or relabelled, and there could be an error in the application of the correct barcode label or in choosing the right medication. One medication error report includes a scenario where a facility that utilized a barcode medication administration system for their inpatients where not all injectables used at the organization had manufacturers' barcodes on the vials or ampules, and pharmacy technicians had to generate computer-printed barcodes for those products. Prior

to the intubation of a patient, a vial of succinylcholine chloride with an incorrect dose label was discovered. The printed label read 20 mg/10 mL, whereas, the manufacturer's label read 20 mg/mL. Had the patient received the incorrect dose, it would have been 10 times the dose needed.

The use of BPOC systems can possibly introduce new types of medication errors. Although, few medication errors have been reported with these systems, it can be hypothesized that some of the following types of errors could occur, especially if the system includes only the most basic of functionality:

- **Wrong dosage form:** Certain drug shortages may force a pharmacy to dispense a different strength or concentration (mg/mL) other than what is entered in the BPOC software.

- **Omissions**: After the patient's barcode armband and medication have been scanned, the dose is inadvertently dropped onto the floor. This results in a time lapse between the documentation that the medication was supposedly administered and the actual administration after obtaining the new dose.

- **Extra dose**: An extra dose may be given when there are orders for the same drug to be administered by a different route. For example, if one nurse gives an oral dose and is called away and the covering nurse administers the dose intravenously (IV). The problem arises when there is no alert between profiled routes of administration indicating that the medication was previously administered by one route that is different than the second route.

- **Wrong drug**: In situations when the nurse received an alert indicating that the wrong medication was selected, but the alert is overridden and the medication is administered.

- **Wrong dose:** These systems are limited in their capability to verify the correct volume (eg, 1 mL) of oral or parenteral solutions to administer. Most systems prompt a nurse to manually enter the volume that was administered.

- **Unauthorized drug:** An order to hold a medication unless a lab value is at a certain level such as an aminoglycoside (ie, elevated gentamicin drug level).

- **Charting errors:** Distinguish the indication for the administration of the medication (Tylenol 650 mg every 4 hours as needed for pain or fever).

Automated Dispensing Cabinets

Traditionally, hospital pharmacies provided medications for patients by filling patient-specific bins of unit-dose medications, which were then delivered to the nursing unit and stored in medication carts. The ADC is a computerized point-of-use medication-management system that is designed to replace or support the traditional unit-dose drug delivery system. The devices require staff to enter a unique logon and password to access the system using a touch screen monitor or by using finger print identification. Various levels of system access can be assigned to staff members, depending on their role in the medication-use process. Once logged into the system, the nurse can obtain patient-specific medications from drawers or bins that open after a drug is chosen from a pick list.

Many healthcare facilities have replaced medication carts or open unit-stock systems with ADCs. The results of an ISMP survey showed that 94% of respondents stated that they were utilizing ADCs in their facilities; of those, more than half (56%) are using the technology as the primary means of drug distribution (ISMP, 2008a).

The results of an ASHP survey of 1066 pharmacy directors showed that hospitals are split between centralized and decentralized drug distribution systems. For maintenance doses, about half of hospitals used ADCs, about 40% of hospitals used a manual unit-dose system, and about 10% of hospitals used a robot. Although over 80% of hospitals had ADCs, about half of hospitals used ADCs to provide maintenance doses on nursing units, and 30% of hospitals with ADCs used them to provide first doses in procedure areas to provide as-needed medicines, and for other uses (Pedersen, 2007).

The rationale behind the wide acceptance of this technology may include:

- **Improved pharmacy productivity**: The streamlining of the dispensing process due to the reduced number of steps from filling each patient's individual medication bins to filling a centralized station. It also has the potential to reduce time needed to obtain missing medications.

- **Improved nursing productivity**: In a study that was designed to assess how nurses spend their time, nurse location and movement, and nurse physiologic response, approximately two-thirds of all time spent on medication administration was related to drug delivery to the patient (46.7 minutes). The other third (24.9 minutes) was spent preparing drugs for administration. The

authors concluded that process improvements could reduce the time required for this step (Hendrich, Chow, Skierczynski, et al., 2008). Therefore, the time spent gathering or obtaining missing medications could be reduced. Also, the turnaround time in obtaining newly ordered medications is decreased.

- **Reduced costs**: Increased pharmacist and nursing productivity, which frees them from time-consuming processes and allowing more time for patient and clinical interactions. There also is a reduction in inventory and containment costs associated with expired medications.

- **Improved charge capture**: ADCs that are interfaced with the accounting department allow for the capture of all patient charges associated with administered medications (CardinalHealth, 2003).

In addition, some systems allow for organization-specific, user-generated warnings to prevent medication errors such as warnings of potential errors from look-alike/sound-alike medication names. ADCs can also be used to comply with regulatory requirements by tracking the storage, dispensing, and use of controlled substances.

However, such systems cannot improve patient safety unless cabinet *design* and *use* are carefully planned and implemented to eliminate opportunities for wrong drug selection and dosing errors. More than 356 medication error reports involving the use of ADCs have been submitted to the Institute for Safe Medication Practices Medication Errors Reporting Program (MERP). According to the Pennsylvania Patient Safety Authority, nearly 15% of all medication error reports cited ADCs as the source of the medication, and 23% of those reports involve high-alert medications. Many of the reports described cases in which the design and/or use of ADCs has contributed to the errors. The types of errors reported included wrong drug errors, stocking/storage errors, and medications being administered to patients with a documented allergy (PSA, 2005).

Some documented unsafe practices with the use of these devices include **the lack of pharmacy screening of medication orders prior to administration**, which negates an independent double-check of the original order. At a minimum, medication orders are screened by the pharmacy for the appropriateness of the drug, dose, frequency, and route of administration, therapeutic duplication, real or potential allergies or sensitivities, real or potential interactions between the prescription and other medications, food, and laboratory values, and other contraindications.

This is particularly problematic when medications, which are considered "high-alert" medications, are stored in these devices[1] (Table 22.1). For example, one medication error occurred in a small hospital after the pharmacy was closed. An order was written for "calcium gluconate 1 g IV," but the nurse misread the label and believed that *each 10 mL* vial contained only 98 mg. Thus, she thought she needed 10 vials when actually each mL actually contained 98 mg, or 1 g/10 mL vial. A 10-fold overdose was avoided because the drug cabinet contained only six vials of calcium gluconate. Fortunately, this error was detected when the nurse contacted a pharmacist at home to obtain additional vials.

Choosing of the wrong medication from an alphabetic pick list is a common contributing factor in medication errors, which arises from medication names that look alike. For example, one organization reported three errors regarding mix-ups between diazepam and diltiazem removals from their ADCs in their intensive care units. In one case, diazepam was given at the ordered diltiazem dose and, in another case, a physician noted the amber color of the diazepam vial as the nurse was drawing up the dose (meaning to obtain diltiazem). The organization concluded that once the wrong drug was chosen, the cabinet seemed to "confirm" that the correct drug was selected since the nurse assumed the correct drug was chosen from the menu and thought the correct drug was in the drawer that opened. The nurse "relied" on her ability to choose the right drug from the pick list and, in these cases, no physical check of the product was made or reading of the label was done.

Medications, especially high-alert drugs, placed, stored, and returned to ADCs are problematic. The process of placing and restocking medications into an ADC is primarily a pharmacy function. Unfortunately, studies have indicated that an independent double-check (one individual supplies the cabinet with the medication and a second individual independently checks that the correct medication was placed into the correct location) does not occur. A survey by ISMP of more than 800 practitioners revealed the following:

- The requirement for a pharmacist to check ADC stock medications before they leave the pharmacy increased from 65% in 1999 to 75% in 2007.

TABLE 22.1	Examples of ISMP's High-Alert Medications

Class/Category of Medications

- Adrenergic agonists, IV (eg, epinephrine)
- Adrenergic antagonists, IV (eg, propranolol)
- Anesthetic agents, general, inhaled, and IV (eg, propofol)
- Chemotherapeutic agents, parenteral and oral
- Dextrose, hypertonic, 20% or greater
- Epidural or intrathecal medications
- Glycoprotein IIb/IIIa inhibitors (eg, eptifibatide)
- Hypoglycemics, oral
- Inotropic medications, IV (eg, digoxin, milrinone)
- Liposomal forms of drugs (eg, liposomal amphotericin B)
- Moderate sedation agents, IV (eg, midazolam)
- Moderate sedation agents, oral, for children (eg, chloral hydrate)
- Narcotics/opioids, IV and oral (including liquid concentrates, immediate and sustained release)
- Neuromuscular blocking agents (eg, succinylcholine)
- Radiocontrast agents, IV
- Thrombolytics/fibrinolytics, IV (eg, tenecteplase)

Specific Medications

- IV amiodarone
- Colchicine injection
- Heparin, low-molecular-weight, injection
- Heparin, unfractionated, IV
- Insulin, subcutaneous, and IV
- IV lidocaine
- Magnesium sulfate injection
- Methotrexate, oral, nononcologic use
- Nesiritide
- Nitroprusside, sodium, for injection
- Potassium chloride for injection concentrate
- Potassium phosphates injection
- Sodium chloride injection, hypertonic, >0.9% concentration
- Warfarin

---

[1]High-alert medications can be defined as medications that, when involved in medication errors, have a high risk of injury or death. There is no documentation that the occurrence of medication errors is more common with high-alert medications than with the use of other drugs but the consequence of the error may be far more devastating (Cohen, 2007). Examples of high-alert medications can be found in Table 22.1 (ISMP will provide list as a side table).

- No improvement was seen between 1999 and 2007 regarding verification processes *after* restocking the ADCs; in both years, only 18% of respondents reported that another person verifies drug placement in the ADC.

- Requiring another practitioner to double-check a drug removed from an ADC via override, before pharmacy review, only increased from 10% in 1999 to 29%

- While these checking functions could be performed with barcoding, only 25% of hospitals use this technology to verify the accuracy of drugs that have been selected to restock the ADCs or to verify accuracy when placing them in the cabinets (ISMP, 2008a).

Even when the barcode on a drug container is matched with the proper location of an ADC, loading the equipment is a manual operation. In one case, a patient had orders for both MS Contin (morphine sulfate *controlled* release) 15 mg tablets and for morphine sulfate *immediate* release 15 mg tablets. A pharmacy technician loaded both medications in the ADC in the patient care unit. The person loading the medications inadvertently loaded the MS Contin in the pocket for the morphine sulfate immediate release and the morphine sulfate immediate release in the pocket for the MS Contin. Some doses of each medication were actually administered to a patient. Fortunately, the patient suffered no apparent adverse effects from this incident. A second nurse discovered the error when removing the medication for the next dose.

Another report involved the need to refill unit stock in an ADC with furosemide 40 mg/4 mL. A pharmacy technician pulled what was thought to be vials of furosemide 40 mg/4 mL from the stock in a satellite pharmacy and then, without a pharmacist double-check, left the pharmacy and filled the ADC. A nurse on the unit went to the cabinet to fill an order for furosemide 240 mg. She obtained six vials out of the ADC and drew them into a syringe. After drawing up the sixth vial, the nurse noticed a precipitation. At that point, the nurse checked the vials to find that she had five vials of furosemide 40 mg/4 mL and one vial of phenylephrine 1% 5 mL. Both these medications were available in the same size amber vials with very little color or marking differentiation.

Storage of medications with look-alike names and/ or packaging next to each other in the same drawer or bin is one of the root causes of more than half the errors reported through the MERP (ISMP, 1999). A common cause of these mix-ups is what human factors experts call "confirmation bias," where a practitioner reads a drug name on an order or package and is most likely to see that which is most familiar to him, overlooking any disconfirming evidence. Also, when confirmation bias occurs, it is unlikely that the practitioner would question what is being read. This can occur both in the restocking process of the ADC and in the removal of medications. One example includes a situation where a physician asked for ephedrine, but a hurried nurse picked epinephrine from

the ADC, drew up the medication into a syringe and handed it to the primary nurse who administered the epinephrine. The patient suffered a period of hypertension and chest pain but eventually recovered. In another example, a prescriber wrote an order for morphine via a patient-controlled analgesia (PCA) pump. The nurse used the override function (the manual action taken to counteract or bypass the normal operation) to remove a PCA syringe containing meperidine from the ADC. When pharmacy reviewed the override medication removals report the next morning, the error was discovered. The PCA pump still had the meperidine cartridge in place, but the pump settings were for morphine, resulting in an inappropriate dose. An example that made national news involved three premature infants who died in a Midwestern hospital after receiving an overdose of heparin. Vials of heparin 10,000 unit/mL 1 mL were placed incorrectly into a unit-based automated dispensing cabinet where 1 mL, 10 units/mL vials were normally kept. Several nurses requested 10 units/mL vials to prepare an umbilical line flush and were directed to that drawer, but did not notice that the vials contained the wrong concentration (ISMP, 2006).

The development of "workarounds" for ineffective or inefficient systems can be devastating to patient safety. The interaction between a nurse and technology is very important and often is not considered when various forms of automation, including ADCs, are purchased, installed, and employed on the nursing unit. When the device does not respond as expected, nurses often find various ways of working around the system to obtain medications. In the error previously mentioned, overrides were established by the organization that allowed nursing to obtain medications without the approval or review by a pharmacist. Overrides usually are needed with medications used in emergency situations. Unfortunately, when overused, overrides also serve as an "extended" pharmacy in order to obtain and administer medications prior to verification by the pharmacy. Additional error reports involving workarounds include the removal of medications using the inventory function (used to determine the number of doses on hand of a particular medication) to obtain medications for patients without pharmacy screening, removal of a larger quantity of medications than ordered for one patient, and removal of medications for multiple patients while the cabinet is open.

One study involving the use of an expert panel who developed criteria for override access and revised the override medication list by reducing the number of medications and dosage forms on the override list by 42%, from 119 different medications (in 244 different dosage forms) to 92 different medications (in 163 different dosage forms), resulting in a significant decrease in opioid override rates (Kowiatek, Weber, Skledar, et al., 2006).

In spring 2007, the ISMP convened a national forum of stakeholders to create interdisciplinary guidelines for ADCs. These guidelines are intended to be universally incorporated into practice in an effort to promote safe ADC use and subsequently improve patient safety. This lead to the development of core processes, listed below, including a description of the element of practice and a rationale for the process.

1. **Provide Ideal Environmental Conditions for the Use of ADCs.** The physical environment in which the ADC is placed can have a dramatic effect on medication errors. Specifically, the work environment and a busy, chaotic work area were cited as the top two contributing factors in medication errors

2. **Ensure ADC System Security.** Security processes must be established to ensure adequate control of medications outside of the pharmacy and to reduce the potential for medication diversion from ADCs.

3. **Use Pharmacy-profiled ADCs.** The use of a "profiled" ADC ensures that the pharmacist will validate the new medication order, including first doses, in the pharmacy computer system prior to the medication being dispensed or accessed by the nurse or other healthcare professional.

4. **Identify Information That Should Appear on the ADC Screen.** Having sufficient patient information and drug information when dispensing and administering medications is key to the safety of the medication use process. Because there is limited space available on the ADC screens, it is important to focus on presenting the information that is of the greatest value to practitioners, allowing for the clear identification of specific patients, their active medication profiles, and supporting information for safe drug use.

5. **Select and Maintain Proper ADC Inventory.** The ADC inventory should be determined based on the needs of the patients served and replenished on a regular basis. Medications should be routinely reviewed and adjusted based on medication prescribing patterns, utilization, and specific unit needs (taking into account typical patient ages and diagnoses). Standard stock medication should be identified, and approved, for each patient care area.

6. **Select Appropriate ADC Configuration.** Restricting access to medications limits the potential for inadvertently selecting the wrong medication. Medications stocked in ADCs may be high alert or high cost, and it is important to ensure that only the right drug is selected. For these reasons, it is important that each drug have its own unique and segregated location within the ADC, so only the specific drug needed is accessible.

7. **Define Safe ADC Restocking Processes.** The restocking process encompasses a number of sub-processes that can involve both pharmacy and nursing staff. It is important that the process contain redundancies to ensure that the correct medication is placed in the correct location within the ADC. It is also important that the process be defined and organized so staff involved can only follow the correct pathway and the potential for process variation is limited.

8. **Develop Procedures to Ensure the Accurate Withdrawal of Medications From the ADC.** Processes must be developed that reduce the risk or mitigate the harm associated with the administration of the wrong medication, dose, route, or frequency due to retrieval errors of medications from the ADC. The contents (variety, concentrations, and volume) and configuration of the ADC play a large role in the practitioner's ability to safely select and remove medications from the ADC.

9. **Establish Criteria for ADC System Overrides.** Use of ADC overrides should be situationally dependent, and not based merely on a medication or a list of medications. Criteria for system overrides should be established that allow emergency access in circumstances in which waiting for a pharmacist to review the order before accessing the medication could adversely impact the patient's condition.

10. **Standardize Processes for Transporting Medications From the ADC to the Patient's Bedside.** A process should be developed that reduces the risk of medications being administered to the wrong patient at the wrong time during the transportation of medications from the ADC to the patient. Supporting safety may require the availability of additional ADCs or the placement of ADCs in strategic locations to prevent workarounds. Not having sufficient ADCs, or having them located far from patient

rooms, fosters the at-risk behavior of taking medications for more than one patient at a time or taking medications for more than one scheduled administration time. The safety of this practice also is impacted by the organization's ability to secure medications during transport between the ADC and the patient's bedside.

11. **Eliminate the Process for Returning Medications Directly to Their Original ADC Location.** One source of incorrectly stocked items is allowing practitioners to return a medication directly to the ADC bin or pocket. Occasionally medications are inadvertently returned to the wrong pocket, either because of user distraction, look-alike and sound-alike medications in a matrix bin, or a slip in procedure.

12. **Provide Staff Education and Competency Validation.** All users of the ADCs must be educated and have regular competency validation in the safe operation of the device in order to meet expectations for safe use. Most often this education occurs during the practitioner's orientation period, or upon ADC installation, but an annual update may be required in order to ensure ongoing appropriate use. Users who are not properly oriented to the device may develop practice habits and device workarounds that are considered unsafe (ISMP, 2008b).

Regardless of an organization's steps to purchase or implement ADCs, the following issues should be considered to ensure safe medication practices:

- Consider purchasing a system that allows for patient profiling so pharmacists can enter and screen drug orders prior to their removal from the ADC and subsequent administration. Also, consider purchasing a system that utilizes barcode technology during the stocking, retrieval, and drug administration processes.

- Carefully select the drugs that will be stocked in the cabinets. Consider the needs of each patient care unit as well as the age and diagnoses of patients being treated on the units. If possible, minimize the variety of drug concentrations avoiding bulk supplies, and stock drugs in ready-to-use unit-doses.

- Place drugs that cannot be accessed without pharmacy order entry and screening in individual matrix bins. Store all drugs that do not require pharmacy screening together so that access to these medications does not also allow access

to other drugs, which do require pharmacy screening.

- Use individual cabinets to separate pediatric and adult medications.

- Periodically reassess the drugs stocked in each unit-based cabinet. As appropriate, remove low-usage medications and those with multiple concentrations.

- Remove only a single dose of the medication ordered. If not administered, return the dose to the pharmacy or ADC return bin and allow pharmacy to replace it in the cabinet.

- Develop a check system to assure accurate stocking of the cabinets. Another staff member from pharmacy or nurse on the unit can verify accurate stocking by having pharmacy provide a daily list of items added to the cabinet.

- Routinely run and analyze override reports to help track and identify problems.

- Periodically assess the medication safety practices in your institution surrounding the use of automated dispensing cabinets, identifying opportunities for improvement.

Smart Infusion Pump Delivery Systems

Infusion pumps are primarily used to deliver parenteral medications through IV or epidural lines and can be found in a variety of clinical settings ranging from acute-care and long-term care facilities, patient's homes, and physician's offices. Among ADEs, the significant potential for patient injury and death related to IV medication errors is well known (ASHP, 2008; Aspden, Wolcott, Bootman, & Cronenwett, 2006; Cohen, 2007).

Medication errors with infusion pumps can occur due to incorrect or inappropriate order, or miscalculation of a drug order. Studies have shown that medications intended for IV or epidural use are involved in many serious mishaps. In a study of pediatric inpatients, IV medications were associated with 54% of potential ADEs, and 60% of serious and life-threatening errors were associated with IV therapy (Kaushal et al., 2001). One study showed that the most common reason for the administration of wrong doses of intravenous medications was an error in programming IV infusion pumps (41%), and this step in the medication-use process was associated with the highest impact (Adachi & Lodolce, 2005). An Australian study designed to identify the prevalence of medication administration errors and their related causes found that errors in the administration of continuous IV infusions occurred in almost one out of five infusions, and the most common error (79.3%) was wrong administration rate (Han, Coombes, & Green, 2005). Husch and colleagues (2005) examined IV administration errors specifically associated with IV pumps and of the 426 medications observed infusing via an IV pump, 66.9% had one or more errors related to their administration. Causes of these IV administration errors were diverse in nature. Infusion pumps with dose calculation software, often referred to as smart pumps, could reduce medication errors, improve workflow, and provide a new source of data for continuous quality improvement by identifying and correcting pump-programming errors.

The administration of parenteral medications has traditionally been based on a calculation of a volume to be infused per hour of delivery. Infusion pumps are capable of delivering a wide range of delivery rates, ranging from 0.01 mL/h to as much as 1 L/h, which could result in the device being programmed all too easily in error to deliver a 10- or 100-fold overdose. Confusion with dosing nomenclature has been another source of error. A medication may be inadvertently programmed to be administered as micrograms per kilogram per minute (mcg/kg/min) instead of micrograms per minute (mcg/min), a 24-hour dose may be delivered over 1 hour, or a missing decimal point or an additional zero may result in a 10-fold overdose. Infusion pumps are specifically designed to have maximum flexibility, so they can be used in multiple areas of the facility. Consequently, a pump used today for a 200-kg patient in the adult ICU may also be used on a 1 kg premature infant. Errors of 10, 100, or even 1000 times the intended dose can easily be programmed, since there are no limits in devices. Basically, the safe use of infusion pumps requires perfect performance by the practitioner programming the pump.

There are numerous published reports of fatal errors involving infusion pumps, such as when a nurse attempted to program an infusion pump for a baby receiving total parenteral nutrition (TPN) by inputting 13.0 mL/h. The decimal point key on the pump was somewhat worn and difficult to engage. Without realizing it, the nurse programmed a rate of 130 mL/h. Fortunately, the error was discovered within 1 hour. The baby's glucose rose to 363, so the rate of infusion for the TPN was decreased for a while and the baby was fine.

In other cases, morphine was entered as 90 mg/h instead of 9 mg/h, causing delivery of 10 times the intended dose. Nitroglycerin ordered to be administered in mcg/min was inadvertently programmed as mcg/kg/min, resulting in administration of 60 times the

intended dose, and in a neonatal ICU, an infusion rate was reprogrammed from 3.2 to 304 mL/h, when the intention was 3.4 mL/h.

In addition, many of the tragic errors occurring with PCA pumps have resulted from incorrect programming of the drug concentration, leading to 10-fold overdoses. In terms of rate, any IV solution ordered for administration over a 24-hour period can be easily programmed incorrectly to infuse in 1 hour (Reves, 2004).

The common denominator in many of these and other cases was a single wrong entry or button pressed. The use of a smart infusion pump, programmed with patient and drug parameters, would have been able to recognize the error before the infusion even began since a practitioner would no longer have to rely on memory to determine correct dosing, or on keystroke accuracy to ensure correct programming. Instead, a practitioner could rely on the technology of the smart pump, which is programmed according to institution-established best practices. In a study to assess the impact of infusion pump technologies, comparing traditional infusion pumps with smart pumps, the number of nurses who remedied "wrong dose hard limit" errors was higher when using the smart pump (75%) than when using the traditional pump (38%) (Trbovich, Pinkney, Cafazzo, et al., 2010).

The introduction of smart infusion technology has changed the paradigm of infusion therapy by removing the reliance on memory and human input of calculated values to a software-enabled filter to prevent keystroke errors in programming infusion devices for delivery of parenteral medications. Smart pumps can include comprehensive libraries of drugs, usual concentrations, dosing units (eg, mcg/kg/min, units/h) and dose limits as well as software that incorporate institution-established dosage limits, warnings to the practitioner when dosage limits are exceeded, and configurable settings by patient type or location in the organization (ie, ICU, pediatric ICU [PICU]). Such systems make it possible to provide an additional verification at the point-of-care to help prevent medication errors. Although not widely available at the present time, smart infusion systems could also integrate barcode technology to provide additional checks and balances in the drug administration process. This would ensure that the correct medication intended for parenteral administration is reaching the correct patient at the right dose, prior to the initiation of the infusion.

Current smart pump software enables the infusion system to provide an additional verification of the programming of medication delivery. The user receives an alert when the dose is below or above the organization's preestablished limits. Depending on the drug, these alerts can be warnings that must be confirmed or stops that require the nurse to reprogram the pump for a different infusion rate. The limits can be set as either "soft" (can be overridden) or "hard" (one that will not let the nurse go any further without reprogramming the pump). The drug library in the system generally requires the practitioner to confirm the patient care area, drug name, drug amount, diluent volume, patient weight (as appropriate), dose, and rate of infusion. The system can allow organizations to configure unit-specific profiles, which include customized sets of operating variables, programming options, and drug libraries.

Access to transaction data from the infusion device can be obtained for quality improvement efforts. Continuous quality improvement logs in the software record the close calls (programming errors) averted by the new system. Practitioners can use this tool to assess current practices and identify ways of improving safe use of medications. This provides data on transactions at the bedside that are not currently available with traditional infusion devices. For each safety alert, a record can be generated with the time, date, drug, concentration, programmed rate, volume infused, and limit exceeded, as well as the clinician's response to the warning (ie, continue at the current settings or change the programming). Similar data for infusions delivered with traditional settings for rate and volume can also be captured, along with other transactional data generated as a result of pump use (eg, alarms, air in line). Thus, the system can be used to show whether potential infusion errors were detected and to assess current practice to determine if improvements can be made to optimize care and reduce costs.

Documented examples of errors prevented using smart pump technology have been published. For example, a physician in the emergency department wrote an order for Integrilin (eptifibatide) but inadvertently prescribed a dose appropriate for ReoPro (abciximab). The Integrilin infusion was initiated and continued for approximately 36 hours after the patient was transferred to a medical/surgical unit. During this time, the patient's mental status was deteriorating. Coincidentally, at that time, the hospital was switching to a smart pump infusion system, which performed a "test of reasonableness" before allowing the infusion to begin. As the nurse was transferring the infusion parameters from the old infusion system to this new system, safety software incorporated in the device alerted the nurse that there was a "dose out of range." The pump would not allow the nurse to continue until a pharmacist was called and the mistake was corrected.

In another case, a hospital's heparin protocol called for a loading dose of 4,000 units followed by a constant infusion of 900 units/h. The loading dose was administered correctly, but the nurse inadvertently programmed the continuous dose as 4,000 units/h. Since the pump limit for heparin as a continuous infusion was set at 2,000 units/h, the infusion device would not start until the dose was corrected. In both cases, these mistakes may have gone undetected without preprogrammed limits and patient harm might have resulted (ISMP, 2002).

Prior to implementation, it is important to use a proactive technique (eg, FMEA) to assess for the risk of error and determine potential issues with IV drug administration utilizing smart infusion pumps. Implementation should be coordinated by a multidisciplinary team that can determine best practices. This team should institute changes in policies and procedures that reflect the installation of smart infusion technology. Asking a nurse to choose from among many concentrations, dosing units, or remembering several possible drug names will increase the risk of error with smart pump use. Therefore, standardization of IV-related policies and procedures, standardization of concentrations, dosing units (eg, mcg/min vs mcg/kg/min) and drug nomenclature is essential. These items should be consistent with those used on the MAR, CPOE system, pharmacy computer system, electronic medical record and pharmacy labels, if applicable. The effective implementation of smart technology thus changes the role of the nurse from that of looking for or memorizing data and rules to that of a clinical decision maker.

Many drug references provide information on the maximum dose over a 24-hour period but do not provide the minimum and maximum doses that can be administered over 1 hour so the team should determine dosage limits for infusions and boluses based on current policy and practice, the literature, and common references used in medical practice. In addition, there needs to be a determination of which dose limits require a "soft" or a "hard" stop. Existing best practices and policies and unit-based dosage limits should then be used to developed data sets based on patient care areas, for example, adult ICU, adult general care, neonatal intensive care unit (NICU), PICU, pediatric general care, labor and delivery, and anesthesia. Different configurations can be developed for each area. Lastly, a procedure for the nursing staff to follow in the event a drug must be given which is not in the library or if a nonstandardized concentration must be used, should be created (Institute for Healthcare Improvement, 2004).

Smart pump technology is also not without limitations. If the smart pump drug library is bypassed, and the infusion rate and volume is manually entered, the dose error reduction software will not be in place to prevent a potential error. Engaging in this at-risk behavior reduces the likelihood that an error will be identified since no alerts will be triggered (ISMP, 2009). In a prospective, randomized time-series trial, Rothschild and colleagues (2005) noted that intravenous medication errors were frequent and could be detected using smart pumps. The authors found no measurable impact on the serious medication error rate with smart infusion pumps, likely in part due to poor compliance. Violations of infusion practice during the intervention periods included bypasses of the drug library (25%). Numerous events were reported to the Pennsylvania PSA that includes examples of errors associated with the use of smart infusion pumps. Some examples include similar types of errors that may occur with the use of general infusion pumps.

- Organizations that did not standardize the concentrations of high-alert medications.

- Practitioners inadvertently switching IV lines between separate infusion pumps or dual-chambered infusion pumps.

- Wrong-dose errors when inaccurate patient weights were used to calculate and program weight-based doses.

- Inadvertent selection of a wrong drug or the wrong unit of measure in the smart pump's library (PSA, 2007).

IMPLEMENTATION OF TECHNOLOGY

Implementing any form of technology in a healthcare organization can be an imposing task. Many organizations have purchased various forms of automation, with little or inadequate planning and/or preparation, which can lead to errors as well as the development of serious problems. Therefore, it is vitally important to thoroughly plan for the workflow changes and to remember your goal is to improve clinical processes, which can be facilitated by technology. Foremost, the process will require total commitment from the organization's executive and medical leadership as well as all staff members who will be affected by the implementation. It is essential that leadership sends a clear message that the new technology is important to patient safety and that they provide their unwavering support and financial backing as the project evolves. Providing this

level of commitment will greatly increase the success of the project.

Identifying physician champions at a very high level in the organization is crucial and involving them in the decision making and planning process will help to persuade practitioners to "buy into" technology. In addition, an interdisciplinary team of key individuals who can collaborate on an effective and realistic plan for implementation, including front-line clinical staff should be organized to provide ongoing project direction and oversight. Important key players such as the chief information officer, information technology, risk managers, medical staff, front-line practitioners, and other support staff who may interact directly with the technology (ASHP, 2001). The multidisciplinary implementation team will need to address the following issues:

- Outline goals for the type of automation to be implemented (eg, to improve safety, decrease costs, eliminate handwritten orders). Consider identifying primary and secondary goals.

- Develop a wish list of desired features and determine which, given budgetary constraints, are practical.

- Investigate systems that are presently available. Find out about successes and failures by talking with or visiting individuals from other organizations who have implemented similar systems. Determine whether the new system will interface with your current information systems and to what extent will customization be required.

- Analyze the current workflow and determine what changes are needed. This may include any changes that will occur in the current processes as well as the organizational culture. A lack of fit with clinical process and practice can be a downfall because healthcare practitioners tend to resist process changes that produce inefficiencies, complicate their work, or do not provide clear benefits.

- Policies and procedures for both the implementation and ongoing use must be defined prior to rollout. There will be numerous workflow changes that must be carefully planned to address the multiple operational transitions during the rollout such as:

  ○ When each care area transitions from a paper-based system to an automated system

- When patients are transferred from the automated units to areas with no automation
- Healthcare providers working in areas with automation to areas without automation (California HealthCare Foundation, 2000)

- Identify the required capabilities and configuration of the new system. If the system allows for the creation of rules, protocols, guidelines, or drug dictionaries, individuals that will be affected by these changes need to develop these items before the system is implemented.
- "Sell" the benefits and objectives of automation to staff. Do not try to justify the new system by promising that it will allow the institution to decrease the number of staff members, because it most likely will not. A good system, though, should enhance safety and improve efficiency by decreasing the number of repetitive and mundane tasks. You may see the number of steps in the medication-use process decrease, but the remaining steps will require highly educated, competent personnel who understand and can deal with the complexity and importance of those steps.
- Develop an implementation plan. Set realistic timeframe expectations. Extensively test the system for accuracy and safety before implementation. Focus on efficiency and safety. Healthcare practitioners will not use a system, which is perceived as less efficient than the existing system.

Once the system has been implemented within the organization, there are still many issues that need to be considered. Plan on many years of system development and enhancement after the product is initially piloted. As soon as the system is installed, it is important to commit in a meaningful way to its continual monitoring and improvement. The healthcare environment is a dynamic one in which opportunities for new (and some old, but as yet unidentified) errors will likely arise. Identify key measures that will help you determine whether your systems are really improving safety and quality and reducing costs. Beware of cumbersome features that may provoke users to override features or develop workarounds with the system. Finally, do not be discouraged by initial dissatisfaction among staff members, and do not interpret initial negative reactions as failures.

CONCLUSION

Nurses have the responsibility to become familiar with the availability of "safety" technology, its advantages and disadvantages, and to work in collaboration with other healthcare stakeholders in the search for new and innovative technologic solutions to improve patient safety.

REFERENCES

Adachi, W., & Lodolce, A. E. (2005). Use of failure mode and effects analysis in improving the safety of i.v. drug administration. *American Journal of Health-System Pharmacy*, 62, 917–920.

American Hospital Association. (2000). *AHA guide to computerized physician order-entry systems.* (2000). Retrieved on 9 August, 2010 from http://www.hospitalconnect.com/aha/key_issues/medication_safety/contents/CompEntryA1109.doc

American Hospital Association. (2007). *Continued progress hospital use of information technology.* Retrieved on 10 August, 2010 from http://www.aha.org/aha/content/2007/pdf/070227-continuedprogress.pdf.

American Society of Health-System Pharmacists. (1993). ASHP guidelines on preventing medication errors in hospitals. *American Journal Hospital Pharmacists, 50,* 305–314.

American Society of Health-System Pharmacists. (2008). Proceedings of a summit on preventing patient harm and death from i.v. medication errors. *American Journal of Health-System Pharmacy, 65,* 2367–2379.

American Society of Health-System Pharmacists. (2001). *Computerized prescriber order entry systems.* Retrieved on 9 August, 2010 from http://www.ashp.org/patientsafety/genprinciples.cfm?cfid=11647716&CFToken=88898100.

Aspden, P., Wolcott, J. A., Bootman, L., & Cronenwett, L.R. (Eds.) (2006). *Preventing medication errors: quality chasm series.* Washington, DC: The National Academies Press.

Barker, K. N., Flynn, E. A., Pepper, G. A., et al. (2002). Medication errors observed in 36 healthcare facilities. *Archives of Internal Medicine, 162,* 1897–1903.

Bartlett, B. (2009). Healthcare: Costs and reform. Forbes. Retrieved on 12 August, 2010 from http://www.forbes.com/2009/07/02/health-care-costs-opinions-columnists-reform.html

Bates, D. W., Leape, L. L., Cullen, D. J. (1998). Effect of computerized physician order entry and a team intervention on prevention of serious medication errors. *Journal of American Medical Association, 280,* 1311–1316.

Bates, D. W., Teich, J. M., Lee J.,Leape LL, Cullen DJ, et al. (19998). The impact of computerized physician order entry on medication error prevention. *Journal of the American Medical Informatics Association, 6,* 313–321.

Brodell, R. T. (1997). Prescription errors. Legibility and drug name confusion. *Archives of Family Medicine, 6,* 296–298.

Cabral, J. D. T. (1997). Poor physician penmanship. *Journal of American Medical Association, 278,* 1116–1117.

CardinalHealth. (2003). *Healthcare technology: innovating clinical care through technology.* Retrieved on 12 August, 2010 from http://www.pyxis.com/products/Automation_Pharmacies.pdf

Case, J., Mowry, M., Welebob, E. (2002). The nursing shortage: Can technology help? Oakland, CA: California HeathCare Foundation.

California HealthCare Foundation. (2000). *A primer on physician order entry.* Retrieved on 12 August, 2010 from http://www.chcf.org/documents/hospitals/CPOEreport.pdf

Centers for Medicare & Medicaid Services. (2010). *Fact Sheets. Details for: CMS proposes definition of meaningful use of certified electronic health records (EHR) technology.* Retrieved on 12 August, 2010 from http://www.cms.gov/apps/media/press/factsheet.asp?counter=3564

Cohen MR. (1999) Preventing Medication Errors Related to Prescribing. In: Cohen MR. *Medication errors.* Washington (DC): American Pharmaceutical Association; 8.2.

Cohen MR. (2007) Preventing Prescribing Errors. In: Cohen MR. *Medication errors,* 2nd ed. Washington (DC): American Pharmaceutical Association; 189.

Garbutt, J. M., Highstein, G., Jeffe, D. B., et al. Safe medication prescribing: training and experience of medical students and housestaff at a large teaching hospital. *Academic Medicine, 80,* 594–599.

Goon, E. G., Keohane, C. A., Yoon, C. S., et al. (2010). Effect of bar-code technology on the safety of medication administration. *New England Journal of Medicine, 362,* 1698–1707.

Han, P. Y., Coombes, I. D., & Green, B. (2005). Factors predictive of fluid administration errors in Australian surgical care wards. *Quality and Safety in Healthcare, 14,* 179–184. Retrieved November 30, 2008 from http://qshc.bmj.com.ezproxy.library.drexel.edu/cgi/reprint/14/3/179

Hendrich, A., Chow, M., Skierczynski B, et al. A 36-hospital time and motion study: How do medical-surgical nurses spend their time? *Permanente Journal, 12,* 25–34.

Healthcare Information and Management Systems Society. (2002). Gaining MD buy-in: Physician order entry. *Journal of Healthcare Information Management, 16,* 67.

Hurley, A.C., Bane, A, Fotakis, S. et al. (2007). Nurses' satisfaction with medication administration point-of-care technology. *Journal of Nursing Administration, 37,* 343–349.

Husch, M., Sullivan, C., Rooney, D., et al. (2005). Insights from the sharp end of intravenous medication errors: Implications for infusion pump technology. *Quality and Safety in Healthcare, 14,* 80–86.

Institute for Healthcare Improvement. (2004). *Reduce adverse drug events (ADEs) involving intravenous medications: implement smart infusion pumps.* Retrieved on 16 August, 2010 from http://www.qualityhealthcare.org/IHI/Topics/PatientSafety/MedicationSystems/Changes/IndividualChanges/ImplementSmartInfusionPumps.htm

Institute of Medicine. (2004). Keeping patients safe: transforming the work environment of nurses. Washington, DC: National Academies Press. http://www.nap.edu/catalog.php?record_id=10851

Institute for Safe Medication Practices. (1999). "Prescription mapping" can improve efficiency while minimizing errors with look-alike products. *ISMP Medication Safety Alert!, 4*(20),1.

Institute for Safe Medication Practices. (2000). *A call to action: eliminate handwritten prescriptions within 3 years.* Retrieved on 9 August, 2010 from http://www.ismp.org/MSAarticles/Whitepaper.html

Institute for Safe Medication Practices. (2002). "Smart" infusion pumps join CPOE and bar coding as important ways to prevent medication errors. *ISMP Medication Safety Alert!, 7*(3), 1.

Institute for Safe Medication Practices. (2004). *ISMP Medication Safety Alert!, 9*(4), 1.

Institute for Safe Medication Practices. (2006). Infant heparin flush overdose. *ISMP Medication Safety Alert!, 11*(19), 1–2.

Institute for Safe Medication Practices. (2008a). ADC survey shows some improvements, but unnecessary risks still exist. *ISMP Medication Safety Alert!, 13*(1), 1–2.

Institute for Safe Medication Practices. (2008b). *Guidance on the interdisciplinary safe use of automated dispensing cabinets.* Retrieved August 18, 2010 from http://www.ismp.org/Tools/guidelines/ADC_Guidelines_Final.pdf

Institute for Safe Medication Practices. (2009). *Proceedings from the ISMP Summit on the use of smart infusion pumps: guidelines for safe implementation and use.* Retrieved August 18, 2010 from http://www.ismp.org/Tools/guidelines/smartpumps/comments/printerVersion.pdf

Kohn, L., Corrigan, J., and Donaldson, M. (Eds.). (1999). *To err is human: Building a safer health system.* Washington, DC: National Academy Press.

Johnson, C. L., Carlson, R. A., Tucker, C. L., and Willette, C. (2002). Using BCMA software to improve patient safety in Veterans Administration Medical Centers. *Journal of Healthcare Information Management, 16*(1), 46–51.

The Joint Commission. (2010). *2010 accreditation program: Hospital national patient safety goals.* Retrieved on

10 August, 2010 from http://www.jointcommission. org/NR/rdonlyres/868C9E07-037F-433D-8858- 0D5FAA4322F2/0/July2010NPSGs_Scoring_HAP2.pdf

Kaushal, R., Bates, D. W., Landrigan, C., et al. (2001). Medication errors and adverse drug events in pediatric inpatients. *Journal of American Medical Association, 285*, 2114–2120.

Koppel, R., Wetterneck, T., Telles, J. L., & Karsh, B-T. (2008).Workarounds to barcode medication administration systems: Their occurrences, causes, and threats to patient safety. *Journal of the American Medical Informatics Association, 15*, 408–423.

Kowiatek, J. G., Weber, R. J., Skledar, S. J., et al. (2006). Assessing and monitoring override medications in automated dispensing devices. *Journal on Quality and Patient Safety, 32*, 309–317.

Leape, L. L., Bates, D. W., Cullen, D. J., et al. (1995). Systems analysis of adverse drug events. *Journal of the American Medical Association, 274*, 35–43.

Leapfrog. (2010). *Leapfrog Group report on CPOE evaluation tool results June 2008 to January 2010.* Retrieved on 16 August, 2010 from http://www. leapfroggroup.org/news/leapfrog_news/4778021

Metzger, J., Welebob, E., Bates, D. W., et al. (2010). Mixed results in the safety performance of computerzied physician order Entry. *Health Affairs, 29*, 655.

Nebeker, J. R., Hoffman, J. M., Weir, C. R., et al. (2005). High rates of adverse drug events in a highly computerized hospital. *Archives of Internal Medicine, 165*, 1111–1116.

Osheroff J, ed. (2009) Improving medication use and outcomes with clinical decision support: a step-by- step guide. Chicago: Healthcare Information and Management Systems Society.

Paoletti, R. D., Suess, T. M., Lesko, M. G., et al. (2007). Using bar-code technology and medication observation methodology for safer medication administration. *American Journal of Health-System Pharmacy, 64*, 536–543.

Pennsylvania Patient Safety Authority. (2005). Problems associated with automated dispensing cabinets. *Pennsylvania Patient Safety Advisory, 2*, 122–126.

Pennsylvania Patient Safety Authority. (2007). Smart infusion pump technology: don't bypass the safety catches. *Pennsylvania Patient Safety Advisory, 4*, 139–143.

Pennsylvania Patient Safety Authority. (2008). Medication errors occuring with the use of bar-code administration technology. *Pennsylvania Patient Safety Advisory, 5*, 21–23.

Patterson, E. S., Cook, R. I., & Render, M. L. (2002). Improving patient safety by identifying side effects from introducing bar coding in medication administration. *Journal of the American Medical Informatics Association, 9*, 540–553.

Pedersen, C. A., & Gumpper, K. A. (2007). ASHP national survey on informatics: Assessment of the adoption and use of pharmacy informatics in U.S. hospitals—2007. American *Journal of Health-System Pharmacy, 65*, 2244–2264.

Poon, E. G., Keohane, C. A., Bane, A., et al. Impact of barcode medication administration technology on how nurses spend their time providing patient care. *Journal of Nursing Administration, 38*, 541–549.

Potts, A. L., Barr, F. E., Gregory, D. F., Wright, L., & Patel, N, R. (2004). Computerized physician order entry and medication errors in a pediatric critical care unit. *Pediatrics, 113* (1 pt 1), 59–63.

Reves, J. G. (2004). *"Smart pump" technology reduces errors.* Retrievedon 16 August, 2010 from http://www.apsf. org/newsletter/2003/spring/smartpump.htm

Rothschild, J. M., Keohane, C. A., Cook, E., F., et al. (2005). A controlled trial of smart infusion pumps to improve medication safety in critically ill patients. *Critical Care Medicine, 33*, 533–540.

Shamliyan, T. A., Duval, S., Du, J., et al. (2008). Just what the doctor ordered. Review of the evidence of the impact of computerized physician order entry system on medication errors. *Health Services Research, 43*, 32–53.

Stefanacci, R. (2004). Public reporting of hospital quality measures. *Health Policy Newsletter, 17*, 4.

Trbovich, P. L., Pinkney, S., Cafazzo, J. A., et al. (2010). The impact of traditional and smart pump infusion technology on nurse medication administration performance in a simulated inpatient unit. *Quality & Safety on Healthcare, 19*, 430–434. .

Wang, J. K., Herzog, N. S., Kaushal, R., Park, C., Mochizuki, C., Weingarten, S. R. (2007). Prevention of pediatric medication errors by hospital pharmacists and the potential benefit of computerized physician order entry. *Pediatrics, 119*, e77–e85.

23

Planning, Design, and Implementation of Information Technology in Complex Healthcare Systems

Thomas R. Clancy

• OBJECTIVES

1. Define complex systems in the context of general systems theory (GST).
2. Describe complex adaptive systems, a special case of complex systems.
3. Illustrate challenges and solutions for planning and designing information technology in complex healthcare systems.
   i   Wicked problems
   ii High reliability organizations
   iii Structured and agile design methods
4. Provide examples of tools and methods used to plan and design information systems in complex healthcare processes.
   i   Computer-aided software engineering
   ii Discrete event simulation
   iii Network analysis tools

• KEY WORDS

Complex adaptive systems
Wicked problems
Agile design
Discrete event simulation
Network science
Nurse informaticist
Electronic medical record
Systems analyst

INTRODUCTION

The introduction of information technology into the workflow of clinicians requires thoughtful planning, design and implementation. Healthcare organizations of today are among some of the most complex systems in the world. They are composed of diverse specialties and multiple providers linked through a complex information network. Understanding and predicting the impact of new technology on healthcare system behavior is an ongoing challenge for nurse informaticists. That is because complex systems are unpredictable and what works in one organization does not guarantee success in another.

Nurse informaticists play a critical role in the successful deployment of healthcare information technology. Their unique blend of clinical knowledge and information systems expertise make them ideal systems analysts. As complex systems research discovers new findings, nurse informaticists must remain informed on how new knowledge can be translated into practice settings. The objective of this chapter is to provide a review of complex systems from the context of a general systems theory and then provide an overview of new strategies to plan, design and implement information systems in healthcare organizations.

GENERAL SYSTEMS THEORY

A system can be defined as a set of interacting units or elements that form an integrated whole intended to perform some function (Skyttner, 2001). An example of a system in healthcare might be the organized network of providers (nurses, physicians, and support staff), equipment and materials necessary to accomplish a specific purpose such as the prevention, diagnosis and treatment of illness. General systems theory provides a general language which ties together various areas in interdisciplinary communication. It endeavors toward a universal science that joins together multiple fields with common concepts, principles, and properties. Although healthcare is a discipline in and of itself, it integrates with many other systems from fields as diverse as biology, economics, and the physical sciences.

Systems can be closed, isolated, or open. A closed system can only exchange energy across its borders. For example, a green house can exchange heat (energy) but not physical matter with its environment. Isolated systems cannot exchange any form of heat, energy or matter across their borders. Examples of closed and isolated systems are generally restricted to physical sciences such as physics and chemistry. An open system is always dependent on its environment for the exchange of matter, energy and information. Healthcare systems are considered open and are continuously exchanging information and resources throughout their many integrating subsystems. Some fundamental properties collectively comprise a general systems theory of open systems.

Open Systems

All open systems are goal seeking. Goals may be as fundamental as survival and reproduction (living systems) to optimizing the flow of information across computer networks. To achieve goals, systems must transform inputs into outputs. An input might include the entry of information into a computer where it is transformed into a series of binary digits (outputs). These digits can then be routed across networks to end users more efficiently than other forms of communication. As simple systems interact, they are synthesized into a hierarchy of increasingly complex systems, from subatomic particles to entire civilizations (Skyttner, 2001). Levels within the hierarchy have novel characteristics that apply universally upward to more complex levels but not downward to simpler levels. In other words, at lower or less complex levels, systems from different fields share some characteristics in common. For example, both computer and biological systems communicate information by encoding it; either through computer programs or via the genome, respectively. It is the interrelationships and interdependencies between and across levels in hierarchies that creates the concept of a holistic system separate and distinct from its individual components. As commonly noted, a system is greater than simply the sum of its individual parts.

Complex Systems

System behavior can be related to the concept of complexity. As systems transition from simple to complex it is important for nurse informaticists to understand that system behavior also changes. This is especially important in the management of data and information for clinical and administrative decision-making. Table 23.1 presents some examples of differences between simple and complex systems in healthcare.

As healthcare systems become increasingly complex it becomes progressively more difficult to predict how changes in provider workflow are impacted by new information technology. This is especially important for those individuals responsible for planning, designing, and implementing information systems in the healthcare environment of today.

TABLE 23.1	Simple versus Complex Healthcare Systems		
Simple System	**Example**	**Complex System**	**Example**
There are a small number of elements in the system. Elements are parts of the system (people, places, and things)	A one physician, one nurse practice	There are a large number of elements in the system	A large academic health center with multiple providers and specialties
There are few interactions between the elements	Interactions occur primarily between the nurse and physician and patient	Many interactions between elements	Thousands of interactions occur daily between patients, providers, and machines (computers)
Interaction between elements is highly organized. The number of subsystems is small and fixed. Information flows primarily in two or three directions	There is direct communication between the nurse, physician and patient. These interactions may be enabled through a single, practice based EMR	Interactions between elements are loosely organized. There are multiple levels in the hierarchy of subsystems where information flows in many directions	Interactions occur between multiple providers. The medical center may have a sophisticated EMR with many applications integrated within it
System behavior varies little. Day-to-day activities are highly predictable	Because patient acuity varies little, provider workload remains the same from day to day	System behavior is probabilistic and it is impossible to predict with certainty	Because patient acuity can vary considerably. Provider workload can change significantly from day to day
The system does not evolve over time, is largely closed and is slow to adapt to environmental changes	The practice is mature and is not accepting new patients	The system evolves over time. The system is largely open and constantly adapting to the external environment	The medical center has multiple specialties that accept diverse disease conditions that require on-going research and new knowledge
The system is not robust to environmental shocks	Changes in reimbursement or competitive pressures can quickly eliminate the practice in the marketplace	Because of its diversity of services, the system can withstand environmental shocks	Because there are many providers with multiple specialties, the system can withstand significant environmental changes that may impact one area

The evolution of information systems in healthcare is replete with failed implementations, cost overruns and dissatisfied providers. It is important to understand, however, that healthcare systems of today are some of the most complex in the world. The unpredictable nature of complex healthcare systems results from both structural and temporal factors. The structure of complex systems is composed of numerous elements connected through a rich social network. In hospitals, those interactive elements include both internal entities such as patients, nurses, physicians, technicians, and external entities, such as other hospitals, insurance payers, and regulatory agencies. The way information flows through this complex web of channels depends on the technology used, organizational design, and the nature of tasks and relationships (Clancy & Delaney, 2005).

As systems evolve from simple to complex systems a hierarchy of levels emerges within the organization. From a theoretical standpoint, complex systems form a "fuzzy," tiered structure of macro-, intermediary, and microsystems (Clancy & Delaney, 2005). In hospital environments, for example, nursing units can be understood as microsystems within the health system. When nursing units are combined into divisions (eg, critical care, medical-surgical, or maternal-child), the nursing units' internal processes expand beyond their boundaries (eg, the medication usage process) to create intermediary or meso-systems. Major clinical and administrative systems emerge at the macro level through the aggregation of interactions occurring at lower levels.

At the micro-system level, the relationship between cause and effect is somewhat predictable. However, as the organizational structure expands to include meso- and macro-system levels, causal relationships between stimulus and response become blurred. With increasing levels of complexity, the rich network of interactions between nurses, physicians, pharmacists, and other providers at multiple levels within the organization, quickly expands the variability and range of potential states a system might exhibit. This is the driving force behind the unpredictability in complex system behavior.

Complex Adaptive Systems

Complex adaptive systems (CAS) are special cases of complex systems; the key difference being that a CAS can learn and adapt over time (Clancy, Effken, & Persut, 2008). From biologic to man-made systems, CAS's are ubiquitous. The human body, composed of its many subsystems (cardiovascular, respiratory, neurologic) is a CAS and continuously adapts to short- and long-term changes in the environment. The same principles can be applied to social organizations such as clinics or hospitals. Organizational learning is a form of adaptation and it has the capacity to change culture. New reporting relationships can alter the structure of a social network and act as the catalyst for adaptation to environmental change. For example, the movement from hierarchical organizational structures to quasi-networked reporting relationships can improve communication both vertically and horizontally.

Complex adaptive systems exhibit specific characteristics that are different than simple systems and the terminology used to define them may be unfamiliar to healthcare providers. Table 23.2 provides a description of terminology used to describe complex system behavior. Each term in the table builds on the previous term to demonstrate how system behavior becomes unpredictable.

As healthcare systems become increasing complex, those individuals challenged with planning, designing and implementing information technology must be knowledgeable of complex adaptive system principles as well as the tools and methods to analyze their behavior.

INFORMATION SYSTEM PLANNING

The interrelatedness of subsystems characteristic of complex healthcare processes requires participation by many different stakeholders in the planning cycle. In complex systems, outputs from one process often become inputs to many others. A new admission on a nursing unit (input) can generate orders (output) to pharmacy, radiology, respiratory care as well as many other departments. As various levels of care (clinic, hospital, long-term care) become increasingly connected, interoperability of computer systems becomes crucial. In addition, as clinical and administrative areas become more specialized, it is essential that domain experts participate in the planning process.

Wicked Problems

Problems encountered in complex systems are commonly described as "wicked". A wicked problem is difficult or impossible to solve because of incomplete, contradictory, and changing requirements that are often difficult to recognize (Rittel, Horst and Webber, 1973). Wicked problem are:

- Very difficult to define or formulate
- Not described as true or false, but as better or worse
- Have an enumerable or exhaustive set of alternative solutions
- Inaccessible to trial and error; solutions are a "one-shot" deal
- Unique and often a symptom of another problem

Provider order entry (POE) systems often exhibit wicked problem behavior because stakeholders have incomplete, contradictory and changing requirements. For example, although POE systems have been shown to reduce cycle time for the entire medication management process on a *global* level, individual providers may spend more time *locally*, having to enter orders via a keyboard. Here global and local benefits contradict each other. In addition, commercial vendors cannot allow "test driving" their application before purchase (trial and error). Because of the enormous expense associated in implementation of POE applications, once a system has been installed it is very difficult and costly to remove it (a one-shot deal). Finally, because practice patterns vary, each provider wants the system customized to their workflow (each problem is unique). But because there are many providers there are an enumerable number of alternative solutions.

Wicked problems cannot be solved by the common rubric of defining the problem, analyzing solutions and making a recommendation in sequential steps; the reason being, there is no clear definition of the problem. By engaging all stakeholders in problem solving, those people most affected participate in the planning

TABLE 23.2	Complex Adaptive Systems Terminology	
Term	**Description**	**Example**
Combinatorial complexity	A system with a large number of alternative states	The medication management process involves many different providers, medications, times, routes and patients. The many potential combinations of these at any one time can be enormous
Dynamic complexity	The degree to which system behavior becomes more complex over time	Computer provider entry systems can create a network of interactions between the prescription, transcription, dispensing and administration process that is so complex that errors may become lost in the system. *Over time*, if not discovered, the effects of the error can amplify and result in serious harm to a patient
Feedback	The iterative process where system outputs loop back and impact system inputs	Growth in the complexity of CPOE systems is driven by feedback. Since CPOE systems are composed of combinations of many different applications, new combinations of them create new features adding to overall complexity. Technology actually creates itself out of itself
Exponential growth	The doubling of an output in a fixed period of time. Exponential growth can be positive or negative	The computational processing capacity of computers doubles about every 18 months. This phenomenon, known as Moore's law, has held steady for many years
Nonlinearity	When stimulus and response are unequal. A large stimulus may have little effect on outcomes while a small stimulus may generate a large response	The introduction of information technology into the traditional workflow of providers can elicit a significant backlash if not carefully managed. The long-term negative effects of provider resistance can far exceed the initial costs of purchasing the system
Self-organization	The "coming together" of system entities (providers) to achieve a goal without the guidance or influence of a central authority	Work-arounds are a form of self-organization. For example, if a new barcode medication management system interferes with the workflow of nurses, they may self-organize and apply short-cuts without knowledge by the manager.
Emergence	New patterns of behavior arising from self-organization	A spike in medication errors from work-arounds may emerge as a new pattern on managerial reports
Stochastic	The distribution of events is a mixture of deterministic and random processes	The sequence of times between medication administrations is a mixture of scheduled (deterministic) and PRN (random) processes. The distribution is neither fully deterministic nor random
Chaos	Chaos describes a class of systems in which small changes to the initial conditions of the system create deterministic (nonrandom), but very complex behavior	The behavior of a system, from simple to complex lies on a continuum from fully deterministic to fully random. Chaos appears random but in fact is deterministic. It is found primarily in natural systems (weather patterns, biologic systems, chemistry) but also in man-made systems. Chaotic behavior often shows itself in the sequence of events in a process, ie, inter-arrival rate of admissions to a nursing unit
Power law distributions	A power law distribution is characterized by a few events of enormous magnitude disbursed among many events with much smaller impact	Pareto's law where 80% of the output is caused by 20% of the input is an example of a power law distribution. For example, 80% of the complaints surrounding a new information systems may be verbalized by only 20% of the users

process and a common, agreed approach can be formulated. Of utmost importance is understanding that different problem solutions require different approaches. For example, barcoded medication management is one strategy for reducing medication errors. However, to be effective, this strategy must be implemented as part of an overall strategy for reducing medical errors. This strategy might be adopting concepts and principles from High Reliability Organizations (HRO). A high reliability organization assumes that accidents (or errors) will occur if multiple failures interact within tightly coupled, complex systems. Much of the research regarding HRO has been fueled by well-know catastrophes, such as the Three Mile Island nuclear incident, the space shuttle Challenger explosion, and the Cuban Missile Crisis (Weick & Sutcliff, 2001).

High Reliability Organizations

Key attributes of HROs include a flexible organizational structure, an emphasis on reliability rather than efficiency, aligning rewards with appropriate behavior, a perception that risk is always present, sense making (an understanding of what is happening around you), heedfulness (an mutual understanding of roles), redundancy (insuring there is sufficient flex in the system), mitigating decisions (decision making that migrates to experts), and formal rules and procedures that are explicit. Employing information technology, such as barcoded medication administration, must be implemented in the context of an overall strategy to become an HRO. For example, Bar Code Medication Administration (BCMA) emphasizes reliability over efficiency and integrates formal rules and procedures into the medication management process. Collectively, these features reduce the probability of multiple failures converging simultaneously.

On the other hand, planning for clinical decision support (CDS) applications may require a different approach than implementation of BCMA. CDS systems link health observations with health knowledge to influence health choices by clinicians for improved healthcare (Garg, Adhikari, McDonald, et al., 2005). These applications cover a broad range of systems from simple allergy alerts to sophisticated algorithms for diagnosing disease conditions. The cognitive sciences inform and shape the design, development, and assessment of information systems and CDS technology. The subfield of medical cognition focuses on understanding the knowledge structures and mental processes of clinicians during such activities as decision making and problem solving (Patel, Arocha, & Kaufman, 2001).

Optimizing the capabilities of CDS systems to allow better decision-making requires an understanding of the structural and processing patterns in human information processing. For example, knowledge can be described as conceptual or procedural. Conceptual knowledge refers to a clinicians understanding of specific concepts within a domain while procedural knowledge is the "how to" of an activity. Conceptual knowledge is learned through mindful engagement while procedural knowledge is developed through deliberate practice. If CDS planners are not careful, they may inadvertently design a system that transforms a routine task such as checking a lab value (procedural knowledge) into a cumbersome series of computer entries. If the clinician is simultaneously processing conceptual knowledge (problem solving and decision making) and complex procedural tasks, it will place an unnecessary burden on working memory and create frustration.

In summary, the frequent occurrence of wicked problems in complex healthcare systems highlights the challenges faced by information system planners today. Successful planning for the introduction of information technology requires participation by a diverse group of stakeholders and experts. There is no "cookie cutter" solution in system planning. Each application must be aligned with an overall organizational strategy which drives the implementation approach.

INFORMATION SYSTEM DESIGN

The characteristic behavior of complex systems and the emergence of wicked problems have prompted system planners to search for new methods of system design and implementation. The introduction of new information technology in healthcare organizations involves the integration of both new applications and incumbent legacy systems. For example, a new POE application will need to interface with existing pharmacy, radiology, and laboratory systems. Although, an initial "starter set of orders" usually accompanies the POE application, the task of interfacing it with appropriate departmental systems, creating new order sets, and developing CDS generally falls to an internal implementation team with vendor support. Over time, this development team will design and build a POE system that is much different than the original application.

Structured Design

Historically, design and implementation of healthcare information systems relied heavily on structured methods. The most common structured design and

TABLE 23.3	System Design and Life Cycle
Step	**Description**
1	Identify problems, opportunities, and objectives
2	Determine human information requirements
3	Analyze system needs
4	Design the recommended system
5	Develop and document software
6	Test and maintain the system
7	Implement and evaluate the system.

implementation method used is the Systems Design Life Cycle (SDLC). The SDLC acts as a framework for software development, implementation, and testing of the system. Table 23.3 presents the broad steps in the SDLC (Kendall & Kendall, 2006).

A SDLC approach prescribes the entire design, testing and implementation of new software applications as one project with multiple subprojects (see Table 23.3). Project deadlines can extend over many months and in some cases years. The method encourages the use of standardization (eg, programming tools, software languages, data dictionaries, data flow diagrams, and so forth). Extensive data gathering (interviews, questionnaires, observations, flow charting) occurs before the start of the project in an effort to predict overall system behavior, after full implementation of the application.

Agile Design

As healthcare systems have become increasingly complex, the SDLC approach has come under fire as being overly rigid. Behavior, characteristic of complex systems, (sensitivity to initial conditions, nonlinearity and wicked problems) is often unpredictable, especially after the introduction of information technology in clinical workflow. Equally challenging is the difficulty of trialing the impact of new information systems before having to actually purchase them. Site visits to observe a successful application in one facility are no guarantee of success in another. Many healthcare organizations have spent countless millions in failed system implementations.

To overcome these problems, healthcare organizations are turning to "agile" methods for design and implementation of information systems (Kendall & Kendall, 2006). Agile design is less prescriptive than structured methods and allows for frequent trial and error. Rather than mapping the entire project plan up front, agile

methods clearly define future milestones but focus on short term successes. To do so the implementation team and software developers collaboratively evaluate and prioritize the sequence of task to implement first. Priority is assigned to tasks that can be accomplished within a short time frame, with a minimum of cost while maintaining high quality standards. This "time boxing" of projects forces the team to search for simple, but elegant solutions. Developers often work in pairs to cross check each others work and distribute the workload. Communication is free flowing between developers and the implementation team. Once a solution is developed it is rapidly tested in the field and then continuously modified and improved. There is a philosophy that the interval between testing and feedback be as close as possible to sustain momentum in the project.

Agile design is one example of how to manage information technology projects in complex systems. Rather than trying to progress along a rigid project schedule, simple elegant solutions are rapidly designed, coded, and tested on a continuous basis. Over time, layer upon layer of elegant solutions evolve into a highly integrated, complex information system. Ironically, this is the same process that many natural systems have used to evolve into their current state.

THE SYSTEMS ANALYST TOOLBOX

Whether structured or agile design methods are used during project implementation, systems analysts rely heavily on various forms of modeling software. Modeling applications visually display the interaction and flow of entities (patients, providers, information) before and after implementation of information technology. Models link data dictionaries with clinical and administrative workflow through logical and physical data flow diagrams. Models can be connected through a hierarchy of parent and child diagrams to analyze system behavior locally (at the user level) and globally (management reports). There are many commercial modeling tools available. Table 23.4 presents various types of modeling software and how they are used.

Discrete Event Simulation

Two software applications that are well suited for the analysis of complex systems are discrete event simulation (DSA) and network analysis (NA). DSA is a software application that allows analysts to flow chart processes on a computer and then simulate entities (people, patients, information) as they move through individual steps. Simulation allows analyst to quickly

TABLE 23.4	The Systems Analyst Toolbox	
Simulation Method	**Description**	**Healthcare Example**
Flow charts	Flow charts represent one of the most basic tools used by system analysts to describe the flow of entities (information, patients, and providers) in a process. Flowcharting software can be found as a stand-alone commercial product or as a feature in word processing, spreadsheet and project management software	Prior to the installation of a new clinical documentation system, the current paper documentation process was flow-charted and then compared with the new automated process using standard flow chart symbols
CASE tools	Computer-aided software engineering is a suite of software applications used for systems design and analysis. CASE tools improve communication, integrate life cycle activities and are used extensively in the design and implementation of new applications	CASE tools could be used to develop and implement a package of software application used in the development of an electronic medical record
Discrete event simulation	Discrete event simulation utilizes mathematical formulas to show how model inputs change as a process evolves over time. Typically the model is built visually using standard flow-chart symbols. For example, rectangles may represent processes and diamonds, decision points	Analyzing cycle time, patient flow, bottlenecks and nonvalue-added activities before and after installation of a computerized clinical documentation system in an emergency department. Simulation can be easily incorporated into popular methods of performance improvement such as Six Sigma and Lean
Network analysis	The unit of measure in network analysis is the pattern of relationships that exist between entities and the information that flows between them. Network analysis combines theories from sociology and information science (network theory). The field characterizes entities as "nodes" and the relationship or link between them as "ties." The pattern and strength of ties between nodes is then plotted on a graph where the flow of information can be analyzed	Network analysis tools could be used to quantify access to computer help desks for providers are by showing how centralized or decentralized the distribution of centers are for organizations within a health system

communicate the flow of entities within a process and compare differences in workflow after the introduction of new technology. DSA applications contain statistical packages that allow analysts to fit empirical data (process times, inter-arrival rates) to theoretical probability distributions to create life like models of real systems. Pre- and post-implementation models can be compared for differences in cycle time, queuing, resource consumption, cost, and complexity. DSA is ideal for agile design projects because processes can be quickly modeled and analyzed prior to testing. Unanticipated bottlenecks, design problems and bugs can be solved ahead of time to expedite the agile design process.

Network Analysis

Network analysis applications plot the pattern of relationships that exist between entities and the information that flows between them. Entities are represented as network nodes and can identify people or things (computers on nursing units, handheld devices, servers). The information that flows between nodes is represented as a tie and the resulting network pattern can provide analysts with insights on how data, information and knowledge move throughout the organization. Network analysis tools measure information centrality, density, speed and connectedness and can provide an overall method for measuring the accessibility of information to providers. NA graphs can uncover power laws (see Table 23.2) in the distribution of hubs in the organizations network of computers and servers. This can be beneficial in investigating the robustness of the computer network in the event a key hub crashes.

SUMMARY AND CONCLUSIONS

Healthcare complexity is growing at an exponential rate (Clancy, 2010). This, in part, is because new technology itself is composed of combinations of existing technologies. For example, POE systems interface with existing applications (technologies) in pharmacy, laboratory, and radiology. Each individual departmental application is composed of further subcomponents that are themselves technologies. This recursive process continues until it reaches the most basic parts of the system. If each component of this hierarchical tree is considered a technology, then new technologies form from new combinations. For example, voice activated clinical documentation recently emerged by combining Voice over Intranet, or VoIP, technology from other industries with existing electronic medical record (EMR) systems. Thus as we see new technologies grow at a linear rate, the potential combinations grow exponentially. The more potential combinations of technologies there are (combinatorial complexity), the higher the probability of discovering novel uses for them. Thus, technology actually creates itself out of itself (Arthur, 2009).

The relentless march of technology creates both benefits and challenges for nurse informaticists. As the sheer number of technologies grows, the combinations of them become ever more complex. Simply look at the complexity of EMR systems in hospitals today. These systems are a mixture of new and legacy systems connected through a complex network of customized interfaces. Equally complex is the acceleration in how quickly the underlying processes these technologies execute changes. New knowledge supporting evidence based practices is growing so fast that new CDS algorithms programmed into today's EMs can become outdated in a matter of weeks.

The potential impact of growing healthcare complexity is enormous. Beyond a certain level, organizational complexity can decrease both the quality and financial performance of a health system. Nurse informaticists play a vital role in the successful planning, design and implementation of information technology. However to achieve that success, nurse informatics must have an in-depth knowledge of complex systems and strategies to manage its behavior.

REFERENCES

Arthur, B. (2009). *The Nature of technology: What it is and how it evolves*. New York: Simon & Schuster.

Clancy, T. R., & Delaney C. (2005). Complex nursing systems. *Journal of Nursing Management, 13*(3), 192–201.

Clancy, T. R., Effken, J., & Persut, D. (2008). Applications of complex systems theory in nursing education: Research and practice. *Nursing Outlook, 56*(5), 248–256.e3.

Clancy T. R. (2010). Technology and complexity: Trouble brewing? *Journal of Nursing Administration, 40*(6), 247–249.

Garg A. X., Adhikari, N. K., McDonald H., Rosas-Arellano, M. P., Devereaux, P .J., Beyene, J. et al. (2005). Effects of computerized clinical decision support systems on practitioner performance and patient outcomes: a systematic review. *JAMA, 293,* 1223–1238.

Kendall, K. E. & Kendall, J. E. (2006). *Systems analysis and design* (6th ed.). Upper Saddle River, NJ: Pearson Prentice Hall.

Patel, V. L., Arocha, J. F., & Kaufman, D. R. (2001). A primer on aspects of cognition for medical informatics. *Journal of the American Medical Informatics Association, 8*(4), 324–343.

Rittel, Horst, & Webber, M. (1973). Dilemmas in a general theory of planning. Amsterdam: Elsevier Scientific Publishing, *Policy Sciences, 4,* 155–169. [Reprinted in N. Cross (Ed.), *Developments in design methodology.* Chichester, UK: J. Wiley & Sons, 1984, 135–144.]

Skyttner, L. (2001). *General systems theory: Ideas & Applications*. Singapore: World Scientific.

Weick, K. E., & Sutcliffe, K. M. (2001). *Managing the unexpected – assuring high performance in an age of complexity* (pp. 10–17). San Francisco: Jossey-Bass.

24

The Integration of Complex Systems Theory Into Six Sigma Methods of Performance Improvement: A Case Study

Thomas R. Clancy

• OBJECTIVES

1. Understand the conceptual framework of the Six Sigma method.
2. Recognize how to identify critical to quality indicators.
3. Identify traditional methods of measurement in Six Sigma using process capability.
4. Understand how to integrate complex system metrics, such as power law distributions into the Six Sigma framework.
5. Learn the benefits of discrete event simulation as a tool to explore problem solutions through scenario analysis.
6. Provide information technology solutions to the problem.

• KEY WORDS

Six Sigma
Complex systems theory
Power laws
Bursts
Nurse informaticists
Computer simulation

INTRODUCTION

Health systems often utilize a formal method of continuous performance improvement to identify, analyze and recommend solutions to problems. These may include such popular methods as Six Sigma, Lean Six Sigma, FOCUS-PDCA (find, organize, clarify, understand, select, plan, do, check, act) and high reliability organizations. Information technology is often introduced,

in part, as a recommended solution to a problem; for example, reducing medical errors or improving documentation. Nurse informatacists play a critical role as participants on performance improvement teams by providing expert knowledge regarding the capacity of information technology to solve the problem.

The objective of this chapter is to provide a case study of an actual performance improvement project unit using a Six Sigma framework.

CASE STUDY

A large community hospital was experiencing declining patient satisfaction scores on a 24-bed medical/surgical unit. Specifically, scores indicated many patients were experiencing long admission and discharge delays. To study and recommend solutions to the problem, the hospitals chief nursing officer (CNO) convened a task force made up of the director of nursing, nurse manager, charge nurse, director of performance improvement for the hospital, and staff nurses from the unit. The director of performance improvement was assigned the role of group facilitator and decided to utilize a Six Sigma process as a framework for the project.

SIX SIGMA

Six Sigma methods of performance improvement were developed by Motorola in the late 1970s. Six Sigma is a philosophy that assists organizations improve process capability and reduce variation. The focus is on process outcomes and the method uses a disciplined approach known as DMAIC (Table 24.1).

Key metrics in Six Sigma are critical to quality indicators, or CTQs. Critical to quality metrics are those factors that cause customer expectations (voice of the customer) to vary. Using the DMAIC steps, the team first identified key stakeholders and defined their expectations in the admission and discharge process on the unit. Key stakeholders were patients and

TABLE 24.2	Admission Sources to the Unit	
Admission Source	**Cases**	**% Cases**
Emergency outpatient	400	73%
Other facility	65	12%
Routine - unscheduled	31	6%
Routine - scheduled	22	4%
Outpatient service	17	3%
Nursing home or snf	11	2%
Other acute care hospital	5	1%
Family physician referral	0	0%
Intermed. Care facility	0	0%
Rehab center	0	0%
Total cases	**551**	**100%**

families as well as clinical providers on the unit. A 3-month sample of data revealed the following referral sources (stakeholders and customers) to the unit (Table 24.2).

Team members also reviewed comments on patient satisfaction surveys and interviewed patients and families regarding delays in the admission and discharge process to the unit. Key referral sources were the emergency room and sub-acute care facilities while key clinical specialties were internal medicine, cardiology and family medicine (Table 24.3). Table 24.4 presents the percentage of admissions to the unit by diagnosis related group; Table 24.5, the severity by subclass; and Table 24.6, discharge status.

TABLE 24.1		The DMAIC Framework for Six Sigma
Step	**Phase**	**Description**
D	Define	Define customer expectations
M	Measure	Measure the gap between the current and desired state and whether or not the existing process is capable of meeting expectations (process capability)
A	Analyze	Analyze cause-and-effect relationships and conduct scenario analysis on potential performance improvement activities
I	Improve	Intervene with recommended performance improvements
C	Control	Control process variation and sustain the improvements

THE DMAIC PROCESS

Key Stakeholders and Expectations

A review of the initial data indicated that the typical patient was over 60 years of age, was admitted from the emergency room (ER) with a high acuity, cardiac disease condition and was treated by either a cardiologist, hospitalist, or family medicine physician. The average length of stay was 4.97 days and 60% of the patients were discharged to home. The remaining 40% were transferred to a long-term care facility or home health. Key stakeholders were thus identified as patients and their families, cardiologists, family medicine physicians and internists (hospitalists), emergency room staff, and subacute care facilities.

TABLE 24.3	Admissions by Clinical Specialty	
Attending Physician Specialty	**Cases**	**Days**
Internal medicine	367	1242
Cardiology	107	301
Family practice	29	138
Surgery-general	11	47
Nephrology	10	42
Orthopedic surgery	10	31
Hematology & oncology	4	11
Gastroenterology	3	14
Surgery-thoracic & cardi	3	15
Surgery, colon & rectal	2	4
Emergency medicine	1	2
Neurological surgery	1	6
Neurology	1	1
Obstetrics & gynecology	1	1
Urology	1	8
Total cases/days	**551**	**1863**

Critical to Quality Indicators

Patient dissatisfaction with long delays prior to admission and discharge from the unit had prompted the CNO to originally convene the task force. Two CTQs indicators that measured admission and discharge delays included:

1. The time between when orders were written and the patient was actually admitted or discharged from the floor

2. Scores from patient satisfaction surveys

A review of available historical data revealed that the average wait time for patients being admitted to the unit from the ER was 4 hours and 30 minutes and the average discharge wait on the unit was 5 hours and 45 minutes. Patient satisfaction scores for admission delays were at the 75th percentile (benchmark was 90th percentile) and for discharge delays was at the 72nd percentile (benchmark was 93rd percentile). The team set a goal to reduce the average wait by 75% by the end of the first year and to be in the 90th percentile for patient satisfaction scores.

TABLE 24.4	Top Diagnosis Related Groups (DRG)			
Drg Distribution		**Cases**	**% Cases**	**Avg Los**
DRG 291 Heart failure & shock w MCC		27	5%	8
DRG 871 Septicemia or severe sepsis w/o MV 96+ hours w MCC		27	5%	6
DRG 682 Renal failure w MCC		23	4%	5
DRG 292 Heart failure & shock w CC		21	4%	3
DRG 313 Chest pain		18	3%	1
DRG 287 Circulatory disorders except AMI, w card cath w/o MCC		17	3%	2
DRG 310 Cardiac arrhythmia & conduction disorders w/o CC/MCC		16	3%	2
DRG 193 Simple pneumonia & pleurisy w MCC		13	2%	6
DRG 190 Chronic obstructive pulmonary disease w MCC		12	2%	3
DRG 377 G.I. hemorrhage w MCC		11	2%	4
DRG 378 G.I. hemorrhage w CC		11	2%	4
DRG 641 Nutritional & misc metabolic disorders w/o MCC		11	2%	2
DRG 247 Perc cardiovasc proc w drug-eluting stent w/o MCC		10	2%	1
DRG 312 Syncope & collapse		10	2%	2
Others with 9 cases or less (138 drgs)		324	59%	
Total cases		**551**	**100%**	

TABLE 24.5	Patient Severity by Subclass	
Severity Subclass Distribution	**Cases**	**% Cases**
No assignment	1	0%
Patient severity 1 minor	66	12%
Patient severity 2 moderate	156	28%
Patient severity 3 major	228	41%
Patient severity 4 extreme	100	18%
Total cases	**551**	**100%**

Measure Phase

The measure phase in the DMAIC process focuses on analyzing the gap between the current and desired state and whether or not the existing process is capable of meeting CTQ expectations (process capability). In this case, the boundaries of the process started when orders were written for admission to the floor and ended when the patient was discharged. Process capability represented the ability of the unit to "process" (care and treat) patients, given the number of admissions. In other words, are the current clinical and administrative processes on the unit capable of moving patients from admission to discharge (length of stay) while meeting or exceeding CTQ indicators?

A broad measure of process capability is the unit census. If the unit census is at 100% occupancy when an admission is ordered the patient must wait until a bed

TABLE 24.6	Discharge Status	
Discharge Status	**Cases**	**% Cases**
Home, self-care	335	61%
Snf	107	19%
Home health service	45	8%
To another rehab facility	24	4%
Hospice, medical facility	10	2%
Expired	9	2%
Hospice, home	9	2%
Intermediate care facility	4	1%
Short-term hospital	3	1%
Against medical advice	2	0%
To long term care facility	2	0%
To a psychiatric hospital/unit	1	0%

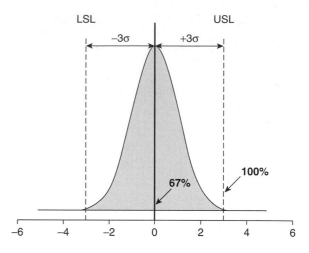

• **FIGURE 24.1.** Histogram of percentage occupancy using midnight census.

becomes available (for example, in the ER). Thus the "true census" is both the patients physically on a unit and the patients waiting to be admitted. Unfortunately, unit census is usually analyzed in hospitals by using the midnight census which grossly underestimates the true census at any point in time. For example, a histogram of the midnight census for each of the 365 days in the previous year showed a normal distribution with the mean at 67% occupancy and a standard deviation of 10% (Figure 24.1).

Using a Six Sigma methodology, if the percentage occupancy follows a normal distribution, 99.73% of the midnight occupancy rates will fall between ±3 standard deviations (SD) and only 0.27% of the values will fall outside of the limits. Since the process limits extend from −3 SD to +3 SD, the total spread is 6 SD (hence the name, Six Sigma). This total spread is the process spread and is used to measure the range of process variability. Statistics using midnight census would indicate that the unit rarely (<1% of the time) exceeded a percent occupancy of 100% (>3 SD) and that process capability should be sufficient to accommodate the current number of admissions.

Determining process capability by using the midnight census is one example of the problems encountered when using traditional statistical measures to measure complex system behavior. The average midnight census is a point estimate and does not account for the dynamic behavior of the system. A better measure of process capability is the true unit census whenever an admission occurs. True unit census can be obtained by

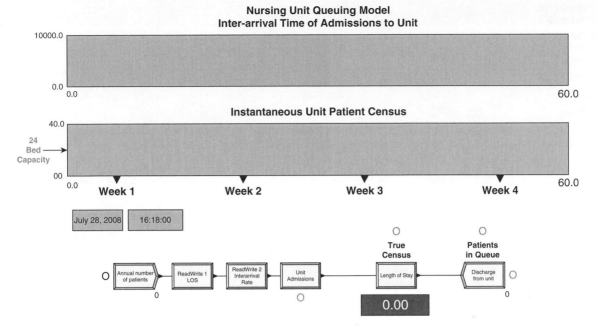

• **FIGURE 24.2.** Discrete event simulation queuing model.

building a queuing model in discrete event simulation software (Figure 24.2).

By entering the chronological admission and discharge times into discrete event simulation software (Table 24.7), the number of patients in the queue (waiting to be admitted) is continuously calculated and added to the current unit census to measure the true census at any point in time.

Figure 24.3 presents a histogram of the true percentage occupancy each time a patient is admitted for the previous 1-year period. Note that the true percentage occupancy is also normally distributed, but the mean occupancy is 95% with a SD of 5%. This indicates that the unit *frequently* exceeds 100% occupancy and current process capability is not sufficient to accommodate the number of admissions to the unit. Group members surmised that at the busiest times of the day, the unit was at 100% capacity for short periods until all discharged had been completed (usually by midnight).

To further investigate process capability, the team developed time-sequence plots that compared the interarrival rate of admission with the unit census (Figures 24.4 and 24.5).

The time-series plots demonstrated that the unit census frequently exceed 100% occupancy (≥24 beds) for short periods nearly every day. Of note was that when unit census exceeded 100% occupancy it was usually

after a "burst" of admissions with short interarrival rates. Bursts are represented in Figure 24.4 as periods where a cluster of admissions occur in rapid succession. There are two bursts noted in Figure 24.4 (on the x axis); the first is from admission 12–26 and the second is from admission 56–61.

To validate the annual number of admission bursts onto the unit, the team plotted a histogram of the time between admissions (in minutes) for the prior year (Figure 24.6).

Figure 24.6 confirms there is a high frequency of admissions with a very short interarrival rate (the tall columns on the left) interspersed with long periods without an admission (the short columns on the far right). In other words, there are "bursts" of admissions (during the day and evening shifts) followed by long periods of few admissions (the night shift).

Figure 24.6 can be transformed (Figure 24.7) to show the admission interarrival rate follows a power law distribution. Power law distributions are suggestive of a complex mix of underlying random and nonrandom mechanisms that drive system behavior. Figure 24.5 is a log-log graph of Figure 24.2, and the solid curve represents the best fit to the histogram data (a hyperbolic distribution) and asymptotically becomes inverse power law. Of note is that power law distributions also occur in many other complex systems such as the magnitude of

TABLE 24.7	Discrete Event Simulation Model Inputs			
Adm Date	**Adm Time**	**Dsch Dt**	**Dsch Tm**	**Dsch Disposition**
9/9/2008	1118	9/13/2008	1339	ARS
9/9/2008	1118	9/13/2008	1339	ARS
9/3/2008	1012	9/4/2008	1344	AHR
9/3/2008	1012	9/4/2008	1344	AHR
9/3/2008	1724	9/9/2008	1358	AHR
9/3/2008	1724	9/9/2008	1358	AHR
9/19/2008	725	9/25/2008	1553	ATR
9/19/2008	725	9/25/2008	1553	ATR
9/5/2008	1815	9/15/2008	1054	ATE
9/5/2008	1815	9/15/2008	1054	ATE
9/8/2008	1422	9/10/2008	1710	AHR
9/8/2008	1422	9/10/2008	1710	AHR
9/15/2008	0	9/20/2008	1444	AHR
9/15/2008	0	9/20/2008	1444	AHR
9/9/2008	1230	10/3/2008	6	DBN
9/9/2008	1230	10/3/2008	6	DBN
9/10/2008	1055	9/12/2008	1818	AHR
9/10/2008	1055	9/12/2008	1818	AHR
9/10/2008	1535	9/12/2008	1817	AHR
9/10/2008	1535	9/12/2008	1817	AHR
9/16/2008	1215	9/29/2008	1843	AHR
9/16/2008	1215	9/29/2008	1843	AHR
9/12/2008	1359	9/15/2008	1413	AHR
9/12/2008	1359	9/15/2008	1413	AHR
10/13/2008	600	10/17/2008	1754	ARS
10/13/2008	600	10/17/2008	1754	ARS
9/24/2008	213	10/7/2008	1143	AHR
9/24/2008	213	10/7/2008	1143	AHR
9/15/2008	1601	9/19/2008	1148	AHR

ARS, Intermediate Rehabilitation Facility; AHR, Acute Hospital Rehabilitation Facility; ATE, Expired; ATR, Long Term Care Facility; DBN, Discharge to Home.

natural disasters (earthquakes, hurricanes, and floods). They also emerge in complex man-made systems such as financial markets (stock price fluctuations) and the distribution of Intranet Websites.

A power law distribution is characterized by many small events interspersed with a few events of enormous magnitude. If plotted as a graph, a power law is in the form of a Pareto distribution (also known as the 80–20 rule) where 80% of the effects come from 20% of the causes.

In the case of the unit, 80% of the admissions were in bursts with very short interarrival rates followed by long periods of no admissions (the night shift). Bursts of admissions to the floor draw nurses away from other responsibilities such as discharging patients and freeing up beds. In fact, data showed that admissions onto the unit peaked between 12 and 2 PM but discharges peaked between 3 and 4 PM. To maximize patient flow, peak discharges should occur before peak admissions. It

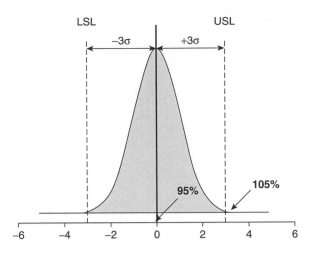

• **FIGURE 24.3.** True percentage occupancy measured at each admission (1 year).

appeared that admission busts were, in part, contributing significantly to the delays patients were experiencing related to admissions and discharges.

The discovery that admissions to the unit were distributed as a power law provided a key insight to the team. Power law distributions are indicative of the increasingly complex and interdependent nature of interactions woven into healthcare systems today. Power laws indicate that admissions to the floor are not purely random but that there is an underlying mechanism driving the behavior. If the team could discover what that mechanism was, it should provide some relief to the problem. In the case of admission bursts, new evidence suggests that this mechanism might result from simply setting priorities.

In his new book *Bursts*, Barabasi (2010), describes the flow of entities (people, information, things) in human systems as having a natural rhythm that is "bursty." Whether it is the frequency of e-mails, automobile traffic, or patients arriving at an emergency room, human activity usually occurs in bursts. And these busts often occur in a power law distribution. Barabasi suggests that these bursts result from having to prioritize activities. For example, if there are a limited number of vacant beds on a nursing unit, those patients with the most critical needs are admitted first while those with less critical needs must wait. This results in busts of activities (critical admissions) with long periods without activity (no admissions). What is most amazing about this phenomenon is the ubiquity of power law distributions, regardless of the area. There seems to be an underlying principle at work when prioritization takes place in complex human systems (such as in a hospital).

Analyze Phase

The analyze phase in Six Sigma methods focuses on identifying cause and effect relationships and conducting scenario analysis on potential performance improvement activities. Using a brainstorming methodology the team developed a list of possible causes for admission and discharge delays on the unit (Table 24.8).

A key factor in the analysis of potential causes for delays was the percentage of patient admissions that were unscheduled. Table 24.2 shows that nearly 80% of patient admissions were either from the ER or unscheduled direct admits. A high percentage of unscheduled admissions creates an environment where prioritization of critical needs will occur. Prioritization of critical needs can lead to bursts of activities and delays in admissions and discharges. Therefore a key solution would be to

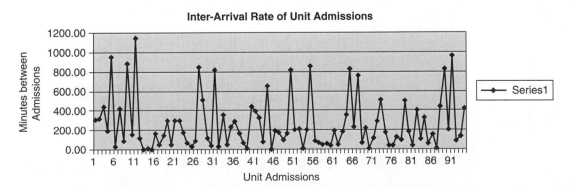

• **FIGURE 24.4.** Time series plot of minutes between admissions over a 2-week period.

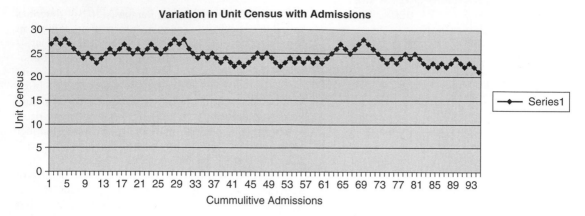

• **FIGURE 24.5.** Time series plot of a medical unit's census after every admission over a 2-week period.

balance the interarrival rate of admissions and transfers to the floor.

The team brainstormed potential solutions that could potentially reduce admission and discharge delays on the unit (Table 24.9).

Although each idea appeared viable, the team was unsure of which alternative would provide the most effective solution first. Implementing process changes in an existing workflow can be challenging and costly. One solution is to conduct scenario analysis using computer simulations. Simulations are a safe and effective method to test various alternatives without having to actually implement them. Using the discrete event simulation model previously developed for admission queues, the team ran multiple alternative scenarios from Table 24.8. Two simulated alternatives appeared to provide significant reductions in the wait times for patient admission and discharges; they were discharging patients earlier in the day and developing a robust bed management system. For example, having the peak discharge hour at 9 AM rather than 1 PM improved the wait time by 33%. However, strategically redistributing admissions to other units using a bed management system eliminated bursts and reduced waiting time to nearly zero.

The results of the simulation provided validation that admission bursts were a significant cause of admission and discharge delays and that balancing the interarrival rate through a bed management system was a key strategy for eliminating the problem. As of this writing, the performance improvement team is just beginning the intervention phase and will be recommending the adoption of a bed management system as well as a number of other alternative solutions.

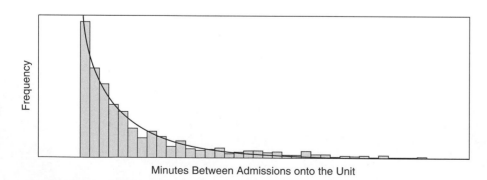

• **FIGURE 24.6.** Minutes between admissions onto the medical nursing unit for the prior year.

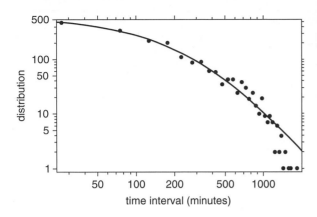

• **FIGURE 24.7.** Inverse power law distribution minutes between admissions to medical unit.

DISCUSSION

This case study highlights the usefulness of tools and metrics used in the analysis of complex healthcare system behavior. As shown in the case study, these tools can easily be integrated into popular performance improvement methodologies such as Six Sigma. Events within complex systems often appear independent, random and normally distributed when in fact they are not. Power law distributions are one example of how metrics used in other fields (such as physics) can be used to discover hidden patterns of interdependence between system factors. These clues can help teams better analyze cause and effect relationships and develop effective solutions. However, implementing potential solutions into the actual workflow of clinicians is challenging and costly. Discrete event simulation allows analysts to test various solutions on a computer before actually having to implement them.

QUESTIONS

As the nurse informaticist on the unit's performance improvement team what expert opinion would you provide in regards to the following questions;

1. What information system applications would best enable the solutions the team is recommending?

2. Describe how you would implement the application and the barriers you might expect to encounter.

3. How would you measure whether or not you had successfully solved the problem?

4. Are there additional solutions you would recommend to solve the problem?

REFERENCE

Barabasi, A. L. (2010). *Bursts: The hidden pattern behind everything we do*. New York: Penguin Publishing.

TABLE 24.9	Brainstorming List: Alternative Solutions for Admission and Discharge Delays
	Description
1	Have hospitalists begin the discharge process earlier in a patients stay
2	Work closely with subacute care centers for earlier bed placement
3	Implement a hospital-wide bed management program that balances admissions and transfers to nursing units
4	Develop a robust pool of nurses to flex staffing when bursts occur
5	Better align core staffing with historic patterns of inter-shift activity
6	Review the admission and discharge process for efficiency
7	Increase bed capacity and staffing to better accommodate fluctuations in census

TABLE 24.8	Brainstorming List: Causes for Admission and Discharge Delays
	Description
1	Timing of hospitalist rounds for discharge and admission orders
2	Placement of patients transferring to nursing homes
3	Timing of transfers from other units
4	Admission policies for the unit (who makes the decision for bed placement)
5	Lead time for the admission and discharge process
6	Alignment of staff with peak workload on the unit
7	Bed capacity on the unit and ER
8	Acuity of the patients
9	Staff training and competency

25

Workflow and Healthcare Process Management

Mical DeBrow / Cynthia M. Mascara

- ## OBJECTIVES

  1. Describe the concepts of workflow[1] and healthcare process management (HPM) (an adaptation of business process management to the needs of healthcare organizations)
  2. Relate the implications of workflow and HPM to the clinical arena.
  3. Relate the potential of workflow and HPM to the future of clinical care.
  4. Briefly relate the future potential of workflow.

- ## KEY WORDS

  Workflow
  Healthcare process management
  Advanced workflow
  Integrated electronic medical record
  Workflow applications

INTRODUCTION

Have you ever thought about how much time and money a healthcare organization spends looking and waiting for information? Manually routing data and paper documents in and out of a healthcare organization is not only expensive, it is risky. Automated workflow and healthcare process management (HPM) can help support a more efficient, safer, and cost-effective information flow. Tasks that require an army in a paper-based world are completed quickly and

free up costly, highly skilled nurses from manual tasks. More than just routing documents, workflow provides ready, near real-time information in order for nurses to focus on their highly skilled and knowledge-based patient care—not chasing paper. Additionally, workflow enables improvement in the quality of healthcare processes and faster turnaround times, reduces cost by freeing staff from low-value manual tasks and enforces consistent knowledge- and evidence-based practice and ensures accountability and compliance. This chapter will examine concepts of workflow and healthcare process management as an adaptation of business process management. We believe that workflow management systems can manage repetitive activities and large amounts of data into actionable clinically relevant information (Dwivedi, Bali, James, & Naguib,

---

[1]Note: For purposes of this chapter, workflow means the series or sequence of tasks engaged by a workflow engine as part of the electronic health record and not the work done in the head or by the hands of clinicians.

2007). This capability to manage entire processes, rather than simply triggering or prompting clinicians to perform a specific task is what drives the value of workflow in healthcare. Many types of information systems notify clinicians of interventions that need to be performed but workflow management helps guide the healthcare processes to completion. Workflow involves the management of healthcare processes in order to support and complement the translation of information and tasks between healthcare providers. Workflow has become essential in the healthcare industry which manages vast amounts of information, all of which may be critical to the patient's outcome. The difference in the rate of dissemination of information and the healthcare provider's action upon that information can make the difference in the crucial step between life and death or serious injury. A workflow consists of a sequence of connected steps. It is a depiction of a sequence of operations, declared as work of a nurse, or group of clinicians, and one or more functions. A workflow is a model to represent real work for further assessment—a reliably repeatable sequence of operations or tasks. In today's healthcare world, workflow is used in information systems to capture and enhance human-to-data technology interactions. Workflow has tremendous potential to enable the delivery of an array of healthcare services at a significantly lower cost while enhancing the quality of those services. At its most basic level, workflow can streamline complex administrative tasks, leaving clinical staff with time for real, potentially life-saving clinical procedures and interventions. The application of business process management to healthcare or HPM involves 4 steps:

Design: Design is process modeling for efficient and effective healthcare workflows.

Synchronize: Synchronization is the use of a workflow engine (manager) to help track and direct organizationally defined processes while driving process compliance.

Analyze: Analysis and monitoring is done via embedded analytics or log steps with business activity monitoring (BAM).

Adapt: Service-oriented architecture helps the organization prepare for future changes in healthcare and the delivery of benefits throughout the healthcare enterprise

Accordingly, this chapter is the examination of concepts related to workflow and healthcare process management.

DEFINITIONS AND HISTORY

Workflow, in healthcare, is a sequence of connected steps or operations typically performed by the healthcare staff and is a model representing the manual work performed to help improve patient care. It is a pattern of activity enabled by a systematic organization of resources with defined roles and information flows into a work process that can be documented and learned. Workflows are designed to achieve processing of events such as physical changes, service provision or information processing. The modern history of workflows can be traced to the study of the deliberate, rational organization in the context of manufacturing. These typically involved mass and energy flows and were studied and improved using time-and-motion studies. The assembly line remains the most common example of workflow in the early work but is an example of the simplest notion of workflow optimization: throughput and resource utilization. However, workflow has grown and matured in healthcare. Rather than utilize clinicians to simply repeat manual processes and function as data input and output sources, workflow has allowed for the clinician to work on more knowledge and skill driven functions. The quality movement transformed the nature of work through a variety of movements, including Total Quality Management (TQM), Six Sigma, and Lean Six Sigma. In many ways, TQM gave birth to both Six Sigma and Lean. Table 25.1 identifies the key components of both Six Sigma and Lean. Essentially, Six Sigma was designed to identify and remove the causes of defects and minimize variability and Lean was designed to eliminate the expenditure of resources for any goal other than the creation of value. Workflow in healthcare supports both quality methods by reducing variability and eliminating activities that do not produce value.

WORKFLOW COMPONENTS AND TECHNICAL OVERVIEW

The components of a workflow management system can be categorized as input, throughput, and output, as defined by traditional information processing theory. Input refers to the clinical or event data that are received by the system. Processing in the form of data evaluation and formation of conclusions occurs during throughput. Finally, the system produces output in the form of an action or notification.

Specific input data are often used to trigger or start the workflow. Examples include certain events such as patient admission, the entry of an order in the clinical information system, or the posting of results to the

TABLE 25.1	Key Components of Six Sigma and Lean Six Sigma

Six Sigma
- Concentrates on measuring quality
- Drives process improvement and savings
- Dedicates resources to process improvement
- Focuses team efforts on most important projects
- Use DMAIC method (define, measure, analyze, improve, and control)

Lean Six Sigma
- Focuses on maximizing value and reducing waste
- Eliminates waste along the entire value stream of a process or product
- Requires understanding of customer value and focuses key processes to continuously improve that value
- Underlying principles are continuous improvement, respect for people and focus on a long-term philosophy
- Works best if all employees are involved

Both Six Sigma and Lean Six Sigma
- Use teams to make improvements
- Involve taking waste out of processes
- Intend to make processes more effective
- Involve learning tools
- Require redesign for success

clinical database. The workflow may also wait for other events or data to be received as additional input. Typical inputs in a clinical workflow management system may include lab or diagnostic test results, data from clinical documentation, physician orders, patient demographic data, and hospital registration or admission, discharge, and transfer (ADT) data.

During throughput clinical data are evaluated using rules or algorithms in order to detect trends or abnormal conditions. If required data has not already been received as input, the workflow may query clinical databases to obtain it. Other processing may include setting timers and evaluation of due dates. It is important to understand that workflow processing is not a linear process. That is, various threads or branches of the workflow may be occurring simultaneously and independently of each other. Just as a nurse may multitask and perform patient assessment and dressing changes simultaneously, the workflow can also process more than one set of data simultaneously using different algorithms and rules.

The output of this evaluation process may be seen as notifications of actions by the healthcare process management system. The goal is to provide information to clinicians when and where it is needed. The right information should be communicated to the right person at the right time. Notifications may be provided in a number of formats, including online notifications, online work list entries, e-mail messages, pager notifications, printed documents, and even wireless voice communication system messages. Regardless of the type of notification, the message content that should include timely notifications of potential issues, communication of essential patient information and escalation of overdue activities and interventions. Notification characteristics that make the message more meaningful are inclusion of the date and time of message generation, inclusion of pertinent patient data, communication of message urgency and recommendations for action (Nguyen & Sailors, 2003). An effective workflow management system should provide the ability to track the notifications that have been sent and when indicated, the action taken in response by the user.

A workflow management system that is embedded in the clinical information system will ideally allow the system output to include the capability for actions. Some example actions include placing orders or valuation of assessment fields. It is this capability that supports streamlining the work of the physician and nurse so that less time is spent in repetitive administrative tasks. Studies have shown that clinical support systems that were integrated with the clinical information system were significantly more likely to succeed than stand-alone systems (Kawamoto, Houlihan, Balas, & Lobach, 2005). In addition, systems that provide a suggested action and require users to document reasons for not following the suggestion were most effective.

An example of a workflow may be seen with processing related to the nursing admission assessment. This workflow would be triggered or started when the patient is admitted, with the input of data related to the admission event such as the date and time of admission. During throughput a timer may be set for 4 hours after admission. When the timer expires the workflow will check to see if the nursing admission assessment has been entered into the clinical information system. If not, the workflow will provide output in the form of a notification to the nurse within the clinical information system. At the same time, a new timer is set for 2 hours. If the admission assessment has not been entered when this timer expires, the workflow generates an escalation notification to the nurse. This notification should be displayed with a greater urgency, perhaps indicated by changing the font color to red. Once the notification is generated the workflow waits for the nursing admission assessment to be saved. When this occurs, the workflow removes any relevant notifications from the nurse's worklist.

This same workflow might also have a logic branch that waits for the nursing admission assessment to be saved and then evaluates the assessment data. If certain values are documented that indicate the need for consults to various departments such as social services or the chaplain the workflow management system helps streamline this action in the clinical information system. In addition, notifications in the form of alerts, e-mails, or text pages can be sent to various clinicians or ancillary departments if certain data are documented, such as history of certain infectious diseases or food allergies. Such functionality can result in significant time savings for clinicians as well as improved communication of essential patient information.

WORKFLOW IMPLEMENTATION

The effectiveness of the workflow is dependent upon the quality of the design effort. Complete and detailed analysis of the current process and patient data available is essential for designing a workflow that is comprehensive and provides new processes that best meet the needs of the users and also helps improve patient care. It is imperative to understand that the best workflows do not just automate existing manual processes, but take advantage of the opportunity to redesign processes to best utilize workflow management and clinical information system capabilities.

The design process is not usually accomplished by just one individual. Instead, the use of a team or committee of appropriate staff will be most effective in designing a successful workflow. The coordinator of this team may be a staff member such as a nursing informatics

specialist who has both a clinical background as well as some technical understanding of the clinical information system and how the healthcare process management system operates. Other team members should include representatives of clinicians or hospital department groups who are stakeholders in the process being automated. In the example of the admission assessment workflow described previously, the team might include representatives for staff nurses, unit secretaries and nursing management. Ad hoc committee members may be contacted as needed for information regarding the pertinent patient data to be evaluated and the notifications that will be produced as output. For example, a dietician may be included when the discussion revolves around communication of dietary allergies and preferences.

Workflow design begins with documentation of the current processes, including policies and procedures. This information is then used to define future workflow requirements in an activity called process modeling. Typically a flow diagram defining the desired process steps and decision points is created using flow chart or process modeling software. Figure 25.1 shows a flow diagram example for a section of an admission assessment due workflow. Flow diagrams are often accompanied by a textual description of how the workflow should operate. In addition, documentation must include specific definitions of the workflow input data, any algorithms or rules for data evaluation during throughput, and the format for notifications or other output. It is helpful if the workflow design committee is provided with key items to address during worklfow design such as such as those listed in Table 25.2.

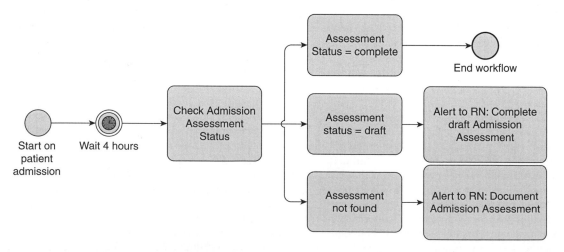

• **FIGURE 25.1.** Flow diagram example for a section of the admission assessment workflow.

TABLE 25.2	Key Items to Address During Workflow Design

- Review any policies or procedures related to the current process
- Identify the patient population affected by the workflow
  - Should any patients be included or excluded based on factors such as age, gender, diagnosis or history, or nursing unit?
- What event or data should trigger the workflow to start?
- What data are needed by the workflow, and is it available in a clinical information system?
- What decisions need to be made based on the data?
- Who gets notified, when, and how (eg, alert, e-mail, page)?
  - Identify all characteristics and data included in the notification
  - Should the notification suggest actions to the clinician?
- Will the workflow perform any automatic actions?
- What happens if the actions aren't taken? Are escalations needed?
- How does the workflow end?

The workflow design team should also develop use cases related to the workflow. Use cases are scenarios that can be used to describe the workflow's desired behavior based upon certain scenarios, including details about what the user will see and do. These scenarios should be written using common language that can be understood by users and should not contain technical jargon or descriptions. Use cases are effective tools for describing the desired workflow behavior to the technical staff that will configure the workflow in the workflow management system. In addition, use case scenarios can be used during the workflow testing process to ensure that the completed workflow fulfills the design requirements. A typical workflow will have multiple use cases to describe all scenarios that might occur, with scenario variations related to patient data and user actions.

The development of use cases is one aspect of the Rational Unified Process (RUP) approach to software design and implementation. This software engineering model outlines a disciplined approach to assigning roles and responsibilities toward the goal of developing software that meets end-user requirements while honoring schedule and budget controls (Saqib, Ahmad, Hussain, et al., 2010). Following the four phase RUP model, workflow design would begin in the first phase, known as inception. During this phase the requirements of the stakeholders are identified and documented in detail, including use cases. Refinement of the requirements takes place during the elaboration phase. These requirements are configured in the software and tested during

the construction phase, then implemented with users during the transition phase. Each phase ends at a milestone, or point in time where critical decisions must be made and key goals achieved (Rational Software White Paper, 2001). Rational Software was developed by IBM, and is continuously updated to reflect recent experiences and proven best practices. This process describes how to effectively deploy processes, tools, and guidelines to software development teams with a focus on the following best practices:

1. Develop software iteratively
2. Manage requirements
3. Use component-based architectures
4. Visually model software
5. Verify software quality
6. Control changes to software

Finally, the design committee should consider how the success of the workflow can be measured. Metrics collection can be used to evaluate the impact of the workflow on care providers as well as patient outcomes. If any data related to the workflow process are already being collected, the group should review this to identify opportunities for improvement that the workflow might address. A plan for capturing baseline data should be developed if none exists, as well as a method for measuring the effectiveness of the workflow after implementation. Post-implementation data may provide useful information for the organization as they embark on future workflow design efforts.

WORKFLOW APPLICATIONS

A workflow management system that supports aspects of clinical workflow may be classified as a clinical decision support system. Healthcare organizations use these information systems to assist clinicians as they evaluate clinical data and exchange information in the form of clinical documentation and work handoffs to other clinicians, often while multitasking. Automated workflows are most often developed using XML process definition language, or XPDL, the industry standard language for business process management.

A number of independent workflow management systems are used across many industries and are now being introduced into the healthcare arena. An important consideration when implementing a workflow management system is the degree to which it can be integrated with the clinical information system. This ensures a seamless view to the clinical users, who should not be aware that multiple systems are in place as they interact with the clinical information system. The clinical information system must be able to support the workflow process by including the capability for displaying notifications and worklists to clinicians. The notification capability should include the display of organizationally defined recommended actions, such as documentation forms to be completed or orders to be placed, and provide links to allow the user to easily complete these actions.

Another essential feature of the integration between the workflow management system and the clinical information system is the ability to route data and information such as notifications to the appropriate users. In the design phase, the organization can assign a role to the notification, but the clinical information system must have security capabilities to display notifications or other output based upon user role. This supports the goal of delivering the right information to the right user and prevents "alert fatigue" for other users.

Business activity management (BAM) refers to the monitoring and reporting of real-time information related to critical business activities and indicators (McCoy, 2002). Events and data from the workflow management system provide an essential contribution to BAM, which utilizes information from multiple systems to support the measurement and reporting of key performance indicators (KPIs) (Wetzstein, Leitner, Rosenberg, et al., 2009). Since patient care activities can be evaluated by a workflow, integration of this event data can be utilized by the BAM system to track the organization's progress in the form of KPIs that address business and patient outcome goals. These data are often displayed in the form of a dashboard that can be accessed on demand by hospital executives and clinical leadership. The implications for the KPI dashboard should be considered when identifying metrics and outcome measurements during workflow design.

A growing trend in the development of information systems is the use of open source software (OSS). This is software that you can freely use, modify, or distribute (Ebert, 2008). The use of OSS components that are distributed by software vendors when building software applications, such as workflow process management, can help to reduce costs and also support integration. Some information systems that include open source coding are more easily integrated with other systems, and support the transfer of data between systems.

Example of Embedded Workflow

One example of an advanced workflow technology system embedded within a healthcare information system is seen with the Soarian Clinicals solution.

Soarian Clinicals is a hospital information system developed by Siemens Healthcare to help healthcare organizations manage patient data and processes through coordination of activities and interventions, synchronizing handoffs, expediting communications and providing streamlined assistance for completing process steps. Soarian Clinicals utilizes healthcare process management to help organizations coordinate and monitor critical aspects of patient care, enhance collaboration among care providers, and provide notifications to clinicians based on role and patient responsibility. Healthcare Process Management is embedded within Soarian Clinicals, and end users are presented with a seamless view which combines clinical information, notifications, and suggested actions. Starter set workflows that are predefined by Siemens, such as those addressing infection control or acute myocardial infarction, can be adapted and implemented by organizations, as well as custom-designed workflows that address hospital specific processes and priorities. Figure 25.2 shows an example of several notifications generated from a workflow in Soarian Clinicals using healthcare process management.

The Chester County Hospital in Pennsylvania has also used Soarian Clinicals and its embedded workflow engine to develop workflows that have had a positive impact on clinical outcomes (Hess, 2009). Using this technology, the hospital was able to demonstrate significant decreases in hospital acquired Methicillin-Resistant *Staphylococcus aureus* (MRSA). This workflow is triggered on hospital admission and checks for a history of positive MRSA cultures as well as any notations of MRSA history in clinical documentation. If a patient has a past history of MRSA, the information system sends notifications to the bed manager,

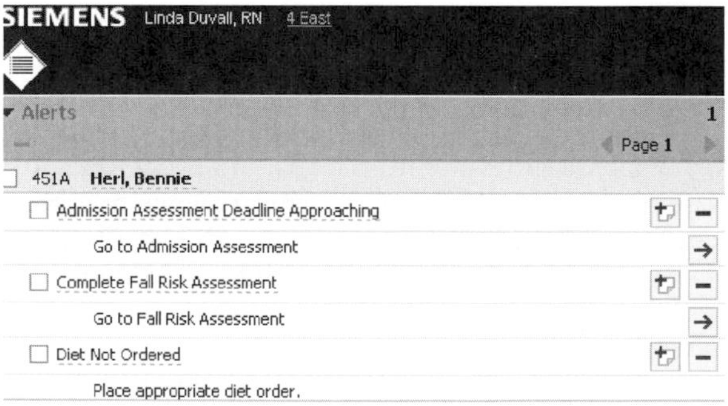

• **FIGURE 25.2.** Notifications from a workflow in the Siemens's Soarian Clinicals's information system.

physician, nurse, and infection control department. The system also evaluates current MRSA screen results to help clinicians determine if the patient should stay in isolation. This workflow was implemented in 2005 and over the next 2 years the number of new MRSA cases at admission continued to rise, but the incidence of hospital acquired MRSA infections at Chester County Hospital dropped by 38%. This key indicator of the success of this workflow demonstrates the powerful impact that an automated workflow can have on clinical outcomes.

CLINICAL TRIALS AND ADVANCED PRACTICE IMPLICATIONS

The use of Workflow and HPM in clinical trials is a relatively new advance in the science of clinical trials. Understanding the workflow of clinical trials is critical to development of reengineering strategies. The use of workflow in clinicals trials can also improve organizational efficiency by streamlining and standardizing procedures, ensuring accountability and providing audit trails. The use of workflow enables the definition of observational criteria for clinical trials and ensures the use of concrete and observable activities. Such modeling for clinical trials focuses on the individual and is similar to models used in comparable systems research, such as Marshak's (1993) identification of work as being composed of sequences of actions, tools, and information sources and Norman's (1988) seven-stage theory of action, which has been widely used to define human-computer interaction models. Advanced practice nurses are charged with direct and indirect patient care that achieves the goal of optimal outcomes for patient populations in a cost-effective manner. They maintain 24/7 accountability for achieving quality patient care outcomes. Workflow supports the advanced practice nursing roles of practitioner, educator, consultant, change agent, investigator, role model, and patient advocate. The Advanced Practice Nurse has the additional responsibility of fostering and advancing the professional practice of nursing through an advanced body of knowledge and operationalization of quality nursing care. Workflow supports those roles and knowledge.

WHERE DO WE GO FROM HERE?

We believe that in the near future, workflow-based, patient-centric systems will become the norm for healthcare organizations. The development and acceptance of regulation and outcomes for patient systems is likely to increase the problem of healthcare organizations being deluged with large amounts of clinical data. Many of the clinical processes and procedures relating to patient management are repetitive and can reasonably be automated. We believe that workflow will enable healthcare organizations to face the challenge of transforming large amounts of clinical data into contextually relevant clinical information to improve quality of care and reduce healthcare cost.

REFERENCES

Dwivedi, A., Bali, R. K., James, A. E., Naguib, R. N. G. (2007). How workflow management systems enable the achievement of value driven healthcare delivery. *International Journal of Electronic Healthcare*, 3(3), 382–393.

Ebert, C. (2008). Open source software in industry. *IEEE Software*, May-June, 52–53.

Hess, R. (2009). The missing link to success: Using a business process management system to automate and manage process improvement. *Journal of Healthcare Information Management*, 23(1), 27–33. Retrieved 6 June, 2010 from http://www.himss.org/content/files/jhim/23-1/JHIM_9Hess.pdf

Kawamoto, K., Houlihan, C. A., Balas, E. A., Lobach, D. F. (2005). Improving clinical practice using clinical decision support systems: a systematic review of trials to identify features critical to success. *British Medical Journal*. doi:10.1136/bmj.38398.500764.8F

Marshak, R. (1993). Young and Rubicam improves productivity with workflow. *Workgroup Computing Report*, 16, 12–20. Boston: Seybold Group.

Norman, D. (1988). *The Psychology of everyday things*. New York: Basic Books.

McCoy, D. (2002). *Business activity monitoring: calm before the storm*. Gartner Publication LE-15-9727.

Nguyen, A., & Sailors, R. M. (2003). *A proposed clinical decision support system (CDSS) output message*. Proceedings of American Medical Informatics Association, 2003; Washington, DC.

Rational Software White Paper. (2001). *Rational Unified Process: Best practices for software development teams*. Publication TP026B.

Saqib S. M., Ahmad, S., Hussain, S., Ahmad, B., & Bano, A. (2010). Improvement in RUP project management via service monitoring: best practice of SOA. *Journal of Computing*, 2, 38.

Wetzstein, B., Leitner, P., Rosenberg, F., Brandic, I., Leymann, F., & Dustdar, S. (2009). *Monitoring and analyzing influential factors of business process performance*. Proceedings of the 13th IEEE International Enterprise Distributed Object Computing Conference; Auckland, New Zealand.

26

Translation of Evidence Into Nursing Practice

Lynn McQueen / Heather Carter-Templeton / Kathleen A. McCormick

- ## OBJECTIVES

  1. Define evidence and when the term "evidence-based practice" (EBP) was first used.
  2. Define meaningful use and indicate how it influences incentives to use evidence, as well as how it is expected to impact healthcare and nursing.
  3. Identify evidence-based approaches, models, and frameworks used in translation of evidence into practice.
  4. Define evolving trends in the translation of evidence into practice.
  5. Describe how informatics is used as a tool to promote EBP and improve performance metrics.
  6. Describe innovative implementation and evaluation efforts involving nurses.
  7. Discuss how nursing education can promote EBP.

- ## KEY WORDS

  Evidence
  Clinical practice guidelines
  Evidence-based practice tools
  Meaningful use
  Performance metrics
  Quality and safety of patient care

INTRODUCTION

The time for evidence has arrived in the translation of evidence into measurable improvements in the quality and safety of patient care. In recent decades, technology and healthcare have fuelled each other's advancement. E-prescribing, the electronic health record (EHR), personal health records (PHRs), and any other imaginable form of e-Health is likely to now appear just as

micro/nanosystems continue to impact the availability of integrated systems (RAND, 2001). The impact of these trends on genomics, individualized medicine (including gene-based personalized treatments), telehealth, and the application of electronic tools will depend on how nursing science and practice evolve and also on how effectively we interact with other professions and groups. Practical applications will lag behind advancements unless relationships and systems keep pace. The union of information science with nursing science and practice will be part of what promotes development of

Acknowledgement: Cheryl Stetler

technology infrastructures. Within these infrastructures, nurses competent in core informatics skills will be able to apply technology in ways that systematically help patients and advance knowledge.

Automated health information is now central to new U.S. healthcare reform legislation and to national efforts to restructure primary and specialty care. Advice from Sir William Osler (Canadian Physician, 1849–1919) to "Learn to see, learn to hear, learn to feel, learn to smell, and know that by practice alone you can become expert" is gradually meshing with our collective understanding of what evidence-based practice (EBP) means. Health Information Technology (HIT) advances our focus to how we apply evidence using computers, not whether it is a good idea.

The desire for rational choice is not new nor is the complexity of pursuing truth amidst gaps in knowledge and practice. Needed linkages are impacted by social factors, emotions, preferences, and limited resources. Despite these complexities, the exponential rate of HIT advancement has rapidly promoted use of evidence in healthcare decision making. HIT applications are profoundly impacting nursing roles with dramatic changes in how nurses accomplish their work. Similarly, recent evidence put forth in design theory impacts patient safety and the quality of care delivered by nurses. Skills once deemed "advanced" are now basic. Many nurses enter their formal nursing education with more experience using technology than some of their professors. More than ever, all nurses must know how to access, evaluate, use, teach, and pursue the evidence needed to make scientifically grounded decisions in real time, often at the point-of-care. The skills needed to combine automation and evidence-based healthcare are now as central to professional practice as any patient care or administrative skill.

Nurses require standardized language embedded into integrated systems that promote processing activities and information creation. Data driven systems of care provided through integrated workstations or on handheld devices provide the power needed at the point of decision making. Of particular interest are handheld clinical decision support (CDS) tools that promote prognosis, diagnosis, treatment, discharge, and care planning. With growing availability of powerful and convenient tools like this, it is becoming impossible to avoid routine use of evidence in practice. What is still coming into focus is how relationships and teams can most effectively and efficiently help us advance.

As evidence brokers, computer-literate nurses must know not only how to critically appraise the best available evidence, but they must also know how to explain their thoughts about this evidence to many different partners, groups, and teams. Requisite skills include knowing how to explain uncertainty when evidence is incomplete, misleading, contradictory or simply hard to apply in real situations.

This chapter will identify evidence-based approaches, models and frameworks used in translation of evidence into practice for quality, patient safety, design, access and disparities, translational health, and personalized health.

THE EVOLUTION OF EVIDENCE-BASED PRACTICE

Much has been written since the 1990s about the history of EBP, including chapters in two previous editions of Saba and McCormick (2001 and 2006). While the pursuit of evidence is not new, burgeoning notions about "meaningful use," patient-centered medical home (PCMH), knowledge transfer, comparative effectiveness research (CER) and practice-based research networks (PBRN) can be linked directly back to events occurring less than 20 years ago. The term "evidence-based practice" only became popular after 1992 when used by Gordon Guyatt and a group he led at McMaster University (Guyatt, 2002). David L. Sackett soon after described EBP as, "the conscientious, explicit, and judicious use of current best evidence in making decisions about the care of individual patients. The practice of EBP means integrating individual clinical experience with the best available external clinical evidence from systematic research" (Clinical Linkages, 2009). Quickly, EBP became a practical way to organize, collect, and use information. EBP employs a systematic approach to clinical decision using the best evidence available relevant to specific decisions about patient care (Sackett, Straus, Richardson, et al., 2000). As automation advanced, the ideas underlying EBP provided common ground for conceptualizing about rational processes. PBRNs (and similar structures) began to evolve as a way to promote collaborations that generate research knowledge. Terminology, language, coding, and the definitions surrounding rational choice began being shared and gradually standardized. Among other benefits, this helps nurses capture and quantify their own work.

Shortly after EBP began to appear in peer-reviewed scientific journals, ideas about how evidence can be used as the basis for decisions expanded globally. Use of the term "evidence-based" has been generalized across professions and is now routinely used by the popular media. Yet we are still in the early stages of these advancements. As hardware and software become visible tools of clinical proficiency and judgment, core notions surrounding EBP quickly evolve. Nowhere is this more important than reducing the time needed to translate evidence into practice. Despite many advances, it is widely understood that knowledge generation leaps far ahead of practical use. It takes approximately 17 years for research to find its way into routine practice (Balas & Boren, 2000). Studies and theories proliferate about how EBP can be implemented. New sources of funding and professional development are appearing so that EBP tools can more often be tested in practice. Largely due to the Internet, innovative new dissemination avenues flourish. The next leap will be in finding ways to expand communication and strengthen relationships in ways that shorten the time taken to move knowledge into practice and then evaluate what happens.

"Meaningful Use" Arrives

Figure 26.1 is a framework depicting the multiple types of evidence that collectively provides the structure giving incentive to evidence through meaningful use. There are no required dependencies upon any of the components and each will be described in subsequent parts of this chapter.

The U.S. Centers for Medicaid & Medicare Services (CMS) defines "meaningful use" in ways that tighten links between evidence and practice. Currently, the 2011 and 2013 Objectives are to "electronically capture in coded format and to report health information and use that information to track key clinical conditions." The 2015 goal is to "achieve and improve performance and support care processes on key health system outcomes" (Centers for Medicare & Medicaid Services, 2007). To qualify for incentive payments during the initial year, eligible providers must meet established 2011 standards, including the ability to report quality measures about diabetes, hypertension, cholesterol, smoking cessation, and obesity directly to CMS, and report the percentage of orders entered directly by physicians through computer physician order entry (CPOE) and specific screening measures. Because EBP involves applying the best available research results to healthcare decision making, the legislation authorized meaningful use as a way to improve quality through EHR incentives (Hogan & Kissam, 2010).

The meaningful use provision in current legislation prioritizes use of EHR in ways that promote EBP. As U.S. healthcare reform efforts evolve over the coming decade and beyond, ideas surrounding meaningful use,

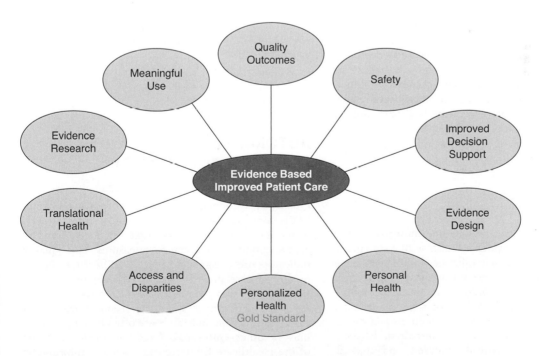

FIGURE 26.1. Multiple types of evidence leading to improved patient care.

including certification of EHR technology, will center on how teams, organizations, and systems interpret the meaningful use requirements. If incorporated in ways that make it easier to use evidence, the larger health information infrastructure will become more manageable while systematically linking evidence as well as quality and performance data to ongoing quality improvement, efficiency, and safety efforts. Incentives that support effective practices will gradually become stronger and organizational alignments will be enhanced. It is hoped that meaningful use helps us collectively address traditional hurdles related to uncertain standards, privacy, workflow, and the use of technology itself (Kane, 2010). But gaps between potential and actual use need to be understood across professions if they are to be systematically addressed (Baron, 2010). As standards are adopted and specifications implemented, certification of health information technology will largely be based on the degree to which evidence from both scientific knowledge and clinical practice can be applied.

THE RISE OF AUTOMATED EVIDENCE-BASED TOOLS

EBP tools provide a convenient way to present vast, complex data about outcomes, efficiency, effectiveness, patient preferences, policy, and sometimes cost. Over the past 5 years, there has been a proliferation in different types of automated EBP tools or "evidence-based quality tools" because, when implemented effectively, they promote improved processes and outcomes, contributing to reductions in unexplained variation. Much research has been done (and is underway) to study how and under what conditions specific EBP tools impact structures, processes, and outcomes. This chapter includes descriptions of only a few of the many common automated EBP tools.

Evidence: The Cornerstone of Systematic Approaches to Quality Improvement

The seamless translation of data and information into what we think of as "evidence" starts with a systematic approach to integrating scientific and clinical knowledge then considering its intersection with ongoing quality improvement efforts. As tradition and anecdote continue to be replaced by automated support for scientifically grounded decisions, reconceived definitions and methods alter how such evidence is discussed, labelled, accessed, stored, synthesized, analyzed, and applied. As ideas about what does and does not constitute

"evidence-based practice" evolve, system-level thinking leads to embedded and redundant practices believed to promote optimal processes and outcomes. Terminology and emphasis vary, but current trends in patient safety, risk management, and utilization management based on quality improvement, systems redesign, PCMH, CER, meaningful use, PBRN, and telehealth are all consistent with current system-level approaches.

As our best scientific information is now inserted into the sometimes messy realities of real practice, new applications (sometimes invisible) make it easier to provide good and safe care while making it harder to harm a patient. Evidence-based tools, including electronically available clinical practice guidelines, automated performance measures, and computerized reminders, are now embedded into routines of care with feedback provided "just in time" to impact processes, intermediate outcomes, and outcomes. Evidence-based practice is now successfully partnering with engineering to form "systems redesign" and related ideas leading to ever-more powerful ways of thinking about what we do and how we do it. As the capabilities of evidence-based applications become more affordable and accessible, changes occur in the inevitable controversies surrounding appraisal of different forms of knowledge. As evidence becomes more available in ways that naturally foster the integration of science and practice, greater discernment is required regarding the validity and reliability of this evidence. Identification of accurate evidence is central as investigators work to close gaps in clinically relevant knowledge while clinicians champion the use of evidence in real situations. The pace of progress will be influenced by how easily we can communicate about these changes.

AUTOMATED PERFORMANCE MEASURES AND QUALITY INDICATORS

Quality measurement takes on many forms and names but is consistently driven by a desire to integrate evidence into practice in ways that can be understood across groups. Performance measures and quality indicators are designed to identify differences in the quality of care provided by individuals, plans, facilities, organizations, or networks. Effectiveness data measures performance about important dimensions of care. Measures and indicators are often based on guidelines or other synthesized (credible) evidence. Some of the Healthcare Effectiveness Data and Information Set (HEDIS) measures developed by the National

Committee for Quality Assurance (NCQA) are now considered standards and used by more than 90% of U.S. healthcare insurance plans to measure performance on specific dimensions of care (National Committee for Quality Assurance, 2010).

A performance measure is often derived from administrative data that is pulled from abstracted (sometimes automated) records. An example would be electronic measurement (using EHR) of the number of patients who appropriately received antibiotics for pneumonia within a 4 or 6 hour window after arriving at a specific care setting, such as an emergency department. Such measurement is meant to assess provider and organizational performance and more specifically to be used in benchmarking, quality improvement efforts, and financial decisions.

The Patient Protection and Affordable Care Act (PPACA) established new requirements for the Secretary of Health and Human Services (HHS) to request feedback about quality measures to be used for public reporting and payment programs (HR 3590; Sections 3011 and 3012–3015.). These entities are to include Medicare payment programs. Debate is likely to include consideration of the "unintended consequences" that accompany attention and prioritization (through measurement and feedback) of some interventions at the expense of others.

The National Quality Forum (NQF) is a key group working to promote quality measurement and reporting. They have developed many performance measure sets, including a "never practice" set, which measures adverse events that would ideally never happen. NQF is also working to create partnerships that address measures routinely used for quality improvement. An evidence-based and patient-centered approach has been proposed to create a consensus-based partnership that would report to the NQF Board. This partnership would serve to generate input for the Secretary of HHS about the selection of public measures (www.qualityforum.org).

Key to building an informatics infrastructure that supports EBP is developing electronic linkages between the evidence generated through research and the data generated through performance, QI, and safety activities. The Joint Commission, the National Quality Forum, the Commonwealth Fund, the Robert Wood Johnson Foundation, Agency for Healthcare Research and Quality (AHRQ), Centers for Disease Control and Prevention (CDC), CMS, MD Consult, and many other public and private groups provide online resources that assist nurses in translation activities designed to link research and internal quality-related data to practice change.

Automation and methodological advances are changing how performance measurement is conducted but much work remains. This area of inquiry requires prioritization among agencies, organizations, and professional groups. Due to links with meaningful use and other legislation, performance measurement is more popular than ever. But accuracy is needed and this type of measurement belongs within an overall vision of quality improvement rather than simply measuring for the sake of measurement. The gains associated with measurement are maximized when conceived with a broad approach. A narrow focus on only a few measures (or many measures that do not impact practice) may influence other components of care in unforeseen ways.

While automation is fuelling the use and availability of performance measures and there is tremendous capacity for benefit, concerns about specific aspects of metrics development, use, and implementation are generating healthy debate within and between professional groups (Selby, Uratsu, Firemanm, et al., 2009; Hayward, Kent, Vijan, & Hofer, 2007; Pogach, Rajan, Maney, et al., 2010; Kerr, Smith, Hogan, 2003). Concerns about methodological issues and how performance information is used are rising as measurement is promoted. Key points of discussion include an ongoing need to improve the accuracy of the epidemiological evidence used in EBP, generally, and applied to performance measures, specifically. The traditional analysis and reporting of randomized controlled trials (RCTs) is thought by some to over-estimate benefits and under-estimate costs (Hayward, Kent, Vijan, & Hofer, 2005; Hayward et al., 2007; Pogach, Tiwari, Maney, et al., 2007; Pogach et al., 2010). Vigilance is especially needed to assure that national performance standards do not systematically spread misinformation.

Providers need to be careful that the influence of industry-funded "experts" and advocates does not contribute to misuse of evidence, including over-treatment. Although performance measurement and other EBP tools were designed to promote value and efficiency, it is important to remember that they hold potential for promoting both benefit and harm. One cannot simply implement a measure or other EBP tool and walk away. Ongoing monitoring, assessment, and feedback about effectiveness and safety are needed, long term. Dr. Rod Hayward has spoken and published widely on this topic and wrote in 2007, "It is simply magical thinking to believe that performance measures will do good regardless of how haphazardly they are constructed and that they will not do harm even when the measures adopted provide strong incentives for overtreatment" (Hayward et al., 2007).

Ongoing issues about the potential for bias and other aspects of rigor may influence motivation to develop, use, refine, update, or respond to performance feedback.

In some cases, these discussions lead to positive change. For example, the need to better integrate and address risk is contributing to methodological advances. A new and more statistically robust generation of performance measures are now being developed and tested by many groups. Advances in performance measurement include testing of composite (combined) and "tightly linked" measures for specific conditions. This promotes measurement that better captures the complexity of real situations and aligns incentives. Nurses help their organizations and professional groups when they work to assure that measures are valid and reliable, and also promote quality rather than punitively punish or overburden providers.

EVIDENCE FOR IMPROVING PATIENT SAFETY

Since the 1999 publication of *To Err Is Human: Building a Safer Health System* and the subsequent 2001 publication of *Crossing the Quality Chasm: A New Health System for the 21st Century*, nurses have worked across practice, education, administration, and research domains to expand the evidence base needed to systematically prevent errors and promote ongoing safety initiatives (Institute of Medicine, 1999, 2001). These efforts are often thought of as systems approaches to analysis and prevention of errors. The term "patient safety" often encompasses analysis of human factors combined with engineering concepts then integrates these ideas into the realities of clinical practice, for example, by promoting the integration of evidence into the EHR, HIT, and overall decision support (Bakken, Currie, Lee, et al., 2008; Rich & Day, 2008).

As the evidence needed to sustain a safety culture matures, a growing number of evidence-based tools and approaches are being developed, implemented, and evaluated. Over the past decade, these trends have merged patient safety efforts with overall EBP. As part of the evolution of Implementation Science, CER and similar approaches, the results of patient safety evaluations can now be fed back both to those who build new knowledge and close gaps in practice. Current trends in how care is structured, such as reorganization of primary care through PCMH, are often central to promoting safety. For example, significant reductions in diagnostic error can be systematically pursued while EHR is promoted as a component of restructuring of primary care (Singh, H., & Graber, M., 2010).

Understanding how to proactively (rather than reactively) protect patients and manage risk from a quality perspective is leading to rapid advancements in patient safety, often requiring strong collaboration. HIT is used in a myriad of ways to impact what information is provided to decision makers, how it is provided, the factors that promote uptake, and barriers that interfere with use. A dynamic patient safety culture requires that nurses continually reconsider how to link knowledge and practice. Patient safety tools available to nurses abound, including barcoded patient wrist bracelets that match automated records to prevent patients from receiving the wrong medication; surveillance systems designed to detect healthcare–acquired infections; and automated systems in Operating Rooms that reduce the risk of reading an x-ray backwards, losing count of sponges and instruments, or operating on the wrong patient. Simulation is increasingly used to prepare nurses for complex procedures, especially when the margin for error is small and options for training are limited.

In the past decade, use of patient safety indicators (PSI) has risen sharply and helped quantify risk, thus revealing opportunities for improvement and prevention. PSIs are typically used to feed back abstracted administrative data to providers, patients, teams, organizations and systems. These data increasingly are transparent and publicly reported on the Internet. This results in patient safety data being used in a wide variety of ways, including powerful feedback about morbidity and mortality. For example, when patients unexpectedly die or are identified after unexpected readmission within a designated time period (such as 2 weeks or 30 days) after a surgical or other intervention, patient safety tools, such as Root Cause Analysis, can be employed to reveal what occurred and how to mitigate future risk.

Patient safety is inherently multidisciplinary. Nowhere in healthcare are team work and patient activation more important than in patient safety. The importance of communication factors, such as civility and interpretation between and across disciplines, are being measured and reported by nurses (Covell, 2010; MacEachin, Lopez, Powell, & Corbett, 2009). National and international patient safety efforts are underway with different target audiences, using varying approaches with different degrees of scientific rigor. Partnerships between groups are resulting in large-scale investigation of errors and exploration of options for improvement. Through these efforts, nurses and other health professionals often receive training about the use of HIT and other patient safety tools, data, and analysis techniques.

Specific attributes can be identified as important for a HIT infrastructure that promotes safety (Doebbeling, Chou, &Tierney, 2006). These attributes lead to flexible, transparent, nonintrusive, reliable, sustainable, secure, timely, standardized, compatible, and easily updated systems. To promote such attributes, nurses and others are developing an international classification for patient safety with an accompanying conceptual framework (Sherman, Castro, Fletcher, et al., 2009) and evaluating use of the Nursing Management Minimum Data Set so that nurse-relevant contextual data are available to promote improved safety (Westra, Subramanian, Hart, et al., 2010). Natural language processing is also evolving so that information and knowledge sharing from text and speech can be extracted or generated accurately (Sarkar, 2010). These and related activities are expected to proliferate as the biomedical informatics field exponentially advances.

EVIDENCE FOR ENVIRONMENTAL DESIGN

There is new evidence that environmental design enhances safety and quality in healthcare environments (AHRQ, 2007). The physical environment is a critical component in programs to improve safety and quality for patients. The evidence demonstrates that with ceiling lifts there is an 83% reduction in annual work injuries and costs related to patient lifting (Joseph & Fritz, 2006). Research also supports building centralized nursing stations in order to increase the time nurses spend in direct patient care (Howard, 2007). These recent evidence reports come from the Institute for Healthcare Improvement (IHI), where Dr. Don Berwick, now at the helm at CMS, was previously the president and CEO. He has stated that the hospital will be a better managed environment when we make the environment more like home and focus the science on the technological enterprise that uses knowledge and machines and drugs correctly (Berwick, 2007).

PERSONAL HEALTH EVIDENCE

Evidence needs to be provided at the level understood by each patient. Pipe and colleagues (2005) describe the importance of nurses using an "empiric way of knowing, focusing on methods of critically appraising and applying available data and research to understand and inform clinical decision-making better." Nurses must also take into account a vast array of factors when applying evidence, including culture and literacy. For example, consider the different approaches to diabetes education that might be needed when teaching a patient who routinely uses technology to talk, transmit, and text versus another patient who rarely (or never) sees a computer. Age, language, exposure, and comfort with technology often need to be considered before discussions about evidence and care can even begin with a patient or family member.

As activated patients increasingly bring their own information to nurses, the skills needed to foster the best possible choices expand. Fuelled by technology, expectations are changing. Watching a nurse scan a patient's identification information to double-check that the correct leg is about to receive surgery is linked to evidence about how to manage risk. Nurses must know how to explain such actions and help a patient explore options in terms of weighing benefits and harms.

Activated patients and families can facilitate change in processes of care, for example, through partnerships that promote communication about follow-up of important test results. Automated training materials can be conveniently provided at a reasonable cost, either by sending materials electronically to the patients at home or making them available at point-of-care. E-mail, texting, and other electronic media can be used to facilitate communication but only to the degree that the healthcare system and providers themselves adapt. For example, when reimbursement structures do not keep pace, providers are less motivated to communicate using a specific technology.

A significant limitation of evidence-based tools is the absence of published findings relevant to patient and community preferences. The absence of cost information and data about societal values is common. While many would agree that active patient participation in decision making contributes to improved patient satisfaction and other positive outcomes, the perspective of patients is especially relevant when the condition is chronic and non–life-threatening, such as cataract extraction. In these instances, the patient's preferences become the focus of the decision. Studies with measurable output relevant to patient and community preferences are needed by nurses who typically bring a patient-focused perspective to research and evaluation.

EVIDENCE FOR ACCESS AND DISPARITIES

Nurses are among the most trusted of health professionals and seen as the patient advocates for access. Nursing leaders are needed as we forge into an era of rapid globalization where we care for an aging population with increasing chronic illness and complex comorbidities. In areas most directly related to evidence (such as telehealth), the nursing profession has an obligation to assure access to evidence for all patients and for groups identified at risk. Leadership is needed, for example, in assuring that groups, such as women, minorities, homeless, those living in poverty, those living in rural areas, and those requiring specialty care, benefit from increased availability of evidence through HIT.

Nurses must know how to promote health with patients young enough to only know life surrounded by hardware tools as well as patients without computer literacy or technology access. As the links needed between science and practice come into sharper focus, doors open to new ways to facilitate use of evidence. Systematic use of evidence to weigh for and against decisions is better understood within our culture, but addressing the use of such evidence in a specific patient situation can be challenging. Nurses are aided in these pursuits by working effectively within partnerships, teams, groups, and systems.

TRANSLATIONAL OF EVIDENCE INTO HEALTHCARE

It is now far easier to find clinically minded scientists/researchers as well as clinicians interested in translation of evidence into practice. Clinical researchers have even been known to change their career goals so that they can focus on EBP. This comes as we recognize that peer-reviewed publications do not, by themselves, help patients. Translating evidence into practice can be complicated but it comes with the motivation that care may potentially improve. As the chorus of "so what?" comes from those staring at the vast amounts of published scientific information that is expensive, time consuming, and often barely used, a growing theoretical base and knowledge base is now available to those who pursue adoption of evidence.

Many terms, including "translation," "translational research," "implementation science," "knowledge to practice transfer," "knowledge translation," "action research," "evidence-based practice," "research utilization," "evaluation research," and many others focus on a desire to promote use of evidence in practice. Individuals and groups working on translation cross a continuum and may focus on hypothesis testing (research) or less tightly controlled quality improvement (evaluation of clinical care). There is no one contribution that defines "translation" and no hard line between research and quality improvement. Yet success often comes (under different terms and frameworks) when evidence-based tools are married with data generated through performance and quality improvement activities.

The specific goals of differing approaches to EBP share a desire to promote use of evidence (from both science and from quality improvement activities) to support clinical decision making. The specific terms are less important than use of a systematic approach. Such an approach allows for implementation of evidence-based strategies and tools. Once implemented, results can be measured then fed back to both investigators and clinicians. This feedback will be available as new or refined research questions are developed to promote ongoing clinical quality improvement.

FINDING EVIDENCE IN ELECTRONIC HEALTH RECORDS

Making complex information useful requires tools and most today are automated and often linked to the EHR. By examining the EHR, there may be evidence of clinical and nursing interventions that are leading to quality care and positive patient outcomes. It is also in the EHR that adverse reactions and patient complications to procedures can be found. Considerations about strength of evidence are tied to analysis of the level of certainty regarding overall benefit. The data generated may become expert opinion. While expert opinion may be necessary to fill in gaps in the evidence, over-reliance on expert opinion raises issues of credibility.

When EHR observation data are peer reviewed, published, and reported to the broader healthcare community, they add to the body of evidence and can change the next version of a guideline or other evidence-based tool. If the best available evidence is adequate to accurately assess the effects of an intervention or service on processes, intermediate outcomes, or outcomes, confidence in the recommendation is generally high. Certainty about overall benefit is impacted by many factors, including how many studies were of high enough quality for inclusion in a systematic review, whether or not there was generalizability across the findings, identification of gaps and inconsistencies in the evidence, and face validity.

When evidence is not strong or is conflicting, the likelihood of inconsistencies between recommendations and an organization's policy increases. While guidelines and evidence-based tools are never a substitute for a nurse's judgment, nurses need the confidence and skills to use their own judgment about how evidence and evidence-based tools should be applied or not applied within a specific circumstance.

MODELS AND FRAMEWORKS TO FOSTER EVIDENCE RESEARCH

Although EBP and Donabedian's (1980) structure, process, and outcomes framework are, themselves, approaches to problem solving, additional prescriptive, criteria-based structures can foster transparent implementation of evidence into practice. Models and frameworks link theory to expectations while making decision-making processes and assumptions about contextual influences explicit. Critical thinking is supported through step-wise processes designed to engineer change and lead to measurable results. A key benefit of "planned action theory" (Graham & Tetroe, 2009) is better understanding of how interactions across disciplines influence change. Nurses are working to test the most common models and evaluate their benefit when used in patient care, including evaluation and ranking of how easy models are to use by clinicians (Mohide & King, 2003). Nurses also use models to address specific aspects of EBP, such as the use of terminology models that promote integration of nursing diagnosis with clinical terms (Bakken, Warren, Lundberg, et al., 2002).

The term "model" is often used to explain links to disciplinary theories, such as theories from the nursing, social, or physiological sciences. "Frameworks" are typically more practical structures that link ideas or concepts to each other or to interventions themselves. Models are often used as frameworks. They are useful when planning either a research proposal relevant to EBP or when considering an implementation project that moves evidence into clinical situations or uses internally generated quality improvement findings to continually improve care. Both models and frameworks define a step-wise path to expected success and are especially important when trying to explain belief in the potential benefit of what is being tested. They can also be used to demonstrate the strength of evidence or to justify changes or expenditures.

Because evidence-based practice involves application of evidence with real people outside the tightly controlled world of RCTs, models and frameworks account for contextual factors, assumptions, and influences on barriers and facilitators. Theory can help plan from the start how to address measurement of the eventual impact of the project on output that matters to patients, providers, families, caregivers, managers, or policy makers. In addition to measuring changes in structures, processes and outcomes, measurable change in risk, safety, collaboration, value, costs, utilization, efficiency and other factors can also be significant. Models and frameworks are often used by teams to match the research or project questions to the initiative being tested. This helps a group collectively understand how they will try to improve practice and makes it easier to define clear goals about complex clinical actions, such as how to foster changes in provider behaviour. Nursing leaders across the world have been instrumental in

development of the theoretical base for knowledge translation that advances use of evidence. Nurses have led the way in development of EBP models that focus on implementation of research findings with integration of supplemental information, such as quality and performance feedback. Over time, this work has created packages of resources and tools for those seeking to link evidence and practice.

While models developed by nurses can be thought of as practitioner oriented, their use also captures actions and interactions with patients, managers, educators, and specialists. Key models used in translation and implementation science include Rogers' Diffusion of Innovations model, the Funk Model, the PRECEDE Model, the Chronic Care Model, the PARIHS Model, the Stetler Model, the Iowa Model, the ARCC model, Kitson's Framework, Melnyk and Fineout-Overholt's Model of EBP, the Lean Framework, the PICO model, the QUERI model, and IHI's Breakthrough Series Collaborative Model. Over time, these approaches and ideas have greatly promoted optimal practice by making it easier to capture complex factors, plan actions, and evaluate the results.

There are now many nursing leaders throughout the world who work diligently to expand and test theories relevant to EBP. Much of this work can be linked back to Roger's understanding of "attributes," such as complexity, that need to be accounted for when change is planned (Rogers, 1995). More than a decade ago, Carole Estabrooks asked nurses to define what our profession sanctions as legitimate evidence (Estabrooks, 1998). Alison Kitson and her colleagues in the United Kingdom have long emphasized the need to marry the nature of the evidence to understanding of context/environment and the ways in which processes are facilitated (Kitson, Harvey, & McCormake, 1998). The PARIHS framework helps define and measure key factors leading to successful implementation (Rycroft-Malone, Kitson, Harvey, et al., 2002). Marita Titler and her collaborators developed and tested the Iowa Model in multiple settings and across diagnoses. This work helped standardize nursing triggers, promote use of the Nursing Interventions Classification and standardized nursing treatment languages in EHR, and quantify clinical relevance in ways that guide measurement of impact (Titler, 2004; Titler & Moore, 2010). Among Dr. Titler's contributions to the evolution of EBP and Implementation Science is synthesis of the evidence base supporting evidence-based practice implementation (Titler, 2008). Melnyk and Fineout-Overholt (2004) have contributed to our theoretical knowledge base, for example, by emphasizing how

research evidence can be merged with clinical expertise, and patient preferences/values within a context
of caring. Cheryl Stetler updated her practitioner-ori-
ented Stetler Model in ways that helped shape EBP in
recent decades (Stetler, 2001; Stetler, Legro, Wallace, et
al., 2006; Stetler & Caramanica, 2007; Stetler, 2010).
Initially developed in 1976 with Marram, the Stetler
Model was refined and expanded to include conceptual details, an underlying set of assumptions, a utiliza-
tion-focused integrative review methodology, targeted
evidence concepts, and continuing experience. The
revised model focuses on judgments about the appropriateness, desirability, and feasibility of using research
findings in practice. Dr. Stetler has also actively promoted use of formative evaluation within translation
efforts (Stetler et al., 2006).

INTEGRATION OF COSTS, PATIENT PREFERENCES, AND COMMUNITY PREFERENCES

The complexity of integrating patient and community
preferences and including considerations of value and
cost are real. EBP is based on the recommendations
using the best available evidence. The cost of the highest quality care may be expensive or comparatively
expensive. It is often said that quality leads to cost
reductions, over the long term. But this is not always
the case and varies by disease and condition. CER and
other methods are evolving to address complex trade-
offs. Values surrounding outcomes and risk need to
be openly addressed. From the start, teams pursuing
EBP need to clarify how quality and cost tradeoffs will
be approached. For example, for many groups, issues
of quality are considered a priority. Cost factors are
important but secondary.

Risk: One Size Rarely Fits All

In addition to considering risk more carefully in the
application of performance measures, risk, risk-ad-
justment, and how risk applies to the needs of special populations are often methodologically difficult
across EBP products and applications. Patients and
their preferences vary such that one size rarely (accurately) fits all applications. Options exist so that EBP
operates at a high level of accuracy and benefit but
thought is required (Hayward et al., 2007; Hayward et
al., 2005; Perlin & Pogach, 2006; Pogach et al., 2007,
2010). For example, vigilance is needed as we address
how to cope with gaps in knowledge across groups

with differing degrees of risk. If data is not available
about a specific subgroup (that may be at higher risk
than others with the same condition) or if there is bias
suspected in existing sources of evidence, it is important to take this into account when planning translation rather than rushing to apply evidence. Gaps in the
evidence are sometimes not well understood, leading
to leaps in interpretation. Nurses can assure that these
concerns link back to overarching principals of EBP,
such as the need to avoid bias. Nurses can also assure
that the profession has active input in how the evidence is synthesized and used as the basis for products
and tools. Credible groups know the limitations of evidence well and often invite public review, comment,
and the input of professional groups—not only about
their draft products but also about their methodology.
The direct involvement of nurses and nursing groups
in these review and comment activities strengthens the
final products. Nurses can also work to advance methods that address risk, including development of predictive modeling tools that translate automated patient
information in ways that predict healthcare needs,
risks, and outcomes (Celebi, 2003).

Personalized Evidence

The penultimate evidence of a possible condition,
diagnosis, or disease is unfolding through the genetic
makeup of the person, the treatments tailored for
that person, and the preventative strategies that can
be enlisted if one is susceptible to a condition or disease. These types of new evidence will be discussed in
Chapter 51.

Informatics Tools That Promote Evidence-Based Practice

Since the publication of the 4th edition of *Essentials
of Nursing Informatics*, the GELLO tool described
by McCormick in that chapter has been balloted and
is included in HL7 recommended standards found at
www.HL7.org (McCormick, 2006). Other tools for
incorporating evidence into automated clinical decision
support tools have also advanced. Innovative new technologies are now broadening the use of evidence in new
automated ways.

Clinical Decision Support (CDS) Tools

CDS tools are interactive automated programs that
assist nurses and other clinicians with decisions, usually
at point-of-care. The term "active knowledge system"

refers to similar ideas. The spectrum of what can be categorized as CDS is growing. CDS comes in many forms, including automated templates for both orders and referrals. CDS comes from a number of applications developed for the EHR to facilitate prognostic, diagnostic, and treatment interventions. These tools include links to reminders or other forms of evidence. Decision analysis and CDS offer ways to link the probability of a clinical course to the likelihood of specific outcomes. The results of clinical decisions can then be predicted, and the probability of alternative strategies quantified. Decision models, data, and complex analyses are required. Most decision support tools work in consort with the EHR. Many are designed to promote the timeliness of a diagnosis or treatment intervention or to promote movement from diagnosis into treatment. Computerized prescriber order entry is an example of a CDS tool embedded in the EHR. Prescriptions can then be filled quickly and risks are more easily managed.

Computerized Pathways, Flow Charts, Algorithms, and Critical Paths

Many guideline-based tools are now available to facilitate implementation of guidelines in seamless ways that simultaneously reduce errors while promoting compliance. Many of these tools can also be categorized as CDS tools. Available tools include those that focus on the prescribing and administration of medications. Checks and triggers are embedded in ways that guide clinicians through diagnostic and treatment interventions based on guideline recommendations. Algorithm-based decision systems can be used, for example, to reduce laboratory testing by prompting clinicians about the correct interval for testing.

Point-of-Care Tools: Cards, Pre-Printed Order Sets, Flags, Checklists, Reminders

Point-of-care refers to healthcare setting where patient care is provided, such as at the bedside, in an emergency room, or within an ambulatory care setting. EBP tools are proliferating but vary widely in complexity and ease of use. Many vendors offer these tools commercially and they come in many formats. Due to wide variations in the types of searches, questions addressed, usability, grading of evidence, and presentation of results, the benefits of each individual tool needs to be appraised carefully. Assumptions should not be made that any specific point-of-care tool is credible. These tools will likely proliferate as meaningful use, PCMH, EHR, and CDS expand.

Many common reminder systems are not automated. Laminated cards, posters, pre-printed forms within charts, and pocket guides are all reminders familiar to most providers. Automated reminders are infinitely more powerful and are gaining popularity as EHR spreads. Reminders are sometimes used in "real time" and at the point of patient contact. For example, an automated system can analyze a patient's age, risk factors, and other data to generate a screen reminder when an evidence-based intervention is not performed. A Computerized Patient Reminder System (CPRS) can also be a decision support system used to guide nurses and other clinicians through the stages of decision making and prompt them regarding the need for a specific evidence-based intervention. A patient's data or characteristics determine what documentation is captured on the template. A CPRS template can be used to document patient symptoms or trigger a consult as early as possible.

Care Coordination and Continuum of Care Mapping

Case management and care coordination are key roles for nurses who follow a panel of patients in order to assure EBP, including monitoring whether or not appropriate diagnostic and treatment interventions were completed and generating follow-up actions for any tasks not completed. Communication is promoted electronically and verbally across providers so that patients are guided through the system in ways that promote efficiency as well as effectiveness.

Automated GIS

Geographic Information Systems or Geographic Information Science (GIS) refers to Websites or services that connect data from different sources and share, remix, repurpose, and reconnect them. Once only available to elite experts, neogeography, GeoWeb technologies, and online services provide a wave of innovation that expands our ability to store, analyze, and display a vast amount of information about the entire Earth. This is leading to a growing number of healthcare and research tools based on GIS. GIS enables "mashing up" of various data and provides map layers and themes from different sources which converge into a map which can then be geo-referenced, meaning that a reference can be made to a specific place on the planet (Boulos, Scotch, Cheung, & Burden, 2008). Visualization of multiple datasets that have been integrated into a common format enhances understanding of how evidence is already being used across geographic areas or where it may be needed (Google, 2007). For example, rural health experts can enhance their understanding of gaps in services by reviewing maps. In addition to using GIS to depict gaps in healthcare service, practice, or outcomes, GIS tools are also being used in public health for infectious disease surveillance, epidemiology, and planning and are gradually gaining popularity with those pursuing translation of evidence (Boulos, 2004; Yu, Cowper, Berger, et al., 2004). The power and potential of GIS brings with it concerns about privacy, accuracy, and national threat. In addition, because extensive statistical and epidemiological sophistication is needed, vigilance about the validity of what is produced is especially warranted.

Trigger Tools, Bundles, and Rapid Cycle Testing

IHI and other groups use many different automated tools that often work in tandem, either together or separately, depending on what change is needed. "Triggers" measure harm through retrospective review of records that reveal clues about adverse events. IHI's Global Trigger Tool supports estimated harm levels across a system (Institute for Healthcare Improvement, 2010). A bundle is a group of 3 to 5 evidence-based practices linked together. A bundle is used to promote adoption of specific interventions. Impact can then be measured.

Automated Toolkits and Evaluation Guides

Automated resources that package translational and evaluation tools together into a "toolkit" or are synthesized into a "guide" help individuals, teams or entire systems as they systematically approach changing practice and measuring impact. A collection of automated tools can support team-based problem solving by making it easier to incorporate what is learned into what is practiced. Through use of a toolkit or guide, goals and systematic processes are more easily planned and organized. Toolkits or guides may contain measures for monitoring, improvement, and/or accountability or may be evaluative tools used in larger quality improvement or systems redesign efforts. Evaluation guides will often provide information about formative evaluation (which is used to guide the ongoing development of a project) and summative evaluation (which provides information about effectiveness and impact). Summative evaluation is often used in projects that use quantitative data tracking of progress or address the flow of patients through the organization. Using a guide or toolkit, it is often easier to focus on specific issues related to quality, risk, or cost.

Email, Social Networking, and Twitter Alert Systems

Personal and social communication can efficiently be used to provide evidence to those who voluntarily register based on personal, professional, or clinical interest. For example, users on a condition-specific list may receive e-mail alerts related to new evidence about interventions of interest. These tools are ideal for receiving information about new publications or to be quickly alerted about a safety concern, such as new evidence that a medication has been found dangerous. There is sometimes a charge for alert services. Alerts are often linked to resources that allow searching access for literature matched to clinical interest. Alerts deliver pre-rated information so the source needs to be appraised by the nurse.

Electronic Screening, Assessment, Tracer, and Self-Assessment Tools

One of the first steps in quality improvement is assessment of current practice. For many diseases and conditions, systems redesign and other frameworks promote use of assessment tools for tracking performance and gauging where to begin. Tracer and self-assessment tools are available for nearly all aspects of health operation and facilitate moving from self-evaluating through improvement and onto impact measurement and feedback.

Health Risk Calculators

Because risk is inherently integrated with use of evidence and because activated patients are partners in use of evidence, health risk calculators will likely proliferate and become more convenient. Electronic calculators provide immediate information relevant to specific personal risk or condition, such as data about Body Mass Index or feedback about a health condition such as pregnancy. Like many other tools, health risk calculators may be most useful when used together with other patient and provider tools or as part of the EHR or other automated documentation system that facilitates tracking.

Web 2.0 and Health 2.0

As described by Van de Belt and colleagues (2010), the term "Web 2.0" has been used since 2004 to describe the economic and social trends that are collectively contributing to the next Internet generation. Although there are different definitions and thoughts about whether or not Web 2.0 is real (many say it is not a new generation because it uses HTML), some believe that it will improve communication and collaboration through enhanced interactions, including expansion of social networking capability. For example, it is possible that Web 2.0 will allow users to more easily add their own content to the Web, thereby creating greater interaction capability. The impact on EBP can only be speculated. The amount of "user-generated content" has already increased via sites like YouTube, Facebook, Twitter, and various health sites. Few studies have explored the impact or risks. When applied to healthcare, the term Medicine 2.0 also appears. Like its cousin, Web 2.0, the term Health 2.0 lacks a consistent definition. It is openly assumed that both Health 2.0 and Medicine 2.0 will contribute to more activated and empowered patients (using new and more advanced versions of existing personal health sites) since it will be even easier to access health information and discuss it (either verbally or through electronic means) with providers. But this also increases opportunities for patients (and all of us) to be misled, misinformed, or manipulated.

There are many assumptions being made about what information will be coming to us and in what format, yet few studies address practical application and risk. For example, what will Health 2.0 mean in terms of processes and outcomes? If a manufacturer, individual, or advocate initiates a global campaign to mislead decision makers, how easy will it be for us to identify the risks and dialog about it with our colleagues and patients? These are questions to address within our own countries but also globally. As scientific resources on the Internet evolve quickly, caution and new criteria for critical appraisal are needed.

Standardization of related terms and definitions will facilitate dialog about this type of evidence across professions. For example, while it is within the bounds of traditional scientific rigor to use online, "open access" journals when basic scientific standards are met, a more conservative approach is merited when considering use of evidence from social media. Until we understand what we are seeing and have time to reach consensus about appraisal, caution is needed.

Teamwork: No Longer Simply a Good Idea

While teamwork in healthcare is not new, the critical importance of shared decision making is more essential than ever before. Nurses do not use automated evidence in isolation. Evidence is used by nurses with their clinical peers, patients, families, caregivers, managers, and policy makers. A characterizing trait of the current age is the requirement for collaboration. Nurses not only use evidence to support their own decisions and the decisions of their patients, but also to facilitate evidence-based decision making across professions and within groups. Online groups, like Nursing Knowledge International (Excellence in Nursing Knowledge), provide a forum for interactive discussion about "where research and reality are engaged in a lively debate" (www.nursingknowledge.org). The rapid expansion of PBRNs fuels the importance of social support when information is sought and considered. This is especially true for providers inclined to seek useful information regardless of format (Andrew, Pearce, Ireson, & Love, 2005).

ONLINE SOURCES OF EVIDENCE

Online communication provides a convenient, cost-effective vehicle for information dissemination and exchange. Online tools are more powerful when integrated within an overall communication strategy and targeted to specific information needs. Simple automated Internet searches using common search engines reveal many sources of synthesized evidence. There are far too many credible sources of information relevant to nurses interested in EBP to provide a comprehensive review. New sites and services appear frequently. Included in this chapter are only a few examples of the resources now available online.

The U.S. government has provided valuable access to guidelines on the Internet since the early 1990s. Credibility is supported through legislation and transparency. This is described on AHRQ's Website found at http://www.ahrq.gov/news/infoqual.htm (Agency for Healthcare Research and Quality, 2010). Section 515 of the Treasury and General Government Appropriations Act for Fiscal Year 2001 (Public Law 106-554; H.R. 5658) directed the Office of Management and Budget to issue government-wide direction to Federal agencies in order to assure the quality, objectivity, utility, and integrity of information disseminated by Federal agencies. In October 2002, Federal agencies issued their own individual guidelines about the integrity of the information they disseminate. For this reason, the quality review procedures used by AHRQ and other Federal agencies applies to information disseminated on or after October 1, 2002.

The National Guideline Clearinghouse (NGC) is an Internet resource for evidence-based clinical practice guidelines. NGC can be found at www.guideline.gov. AHRQ is part of the U.S. Department of Health and Human Services. NGC provides guideline syntheses as well as expert commentary. Significant changes are currently underway for NGC and a similar site, National Quality Measures Clearinghouse (NQMC). Updated designs and displays are expected as well as enhanced functionality, such as easier access to content.

AHRQ also administers an Evidence-based Practice Centers (EPC) Program, which includes funding and oversight of 5-year contracts awarded to U.S. and Canadian institutions that serve as EPCs. Each EPC reviews all peer reviewed scientific literature on specific clinical, behavioral, organizational and financing issues in order to produce evidence reports and technology assessments related to a topic. These reports are used in development of clinical practice guidelines, quality measures, performance measures, educational materials, clinical tools, policies, and research agendas. The EPCs go beyond developing these products by investigating the methodology of systematic reviews and continuously improving related methods.

Systematic reviews are also available through Cochrane Database of Systematic Reviews and Evidence Reports published on www.thecochranelibrary.com. Cochrane uses its own databases as well as MEDLINE/PubMed (www.pubmed.gov), ClinicalTrials (www.clinicaltrials.gov), the FDA's MAUDE Database (http://www.accessdata.fda.gov/scripts/cdrh/cfdocs/cfMAUDE/search.CFM), and other sources to conduct systematic reviews. Cochrane reports include searches of nursing literature through sources like the Cumulative Index to Nursing and Allied Health Literature (CINAHL), which is the largest index for nursing and allied health literature. CINAHL is available through OVID or EBSCOHost interfaces. The increased availability of resources like OVID and Library Information Science & Technology Abstracts (LISTA), improves research productivity and makes it easier to link research and practice. The National Library of Medicine, Clinical Evidence resources offered by the British Medical Journal, Knowledge Transfer + (McMaster University), Research into Action (University of Texas), Center for Evidence-Based Medicine (Oxford), and JAMAevidence are among the growing list of information sources readily available to most nurses. These online sources provide a wide array of information relevant to EBP, including glossaries, online discussions, automated tools, and support for hand-searched journals.

A vast array of online websites makes many journal articles and synthesized evidence reviews available to nurses and others interested in EBP. The use of electronic databases using pre-appraised evidence expedites searches and enhances the ability of clinicians to apply evidence in ways that individualize care (Krupske, Dahm, Fesperman, & Schardt, 2008). Only a few are described here; there are many others and new resources appear all the time. Searching using terms such as "evidence-based nursing" along with the condition or disease of interest reveals a growing list of sites.

Examples of useful sites includes filtered articles provided through abstraction journals and databases, such as Evidence-Based Nursing (http://ebn.bmj.com/), which is published quarterly in order to provide nurses with information about scientific advances in prevention, diagnosis, and treatment. *Evidence-Based Nursing* reviews a large number of international clinical journals, then applies criteria to rate the quality and validity of the research. Clinicians then evaluate the clinical relevance of those rated highest. The selected studies are then posted along with expert commentary about clinical application. Abstraction journals provide electronic access to both articles that the journal abstracts but also to other articles that meet quality criteria and are made available on a searchable database.

Together with the British Medical Journal Publishing Group, a product called "bmjupdates" is produced by the Health Information Research Unit at McMaster University (which also serves as the Editorial Office for *Evidence-Based Nursing*). This service is free and provides a searchable database of the evidence from published literature. The evidence is pre-rated for quality by researcher experts and includes over 100 clinical journals. Articles are rated for clinical relevance and newsworthiness. The service also provides an e-mail alert system.

Knowledge Translation+ (KT+) is provided by McMaster University's Health Information Research Unit and provides access to the current evidence on "T2" knowledge translation, which refers to research addressing the knowledge to practice gap. The purpose is to provide current information for those working in areas relevant to translation. The information provided includes peer reviewed articles and systematic reviews, information about QI, continuing education, and patient information. KT+ provides two types of articles, those that are relevant to knowledge translation and have been filtered for quality and non-filtered KT+ articles. KT+ also offers a cumulative searchable database of healthcare literature and an email alert system (Knowledge Translation+, 2010).

Another online journal of interest to many nurses is called *Implementation Science (IS)*. This journal is useful to nurses who see EBP as an inherently interdisciplinary research arena. *IS* does not embrace any particular research method but seeks publication of articles of high scientific rigor using methods that promote the generalizability of findings. In addition to hosting papers describing the effectiveness of interventions, *IS* publishes articles describing intervention development, evaluations of the process by which effects are achieved, and the role of methods and theory development. The journal also publishes debate and discussion articles that present novel methods, particularly those that capture theoretical issues (*Implementation Science*, 2010). *IS* is one of many online open access journals that includes an impact factor that measures the average citation count in science and social science journals. For journals that are indexed in Thomson Reuter's (2010) *Journal Citation Reports*, an impact factor is calculated annually and thought to reflect the relative importance of a specific journal within its own field (higher impact factors are seen as more important).

NURSING INFORMATICS EDUCATION TO PROMOTE EVIDENCE-BASED PRACTICE

This section describes innovative ways that education can promote EBP in such areas as academic detailing, automated training, and tracking databases.

Academic Detailing (AD). AD is an acronym used to describe customized "educational outreach." Individual providers are targeted for education. Computers can supplement AD in a variety of ways. For example, computer-assisted instruction or videodisc technology can be used to convey information about a guideline and allow the provider to explore this information safely prior to applying it to real patients. Unlike conferences or workshops, which are often passive, computerized AD provides focused, individualized education that can be highly interactive. The stimulating and engaging nature of computer-facilitated AD promotes success.

Automated Training and Support for Clinical Champions. Individual practitioners, multidisciplinary teams, managers and others are supported through ongoing conferences and communication from experts. Webinars and electronic media now make education easier and more consistent. New or revised evidence can more readily be communicated and encouraged. These communication devices can often be streamed to work areas or conference rooms or made available 24/7 for ready access.

Tracking Databases or Registries. Tracking panels of patients with the same disease or condition can be a powerful automated tool that enhances monitoring of progress and impact. Expanded use of tracking data enhances implementation by helping to organize vast amounts of complex information.

Leadership and Organizational Support for EBP

For the ongoing education required to expand competency and knowledge in EBP, leadership and organizational commitment is required. Nurses at all levels require dedicated (protected) time to support advancement of their skills and knowledge. Mentoring relationships and coaches can help a nurse learn the skills needed for EBP. This education will include learning the communication and social skills needed to promote team work and help break down silos that impede EBP. For example, negative attitudes towards research "silos" as well as feelings of intimidation regarding working with some clinicians needs to be openly addressed. Common terminology is needed so that team members easily understand each other as they determine how to move evidence into practice.

The time and resource constraints associated with EBP can be daunting. If implementing an evidence-based tool is not feasible or adds stress in a clinical setting, the best evidence or evidence-based tools may be ignored by busy providers. The change being pursued may be "the right thing to do," but achieving it may generate chaos in the short term. Ongoing communication is needed so that providers understand the rationale for change and have an idea of what to expect when change is coming. Communicating options for control and ongoing positive improvements to those working to implement evidence in practice seems obvious but might be overlooked. Online Journal Clubs, online and open access journals, mentoring, blogging, social networking, and professional/academic activities can generate enthusiasm. The benefits of using an evidence-based tool need to be clear and concerns addressed openly. Motives and incentives need to be taken into account. Rather than simply telling a provider that they must use a specific tool, the value to the patient needs to be addressed and discussed in respectful and nonpunitive ways.

Limitations

EBP is increasingly found in ambulatory settings, in patient homes and primary care homes, and in highly specialized settings with activated patients who desire a role in decisions relevant to their care. Tools that embed evidence in the form of robotic aids, reminders, performance measures, and guidelines promote interaction at the time of a decision, but also demand accountability for how securely evidence is accessed, transmitted, used, and protected. As the demand for evidence grows and formats for providing this evidence are ever-more dynamic and interactive, demands for protective restriction evolve. Nurses are positioned to play a key role in protecting the privacy of patients and the confidentiality of health information. As patient advocates, nurses play a key role in assuring that confidentiality is protected when personally identifiable information is involved. Nurses also protect their patients and the system when they help navigate the unclear line between research and quality. When there are questions about how evidence and data are being used, nurses are in a good position to assure that ethics regulations regarding oversight and monitoring are addressed.

No limitation is more significant than the risks posed by practitioners, patients, and others who do not know how to access and appraise the best available evidence. When sources of opinion and anecdote are mistaken for scientific knowledge, the risks to patients can be high. Nurses need to not only appraise evidence, they need to know how to communicate with others about evidence in constructive ways that benefit and protect patients.

Innovative Evidence Implementation Efforts Involving Nurses

Examples of nurses applying theoretical knowledge to EBP are, fortunately, growing. Nurses are actively contributing to a growing body of literature about translation and implementation science. For example, nurses have been an instrumental part of EBP teams promoting ongoing improvements in mental health within the Department of Veterans Affairs (VA) for more than 2 decades. There is no better example of the commitment required to embrace EBP than these extensive and integrated endeavors (Luck, Hagigi, Parker, et al., 2009; Rubenstein, Mittman, Yano, & Mulrow, 2000; Rubenstein et al., 2002; Smith, Williams, Owen, et al., 2008). Nurses have participated in teams of investigators and clinicians, led by Dr. Lisa Rubenstein in collaboration with the VA Mental Health Quality Enhancement and Research Initiative (QUERI) group. Integrated multidisciplinary efforts optimize the quality of depression care based on evidence from VA and non-VA studies of effectiveness, cost-effectiveness, and quality improvement. A collaborative care model helps systematically unite mental health specialists with primary care activities. Through implementation of this model, patients diagnosed with depression are systematically assessed, educated, and followed for symptoms and treatment compliance, consistent with AHRQ guidelines. This approach requires ongoing collaboration and communication between the depression care manager and others. Many EBP tools have been used. Although results

are still being calculated by Rubenstein and her colleagues, she has already reported that a great deal is being learned about how knowledge spread occurs. In addition to the significance of performance measurement, Rubenstein reports that "care model 'tweaking' is continuous," and that roles that tighten links within the evidence base are important. Social marketing has also been found to be a promising implementation strategy (Luck et al., 2009).

In a separate endeavor, also related to the QUERI program, Dr. Denise Hines, a nurse scientist who leads the VA's Information Resource Center, evaluated the role of HIT across 83 individual QUERI implementation projects. She addressed how HIT impacted implementation of research findings into practice and also evaluated barriers and facilitators (Hynes, Weddle, Smith, et al., 2010). Hines and her team reported interdependency on a well-established HIT infrastructure. She identified relationships with key stakeholders as a positive factor in successful implementation. In the next section, a more detailed application of EBP in a real situation is described.

The LISTEN Project: Helping Nurses to Obtain and Use Evidence-based Information in the Clinical Setting

As a nurse in a clinical setting you may often find yourself in situations where you need more information or data. Where do you go? Often our initial reaction may be to turn to a colleague; however, this may not always be the right choice since they may not be updated on current research or new practice guidelines. What about turning to available texts? This might be a good option, but texts are often outdated by the time they are published and may not have the most current information. What about looking online for answers to your question? This is another good choice, but how do you know the information you are reviewing is valid and trustworthy and derived from an authority on the subject matter? The LISTEN (Learning Information Seeking and Technology for Evidence-based Nursing) Project (www.listenuphealth.org) works to help nurses gain information literacy skills to combat the uncertainty and questions related to finding and using new information as they practice evidence-based nursing and to support lifelong learning.

While EBP relies on observation and past nursing experience to make decisions, we must also use research literature to validate or corroborate the decisions made for patient care. The upsurge of information available to nurses today has made it increasingly challenging for nurses at all levels to process relevant literature and available information. Information literacy skills are essential to nursing practice based on evidence, and according to some EBP is not possible without possession of these skills (Tanner, Pierce, & Pravikoff, 2004; Tarrant, Dodgon, & Law, 2008). By gaining skills to efficiently and effectively locate, retrieve, evaluate, and apply information, nurses can be more poised to provide care based on evidence (Newhouse, Dearholt, Poe, et al., 2007). The LISTEN Project works with nurses at all levels to improve information seeking, information application and information technology competencies in student and professional nurses. The LISTEN Project, an educational intervention, was a Health Resources and Services Administration funded project from 2007 to 2010 (Russell, 2006).

Educational content delivered on behalf of the project was designed and developed by nurses and health sciences librarians along with consultants in the areas of information literacy, evidence-based practice, and nursing informatics. Project content development was guided using up-to-date and modern guidelines in the areas of information literacy, information technology, and nursing informatics. The project team worked together to develop 24 learning outcomes that addressed recognizing and prioritizing information needs, seeking and accessing information, evaluating information, evidence-based nursing practice concepts and resources, evidence-based nursing practice searching and evaluating, and evidence-based nursing practice application. Within these areas participants gained specific and guided instruction about creating clinical questions, using Boolean operators, accessing and searching in specific databases such as CINAHL or PubMed, how to evaluate information, and lifelong learning techniques, to name a few.

Due to variations in workflow in nursing, the LISTEN Project was offered to participants a number of ways. Participants could opt to participate in the project via a face-to-face workshop or one of two online options. The face-to-face option offered participants the opportunity to progress through a two-part scenario where they were prompted to answer questions related to information seeking, information application, and information technology. The face-to-face environment offered comfort and support to many participants that were not as computer savvy. Participants were given the opportunity to ask questions and progress as a group. The online scenario option offered the same scenario as the face-to-face but in a self-paced, asynchronous style. The other online option, the Brief Online Learning Tutorials,

or BOLTs, addressed the same content and learning outcomes as the module but provided the information in brief segments of instruction, often very compatible with those working in the clinical setting.

Nursing will continue to be practiced in ever changing environments. Possessing skills that enable EBP and lifelong learning will be required of every nurse to maintain competence in the field. Programs such as LISTEN will become vital to nurses' success in learning about EBP and applying evidence to practice for the betterment of patient care.

SUMMARY AND CONCLUSIONS

As debates about whether or not clinical practice guidelines are appropriate is gradually replaced with measuring the impact of their use and conditions that promote change, our hardware is shrinking, broadband is spreading, wireless systems are proliferating, and e-mails and all imaginable electronic communication are flourishing. We watch as our patients start accessing their medical records at home and then bring us data comparing the quality of their neighbourhood hospital to others nearby. Nurses deal with these realities and uncertainties using rational processes, now thought of as EBP. Nurses are pivotal part of EBP at the international level while strongly contributing to local efforts to build relationships, teams, organizations, and systems capable of effectively addressing meaningful use, the expansion of practice networks, the restructuring of primary care, growing use of CER and other methods, and the application of many powerful electronic EBP tools. Strong skills in the appraisal of evidence are needed at each turn. Although nurses use different terms when thinking about evidence, we share similar challenges. Specific action steps for nursing include:

- Continue to question the accuracy of the scientific information that influences healthcare decisions, EBP tools, methods and policies. Specifically, there is an ongoing need to improve the accuracy of the epidemiological evidence used in EBP, generally, and when applied to performance measures, specifically.

- EBP's central place in ideas about meaningful use heightens awareness that evidence and other information are not transmitted without risk. These risks must be understood and addressed.

- Much work remains in defining EBP in ways that are meaningful to nursing and accurately reflect nursing practice. Additional work in measurement, methodology, standardization, coding, documentation, and communication lies ahead.

- Customizing EBP to individual patients is not automatic and requires consideration of risk. Handheld devices and other hardware can be used, even at the bedside, to work with other members of the team to apply EBP tools.

- Methods, analysis, and reporting that is transparent and user-friendly can help teams stratify by risk and thoughtfully explore benefits and harms.

- EBP tools need to be evaluated in order to understand system-level barriers and facilitators, especially as they apply to patients facing complex chronic illness and comorbidities. Nurses need to be able to help patients understand evidence and use it to make decisions, particularly when evidence is missing, conflicting, or hard to understand.

- Leadership and management support are needed to assure that nurses are able to access and use the best available information. Ongoing skill development hinges on cultivating specific critical appraisal skills over time. Development of skills related to EBP needs to begin early in a nurse's education and continue throughout a career. Without the prerequisite skills, computers are only machines. Regardless of how the evidence is accessed, peer review and transparent reproducibility stand out as essential components of scientific evaluation. Nurses need to mentor and teach each other in order to assure that the skills associated with critical appraisal are understood and remain current. Incentives should be provided for those who keep their skills current and teach others. Learning time needs to be protected and social events used to foster a positive association with EBP.

- Investigation is needed as we grapple with how and under what conditions interactive Internet communication and information sharing benefits patients and makes it easier for healthcare professionals and consumers to access and use evidence. Protection of patient information and the security of HIT will rise in importance and requires vigilance.

- There is lack of agreement about the credibility of online sources. Professional nursing groups need to consider the criteria needed to evaluate resources obtained from the Internet. Nurses need to work with colleagues and patients to define what evidence is grounded in science and how to deal with less credible resources.

REFERENCES

Agency for Healthcare Research and Quality. (2007). Transforming hospitals: Designing for safety and quality. Rockville, MD.

Agency for Healthcare Research and Quality. (2010). U.S. Preventive Services Task Force. Retrieved June 1, 2010 from http://www.ahrq.gov/clinic/uspstfix.htm

Andrew, J. E., Pearce, K. A., Ireson, C., & Love, M. M. (2005). Information seeking behaviours of practioners in a primary care practice-based research network (PBRN). *Journal of the Medical Librarians Association, 93*(2), 206–212.

Bakken, S., Currie, L. M., Lee, N.J., Collins, S. A., & Cimino, J. J. (2008). Integrating evidence into clinical information Bates systems for nursing decision support. *International Journal of Medical Informatics, 77*(6), 413–420.

Bakken, S., Warren, J. J., Lundberg, C., Cassiey, A., Correia, C., Konicek, D., et al. (2002). An evaluation of the usefulness of two terminology models for integrating nursing diagnosis concepts into SNOMED clinical terms. *International Journal of Medical Informatics, 68*(1–3), 71–77.

Balas, E., & Boren, S. (2000). Managing clinical knowledge for healthcare improvement. In M. Bemmel, J. A. (Ed.), *Yearbook of medical informatics: Patient Centered Systems* (pp. 65–70). Stuttgart, Germany: Verlagsgesellschaft.

Baron, R. J. (2010). Meaningful use of health information technology is managing information. *Journal of the American Medical Association, 304*(1), 89–90.

Berwick, D. (2007). Eating Soup with a Fork. 19th National Forum Keynote, http://www.ihi.org/IHI/Programs/AudioAndWebPrograms/OnDemandPresentationBerwick.htm

Boulos, M. N. (2004). Towards evidence-based, GIS-driven national spatial health information infrastructure and surveillance services in the United Kingdom. *International Journal of Health Geographics, 3*(1).

Boulos, M. N., Scotch, M., Cheung, K., & Burden, D. (2008). Web GIS in practice V1: A demo playlist of geo-mashups for public health neogeographers. *International Journal of Health Geographics, 7*(38).

Celebi, D. (2003). The pwoer of predictive modeling. *Healthcare Informatics, 20*(8), 56.

Centers for Medicare & Medicaid Services. (2007). Fact Sheet. Retrieved June 1, 2010, from http://www.cms.gov/apps/media/press/factsheet.asp?Counter=3564

Clinical Linkages. (2009). Retrieved June 1, 2010, from http://www.clinical-linkages.com

Covell, C. L. (2010). Can civility in nursing work environments improve medication safety?. *Journal of Nursing Administration, 40*(7/8), 300–301.

Doebbeling, B. N., Chou, A. F., Tierney, W. M. (2006). Priorities and strategies for the implementation of integrated informatics and communications technology to improve evidence-based practice. *Journal of General Internal Medicine, 21*, S50–S57.

Donabedian, A. (1980). *Explorations in quality assessment and monitoring* (Vol. 1). Ann Arbor, MI: Health Administration Press.

Estabrooks, C. A. (1998). Will evidence-based nursing make practice perfect? *Canadian Journal of Nursing Research, 30*, 15–36.

Google. (2007). Official Google maps API blog: Introduction and Yahoo! pipes. Retrieved June 1, 2010, from http://googlemapsapi.blogspot.com/2007/04/introduction-and-yahoo-pipes.html

Graham, I. D., & Tetroe, J. (2009). Theories of knowledge to action: Planned action theories. In S. Straus, J. Tetroe, & I. Graham (Eds.), *Knowledge translation in healthcare*. London: Wiley-Blackwell.

Guyatt, G. R. D. (2002). *Users' guide to the medical literature*. Chicago: AMA Press.

Hayward, R., Kent, D. M., Vijan, S., & Hofer, T. P. (2005). Reporting clinical trial results to inform providers, payers, and consumers. *Health Affairs, 24*(6),1571–1581.

Hayward, R., Kent, D. M., Vijan, S., & Hofer, T. P. (2007). All-or-nothing treatment targets make bad performance measures. *American Journal of Managed Care, 13*(3), 126–128.

Hogan, S. O., & Kissam, S. M. (2010). Measuring meaningful use. *Health Affairs, 29*(4), 601–606.

Howard, L. M., K. (2007). Centralized and decentralized nurse stations design: An examination of caregiver communication, work activites, and technology. *Health Environments Research and Design Journal, 1*(1), 44–57.

Hynes, D. M., Weddle, T., Smith, N., Whittier, E., Atkins, D., & Francis, J. (2010). Use of health information technology to advance evidence-based care: Lessons from the VA QUERI program. *Journal of General Internal Medicine, 25*, 44–49.

Institute for Healthcare Improvement. (2010). Retrieved 2010 from http://www.ihi.org

Implementation Science (2010) http://www.implementationscience.com

Institute of Medicine. (1999). *To err is human: Building a safer health system*. Washington, DC: National Academies Press.

Institute of Medicine. (2001). *Crossing the quality chasm: A new health system for the 21st century*. Washington, DC: National Academies Press.

Joseph, A., & Fritz, L. (2006). Ceiling lifts reduce patient-handling injuries. *Heatlhcare Design, 6*(1), 10–13.

Kane, L. (2010, June 15). EHR meaningful use – so easy, even a caveman could do it.

Retrieved from http://boards.medscape.com/oforums?14@@.2a00a190!comment=1

Kerr, E. A., Smith, D. M., Hogan, M. N., Hofer, T. P., Krein, S. L., Bermann, M., Hayward, R. A. (2003). Building a better quality measure: Are some patients with 'poor quality' actually getting good care? *Medical Care, 41*(10), 1173–1182.

Kitson, A., Harvey, G., & McCormake, B. (1998). Enabling the implementation of evidence-based practice: A conceptual framework. *Quality in Healthcare, 7*, 149–158.

Knowledge Translation +. (2010). Retrieved June 1, 2010, from http://plus.mcmaster.ca/kt/Default.aspx

Krupske, T. L., Dahm, P., Fesperman, S. F., & Schardt, C. M. (2008). How to perform a literature search. *Journal of Urology, 179*(4), 1264–1270.

Luck, J., Hagigi, F., Parker, L. E., Yano, E. M., Rubenstein, L. V, & Kirchner, J. E. (2009). A social marketing approach to implementing evidence-based practice in VHA QUERI: The TIDES depression collaborative care model. *Implementation Science, 28*(4), 64.

MacEachin, S. R., Lopez, C. M., Powell, K. J., & Corbett, N. L. (2009). The fetal heart rate collaborative practice project situational awareness in electronic fetal monitoring – A Kaiser Permanente patient safety program initiative. *Journal of Perinatal & Neonatal Nursing, 23*(4), 314–323.

McCormick, K. A. (2006). Translation of evidence into nursing practice: Evidence, clinical practice guidelines, and automated implementation tools. In V. K. Saba, & K. A. McCormick (Eds.), *Essentials of nursing informatics* (4th ed.). New York: McGraw-Hill.

McQueen, L, McCormick, K.A. (2001). Translating evidence into practice: Guidelines and automated implementation tools. In V.K. Saba, & K.A. McCormick (Eds.), *Essentials of Nursing Informatics* (4th ed.). New York, McGraw-Hill.

Melnyk, B. M., & Fineout-Overholt, E. (2004). *Evidence-based practice in nursing and healthcare*. Philadelphia: Lippincott Williams & Wilkins.

Mohide, E. A., & King, B. (2003). Building a foundation for evidence-based pracitce: Experiences in a tertiary hospital. *Evidence-Based Nursing, 6*, 100–103.

National Committee for Quality Assurance. (2010). Retrieved July 20, 2010, from http://www.ncqa.org/tabid/59/default.aspx

Newhouse, R., Dearholt, S., Poe, S., Pugh, L., White, K. (2007). *Johns Hopkins nursing evidence-based practice model and guidelines*. Indianapolis, IN: Sigma Theta Tau International.

Perlin, J. B., & Pogach, L. (2006). Improving the outcomes of metabolic conditions: Managing momentum to overcome clinical inertia. *Annals of Internal Medicine, 144*(7), 525–527.

Pipe, B. P., Wellik, K. E., Buchda, V. L., Hansen, C. M., & Martyn, D. R. (2005). Implementing evidence-based nursing practice. *Urologic Nursing, 25*(5), 365–370.

Pogach, L. M., Rajan, M., Maney, M., Tseng, C. L., & Aron, D. C. (2010). Hidden complexities in assessment of glycemic outcomes: Are quality rankings aligned with treatment? *Diabetes Care, July*(9).

Pogach, L. M., Tiwari, A., Maney, M., Rajan, M., Miller, D. R.,& Aron, D. (2007). Should mitigating comorbidities be considered in assessing healthcare plan performance in acheiving optimal glycemic control. *American Journal of Managed Care, 13*, 133–140.

RAND. (2001). *The global technology revolution* (No. MR-1307-NIC).

Rich, C. R., & Day, T. D. (2008). Integrating electronic health records in the physical environmentL A system's approach. *Herd-Health Environments Research and Design Journal, 2*(1), 48–65.

Rogers, E. M. (1995). *Diffusion of Innovations* (4th ed.). New York: Free Press.

Rubenstein, L. V., Mittman, B. S., Yano, E. M., & Mulrow, C. D. (2000). From understanding healthcare provider behavior to improving healthcare: The QUERI framework for quality improvement. *Medical Care, 38* (S 6), 129–141.

Rubenstein, L. V., Parker, L. E., Meredith, L. S., et al. (2002). Understanding team-based quality improvement for depression in primary care. *Health Services Research, 37*(4), 1009–1029.

Russell, C. K. (2006). LISTEN: Learning information seeking and technology for evidence-based nursing. Unpublished Grant Proposal. The University of Tennessee Health Science Center.

Rycroft-Malone, J., Kitson, A., Harvey, G., et al. (2002). Ingredients for change: Revisiting a conceptual framework. *Quality in Safety and Healthcare, 11*, 174–180.

Sackett, D. L., Straus, S. E., Richardson, W. S., Rosenberg, W., & Hayes, R. B. (2000). *Evidence-based medicine: How to practice and teach EBM*. London: Churchill Livingstone.

Sarkar, I. N. (2010). Biomedical informatics and translational medicine. *Journal of Translational Medicine, 8*, 22.

Selby, J. V., Uratsu, C. S., Fireman, B., Schmittdiel, J. A, Peng, T., Rodondi, N., Karter, A.J., & Kerr, E. A. (2009). Treatment intesification and risk factor control: Toward more clinically relevant quality measures. *Medical Care, 47*(4), 375–377.

Sherman, H., Castro, G., Fletcher, M., et al. (2009). Towards an international classification for patient safety: The conceptual framework. *International Journal for Quality Improvement, 21*, 2–8.

Singh, H, & Graber M. (2010). Reducing diagnostic error through medical home-based primary care reform. *Journal of the American Medical Association, 304*(4), 463–464.

Smith, J. L., Williams, J. W., Owen, R. R., Rubenstein, L. V., & Chaney, E. (2008). Developing a national dissemination plan for collaborative care for depression: QUERI series. *Implementation Science, 31*(3), 59.

Stetler, C. (2001). Updating the Stetler Model of research utilization to facilitate evidence-based practice. *Nursing Outlook, 49*, 272–279.

Stetler, C., Caramanica, L. (2007). *Evaluation of an evidence-based practice initiative: Outcomes, strengths and limitations of a retrospective, conceptually-based approach. Worldviews on Evidence-Based Nursing, 4*, 187–199.

Stetler, C. (2010). Stetler Model. In J. Rycroft-Malone, & T. Bucknall (Eds.), *Evidence-based practice series: Models and frameworks for implementing evidence-based practice: Linking evidence to action.* Oxford, UK: Wiley-Blackwell.

Stetler, C., Legro, M., Wallace, C., et al. (2006). The role of formative evaluation in implementation research and the QUERI experience. *Journal of General Internal Medicine, 21*, S1–S8.

Tanner, A., Pierce, C., & Pravikoff, D. (2004). *Readiness for evidence-based practice: Information literacy needs of nurses in the United States.* Paper presented at MEDINFO.

Tarrant, M., Dodgson, J., Law, B. (2008). A curricular approach to improve the information literacy an academic writing skills of part-time post-registration nursing students in Hong Kong. *Nurse Education Today, 28*, 458–468.

Titler, M. G. (2004). Understanding synergy: the model from the perspective of a nurse scientist. *Excellence in Nursing Knowledge: Voices of Evidence in Nursing, 1*(1).

Titler, M. (2008). The evidence for evidence-based implementation (Chapter 7). In *Patient Safety and Quality: An Evidence-Based Handbook for Nurses.* AHRQ Publication No. 08-0043. Rockville, MD: Agency for Healthcare Research and Quality. Retrieved from http://www.ahrq.gov/qual/nurseshdbk/

Titler, M. G., & Moore, J. (2010). Evidence-based practice: a civilian perspective. *Nursing Research, 59*(1), Suppl S, S2–S6.

Thomson Reuter. (2010). *Journal Citation Reports.* Introducing the impact factor. Retrieved from http://thomsonreuters.com/products_services/science/academic/impact_factor/

Van de Belt, T. H., Engelen, L., Berben, S., & Schoonhoven, L. (2010). Definition of health 2.0 and medicine 2.0: A systematic review. *Journal of Medical Internet Research, 12*(2), e18.

Westra, B. L., Subramanian, A., Hart, C., et al. (2010). Achieving "meaningful use" of electronic health records through the integration of the nursing management minimum data set. *Journal of Nursing Administration, 40*(7/8), 336–343.

Yu, W., Cowper, D., Berger, M., Kuebeler, M., Kubal, J., & Manheim, L. (2004). Using GIS to profile healthcare costs of VA Quality-Enhancement Research Initiative diseases. *Journal of Medical Systems, 28*(3), 271–285.

27

Evidence-based Practice

Joanne M. Seasholtz / Bernadette Mazurek Melnyk

- OBJECTIVES
  1. Define evidence-based practice.
  2. Discuss how evidence-based practice impacts healthcare quality, safety, and cost reduction.
  3. Discuss barriers and facilitators for successful implementation of evidence-based practice in clinical practice.
  4. Discuss the evidence-based practice paradigm and process
  5. Identify technology tools in clinical practice that support evidence-based practice.
  6. Discuss the role of clinical decision support systems in evidence-based practice.
  7. Discuss process changes and supporting processes for integration of evidence-based practice in clinical areas.
  8. Discuss a professional practice model that supports evidence-based practice.

- KEY WORDS

  Evidence-based practice
  Decision support
  Clinical decision support
  Evidence-based adaptive clinical decision support
  PICOT
  Nursing informatics
  Clinical terminology
  Technology tools
  Evidence-based practice tools
  Professional practice model
  Magnet

IMPROVING HEALTHCARE QUALITY AND PATIENT OUTCOMES THROUGH THE INTEGRATION OF EVIDENCE-BASED PRACTICE AND INFORMATICS

There is mounting evidence that implementation of evidence-based practice (EBP) by nurses and other health professionals results in higher quality healthcare, improved patient outcomes, less variation in care, and reduced costs compared with care that is steeped in tradition or based on outdated policies and practices (McGinty & Anderson, 2008; Melnyk & Fineout-Overholt, 2011; Williams, 2004). In addition, findings from studies have supported that when nurses believe in the value of EBP and are able to implement evidence-based care, they have higher job satisfaction and better group cohesion, which are key determinants of job turnover guide best practices (Block, 2006; Krumholz, 2008). In contrast to research that generates new knowledge and evidence for practice, EBP translates evidence from research into clinical practice to improve healthcare quality and patient outcomes. (Maljanian, Caramanica, Taylor, et al., 2002; Melnyk, Fineout-Overholt, Giggleman & Cruz, in press). Because of the known positive outcomes associated with EBP, the Institute of Medicine set a goal that 90% of healthcare decisions will be evidence-based by 2020 (McClellan, McGinnis, Nabel, & Olsen, 2007). Despite its positive outcomes and recent mandates by leaders, professional organizations, and policy makers to base and reimburse care on the best and latest evidence, EBP is not consistently implemented by numerous healthcare systems and clinicians across the United States (Bodenheimer, 2008; Melnyk & Fineout-Overholt, 2011).

There is no doubt that the use of technology with clinical decision support systems can enhance the delivery of evidence-based care. However, technology must be used by clinicians who implement the steps of EBP and healthcare organizations that cultivate system-wide cultures of EBP if high quality evidence-based care is to be sustained.

In 2000, Sackett and colleagues defined EBP as the conscientious use of current best evidence in making decisions about patient care. Since then, EBP has been broadened and described as a problem solving approach to the delivery of care that integrates the best evidence from well designed studies with a clinician's expertise and patient preferences and values in making clinical decisions (Melnyk & Fineout-Overholt, 2011). Both external evidence (ie, findings from research) and internal evidence (ie, evidence that is generated from outcomes management or quality improvement projects) should be used in evidence-based decision making. When clinicians deliver EBP in a context of caring and an organizational culture that supports EBP, the highest quality of care and best patient outcomes are achieved (Figure 27.1). If healthcare systems are to be redesigned to improve the quality of care and patient outcomes as well as reduce costs, clinicians must translate internal and external evidence that is collected, analyzed and critically appraised into useful information to guide best practices (Block, 2006; Krumholtz, 2008).

The 7 Steps of Evidence-based Practice

There are 7 steps in the EBP process (Melnyk & Fineout-Overholt, 2011) (Table 27.1). In the first step, which is step 0, a spirit of inquiry in clinicians and a culture of EBP must be cultivated in order to stimulate the asking of burning clinical questions to improve patient care. Once a clinical question is generated, step 1 in the EBP process involves formatting clinical questions into PICOT format (P = patient population, I = intervention or interest area, C = comparison intervention or group, O = outcome, and T = time). Formatting clinical questions in PICOT format is necessary to streamline the search for evidence to answer the question. An example of a PICOT question about a treatment is: In depressed adolescents (P), how does the delivery of cognitive behavior therapy in person (I) versus delivery of web-based cognitive behavior therapy (C) affect depressive symptoms (O) three months after treatment (T).

In Step 2 of the EBP process, a search for the evidence is conducted by entering each key word from the PICOT question into the database that is being searched (e.g., Medline, CINHAL) and then combining the search words together to reveal the studies that may answer the question. Reliable resources that should be used to find an answer to the PICOT question include systematic reviews, clinical practice guidelines, pre-appraised literature, and studies from peer-reviewed journals.

In Step 3 of EBP, a rapid critical appraisal of the studies from the search is conducted followed by an evaluation and synthesis of the research evidence.

In Step 4, evidence is integrated with the clinician's expertise and patient preferences and values to make a decision regarding whether a practice change should be made. Once a practice change is made based on the best evidence, outcomes should be measured to determine positive outcomes of the change (i.e., Step 5). Evaluation of outcomes is an essential step in EBP as

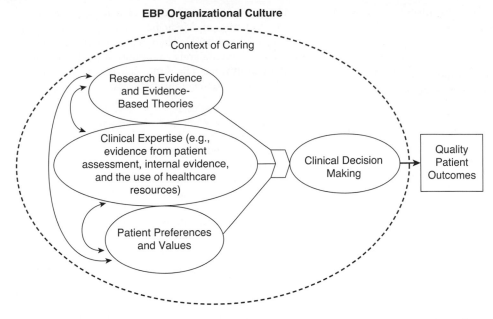

it helps to determine if the EBP practice change was successful, effective, equitable, timely, and needs to be modified or discarded (Gawlinski, 2007). The last step in the EBP process, Step 6, is disseminating the outcome of the practice change through presentation or publication so that others can benefit from the process.

TABLE 27.1	The Steps of the Evidence-based Practice (EBP) Process

0. Cultivate a spirit of inquiry.

1. Ask the burning clinical question in PICOT format.

2. Search for and collect the most relevant best evidence.

3. Critically appraise the evidence (ie, rapid critical appraisal, evaluation, and synthesis).

4. Integrate the best evidence with one's clinical expertise and patient preferences and values in making a practice decision or change.

5. Evaluate outcomes of the practice decision or change based on evidence.

6. Disseminate the outcomes of the EBP decision or change.

From: Melnyk, B. M., & Fineout-Overholt, E. (2011). *Evidence-based practice in nursing & healthcare. A guide to best practice* (2nd ed.). Philadelphia: Wolters Kluwer/Lippincott, Williams & Wilkins.

Barriers and Facilitators of Evidence-Based Practice

There are multiple barriers to advancing EBP in healthcare systems, including: (a) misperceptions by clinicians that it takes too much time, (b) lack of EBP knowledge and skills, (c) organizational cultures that do not support EBP, (d) lack of resources, including clinical decision support tools, (d) executive leaders and managers who do not model EBP, (e) lack of EBP mentors to work with point-of-care staff on implementing evidence-based care, (f) inadequate access to databases by clinicians in order to track patient and system outcomes, and (g) negative attitudes toward research (Fineout-Overholt, Melynk, & Schultz, 2005; Hannes, Vandersmissen, De Blaeser, et al., 2007; McGinty & Anderson, 2008; Melnyk, Fineout-Overholt, Feinstein, et al., 2004; Melnyk, Fineout-Overholt, Feinstein et al., 2008).

Findings from studies also have established key facilitators of EBP that include: (a) strong beliefs about the value of EBP and the ability to implement it, (b) EBP knowledge and skills, (c) organizational cultures that support EBP, (d) EBP mentors who have in-depth knowledge and skills in evidence-based care as well as individual and organizational change, (e) administrative support, (f) clinical promotion systems that incorporate EBP competencies, and (g) EBP tools at the point-of-care, such as clinical decision support systems

(Melnyk, 2007; Melnyk, Fineout-Overholt, & Mays, 2008; Melnyk et al., 2004; Newhouse, Dearholt, Poe, et al., 2007).

Cultivating a Culture That Supports and Sustains Evidence-based Practice

In order to cultivate a culture that supports and sustains EBP, an organization must provide system-wide support for evidence-based care. This support begins with a vision, philosophy and mission that incorporate EBP as a key component, which are made visible to all throughout the organization. High level administration and nurse managers must not only "buy-in" to this vision, but also model EBP themselves as much of how clinicians perform is learned through observation of their key leaders and managers. Integrating EBP throughout the clinical ladder system if one exists also establishes the importance of evidence-based care for staff advancement. Furthermore, ample resources and supports must be provided to clinicians that enhance their ability to provide evidence-based care, including: (a) regular EBP education and skills building sessions; (b) tools at point-of-care, including EBP designated computers, clinical decision support tools, evidence-based policies and procedures; (c) EBP journal clubs and fellowship opportunities; (d) EBP mentors, who are typically advanced practice nurses who have excellent EBP skills along with knowledge in individual and organizational change strategies; (d) access to databases to track outcome data; and (e) funding for EBP implementation and outcomes management projects. Regular recognition of EBP accomplishments through such events as annual EBP poster or conference events also encourages staff to continue their efforts in evidence-based care and shows appreciation for their efforts.

THE ROLE OF TECHNOLOGY IN SUPPORTING EVIDENCE-BASED PRACTICE

Technology Tools in Clinical Practice which Support Evidence-based Practice

Nurses, nurse practitioners, and healthcare providers today are very cognizant of the push for cost containment, improved patient safety, improved quality of care, and reduced variation in care throughout not only the United States but the world. It is readily observed that healthcare choices are being made based on quality and outcomes, not cost.

The Committee on Quality of Healthcare in America of the Institute of Medicine published *Crossing the Quality Chasm* (2001). Their report and other sources have demonstrated significant opportunities for improvement in healthcare. The American Nurses Association (ANA) defines nursing informatics as:

> Nursing informatics is a specialty that integrates nursing science, computer science, and information science to manage and communicate data, information, and knowledge in nursing practice. Nursing informatics facilitates the integration of data, information and knowledge to support patients, nurses, and other providers in their decision making in all roles and settings. This support is accomplished through the use of information structures, information processes, and information technology. (ANA, 2001. p. viii)

Graves and Corcoran define nursing informatics as a combination of computer science, information science, and nursing science that is designed to assist in the management and processing of nursing data, information, and knowledge to support the practice of nursing and the delivery of nursing care (Graves & Corcoran, 1989).

Information technology (IT) has brought to healthcare a compendium of new tools, information, and data which support EBP. As a consequence, information technology has not only improved, but also complicated, many currently existing processes. A goal of informatics is to use technology to bring critical and essential information to the point-of-care to increase efficiency, make healthcare safer and more effective, and improve quality and outcomes (National Quality Forum, 2008). However, despite the advancement in information technology the most effective, evidence-based care remains evasive (Glaser, 1978; Benoliel, 1996). This is due to a lack of translation of research into clinical practice settings. (Nemeth, Wessell, Jenkins, et al., 2007).

Competencies

Nursing professionals range in age from their early 20s to their 60s, with the average age of a registered nurse in their early 50s. This range presents a significant range of learning skills and comfort with technology.

Today's nursing students are very adept with using iPODs, iPADs, Blackberrys, PDAs, IPhones, laptops, and other technology devices. They have been using them in school and college, in fact, many used computers in kindergarten and preschool. In her work reviewing the challenges of making IT work across generations, Geisen (2009) found "the key danger with this group is staying focused on using technology consistently and correctly" (p. 42). Becky Quammen, CEO and founder of Quammen Group, a healthcare information technology consulting firm states:

> Young nurses know how to use technology but they don't know how to use it in a healthcare environment. They often go too fast in and out of applications, skipping necessary data fields, and relying on technology to do their thinking instead of relying on their nursing skills. (Geisen, 2009, p.42).

Even though nurses at the point-of-care are being held accountable for basing their practice on evidence, studies demonstrate that they are not ready for EBP. Pravikoff, Tanner, and Pierce (2005) found that the largest barrier for nurses using EBP is deficits in computer and information literacy or the ability to recognize the need comment locate, retrieve, evaluate, and use the information.

In 2006, a National League of Nursing (NLN) study revealed 60% of nursing programs had a computer literacy requirement and 40% had an information literacy requirement. Less than 50% of the respondents stated informatics was integrated into the curriculum and experience with information systems provided during clinical experiences (National League Nursing, 2008). As an outcome of the study, the NLN published a position statement recommending nursing schools to require all nursing students graduate with knowledge and skills in each of three critical areas: computer literacy, information literacy, and informatics.

Sigma Theta Tau (2006) also conducted a survey of nurses' knowledge of EBP in 2006. They found 69% of the respondents indicated low to moderate levels of familiarity with the EBP processes. Nurses reported difficulty translating research into their daily practice. The difficulties were related to their inability to understand statistical analysis and the lack of links into their day to day practice. Sigma Theta Tau's recommendation also was to incorporate EBP into the nursing curriculums.

Secco and colleagues (2006) completed a survey study which explored the use of different information sources among pediatric nurses. The study was guided by three interrelated concepts: types of information sources, levels of evidence, and computer skill. The survey findings demonstrated the use of traditional, noncomputer information sources such as textbooks and printed journals was higher among baccalaureate-prepared nurse when compared with diploma-prepared nurses. They also documented nurses with greater computer and online searching skills utilized more computer based information. They concluded improving nurses' computer and information seeking skills should promote use of higher-level evidence in planning nursing care.

Pravikoff, Tanner, and Pierce (2005) found that nurses use experientially acquired information from interactions with peers, patients, colleagues, and physicians greater than scientific evidence from medical and research journals. This finding still exists today.

It is imperative for nurses today to have the skills required to engage in EBP. Preparing undergraduate nursing students for EBP has great significance for advancing evidence based practice in nursing. It is imperative nurses learn to search for evidence and evaluate evidence as undergraduates. Coinciding with the skill set is the use of the proper technology to prepare nurses for use of EBP at the point-of-care. Rush (2008) states, "the preparation of undergraduate nursing students for using evidence to guide practice is no longer optional. Evidence Based Practice is imperative for insuring quality, cost-effective, safe care and more predictable outcomes for healthcare consumers" (p. 190).

DECISION SUPPORT AND EVIDENCE-BASED PRACTICE

Decision Support

Decision support systems (DSS) are systems or tools which support decision making activities and improve the decision making process and decision outcomes (Androwich & Kraft, 2006, p. 167).

Clinical decision support systems (CDSS) are systems designed to support healthcare providers in decision making regarding the delivery of patient care. "A CDSS program's goals may include patient safety and improved outcomes for specific patient populations as well as compliance with clinical guidelines, standards of practice, and regulatory requirements" (Androwich & Kraft 2006, p. 167).

Evidence-based adaptive clinical decision support systems are systems designed with multiple rules and access to multiple databases for information. They are complex systems and contain mechanisms to incorporate new findings and evidence (Sim, Gorman, Greenes, et al., 2001).

Three factors which play a significant role in increasing the availability of evidence at point-of-care are: clinical terminologies, referenced terminologies, and vocabulary servers.

1. *Clinical terminologies* have improved in recent years, however, they are not matured to a level to be used in clinical information systems (CIS). Standardized

clinical reference terminology is a necessity for evidence (in plans of care, order sets, rules, alerts, etc.) to be both computable and interoperable with other systems. Gugerty (2006) states, "It's in these forms–plans of care, order sets, standardized rules and alerts, and the like–that evidence will finally be widely, consistently, and reliably used at the point of care" (p. 23). The next step is to facilitate EBP by increasing the transparency to the healthcare provider or end user.

2. *Referenced terminologies* are now being incorporated into electronic health record databases.

3. *Vocabulary servers* that are application independent are being built and integrated into the architecture of electronic health records today.

To be efficient, the evidence for EBP must be incorporated into the everyday workflows and care processes used by nurses and other healthcare providers. The data must be integrated with the clinical systems used by the providers and provide readily accessible evidence-based knowledge for the end user at the point-of-care when needed. To be successful it is imperative to link evidence to assessments, results, documentation, orders, and plans of care.

Colera (2003) defines clinical decision support as a system which augments human performance and provides assistance for healthcare providers, especially for tasks subject to human error.

All decision support systems are based on rules or "what-if" scenarios. "If-then" rules recommend what actions to be implemented. Information is both accessed and stored within the knowledge base of the system. It is important that any information which is used in the clinical arena should be evidence based, current, and able to be continuously updated to assist in effective decision support. The evidence needs to be continuously reviewed and updated. This requires consistent monitoring and change processes to be in place.

The functions of clinical decision support systems include alerting, reminding, critiquing, interpreting, predicting, diagnosing, image recognition, assisting, and suggesting (Lyerla, 2008). One of the benefits of clinical decision support systems is the evidence can be driven into practice in a timely manner. Garg and colleagues (2005) reported that 76% of reviewed studies indicated that clinician performance was improved through the use of reminders. Diagnostic aiding systems were found to be beneficial in 40%. Automatic prompts to the end user were more effective than the end user needing to activate a system with changes in physician performance 73% with auto prompts and 47% when required

to activate a system. The highest success function was the use of reminders and alerts.

Decision support systems are passive or active. A passive system will notify an individual of an event, such as an abnormal finding where an active system will offer suggestions or take actions such as place a specific order when specific identified criteria are met. A topic of frequent discussion is the concept of "cookbook" medicine. Decision support systems are not "cookbook" medicine. The individual provider has the option to ignore alerts, override alerts, or inactivate alerts after his or her synthesis of the information and suggested actions is presented. The provider is the final decision maker.

Clinical decision support systems allow for optimization of both the efficiency and effectiveness with which clinical decisions are made and care is delivered. By providing support at the bedside, they reduce time and improve the decision-making process. The costs of clinical decision support systems can be high; however, the savings occur in the improved decision making at the bedside, improved outcomes, and reduction of errors.

Disparities have been documented by Medicare and other agencies in the treatment of heart disease and congestive heart failure. This was one of the incentives behind the CORE measures to reduce variation in practices when evidence has proven the impact of procedures and medications. The goal is to reduce variations, cost and improve quality. With point-of-care clinical decision support systems, clinical care and cost management do improve. One example is a study by InterMountain Healthcare which demonstrated that inpatients at Salt Lake City LDS Hospital who were treated by physicians with bedside computers got well quicker, suffered fewer complications, and were discharged sooner (Cochrane, 1998).

WHAT CAN OUTSIDE REFERENCE SOURCES (VENDORS) BRING TO THE TABLE?

The amount of evidence available at the point-of-care has grown exponentially in recent years. Fineout-Overhold, Malynk, and Schultz (2005) found it can be as long as 17 years for a research finding to be adopted in practice. Gugerty (2006) explains the tools for EBP have evolved from paper and pencil to EBP embedded in clinical information systems and decision support systems at the point-of-care. Technology has made tremendous advances from paper to icons to links available within healthcare information systems in 1996 to reference terminology and vocabulary servers tightly linked to electronic health records in 2010. The utilization of technology has also moved the amount of evidence available at the point-of-care from low to high and provided the venue for actionability/utility to also advance significantly.

Not only have the methods for using evidence changed but also the producers or originators of EBP have changed during the past 20 years. In the 1980s, hospitals, the government, and professional societies and standards organizations provided the information. Clinical practice guidelines were developed by individual hospitals. Nurses and staff spent hours in committees developing practice guidelines on paper which were printed and copied to be placed in paper charts. Textbooks were purchased with clinical pathway guidelines and the content was used directly or modified by each hospital. The responsibility was on the hospitals, who assumed that the textbooks had the latest evidence identified in their pathways and guidelines. They formed committees to review their standards and procedures in accordance with The Joint Commission and purchased new texts for reference periodically. During the 1990s, the research value of evidence and decision support was demonstrated through funded research. That trend changed in the 2000s to eliminate healthcare delivery organizations from building their own to their use of commercial vendors for information and incorporation into their practice. After the Institute of Medicine report *To Err Is Human* (Kohn, Corrigan, & Donaldson, 2000) indicated 48,000 to 98,000 deaths occur annually in the United States because of medical mistakes, the Institute of Medicine recommended that evidence be driven into practice in a more timely fashion to decrease mortality and morbidity from medical mistakes. In essence, they want the evidence to be driven to the point-of-care so it is available when needed.

The evolution of technology in the provision of information and data has led to changes in EBP. As stated earlier, healthcare organizations are no longer building their own EBP packages. They are now partnering with governmental agencies (Medicare), professional societies, and companies such as Zynx, Wolters-Kluwer, Thomson, Clin-eguide, Micromedex, and others who are now in the business of providing evidence based packages. The costs for current evidence are perceived by many as expensive, however, if one examines the hours spent in completing research literature reviews, evaluating the research, developing the guidelines, having all of the appropriate bodies approve the guidelines, and maintaining the guidelines, the costs are relatively low to a unit of evidence being delivered in a usable form.

The vendor provides the evidence; however, they do not decide what evidence you choose to incorporate into your facilities' practice. With vendors maintaining the responsibility for reviewing the research and presenting the best practices to the facilities the information can be incorporated into bedside care in a more expeditious manner.

PROCESS CHANGES AND SUPPORTING PROCESSES FOR INTEGRATION OF EPB IN THE CLINICAL AREAS: A CONTINUOUS PROCESS

Evidence-based practice has been defined in the nursing literature as "a problem solving approach to clinical practice that integrates a systematic search for, and critical appraisal of, the most relevant evidence to answer a burning clinical question, one's own clinical expertise, and patient preferences and values" (Melynk & Fineout-Overhold, 2005, p. 6). LoBiondo-Wood and Haber (2006) state what many believe that all nurses, regardless of the educational preparation, are responsible for research review and participation in EBP. The barriers to research implementation that were identified 3 decades ago—lack of time, insufficient administrative support, and limited access to information—still remain today (Rauen, Makic, & Bridges, 2009). Granger (2008) explains an additional limiting factor today is the actual transformation of the research findings into clinical practice at the point-of-care. In an integrative review of the literature, Funk, Tornquist, and Champagne (1995) identified four barriers to EBP: lack of knowledge, difficulty interpreting findings and applying them to practice, lack of time, and lack of autonomy to implement change. Simpson (2005) also defined five barriers to EBP: lack of nurses and demands on time, inability to access research and difficulty synthesizing the information online, occasional links to "cookbook" nursing, lack of formalized evidence-based training and undergraduate education, and a need for postgraduate training. When reviewing these reports one can easily identify similarities in their findings.

Lack of Time

The bedside caregiver can offer great insight into what is working and what is not working in the care of patients. Many organizations continue to make decisions about practice without the bedside caregiver present in the conversation. To be effective, nursing must make it a priority to include caregivers in the discussions when practices are changed.

Insufficient Administrative Support

A common error in developing IT systems and decision support systems is the lack of input into the design and functionality by the end users such as the nurses. In addition to the end user input there needs to be adequate administrative support to provide minutes, type documents, set up meetings, and complete the tasks which the end users, such as nurses do not have time to perform.

> As the single constant professional presence with hospitalized patients, nurses uniquely gather, filter, interpret and transform data from patients and the system into the meaningful information required to diagnose, treat, and deliver care to a patient. This data management role of nurses is a vital link in the decision making activities of the entire healthcare team. Failure to incorporate the experienced perspective of nurses in clinical and operational decisions may result in costly errors, jeopardize patient safety and threaten the financial viability of healthcare organizations. (American Association of Critical-Care Nurses [AACN], 2005, pp. 187–197)

Limited Access to Information

Where do Nurses look for information? There are more than 150,000 medical articles published each month (Matter, 2006). The following are many of the sources of information utilized by nurses.

- MEDLINE. Indexes over 5200 journals worldwide from 1966 to present. It is accessible free at www.nlm.nih.gov/databases_medline.html.
- CINAHL (Cumulative Index to Nursing and Allied Health Literature). Abstracts of journals, books, pamphlets, dissertations, software, and other forms of education for nursing and allied health professionals since 1982. CINAHL is not free; however, most educational libraries have a subscription to this service.
- CRISP (Computer Retrieval of Information on Scientific Projects). A searchable database of federally funded biomedical research projects conducted at universities, hospitals, and other research institutions that have been supported by the Department of Health and Human Services since 1972.

- EMBASE. A bibliographic database which covers drug research including side effects and drug interactions. A free demo contains approximately 30,000 records. There is a fee for this service.
- OVID. Provides access to a variety of resources including bibliographic databases (such as MEDLINE, EMBASE, and CINAHL); full-text journals; and other clinical information products such as Evidence Based Medicine Reviews. There is a fee for this service.
- Cochrane Reviews (http://www2.cochrane. org/reviews/). The Cochrane Collaboration prepares, maintains, and disseminates systematic reviews of healthcare interventions focusing primarily on systematic reviews of controlled trials of therapeutic interventions. Access to the Cochrane Library is available by subscription; however, the abstracts of Cochrane Reviews are freely available and can be searched.
- The Joanna Briggs Institute (www.joannabriggs. edu.au). An international collaborative of nursing medical and allied health researchers, clinicians, academics, and managers which provide best practice information sheets.
- BMJ Clinical Evidence. (http://clinicalevidence. bmj.com/ceweb/index.jsp). A free service. They also provide an annual edition of *Clinical Evidence Concise* which provides current comprehensive and user-friendly, evidence-based literature for clinicians.
- The Agency for Healthcare Research and Quality (AHRQ). A U.S. government agency which focuses primarily on medical healthcare services
- National Quality Measures Clearinghouse. NQMC is sponsored by AHRQ to promote widespread access to quality measures by the healthcare community and other interested individuals. It is a public resource for evidence-based clinical practice guidelines.
- The National Institute of Nursing Research. One of 27 institutes at the National Institutes of Health. Supports research to establish the scientific knowledge for the care of individuals across the life span for nursing.
- The Sarah Cole Hirsh Institute for Best Nursing Practices Based on Evidence. The institute is affiliated with the Frances Payne Bolton School of Nursing at Case Western Reserve. Systematic

reviews are published in the open access publication, *Online Journal of Issues in Nursing*.

- The National Comprehensive Cancer Network (www.nccn.org). Online network for oncology specific guidelines.

- Professional organizations such as Oncology Nurses Society, Emergency Nurses Association, American Association of Critical-Care Nurses, and others publish in their journals' evidence-based guidelines for nursing. There are available in digital format:
  ○ AACN Fast Facts: Evidence Based Practice Habits: Transforming Research into Bedside Practice. Published in Critical Care Nurse
  ○ Putting Evidence into Practice (PEP) addresses nursing sensitive patient outcomes which are significantly impacted by nursing interventions and within the scope of nursing practice and integral to the processes of nursing care. These are in the *Clinical Journal of Oncology Practice*

Technology is only a tool for the implementation of EBP in nursing. Evidence-based practice is not only valuable for clinicians but also plays a vital role in healthcare management. As agencies, payers, and consumers require quality care and disparities between hospitals are identified, there is a drive for evidence-informed managerial decision making. Numerous barriers to managers' use of evidence in decision making exist, including time pressures, perceived threats to autonomy, preference for anecdotal knowledge based on individual experiences, difficulty accessing the relevant evidence, reliance on external consultants (and others) to determine the quality of the information, and lack of resources (Rundall, Martelli, Arroyo, et al., 2007). These barriers are similar to those identified for the clinical areas.

MORE EVIDENCE AND ALERTS IS NOT NECESSARILY BETTER QUALITY CARE

Data, Information, Knowledge, Wisdom

Worthley (2000) defines data as the raw materials from which information is generated and information is the relevant, usable commodity needed by the end user. Healthcare produces an enormous amount of data, however, a significantly smaller amount of information. "Information is born when data are interpreted" (Bylone, 2010, p. 130) and in order for information to be useful it needs to be accurate, timely, complete, concise, and relevant (Worthley, 2000). Englebardt and Nelson (2002) explain in the Nelson Data to Wisdom Continuum the complete path of data as follows: data generates information, information generates knowledge and the interpretation, integration, and understanding of knowledge leads to wisdom. "Once you have all this data centralized, you can use value-added tools, such as decision support to provide caregivers with the information they need to make decisions" (Worthley, 2000, p. 28).

An important differentiator today is the use of clinical information systems (CIS). Clinical information systems provide both information and data. As a result, they are designed to assist in decision-making needs. To accomplish this task, it is necessary to bring together in one system various data relevant for the decision making process. In 2001, HIMSS (Health Information Management Systems) conducted its leadership survey. The five information technology applications considered most important for the next 2 years were CIS, Web-based applications, a clinical data repository, computer-based patient records, and point-of-care decision support. It is now 2010 and the focus had changed. The ARRA (American Recovery and Reconciliation Act) and Centers for Medicare and Medicaid Meaningful Use regulations published July 13, 2010 (Blumenthal & Tavenner 2010) have significantly altered the applications and functionality emphasized. These acts and regulations have deadlines and monetary incentives and penalties in place for healthcare providers and institutions. Although we are making strides, we still continue to have many disparate systems lacking in interoperability and face a long road ahead.

Prerequisites for a Successful Real-Time Clinical Decision Support System

Sittig (1999) identified five elements as prerequisites for a real-time, point-of-care clinical decision support system:

1. INTEGRATED, REAL-TIME PATIENT DATA BASE

Such a data base integrates data under a common patient identifier from a variety of clinical and administrative sources including the pharmacy, clinical laboratory, admissions, discharges, transfers, nursing notes, and radiology reports. It stores and updates all data as soon as laboratory results are available, forming the basis of any real-time CDSS effort and enabling the knowledge engineer to implement logic that involves patient-specific data from multiple data sources. For example, to develop a CDSS that helps a clinician interpret blood gas data, the patient's level of respiratory support at the time of the measurement is essential.

2. DATA-DRIVE MECHANISM

A data-drive mechanism in a computer system enables a knowledge engineer to set a flag so that a program can be activated when a particular type of data or data item (e.g., clinical laboratory results or a chest radiograph report) is stored in the database. Such a "triggering" event enables a KE to create automatic, real-time, asynchronous, clinical decision support systems. They are automatic in the sense that the clinician does not have to ask the computer to execute a particular program, rather the simple act of storing data in the patient's medical record starts the CDSS. Such systems are real-time in that they run as soon as the data is stored, instead of at a specified time of day.

3. KNOWLEDGE ENGINEER

The knowledge engineer is an informatics expert who is responsible for extracting and then translating the clinical knowledge into machine executable logic. The knowledge engineer must have in-depth knowledge of the structure and meaning of the data recorded in the patient's electronic medical record, a thorough understanding of the various knowledge representation schemes, and the analytical and social ability to discuss and help others choose between complex options in clinical and patient care scenarios. It is not necessary that the knowledge engineer is a clinician or a computer programmer, although either skill set would be useful.

4. TIME-DRIVE MECHANISM

The time-drive mechanism on a computer allows the knowledge engineer to develop programs that will be executed automatically at a specific time in the future (e.g., 2 am) or after a specific time interval has passed (24 hours after ICU admission). By running a program based on time, the knowledge engineer can create logic to remind clinicians to perform specific activities or to check that the appropriate action has been performed.

5. LONG-TERM, CLINICAL DATA REPOSITORY

The long-term clinical data repository contains patient-specific data from a variety of clinical sources collected over a period of several years. It allows the knowledge engineer, in conjunction with the clinical advisory group, to develop reliable statistical predictors of specific events. For example, one could develop a logistic regression equation that identifies the pathogen most likely to be found in a particular specimen and recommends the least expensive antibiotic. The database could also be used to identify potential problem areas, such as the percentage of patients with diabetes who have not had an HBA1C test performed within the last six months. Finally, one could use the database to test the newly created logic, a crucial step in the development of any CDSS.

The success of a clinical decision support also depends on the end user satisfaction with the system. A system for which the end user builds workarounds or ignores does not provide any use to the patients or clinicians. Three barriers have been identified: (1) excessive use of alerts and reminders, (2) outdated, or inaccurate information within the system, and (3) inappropriate level of the alerts. Many computerized physician order entry projects have been stalled related to excessive use of alerts. It can be a fine line to work with the clinical staff to identify the proper level of alerts and reminders. Lyerla (2008) explains "a reminder or alert that is too general may produce too many messages and result in clinician frustration, causing the reminder to be ignored, whereas a system that is too specific may not produce enough messages resulting in missed appropriate messages" (p. 229).

In a study by Im and Chee (2006), they describe nurses' acceptance of a decision support computer program for cancer pain management. Their results strongly supported that nurses welcomed the decision support computer program; however, there were some sociodemographic and professional characteristics which were significantly associated with the level of acceptance. "Many information systems, including decision support systems, have failed because developers have neglected users' judgments about a system's feasibility, time requirements, and usefulness in clinical practice" (Im & Chee, 2006, p. 103). Involvement of the end clinical users is imperative in the development process for a successful system. "It is much more important to develop a decision support system that the target users really consider necessary and useful for their practice and one that is easily applicable in their clinical practice" (Im & Chee, 2006, pp. 103–104).

It is imperative technology assists in getting evidence to nurses at the point-of-care. Again, this can be via various methods such as hyperlinks, text, and icons. Nurses need access to the information during their care provision, not 3 hours later. Information technology needs to integrate the evidence into their workflows so clinicians move readily from task based care to managing care and knowledge based decisions. When this is achieved, Matter (2006) explains the clinicians will be functioning at an elevated level of critical thinking and incorporate EBP into their daily work to improve efficiency, effectiveness, and patient outcomes.

A PROFESSIONAL PRACTICE MODEL TO SUPPORT EBP: TECHNOLOGY IS ONLY A TOOL

There are examples in the literature of hospitals implementing evidence based practice however many do not incorporate information technology as a tool. Matter (2006), Brokel, Shaw, and Nicholson (2006), and Lyerla (2008) present cases using clinical decision support to support EBP.

Implementing EBP, with the use of information technology or not, requires a transformation within nursing practice. Eastwood, O'Connell, and Gardner (2008) and Sanares, Waters, and Marshall (2007) present strategies to integrate research into practice. Vanhook (2009), Ogiehor-Enoma, Taqueban, and Anosike (2010), and Pipe, Cisar, Caruso, Wellik (2008) discuss approaches to overcome the barriers, transform the organization to support EBP, and inspire EBP. Through all of these scenarios there remains a constant thread for the establishment of strong nursing leadership which supports and empowers nursing to research and create change by the integration of EBP into their daily lives. This involves providing the educational resources, time, and informational technology support for nursing at the point-of-care.

Magnet Status and Shared Governance

The Magnet Model was developed by the American Nurses Credentialing Center in the 1990s. In 2007, the program evaluated 164 sources of evidence to evaluate how they interplay to create a work environment that supports excellence in nursing practice. The revised model in 2009 "reflects a shift in focus to measuring empirical quality results or outcomes to demonstrate excellence and places emphasis on new knowledge and innovation to advance nursing practice" (Morgan, 2009, p. 105). The five pillars of the Magnet model are (1) transformational leadership; (2) structural empowerment; (3) exemplary professional practice; (4) new knowledge, innovations and improvements; and (5) empirical outcomes. This model communicates the value or measuring results and using evidence to promote improvements, changes

in processes, innovations in practice, and the nursing work environment (Morgan, 2009, p. 105). Nursing, as medicine and other clinical disciplines, is a practice discipline which is supported by standards, research, and the application of the evidence. New knowledge, innovations, and improvements encompass both the quality of care (research and evidence-based practice) and outcomes. Day (2009) clearly identifies that today it is an expectation that Magnet organizations both transform and expand knowledge to provide effective and efficient patient centered care. Nurses evaluate research and utilize research findings daily. It is an expectation they evaluate their current nursing practice against the practice based evidence and make appropriate changes in their practice. In this way nurses can demonstration translation of new knowledge into nursing practice and the positive impact on patient outcomes.

Opportunities are present in empowering nurses with information technology tools to leverage the vast clinical knowledge base to improve care, increase patient safety, and meet regulatory requirements. To maximize the potential of evidence based practice. Challenges abound in synthesizing the latest most current research, making the research actionable, and finally putting the research into practice.

Practice guidelines are systematically developed standards to assist practitioners and patients in decisions regarding specific clinical situations. The rapid pace of knowledge expansion presents a challenge to nurses to provide care that is based on current research and evidence. This is one reason more and more facilities use outside vendors to provide the current evidence-based information. Providing practice guidelines at the point-of-care is one way of supporting nurses to provide optimal care based on current best evidence and research.

The Joint Commission recommends in the accreditation standards and elements of performance for hospitals that there are guidelines which have been scientifically developed based on recent literature reviews. This mandates that nursing policies and procedures based on current research be available to nurses on every unit (The Joint Commission, 2010); however, the literature shows nurses' adherence to evidence-based guidelines is low and significant variations in practice continue to occur (Anthony, 2008).

Support from Nursing Administration has been linked to successful use of research for many years and it still remains a vital link in the chain for success. The Magnet Status programs assist in promoting environments supportive of autonomy and inquiry which lead to professional practice and high quality care reflected in empirical outcomes.

Integration of Evidence into Healthcare Decisions

When nursing seeks to integrate the evidence into healthcare decisions, they face various rating systems for rating the strength of the evidence. This makes comparisons difficult when different systems are utilized. *Worldview on Evidence-Based Nursing* contains a section called Evidence Digest. The purpose is to provide concise summaries of well-designed and/or clinically significant studies, along with implications for healthcare. The level of evidence generated by the study is included with each study to enable readers to integrate the strength of the evidence into their own healthcare decisions. They utilize a 7-level rating system for the hierarchy of evidence from Melynk and Fineout-Overhold (2005) and modified from Guyatt and Rennie (2002).

The American Association of Critical-Care Nurses has published resources such as practice alerts, protocols for practice, and procedure manuals to provide recommendations for clinical practice based on comprehensive and scientific review of the evidence. In 2009, they revised their hierarchy system to grade the level of evidence in 6 levels.

Vendors such as Zynx also use rating systems to rate the strength of the evidence. It is important to note that the evidence hierarchies are not consistent between agencies, organizations, and vendors. The use of multiple systems has been a challenge to nurses.

Fineout-Overhold, Melnyk, and Schultz (2005) discuss that many professional organizations, healthcare organizations, and federal and state agencies are emphasizing the value of evidence-based practice (EBP). This value is related to the problem solving approach including well designed studies, clinical expertise, and patient values. As a result healthcare providers such as nurses can provide care which results in improved outcomes.

The transition to evidence based practice is a cultural change process. Nursing leadership needs to support nursing and empower them to question nursing practices and have available resources and time to support their searches for evidence to guide their delivery of care.

Brokel, Shaw, and Nicholson (2006) found in implementing clinical rules to automate steps in delivering evidence based care that to be successful there must be (1) use of uniform coded terminologies, (2) a culture to transform care with the use of evidence based practices, (3) processes in place to guide the organization and staff, and (4) interdisciplinary involvement is required to be successful (Brokel et al., 2006, p. 203). "The transformation from paper checklist, which prompted evidence-based practice, to the expert rules in an electronic health record in the health system of hospitals and clinics required an organizational culture to redesign workflow processes to improve the use of evidence based guidelines" (Brokel et al., 2006, p. 203).

Pennington, Moscatel, Dacar, and Johnson (2010) present a partnership model which paired undergraduate honors nursing students with seasoned staff nurses to implement evidence based practice changes over a two year period. They identified some of the barriers encountered as staff shortages, class constraints, inability to physically meet as teams, and a lack of clear delineation of leadership and timelines.

Pipe, Cisar, Caruso, and Wellik (2007) evaluated leadership strategies to engage evidence based practice by the nurses. One of their lessons learned was "find new ways to engage imagination...a virtual evidence based practice (EBP) toolkit.... The approach was to find out what direct care nurses need and to develop creative ways to meet their information needs. An internal online toolkit was started which includes tutorials on EBP, glossary of terms, links to external resources and organizations, links to internal resources, and descriptions of the unit based projects. The major challenge is keeping the toolkit current." (p. 270).

Rundall, Martelli, Arroyo, et al. (=2007) developed an Informed Decisions Toolbox to assist managers overcome the barriers, be less reliant on colloquial evidence and consultants, and be better able to improve the performance of their organizations. It provides six steps in the evidence informed approach to decision making. The complete toolbox is available at www.ache.org/pubs/jhmsub.cfm. The six steps are:

1. framing the management questions
2. finding the sources of information
3. assessing the accuracy of the information
4. assessing the applicability of the information
5. assessing the actionability of the evidence
6. determining if the information is adequate

To build an organizational environment conducive to evidence informed decision making Rundall, Martelli, Arroyo, et al. (2007) also suggest four leadership-driven strategies:

1. recognize and respond to the growing demand for accountability as a strategic issue
2. establish organizational structures and processes for knowledge transfer

3. build a questioning organizational culture

4. build organizational research capabilities

Each of Rundall, Martell, Arroyo, et al.'s (2007) strategies is a method for dealing with bounded rationality decision making which is common in healthcare decision making. Herbert Simon identified the bounded rationality decision making process in managerial behavior (Simon 1947) as a means whereby a manager's search for alternative solutions to problems is limited by their cognitive, informational, and resource constraints. Bounded rationality decision making occurs within healthcare where the approaches to care are limited by individual cognitive information, information from peers and verbal sources, and resource constraints which limit their ability to search outside a limited sphere such as written policies and protocols located on a clinical unit. Information technology can expand that limited sphere and assist in providing the evidence for evidence based practice at the point-of-care.

Karlene Kerfoot (2009) states, "Nurses are either professional owners of their practice or merely renters" (p. 36), "Nurses who own their practice adopt the mission, vision, philosophy of the unit/organization. They are personally involved in and personally care about the outcomes their team creates. They feel accountable for their practice and treat it like an owner would.... Nurses who own their practice are equally concerned about the outcomes their team produces" (p.36) Tim Porter O'Grady notes ownership must be embedded into the fabric of the organization. Ownership must be an expectation not an option. (Porter-O'Grady T 2009). Shared governance structures have been proven to be effective in building partnership models that have created excellence in outcomes.

> In order to successfully implement an accountability-based practice model, management must institute structures that support the core business of patient care delivery and, in doing so, create empowering workplaces. In fact, to be recognized as a Magnet hospital, elements of a shared governance structure must be in place because the evidence has consistently shown this effectively creates excellence in patient care. The roles in an effective shared governance structure are clear, and the roadmap to effective collaboration and decision-making is clear. (Kerfoot, 2009, p. 370)

It is necessary to create transparency. Nurses who own their practice need information to take the correct actions and make the right decisions. To support this model nurses need access to real time information they can use to intervene and analyze care. This includes information from both internal and external sources. They need to be able to use the power of information effectively with the help of information technology, decision support systems, and EBP to change their practice and be responsible for their outcomes. The Chief Nursing Officer and Chief Nursing Informatics Officer need to support the building of systems to support a professional practice through the engagement of a shared governance structure, education, support, and time for research and meetings.

Evidence-based practice is not just about connecting nurses with the evidence; it is also about transforming the structures and culture of healthcare organizations to enable staff nurses to use research evidence to make more effective decisions. The evidence does not, make the decisions—people do and people work in environments which can encourage or discourage an EBP approach.

Novice to Expert?

Technology is only a tool. Technology can help provide evidence at the point-of-care and clinical systems can provide information, however, the nurse is still the decision maker.

Patricia Benner, in her book *Novice to Expert*, explains that expertise develops when the clinician tests and refines propositions, hypotheses, and principle-based expectations in actual practice situations (Benner, 1984, pp. 2–3). As nurses grow, their experience helps them acquire expertise and experience is a requisite for expertise.

While examining professional practice models, Day (2009) argues that

> as a form of rule-following, practice based on research evidence is limited in its ability to capture essential domains of nursing practice and that reducing the practice to sets to rules to be followed precludes expertise. There is a place for rule-following in expert practice but we must be careful not to let rules take over to the point that existing experts are deskilled and expertise is no longer fostered. (p. 479)

As evidence-based practice expands and takes on more areas of nursing practice, and as the patient safety movement demands more standardization of nursing interventions, nurses find fewer situations in which they are called on to use clinical judgment. The situations in which nursing judgment results in a worsening of the patient's situation often create a new set of institutional rules to be followed in the next, similar situation. By following the rules next time, the nurse does not gain from her experience, and if the system response to getting it wrong is always to make new rules the development of clinical expertise is impeded. (p. 481)

Healthcare is continually being changed by medical science and the pace of change is rapidly increasing exponentially. Challenges remain in empowering nurses with the needed information technology tools to leverage an ever-growing clinical knowledge base to improve practice, increase patient safety, and meet regulatory and credentialing standards. These can be accomplished with the use of evidence based practice (Matter, 2006). Technology can readily support evidence-based practice; however, it is only a tool.

SUMMARY

Florence Nightingale (1859) wrote: "Let whoever is in charge keep this simple question in her head. Not how can I always do the right thing myself, but how can I provide for this right thing to always be done?" (p. 24).

The electronic health record and evidence-based practices have made great strides in the past 20 years. We are moving forward with providing evidence-based usable information at the point-of-care in a transparent format to not only improve quality and outcomes but also reduce costs and variations in care. But we are only at the tip of the iceberg when we look at what research is currently available for nurses and healthcare providers and what is actually incorporated into our daily practice. Where the path will take us we do not know, but in 5 years the path will lead to a use of EBP with information technology different from current day use, a more enhanced use, more transparent, comprehensive, and more individualized use. And as we follow the path it will lead us to safer, more effective, quality, individualized care for our patients.

REFERENCES

Androwich, I., & Kraft, M. (2006). Incorporating evidence: use of computer based clinical decision support systems for health professionals. In V. Saba & K. McCormick, *Essentials of nursing informatics* (4th ed.) (p. 167). New York: McGraw-Hill.

Anthony, M. (2008). Relationships among nurse staffing, adherence to practice guidelines, and patient outcomes in the treatment of hypoglycemia. *Quality Management Healthcare, 17*(4), 312–319.

Benner, P. (1984). *From novice to expert. Excellence and power in clinical nursing practice* (pp. 2–3). Menlo Park, CA: Addison-Wesley Publishing Company.

Benoliel, J. (1996). Grounded theory and nursing knowledge. *Quality Health Research, 6*(3), 40.

Block, D. (2006). *Healthcare outcomes management: Strategies for planning and evaluation.* Sudbury, MA: Jones & Bartlett.

Blumenthal, D., Tavenner, M. (2010). The "meaningful use" regulation for electronic health records. *New England Journal of Medicine, 363*(6), 501–504.

Bodenheimer, T. (2008). Transforming practice. *New England Journal of Medicine, 359* (20), 2086, 2089.

Brokel, J., Shaw, M., Nicholson, C. (2006). Expert clinical rules automate steps in delivering evidence-based care in the electronic health record. *CIN: Computers, Informatics, Nursing, 24*(4), 196–205.

Bylone, M. (2010). Effective decision making: data, data, & more data!. *AACN Advanced Critical Care, 21*(2), 130–132.

Cochrane, J. (1998). 1998 Information systems priorities. *Integrated healthcare report, 5*(1), 17–19.

Colera, E. (2003). *Guide to health informatics* (2nd ed.). Oxford, UK: Oxford University Press.

Committee on Quality of Healthcare in America, Institute of Medicine. (2001). *Crossing the quality chasm: A new health system for the 21st century* (p. 145). Washington, DC: National Academies Press.

Day, L. (2009). Evidence-based practice, rule-following, and nursing expertise. *American Journal of Critical Care, 18*(5), 479–451.

Eastwood, G., O'Connell, B., Gardner, A. (2007). Selecting the right integration of research into practice strategy. *Journal Nursing Care Quality, 23*(3), 258–264.

Englebardt, S., & Nelson, R. (2002). *Healthcare informatics: An interdisciplinary approach* (p. 13). St. Louis, MO: Mosby Elsevier.

Fineout-Overholt, E., Melnyk, B. M., & Schultz, A. (2005). Transforming healthcare from the inside out: Advancing evidence-based practice in the 21st century. *Journal of Professional Nursing, 21*(6), 335–344.

Funk, S., Tornquist, E., & Champagne M. (1995). Barriers and facilitators of research utilization. An integrative review. *Nursing Clinics of North America, 30*(3), 395–407.

Garg, G., Adhikari, N., McDonald, H., Rosas-Arellano, M., Devereaus, P., Beyene, J., Sam, J., & Haynes, R. (2005). Effects of computerized clinical decision support systems on practitioner performance and patient outcomes: a systematic review. *Journal of American Medical Association, 293*(10), 1223–1238.

Gawlinski, A. (2007). Evidence-based practice changes: Measuring the outcome. *AACN Advanced Critical Care, 18*(3), 320–322.

Geisen, C. (2009) Teaching tech: The challenges of making IT work across generations. *Nurse Leader, October,* 41–43.

Glaser, B. (1978) *Theoretical sensitivity: advances in the methodology of grounded* theory. Mill Valley, CA: Sociology Press.

Granger, B. (2008). Practical steps for evidence-based practice: putting one foot ahead of the other. *AACN Advanced Critical Care, 19*(3), 314–324.

Graves, J., & Corcoran, S. (1989). The study of nursing informatics. *IMAGE: Journal of Nursing Scholarship, 21*(4), 227–231.

Gugerty, B. (2006). The holy grail: Cost-effective healthcare evidence transparently and consistently used by clinicians. *Journal Healthcare Informatics Management, 20*(3), 21–24.

Guyatt, G., & Rennie, D. (2002). *Users' guide to the medical literature.* Washington, DC: American Medical Association.

Hannes, K., Vandersmissen, J., De Blaeser, L., Peeters, G., Goedhuys, J., & Aertgeerts, B. (2007). Barriers to evidence-based nursing: A focus group study. *Journal of Advanced Nursing, 60*(2), 162–171.

Health Information Management Systems. (2001). *12th Annual HIMSS Leadership Survey. Preliminary results* (pp.1–28). Chicago: HIMSS.

Im, E., & Chee, W. (2006). Nurses' acceptance of the decision support computer program for cancer pain management. *CIN: Computers, Informatics, Nursing, 24*(2), 95–104.

Kerfoot, K. (2009). The CNO's role in professional transformation at the point of care. *Nurse Leader, October,* 34–38.

Kohn, L., Corrigan, J., & Donaldson, M. (Eds.). (2000). *To err is human: Building a safer health system.* Committee on Quality of Healthcare in America. Washington, DC: National Academy Press.

Krumholz, H. M. (2008). Outcomes research: Generating evidence for best practice and policies. *Circulation, 118,* 309–318.

LoBiondo-Wood, G., & Haber, J. (2006). *Nursing research: methods and critical appraisal for evidence-based practice.* St. Louis, MO: Mosby Elsevier.

Lyerla, F. (2008). Design and implementation of a nursing clinical decision support system to promote guideline adherence. *CIN: Computers, Informatics, Nursing, 26*(4), 227–233.

Maljanian, R., Caramanica, L., Taylor, S. K., MacRae, J. B., & Beland, D. K. (2002). Evidence-based nursing practice, Part 2: Building skills through research roundtables. *Journal of Nursing Administration, 32*(2), 85–90.

Matter, S. (2006) Empower nurses with evidence-based knowledge. *Nursing Management, December,* 34–37.

McClellan, M. B., McGinnis, M., Nabel, E. G., & Olsen, L. M. (2007). *Evidence-based medicine and the changing nature of healthcare.* Washington, DC: National Academies Press.

McClellan, M. B., McGinnis, M., Nabel, E. G., & Olsen, L. M. (2007). *Evidence-based medicine and the changing nature of healthcare.* Washington, DC: National Academies Press.

McGinty, J., & Anderson, G. (2008). Predictors of physician compliance with American Heart Association Guidelines for acute myocardial infarction. *Critical Care Nursing Quarterly, 31*(2), 161–172.

Melnyk, B. M. (2007). The evidence-based practice mentor: A promising strategy for implementing and sustaining EBP in healthcare systems. *Worldviews on Evidence-Based Nursing, 4*(3), 123–125.

Melynk, B., & Fineout-Overhold, E. (2005). *Evidence-based practice in nursing and healthcare* (p. 6). Philadelphia: Lippincott Williams & Wilkins.

Melnyk, B. M., & Fineout-Overholt, E. (2011). *Evidence-based practice in nursing & healthcare. A guide to best practice* (2nd ed.). Philadelphia: Wolters Kluwer/ Lippincott, Williams & Wilkins.

Melnyk, B. M., Fineout-Overholt, E., & Mays, M. (2008). The evidence-based practice beliefs and implementation scales: Psychometric properties of two new instruments. *Worldviews on Evidence-Based Nursing, 5*(4), 208–216.

Melnyk, B. M., Fineout-Overholt, E., Feinstein, N. F., Li, H., Small, L., Wilcox, L., et al. (2004). Nurses' perceived knowledge, beliefs, skills, and needs regarding evidence-based practice: Implications for accelerating the paradigm shift. *Worldviews on Evidence-Based Nursing, 1*(3), 185–193.

Melnyk, B. M., Fineout-Overholt, E., Feinstein, N. F., Sadler, L. S., & Green-Hernandez, C. (2008). Nurse practitioner educators' perceived knowledge, beliefs, and teaching strategies. *Journal of Professional Nursing, 24*(1), 7–13.

Melnyk, B.M., Fineout-Overholt, E., Giggleman, M., & Cruz, R. (2010). Correlates among Cognitive Beliefs, EBP Implementation, Organizational Culture, Cohesion and Job Satisfaction in Evidence-based Practice Mentors from a Community Hospital System. *Nursing Outlook, 58* (6), 301-308.

Morgan, S. (2009). The Magnet Model as a framework for excellence. *Journal Nursing Care Quality, 24*(2), 105–108.

National League for Nursing. (2008). *Position statement. Preparing the next generation of nurses to practice in a technology-rich environment: An informatics agenda.* Retrieved June 23, 2008 from http://www.nln.org. aboutnln/position Statements/informatics_052808.pdf

National Quality Forum. *Wired for quality: The intersection of health IT and healthcare quality.* Retrieved June 23, 2008 http://216.122.138.39/news/ Issuebriefsandnewsletters/ibhitMar08.pdf

Nemethm, L., Wessell, A., Jenkins, R ., Nietert, P., Liszka, H., & Ornstein, S. (2007). Strategies to accelerate translation of research into primary care within practices using electonic medical records. *Journal Nursing Care Quality, 22*(3), 343–349.

Newhouse, R. P., Dearholt, S., Poe, S., Pugh, L., & White, K. M. (2007). Organizational change strategies for evidence-based practice. *Journal of Nursing Administration, 37*(12), 552–557.

Nightingale, F.(1859). *Notes on nursing: What it is and what it is not* (p.24). London: Harrison & Sons.

O'Rourke, M. (2007). Role-based nurse managers; linchpin to practice excellence. *Nurse Leader, 5,* 44–53.

Ogiehor-Enoma, G., Tagueban, L., & Anosike, A. (2010). 6 steps for transforming organizational EBP culture. *Nursing Management, May,* 14–20.

Pennington, K., Moscatel, S., Dacar, S., & Johnson, C. (2010). EBP partnerships: Building bridges between education and practice. *Nursing Management, April,* 19–23.

Pipe, T., Cisar, N., Caruso, E., & Wellik, K. (2008). Leadership strategies: Inspiring evidence-based practice at the individual, unit and organizational levels. *Journal Nurse Care Quality, 23*(3), 265–271.

Porter O'Grady, T. (2009). *Interdisciplinary shared governance: Integrating practice, transforming healthcare* (2nd ed.). Sudbury, MA: Jones & Bartlett.

Pravikoff, D., Tanner, A., Pierce, S. (2005). Readiness of US nurses for evidence-based practice. *American Journal Nursing, 105*(9), 40–51.

Rauen, C., Flynn, M., & Bridges, E. (2009). Evidence-based practice habits: Transforming research into bedside practice. *Critical Care Nurse, 29*(2), 46–60.

Rundall, T., Martelli, P., Arroyo, L., McCurdy, R., Graetz, I., Neuwirth, E., et al. (2007). The informed decisions toolbox; Tools for knowledge transfer and performance improvement. *Journal of Healthcare Management, 52*(5), 325–342.

Rundall, T., Martelli, P., McCurdy, R., Arroyo, L., Neuwirth, E., Curtis, P., et al. (2008). Using research evidence when making decisions: views of health services managers and policy makers. In A. Kovner, R. Aguila, & D. Fine (Eds.), *The practice of evidence-based management.* Chicago: Health Administration Press.

Rush, K. (2008). Connecting practice to evidence using laptop computers in the classroom. *CIN: Computers, Informatics, Nursing, 26*(4), 190–196.

Sackett, D. L., Straus, S. E., Richardson, W. S., Rosenberg, W., & Haynes, R. B. (2000). *Evidence-based medicine: How to practice and teach EBM.* London: Churchill Livingstone.

Sanares, D., Waters, P., & Marshall, D. (2007). Mainstreaming evidence based nursing practice. *Nurse Leader, June,* 44–49.

Secco, M., Woodgate, R., Hodgson, A., Kowalski, S., Plouffe, J., Rothneym, P, et al. (2006). A survey study of pediatric nurses' use of information sources. *CIN: Computers, Informatics, Nursing, 24*(2), 105–112.

Sigma Theta Tau. (2006). *Evidence-based practice research study.* Sigma Theta Tau International, 2006.

Simon, H. (1947). *Administrative behavior.* New York: Macmillan.

Simpson, R. (2005). Practice to evidence to practice: Closing the loop with IT. *Nursing Management, Sept,* 12–17.

Sims, I., Gorman, P., Greenes, R., Haynes, B., Kaplan, B., Lehman, H., Tang, P. (2001). Clinical decision support systems for the practice of evidence-based medicine. *Journal of the American Medical Informatics Association, 8*(6), 527–534.

Sittig, D. (1999). Prerequisites for a real time clinical decision support system. Retrieved June 25, 2010 from http://www.informatics-review.com/thought/prereqs.html

The Joint Commission. (2010). *2010 Joint Commission hospital standards for accreditation.* Retrieved from July 14, 2010 http://e-dition.jcrinc.com

Vanhook, P. (2009). Overcoming the barriers to EBP. *Nursing Management, August,* 9–11.

Williams, D. O. (2004). Treatment delayed is treatment denied. *Circulation, 109,* 1806–1808.

Worthley, J. (2000). *Managing information in healthcare: Concepts and cases.* Chicago: Health Administration Press.

28

Incorporating Evidence: Use of Computer-based Clinical Decision Support Systems for Health Professionals

Ida M. Androwich / Margaret Ross Kraft

• OBJECTIVES

1. Describe computerized clinical decision support systems (CDSS), including types, characteristics, and the levels of responsibility implicit in the use of each type.
2. Describe effects of CDSS on clinician performance and patient outcomes in healthcare.
3. Understand the features, benefits, and limits of CDSS.
4. Discuss how wide use of the electronic health record impacts CDSS.
5. Develop a future vision for CDSS within nursing.

• KEY WORDS

clinical decision support
decision support systems
information systems
knowledge and cognition

INTRODUCTION

Decision support systems (DSS) are automated tools designed to support decision making activities and improve the decision-making process and decision outcomes. Such systems are intended to use the enormous amounts of data that exist in information systems to facilitate decision processes. A clinical decision support system (CDSS), designed to support healthcare providers in making decisions about the delivery and management of patient care, has the potential to improve patient safety and outcomes for specific patient populations, as well as compliance with clinical guidelines and standards of practice and regulatory requirements.

Within the complexity of today's healthcare environment, there is an increasing need for accessible information that supports and improves the effectiveness of decision making and promotes clinical accountability and the use of best practices. Clinical tasks to which CDSS may be applied include alerts and reminders, diagnostic assistance, therapy critiques and plans, medication orders, image recognition and interpretation, and information retrieval. The primary goal of clinical decision support systems is to optimize the efficiency and effectiveness with which clinical decisions are made and the manner in which care is delivered. Without the ability to recall and process all available complex information, decisions in healthcare often cannot be justified on

427

the basis of available knowledge, costs, benefits, possible risks, and patient preferences (Weed & Weed, 1999).

Clinicians depend on timely, reliable, and accurate information to make clinical decisions. Availability of such information depends on how data are collected, stored, retrieved, and transformed into meaningful information. Improving the efficiency and effectiveness of nursing practice supports the demand for more and more professional accountability for practice. Consequently, CDSSs, tools that aid nurses in improving their effectiveness in care delivery, identifying appropriate interventions, determining areas in need of policy or protocol development, and supporting patient safety initiatives and quality improvement activities are increasingly needed. Accuracy, timeliness, availability, and reliability of information are just as important to nursing as they are to other healthcare providers. Nurses as knowledge workers need access to current knowledge where it is useful: in clinics, at the bedside, in homes, offices, and in research that makes contributions to evidence-based nursing practice.

A CDSS includes a set of knowledge-based tools that can be fully integrated with the clinical data embedded in the computerized patient record (electronic health record, or EHR) to assist providers by presenting information relevant to the healthcare problem(s) being faced. This means the delivery of the right information to the right person at the right point within the workflow. Ideally, the CDSS is available at the point of care with quick (real time) responses, requires minimal training, is easily integrated into the workflow of practice, and is user friendly. It should have a powerful search function that can access useful and reliable information from knowledge sources that may include electronic libraries, medical dictionaries, drug formularies, expert opinion and database access. A CDSS is only as effective as its underlying knowledge base. Knowledge sources can provide simple facts, relationships, evidence-based best practices, and the latest in clinical research. CDSS may focus on treatment, diagnosis, or specific patient information. Systems may be passive, requiring the clinician to access the advice or with a higher level of information processing, systems may be active, giving unsolicited advice.

The availability of reliable clinical information and the propagation and management of clinical knowledge within CDSS has the potential to transform healthcare delivery but it is important to remember that the clinical user's experience, understanding of context and knowledge base are not replaced but, rather, supported in the decision-making process. Implementation of CDSS requires the development of a strategy built on an understanding of available CDSS tools, clinician readiness to adopt and use CDSS, and areas within the organization that carry significant risk to patient safety. Attention is paid to delivery of the right information at the right time and place to enable decision making. CDSS is a "tool" system, not a "rule" system. In no way does a CDSS usurp the clinician's decision-making role. Final decisions are always made by the clinicians who can accept or reject the CDSS information within the context of the healthcare situation.

As decision making is optimized, the expectation of compliance with guidelines increases. Choices for diagnostics or therapy are increasingly supported by evidence. Chronic condition management and patient workups will be more focused.

CDSS DEFINED

A CDSS may be defined as any computer program which helps health professionals make clinical decisions. "A clinical decision support system provides clinicians or patients with clinical knowledge and patient-related information ,intelligently filtered and presented at appropriate times to enhance patient care" (Jenders & Sittig, 2007). CDSS software has a knowledge base designed for the clinician involved in patient care to aid in clinical decision making. Johnston and colleagues (1994) defined CDSS as "computer software employing a knowledge base designed for use by a clinician involved in patient care, as a direct aid to clinical decision-making." In 2001, Sims, Gorman, Greenes, et al. broadened the definition to "CDSS are software designed to be a direct aid to clinical decision-making, in which the characteristics of an individual patient are matched to a computerized clinical knowledge base and patient-specific assessments or recommendations are then presented to the clinician or the patient for a decision." Coiera (1994) discussed the role of CDSS as augmenting human performance and providing assistance for healthcare providers especially for tasks subject to human error. Whatever definition chosen, it seems clear that healthcare is being transformed through information and knowledge management and technology is being used to "tame data and transform information" (Hannah & Ball, 1999). It is impossible for the unaided human mind to stay current when medical knowledge has exploded, the number of drugs has increased 500% in the past 10 years and approximately 20,000 new articles appear in biomedical literature annually. Genomic healthcare and interaction between genetic factors and environment require new understandings of types of information needed to meet decision needs—characterized as a "Data Tsunami" (NLM Strategic Plan) (Bakken, Stone, & Larson, 2008). Consequently, the application of CDSS is necessary to help clinicians access and use what science has learned.

The computer has virtually unlimited capacity for processing and storage of data. The human, on the other hand, has limited storage (memory) and processing power, but does have judgment, experience, and intuition. Decision support systems integrate and capitalize of the strengths of both. The three key purposes of a DSS are to:

1. Assist in problem solving with semistructured problems

2. Support, not replace, the judgment of a manager or clinician

3. Improve the effectiveness of the decision-making process

Highly structured or deterministic problems, which can be solved with existing facts, and completely unstructured problems, which are highly dependent on values and beliefs, are generally not well suited for decision support.

History of CDSS

One of the earliest known CDSS designed to support diagnosis of acute abdominal pain was developed by de Dombal in 1972 at Leeds University. By 1974, INTERNIST I was developed at the University of Pittsburgh to support the diagnostic process in general internal medicine by linking diseases with symptoms. Its medical knowledge base later became the basis of successor systems, including Quick Medical Reference (QMR). MYCIN, a rule-based expert system to diagnosis and recommend treatment for certain blood infections was functional in 1976. Next came the development of a series of systems addressing specific clinical issues. These included ONCOCIN developed for oncology protocol management at Stanford; CASNET developed at Rutgers University for diagnosis and treatment of glaucoma; and ABEL, an expert system developed at MIT that used causal reasoning to manage acid-base and electrolyte imbalance (www. openclinical.org/dss.html). Several websites addressing CDSS in routine clinical use with entries ranging from simple expert or knowledge-based systems to advanced systems capable of complex inferences are available. These sites contain links to specific CDSS (Table 28.1).

CDSS IMPACT ON CLINICIANS

There is growing pressure for clinicians including nurses to use knowledge at the point of care that is based on researched evidence. This became especially true after human error was widely recognized as a major source of patient care morbidity and mortality. Studies have been done to determine whether access to information in a variety of forms would impact patient care. One early study showed that MEDLINE access did have a significant effect on physician resolution of diagnostic and treatment problems (Lindberg, Siegel, Rapp, et al., 1993). Gorman, Ash, and Wykoff (1994) found that availability of information at the time of a patient visit would definitely impact care. The use of CDSS to find and prevent errors related to gaps between optimal and actual practice can result in improved quality of care. Applications of CDSS suggest the ability to lessen the incidence of adverse drug events, nosocomial infections, and the inappropriate use of antibiotics. Prevention of prescription errors is a valuable and widely used function of CDSS. Bates, Kuperman, Wang, et al. (2003) have determined that effective clinical decision support depends on CDSS speed, anticipation of information needs, real-time delivery, usability, simplicity, and the maintenance of the knowledge-based system. They also identified that successful use of a CDSS requires integration of the system with the user's normal workflow. CDSS must be designed to support clinician requirements rather than dictate clinician workflow practices.

The move to the electronic medical record (EHR) provides tremendous opportunities to improve care. This has led to an understanding of the dual nature of information needs for decision support. First, evidenced-based information (content) needs to be available at the point-of-care to inform the **present** patient encounter. Second, systems need to be designed so that key data entered in the process of documentation needs is entered in a manner that it can be able to be aggregated to inform **future** patient encounters. In the latter, new knowledge becomes a transparent by-product of care (Perlin, 2009). We move from *"TRIP"—translating research into practice to "TPIR"—translating practice into research* (new knowledge and evidence of value and quality).

According to Sims, Gorman, Greenes, et al. (2001), only about half of treatments used for patient care in internal and family medicine are supported with research evidence of efficacy. Bates, Kuperman, Wang, et al. (2003) suggest that practice lags behind knowledge by at least several years. This lag could be shortened if not eliminated by the availability of current knowledge to support the decision-making process. A systematic

TABLE 28.1	Examples of Clinical Decision Support Systems
CDSS Sources	**Descriptions**
Clin-eguide	A point-of-care CDSS designed for integration with electronic health records that makes recommendations on diagnosis, management and treatment of specific diseases
Clinical Pathway Constructor	Zynx Health's Web-based tool with a compendium of evidence-based guidelines. Available by subscription
CURE (Carotid US Report Enhancement, Washington University, St. Louis)	Augments carotid ultrasound reports with treatment-specific prognostic information
DiagnosisPro	Contains a database of 9000 disease and drug terms and 16,000 symptoms, signs, lab, and x-ray findings linked with 120,000 relationships to suggest diagnoses and treatment
DXplain (Harvard/MIT)	A system using a set of clinical findings including signs, symptoms, and lab data to produce a ranked list of diagnoses that might explain the clinical signs and symptoms
Healthaction (Health Development Agency [HAD])	A Website that is a knowledge management service for primary care; shares approaches to reduce health inequalities and facilitated interactive learning exchange
HDP (The Heart Disease Program)	A system to assist in the diagnosis of cardiovascular disease
HELP (Salt Lake City LDS Hospital)	
Iliad	A system that provides expert diagnostic consultation with more than 900 diseases and 1500 symptoms; includes ICD-9 codes for each diagnosis
IMKI (Institute for Medical Knowledge Implementation)	Has developed and maintains a library of medical knowledge applications and is developing a process for development, evaluation, and dissemination of CDSS rules
InfoRetriever (InfoPOEMS)	Contains seven evidence databases, clinical decision rules, practice guidelines, risk calculators, and basic information on drugs; can be loaded on a PDA
ISABEL	A diagnostic reminder system from the United Kingdom that covers the spectrum of pediatric medicine and is designed to integrate with electronic medical record systems
Logiciana	MedicaLogic's electronic record system that checks medications and formulary compliance and includes clinical reminders and patient education material
Micromedex	A system designed to provide clinicians with alerts, recommendations, and evidence-based references
Misys Insight	A open CDSS designed to work with a broad spectrum of clinical information systems
NEONATE (Salt Lake City Children's)	
ORAD (Oral Radiographic Differential Diagnosis)	A system designed to evaluate radiographic and clinical features of patients with intrabony dental problems
Oxford Clinical Mentor (Oxford)	A UK electronic medical knowledge support system with details on more than 2000 diseases cross-referenced with 26,000 commonly used terms and synonyms
Pathmaster (Yale)	
PIER (Physicians' Information and Education Resource)	American College of Physicians–American Society of Internal Medicine Web-based DSS tool which combs medical literature and provides bullet lists under six different topics. Available to members only
PlanAlyzer (Darthmouth)	

TABLE 28.1	Examples of Clinical Decision Support Systems *(continued)*
CDSS Sources	**Descriptions**
PKC (Problem Knowledge Couplers) (Weed, 2001)	A system of data capture and clinical guidance that provides decision and management support to clinicians
PRODIGY(Prescribing RatiOnally with Decision Support in Genera-Practice study)	A UK initiative for evaluation of a prescribing practices in general practice
QMR (Quick Medical Reference) (University of Pittsburgh/First Databank)	A system with a knowledge base of close to 700 diseases, signs, symptoms, and lab information to suggest relevant diagnosis
TraumAID	A system of decision support for emergency center management of multiple trauma that produces diagnostic and therapeutic plans for patient management
VisualDx	An image based system that serves as a reference to support diagnosis and treatment

review of CDSS studies (Hunt, Haynes, Hanna, & Smith, 1998) showed that in 43 of 65 investigated studies some benefit was found in either the process of care or in patient outcomes.

In the Veterans Health Administration (VHA), electronic patient record decision support includes alerts that may address order checking, allergies and medication interactions. This system also includes reminders for such things as preventative health services. One study of VHA reminders identified that 10 of 15 national performance measures had reminders in their clinical information system for conditions such as smoking cessation and immunizations (Fung, Woods, Asch, et al., 2004).

In instances where CDSS implementation has not been successful, barriers identified included lack of noticeable benefits, insufficient cost benefits, inadequate staff training, and lack of system support. The involvement of healthcare professionals in CDSS selection is essential to system acceptance. It is also important to consider how a CDSS will affect organizational culture, practice, and personnel attitudes.

TYPES AND CHARACTERISTICS OF DSS

Included in the field of healthcare decision support are systems that support organizational, executive/managerial, financial, and clinical decisions. Administrative systems, including those designed for finance or quality, generally support the business decision-making process. These systems encompass decision processes other than direct patient care delivery, and even if clinical in nature, such as quality improvement systems, are mainly used for strategic planning, budgeting, financial analysis, quality management, continuous process improvement, and clini-

cal benchmarking. In these systems, decisions occur at the strategic, tactical, population or aggregate and operational levels, not at the individual level.

These systems tend to be batch oriented in nature, ie, not real-time, mostly concerned with aggregations of many data elements largely for purposes of intelligence gathering. These systems tend to be unstructured, goal seeking/searching, and long range in nature. In contrast, the clinical decision support systems discussed in this chapter tend to be focused on real-time decision support, goal orientation, and intelligence gathering, and are designed to be used at the point of care by clinicians. More recently, healthcare agencies have begun to understand that combination systems offer optimal value to the organization. Such systems are able to support outcomes performance management by integrating operational data (the business side)—budgeting, executive decision making, financial analysis, quality management, and strategic planning data—with clinical data (the clinical side)—clinical event tracking, results reporting, pharmaceutical ordering and dispensation, differential diagnoses, real-time clinical pathways, literature research, and clinical alerts. The intent, the content, and the methods may differ but both business and clinical approaches to DSS have common elements and the integration of the two can increase effective decisions (Perreault & Metzger, 1999). The goals of a CDSS implementation are variable but address the use of best clinical practices, patient safety, and patient empowerment as well as the financial well-being of the institution (Jenders & Sittig, 2007).

Just as there are many types of decision support systems, there are also a number of ways to examine the characteristics of a given DSS. These systems can be studied based on their structure, their organization, their content, or their purpose. Shortliffe (1990) uses function, mode of advice, consultation style, underlying decision-science methodology, and user-computer interactions to categorize systems. Teich and Wrinn (2000) examine DSS from the aspect of *functional and logical classes*. Functional classes include feedback as provided to the clinician, the organization of the data, the extent of proactive information provided, the intelligent actions of the system, and the communication method; logical classes include substitute therapy alerts, drug family checking, structured entry, consequent actions, parameter checking, redundant utilization checking, relevant information display, time-based checks, templates and order sets, and profile display and analysis, rule-based event detection, and aggregate data trending. CDSS *structural elements* according to Teich and Wrinn include triggering, dispatching, rule logic, process control, notification/acknowledgement, action choices, action execution and rule editor. In 1999 Perreault and Metzger organized key CDSS functions as:

Administrative—support for clinical coding and documentation

Management of clinical complexity and details— keeping patients on research and chemotherapy protocols, tracking orders, referrals, follow-up, and preventive care

Cost control—monitoring medication orders and avoiding duplicate or unnecessary tests

Decision spport—supporting clinical diagnostic and treatment plan processes promotion of best practices, use of condition-specific guidelines, and population-based management

Shortliffe (2006) has addressed what he labels the myths of CDSS and specifically notes that diagnosis is not the dominant decision made in medicine, clinicians may not use CDSS even if the knowledge base is at the level of experts. He also believes that clinicians will not use stand-alone DSS tools.

If one were to consider ontology (Tan & Shep, 1998), DSSs could be divided into data based (population based), model based (case based), knowledge based (rule based) and graphics based. In this view, a *data-based* system provides decision support with a population perspective and uses routinely collected, longitudinal, cohort, and cross-sectional databases. Population-based information is used to enhance clinical decision making, "funnel" patients to medical care, and enhance medical practice.

A *model-based* DSS is driven by access to and manipulation of a statistical, financial, optimization, and/or simulation. The data in this instance is compared to various decision-making and analytic models. A model is a generalization that can be used to describe the relationships among a number of observations to represent a perception of how things fit together. The models may be pathophysiologic, statistical, or analytic. Some model-based examples are lineal programming, such as scheduling nurses or physicians or resource allocation, simulation, such as emergency department or operating room scheduling or provider profiling.

A *knowledge-based* system relies on expert knowledge that is either embedded in the system or accessible from another source and uses some type of knowledge acquisition process to understand and capture the cognitive processes of healthcare providers. Much of what we consider evidence-based practice refers to knowledge based decision support. Yet there are many issues with maintaining current evidence in DSS. Sims, Gorman, Greenes, et al. (2001) identify the policy and research challenges in developing and maintaining practice evidence in machine readable repositories. They have coined a term "evidence-adaptable CDSSs" to describe a new type of CDSS that has a knowledge base that is constantly updated with the most current evidence available and is viewed as both a goal and necessity.

Some examples of CDSS applications include:

- Computer tools for focusing attention such as "flags" for abnormal values

- Care maps, guidelines, protocols, etc.

- Patient-specific consultations using diagnostic or management tools, such as Problem Knowledge Couplers (PKC) (Weed, 2001)

- Lab systems with interpretation of measured values and automated preparation of reports, as well as physician guidance as to which tests to order

- Drug advisory systems used for advising on drug–drug interactions, side effects, selecting most cost-effective drug

- Clinical workstations with online literature, e-tools for calculation, patient guidelines

- Image recognition and interpretation with capabilities of mass screening, eg, mammography, assistance with expensive and complex investigations, eg, MRI

- Signal interpretation such as interpretive alarms for real-time clinical signals in ICU, automated ECG interpretation, retinal scans, voice recognition

- Natural language/speech recognition offering interpretation of freely entered clinical notes and archiving to make electronically accessible in future

- Evidence-based quality improvement with using up to date and consistent tools
- Multitask tools for assessment, diagnosis, and management

When CPOE (computer provider order entry) is in use, CDSS types can include facilitators for order creation, relevant data display, pathway support, context sensitive reference information, and reactive alerts (Jenders, Sittig, Desai, et al., 2007). Some projections indicate that CPOE with a CDSS could create a significant reduction in medication errors.

The construction and upkeep of clinical protocols or guidelines is not easy. Often there are multiple authors, protocol selection is not always straightforward, multiple protocols may be available or there is a situation that demands a departure from protocols assumptions. Some early expert systems were referred to as using the "Greek Oracle" approach, where the DSS provided a solution from "on high," but others have called for a "catalyst" approach, whereby the DSS serves as a catalyst and provides guidance, but the user remains in control.

Demand management centers (telephone call centers) often use decision tree or rule-based logic for patient management. Decision tree logic (DTL) is useful for specific straightforward tasks. User training is easily accomplished because DTL is often based on probabilities. When cases are more complex with more variables to consider, DTL requires a tremendous amount of programming and has limited data specificity and rigidness in solution options. An example of DTL: if A, then B.

Rule-based logic (RBL) has complex decision capacities, is more flexible with answers, provides consistent outcomes and is adaptable to change. But RBL also has rigid solutions and allows little or no clinician autonomy. Typical RBL would be a statement: if 1, 4, and 7 apply, then do A; if 2, 5, and 8 apply, then do B. Both DTL and RBL are forms of electronic algorithms using step-by-step problem solving and the evidence from which decisions are made comes from best practice guidelines. In a well-designed system, the clinician has an opportunity to override a solution with an explanation or justification.

In many ways, CDSS distinctions are somewhat artificial and are increasingly blurring. A very simplistic, broad view of DSS is a "push-pull" distinction. In a "pull" system, the provider needs to take some action independent of the usual workflow to initiate a request for support or to query the system for additional information; whereas in a "push" system the system automatically generates the alert in response to a clinician action such as a medication order for which the patient has reported an allergy.

CDSS Development. CDSS development requires a team approach. The first step in the development process is identification of the information needs that leads to the question of whether a CDSS would be helpful. Next is the need to identify the stakeholders with interest in the topic. Stakeholders can include physicians, nurses, administrative staff, Quality and Safety Education in Nursing (QSEN) staff, and even patients. As a group, the stakeholders must address CDSS goals. It is important to synthesize and validate a unified working list of goals and objectives. As the specific clinical issue is addressed, determination of potential frequency of use is necessary to determine whether assignment of resources to a development project is justified. Is this a frequently encountered unstructured or semistructured problem? Is there sufficient evidence that justifies the assignment of necessary resources for development? Is the proposed CDSS to be built to address process and outcome data, departmental needs, the needs within the community of service, or a result of reporting and accreditation issues? Will the proposed system address a strategic target such as medication safety? If the decision is to move forward, an inventory of all available information systems such as laboratory, radiology, and pharmacy systems as well as the clinical record system, order systems, and administrative systems may be data and information sources. CDSS capabilities depend on availability of coded data, use of standard vocabularies, and the ability to aggregate data from multiple sources.

The knowledge bass of the CDSS must be clearly defined and a system for knowledge update must be in place. After the system inventory, it is necessary to select CDSS interventions as part of the process of developing specifications for the system build. Building the CDSS requires an identification of when and how interventions are triggered, the data source and content of the intervention, how the information is delivered to the recipient, and also needs a feedback mechanism. After a CDSS is built, it must be tested and only then should it "go live." The system launch requires planning that addresses not just a date but all the necessary educational preparation of the end users. The final step of CDSS development is evaluation and system enhancement as needed. Ongoing assessment of intervention use and usability, evaluation of intervention performance against objectives, and continuous enhancement of CDSS provides value to users.

A successful CDSS emerges from and supports performance improvement initiatives (Osheroff, Pifer, Teich, et al., 2005). The choice of a CDSS target may be related to a patient benefit that outweighs any possibility of harm, practices supported by evidence, physician practice patterns, disease management, chronic care management, and national quality measures. Also considered is the gap that exists between what is ideal and what is real. The CDSS development looks at preventing errors, optimizing decision making, and improving the care process.

Remember that the principal purposes for CDSS are to answer questions, which may mean a direct hyperlink to information sources, to make decisions after gathering, and analyzing data and providing information related to diagnosis, diagnostics, and treatment, and to optimize process flow and workflow, to monitor actions, and to focus attention through the presentation of items or reporting applications.

CDSS governance involves executive leadership, management oversight, project managers, and the end users. Successful development and implementation depends on strong executive support for clinical quality improvement and belief in information technology (IT) as a tool to achieve desired quality. A history of previously successful IT projects has a positive impact. Communication with the stakeholders must be successful and the key end users must be involved in implementation.

KNOWLEDGE AND COGNITIVE PROCESSES

Knowledge engineering is the field concerned with knowledge acquisition (extracting or eliciting knowledge from experts) and the organization and structure of that knowledge within a computer system. Building a knowledge-based or expert system requires an understanding of the cognitive processes of healthcare providers and how they deal with complexity. Most DSS take advantage of the research on human reasoning and decision-making.

How do nurses solve problems? Or even determine that there is a problem? What information seeking behaviors do nurses use? Is "intuition" really a case of statistical pattern recognition. When an expert nurse claims that the patient "just didn't look right," is it intuition or do years of nursing experience that place that patient three standard deviations from the mean of all the patients cared for? Answering these questions requires an understanding of the decision-making process, human diagnostic reasoning, and critical thinking. The formulation of a problem does have an impact on the solution selected. Nurses recognize various types of knowledge such as declarative knowledge and procedural knowledge. Declarative knowledge can be considered the "know what" or descriptive knowledge, procedural knowledge is the "know how," and the processes of reasoning and inference produce the "know why." There are a number of methods of reasoning: rule based, Bayesian, causal, probabilistic, decision-theoretic, "possibilistic," common sense, and case based.

A variety of methods have been used to elicit knowledge from expert clinicians. Some knowledge elicitation techniques require clinicians to "think aloud." Some use observations of clinician behavior in practice settings. Interviews with experts has been the most commonly used method of eliciting knowledge. The expert clinician is directly asked in a structured interview to describe a typical case and how aspects of the case influence care decisions. The advantages of this method are ease of use and the ability to draw out important information; however, a potential problem may be that the experts tend to say what they *think* that they do, but may be unaware of what they are actually doing or they may be unable to break down their thought processes into steps. Benner (1984) described this phenomena in *Novice to Expert*. Cognitive Task Analysis (CTA) refers to a set of methods that capture the skills, knowledge and processing ability of experts in dealing with complex tasks. The goal of CTA is to tap into "higher order" cognitive functions. This technique is beneficial in comparing an "expert performance" with the performance of "less than experts" (Tan & Sheps, 1998). CTA attempts to identify pitfalls or trouble spots in the reasoning process of the beginner or intermediate level practitioner while comparing the reasoning process with that of the expert. In one study using nonexperts and experts, the nonexperts used more interventions such as ordering additional tests and tended to rely on the test results. The experts, on the other hand, used increased assessment and were more apt to consider the context when determining a course of action. Tan and Sheps (1998) describe a six-step approach to cognitive task analysis as follows:

1. Identify the problem to target in the analysis, eg, pulmonary embolus with symptoms of shortness of breath, chest pain, and hemoptysis

2. Generate cases (decision tasks) that vary on key factors

3. Observe a record of an expert problem solving for the case using "think aloud"

4. Observe the novice and the intermediate problem solving

5. Analyze expert vs "less than expert"

6. Recommend systems needs, design specs, and knowledge base components

Computer-based techniques which use interactive tools are also used to assess decision making. These tools have the advantage of not needing to interact directly with the clinician but also tend to be overly simplistic for complex decision analysis. Rating and sorting methods, borrowed from the social sciences and protocol analysis are also methods used. Each has advantages and disadvantages.

RESPONSIBILITY OF USER: ETHICAL AND LEGAL ISSUES

CDSS are considered similar to medical devices but the legal responsibility for treatment and advice given to a patient rests with the clinician regardless of whether a CDSS is used (Hunt, Haynes, Hanna, & Smith, 1998). Still unknown are the legal ramifications of not following CDSS advice. Courts seem to believe that cost should have no role in clinical decision making. Attempts to save money by reducing treatment below an undisputed standard of care are not acceptable. If a treatment plan is based on anything but the best available medical evidence and standards of practice it may be considered malpractice even though legal reasoning is often seen as more compatible with the old clinical decision paradigms based on anecdote, custom, and algorithms than with new statistical models.

One must always consider the potential of adverse consequences but there seems to be no major adverse effect from the use of a CDSS; however, such systems must be developed with high standards of quality. The provision of erroneous information and/or guidance does have the potential for harmful impact. There must be some way to provide a high degree of assurance that a CDSS has been developed according to quality and safety standards. CDSS will be expected to comply with a "duty of care" if CDSS is to become safely integrated into routine patient care. The knowledge base of healthcare changes frequently and often past practices are proved ineffective and perhaps even hazardous. Healthcare knowledge may also be based on professional judgment without objective scientific evidence. Therefore, the knowledge base of a CDSS must be as reflective as possible of the current state of professional and scientific opinion and evidence and must draw upon traditional knowledge sources such as journals and textbooks to maintain currency. Safe use of CDSS may include such techniques as limiting access, developing audit trails, use monitoring, and clinical hazard alerts. Rector (2002) suggests the risk of system harm should be weighed against the risks associated without the system.

CDSS documentation should address the purpose of the system, the population for which the application is intended along with inclusion/exclusion criteria, the context for use, the expected user skill level, evidence source(s), and review and update methods. Keeping a CDSS current requires a commitment of technical, professional, and organizational dimensions. Any CDSS will be only as effective as the strength and accuracy of underlying evidence base.

FUTURE OF CDSS

Despite the many challenges of developing and implementing CDSS, it is clear that the use of decision support will increase. Today's healthcare environment is complicated by diverse priorities, providers, and practice modes. Acceptance depends largely on organizational culture, leadership attitudes, and provider involvement. Barriers to CDSs include costs, lack of exposure to technology, lack of training, system support. Barriers to the use of CDSS have been identified as:

- Limited implementation of EHRs and PHRs
- Lack of standards
- Absence of a central repository or knowledge resource
- Poor support for CDS in commercial EHRs
- Alert fatigue
- Challenges in integrating CDS into clinical workflow
- Limited understanding of organizational and cultural issues relating to clinical decision support

With increased focus on the EHR, an improved understanding of the potential benefits of good CDSS, and implementation of meaningful use, these barriers are starting to be overcome.

CDSS AND MEANINGFUL USE

The U.S. Department of Health and Human Services's final definition of meaningful use will likely include an organization's ability to use health IT to improve quality and *"inform clinical decisions at the point of care."* (Retrieved June 1, 2011 from healthit.hhs.gov/...pt/.../ federal_hit_strategic_plan_public_comment_period.) The CDSS Taskforce of HIMSS (Health Information Management Systems Society) is working on developing a link between CDS and specific meaningful use. A CDSS deployed effectively can optimize its value in targeted clinical outcome measures. A CDSS can assist in the management of chronic conditions. It could also address the meaningful use objectives of drug, drug–drug, drug–allergy, and drug formulary checks, and support the maintenance of a medication allergy list. Weingarten (2010) believes CDS will feature prominently in defining meaningful use.

Patient Decision Support

Another important area is patient decision support. Given the opportunity, patients may become more engaged in self-care. As telemedicine is used for screening and communication, patients as well as clinicians will have the information needed to make better decisions (mHealth, 2010.)

The development of CDSS requires a huge financial and intellectual investment but also represents the potential of reduction in care costs through improvement of the decision process at the point-of-care and a reduction in the possibility of costly errors. Current evidence indicates that CDSS can improve patient care quality, reduce medication errors, minimize variances in care, improve guideline compliance, and promote cost-savings. Wider adoption of such tools will support clinical care decisions through the provision of additional and current information at the time and place of care delivery while final decision authority will remain with the clinician. Ease of use within existing workflow practice will determine the success of a CDSS. Although no one single CDSS is in widespread use, such systems, whether simple or complex, are becoming ubiquitous and research on their use is growing.

REFERENCES

Bakken, S., Stone, P., & Larson, E. (2008). A nursing informatics research agenda for 2008–18: Contextual influences and key components. *Nursing Outlook, 69*(5), 206–214.

Bates, D., Kuperman, G., Wang, S., Gandhi, T., Kittler, A., & Volk, L. (2003). Ten commandments for effective clinical decision support. *Journal of the American Medical Informatics Association, 10*(6), 523–530.

Benner, P. (1984). *From novice to expert*. Menlo Park, CA: Addison-Wesley.

Coiera, E. (1994). Designing for decision support in a clinical monitoring environment (pp. 130–142). Proceedings of the International Conference on Medical Physics and Biomedical Engineering.

Fung, C., Woods, J., Asch, S., Glassman, P., & Doebbeling, B. (2004) Variation in implementation and use of computerized clinical reminders in an integrated healthcare system. *American Journal of Managed Care, 10*(11 Pt 2), 878–885.

Gorman, P., Ash, J., & Wykoff, L. (1994). Can primary care physicians' questions be answered using the medical journal literature? *Bulletin of the Medical Library Association, 82*, 140–146.

Hannah, K., & Ball, M., In Berner, E. (Ed.). (1999). *Clinical decision support systems K.: Theory and practice*. New York: Springer. *Preface*, ix.

Hunt, D., Haynes, R., Hanna, S., & Smith, K. (1998). Effects of computer-based clinical decision support systems on physician performance and patient outcomes: A systematic review. *Journal of the American Medical Association, 280*, 1339–1346.

Jenders, R., & Sittig, D. (2007). *Improving outcomes with clinical decision support*. Washington, DC: AMIA Conference.

Jenders, R., Sittig, D., Desai, B., Glanter, B., & Garber, M. (2007). *Clinical decision support in context*. Washington, DC: AMIA Conference.

Johnston, M., Langton, K., Haynes, R., & Mathieu A. (1994). The effects of computer-based clinical decision support systems on clinician performance and patient outcome: A critical appraisal of research. *Annals of Internal Medicine, 120*, 135–142.

Lindberg, D., Siegel, E., Rapp, B., Wallingford, K., & Wilson, S. (1993). Use of MEDLINE by physicians for clinical problem solving. *Journal of American Medical Association, 269*, 3124–3129.

mHealth. (2010). *Telemedicine delivers decision support*. Retrieved August 12, 2010 from www.healthimaging.com/index.php

Osheroff, J., Pifer, E., Teich, J. Sittig, D., & Jenders, R. (2005). *Improving outcomes with clinical decision support: An implementer's guide*. Chicago: HIMSS. Retrieved http://www.himss.org/ASP/topics_cds_workbook.asp?faid=108&tid=14

Open Clinical (2011) *knowledge management for medical care*. Retrieved on April 17, 2011 from http://www.openclinical.org/dss.html

Perlin, J. (2009). *Health IT and value-based healthcare*. Personal Electronic Health Records; Biomedical Research to People's Health; Friends of the National Library of Medicine Conference; NIH Natcher Conference Center; May 20–21, 2009.

Perreault, L., & Metzger, J. (1999). A pragmatic framework for understanding clinical decision support. *Journal of Healthcare Information Management, 13*(2), 5-21.

Rector, A. (2002). *Response to quality and safety of clinical decision support systems*. Draft V0.12. Retrieved March 22, 2010 from openclinical.org

Sims, I., Gorman, P., Greenes, R., Haynes, B., Kaplan, B., Lehmann, H., & Tang, P. (2001). Clinical decision support systems for the practice of evidence based medicine. *Journal of the American Medical Informatics Association, 8*, 527–534.

Shortliffe, E. (2006). Myths affecting development of DSS. Medical Thinking Meeting. London; June.

Shortliffe, E. (1990). *Medical informatrics: Computer applications in healthcare*. Reading, MA: Addison-Wesley.

Tan, J. K. & Sheps, S. (1998). *Health decision support systems*. Gaithersburg, MD: Aspen Publishers, Inc.

Teich, J. & Wrinn, M. (2000). Clinical decision support systems come of age. *MD Computing, Jan/Feb*, 43–46.

Weed, L. (2001). Knowledge coupling. New York: Springer-Verlag.

Weed, L., & Weed, L. (1999) Opening the black box of clinical judgment—an overview. *British Medical Journal, 319*,1–4.

Weingarten, S. (2010). *Clinical decision support and meaningful use*. Perspectives from Zynx Health. Podcast interview. Retrieved August 2, 2010 from www.healthbusinessblog.com

29

The Magnet Model

Andrea Schmid-Mazzoccoli

- ## OBJECTIVES
  1. Identify the five components of the ANCC Magnet Model
  2. Describe how technology has influenced the professional practice environment
  3. Describe some ways nursing informatics as a specialty can support the achievement of magnet standards

- ## KEY WORDS
  Transformational leadership
  Structural empowerment
  Exemplary professional practice

The nursing practice environment is continually challenged to respond to internal and external demands. The demand for value-driven, patient-centered healthcare outcomes across the continuum amidst the landscape of increasing complexity of care is essential. The response will require new models of care, innovative education models, and ways in which nursing's contribution to value-based care outcomes can be measured and used to influence the transformation of the delivery system. These new models will be accomplished, in part, through the use of informatics to track and quantify cost of care, improve the process and workflows of care, and more transparently communicate outcomes of care. Incorporating healthcare information technology and the expertise of nursing informatics into future models will assure patient care is safer, more efficient and effective, and promote excellence in nursing practice. Nursing excellence is promoted and recognized through the American Nurses Credentialing Center (ANCC) Magnet Recognition Program. The Magnet Commission has defined a vision for Magnet organizations to serve as the fount of knowledge and expertise for the delivery of nursing care globally by

striving for discovery and innovation to lead the reformation of healthcare and the discipline of nursing (Commission on Magnet Recognition, 2008). Sources of evidence used to define and evaluate the organization's achievment of the magnet standards identifies informatics and technology as necessary components of the structures and processes to achieve the anticipated benefits.

Essential elements for excellence in professional nursing practice are defined within the ANCC Magnet Recognition Program. The Magnet model defines five components that when fully disseminated and enculturated thoughout organization the create professional practice environments that yield positive patient, nurse, and organizational outcomes. The five components are: *transformational leadership, structured empowerment, exemplary professional practice, new knowledge and innovation, and empirical outcomes* (Figure 29.1). The essential elements are described along with the structures and processes known to develop professional nursing practice as a core competency and contribute to patient and provider outcomes for organizational effectiveness. The Magnet Model informs nursing informatics

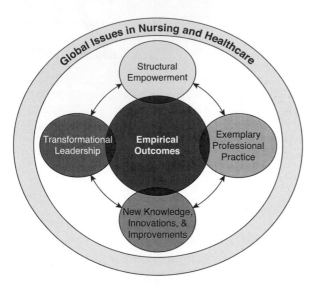

• **FIGURE 29.1.** The Magnet model.

practice to serve as a driver to practice excellence. Nursing informatics fully enculturated in the practice environment supports development of high performing nursing organizations and most importantly, supports the ability to define, measure and report outcomes at a individual, department, population or organizational level. The following paragraphs will define the specific domains defined within the ANCC Magnet Recognition Program Magnet model and describe the influence and relationship between practice and informatics.

TRANSFORMATIONAL LEADERSHIP

Transformational leadership can be defined many ways. The ANCC Magnet Model defines the transformational leader as one who develops a strong vision for the practice and creates an environment where nurses at every level has a voice to advocate for resources, fiscal and technology, to support their practice. The transformational nurse leader articulates a future vision where patient care is supported and accelerated through access to information and interoperability of the technology. The patient care vision supports the alignment of people, process and technology. The leader is accountable to assure the provision of the highest quality of care, which positions the chief nurse executive to serve as a the organization's executive project sponsor for the implementation of technology solutions and electronic health record. Most importantly, the nurse leader is

responsible for the strategic nursing platform, which requires reformation of our care delivery systems and relationships between and among providers, patients, and community.

A strategic vision for practice that is supported by informatics promotes the development of innovative approaches to care by improving the work of the nurse through improved access to information and opportunities and new ways for the nurse to communicate and interact with other providers and the patient. The use of informatics science to drive the design of new models and roles for nursing practice requires a different set of skills and competencies for nursing leaders. The American Organization of Nurse Executives (AONE) has included informatics in its recent update of competencies for nursing executives. The competencies will support the application of informatics to create a new way of thinking and defining practice excellence.

All health systems today are being influenced by the growth in technology. One of the sources of evidence organizations must be able to demonstrate is the work of the nursing leader and department in strategic planning. Specifically, how the nursing mission, vision, strategic and quality plans aligns with the overall organization's strategic goals. This plan must demonstrate the structure and processes used by nursing to improve efficiency and effectiveness. Without the strong influence of informatics, organizations would struggle to meet this standard. Many organizations use their strategic information technology initiatives as evidence of their effort in this aspect of the magnet standards.

The role of the Chief Nursing Informatics Officer (CNIO) has emerged to support and help to translate the science of informatics for all nursing roles. Associated with a specific set of standards for practice in the ANA Scope and Standards for Nurse Informatics, the CNIO role provides a partner to the role of the chief nurse executive. The partnership described by Swindle and Bradley describes an engagement between the roles where the CNIO provides direction and oversight for clinical informatics programs aligned with the vision for practice and operations led by the CNO (Swindle & Bradley, 2010). The area of informatics provides a dimension within our profession for ongoing professional development. The recognition of informatics as a dimension for professional growth and incorporation of informatics the expertise into organizational structures will support the alignment of our people, processes, and technology Through the effective alignment of practice, operational and informatics expertise and leaders, more creative and successful solutions to improve workflow, and process changes that improve communication and care coordination to improve outcomes.

STRUCTURAL EMPOWERMENT AND EXEMPLARY PROFESSIONAL PRACTICE

The voice, autonomy, and decision-making authority of direct care nurses is at the core of the structural empowerment and exemplary professional practice components of the ANCC Magnet model. Structural empowerment is evidenced through flat, flexible organization where the flow of information is fluid between the bedside and leadership. Improvements in practice settings and nurses' involvement in decision-making groups are critical. Magnet organizations are required to demonstrate improvements in practice settings across the continuum that has occurred as a result of the use of data and information. Selection and use of technology that includes the clinical voice at the bedside partnered with information system experts promotes structure and process components defined in the magnet framework. The changes to workflow process that improve care support the evidence of how those structures and processes result in improved outcomes that can be measured and reported.

Exemplary professional nursing practice within the magnet framework is supported through a professional practice model and care delivery system that delineate the role of the nurse as a fully accountable provider responsible for care that is patient centered, safe, effective, efficient, and equitable. Interdisciplinary collaboration within magnet facilities demonstrates the need for collegial and respectful alignment of all disciplines focused on the needs of the patient. This requires new methods to support interdisciplinary planning, communication and coordination. In addition, this will require the effective use of information systems and technology to support clinical care planning, execution, and documentation. The effective use of informatics to improve interdisciplinary care communication and coordination, positions the care team to respond to the growing need to increase patient involvement in their own care.

At the core of achieving exemplary professional nursing practice is the ability to monitor care for effectiveness by having access to data to analyze and evaluate against national benchmarks and respond to improve. There are standards designed to evaluate how nurses investigate, develop, implement, and systematically evaluate standards of nursing practice. This requires evidence that nurses are using a data-driven approach focused on outcomes to evaluate their practice on a regular basis. Technology influences improvements in workflow and care processes associated nursing informatics transcends the areas defined within exemplary professional nursing practice: interdisciplinary care, privacy, security and confidentiality, culture of safety, and quality of care monitoring and improvement. There are many specific patient care initiatives (restraint use, falls, pain) that Magnet organization use to demonstrate their efforts and each organization is required to provide evidence that demonstrates how information systems and technology used for clinical care is integrated and evaluated. Magnet organizations are expected to out perform mean or median benchmark performances and to lead the creation of a new delivery system through continuous improvement and research efforts.

NEW KNOWLEDGE, INNOVATION, AND EMPIRICAL QUALITY OUTCOMES

The demand for exceptional performance and continuous improvement requires Magnet organizations to integrate the current evidence into practice. Nurses at the bedside drive and champion the adoption of new practices in an effort to provide the best care for their patients. The impact of technology to support the use of evidence and decision support at the point-of-care is powerful. The use of data and evidence to drive improvements in care can be found throughout magnet organizations. It is, in part, due to the nurse's involvement in decisions related to technology and information systems that lead to these improvements in care. There are many areas where technology can be used to support improvement in care coordination and outcomes such as medication reconciliation, provider order entry and transition of care management. The magnet framework supports an environment of creating and applying new knowledge to create the future. Nurses involved in system design, selection, implementation, and optimization of information technology will impact patient safety through the redesign of workflows. Their involvement will influence the acceptance and adoption of technology to fully allow for the support of informatics a driver of quality of care and enhanced patient outcomes. Informatics will be critical as hospitals and health systems attempt to leverage their electronic medical records to respond to and achieve the "meaningful use" criteria to receive incentives. Nurses across care settings and roles must be better equipped to understand information technology process to fully optimize to meet the needs of clinicians and patients. Magnet standards unified with the informatics objective to improve nursing practice through the use of technology provide a compelling transformative nursing agenda. Magnet organizations are poised to lead this effort as demonstrated by their ongoing commitment to practice excellence.

REFERENCES

American Nurses Credentialing Center. (2008). *Magnet Recognition Program Application Manual*. Silver Spring, MD: American Nurses Credentialing Center.

Swindle, C. G., Bradley, V. M. (2010). The Newest O in the C-Suite: CNIO. *Nurse Leader, 8*(3), 28–30.

30

Internet Tools for Patient Care in Advanced Practice

Mary Ann Lavin / Laketa Entzminger / Mary Lee Barron

• OBJECTIVES

1. Searches, saves and communicates clinical knowledge and information.
2. Searching, saving, and communicating clinical knowledge and information.
3. Identify.
4. Integrate basic and advanced Internet search skills in the delivery of healthcare to English- and Spanish-speaking populations.
5. Access a variety of clinical practice Internet-available tools, with special sections on vaccination, STIs, and Hispanic resources, organized within nursing process categories.
6. Integrate content on the quality improvement, patient-centered medical home, interprofessional team development, and healthcare reform into advanced practice.

• KEY WORDS

Internet tools
search methods
clinical practice
nursing process
vaccination
sexually transmitted infections
patient-centered medical home
interprofessional practice
Hispanic resources
standardized terminologies
NLINKS

MULTIDIMENSIONAL INFORMATION: REFRAMING KNOWLEDGE AND INFORMATION ACQUISITION

Two reports rank the United States and other countries in terms of information and communication technology (ICT) readiness and information and communication technology as it is related to eHealth. The former is the Global Information Technology Report 2009–2010 (WHO, 2011). This report ranks the US as fifth in terms of its network readiness index; behind Sweden, Singapore, Denmark and Switzerland. (Dutta & Mia, 2011). Although the US ICT Development Index seems respectable, this index number ranks 19th globally due to mobile health. That is defined as the support of medical and public health practices by mobile devices, whether that be for patient monitoring purposes, clinical uses of PDAs, or other wireless applications.

As a developed country, we are not alone in terms of a poor ranking. Canada ranked 21st (Webster, 2011). The President of Canada's National Institute of Health Informatics called for a "watchdog" over the ranking and solution.

Practices must incorporate clinical information in a more systematic and organized manner. Just having one or two formularies on a PDA no longer suffices. The purpose of this chapter is to provide clinicians with a systematic approach to searching and using reliable, online clinical information in a productive manner to promote health, quality of care, and safety.

This chapter presents a variety of Web-based applications that help form the knowledge and clinical information base of advanced nursing practice, indeed of clinical practice in general, whether medical or nursing. Knowledge and information are their communication are important concepts. Before the written word, communication was oral. Its transmission requires being in the presence of the speaker. Before the electronic word, written communication required paper and the transmission of paper (letter, article, book) from person to person. Communication is now oral, written, and electronic. Electronic transmission of the latter simply requires access to the Internet.

Changes in communication change the way in which we think about and organize knowledge and information. Walter Ong wrote of reframing consciousness. He anticipated that Internet communication would reframe consciousness in an analogous but perhaps even greater manner.

The term "reframing" is critical. Frameworks help us organize knowledge and information. The identification

of the nursing process (assessment, diagnosis, intervention, and evaluation) is a unidimensional framework. Even with the addition of the nursing classifications (diagnoses, interventions, and outcomes), it remained, when written in a textbook format, a flat 2-dimensional framework. For example, Table 30.1 frames knowledge so that the reader may grasp that assessment concludes with a diagnosis, which, in turn leads to diagnostic-specific interventions with measurable outcomes.

A third dimension may be added by placing this particular 2-dimensional matrix within a theoretical framework, whether the framework be adaptation, self-care, or a physiological one centering on visual or neurological pathologies. Conceptually, the matrix can be extended even further. The same model could conceivably be viewed within multiple theoretical frameworks.

In the pre-Internet era, this kind of knowledge was acquired and related information was communicated orally by teachers and mentors or in print journals and textbooks. Oral and print media continue to play a vital but increasingly limited role today. With the growth and development of the Internet the reader is no longer confined to the slower thinking of teachers in class or to the works of two or three or more authors writing manuscripts or textbooks. Merely clicking a hyperlink; opens pathways that reframe the way in which we access and organize knowledge and information.

The best Websites provide the reader with an opportunity to develop an information matrix. For example, go to nih.gov and click on Institutes in the tool bar. Scroll down to and click on Center for Complementary and Alternative Medicine. Click on "herbs at a glance." Select St. John's wort. Note that the information on St. John's wort is categorized into: Introduction, What St. John's wort Is Used For, How St. John's wort Is Used, What the Science Says, Side Effects and Cautions, Sources, For More Information. Repeat the search for Valerian, another herb that has been used for depression. Note that the informa-

TABLE 30.1	Simple Matrix Examining Application of Nursing Process to Risk for Fall Diagnosis
Nursing Process	**Diagnosis: Risk for Fall**
Assessment	Fall risk assessment
Diagnosis	Degree of risk
Interventions or treatment	Interventions and related activities, given the degree of risk
Evaluation	Falls prevented or not

tion on Valerian is categorized in the same manner. Thus, within a matter of seconds, the Internet user is immediately capable of comparing two herbs within the same categories and either storing that information mentally or communicating it to others. In the next section, the reader will learn how to conduct advanced searches, save and communicate the information retrieved.

SEARCHING, SAVING, AND COMMUNICATING KNOWLEDGE AND INFORMATION

Regardless of the search engine used, certain search methodologies, if applied correctly, increase the efficiency of retrieval. The following search strategies proceed from basic to advanced. Clinical examples are provided to facilitate learning. The strategies are three: name precisely the information being sought, use search strings rather than single words, and enhance search strings by using Boolean or natural language methods. Each of these strategies is described below.

- Name precisely the information being sought. The Internet is not a book. There is no need to go to a chapter on diabetes mellitus, then find the section on therapeutic management, and then locate the specific pages or paragraphs containing information on insulin dosing. If the search terms used are precisely chosen, the searcher goes directly to the desired information.

- Use a search string (one or more search terms) rather than a single word to increase the preciseness of a search. If information on insulin dosing is needed, then enter "insulin dosing" into the search box and not "insulin." This principle may appear simple, but many fail to apply the principle when searching the Internet. The end result is frustration over time wasted. If tempted to use a single term such as insulin, ask, What is it

about insulin I want to know? Insulin reactions? Insulin resistance? Insulin administration? Insulin dosing? Enter the precise search terms in a string, rather than a single term, eg, insulin.

- Enhance search strings by Boolean or natural language methods. Use the Boolean terms: AND, OR, or NOT. The term AND is used when search terms or strings need to be added together. The term OR is used when equivalent terms or synonyms are used to capture the information required. The following is an example of how AND may be used to create a search string that precisely expresses the intent of the searcher. Suppose the searcher is looking for asthma death rates in children in 2006.

These strategies may be applied in different ways and yield different results. Table 30.2 presents three different search strategies, each attempting to retrieve the same information.

All three searches may be saved and hence available for subsequent use by using the PubMed My NCBI function. The steps are:

- Access pubmed.gov
- Click on My NCBI hyperlink in the upper-right hand corner
- Register for a new account

Save the searches under the new account username and ID.

This section on search methods concludes with tips on the quality of Websites. Quality and Internet domains are directly related. Primarily, there are government (gov), education (edu), organization (org), and commercial (com) domains. Domains are one way in which Internet sites are organized.

When using Websites for clinical decision support purposes, the clinician must understand differences among these domains and evaluate the credibility of the content

TABLE 30.2	Differences in Citations Retrieved Given Changes in Search Term Strategies	
Strategy	**Search Terms**	**Citations Retrieved (May 31, 2010)**
Boolean	asthma AND (death OR mortality) AND rates AND children AND 2006	104
PubMed recommended method, without Boolean terms	asthma death mortality rates children 2006	38
Natural language	asthma death or mortality rates in children in 2006	6564

retrieved. In general, clinical information obtained from governmental domains is likely to be less biased than information obtained from commercial sites. The credibility of content from educational Websites varies and is likely to be directly related to the academic quality of the university the Website represents. An organizational Website is likely to present organizational interests and bias. There is a vast difference in quality among commercial Websites. It is therefore incumbent on the clinician to evaluate the credibility of the information obtained.

When communicating information in writing, one cites references. But, when communicating Web-based information orally, too many merely identify the Internet as their source of information. It only takes slightly more effort to identify the source, eg, "When conducting a PubMed search, I found...." or "When looking up a drug on the FDA Website or on rxlist. com...." or "When checking the cancer risk calculator from Washington University School of Medicine in St. Louis, I found that...."

Case 30.1 presents an exercise in evaluating credibility of information obtained on the topic of drug interactions associated with St. John's wort.

The above search methodology and website quality considerations are applicable when the clinician is using a search engine, eg, the National Library of Medicine's (NLM) PubMed, OVID, or commercial search engines, eg, Google. They are also applicable when conducting a metasearch, ie, a simultaneous search of multiple search engines or databases. They include:

- Digital windmill (http://digitalwindmill.com/)

- eMetasearch (http://emetasearch.com/)

For additional information on Web searches, including metasearches, access the William H. Welch Medical Library Evidence Based Medicine Webpage and scroll down to Meta-Search Engines) (Johns Hopkins Medical Institutions, Welch Medical Library, http://www.welch.jhu.edu/internet/ebr.html#meta-analysis).

Now that we have learned something about searching, saving, and communicating knowledge and information, let's examine ways of organizing information. First, we will organize Internet-available information on practice management tools.

INTERNET-AVAILABLE PRACTICE MANAGEMENT TOOLS: PATIENT-CENTERED MEDICAL HOME (PCMH), PCMH QUALITY IMPROVEMENT (QI), EVIDENCE-BASED GUIDELINES, AND INTERPROFESSIONAL PRACTICE TOOLS

Patient-Centered Medical Home

Certainly, there are more Internet-available practice management tools available than those focused on the PCMH. Yet, the importance of the PCMH to healthcare at this time justifies using it as a focal point in this section. Key PCMH stakeholders define the PCMH in different ways. For example, the College of Physicians defines the PCMH as "a team-based model of care led by a personal physician who provides continuous and coordinated care throughout

Case 30.1. Drug Interactions Associated with St. John's Wort: A Comparison of the Information Obtained from Three Internet Domains

Government Domains. Several government Websites were selected: the Food and Drug Administration (www.fda.gov), the NLM PubMed database (www.pubmed.gov), and the National Center for Complementary and Alternative Medicine (NCCAM) (http://nccam.nih.gov/). The site that provided the quickest access and the most concrete information on drug interactions was the FDA Website with its warning letter to health professionals, dated February 10, 2000 (Food and Drug Administration, http://www.fda.gov/Drugs/DrugSafety/PublicHealthAdvisories/UCM052238). To retrieve this letter, the search terms "St. John's Wort" or "St. John's Wort AND drug interactions" were entered into the FDA home page search box. The letter indicated that St. John's Wort lowers the plasma

concentration and hence decreases the effectiveness of indinavir, a protease inhibitor. The letter postulated that the cause of the interaction is due to the metabolism of the two drugs. St. John's Wort induces the P450 metabolic pathway in the liver that indinavir relies on P450 isoenzymes for its metabolism. Therefore, the metabolism (in this case, inactivation) of indinavir occurs more rapidly than normal. Consequently, its plasma concentration is thereby reduced. The FDA noted that similar interactions are likely to occur between St. John's Wort and other protease inhibitors metabolized by the same P450 subsystem.

The PubMed site provided additional information relevant to clinical decision making. When the search terms "St John's Wort AND P450" were used and results limited to English language articles published within the last 5 years, 31 citations were retrieved. In brief, St. John's wort was found to reduce the plasma concentrations of:

- Alprozolam, amitriptyline, cyclosporine, digoxin, fexofenadine, indinavir, irinotecan, methadone, simvastatis, tacrolinus,verapamil, warfarin, and oral contraceptives (Borrelli & Izzo, 2009; Izzo & Ernest, 2009)

- Dextrometorphane, phenprocoumon (Madabushi, Frank, Drewelow, et al., 2006)

These interactions are secondary to the induction of P450 human isoenzymes, including CYP2C19 (Saxena, Parijat Tripathi, Roy, et al., 2008). CYP2C19 is responsible for the metabolism of drugs, eg, proton pump inhibitors, phenytoin, diazepam, amitriptyline, and warfarin (Indiana University-Purdue University Indianapolis, School of Medicine, 2009 version 5.0, http://medicine.iupui.edu/clinpharm/ddis/)

Other drug interactions with St. John's Wort were mentioned. It was found to:

- Increase P-glycoprotein expression (Nowack, 2008)

- Induce serotonin syndrome when coadministered with selective serotonin reuptak inhibitors (Borrelli & Izzo, 2009)

A second search was conducted using the terms "cyclosporine AND St. John's Wort." This search yielded reports on the effects, mostly of transplant rejection, of St. John's Wort-cyclosporine interaction. These reports included:

- Decreased cyclosporine bioavailability when co-administered with St. John's wort (Yang, Chao, Hou, et al., 2006)

- A pharmacokinetic modeling of the cyclosporine and St. John's Wort interaction (Murakami, Tanaka, Murakami, et al., 2006)

On introducing the search terms "St. John's Wort AND P450" into its search box, an article was retrieved in which NCCAM reported on St. John's Wort and its use to treat depression. The article was written in language addressed to the lay consumer (Article, http://nccam.nih.gov/health/stjohnswort/sjw-and-depression.htm).

The homepage also featured a link to more general information about St. John's Wort under the "Take Charge of Your Health" header. After inserting "St. John's Wort" into the search engine of the clinical trials page of NCCAM (www.clinicaltrials.gov), several studies were found that investigated the effect of St. John's Wort on irritable bowel syndrome, mild to major depression, oral contraceptives, social phobia, and herbal-opioid interactions.

Educational Domains. When the search phrase "P450 drug interactions" was entered into the Google search box, the first site listed with an edu domain was Indiana University, Purdue University Indianapolis P450 Drug Interactions Table (http://medicine.iupui.edu/flockhart/table.htm), where a P450 cytochromosal drug interaction table is provided. To use, enter "St. John's Wort" in the find box. Note that St. John's Wort is listed as a CY 3A4,5,7 inducer. Note the CY 3A4,5,7 substrates and inhibitors as well. As an inducer, St. John's Wort will lower the plasma concentration of substrates and inhibitors within the same P450 isoenzyme subsystem.

Organizational Domains. Very little actual and no new information was found when the search string "St. John's wort AND drug interactions AND organizations" was entered in Google. Of the first 10 sites listed, four were organizational sites, but none represented major professional organizations within medicine or nursing.

Commercial Domains. The credibility of commercial sites was mixed. Known sites were accessed first: medscape.com and rxlist.com. Medscape provided assessable, user-friendly, and updated information. In the search box on the home page, enter the search terms, in this case "St. John's Wort" and then click on "drugs" in the toolbar. When the drug information section appears, click on "drug interactions." A comprehensive listing of the drug interactions appears.

Another pharmacology reference site is rxlist.com. Click on "supplements" in the toolbar. A page appears with lists of major food supplements, among which is listed St. John's wort. A comprehensive listing of the drugs with which St. John's wort interacts is listed on the third page of this report.

Conclusions. Credible information on specific clinical topics is readily available on the Internet. The type and depth of information varies by domain and by the quality of the Websites within the domains. For clinical decision support purposes, it is suggested that a database of sites be kept readily available for use. With this particular search, government and university sites provided the best available information.

a patient's lifetime to maximize health outcomes." A joint statement by four organizations—American Academy of Family Physicians (AAFP), American Academy of Pediatrics (AAP), American College of Physicians (ACP), and the American Osteopathic Association (AOA)—defines the PCMH in a less profession-specific manner. They state that a PCMH is "an approach to providing comprehensive primary care for children, youth and adults. The PCMH is a healthcare setting that facilitates partnerships between individual patients, and their personal physicians, and when appropriate, the patient's family" (http://www.pcpcc.net/node/14).

The term "patient-centered medical home" is relatively new. In 2006, Congress passed legislation approving the Medicare Medical Home Demonstration Project. In 2008, the Senate Finance Committee expanded the Medical Home project. At that time, the American Nurses Association (ANA) expressed concern and encouraged legislators to move away from defining a "medical" home only as physician-led practice but also allow nurse practitioners to lead "medical" homes (http://www.nursingworld.org/HomepageCategory/NursingInsider/Archive_1/2008NI/Apr08NI/NursePractitionersinMedicalHomesDefinition.aspx). In late 2009, the American College of Physicians issued a document titled, *Nurse Practitioners in Primary Care*, in which the ACP formulated principles of parity between nurse practitioners and physicians with regard the patient-centered medical home. Nurse practitioners were to be subject to the same recognition, evaluation, and disclosure of professional credential standards as physicians. The ACP added that practitioner-led PCMH practices considers case mix differences between physicians and nurse practitioners (http://www.acponline.org/advocacy/where_we_stand/policy/np_pc.pdf). On May 28, 2010, the National Committee for Quality Assurance (NCQA) announced that nurse practitioners and physician assistants are now eligible for four NCQA Recognition programs, including the Physician Practice Connections Recognition (PPC), and Physician Practice Connections – Patient Centered Medical Home Recognition (PPC-PCMH) programs (http://www.ncqa.org/tabid/1198/Default.aspx).

The elements of a PCMH are several. They include a primary care clinician-directed practice, a personal primary care clinician who provides for continuity of care over time, a whole person orientation to the patient, care that is coordinated and integrated across the entire system of care, and patient safety and quality. The latter includes evidence-based practice, patient and/or family involvement in decision making and in quality improvement activities, patient advocacy, clinician accountability, electronic health records and information technology,

and office participation in a recognition program. Finally, PCMH enhance access to care through expanded hours, open scheduling, and open communication between patients, clinician and staff, keeping in mind the importance of documenting all communication and closing communication loops (http://www.pcpcc.net/node/14).

Principles require operationalization. A significant step forward in this direction was made by the National Committee for Quality Assurance (NCQA) in its 2008 CMS version, *Standards and Guidelines for Physician Practice Connections – Patient-Centered Medical Home (PPC-PCMH)*. Available at www.ncqa.org, this detailed document is indispensable in the management of any office, whether a PCMH or not. There is also a most useful PCMH Standards and Scoring sheet developed by the Maryland Department of Health (http://dhmh.maryland.gov/mhqcc/materials/pcmh/PPC-PCMH_Standards_Scoring_12-3-07.pdf). Finally, there is a NCQA Frequently Asked Questions Sheet on the PCMH. These online resources serve as an excellent introduction to the following section.

PCMH Quality Improvement

HEDIS measures provide quality improvement criteria for commercial health plans and plans serving Medicare and Medicaid clients. There are also HEDIS measures for the PCMH. The 2010 PCMH HEDIS measures are available at the following user-friendly NCQA Website (http://www.ncqa.org/tabid/59/Default.aspx). They are:

- Adult BMI Assessment
- Weight Assessment and Counseling for Nutrition and Physical Activity for Children/Adolescents
- Childhood Immunization Status
- Immunizations for Adolescents
- Lead Screening in Children
- Breast Cancer Screening
- Cervical Cancer Screening
- Colorectal Cancer

Guidelines for each measure are available through the National Quality Measures Clearinghouse (http://www.qualitymeasures.ahrq.gov/).

The date of HEDIS measure is important insofar as NCMC provides the last updated version of the measure. For example, the 2010 HEDIS breast cancer screening measure indicates "no change in the measure." Therefore, the 2010 HEDIS measure defaults to the 2009 HEDIS measure.

At times, the HEDIS measure assists clinicians regarding guidelines that may vary among professional organizations or governmental agencies. Breast cancer screening is one example. The latest 2009 HEDIS breast cancer screening measure refers to "percentage of women 40 to 69 years of age who had one or more mammograms during the measurement year or the year prior to the measurement year." Health Centers may count themselves as HEDIS compliant if a mammogram has been performed in 2011 or within one year prior to the 2011 visit. (http://www.fchp.org/providers/resources/hedis-measures.aspx)

HEDIS compliance means that the office practice may cite the NCQA as the source of its standards, even as the medical community is resolving the differences in the 2009 mammogram frequency recommendations from the United States Preventive Health Services (annually from age 50), the American College of Obstetricians and Gynecology (every 1 to 2 years from ages 40 to 49 and annually thereafter), and the September 2009 American Cancer Society (annually from age 40).

Evidence-Based Guidelines

Despite occasional differences in their clinical conclusions, government and professional organization are excellent sources of trustworthy evidence-based practice tools. Take, for example, the clinical practice guidelines available through the National Heart, Lung and Blood Institute (http://www.nhlbi.nih.gov). At the time of this printing, the current guidelines are:

- Asthma
  - Guidelines for the Diagnosis and Management of Asthma—2007
  - Managing Asthma in Pregnancy—2004
- High Blood Cholesterol
  - Clinical Guidelines on Cholesterol Management in Adults (ATP III)—2002—(Update in Development)
- High Blood Pressure
  - High Blood Pressure in Children and Adolescents—2004
  - High Blood Pressure Guidelines (JNC 7)—2003—(Update in Development)
- Overweight and Obesity
  - Clinical Guidelines on Overweight and Obesity—1998—(Update in Development)
- von Willebrand Disease

TABLE 30.3	USPSTF Summary Recommendations and Evidence on Breast Cancer Screening

The USPSTF recommends biennial mammography screening for women aged 50–74 years. This is a B recommendation.

The decision to start regular, biennial mammography screening before the age of 50 years should be an individual one and take patient context into account, including the patient's values regarding specific benefits and harms. This is a C recommendation.

The USPSTF concludes that the current evidence is insufficient to assess the additional benefits and harms of mammography screening in women 75 years or older. This is an I statement.

The USPSTF recommends against teaching breast self-examination (BSE). This is a D recommendation.

The USPSTF concludes that the current evidence is insufficient to assess the additional benefits and harms of clinical breast examination (CBE) beyond screening in women 40 years or older. This is an I statement.

The USPSTF concludes that the current evidence is insufficient to assess the additional benefits and harms of either digital mammography or MRI instead of film mammography as screening modalities for breast cancer. This is an I statement.

It is easy to pull up clinical practice guidelines on the Internet. It is more difficult to know how to interpret them correctly. Evidence-based guidelines rank grades of recommendation and levels of certainty. These criteria vary from one governmental agency to another and among professional organizations. Take, for example, the United States Preventive Service Task Force (USPSTF) recommendation statement on breast cancer screening. To access, go to the National Guidelines Clearinghouse (www.ncg.gov) and scroll down to and click on: (1) Screening for breast cancer: U.S. Preventive Services Task Force recommendation statement. (2) December 2009 addendum. 1996 (NCG, revised 2009; addendum released 2009 December). The summary recommendations are presented in Table 30.3.

The B,C,D, and I statements refer to the grades of recommendation. The USPSTF grades of recommendation are presented in Table 30.4.

In the last row of Table 30.4 the authors discuss "uncertainty". Certainty and uncertainty, in this context, refer to the net benefit of the practice in light of the quality of the scientific evidence (Table 30.5).

It is important to realize that HEDIS standards and clinical practice guidelines represent the best clinical

TABLE 30.4	USPSTF Grades of Recommendation	
Grade	Grade Definitions	Suggestions for Practice
A	The USPSTF recommends the service. There is high certainty that the net benefit is substantial.	Offer or provide this service.
B	The USPSTF recommends the service. There is high certainty that the net benefit is moderate or there is moderate certainty that the net benefit is moderate to substantial.	Offer or provide this service.
C	The USPSTF recommends against routinely providing the service. There may be considerations that support providing the service in an individual patient. There is moderate or high certainty that the net benefit is small.	Offer or provide this service only if other considerations support offering or providing the service in an individual patient.
D	The USPSTF recommends against the service. There is moderate or high certainty that the service has no net benefit or that the harms outweigh the benefits.	Discourage the use of this service.
I	The USPSTF concludes that the current evidence is insufficient to assess the balance of benefits and harms of the service. Evidence is lacking, of poor quality, or conflicting, and the balance of benefits and harms cannot be determined.	Read "Clinical Considerations" section of USPSTF Recommendation Statement (see "Major Recommendations" field). If this service is offered, patients should understand the uncertainty about the balance of benefits and harms.

TABLE 30.5	Grading the Quality of the Scientific Evidence
Level of Certainty	Description
High	The available evidence usually includes consistent results from well-designed, well-conducted studies in representative primary care populations. These studies assess the effects of the preventive service on health outcomes. This conclusion is therefore unlikely to be strongly affected by the results of future studies.
Moderate	The available evidence is sufficient to determine the effects of the preventive service on health outcomes, but confidence in the estimate is constrained by factors such as: • The number, size, or quality of individual studies • Inconsistency of findings across individual studies • Limited generalizability of findings to routine primary care practice • Lack of coherence in the chain of evidence As more information becomes available, the magnitude or direction of the observed effect could change, and this change may be large enough to alter the conclusion.
Low	The available evidence is insufficient to assess effects on health outcomes. Evidence is insufficient because of: • The limited number or size of studies • Important flaws in study design or methods • Inconsistency of findings across individual studies • Gaps in the chain of evidence • Findings not generalizable to routine primary care practice • A lack of information on important health outcomes More information may allow an estimation of effects on health outcomes.

and scientific judgments, based on the current available evidence. In the case of HEDIS standards the best available judgment refers to the quality of care being offered within an office or an HMO. In the case of practice guidelines, the best available judgment refers to quality of the evidence supporting the standardization of screening, diagnostic, and treatment plans. This standardization does not mean one shoe fits all. It does mean that the evidence has been examined in a systematic manner and best practices determined given available evidence today. Both standards and clinical practice guidelines change over time as the science underlying each evolves.

Interprofessional Practice Tools

Interprofessional practice is an approach to care that involves a philosophy of office management, dedication to quality improvement, and the integration of clinical practice. It is team-oriented, building upon shared experience, reflection, action, and communication. These components form a matrix which address other team issues: certainty and uncertainty, excellence and need for improvement, conflict and its resolution, and the meaning of team, and team leader and team member responsibilities. All factors interplay dynamically within the practice team, composed of members with varying knowledge, and information bases, skill sets, professional vocabulary, expectations, socialization processes, and personalities. They share, however, a common goal: improvement in patient care and reduction of patient risk. A well-functioning interprofessional practice may even exceed its own performance expectations.

Interprofessional practice is a team activity. Shared experience, reflection, action, and communication preceded by an understanding of the context in which the experience occurs and followed by an evaluation of the actions taken are central to its success. These concepts are pedagogical principles that date back at least 450 years in Jesuit education (http://www.ajcunet.edu/Jesuit-Education-and-Ignatian-Pedagogy). This approach is similar to Lewin's experiential learning and action research approaches in his study of group dynamics (http://www.infed.org/thinkers/et-lewin.htm; http://www.solonline.org/res/wp/10006.html). Both models are conducive to personal, group, and organizational learning and change.

Perhaps equally powerful is effective team communication. One method of facilitating targeted clinical communication among team members is to standardize the method of communication. One example is

SBAR, where the **situation** is described in a sentence, the **background** is presented, concluding with a succinct **assessment** and assessment-specific **recommendations** (http://www.ihi.org/ihi/search/searchresults.aspx?searchterm=SBAR&searchtype=basic&Start+Search.x=0&Start+Search.y=0).

Just as there are quality improvement tools, there are also practical interprofessional practice tools. Many interprofessional practice tools are available on the Internet. The following are a few samples:

- Geriatric Interprofessional Interorganizational Collaboration (http://rgps.on.ca/giic/GiiC/interprofessional-practice.html)
- Regional Geriatric Program of Toronto (http://rgp.toronto.on.ca/issues_teamwork_interpro_practice)
- Center for Effective Practice (for tools, access hyperlinks in left hand margin) (http://www.effectivepractice.org/index.cfm?id=13051)
- Canadian Virtual Hospital: Tools for Practice (http://www.virtualhospice.ca/en_US/Main+Site+Navigation/Home/For+Professionals/For+Professionals/Tools+for+Practice/Interdisciplinary+practice.aspx)

Effective interprofessional practice relies on effective teamwork. The Institute for Healthcare Improvement (IHI.org) has many sites and tools that facilitate teamwork. Subscribe for free and access the following:

- Teams (http://www.ihi.org/ihi/search/searchresults.aspx?searchterm=team&searchtype=basic&Start+Search.x=4&Start+Search.y=9)
- Teamwork (http://www.ihi.org/ihi/search/searchresults.aspx?searchterm=teamwork&searchtype=basic&Start+Search.x=0&Start+Search.y=0)
- Team relations (http://www.ihi.org/ihi/search/searchresults.aspx?searchterm=team+relations&searchtype=basic&Start+Search.x=3&Start+Search.y=8)
- Team meetings (http://www.ihi.org/ihi/search/searchresults.aspx?searchterm=team+meetings&searchtype=basic&Start+Search.x=1&Start+Search.y=3)
- Team evaluation (http://www.ihi.org/ihi/search/searchresults.aspx?searchterm=Team+evaluation&searchtype=basic&Start+Search.x=2&Start+Search.y=8)
- Team graphics (http://www.ihi.org/ihi/search/searchresults.aspx?searchterm=team+graphics&searchtype=basic&Start+Search.x=2&Start+Search.y=9)

Effective interprofessional teamwork improves patient safety. The Agency for Healthcare Research and Quality is highly invested in this aspect. Perhaps the most comprehensive source of online information about the relationship between teamwork and safety is the following: Medical teamwork and patient safety at http://www.ahrq.gov/qual/medteam/

INTERNET-AVAILABLE CLINICAL PRACTICE TOOLS

This section is divided into the most basic components of the nursing process: assessment, diagnosis, treatment, and outcomes evaluation. These components provide the outward structure for the development of a Clinical Information Database for Advanced Practice Nursing. The Internet sites selected are listed within this structure. Although the listing is not exhaustive, it does represent carefully selected examples of the types of clinical information available on the Internet. This structured approach to information database development is clinically useful, helps clinicians organize their own knowledge databases, and facilitates ready access to needed information.

Assessment

Assessment refers to the systematic collection of data needed to arrive at one or more diagnoses. The tools included in this section include forms, miscellaneous screening tools, risk assessment instrument, and information of the manifestation of signs and symptoms. These tools represent a sampling of assessment content available on the Internet. Each category is described briefly.

Nursing assessment is the first step in the nursing process. The following site provides an example of a comprehensive nursing assessment form:

http://www.hospitalsoup.com/public/nursingassess2001.pdf.

Craving, loss of control, physical dependence, and tolerance constitute four cardinal signs and symptoms of alcoholism. This Website of the NIH National Institute on Alcohol Abuse and Alcoholism provides not only a reminder of signs and symptoms but also contain outstanding resource information:

http://www.niaaa.nih.gov

Domestic abuse assessment is an integral part of primary care practice. The following assessment tool, from the Vermont Department of Health, provides informa-

tion on a professional approach to interviewing on the delicate topic and the essential questions to be asked. One additional tip is to have available directions to and the phone number of a safe house. Some domestic abuse counselors recommend that the information be given verbally, asking the patient to memorize it rather than placing the patient at added risk should the abusive partner find the written material and use it as an excuse for further abuse:

(http://healthvermont.gov/family/domestic_abuse/ domestic_abuse.aspx).

The following Web page is from the Connecticut Clearinghouse, a program of the Wheeler Clinic. It consists of multiple assessment and screening hyperlinks, useful in advanced nursing practice:

(http://www.ctclearinghouse.org/Topics/Links/linkCategoryView.asp?LinkCategoryID=7).

Risk assessment is an important part of clinical practice. The following Internet tools are health risk calculators that provide the evidence to support risk diagnoses.

- Body mass index calculator from the NIH National Heart, Lung and Blood Institutes of the (http://nhlbisupport.com/bmi/bmicalc.htm).

- The same cancer risk tool is available on the Web pages of the Siteman Cancer Center, A National Cancer Institute Comprehensive Care Center of the Barnes-Jewish Hospital and Washington University-St. Louis School of Medicine and at Harvard, where the tool was originally developed. Access either of the following http://www.yourdiseaserisk.wustl.edu/ or http://www.diseaseriskindex.harvard.edu/update/ and enter the patient's risk data. Risks may be calculated for breast, prostate, lung (Case 30.2), colon, bladder, melanoma, uterine, kidney, pancreatic, ovarian, stomach, and cervical cancers

- Coronary heart disease risk calculator, a risk assessment tool for estimating 10-year risk of developing hard CHD (myocardial infarction and coronary death), based on age, gender, total cholesterol, high-density lipoprotein (HDL), smoker, blood pressure, and current medication for hypertension for the NIH National Heart, Lung, and Blood Institute (http://hin.nhlbi.nih.gov/atpiii/calculator.asp?usertype=prof)

- Health risk calculators from the University of Maryland Medicine for 24 health conditions, including asthma, depression, diabetes, pregnancy due date, HIV risk, nicotine dependency, teen

Case 30.2. Cancer Risk Assessment

A 73-year-old male, retired insurance agent, who smoked between 14 and 25 cigarettes per day between the ages of 18 and 45 years, but never any cigars, asks you what his chances of developing lung cancer. How would you respond?

To answer this patient's question, the advanced practice nurse with the patient accesses the Washington University or the Harvard risk assessment tools at http://www.yourdiseaserisk.wustl.edu/ or http://www.diseaseriskindex.harvard.edu/update/

Click on "cancer"

Then click, on "Lung Cancer"

Next, click on "Questionnaire"

Enter sex and age

Then, click next and proceed through a list of questions, such as the following

Answer question about any prior diagnosis of cancer and click next

Answer question about diagnosis of cancer in family members

Answer question about smoking history

If yes, answer question about number of cigarettes/day

Answer question about number of cigars/day

Answer questions about living in an urban area and exposure to asbestos

Answer questions about chemical exposure

Answer questions about exposure to various industrial processes

Answer questions about diet

Instruct patient on his risks of other smoking-related illnesses

Provide patient with information on his cancer risk, how he may decrease his risk, and what healthy behaviors he is currently doing well

Results. Based on the answers to these questions, this 73-year-old male patient (who had no prior history of cancer, no family history of lung cancer, smoked 15 to 25 cigarettes perday for more than 20 years but never any cigars, lived all his life in an urban area but had no chemical or pertinent exposure to industrial processes, and eats more than 5 fruit and vegetable servings per day, has a below average risk of developing lung cancer.

---

suicide risk, and more (http://www.umm.edu/healthcalculators/)

Diagnosis

Treatment is diagnostic specific. Hence, diagnosis and treatment information categories are frequently not discreet. Practice guidelines often address assessment, diagnosis, and treatment. Disease directories often do the same. Conceptually, however, it was thought best to divide the content sequentially. In this section, the focus is diagnosis.

The etymology of the word *diagnosis* is based in its Greek roots. *Dia* means "through," and *gnosis* means "knowledge." Diagnosis, therefore, is dependent on the knowledge base of the person diagnosing. Disease represents the knowledge base of physicians. Human responses to illness and health represent the knowledge base of nursing. A classification of functional health and disability terms represents a beginning step toward the elaboration of a unified health professional knowledge base. These knowledge bases are displayed within classification systems specifically,

1. Medical classifications of diseases, eg, the International Classification of Disease (ICD)-10-CM (World Health Organization [WHO], 1992) and the ICD-9 (American Medical Association, 2004). The current version of the ICD-10 is available online at http://apps.who.int/classifications/apps/icd/icd10online. It has not as yet been fully incorporated into use in the United States. This transition must be complete by October, 2019. For more information on the transition, access https://www.cms.gov/ICD10. The ICD-9 codes are available at http://ICD9cm.chrisendres.com.

2. Nursing classifications of human responses to illness and health, e.g., the NANDA Diagnoses: Definitions and Classification (NANDA, 2009–2011).

3. Functional health and disability, eg, the International Classification of Functioning in Health and Disability (WHO, 2002). The online version is available at http://apps.who.int/classifications/icfbrowser.

Classifications display in a systematic manner the array of diagnoses that represent the knowledge bases of the professions represented. Clinicians need to be aware of these classifications for data entry, aggregation, analysis, and reimbursement purposes. For clinical purposes, they need to know how to access information on the diagnoses themselves and how to contribute to their development.

Diagnosis of New Threats to Health. Clinicians today are faced with new threats to health, requiring rapid access to related information. The Center for Disease Control Emergency Response and Prepared webpage (http://www.bt.cdc.gov/), assists professionals to deal with mass trauma, bioterrorism, chemical emergencies, natural disasters and severe weather, radiation emergencies, and recent outbreaks and incidents. In addition, an entirely new section called the 2010 Gulf of Mexico oil spill has been added (http://emergency.cdc.gov/gulfoil-spill2010), with a section for health professionals that covers topics such as hazardous substances information, health surveillance, taking an exposure history, and fact sheets for health providers.

Disease Diagnoses

There are several disease directories, with A–Z lists, that are Internet available. Examples include:

Centers for Disease Control and Prevention (CDC), Diseases and Conditions. The hyperlink is available in the left hand margin of the CDC homepage (www.cdc.gov) or may be accessed directly at *http://www.cdc.gov/node.do/id/0900f3ec8000e035*. A–Z list of cancers from the National Cancer Institute (www.nci.nih.gov).

While the above directories are appropriate for clinicians, there are also disease directories that target a lay audience and that provide outstanding health education information. Examples include: National Institute of Diabetes, Digestive Kidney Diseases, National Digestive Diseases Information Clearinghouse (NDDIC) (http://digestive.niddk.nih.gov/ddiseases/a-z.asp)

New York Online Access to Health (www.noah-health.org). The latter site has an A–Z index, which is especially useful for providing laypersons with information on uncommon illness, for example, lupus erythematosus, Marfan's syndrome, Ehlers-Danlos syndrome.

Many Internet sites provide clinical information on tools useful in the diagnosis of specific diseases. For example, Brain Attack: Stroke Scales, National Institute of Neurological Disorders and Stroke (http://www.stroke-site.org/stroke_scales/stroke_scales.html).

Other sites are devoted to a group of diseases, related in some way. The new field of genomics fits this latter category. For information on genomics and disease prevention, access CDC, Genomics and Disease Prevention (http://www.cdc.gov/genomics/default.htm).

Human Response to Illness/Health Diagnoses

The Internet tools presented in this section are infrastructure tools, because much of the work that needs to be accomplished in the field of nursing diagnosis is at the infrastructure level, especially the expansion of current nursing terminologies. These include NANDA Diagnoses: Definitions and Classification (NANDA, 2009–2011, nanda.org), Clinical Care Classification (Saba, 2004–2010, sabacare.com), the Omaha System (Martin, 2005, omahasystem.org), and Nursing Minimum Datasets (International, USA, and Management). Access: http://www.nursing.umn.edu/ICNP/

These classifications are recognized by the ANA, included in the UMLS of the NLM, and available through the standardized nomenclature of medical terminology—clinical terms (SNOMED CT). The latter is a terminology model approved as the U.S. standard for the entry and aggregation of electronic health record data (Lavin, Avant, Craft-Rosenberg, et al., 2004).

To develop an array of nursing diagnoses that are evidence-based, an infrastructure is needed to facilitate the requisite literature searches reporting primary data results. Primary data refers to data collected at the point of patient contact, whether quantitative or qualitative (Lavin, Krieger, Meyer, et al., 2005). A nursing diagnosis and primary data database that connects to PubMed (NLM, pubmed.gov) is available through the Network for Language in Nursing Knowledge Systems Research Center (http://www.nlinks.org/research_main.phtml); or, to retrieve citations on any single nursing diagnosis, follow these directions:

1. Access nlinks.org.

2. Click on Research Center.

3. Scroll down to the Nursing Diagnosis and Primary Data Database hyperlink and click on it.

4. A PubMed Web page will appear. In the search box is a nursing diagnosis and primary data filter. Do not alter the filter. Rather, place the cursor at the beginning of the filter.

5. Type in the nursing diagnosis of interest and use a Boolean AND to connect it to the filter already present in the search box.

6. Click on limits.

7. Limit the choices to "abstracts only" and, if desired, limit to "nursing journals" by click on "Subsets."

8. Click on "Go" to retrieve the abstracts of interest.

Save the search citations in PubMed's *My NCBI* directly. Simply click on My NCBI in the upper right hand of the pubmed.gov Web page, register free and then save your search. NCBI is an acronym for the National Center for Biotechnology Information at the NLM.

Table 30.6 presents the results of NLINKS nursing diagnosis and primary data searches for three time periods. limited to abstracts only and the nursing journals subset. Notice that primary data research on all diagnoses have increased during the more recent time perior. Other literature databases include PubMed's Clinical Queries and Special Queries. Each may be accessed from the pubmed.gov home page. Because each database relies on its own unique filter or filters, the results will be different even if the same search terms are used.

For example, "SNOMED CT® encoded Nursing Problem List Subset is available from the National Library of Medicine for use in Patient Problem Lists, meeting the mandate of Meaningful Use Stage One" (Warren, 2011; http://www.nlm.nih.gov/research/umls/Snomed/nursing_problemlist_subset.html). The problems are drawn from the UMLS® Metathesaurus.

"Meaningful Use Stage One" is a phrase, which refers to a set of functional/interoperability and clinical measures mandated by the Centers for Medicaid and Medicare Services for eligible providers and hospitals. One of the measures refers to problem list documentation. Problem list entries are to be from the ICD® or from SNOMED CT®. Included now, in the SNOMED CT® is the Nursing Problem List Subset.

The Nursing Problem List Subset is of historical importance to the nursing profession. It also brings to mind the question, asked by Saint Louis University's Joan Carter, RN, PhD (Carter, 1973) and which led to the First National Conference on the Classification of Nursing Diagnoses (Gebbie & Lavin, 1975). This prime question continues to be answered by succeeding generations of nursing informatics leaders in increasingly sophisticated ways. The question was: How is nursing data to be entered into a computer for documentation purposes? (http://www.nursingworld.org/npii/.terminologies.htm)

Treatment

The term "treatment" is used here in lieu of interventions and nursing actions, because it expresses more precisely the broad clinical management focus of this section.

Nursing Treatment. Several Internet sites are available for those who desire more information on:

- Saba's Clinical Care Classification framework and model in addition to a toolkit with downloadable standardized, individualized, and interactive plans of care. Access (Saba, 2003, www.sabacare.com).

- An overview of the Nursing Interventions Classification (NIC) available at the Center for Nursing Classification and Clinical Effectiveness (University of Iowa School of Nursing, http://www.nursing.uiowa.edu/excellence/nursing_knowledge/clinical_effectiveness/index.htm).

- The Omaha System, including case studies (Martin, Elfrink, Monsen, and Bowles, 2006, http://www.omahasystem.org'casestudies.html.)

- Perioperative Nursing Data Set (PNDS) online course (http://www.aorn.org/Education/ContinuingEducation/FREEOnlineEducation/PerioperativeNursingDataSet/)

Calculators

Internet tools are available to facilitate calculations used in planning treatment. Examples include:

- Martindale's Calculators Online Part I: Nutrition (http://www.martindalecenter.com/Calculators1B_4_Nut.html). In addition to the folic acid, calcium, and calorie calculators, there is also a basal metabolism calculator especially applicable given interest in dieting and a surge in the proportion of the population who are overweight or obese. After entering age, sex, height, and weight variables, this calculator computes the number of daily calories required to maintain or lose weight and also provides the number of related grams of protein, fat, and carbohydrate (Cases 30.3 and 30.4).

TABLE 30.6	Results of NLINKS Nursing Diagnosis and Primary Data Database Searches for the Years 1994–1998, 1999–2003, and 2004–2008		
Nursing Diagnosis	**1994–1998**	**1999–2003**	**2004–2008**
Knowledge deficit	6	3	28
Acute pain	73	92	142
Chronic pain	86	133	187
Self-care deficit	16	2	21
Anxiety	166	211	462

Note: Limited to abstracts only and nursing journal subset.

Case 30.3. Coding Nursing Diagnosis in ICD-9

You have recently joined a primary care practice. One of your first patients, a 43-year-old, obese, female, secondary school teacher returns to the office for follow-up type 2 diabetic management. She reports that her fasting blood sugars are between 230 and 255 mg/dL per finger stick. She indicates that she has been avoiding all sugars. For breakfast, she eats a dish of oatmeal with about one-half cup of milk and a little honey, a banana, and about 4 oz of orange juice. For lunch, she usually eats one or two slices of pizza or a pasta dish with the teachers at school along with a diet soda. Every now and then she will eat a small slice of cake, when it is a coworker's birthday. For supper, she will stop by a fast food restaurant for a hamburger and salad on the way home or eat part of a pot roast or stew she had prepared over the weekend. She eats graham crackers and milk at bedtime. Your diagnoses are type 2 diabetes mellitus, obesity, and diabetic diet knowledge deficit. You would like to code all three, but you have been told by your nurse practitioner colleagues that there is no way to code nursing diagnoses for reimbursement purposes. What would you do?

The ninth edition of the ICD-9 (2000), as in previous editions, contains V codes, which allow for the classification of factors influencing health status or contact with health services. The V codes are numbered V01-V89, but the V40-49 codes are designed for conditions affecting a person's health status.

Nursing diagnoses, e.g., "risk" nursing diagnoses, deficient knowledge, and ineffective management of therapeutic regimen, may be coded with the ICD using V codes, especially V49, other specified conditions influencing health status. These codes need to be explored for clinical application and reimbursement purposes. The following site provides free, online access to the codes (ICD-9, http://icd9cm.chrisendres.com). Click on 'Tabular Index" in the left-hand margin and then scroll down to the V40-49 codes. Also note the V85 BMI codes.

Case 30.4. Examples of Websites to Assist in Treatment of Primary Care Health and Wellness/Disease Diagnoses

A 63-year-old woman asks how many calories she needs/day to lose weight. Her height is 63.5 in. and her weight is 173 lb. What would you do?

1. Access Cornell Medical Calculators which includes a formula for Basal Energy Expenditure at http://www-users.med.cornell.edu/~spon/picu/calc/beecalc.htm.

   Enter the patient's criteria

   Gender: female

   Weight: 173 lb (U.S.)

   Height: 63 in. (U.S.)

   Age: 63 years

   Click on "calculate"

   The basal energy expenditure is 1409 kcal/day and the caloric requirement to maintain that weight is 1761 kcal/day. This patient will lose weight on a 1500 kcal/day diet.

2. Food and Drug Administration (www.fda.gov), with an outstanding search capability. Clinicians need to remember that herbal products, even though pharmacologically active, are listed under "Foods" and not under "Drugs." Within the FDA Website, the following are especially useful pages:

   (a) Center for Drug Research and Evaluation (http://www.fda.gov/AboutFDA/CentersOffices/CDER/ContactCDER/default.htm)

   (b) Medwatch: The FDA Safety Information and Adverse Event Reporting Program (http://www.fda.gov/Safety/MedWatch/default.htm)

   (c) Medwatch Adverse Event and Product Problem Forms (http://www.fda.gov/Safety/MedWatch/HowToReport/DownloadForms/default.htm)

   (d) Vaccine Adverse Event Reporting System. Enter VAERS in the fda.gov search box and then click on the Vaccine Adverse Event Reporting System (http://vaers.hhs.gov/resources/vaersmaterialspublications)

3. NLM Clinical Alerts Database, may be accessed in the left hand margin of the www.pubmed.gov Web page or directly (http://www.nlm.nih.gov/databases/alerts/clinical_alerts.html)

4. The National Institutes of Health (www.nih.gov) provide outstanding drug information. See especially the following:

   (a) National Institute on Alcohol Abuse and Alcoholism (www.niaaa.nih.gov/)

(b) National Institute on Drug Abuse (www.nida.nih.gov)

(c) National Center for Complementary and Alternative Medicine (www.nccam.nih.gov)

5. The CDC (www.cdc.gov) provide a wealth of information of vaccines as well as annually updated vaccine schedules for all age groups:

(a) CDC Vaccines and Immunizations (http://www.cdc.gov/vaccines/) with the Pink Book (http://www.cdc.gov/vaccines/pubs/pinkbook/default.htm) are an outstanding resource for vaccine clinic administration

(b) CDC National Immunization Program (http://www.cdc.gov/nip/)

(c) More information on vaccines (http://www.cdc.gov/vaccines/vpd-vac/default.htm)

6. University sites are excellent sources of information as well. Examples include:

(a) Indiana University-Purdue University Indianapolis for its P450 drug interactions table (http://medicine.iupui.edu/flockhart/table.htm)

(b) Johns Hopkins University ABX Guide (http://hopkins-abxguide.org/) categorizes drugs by diagnosis, drugs, pathogens, management, and vaccines

(b) University of Missouri–Columbia, Pharmacy provides an excellent page of pharmacy resources (http://mulibraries.missouri.edu/guides/subjects/pharmacy.htm)

7. There are also commercial sites that provide readily accessible manufacturer's information on drugs, including:

(a) Medscape (www.medscape.com). Enter the drug name in the search box and click on "drug information"

(b) Rxlist (www.rxlist.com)

8. There are other commercial sites that provide excellent online clinical educational information. For example, clinicians and students can sharpen their clinical dosing skills through the Family Practice Notebook, which connects to AIDA, a free diabetes software program for purposes of teaching insulin dosing (http://www.fpnotebook.com/Endo/Pharm/InslnDsng.htm)

• Nursing calculators for drug administration purposes (http://www.manuelsweb.com/nrs_calculators.htm)

• Medical calculators developed by Cornell University Medical College, Pediatric Critical Care Medicine (http://www-users.med.cornell.edu/~spon/picu/calc/medcalc.htm)

Drug Management

There is no shortage of information available on pharmacotherapeutics and the pharmacologic management of patients. The Federal government provides a wealth of information. The Drug Enforcement Agency (www.dea.gov) is excellent source of information on drugs and chemicals of concern (http://www.deadiversion.usdoj.gov/drugs_concern/index.html).

Outcomes

Outcomes measurement is a tradition within nursing practice. When Florence Nightingale arrived in Crimea, she noted that soldiers, said to be dying from "wounds," were actually dying from "conditions," eg, fever, diarrhea,

fatigue, lack of clothing, and lack of shelter. When she initiated condition or diagnostic-specific nursing actions, death rates attributable to zymotic disease fell from 480.3 to 47.5 per 1000 soldiers; deaths attributable to all other causes except wounds fell from 68.6 to 5.0 per 1000 (Nightingale, 1859). Nightingale measured patient outcomes to improve the healthcare of the patients whom she served. Outcomes measurement does the same today.

Many categories of patient outcomes are measured today. This section provides examples of outcome measures within several categories. The categories are patient safety, nursing outcomes, nursing home and home healthcare setting outcomes, health plan outcomes, and the short form (SF) health survey.

Patient Safety

Patient safety is an outcomes issue. There are several patient safety sites, which are of prime importance to advanced practice nurses. They include the following:

• Agency for Healthcare Research and Quality Web Morbidity and Mortality Rounds (Case 30.5), an online forum for presentation

Case 30.5. Quality in Primary Care and a Case from the AHRQ Web Morbidity and Mortality Rounds

You are a nurse practitioner in primary care. You want to increase the consciousness of your staff in measuring patient outcomes to improve the quality of care. You decide that at the first meeting you will present a case from the Agency for Healthcare Research and Quality Web Morbidity and Mortality Rounds. Select a case and indicate how it might best be presented.

First, the nurse practitioner needs to find a case. The steps are:

1. Go to the AHRQ Web Morbidity and Mortality Rounds webpage at http://www.webmm.ahrq.gov/

2. Click on "Case Archives" in the toolbar which leads to http://www.webmm.ahrq.gov/caseArchive.aspx

3. Click on primary care which leads only two (as of this printing) primary care cases: http://www.webmm.ahrq.gov/caseArchive.aspx#25

4. Read the two cases and select the nurse practitioner case: http://www.webmm.ahrq.gov/case.aspx?caseID=133

The case presents the experience as it occurred and a reflection on that experience. The nurse practitioner reads it and takes notes about safety improvements that can be learned from the case and applied within the office.

At the staff meeting, the nurse practitioner elicits further ways from the staff about their insights into patient outcomes that they want to see improved.

An animated discussion ensues. The nurse practitioner thanks the team and suggests that at the next meeting, the team can work on placing one or more of their outcome suggestions into a framework for quality improvement, using the ANA webpage: http://www.nursingworld.org/mods/archive/mod72/ceomfull.htm). The team leaves, enthused about their role in improving care. Note that as the case progress, the nurse practitioner moved from calling her co-workers "staff" to "team.

It is incumbent on the advanced practice nurses within primary care settings to measure the quality of care being delivered and make improvements accordingly.

---

and discussion of medical errors (http://www.webmm.ahrq.gov/)

- The patient safety resource page of Medscape.com, a free subscription service (http://www.medscape.com/pages/editorial/resourcecenters/public/patientsafety/rc-patientsafety.ov?src=hp24.rcbottom)

- Institute for Healthcare Improvement (http://www.ihi.org/ihi) (Case 30.6)

Nursing Outcomes

The Internet sites presented within this section refer to standardized nursing terminologies that either present outcomes in a structured format or data sets that may be used for evaluative purposes.

- ANA Quality Indicators (http://www.nursingworld.org/mods/archive/mod72/ceomfull.htm), with its history (http://www.medscape.com/viewarticle/569395_2)

Case 30.6. Find an Online Colleague

You are a critical care nurse practitioner in a teaching hospital interested in patient safety. Lately, you have noticed increased difficulty in weaning patients from mechanical ventilators. In addition, to seeking input from colleagues within the teaching hospital, you would like to connect with other colleagues, who may be addressing the same issue. Furthermore, you like the efficiency of electronic communication. What would you do?

The Institute for Healthcare Improvement (ihi.org), provides such a service. After subscribing free, click on "Community" in the left hand margin and then click on "Find a Colleague." Sign on as a nurse practitioner, from a teaching hospital, interested in critical care and patient safety.

- Nursing Outcomes Interventions (NOC), with an overview available at the Center for Nursing Classification and Clinical Effectiveness (University of Iowa School of Nursing, http://www.nursing.uiowa.edu/excellence/nursing_knowledge/clinical_effectiveness/index.htm).

- International Nursing Minimum Data Set (i-NMDS) available at the Center for Nursing Minimum Data Set Knowledge and Discovery (University of Minnesota School of Nursing, http://www.nursing.umn.edu/ICNP/i-NMDS/index.htm)

Nursing Home and Home Healthcare Setting Outcomes

Related to nursing outcomes are those measures that evaluate the quality of care within nursing homes and home healthcare settings.

- Minimum Data Set (MDS), used by the Centers for Medicare and Medicaid Services for long-term care. Although there are no downloads, requests can be made at http://www.cms.gov/IdentifiableDataFiles/10_LongTermCareMinimumDataSetMDS.asp

- Outcomes Assessment Information Set (OASIS), used by the Centers for Medicare and Medicaid Services to evaluate quality within home healthcare settings (http://www.cms.gov/OASIS/)

These nursing outcome measures, indeed this entire section, is closely related to the section on Quality Improvement presented earlier in this chapter. This redundancy serves a purpose, however. Beginning with Florence Nightingale, nurses and today's advanced practice nurses are committed to quality improvement and outcomes measurement.

Office Tools

Until the electronic health record is universal, the completeness of the health record or specific aspects of care need to be evaluated manually. The following links provide resources on just some of the tools available at the Institute for Healthcare Improvement (IHI). To retrieve, simply insert the respective keywords in the IHI search box, after you have subscribed (free).

1. Outcomes measurement (www.ihi.org)
2. Patient Satisfaction Form (www.ihi.org)

Short Form (SF) Health Survey. One of the long-lasting outcomes of the Medical Outcomes Study (Kravitz, Greenfield, Rogers, et al., 1992; Ware & Sherbourne, 1992) was the dissemination and use of the 36-item SF health survey (SF-36) and its subsequent versions and redactions. Another outcome was the formation of a nonprofit trust called Medical Outcomes Trust (http://www.outcomes-trust.org) and SF-36.org (http://www.sf-36.org).

After subscribing free at the SF-36 Website, access information on SF-36 and its subsequent versions, SF-12 and SF-8. An SF-8 Internet demo is available. This survey tool is especially useful for population-based intervention studies or in cohort studies. Its eight items survey physical and mental health. Physical health items survey overall health, physical activity, interference with ability to work secondary to physical health problems, and pain. Mental health items survey overall energy, social activity, emotional problems, interference with ability to work secondary to emotional problems.

Outcomes Measurement: Internet-Available Biostatistical and Analytical Tools

Although the biostatistical measurement of outcome variables is not a routine part of clinical practice, it is likely to assume an important role when new programs or initiatives are begun. For this purpose, too, ihi.org is again an outstanding Website. After subscribing free, insert the following words into the search box:

- Qualitative measurement
- Measurement Graphics

Health Information in English and Spanish

There are 300 million people in the United States, as of October 2006. All the health information sites listed in this section are available in English. There are an estimated 46.9 million of Hispanic origin, of whom 35 million speak Spanish. The only other country in the world with a larger Hispanic population is Mexico. The number does not include the 4 million U.S. citizens in Puerto Rico, a self-governing commonwealth (http://2010.census.gov/mediacenter/portrait-of-america/hispanic-origin.php; http://www.infoplease.com/spot/hhmcensus1.html). All the health information Websites listed below are also available in Spanish.

From a public health perspective, it is vital that people have available to them information to help them make healthy choices in life. The Centers for Disease Control and Prevention (www.cdc.gov), therefore, have English and Spanish language Websites. Both Websites possess the same main information categories. In Spanish and English, these are:

Enfermedades y afecciones/Diseases and conditions

Vida saludable/Healthy living

Preparación y respuesta para casos de emergencias/ Emergency preparedness and response

Lesiones, violencia y seguridad/Injury, violence and safety

Salud ambiental/Environmental health

Salud del viajero/Travelers' health

Etapas de la vida y poblaciones/Life stages and populations

Seguridad y salud en el lugar de trabajo/Workplace safety and health

Although the CDC health and safety topics are the same in Spanish and English, the pictorial displays are different. For example, on July 11, 2010, the English-language home page pictured beat the heat, hurricanes, hematochromatosis, health literacy, and the Gulf oil spill. The Spanish language home page pictured:

• Cáncer/Cancer

• Envenenamientos/Poisonings

• Adolescentes latinos/Latin adolescents

• Estreptococo/ Streptococcus

• Medicinas/Medicines

In brief, the CDC provides both common and targeted health and safety information to the English and to the Spanish language populations.

This targeting of information for the population served is analogous to providing individualized patient care. Just as people are not going to have the same health concerns, neither do populations. For example, when the diseases and conditions hyperlink is activated on the English language home page the top 5 most requested conditions are ADHD, arthritis, asthma, autism, and avian influenza. When the corresponding link is activated on the Spanish language homepage the top five most requested conditions are alcoholismo (alcoholism), asma y alergias, autismo, botulismo, and calor extremo (extreme heat). While asthma and autism overlap, the others do not, reflecting the different health concerns of the populations accessing the different language sites.

Other government sites also present Spanish language websites. These include the National Institutes of Health (www.nih.gov) and the majority of its institutes, including the National Library of Medicine (NLM). Medline

Plus is an important part of the NLM. Its outline of health themes in Spanish is available (http://www.nlm.nih.gov/ medlineplus/spanish/healthtopics.html). Not available in Spanish at the time of this printing is the National Human Genome Research Institute (www.genome.gov). Of course, the corresponding sites in English are available when accessing www.nlm.gov/medlineplus.

While some government agencies do not possess a Spanish language version, the health education content they possess is available on other Websites. For example, the Drug Enforcement Agency has health information available for parents, young adults, and teachers, but in the English language only. However, drug abuse information is available in the Spanish language through the Centros para Control y la Prevnción de Enfermedades/Centers for Disease Control and Prevention and the Instituto Nacional sobre el Abuso de Drogas (NIDA, siglas en inglés)/National Institute on Drug Abuse (NIDA).

Some government Websites do not possess a Spanish-language version but have some Spanish language Web pages and documents. For example, the Centers for Medicare and Medicare Services post Spanish-language pages that relate to HIPAA educational material (http://www.cms.gov/ EducationMaterials/06_MaterialEducativoenEspañol. asp#TopOfPageinformation). In summary, there is considerable health information available in Spanish through government Websites.

There are many organizational domains that are devoted to Hispanic healthcare. For example, access the National Hispanic Nurses Association (http:// thehispanicnurses.org/2010conference/NAHN%20 35th%20Annual%20Conference%20Brochure.pdf). Note that the topic of the 2010 conference focuses on transforming policy to support healthy communities for Latinos. Its two keynote speakers are exceptional national and international leaders and consultants. They are Drs. Carmen Portillo and Barbara Aranda-Naranjo.

Other health-related organizations include:

• National Alliance for Hispanic Health, a members only Website, displayed in English, with health related topics (http://www.hispanichealth. org/)

• National Council of La Raza, with a section on health and nutrition (http://www.nclr.org/) and its own Institute on Hispanic Health (http:// www.nclr.org/content/programs/detail/1452/). News notices are in Spanish

Note that in each of the organizations cited, health is addressed as a community issue more than as an individual with a disease issue. Community and policy development are central to the manner in which these organizations address health.

There are several professional organization Websites where health information in Spanish is available. They include:

- NOAH (http://www.noah-health.org/)
- New York Department of Health (http://www. health.state.ny.us/es/index.htm)
- Organización Panamericana de la Salud/ Panamerical Health Organaization (http://new. paho.org/hon/index.php?option=com_content&t ask=view&id=277&Itemid=229), through which is the Organizatión Mundial de la Salud/World Health Organization
- American Diabetes Association (http://www.diabetes.org/ espanol/?utm_source=Homepage&utm_ medium=MainNav&utm_ campaign=ESPANOL)
- American Cancer Society (http://www.cancer. org/Espanol/index)

The above information represents readily available and reliable sources of patient information. Their use is intended to improve the quality of healthcare provided to those who prefer Spanish language literature and Websites.

ADVANCED PRACTICE NURSING EDUCATION AND WEB-BASED ELECTRONIC CLINICAL LOGS

Clinical information systems are integrated into the planning, delivery, and evaluation of patient care. In a parallel manner, clinical education information systems are integrated into clinical coursework. Electronic logs allow advanced practice nursing students to plan, document delivery, evaluate outcomes and track clinical learning. These logs complement graduate nursing education and clinical specialties within allied health fields, dental hygiene, and communication sciences.

The concept of a clinical log is not new. Its transition to electronic media is relatively new. This transition is accompanied by standardization of data entry. Standardization leads to increased ease in communicating, analyzing, and grading student performance. Since data entry is standardized, logs allow for the rapid analysis of information, encounter length and complexity, and type of diagnostic experiences. In turn, this data may be used

to benchmark individual student and program performance (http://www.medscape.com/viewarticle/708590) (Squires, R. Electronic Clinical Logs, 2009).

To maximize the educational utility of the electronic log, faculty need to access it frequently and interact with students about their logged experiences. This interaction enhances student practice. For example, lower than expected adherence to evidence-based guidelines can be noted and corrected.

The benchmark functions of the electronic log help insure that clinical experiences reflect the program's population foci, curriculum and goals. For example, family nurse practitioner students log the number of patients they see within pediatric, young adult, middle, and older adult age ranges. Program-identified age distribution benchmarks for the individual student may be easily evaluated as well as the adequacy of the age distribution benchmarks for the program as a whole. In brief, the electronic log provides an efficient structure for student and program evaluation.

The electronic logs allows for the capturing of data reflecting student experiences within several fields (http://www.medscape.com/viewarticle/708590), including:

- Patient information (eg, demographics, diagnoses/diagnostic work-up, treatment plan/ interventions)
- Student progress (eg, clinical year/track, level of responsibility in the patient encounter, clinical competencies, clinical hours, and evaluations)
- Preceptor information (eg, certification, licensure, specialty, curriculum vitae, contact information, and professional history, and student evaluations of the preceptor)
- Clinical site data (eg, contact information, mission, services, and student evaluations of the clinical site)

Student progression through a curriculum is reflected in evidence-based guidelines:

- Selected advanced assessment information (eg, chief complaint, history of present illness, past medical/health history, family history, social history, review of systems, physical examination)
- Diagnosis (eg, differential diagnoses, diagnoses and coding, diagnostic tests (eg, laboratory, cytology, imaging)
- Treatment plan (eg, medications, lifestyle modifications, activity, symptom management, biopsy, referrals/consultations)

- Outcomes (eg, tracking of physical exam, laboratory, imaging, diet, activity, weight changes)
- Summary clinical competencies (interprofessional collaboration, consultation, patient referral, career development)

For example, a beginning primary care nurse practitioner student in an assessment course focuses on assessment and diagnosis in the healthy patient and in those with acute self-limited conditions and controlled chronic illnesses. An intermediate level student in a clinical management course not only assesses and diagnoses the patient, but also codes the diagnoses, develops a treatment/therapeutic plan, and evaluates outcomes upon the patient's return. An advanced student in a summary clinical practicum conducts a patient visit in an organized, skilled, and independent manner, entering all data points as well as integrating into practice interprofessional collaboration, consultation and sophisticated referral competencies. Aggregation and analysis of the electronic data is useful in developing a professional career portfolio.

An issue with the accuracy of the clinical log arises when students delay data entry. Some students do not use point-of-care entry. They write notes on paper and then enter the data at later time. This:

- Duplicates student work
- Likely decreases satisfaction with learning
- Decreases reliability of the data due to its reliance on recall, even with notes
- May decrease critical and reflective thinking about the actual patient encounter

Ease with data entry and retrieval is important. Software capabilities commonly considered in the selection of electronic logs include (Squires, 2009):

- Individual and aggregate report capabilities
- Data entry ease
- Access options (PDAs, smart phones, laptops, tablets, desktop computers)
- Search and retrieval ease
- Security
- HIPAA-compliance
- Instruction and interaction ease
- Clinical information and decision support capabilities
- Alert capability and architecture of the alert

- Other, e.g, affordability, compatibility, data stewardship

For more complete information on the electronic clinical log, including vendors, access http://www.medscape.com/viewarticle/708590

Not all electronic clinical logs include nursing terminologies. Although taught that advanced practice nursing is different from that of a physician assistant, the nurse practitioner student may be unable to articulate clearly their own discipline's concrete contribution to the clinical encounter. Standardized nursing terminology (eg, NANDA, NOC, and NIC) provide a structure for students to explore the phenomena of concern for advanced practice nursing (what we diagnose), what outcomes we expect to influence, and what interventions/treatment we employ to affect those outcomes.

The electronic clinical log is a useful pedagogic and educational administration tool. It documents growth in clinical performance even as it build competency in informatics and insight into its capability.

REFERENCES

American Medical Association (2004). *International Classification of Diseases*. 9th ed. Clinical Management IDC-9 CM(2004).

Borreli, F., & Izzo, A. A. (2009). Herb-drug interactions with St John's wort (Hypericum perforatum): an update on clinical observations. *The AAPS Journal, 11*(4):10–27.

Carter, J. (1973). Personal communication to M.A. Lavin.

Dutta, S., & Mia, I. (2011). Global Information Technology Report 2009–2010: ICT for Sustainability. Geneva, Switzerland: *World Economic Forum*.

Gebbie, K., & Lavin, M. A. (1975). *First national conference on the classification of nursing diagnoses*. St. Louis: Mosby.

Indiana University-Purdue University. School of Medicine (2009) version 5. http://medicine.iupui.edu/clinpharm/ddis/

Izzo, A. A., & Ernst, E.(2009). Interactions between herbal medicines and prescribed drugs: an updated systematic review. *Drugs, 69*(13):1777–1798.

Kravitz, R. L., Greenfield, S., Rogers, W., Manning, W. G., Jr., Zubkoff, M., Nelson, E. C., Tarlov, A. R., Ware, J. E., Jr. (1992). Differences in the mix of patients among medical specialties and systems of care. Results from the medical outcomes study. *Journal of the American Medical Association, 267*(12):1617–1623.

Lavin, M. A., Avant, K., Craft-Rosenberg, M., Herdman, T. H., Gebbie, K. (2004). Contexts for the study of the economic influence of nursing diagnoses on patient outcomes. *International Journal of Nursing Terminology and Classification, 15*(2):39–47.

Lavin, M. A., Krieger, M. M., Meyer, G. A., Spasser, M. A., Cvitan, T., Reese, C. G., Carlson, J. H., Perry, A. G., McNary, P. (2005). Development and evaluation of evidence-based nursing (EBN) filters and related databases. *Journal of the Medical Library Association, 93*(1):104–115.

Madabushi, R., Frank, B., Drewelow, B., Derendorf, H., Butterweck, V. (2006). Hyperforin in St. John's wort drug interactions. *European Journal of Clinical Pharmacology, 62*(3):225–233.

Martin, K.S. (2005) Omaha System. http://omahasystem. org.

Martin, K. S., Elfrink, V. L., Monsen, K. A., Bowles, K. H. (2006). Introducing standardized terminologies to nurses: Magic wands and other strategies. *Studies in Health Technology and Informtics. 122*:596–599.

Murakami, Y., Tanaka, T., Murakami, H., Tsujimoto, M., Ohtani, H., & Sawada, Y. (2006). Pharmacokinetic modelling of the interaction between St John's wort and ciclosporin A. *British Journal of Clinical Pharmacology, 61*(6):671–676.

NANDA-International (2009–2011). *Nursing diagnoses: Definitions and classification. Indianpolis, IN: Wiley-Blackwell.*

Nightingale, F. (1859). *A contribution to the sanitary history of the British army during the late war with Russia.* London: Harrison and Sons.

Nowack, R. (2008). Review article: cytochrome P450 enzyme, and transport protein mediated herb-drug interactions in renal transplant patients: grapefruit juice, St John's Wort - and beyond! *Nephrology, 13*(4): 337–347.

Ong, W. J. (1982). *Orality and literacy: The technologizing of the word.* London: Methuen.

Saxena A., Tripathi K.P., Roy S., Khan F., & Sharma A. (2008). Pharmacovigilance: effects of herbal components on human drugs interactions involving cytochrome P450. *Bioinformation, 3*(5):198–204.

Ware, J.E., Jr., & Sherbourne, C.D. (1992). The MOS 36-item short-form health survey (SF-36). I. Conceptual framework and item selection. *Medical Care, 30*(6):473–483.

Warren, J. (2011). Electronic mail communication of April 9, 2011 to the Nursing Informatics Working Group of the American Medical Information Association.

Webster, P.C. (2011). Experts call for health infoway "watchdog". *Canadian Medical Association Journal, 183*(3):298–299.

World Health Organization. (1992). International Classification of Diseases (9th ed.).

World Health Organization. (2002). International Classification of Functioning in Health & Disability. http//apps.who.int/classification/icfbrowser.

World Health Organization. (2007). International Classification of Diseases (10th ed.). http://apps.who. int/classifications/apps/icd/icd10online

World Health Organization. (2011). Global Observatory for eHealth Series: Volume 1. Atlas: eHealth Country Profiles. Geneva, Switzerland: WHO.

Yang, C.Y., Chao, P.D., Hou, Y.C., Tsai, S.Y., Wen, K.C., & Hsiu, S.L. (2006). Marked decrease of cyclosporin bioavailability caused by coadministration of ginkgo and onion in rats. *Food and Chemical Toxicology, 44*(9):1572–1578.

Updates to the references can be found at *www.slu.edu/x20050.xml*

31

IT for the Rural Healthcare Market

Susan H. Lundquist / Cathy Delmain

• OBJECTIVES

1. Identify the key challenges facing the rural healthcare market.
2. Relate the implications of these challenges to information technology (IT) acquisition and implementation for small rural hospitals.
3. Describe the impact of industry initiatives, such as ARRA and quality performance measurement, on the rural and critical access hospitals.
4. Describe IT acquisition and implementation options for rural hospitals.

• KEY WORDS

Rural healthcare
Critical access hospitals
Health information technology
IT vendors

INTRODUCTION

Information technology (IT) has become widely recognized as a tool that supports clinicians in day-to-day practice, offering the potential to reduce medical errors and promote quality evidence-based care. In an American Hospital Association (AHA) survey it was noted that IT is assuming a larger and much more influential role in hospitals. Furthermore, it has become central to the national healthcare debate (AHA, 2007). With additional focus on IT as the result of the American Recovery and Reimbursement Act (ARRA) of 2009 and defined meaningful use criteria, organizations are actively looking at how they can accelerate their IT initiatives in an effort to reap financial incentives. Demonstrating meaningful use of healthcare IT is a journey, not a destination, and the ultimate goal is the management and delivery of exceptional, high-quality patient care for all Americans.

Rural hospitals, while faced with numerous challenges, are actively engaged in the adoption and implementation of IT and like their more urban colleagues understand the value and potential to be achieved with a realistic and solid roadmap for IT. They are also very involved in evaluating their organizations' abilities to meet meaningful use criteria in order to receive the outlined incentives. So while distinct differences in rural and urban healthcare settings are very apparent, the rural healthcare provider is very focused on many of the same strategic objectives seen in larger healthcare facilities, including that of the IT initiative.

To consider the applicability of information technology for rural healthcare settings, one must first consider the definition of "rural." The definition of the term rural is often broad and left to interpretation based on where and how it is being used. To most, the term rural implies large and isolated areas of an open space and countryside with a low population density. In today's world of instant communication, social networking, and ubiquitous Internet access, rural communities can now be connected to almost anywhere at anytime, thus changing the view of "isolation" and "remote."

The Rural Assistance Center states that currently three government agencies hold definitions of what is rural in use: the U.S. Census Bureau, the Office of Management and Budget, and the Economic Research Center of the U.S. Department of Agriculture (USDA). They and other organizations continue to strive for more precise definitions to fit new programs as the demographics of the United States are constantly changing. The number of rural counties fluctuates over time, and disparities with old designations continually exist. The need for a clearer definition to meet the needs of new programs and new policies has encouraged other agencies to create more detailed definitions such as found in the collaboration between the WWAMI Rural Health Research Center (2010) and the Economic Research Service of the USDA (2007). Agencies involved with rural health and human services will continue to evolve and adapt themselves, striving to better serve the needs of the rural population, for what is rural today will most likely change as we move on into the new millennium (Rural Assistance Center, 2010a).

The U.S. Census Bureau initially defined specific urban entities. An urbanized Area (UA) has an urban nucleus of 50,000 or more people. Individual cities with a population of 50,000 may or may not be contained in these UAs. Urbanized areas have a core (one or more contiguous census block groups, or BGs) with a total land area less than 2 square miles and a population density of 1000 persons per square mile. They may contain adjoining territory with at minimum 500 persons per square mile and encompass a population of at least 50,000 people. An urban cluster (UC) also has a core as identified above with a total land area of less 2 two square miles and a population density of 1000 persons per square mile. They may contain adjoining territory with at minimum 500 persons per square mile and encompass a population of at least 2500 but less than 50,000 persons. The Census Bureau's classification of "rural" consists of all territory, population, and housing units located outside of UAs and UCs (U.S. Census Bureau, 2009; (Agency for Healthcare Policy and Research, 1996). To further clarify, the USDA states that "rural areas comprise open country and settlements with fewer than 2,500 residents; areas designated as rural can have population densities as high as 999 per square mile or as low as 1 person per square mile" (USDA, 2010).

THE FACE OF RURAL AMERICA

The face of rural America is vastly different than what is typically seen in urban counterparts. To understand the impacts to healthcare, it is important to consider some of the challenges facing rural America.

The USDA's Rural Information Center states that the well-being of America's rural people and places depends upon many things; the availability of good-paying jobs, access to critical services such as education, healthcare, and communication; strong communities; and a healthy natural environment to name a few. And while urban America is equally dependent upon these things, the challenges to well-being look very different in rural areas than in urban. Small-scale, low-density settlement patterns make it more costly for communities and businesses to provide critical services. (USDA, 2010)

The National Rural Health Association states that up to 25 percent of U.S. residents reside in rural areas. Compared with urban populations, rural residents generally have higher poverty rates, a larger elderly population, tend to be in poorer health, and have higher un-insurance rates than urban areas. Rural Americans more often face greater disparities in healthcare. Economic factors, cultural and social differences, educational shortcomings, lack of recognition by legislators and the sheer isolation of living in remote rural areas all conspire to impede rural Americans in their struggle to lead a normal, healthy life. (National Rural Health Association, 2010)

Consider some of the differences in rural and urban demographics in Table 31.1. Healthcare is one area with noted disparities when considering rural versus urban communities. Numerous challenges face rural citizens as they seek access to healthcare services and each can have a direct effect on their overall health status.

Access to healthcare. Rural residents may have transportation challenges, making access to healthcare difficult. Living in remote and often desolate areas, these residents may have to travel great distances to reach the nearest healthcare facility. Many rural healthcare facilities face great financial stressors which may mean facilities closing. This again may necessitate the need to travel longer distances to seek medical care.

Limited Financial Resources. Rural communities have been hard hit during the recent economic downturn. Businesses have downsized and in some instances have closed. Residents of these areas tend to have a higher rate of unemployment and lower income as compared with their urban counterparts, which may mean a lack of or limited access to health insurance, making availability of healthcare even more difficult. Many may rely on Medicare and Medicaid coverage since private insurance coverage is not always widely available (Center for Rural Affairs, 2010).

TABLE 31.1	National Rural Health Snapshot	
	Rural	**Urban**
Percentage of U.S. population	Nearly 25%	75%+
Percentage of U.S. physicians	10%	90%
No. of specialists per 100,000 population	40.1	134.1
Population aged 65 and older	18%	15%
Population below the poverty level	14%	11%
Average per capita income	$19 K	$26 K
Population who are non-Hispanic whites	83%	69%
Adults who describe health status as fair/poor	28%	21%
Adolescents (aged 12–17) who smoke	19%	11%
Male death rate per 100,000 (aged 1–24)	80	60
Female death rate per 100,000 (aged 1–24)	40	30
Population covered by private insurance	64%	69%
Population who are Medicare beneficiaries	23%	20%
Medicare beneficiaries without drug coverage	45%	31%
Medicare spends per capita compared to U.S. average	85%	106%
Medicare hospital payment-to-cost ratio	90%	100%
Percentage of poor covered by Medicaid	45%	49%

Statistics used with permission from Eye on Health by the Rural Wisconsin Health Cooperative (2002), from an article entitled "Rural Health Can Lead the Way," by former NRHA President, Tim Size, Executive Director of the Rural Wisconsin Health Cooperative.

Health Status. As the incidence of chronic illness increases in the United States, it is found to be even greater in rural areas. This combined with other socioeconomic factors such as lower levels of education, higher poverty rates, and an aging population, contribute to an overall poorer health status for these rural residents.

Healthcare Workforce. The supply of healthcare professionals in rural areas is decreasing and recruitment and retention remain an ongoing challenge. About 20% of the U.S. population lives in rural areas, but only 9% of physicians practice there (Institute of Medicine, 2004). Given the demographic factors facing rural communities, this will have a far reaching impact on availability of healthcare services and the overall health of these rural residents.

Types of Rural Healthcare Facilities

Rural hospitals provide essential healthcare services to nearly 54 million people, including 9 million Medicare beneficiaries (AHA, 2007). Within the definition of rural healthcare facilities, there are a number of types of organizations that may provide healthcare services to these populations, including rural healthcare facility or rural health clinic and critical access hospitals.

A **Rural Health Clinic (RHC)** is a clinic certified to receive special Medicare and Medicaid reimbursement. The purpose of the RHC program is improving access to primary care in underserved rural areas. RHCs are required to use a team approach of physicians and midlevel practitioners such as nurse practitioners, physician assistants, and certified nurse midwives to provide services. The clinic must be staffed at least 50% of the time with a midlevel practitioner. RHCs are required to provide outpatient primary care services and basic laboratory services. RHCs must be located within nonurban rural areas that have healthcare shortage designations (Rural Assistance Center, 2010a).

A **Critical Access Hospital (CAH)** is a hospital that provides essential services to the community and receives cost-based reimbursement from Medicare instead of standard fixed reimbursement rates. Some of the requirements for CAH certification include having no more than 25 inpatient beds; maintaining an annual average length of stay of no more than 96 hours for acute inpatient care; offering 24-hour, 7-day-a-week emergency care; and being located in a rural area, at least 35 miles drive away from any other hospital or CAH (fewer in some circumstances). The limited size and short stay length allowed to CAHs encourage a focus on providing care for common conditions and outpatient care, while referring other conditions to larger hospitals. This reimbursement has been shown to enhance the financial performance of small rural hospitals that were losing money prior to CAH conversion and thus reduce hospital closures (Rural Assistance Center, 2010a).

As of July 2009, there were 1305 certified critical access hospitals in the United States. To become a critical access hospital a facility must be licensed as an acute care hospital (Rural Assistance Center, 2010a).

Beyond the reimbursement topic there are specific features and criteria that relate to a Critical Access Hospital:

Emergency Services. For some communities, the CAH may be the only immediate source of emergency medical attention. A CAH must provide 24-hour emergency healthcare services with medical staff onsite or on-call and available onsite within 30 minutes. Staff onsite must meet state licensure requirements. These facilities provide emergency care with the ability to admit a limited number of patients for an average length of stay no longer than 96 hours.

Community Health Needs. Community access hospitals focus on the needs of the community that they serve. For rural communities, the CAH could be the closest most immediate access to healthcare. The community access hospital must have a relationship with an acute care facility. This agreement applies to handling of patient referral and transfer as well as communication and emergency and nonemergency patient transportation. This ability to align with a larger acute care facility provides great opportunities for rural residents to access and seek specialized healthcare as required.

Flexible Staffing. A CAH must have at least one physician who provides direct oversight to care, but he or she is not required to be onsite. Midlevel practitioners may be on staff and also provide direct care and treatment to patients. For some rural areas challenged in recruiting and retaining physicians this may be beneficial. Staffing levels for nursing in community access hospitals have greater flexibility than acute care organizations that are required to have an RN onsite 24 hours a day, 7 days a week. The Federal requirements allow for the hospital to close (and so have no RN on staff) if the facility is empty. State requirements regarding nurse staffing do vary (Rural Assistance Center, 2010a)

The Potential Role of IT for Rural Healthcare

Increasingly it is accepted that information technology has a major role in healthcare delivery and has largely still untapped potential to support reductions in medical errors, lower costs, and improve the overall quality of care delivery. This applies regardless of type or loca-

tion of the healthcare facility. The Health Information Management Systems Society's (HIMSS) position states that lives can be saved, outcomes of care improved, and costs reduced by transforming the healthcare system through the appropriate use of information technology (IT) and management systems (HIMSS, 2008). It is essential that health IT be harnessed as a tool in transforming healthcare, improving quality by delivering information where and when it is most needed, reducing costs, empowering consumers in their healthcare decisions, and providing for the privacy and security of personal health information. Information technology provides access to comprehensive patient medical information and its secure exchange between healthcare consumers and providers. Wide use of health IT has the potential to improve healthcare quality, prevent medical errors, increase the efficiency of care provision and reduce healthcare costs.

In rural communities, the application of health IT enables the coordination of care as well as the maintenance of the continuum of care across the nation. The implementation and adoption of information technology holds great promise for helping rural residents and rural providers overcome some of the challenges they face in regard to distance and workforce shortages. Information technology whether implemented in larger more urban healthcare settings or in a small rural hospitals or critical access hospitals can support improvements in patient care in a number of ways. According to the Department of Health and Human Services (2010), IT can support care delivery with:

- Complete, accurate, and accessible health information, available at the point of care, allowing for more informed decision making to enhance the quality and reliability of healthcare delivery.

- More efficient and convenient delivery of care, without having to wait for the exchange of records or paperwork and without requiring unnecessary or repetitive tests or procedures.

- Earlier diagnosis and characterization of disease, with the potential to thereby improve outcomes and reduce costs.

- Reductions in adverse events through an improved understanding of each patient's particular medical history, potential for drug-drug interactions, or (eventually) enhanced understanding of a patient's metabolism or even genetic profile and likelihood of a positive or potentially harmful response to a course of treatment.

• Increased efficiencies related to administrative tasks, allowing for more interaction with and transfer of information to patients, caregivers, and clinical care coordinators, and monitoring of patient care.

When considering rural healthcare objectives, one can see a direct correlation to specific health IT capabilities (Table 31.2).

Opportunities for IT in Rural Regions

Advances in information technology hold great promise for helping rural residents and rural providers overcome some of the problems of distance and personnel shortages. Paramount among these advances are a variety of telemedicine applications that enable care to be given without the patient and provider being in the same physical space. These applications include opportunities such as remote monitoring of patients' vital signs, video

TABLE 31.2	National Rural Health Snapshot Comparing Rural Health Objectives and Implications for IT
Rural Healthcare Objectives	**Health IT Applications/ Functions**
Treat patients across a wide region	Distance medicine technologies
Provide access to high-quality care in the face of provider shortages	Online access to patient records
Communicate effectively with other clinicians and patients	Electronic referrals, discharge summaries
Reduce duplication and adverse drug events	E-prescribing using built-in formularies
Reduce unnecessary hospitalizations	Automated drug interaction warnings
Maximize third-party reimbursement	Electronic billing
Reduce administrative costs	Clinical decision support at the point of care
Improve patient compliance with prescribed therapies	Automated patient follow-up
	Disease- and population-specific registries

Source: Federal Office of Rural Health Policy (2006). *Roadmap for the Adoption of Health Information Technology in Rural Communities.*

consultations with off-site providers, electronic picture archiving and communications systems and other teleradiology applications, distribution of prescription drugs and oversight by remote pharmacists, and performance of surgical procedures using robotic assistance.

Apart from the applications that are especially well suited to dealing with problems of geographic isolation and provider shortages, many other types of health IT can play a quality improvement role in rural practices. Indeed, in its 2004 report, "Quality through Collaboration: The Future of Rural Health," the Institute of Medicine assigned a pivotal role to health IT as part of a strategy to ensure quality of care in rural areas. Specific prominent examples of these types of applications include electronic medical/health records (EMRs/EHRs)—often complete with clinical decision support software, electronic prescribing and drug interaction monitoring, and electronic ordering and review of tests; bar coding systems for managing medications and other supplies (eg, Pyxis systems); bedside patient charting and point-of-care monitoring systems; and automated patient tracking and reminder systems. Likewise, rural providers are expected to be important partners in Federal and state efforts to foster the exchange of patient health information across providers as part of the National Health Information Network.

In addition to the benefits to the patient through improved access to care, these applications can reduce the burden on rural practitioners by providing support from specialists and linkages to the larger healthcare system. These options have provided much greater opportunity for health and wellness screening as well as diagnosis and treatment. Internet technology also offers the possibility of delivering interactive continuing medical education opportunities directly to rural clinicians' locations, which can help providers to remain current with medical advances without having to travel to distant conferences and training sessions.

Obstacles to Implementation of Health IT in Rural Areas

The adoption and utilization rates of clinical health IT systems tends to be lower in rural areas than in urban areas. A national survey of American Hospital Association members in 2008 found that comprehensive electronic record systems were uncommon and that larger hospitals, major teaching hospitals, system members, and urban hospitals were more likely to have adopted systems (Jha, DesRoches, Campbell, et al., 2009). Over 95% of critical access hospitals use administrative health IT systems but less than one-third use health IT for clinical care. Rural communities face many challenges in adopting clinical health IT, including limited access to capital and infrastructure, lack of workforce expertise in IT, and difficulty in obtaining community buy-in (Agency for Healthcare Research and Quality, 2010). Previous research has shown that smaller hospitals and those located in rural areas are not as likely to adopt health IT applications. An analysis of eight applications related to medication safety found that rural hospitals had about one-third the adoption rates of urban hospitals; larger, private, not-for-profit, teaching, multi-system, accredited hospitals had higher adoption rates (Furukawa, Raghu, Spaulding, et al., 2008).

As we consider the inherent challenges facing rural communities, it is important to acknowledge that these same challenges have a direct impact on the implementation and adoption of health information technology. Industry observers have cited the primary reasons for the lag in healthcare IT implementation in rural hospitals as being financing the IT acquisition and implementation project and workforce recruitment and retention. Either of these may attribute to a decreased rate of adoption of IT and to struggles in maintaining IT implementation efforts and initiatives.

Financing

Financing constraints are most often stated as the main obstacle to achieving widespread adoption of IT. And while financing such initiatives may affect both urban and rural providers in all healthcare settings, rural providers may find it especially difficult to secure the needed financing. Smaller, stand-alone providers often found in rural areas do not have access to the capital that might otherwise come from system partners or parent organizations. Rural providers also traditionally operate on low margins, making them less likely to have significant savings with which to fund a large investment. Finally, the lower volume of most rural providers means that the fixed costs of an investment will be spread over fewer cases, making it more difficult to recover costs and generate a positive return on the investment. In some instances organizations may be faced with financial choices—expenditures related to overhead and construction versus IT advancement.

As the industry has observed the implementation of health IT can be very costly. Financial challenges range from the acquisition of IT to the costs related to implementation and on-going support.

1. Acquisition of the health information system: The cost of acquiring a health information system can be very expensive, including not only software costs but hardware and networking costs. With limited capital and funding this can be a challenge for rural healthcare providers.

2. Implementation Costs: With the implementation comes the requirement for staff involvement and clinical expertise. As stated earlier, with limited resources available in these settings, costs may be specific to needing to rely on existing staff to cover this effort thus taking away from other areas or the need to acquire services or resources outside the organization to assist in the implementation.

3. Ongoing support and maintenance: Health IT as with almost all technology today requires ongoing maintenance; this may involve the technical resources to apply upgrades as well as the cost of new hardware or peripherals. Most IT vendors require ongoing maintenance and support fees and the costs for this are typically monthly. This increases the organization's expense related to the overall IT initiative.

Limited IT Staff and IT Expertise

Limited availability of in-house staff with the necessary IT expertise is also believed to an additional challenge faced by rural providers. Most rural hospitals and critical access hospitals are unlikely to have IT staff with expertise to understand their IT requirements, research product options, select and work with vendors, configure the facility's infrastructure to implement the new system, and maintain and upgrade the system over the long run. After implementation of a system, these providers will often have to rely on outside technical support, which adds to the ongoing maintenance of the operating cost of the system. In this era of rapidly changing technologies many rural providers have been hesitant to make too large a commitment to IT for fear that they may find that the technology or solution is too soon obsolete.

According to the 2006 Roadmap for the Adoption of Health Information Technology in Rural Communities

> Worries about being able to interface efficiently with legacy systems, being able to exchange data with other systems in the absence of national interoperability standards and common data formats, and being able to ensure data security and continuity of operations in the event of system outages

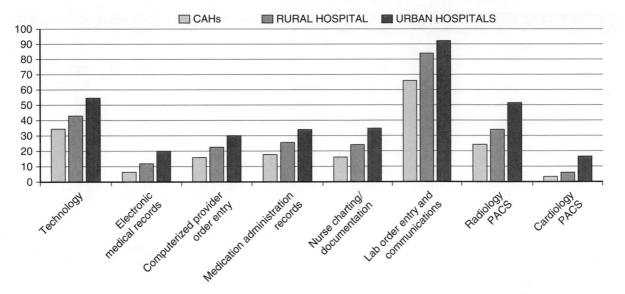

• **FIGURE 31.1.** IT adoption by rural and critical access hospitals. Source: Upper Midwest Rural Health Research Center, Policy Brief, June 2009. Reprinted from *Hospitals & Health Networks*, with permission January 2010. Copyright 2010 Health Forum, Inc.

may all contribute to this hesitancy to make a big investment in health IT at this time. The lack of a convincing business case for many investments – coupled with the fact that providers bear the cost of the investment while the largest benefits accrue to patients and payers – has also slowed the pace of adoption. Although most of these concerns are equally relevant to urban providers, they may cause greater hesitancy among rural providers, who feel that their limited finances afford them only one chance to make the right investment. (Schoenman, Keeler, Moiduddin, & Hamlin, 2006)

A study of health IT use in CAHs concluded that "Medicare cost-based reimbursement has permitted many CAHs to make some initial investments in HIT infrastructure" but found that CAHs had much lower use rates for most clinical applications than larger urban hospitals (Casey, Klingner, Gregg, et al., 2006). Another study found that rural hospitals spend 2% of their annual operating budget on health IT activities, with less activity in smaller rural hospitals (Schoenman et al., 2006). The Institute of Medicine in its 2004 report "*Quality Through Collaboration: The Future of Rural Health*," notes that well-designed health IT systems may open up "many opportunities to improve health and healthcare in rural areas." As you look at the adoption and

implementation of health IT applications (Figure 31.1), note that lab order entry and communications solutions still have the widest use today. Other solutions such as medication administration, nursing documentation, and computerized provider order entry follow with varying degrees of utilization.

To assist in understanding the level of EMR capabilities in U.S. hospitals, HIMSS Analytics created an EMR Adoption Model (EMRAM) that identifies the levels of EMR capabilities. With seven stages, the model ranges from use of a clinical repository to computerized practitioner order entry and closed loop medication administration. Using their EMR Adoption Model, the Healthcare Information and Management Systems Society (HIMSS) found that CAHs had a mean score of 1.89 compared with 3.08 for general medical surgical hospitals and 3.87 for academic/teaching hospitals in early 2010 (HIMSS Analytics, 2010).

In considering trends in EMR adoption, note that HIMSS Analytics provided percentages of CAHs and their progress in meeting the seven-stage EMR Adoption Model (Table 31.3). When comparing all hospitals for 2009 data, HIMSS implies that there is considerable room for growth and IT adoption in community access and rural hospitals still lags behind the general acute care hospitals of more urban settings.

TABLE 31.3	HIMSS Analytics EMR Adoption Model		
2009 EMR Adoption Model Trends			
		2009 Final	**2009 CAH Q4**
Stage 7	Medical record fully electronic; HCO able to contribute CCD as by product of EMR; Data warehousing/mining	0.7%	0.0%
Stage 6	Physician documentation (structured templates), full CDSS (variance & compliance), full R-PACS	1.6%	0.1%
Stage 5	Closed loop medication administration	3.8%	1.8%
Stage 4	CPOE, Clinical Decision Support (clinical protocols)	7.4%	3.8%
Stage 3	Clinical documentation (flow sheets), CDSS (error checking), PACS available outside Radiology	50.9%	33.1%
Stage 2	Clinical Data Repository, Controlled Medical Vocabulary, CDSS inference engine, may have Document Imaging	16.9%	18.0%
Stage 1	Ancillaries–Lab, Rad, Pharmacy–All Installed	7.2%	13.3%
Stage 0	All Three Ancillaries Not Installed	11.5%	30.0%

Source: HIMSS Analytics Database. Used with permission from HIMSS Analytics 2010. Copyright 2009 HIMMS Analytics.

ARRA and the Rural Hospital

With the passage of the American Recovery and Reimbursement Act of 2009 (ARRA), we are seeing even greater emphasis on the use of information technology in healthcare. The program which authorizes the Centers for Medicare and Medicaid Services (CMS) to provide reimbursement incentives for eligible professionals and hospitals who can demonstrate meaningful use of certified EHR technology will occur in stages. It is widely acknowledged that the program, designed to drive greater adoption of IT, is all about increasing the quality of healthcare for American citizens while at the same time reducing the cost of that care.

The legislation requires use of certified electronic health record (EHR) technology that provides for "the exchange of health information to improve the quality of healthcare" and submission of information on clinical quality measures and other measures selected by the Secretary of Health and Human Services. The EHR must include patient demographic and clinical health information and have the capacity to provide clinical decision support, support physician order entry, capture and query information relevant to healthcare quality, and exchange and integrate electronic health information with other sources (American Recovery and Reinvestment Act of 2009).

Meaningful use occurs in three stages with stage 1 beginning in 2011. The proposed stage 1 criteria for meaningful use focus on electronically capturing health information in a coded format, using that information to track key clinical conditions, communicating that information for care coordination purposes, and initiating the reporting of clinical quality measures and public health information (CMS, 2007). Subsequent stages will be defined in future CMS rule making.

As the industry evaluates the definition of meaningful use there are rural advocates that will undoubtedly consider the criteria either too stringent, making it too difficult for many to make any major progress or too lax, with little real impact or effect on the adoption or wider deployment of IT. The criteria and timeline are the same for all hospitals. With little variation in the incentive payments and reimbursement many rural hospitals that have not been actively engaged in the deployment of IT will have an uphill road ahead of them.

Comments issued to the health IT policy committee from the National Rural HIT Coalition, state that "the 2011 meaningful use draft requirements roughly correspond to reaching stage 4 of the 7 stage Healthcare Information Management Systems Society (HIMSS) Electronic Medical Record (EMR) Adoption model and that CAHs and rural acute care hospitals average 1.2 on HIMSS EMR Adoption Scale, whereas general medical-surgical hospitals average 2.5." Furthermore, they emphasize, "Many CAHs and rural acute care hospitals will need to address critical network infrastructure and HIT staff expertise challenges that will also add to the "reasonable" time required" (Wisconsin Office of Rural Health, 2010).

The question at hand is: how successful small rural hospitals will be in meeting identified meaningful use criteria and can they achieve this in the required timeframes? The greatest challenge for rural healthcare providers will be in implementing computerized provider order entry (CPOE). The implementation of CPOE typically occurs later in the IT implementation timeline, and after other prerequisite applications are installed. Given that rural hospitals lag behind in most areas related to the health IT implementation, addressing CPOE within a very short timeframe will become a major challenge for many organizations.

To support the achievement of ARRA health IT initiatives, the Office of the National Coordinator for Health IT has set aside additional funding for regional health IT extension centers to assist small rural hospitals and critical access hospitals set up IT systems. Because of the challenges faced by these providers they require additional support in selecting IT solutions, dealing with vendors and implementing systems. The goal of these centers is to provide the technical support rural healthcare organizations need for not only the initial efforts related to IT deployment but ongoing support as well. The goal is that by offering these types of services for the small rural hospital that they may in fact be able to achieve meaningful use.

Positive Outcomes with IT

The Roadmap for the Adoption of Health Information Technology in Rural Communities published by the NORC Walsh Center for Rural Health Analysis states that

> In addition to their consequences for patient safety and outcomes, health IT projects can address a variety of business needs. For example, distance-shrinking projects, such as telehealth, can expand the organization's potential patient base. This may allow development of economies of scale - for example, a group that has multiple small clinics may be more effectively able to centralize business functions such as IT staff, billing, and human resources. Drawing on a larger base of patients can also help support specialists who otherwise would not have sufficient workload to justify traveling long distances to see patients or working in smaller communities…. Electronic Health Record (EHR) implementation may also affect an organization's business model. Digitizing records can reduce storage needs and allow staff resources to be used in other ways. Electronic billing and prescribing can improve accuracy and compliance. In the longer term, use of EHRs can lead

to better continuity of care, reductions in unnecessary treatment, and other efficiency improvements. (Schoenman et al., 2006)

Considering these examples the use of IT as a tool to support both administrative activities as well as clinical practice can be seen as a positive impact to the overall hospital operations. Technology has the ability to reduce barriers and limitations of specific settings and can also support the delivery of high quality, evidence-based care.

Quality Management—Measuring Success With the Rural Health IT

Numerous studies have assessed the relationship between health information technology and clinical quality. Several studies demonstrate that hospitals experience error reductions subsequent to IT adoption (Kuperman et al., 2003) and suggest that HIT may reduce mortality and improve quality. Some of this may be due to more progressive adoption of health IT in hospitals already demonstrating high quality care.

Critical access hospitals are not required to submit data on Medicare core measures to the CMS, but many are encouraging small hospitals to do so voluntarily (Weinstock, 2010). While critical access hospitals have different reimbursement schemes than the typical prospective payment hospital they too are being scrutinized for their success related to quality measures. It is critical for rural hospitals to meet the requirements of CMS core measures to demonstrate that they are delivering high-quality care. To demonstrate clinical excellence, performance on the CMS core measures must be 100% (Goodspeed, 2006). Small rural and critical access hospitals understand the importance of addressing quality metrics and are increasingly adopting strategies to help them demonstrate their ability to deliver clinical excellence regardless of their location or size.

As hospitals, large and small, look for ways to increase quality, they routinely turn to their IT solutions to assist them in evaluating the effectiveness of their quality initiatives. For most, the evaluation process involves determining which metrics they want to focus on and prioritizing them. Following that, they must carefully consider how well positioned the IT solution is to assist them in; capturing the data they need to monitor, providing analytical tools for measurement and trending and supporting reporting capabilities that can provide dashboards and views for clinicians and leadership who require the ability to review ongoing clinical performance. As a by-product of care delivery,

CAH participation in hospital compare has risen steadily...

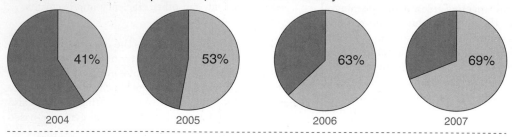

| 41% | 53% | 63% | 69% |
| 2004 | 2005 | 2006 | 2007 |

...and care has improved steadily as well.

Percent of surgical patients receiving preventive initial antibiotic one hour before incision, 2005-2007

	CAHs	Rural PPS	Urban PPS
2005	72.8%	78.0%	82.2%
2006	79.5	81.3	85.4
2007	86.3	87.9	89.2

Percent of heart failure patients receiving discharge instructions, 2005-2007

	CAHs	Rural PPS	Urban PPS
2005	51.0%	57.2%	58.6%
2006	58.4	67.4	69.7
2007	64.5	73.9	77.0

• **FIGURE 31.2.** Critical access hospitals and quality. Source: Flex Monitoring Team (Universities of Minnesota, North Carolina at Chapel Hill and Southern Maine), Critical Access Hospital Year 4 Hospital Compare Participation and Quality Measure Results, September 2009. Reprinted from Hospitals & Health Networks with permission January 2010. Copyright 2010, by Health Forum, Inc.

nurses document patient assessments, clinical observations, the patient plan of care, and evaluation of that care. If documented electronically, IT systems with associated reporting tools can generate reports for periodic review of progress and areas still needing improvement. Information technology as a tool provides the ability to measure quality leading to ongoing processes to monitor and improve clinical performance.

A greater number of rural hospitals do participate in efforts, such as the Centers for Medicare & Medicaid Services, the Department of Health and Human Services, Hospital Compare program, and they recognize the importance of transparent communication of their success with clinical metrics. With this there has also been a positive increase in metrics surrounding care related to specific diagnoses (Figure 31.2). The goal of high-quality care applies to all organizations regardless of size or geographic location.

IT Readiness of the Rural Hospital

As rural and community access hospitals consider their IT initiatives it is important that they first evaluate their readiness for the IT implementation. Before embarking on the implementation of any new system providers should carefully assess any legacy systems that are in place at the organization. Through this evaluation the

organization can determine whether the best strategy will be an upgrade or rebuild instead of starting the evaluation for a new IT solution. This review will include, just like the more urban healthcare providers, an understanding of the regulatory requirements for hospital accreditation as well as those to achieve meaningful use.

And again as with larger more urban hospitals, rural healthcare organizations must take time to plan their IT implementation. This includes the objectives of the effort, priority of the items in the plan, hardware and software costs and requirements, and project timeline and milestones as well as resources. While resources in rural hospitals for this type of effort are very often limited it will be important to include key stakeholders in the process from the beginning promoting a collaborative environment. Leadership engagement in the rural IT effort is just as important as it is in the larger urban hospital organization. These steps, while all similar to IT efforts in larger healthcare organizations, require special focus and attention in more rural settings due to the challenges facing these organizations.

IT Solutions Addressing the Rural Healthcare Market

Selecting a vendor that best fits a rural healthcare setting requires the organization to take the time to become familiar with the company's background and reputation, the types of providers and market it typically serves and the extent of IT support its staff will provide during and after the implementation. There are vendors that are committed to providing services for small and rural clinics as well as hospitals (Table 31.4). Rural healthcare organizations interested in implementing a health IT application should consider participating in forums that discuss the challenges they face in an IT acquisition and implementation. It will also be worthwhile to review solutions that are certified as meeting identified standards for quality, interoperability, and security and privacy. Moving ahead and looking carefully at the requirements for demonstrating meaningful use, hospitals will be required to use a system certified by the Office of the National Coordinator for Health Information Technology.

Clinical IT solutions most often provide a full range of applications to support clinical practice and this is the same whether providing solutions to small rural healthcare providers or larger, complex healthcare organizations. This will include registration, order entry and care provider order entry, access to labs and results, clinical and nursing documentation, pharmacy and medication administration capabilities. However, there are differences in solutions that have been designed specifically for the rural healthcare market. When considering an IT solution for this specific market there are certain characteristics that are typically seen in these product offerings. Some rural IT vendors provide solutions considered turnkey, or "off the shelf," "out of the box." These solutions are often preconfigured and ready to go. They

do not require hours of implementation time nor do they typically allow for extensive customization. Given the challenges with resources and staffing this may be a more desirable solution for small rural healthcare organizations. Another area of difference is in considering system maintenance and support. Solutions designed for the small rural hospital will usually have limited maintenance schedules and will not require large, highly trained, IT resources to manage them. This can be an asset when considering workforce shortages and the often limited number of skilled IT technicians.

Increasingly, the industry is also seeing a greater presence of the larger health IT vendor in the rural hospital market. Decreasing market space and limited opportunity are forcing IT vendors to reevaluate their portfolios and the markets they have traditionally sold into. Additionally, some of the large IT vendors may have a solution to address this specific market, or they have a solution that can be scaled to this market—offering the larger more complex system but adapting it or modifying it to fill the specific need. For instance, the hospital may be able to acquire a more sophisticated system but be able to consider remote access options or other implementations that will meet some of the constraints of the rural hospital IT department.

Opportunities for Rural Hospitals to Meet the Demand for IT

A number of options are available to small rural healthcare providers as they consider their approach to the IT acquisition and implementation. Many organizations are developing creative alternatives that can minimize the challenges and obstacles faced by these facilities. Carefully evaluating these options and considering how the organization is best suited to each will help to determine the best path forward.

Hosted Service

For example, Hospital A is a 40-bed hospital. Due to their location, as well as the financial state of their facility, they sought an option that would provide them with functional, scalable software, while limiting onsite resource requirements. They opted for a hosted option, where their software vendor actually runs the software on hardware located at their main office. The company provides hardware, performs all needed system maintenance, completes all software upgrades, and offers 24/7 support for all hardware-related issues.

The hospital provides the staff required to perform set up and maintenance of the locally definable tables.

TABLE 31.4	IT Vendors for the Rural Healthcare IT Market

Healthland www.healthland.com

NextGen Healthcare Information Systems, Inc. www.nextgen.com/

Quadramed www.quadramed.com

Healthcare Management Systems http://www.hmstn.com/solutions/

CPSI www.cpsinet.com

Meditech www.meditech.com

Siemens MedSeries4 http://www.usa.siemens.com/medseries4

McKesson www.mckesson.com

Cerner www.cerner.com

They perform analysis of workflow and work with clinical staff throughout the facility to refine and tweak the software to meet the facility's needs. They are also responsible, when software updates are made available, to evaluate new functionality and incorporate into the facility workflows where applicable. The hospital staff also performs all user education, site-specific documentation, and system testing.

The benefits gained by the facility in this type of situation are many. Their rural location makes it difficult to attract high-level technical staff, and financially, affording the salaries commanded by those experts is not possible. However, by moving those job responsibilities out of the hospital, and back on the vendor's data center operations, they can benefit from the expertise, without having to maintain the full burden of cost. In addition, due to higher utilization, the systems in the data center are newer, higher performing machines, and maintained at a higher level of security and performance than a rural hospital would be able to acquire and maintain on their own.

With this option, one of the most costly impacts of IT on a small facility, performing routine upgrades and system maintenance is no longer carried by the hospital. The training for and management of those upgrades, both hardware and software, now sits at the data center.

In return, the hospital does incur some less desirable effects. Many of the events surrounding the hospital information system are controlled within the data center, and not in the hospital's control. Scheduled system maintenance and its accompanying downtimes are dictated, not by the hospital's activities and convenience, but by the data center, who must coordinate the events with many hospitals simultaneously. System security, access policies, and hardware management decisions are dictated to the hospital staff, and may not be what the facility would chose, were they in a position to define these practices. However, the trade-off to the facility of not having to hire and maintain the expertise to perform the activities often weighs in the hospital's favor. The ability to free up their resources to focus in hospital initiatives is an invaluable benefit.

Collaborative Hospital to Hospital Partnership

A newer model of shared risk and benefit is emerging where smaller hospitals partner with larger institutions to provide the information technology. A recent report (Reddy, Sandeep, & Kelly, 2008) described an organization where a major referral hospital provided IT services to the three rural hospitals in its referral region. The center provided the hardware, applications and interfaces, and support services. In this instance, the rural hospitals pay for the services received based on a percentage of the regional facility's hardware dedicated to their use, staff time from the regional hospital, as well as discounted rates for software, license, and maintenance fees. In addition to the economic benefits gained from participating in group purchases, the smaller facilities also had access to technical staff and expertise that, on their own, they would not have been able to afford or recruit.

As this type of relationship develops, it will be incumbent on the larger, sponsoring facilities to assume new role not typically performed by healthcare organizations in the past—that of vendor to other healthcare organizations. This will take a refocusing of some effort and perspective within the IT organizations in these facilities.

Shared Services

Another option is shared services organizations. This option was created in response to the need of several rural healthcare organizations to decrease their purchasing costs by creating a purchasing conglomerate. By banding together, they were able to take advantage of economies of scale, reducing costs, and simplifying purchasing. Originally, the scope of these organizations was limited to capital equipment and operational supplies; but as the need for IT continues to grow, IT solutions are also being offered.

Integrated Healthcare Enterprise

Some facilities, by virtue of their membership in an Integrated Healthcare Enterprise (IHE), are able to take advantage of IT investments by their parent company. While these facilities may have less or no autonomy in the purchasing decisions, they obtain significant gains in being able to feed off the expertise and experience of their larger siblings. Efforts to standardize practices across the enterprise also lend to the rural facilities requiring less local resources, if any, to support the implementation, education and support of the supplied systems. One small rural hospital was able to implement a full clinical information system, including nursing documentation, order entry with computer provider order entry capability, and full results review, including online radiology imaging as a result of this arrangement. In the next year, they will incorporate medication management, including bedside barcoding of medication administration, into their clinical workflows.

This degree of automation is possible because of the relationship within the IHE. The organization at large assumes the responsibility for purchasing hardware, software, and related necessary services. This allows the rural facility to "ride the coattails," gaining the benefit of the purchases, as well as the expertise of the IHE technology staff. Financial obligations associated with these services vary, but may include a monthly portion of the software license or maintenance fees, an hourly charge for resources utilized from the IT staff, and fee-per-use after-hours support. Education, local maintenance, and system support may be staffed from the facility, or from the corporate IT staff.

Managed Services

Managed services is another method for minimizing IT cost, while still accomplishing a significant level of automation, is to outsource certain personnel functions, thereby reducing the staff required by the rural facility.

In this environment, the outsourcing partner provides the staff required to perform set-up and maintenance of the locally definable tables. These analysts work with clinical staff throughout the facility to refine and tweak the software to meet the facility's needs. They are also responsible, when software updates are made available, to evaluate new functionality and work with facility staff to incorporate into the facility workflows where applicable. They also typically will perform all user education, site-specific documentation, and system testing. The facility will maintain a small staff of local informaticists whose job it is, in conjunction with the outsourcing partner, to analyze workflow and identify system modifications and refinements needed within the facility. The hardware may reside within the facility, or be hosted, as mentioned previously.

The Role for Nursing Informatics in Rural Healthcare

Regardless of the model assumed by the rural hospitals to ease the cost and resource burden of implementing information systems, certain activities associated with the implementation of these systems still must be managed by the facility itself. As part of this process it is important to consider the role of nursing in the rural IT initiative and the impact that this role can have on achieving a positive outcome. In many rural and small critical access hospitals nursing staff is already stretched and while it may not be feasible to have a clearly defined nursing informatics role in place there are options to consider. It is critically important when planning for the IT initiative, that organizations do not overlook the contribution of nursing and make the effort to include

nursing in a collaborative team approach. Nurses, as the most visible direct care provider, are familiar with clinical workflow processes. Approaches to filling the informatics role may include participation in the IT project from a few identified staff nurses, a nurse working in the IT department or a more formal nursing informatics resource. The important point is to include nursing early on in the acquisition and implementation process of the clinical IT solution. Nurses from rural healthcare organizations are best positioned to understand the specific needs of their setting as well as those of their patients and communities.

SUMMARY: WHAT DOES THE FUTURE HOLD?

As our world becomes more reliant on technology and the healthcare environment advances to embrace IT as a common tool to support clinical practice, we will see greater adoption and implementation in not only large urban hospitals but those in rural settings as well. Healthcare has become a complex and technologically driven workplace and this will grow to even greater proportions in the years ahead. The future of healthcare will be a world where connectivity of systems sharing secure patient medical information can be accessed instantaneously regardless of where the patient or provider may be physically located. Continued advances in connectivity and networking will expand the medical team's abilities to collaborate on providing medical care and services with wide array of technical solutions. With these sophisticated IT solutions providers, patients, and their communities will be connected and expectations for clinical excellence and safe, quality care, whether in a small rural community or a large urban city will be fulfilled.

REFERENCES

Agency for Healthcare Research and Quality. (2010). *Rural health IT adoption toolbox*. Retrieved May 26, 2010 from http://healthit.ahrq.gov/portal/server.p t?open=512&objID=1135&mode=2&pid=DA_112 7036&cid=DA_1189881&p_path=/DA_1251349/ DA_1127036/DA_1189881&pos=

Agency for Healthcare Policy and Research. (1996). *Improving healthcare for rural populations*. AHCPR Publication No. 96-P040. Retrieved May 25, 2010, from http://www.ahrq.gov/research/rural.htm

American Hospital Association. (2007). *Continued progress: Hospital use of information technology*.

Retrieved June 10, 2010 from http://www.aha.org/aha/content/2007/pdf/070227-continuedprogress.pdf

American Recovery and Reinvestment Act of 2009. (2009). Retrieved May 27, 2010 from http://frwebgate.access.gpo.gov/cgi-bin/getdoc.cgi?dbname=111_cong_bills&docid=f:h1enr.pdf

Casey, M., Klingner, J., Gregg, W., et al. (2006). The current status of health information technology use in CAHs. Flex Monitoring Team Briefing Paper No.11. Retrieved May 27, 2010 from http://www.flexmonitoring.org/documents/BriefingPaper11_HIT.pdf

Centers for Medicare and Medicaid. (2007) Fact Sheets. *CMs proposes definition of meaningful use of certified electronic health records (EHR) technology.* Retrieved June 10, 2010 from http://www.cms.gov/apps/media/press/factsheet.asp?Counter=3564

Center for Rural Affairs. (2010). Search page. Retrieved June 2, 2010, from http://www.cfra.org/search?cx=003400857747283632858%3Ayx1mh_cb9og&cof=FORID%3A11&as_q=healthcare+challenges#946

Department of Health and Human Services. (2010). Health Resources and Services Administration. Rural Heath. *Health information technology.* Retrieved May 26, 2010 from http://www.hrsa.gov/ruralhealth/resources/healthit/index.html

Federal Office of Rural Health Policy. (2006). *Roadmap for the adoption of health information technology in rural communities.* Prepared by NORC Walsh Center for Rural Health Analysis. Retrieved May 26, 2010 from, http://www.norc.org/NR/rdonlyres/6A09114C-1B4D-4834-A942-8D6E0EDB799B/0/HIT_Paper_Final.pdf

Furukawa, M. F., Raghu, T. S., Spaulding, T. J., & Vinze, A. (2008). Adoption of health information technology for medication safety in U.S. Hospitals. *Health Affairs (Millwood), 27*(3), 865–875.

Goodspeed, S. W. (2006). Metrics that help rural hospitals achieve world-class performance. *Journal for Healthcare Quality, 185.* Retrieved June 4, 2010 from http://www.nahq.org/journal/ce/article.html?article_id=263

Health Information Management Systems Society. (2008). *Enabling healthcare reform using information technology.* Retrieved May 26, 2010 from http://www.himss.org/2009calltoaction/HIMSSCallToActionDec2008.pdf

HIMSS Analytics. (2010). EMR scores by hospital type, 1st quarter 2010. Retrieved June 8, 2010 from http://www.himssanalytics.org/hc_providers/emr_adoption. asp

Institute of Medicine. (2004). *Quality through collaboration: The future of rural health.* Washington, DC: National Academic Press.

Jha, A. K., DesRoches, C. M., Campbell, E. G., Donelan, K., et al. (2009). Use of electronic health records in U.S. *hospitals. New England Journal of Medicine, 360*(16), 1628–1638.

Kuperman, G., & Gibson, R. (2003). CPOE: Benefits, costs, and issues. *Annals of Internal Medicine, 139,* 31–39.

National Rural Health Association. (2010). Home page. Retrieved June 2, 2010, from http://www.ruralhealthweb.org/

Rural Wisconsin Health Cooperative. (2002). Rural Health Can Lead the Way. *Eye on health tim size, rural health can lead the way, eye on health* (p. 2). Retrieved June 2, 2010, from www.rwhc.com/eoh.02.pdfyEOHSeptember.pdf

Reddy, M. C., Sandeep, P., & Kelly, M. Developing IT infrastructure for rural hospitals: A Case study of benefits and challenges of hospital-to-hospital partnerships. *Journal of the American Medical Informatics Association, 15*(4), 554–558.

Rural Assistance Center. (2010a). Home page. Retrieved May 25, 2010, from http://www.raconline.org/ Rural Assistance Center. (2010b). *What is rural?* Retrieved June 7, 2010, from http://www.raconline.org/info_guides/ruraldef

Schoenman, J., Keeler, J., Moiduddin, A., & Hamlin B. (2006). Roadmap for the adoption of health information technology in rural communities. Washington, DC: NORC Walsh Center for Rural Health Analysis. Retrieved June 4, 2010 from http://www.norc.org/projects/roadmap+for+the+adoption+of+health+information+technology+in+rural+communities.htm.

U.S. Census Bureau. (2009). *Census 2000 urban and rural classification.* Retrieved June 1, 2010, from http://www.census.gov/geo/www/ua/ua_2k.html

U.S. Department of Agriculture. (2007). Economic Research Service. *Measuring rurality: what is rural?* Retrieved June 1, 2010, from http://www.ers.usda.gov/Briefing/Rurality/WhatisRural/

U.S. Department of Agriculture. (2010). National Agricultural Library. Rural Information Center. Home page. Retrieved June 1, 2010, from http://ric.nal.usda.gov/nal_display/index.php?info_center=5&tax_level=1

Weinstock, Matthew. (2010). *Rural IT and quality: Hospital and health networks.* Retrieved June 1, 2010 from http://www.hhnmag.com/hhnmag_app/jsp/articledisplay.jsp?dcrpath=HHNMAG/Article/data/01JAN2010/1001HHN_FEA_GatefoldRuralIT&domain=HHNMAG

Wisconsin Office of Rural Health. (2010). Hospitals / Clinics / EMS page. Retrieved June 7, 2010, from http://www.worh.org/hospitals_clinics

WWAMI Rural Health Research Center. (2010). Home page. Retrieved June 2, 2010, from http://depts.washington.edu/uwrhrc/index.php

32

Ambulatory Care Information Systems

Susan K. Newbold

• OBJECTIVES

1. Understand information issues in ambulatory care, including regulatory requirements.
2. Restate the functions and benefits of information systems in the ambulatory arena and sources for further information.
3. Describe the state of the art in using information systems in ambulatory care.
4. Predict future trends in ambulatory care information systems.
5. Articulate various roles for nurses in the ambulatory care setting.

• KEY WORDS

ambulatory care information systems
computer physician order entry
American Recovery and Reinvestment Act
e-prescribe
electronic medical records
evidence-based medicine
meaningful use
regulatory requirements

INTRODUCTION

On April 27, 2004, President George W. Bush, announced a goal to establish electronic health records (EHRs) for all citizens within a 10-year time frame. He created the position of a National Health Information Technology Coordinator to develop a nationwide interoperable health information technology (IT) infrastructure. One responsibility for the National Coordinator is to improve "the coordination of care and information among hospitals, laboratories, physician offices, and other ambulatory care providers through an effective infrastructure for the secure and authorized exchange of healthcare information" (White House Press Release, 2004).

In July 2004, Health and Human Services Secretary Tommy G. Thompson announced the "Decade of Healthcare Information Technology" and the publication of a report which reveals how vital it is to have automation in the physician's and ambulatory offices.

The report identified four major goals, with strategic action areas for each (Thompson & Brailer, 2004):

- Goal 1 – "Inform Clinical Practice:" Bringing information tools to the point of care, especially by investing in EHR systems in physician offices and hospitals.
- Goal 2 – "Interconnect Clinicians:" Building an interoperable health information infrastructure, so that records follow the patient and clinicians

have access to critical healthcare information when treatment decisions are being made.

• Goal 3 – "Personalize Care:" Using health information technology to give consumers more access and involvement in health decisions.

• Goal 4 – "Improve Population Health:" Expanding capacity for public health monitoring, quality of care measurement, and bringing research advances more quickly into medical practice.

President Barak Obama's American Recovery and Reinvestment Act (ARRA) of 2009 will invest $19 billion in computerized medical records that will help to reduce costs and improve quality while ensuring patients' privacy (www.recovery.gov). For example, $83.9 million in grants were announced in 2010 to help networks of health centers adopt electronic health records (EHR) and other health IT systems. President Obama reaffirmed the goal of electronic health records by 2014.

Although 43.9% of physicians surveyed by the National Center for Health Statistics (Hsiao, Beatty, Hing, et al., 2009) reported all or partial use of EHR systems in their office-based practices, when one looks at the functions, an estimated that 21% of physician practices use a basic EHR and only 6% use a full EHR. A basic system includes the following functions: patient demographic information, patient problem lists, clinical notes, orders for prescriptions, and the ability to view laboratory and imaging results. A fully functioning system includes all functions of basic systems plus the following: medical history and follow-up, orders for tests, prescription and test orders sent electronically, warnings of drug interactions or contraindications, highlighting of out-of-range test levels, electronic images returned, and reminders for guideline-based interventions (DesRoches, Campbell, Rao, et al., 2008).

WHERE AMBULATORY CLIENTS ARE TREATED

As a response to increasing costs of providing healthcare, the healthcare industry has moved away from the expensive inpatient, acute care environment to caring for clients in various ambulatory care settings. There are numerous organizations that fit within the umbrella of ambulatory healthcare. They include ambulatory clinics and surgery centers, single and multi-specialty group practices, diagnostic laboratories, health maintenance organizations, independent physician associations, birthing centers, and college and university health services.

Other organizations that serve the ambulatory population are faculty medical practices, community health centers, prison health centers, Indian health centers, hospital-sponsored ambulatory health services, urgent and immediate care centers, office-based surgery centers and practices, pain management clinics, podiatry offices, networks, mobile clinics, nurse managed centers, and groups of ambulatory care organizations. Many single specialty providers offer care in settings such as birthing centers, cardiac catheterization centers, dental clinics, dialysis centers, endoscopy centers, imaging centers, infusion therapy services, laser centers, lithotripsy services, MRI centers, ophthalmology practices, oral and maxillofacial surgery centers, pain management centers, plastic surgery centers, podiatric clinics, radiation/oncology clinics, rehabilitation centers, sleep centers, urgent/emergency care centers, and women's health centers (The Joint Commission, 2010).

Issues and Trends in Ambulatory Care

Issues surrounding those who work in ambulatory care are similar across the healthcare enterprise, including increased accountability, the need for continuous and documented service improvements, pressures to control utilization, and the protection of confidential information. Effective reimbursement of services is paramount for continued operation. Goals include improving quality, safety and efficiency, engaging patients and their families, improving care coordiantion, improving population and public health, while ensuring privacy and security protections.

Information System Applications in the Ambulatory Environment

Ambulatory care information systems are designed to store, manipulate, and retrieve information for planning, organizing, directing, controlling, and evaluating administrative and clinical activities associated with the provision and utilization of ambulatory care services and facilities. The applications needed in the ambulatory environment are similar to those required in the inpatient arena. Registration, billing, accounts receivable, accounts payable, patient and staff scheduling, and managed care functionality are the major application areas. The emphasis in the past has been on financial and administrative applications, but organizations are now adding automated clinical applications. The benefits that can be achieved by utilizing electronic records encompass the financial, administrative, and clinical areas for physicians, nurses and hospital executives.

Benefits for the Patients

A major reason for automating the records of ambulatory patients is to to provide for quality patient care that is safe, of high quality, while being cost-effective. An electronic record minimizes paperwork, reduces the number of unnecessary treatments, and lowers the risk of drug and medical error.

Benefits for the Physicians and Other Providers

An electronic health record will help the providers by offering clinical data that is easy to read and analyze—from a mobile device, a home computer, or an office computer. Logging in once to a physician portal will allow access to multiple applications. The system can provide warnings of things that should not be done, providing reminders of what should be done and monitoring what is actually done. Malpractice insurance premiums can be reduced by providing documentation for insurance company claims inquiries and malpractice allegations. Evidence-based treatment options can be selected via an EMR.

Billing is facilitated with the use of an EMR which provides a cost-effective and timely bill submission process resulting in decreased days in accounts receivable, and the reduction of rejected claims. In the financial arena, client benefits need to be verified and accurate insurance information obtained. A correct bill must be submitted to the proper payor. Larger ambulatory care organizations utilize electronic data interchange (EDI) to automate the exchange of data (typically between providers and payors) such as claims, submittals and remittances and health plan eligibility information. Some organizations also provide integrated credit card payment applications so that patients may utilize credit cards which are processed immediately. Payments when received, electronically or manually, must be posted to the proper account. If the payor or the client does not pay the bill within a predefined time period, a collections process must be instituted. The electronic or manual system must support adjudication which is the process of determining which payor pays which portion of the bill. The eligibility process needs to be conducted with each instance of service as clients may have changed insurance plans since the last contact with the healthcare organization. Claims submitted to the payor, if electronic, are edited prior to submission so that charges are paid and not rejected which necessitates further processing, costing time and money.

Benefits for the Nurses

The EMR in the ambulatory arena can provide immediate access to the patient record including their medical history. Clinically, the automated healthcare record can provide a problem list, automated ambulatory care provider order entry, a medication record, vital signs, progress notes, results from the laboratory and radiology departments, flow sheets, growth charts, immunization records, medication allergies, profiles, alerts and reminders and a follow-up system. Multiple users can access information and use the patient record simultaneously. Other applications for the clinical area can encompass a clinical decision support system, e-prescribing, and evidence-based medicine.

A patient master index is the basis for collection of all patient related data. If the ambulatory care organization is part of a greater healthcare enterprise then this master patient index must be integrated into an enterprise-wide index. A master patient index is a central repository for patient/member information across the enterprise including sophisticated tools for querying, updating, and managing the index. It must be able to accommodate multiple patient identifiers so that different locations can maintain their current medical record identification system. The registration system collects patient demographics and insurance information.

Benefits for the Executives

The EMR can support compliance with the Healthcare Portability and Accountability Act of 1996 (HIPAA) as well as meet Meaningful Use regulations. Time spent on collecting information for reporting requirements (eg, The Joint Commission and Centers for Medicare & Medicaid Services [CMS]) can be reduced.

Administrative benefits for implementing an automated information system include a reduction in the size of the record room, reduced time spent finding and delivering charts, increase in the privacy of data, formats that are legible and comply with legal regulations, and the promotion of quality assurance and improved patient satisfaction. Additional administrative benefits for automated ambulatory care records are the ability for home access by physicians and nurse practitioners, alerts for incomplete data, and the integration of clinical data.

The patient scheduling system must link existing scheduling systems so that scheduled activities are coordinated across locations to schedule appointment times, providers, resources, and locations throughout the hospital or organization. The patient needs to be seen at the appropriate time with the proper personnel, equipment, supplies, and chart information.

The physicians and nurse practitioners must be credentialed in order to provide services. Credentialing is the exhaustive verification of the medical licenses and qualifications. Healthcare providers must be recredentialed on a regular basis. An automated system can enhance lookup and maintenance of this data.

Other functions of the ambulatory care environment can be enhanced by electronic information technology for data collection and management. Referrals are required by many health plans when a patient is to be seen (or referred) to another healthcare provider. Automatic transfer of these requests will aid patient care and payment of the bill. The multitude of contracts between the healthcare facility and the payor need to be documented and managed through a contract administration function. Reports must be included in any IT application. Beyond standard reports, the user must be able to generate user-specified reports. Medical record location can be tracked automatically with an automated system.

CASE STUDY

A major private, nonprofit healthcare corporation based in the Midwest embarked on a major IT initiative utilizing a commercially available enterprise practice management and an electronic medical record. Within a 2-year period the system will be further developed and standardized according to specialty practice for more than 500 physician practices with more than 2000 employed providers. The first wave of installations will be practice management (medical billing management, accounts receivables, collections, and patient scheduling). The second wave will focus on the EMR which includes order sets and order entry, e-prescribing, and progress notes.

One major reason for implementation of the EMR in addition to the patient benefits is to meet meaningful use requirements. The term meaningful use (MU) came into existence with the passage of the American Recovery and Reinvestment Act (ARRA) of 2009. The term was later defined in January 2010, finalized in July 2010, and made a precondition for receiving reimbursement by physicians who adopted EMRs. There are now incentive payments for the ambulatory community to implement electronic records by October 2011, which will increase the use significantly. Penalties for non–meaningful users will begin in 2015.

Regulatory Requirements, Codes, and Standards

Accounting for costs can be aided by information technology. Systems must support the Resource-Based Relative-Value Scale (RBRVS) and the Relative-Value Unit (RVU). The RBRVS procedure fee pricing is a model designed by the Department of Health and Human Services (DHHS). In this system, each physicians' Current Procedural Terminology (CPT) code has a relative value associated with it. The payor will pay the physician on the basis of a monetary multiplier for the RVS value.

The ambulatory care arena, just like other healthcare sectors, requires data in order to manage care. The Healthcare Portability and Accountability Act of 1996 requires six code sets. Behind the scenes, a database must be maintained of all the current coding schemes utilized for the ambulatory environment. These include Current Procedural Terminology, 4th Edition (AMA, 2011), the 9th revision of the International Classification of Diseases (ICD-9-CM) moving to ICD-10 (CMS, 2010), the Healthcare Common Procedure Coding System (HCPCS) (CMS, 2010), the National Drug Code (NDC), managed by the U.S. Food and Drug Administration (2010), and the Code on Dental Procedures and Nomenclature (CDT).

CPT Codes describe medical procedures performed by physicians and other health providers. The codes were developed by the American Medical Association (AMA) to assist in the assignment of reimbursement amounts to providers by Medicare carriers. A growing number of managed care and other insurance companies, however, base their reimbursements on the values established by HCFA. The most recent version is CPT 2011 (AMA, 2010).

The **International Classification of Diseases, 9th revision, Clinical Modification (ICD-9-CM)** (CMS, 2010) is based on the official version of the World Health Organization's ICD-9 (2010). It is designed for the classification of morbidity and mortality information for statistical purposes, for the indexing of hospital records by disease and operations, and for data storage and retrieval. Diagnoses and procedures coded in ICD-9-CM determine the diagnosis-related group (DRG) that controls reimbursement by CMS programs, and most other payors. The U.S. is currently using the 9th revision although other countries are using the 10th version (https://www.cms.gov/ICD9ProviderDiagnosticCodes/).

The **International Classification of Diseases, 10th revision, Clinical Modification ICD-10-CM** is the new diagnosis coding system developed as a replacement for ICD-9-CM, Volumes 1 and 2. The compliance date for ICD-10-CM for diagnoses is October 1, 2013.

The **HCFA HPCS** (2010) is a collection of codes that represent procedures, supplies, products, and services which may be provided to Medicare beneficiaries and to individuals enrolled in private health insurance programs. The codes are designed to promote uniform reporting and statistical data collection of medical procedures, supplies, products, and services.

The **National Drug Code** (NDC) system identifies pharmaceuticals for human use in detail including the packaging. Its use is required by the FDA for reporting and it is used in many healthcare information systems to aid in reimbursement. At the end of 2001, there were over 1,313,786 NDC codes. The current edition of the NDC Directory is limited to prescription drugs and a few selected over-the-counter products (FDA, 2010). The directory is available at: http://www.fda.gov/cder/ndc/www.fda.gov.

The **Code on Dental Procedures and Nomenclature** (CDT) is HIPAA-mandated for all dental claims filed on or after January 1, 2009. The CDT is the code set for dental services maintained and distributed by the American Dental Association.

Medicare's ambulatory payment classification (APC) system is a prospective payment system for hospital outpatient services. APCs were mandated by Congress as part of the Balanced Budget Act of 1997 (Public Law 105-32). All covered outpatient services are divided into 451 groups called APCs. Software is available to help ambulatory care organizations determine outpatient payment and verify payment received. It also makes it possible for outpatient managers to determine patterns, to predict cost of resource use and to evaluate managed care and physician contracts.

There are a multitude of other federal, state, and local regulations including those from the Centers for Medicare & Medicaid Services (formerly known as the Healthcare Financing Administration).

Another is **Outcome and Assessment Information Set** (OASIS) regulations for the home care industry (CMS, n.d.). OASIS is a data set for use in home health agencies and is an initiative from the Healthcare Financing Administration. The purpose is to provide a comprehensive assessment for an adult home care patient; and measure patient outcomes for purposes of outcome-based quality improvement.

In the ambulatory care environment there is much emphasis on data at the individual patient level. Also, it is important to aggregate data to view patient care and payment trends.

In addition to Meaningful Use, other upcoming regulatory issues include ICD-10, HIPAA 5010, RAC Audits, and other healthcare reform issues. ICD-10 codes must be used on all HIPAA transactions, including outpatient claims with dates of service, and inpatient claims with dates of discharge on and after October 1, 2013 (CMS, 2010). Currently U.S. organizations are using ICD-9 codes. Version 5010 refers to new healthcare electronic HIPAA transaction standards and must be in place by October 1, 2013. CPT codes will still be in use in the outpatient area. Recovery Audit Contractors (RAC) Audits is the the Centers for Medicare and Medicaid Services (CMS, 2010) initiative to combat Medicare fraud in physician overpayment. Other Healthcare Reform issues may solve some problems but cause problems not yet identified.

Implementation Issues and Challenges

There is a long way to go in implementing clinical electronic health records in the ambulatory arena. Statistics vary as to the prevalence of electronic medical records in the ambulatory area. According to a report by Hing, Hall, and Ashman (2010), in 2006, 22.3% of free-standing ambulatory surgery centers and 29.2% of physician's offices had an EMR system. Hospital-based centers fared better with 29.4% of hospital outpatient departments and 62.4% of hospital-based ambulatory surgery centers using any EMR system. In 2010, according to the American Hospital Association, only 43% of the independent physician practices within the "Most Wired" hospitals can electronically document medical records and only 41% have computerized physician order entry (American Hospital Association, 2010). As mentioned in the introduction the diffusion of information systems may actually be less when one defines the functionalities within the systems.

Doctors view improvements in tablet personal computers, hand-held devices, and wireless networks as assisting in the adoption of electronic health records. Physicians are asking national policymakers to assist in the adoption of IT in the clinical area by offering federal loans, grants, tax incentives, and matching funds.

Many of the stratregies for success in the hospital world apply to the ambulatory care arena. When selecting an information system, several products need to be reviewed based on a needs analysis. Use scenarious which emulate use in the actual environment. Involve all stakeholds in the decision-making process. These personnel include clinicians, information technology personnel, administrators, and anyone else who may be affected by the system. Have a clear project strategy and project plan including times lines and outcomes.

THE ROLE OF THE NURSE AND INFORMATION SYSTEMS IN THE AMBULATORY ARENA

First and foremost, the nurse is a user of the data contained in automated systems. The objective is to take the data and put it together in meaningful ways, making information. An automated system can help in this management of data and the transformation from data to information to knowledge. Reports are generated that can be used in the better management of the health of the patient, managing the adminstrative aspects of the practice, generating financial information, or for conducting research. A nurse may be involved in the selection of an automated system based on a needs assessment of the environment. The ambulatory care nurse may be instrumental in the implementation of an automated system whether the emphasis be administration, financial, or clinical. All nurses must be mindful of the impact of the information system on the confidentiality and security of information.

Resources for Education and Networking

There are resources for those embarking upon the implementation of information systems in the Ambulatory arena. There are member associations, journals, conferences, and Websites that may provide value in the journey toward a full set of applications.

Member Associations Involved in Ambulatory Care

As varied as the types of organizations that serve the ambulatory populations are, so are the organizations which serve the professionals that work in those organizations. Major ambulatory care organizations will be highlighted.

The **American Academy of Ambulatory Care Nursing** (**AAACN**) (www.aaanc.org) is a member organization specifically for nurses. The association was founded in 1978 and has more than 2100 members. The AAACN offers networking opportunities for the membership by geographic location through local networking groups and by specialty practice through special interest groups (SIGs). One SIG for informatics, is working to develop an ambulatory care data set for nursing. The organization also represents ambulatory practice to other political advocacy organizations, to government and quasi-government agencies, and in the federal and state legislative arena. They offer education through publications, electronic media, and conferences. Nurses can seek certification in Ambulatory Care Nursing through the American Nurses Credentialing Center (ANCC), a division of the American Nurses Association (ANA). AAACN Headquarters, East Holly AVE, Box 56, Pitman, NJ 08071-0056; 856-256-2350;aaacn@ajj.com;

The **American Medical Informatics Association** (**AMIA**) (www.amia.org) has physicians and nurses amongst their membership. Working groups include

the Primary Care Informatics Working Group. Their purpose is to promote and encourage the appropriate development and use of medical informatics in the practice, research, and teaching of primary-care disciplines. The current membership of more than 600 includes family physicians, internists, nurse practitioners, pediatricians, geriatricians, academicians, managers, psychologists, informaticians and journalists from 18 countries. American Medical Informatics Association, 4915 St. Elmo AVE, Ste. 401, Bethesda, MD 20814; phone: 301-657-1291; fax: 301-657-1296.

The **Medical Group Management Association** (**MGMA**) (www.mgma.com), founded in 1926 and based in Colorado, is a major organization in the United States representing physicians in group practice nationwide. About 13,700 healthcare organizations and 21,500 individuals are MGMA members, representing more than 275,000 physicians. The organization supports education, networking, job recruitment, research, and political action. MGMA Headquarters, 104 Inverness Terrace East, Englewood, CO 80112-5306; phone: 303-799-1111; toll-free: 877-ASK-MGMA (275-6462); fax: 303-643-4439.

The **American Association of Ambulatory Surgery Centers** (**AAASC or ASC**) (www.aaasc.org) is a member organization that promotes advocacy at the national level through relationships with the CMS and Congress, networking and educational opportunities. ASC represents the interests of ambulatory surgery centers in the United States. ASC™ provides member benefits and services including a focus on legislative, regulatory and other challenges at the federal and state level, Assists state ASC associations, and enhances ASC representation at the state and federal level. ASC has established a political action committee. ASC represents the physicians, nurses, administrative staff, and owners industry before the media, Congress, state legislatures, and regulatory bodies. ASC publishes a bimonthly journal and other publications to inform its members and the public. Also ASC conducts educational programs on a variety of topics. ASC, 1012 Cameron ST, Alexandria, VA 22314; phone: 703-836-8808; ASC@ascassociation.org.

The **Association for Ambulatory Behavioral Healthcare** (**AABH**) (www.aabh.org) is an international organization of ambulatory mental healthcare providers dedicated to the delivery of high-quality psychiatric and chemical dependency treatment within a continuum of care. This membership association which started about 1975 is based in Virginia. AABH, 247 Douglas AVE, Portsmouth, VA 23707; phone: 757-673-3741; info@aabh.org.

American Health Information Management Association (AHIMA) (www.ahima.org) with over 46,000 members is a membership organization of health information management professionals. The purpose is to foster the professional development of its members through education, certification, and life-long learning thereby promoting quality information to benefit the public, the healthcare consumer, providers, and other users of clinical data in any healthcare setting. Many resources are available online and in hardcopy documents. AHIMA, 233 N. Michigan AVE, Suite 2150, Chicago, IL 60601-5800; phone 312-233-1100; info@ahima.org.

The **Healthcare Information Management Systems Society (HIMSS)** (www.himss.org), formed an Ambulatory Information Systems Steering Committee for the purpse of "creating pragmatic resources, tools, and education, on health information technology adoption to improve the quality of care in the ambulatory care setting." HIMSS members also initiated is the Ambulatory Community Health Organizations (ACHO) Task force. The mission is to serve as "the national constituency of ambulatory community health organizations encouraging the informed development and adoption of interoperable HIT to improve the quality and cost-effectiveness of healthcare for the underserved."

The HIMSS Ambulatory Care Initiative was created in response to trends such as the aging population, the increasing prevalence of chronic diseases, and the development of minimally-invasive procedures that can be performed without hospitalization. HIMSS, 230 East Ohio ST, Suite 500, Chicago, IL 60611-3269; phone: 312/664-4467; himss@himss.org.

Journals, Conferences, and Websites as Sources for Education

Healthcare professionals who work in the ambulatory care arena need to keep up with regulatory and practice changes in the environment. Among the ways to obtain an education include journals, conferences, and Websites, as well as membership in organizations.

The *Journal of Ambulatory Care Management* is a quarterly peer-reviewed publication. Each issue focuses on one topic of interest related to ambulatory care. The *Ambulatory Pediatrics* is a publication of the Ambulatory Pediatric Association. The journal, started in 1999, is available online and as a print copy for a fee. *The Journal for Healthcare Quality* is a publication started in 1979 by the National Association for Healthcare Quality.

The *Journal of Healthcare Information Management (JHIM)* is a quarterly, peer-reviewed journal edited specifically for healthcare information and management systems professionals. Each issue of JHIM examines a specific topic in the areas of clinical systems, information systems, management engineering and telecommunications in healthcare organizations. It is published by HIMSS.

Several conferences focus on information technology needs of the ambulatory care arena. One of the best known with the largest attendance is the MGMA (Medical Group Management Association) (www.mgma.com), which provides a wide range of educational programs on topics that medical group practices need to be aware of.

The American Medical Informatics Association (AMIA) (www.amia.org) meets twice yearly, primarily in the Washington, DC area. Over 3000 attendees meet primarily to discuss hospital and clinic use of technology. HIMSS hosts a huge Annual Conference and Exhibition with over 26,000 attendees and 900 exhibitors (www.himss.org). Although HIMSS is primarily focused on hospitals, there is much benefit for those in ambulatory care to attend.

One helpful web site is a U.S. Government site, Health Information Technology: For the future of Health and Care (http://healthit.hhs.gov). This site contains funding opportunities, HITECH programs, Federal Advisory Committees, Regulations and Guidance, ONC initiatives and even a blog. Vendor Websites can also be a useful source of information.

Accreditation Organizations in Ambulatory Care

Accrediting organizations validate standards of practice and promote quality care. A private, nonprofit organization was formed in 1979 called the Accreditation Association for Ambulatory Healthcare (AAAHC) (http://www.aaahc.org). Their mission is to develop standards, and conduct a survey and accreditation program. In 2009, the AAAHC added the Medical home to the types of organizations that it accredits. It is the only accrediting body to offer onsite surveys for organizations seeking medical home accreditation.

COLA (http://www.cola.org), headquartered in Columbia, Maryland, is a nonprofit, physician-directed, national accrediting organization. The purpose of COLA is to promote excellence in medicine and patient care through programs of voluntary education, achievement, and accreditation.

The **National Committee for Quality Assurance (NCQA)** (http://www.ncqa.org) is a private, nonprofit organization dedicated to assessing and reporting on the quality of managed care plans. The NCQA is governed by a board of directors that includes employers, consumer and labor representatives, health plans, quality experts, policy makers, and representatives from organized medicine. The Health Plan Effectiveness Data and Information Set (HEDIS) by NCQA is a standardized, comprehensive set of indicators used to measure the performance of a health plan. It is a tool used by more than 90% of health plans to measure performance on dimension of care and service. NCQA, through the PPC-PCMH program, identifies and recognizes medical practices that demonstrate the standards for patient-centered medical homes.

The Joint Commission (www.jcrinc.com) published the *2010 Standards for Ambulatory Care*. Standards are updated yearly and contain rationales, elements of performance, National Patient Safety Goals, and accreditation policies and procedures for all types of ambulatory care settings. In 2010 more than 1600 free-standing ambulatory care organizations were accredited by The Joint Commission.

Awards for Excellence in Ambulatory Care Informatics

Since 1994, the Davies Awards of Excellence sponsored by the HIMSS has recognized successes, lessons learned, and best practices in EHR implementation and value within the healthcare industry. For example, the 2009 Davies Ambulatory Care Award Recipient was the Virginia Women's Center in Richmond, Virginia (Stout, 2009). The systems used help meet their goals to improve patient care and patient safety as well as financial goals. The EHR changed their practice. It is now easier to provide care with ready access to the patient history and current information. The system changed the team process of taking care of patients as opposed to illegible, nonaccessible patient care record. They are able to utilize digital information to make sure patients have received routine care provided at the right time. This changed the work flows and communication in the practice. By instituting the EHR, the Virginia Women's Center estimated they could reduce the number of full time equivalent per provider and transcription costs by $300,000. Other advantages they anticipated included savings through efficiencies in workflow that would allow increased patient volume and reduce redundancy in paper handling, enhanced revenue cycle management from improved coding, charge entry and billing, better access to utilization data for quality assurance and third-party payor negotiations, as well as database features to maximize the success of their clinical research program. All in all they hope to improve patient satisfaction owing to simplified registration, flexibility in choice of office

location and additional time spent with the provider. They expect a greater job satisfaction among the staff with easier access to charts, streamlined tasks and additional time available to be with the patient. They expect greater physician satisfaction with improved patient safety and flexibility. The ability to complete office work from a remote site was a growing concern among physicians with young families, as well as the obstetrician-on-call who spends many hours in Labor and Delivery.

FUTURE DIRECTIONS FOR THE ADOPTION OF IT IN AMBULATORY CARE

The goals set by President Bush and continued by President Obama with the appointment of Dr. David Blumenthal as the National Coordinator for Health Information Technology has injected momentum into the adoption of automated information systems into ambulatory care. There are financial and quality incentives to utilize computer provider order entry (CPOE) systems in ambulatory care. The biggest area of impact is that of medication safety where it is thought that adverse drug events can be prevented.

Some ambulatory practices are using e-mail, computer interviewing, voice recognition, handwriting recognition, smart card technology, wireless devices, and biometrics. Most are working toward the goal of a paperless record. Automating the physician's offices and ambulatory care practices is a primary step in meeting the goal of electronic health records for all citizens.

There is a major impact on the use of electronic health records due to the billions of dollars in federal stimulus money. The current administration is encouraging thousands of primary care physicians using paper-based medical records to become users of electronic medical records.

SUMMARY

This chapter discussed many concepts for the use of information systems in ambulatory care. The discussion ranged from what applications are helpful in ambulatory care for the patient, physician, nurse, and administration. A case study was used to highlight the implementation of an automated system. Regulatory issues and implementation challenges were discussed. Resources for further education and network were listed. Future directions for the adoption of information technology in ambulatory care are highlighted.

REFERENCES

2010 Standards for Ambulatory Care. (2009). Chicago, IL: The Joint Commission.

American Academy of Ambulatory Care Nursing (AAACN). Retrieved 04/19/2011 from www.aaanc.org.

American Hospital Association News Now. (2010, July 7). *Survey: Hospitals increasing health IT use, but barriers remain.* Retrieved August 15, 2010 from www.aha.org

American Medical Association. (2010). CPT® 2011 *professional edition.* Chicago, IL: AMA.

American Recovery and Reinvestment Act of 2009 (ARRA or Recovery Act) (P.L. 111-5), (2009). Retrieved XX XX, 2010 from http://www.recovery.gov/

Centers for Medicare and Medicaid Services. (n.d.a). HIPAA *overview.* Retrieved August 15, 2010 from http://www.cms.gov/HIPAAGenInfo/

Centers for Medicare and Medicaid Services. (n.d.b). *Healthcare Common Procedure Coding System (HCPCS) code set.* Retrieved August 15, 2010 from http://www.cms.gov/MedHCPCSGenInfo/

Centers for Medicare and Medicaid Services. (n.d.c). *ICD-9-CM Provider and Diagnostic Codes.* Baltimore, MD. Retrieved August 15, 2010 from http://www.cms.gov/ICD9ProviderDiagnosticCodes/

Centers for Medicare and Medicaid Services. (n.d.d). *ICD-10 Overview.* Retrieved August 15, 2010 from http://www.cms.gov/ICD10/

Centers for Medicare and Medicaid Services. (n.d.e). *Outcome and Assessment Information Set.* Retrieved August 15, 2010 from http://www.cms.gov/oasis/

Centers for Medicare and Medicaid Services. (n.d.f). RAC audits home. Retrieved August 15, 2010 from http://www.racaudits.com/Medicare_Fraud_Services_SKD.html

DesRoches, C. M., Campbell, E. G., Rao, S. R., Donelan, K., Ferris, T. G., Jha, A., et al. (2008). *Electronic health records in ambulatory care: A national survey of physicians. New England Journal of Medicine,* 359(1), 50–60. http://www.hhs.gov/recovery/index.html

Hing, E., Hall, M.J., & Ashman, J. J. (2010). *Use of Electronic Medical Records by Ambulatory Care Providers: United States, 2006.* National Health Statistics Report. No. 22. Atlanta, GA. US Department of Health and Human Services, Centers for Disease Control

Hsiao, C-J., Beatty, P. C., Hing, E.S., Woodwell, D. A., Rechtsteiner, E. A., and Sisk, J. E. (2009). *Electronic Medical Record/Electronic Health Record Use by Office-based Physicians: United States, 2008 and Preliminary 2009.* National Center for Health Statistics. Retrieved August 15, 2010 from http://www.cdc.gov/nchs/data/hestat/emr_ehr/emr_ehr.htm

Medical Group Management Association(MGMA). (n.d.). Retrieved 04/19/2011 from www.mgma.com.

National Committee for Quality Assurance. (2010). *HEDIS®.* Washington, D.C.

Stout, K. (2009). 2009 *Davies Ambulatory Care Award Application for Virginia Women's Center Davies.* Richmond, VA. Retrieved August 15, 2010 from http://www.wohit.org/davies/docs/2009_RecipientApplications/VirginiaWomensCenter_Davies09Amb.pdf

The Joint Commission. (2010). *Joint Commission Resources – Ambulatory Care.* Retrieved August 15, 2010 from http://www.jcrinc.com/AC-Resources/

Thompson, T.G., Brailer, D.J. (2004). *The Decade of Health Information Technology: Delivering Consumer-centric and Information-rich Healthcare Framework for Strategic Action.* Washington, DC: Department of Health and Human Services.

U.S. Department of Health and Human Services. (n.d.). HHS.gov/Recovery. Retrieved April 19, 2011 from http://www.hhs.gov/recovery/index.html

U.S. Food and Drug Administration . (2010). *National Drug Code Directory.* Washington, DC. Retrieved August 15, 2010 from http://www.fda.gov/cder/ndc/

White House Press Release. (2004, April 27). *President creates position of National Health Information Technology Coordinator.* Washington, DC: White House.

World Health Organization. (n.d.). *International Classification of Diseases and Related Health Problems: Tenth Revision (ICD-10).* Geneva, Switzerland. Retrieved August 15, 2010 from http://www.who.int/whosis/icd10/

Overview of Post Acute Services

Susan J. Quinn

• OBJECTIVES

1. Describe the current use the Electronic Health Record (EHR) in the post acute service area.
2. Discuss current data set used in home health.
3. Describe two nursing languages used in the post acute service area.
4. Identify potential trends in the post acute service area.
5. Discuss the concept of interoperability related to the EHR.

• KEY WORDS

post acute service area
home care
point of care devices
data sets
interoperability

INTRODUCTION

The delivery of healthcare in the post acute service areas is changing rapidly. Advancements in technology are enablers to the provision of care. As with many recent changes in healthcare, one of the main drivers is reimbursement. The adage that change follows the money is certainly true as a driver for healthcare technology improvements. Healthcare reimbursement is at the forefront of many current and proposed changes. This chapter will provide an overview of both the current uses of technology in the post acute service arena as well as exploring where proposed reimbursement may lead the industry. For the purpose of this chapter, post acute services will be limited to those services provided in the community and not in a facility.

CURRENT STATUS OF TECHNOLOGY IN POST ACUTE SERVICES

The largest segment of the post acute service area is home care. Currently there are approximately more than 9000 Medicare-certified agencies in the country (http://www.chhh.org/awards.html) (last retrieved May 20, 2011). These agencies provide skilled care in the home setting. Hospice is a component of home care that provides palliative and supportive care to patients with a life expectancy of 6 months or less to live. Additionally, large proportions of home care companies provide nonskilled care to patients in their homes by offering aide and companion services. Often these companies also provide private duty nursing in the home as well. Other home care companies provide Home Medical Equipment and Home Infusion. The majority of these companies employ technology to some extent to document care and bill for services rendered.

Home Health

Home health is a subset of home care. Although home Health has been provided in this country by visiting nurse agencies since the late 1800s, it was not until Medicare was established in the mid-1960s that the industry became regulated. Home health companies began to use technology in the 1980s. Initial systems used a DOS-based operating system and were used primarily to track patient diagnosis, admissions, discharges, demographics, physician orders, and staff visit activity. This information was primarily collected to meet reporting requirements and to generate a bill. Using database-reporting tools, home health agencies could produce required statistics.

Changes in legislation and regulations as well as advances in technology expanded the use of technology used in home health. The Balanced Budget Act of 1987 was a major force in promoting changes in the use of technology. This legislation provided the basis for a change in payment methodology from fee for service (payment by the visit) to a prospective payment structure for Medicare recipients. Integral to the payment proposal was the requirement for home health agencies to utilize a standardized assessment tool which would be used to calculate case weight and to monitor and report clinical outcomes.

To measure outcomes, a 90-plus question assessment, Outcome and Assessment Information Set (OASIS), was to be used that would not only be the basis for publically reported outcomes, but it would also enable a case weight to be obtained for each Medicare care recipients' admission. This case weight would then serve as a major component in determining payment for the patient's episode of care.

According to the Centers for Medicare & Medicaid Services (CMS) Website, the focus of collecting data using OASIS is to collect and report performance data by home health agencies. Since Fall 2003, CMS has posted on www.medicare.gov, a subset of OASIS-based quality performance information showing how well home health agencies assist their patients in regaining or maintaining their ability to function. The publically reported outcomes include:

- Improvement in Ambulation/Locomotion
- Improvement in Bathing
- Improvement in Transferring
- Improvement in Management of Oral Medication
- Improvement in Pain Interfering with Activity
- Acute Care Hospitalization
- Emergent Care
- Discharge to Community
- Improvement in Dyspnea (Shortness of Breath)
- Improvement in Urinary Incontinence
- Improvement in Surgical Wound Status
- Emergent Care for Wound Deterioration

OASIS data is risk adjusted based on a complex mythology that allows patients to be compared across home health agencies. The outcomes for each Medicare certified agency are provided and are compared to both state and federal averages. Agencies are to utilize Outcomes Based Quality Improvement (OBQI) approach to improve the individual performance on selected indicators as part of the overall Quality Plan for the agency.

The current version of OASIS (OASIS-C) was implemented in 2010. With the implementation of OASIS-C the focus of the instrument has changed from a tool used to measure outcomes to one that also evaluates the process used to obtain the desired outcomes. Outcomes related to chronic disease are now collected as well. The newly developed items measure the process for immunization, medication management, pain management, fall prevention, depression screening, intervention, care coordination, risk assessment, heart failure, and diabetes. From the focus of the new items, it is clear the CMS is moving towards increased emphasis on chronic care initiatives. Further, it is anticipated that in future years the publicly reported outcomes will serve as a baseline for financially motivating home health providers. Those providers that have the best outcomes will receive a higher reimbursement than those providers that have poor outcomes.

As part of the requirements to use the OASIS, Medicare-certified home health agencies are required to transmit the OASIS data to CMS through their respective state agencies. For home health agencies that did not utilize a commercial software vendor, a state supported tool is provided. This tool is named HAVEN. To utilize HAVEN, agencies would enter the OASIS responses into the software and transmit them to the state on a regularly scheduled basis.

For many agencies, especially the larger ones, the requirement to utilize the OASIS tool as a means to calculate reimbursement and to report finding to CMS, lead agencies moved to an electronic record for both billing and clinical data. Advances in software development that allowed information to be stored in a relational database provided another driver for the use of an automated patient record. In the last decade more and more home health agencies have moved to an electronic medical record (EHR). To that end, a larger percentage of home health agencies have an EHR than have their hospital counterparts. Stolle reviews an in-depth description of barriers and facilitators in an article on the uses of an EHR (Stolle, Steeves, Glenny, & Filsinger, 2010).

A number of home health software vendors provide an EHR system that can be used in home health. Most vendors offer a baseline product of similar features and capabilities. Included in the program are the following modules: referral and admission, scheduling and service utilization, clinical assessment including the OASIS tool, clinical documentation, medication management including the use of a medication formulary which is updated generally on a quarterly basis, billing, which includes aging of accounts, collections and reporting. The systems are used by all home health disciplines that may include nursing, physical therapy, occupational therapy, speech therapy, medical social workers, and home health aides. Most systems have the capabilities to provide the functions that are required by state and federal regulations (CMS, Conditions of Participation). Additional features and functions may also be available to enhance the product. These include the use of additional modules to track payroll, accounts receivable and supply usage. Other enhancements include the use of telephony and wound care-imaging software. Tele-health or remote patient monitoring is also a module provided by the vendors. This capability will be discussed in a separate section of the chapter.

The software application can be hosted on a server located at either the home health agency or at a remote site, or it can be web enabled and hosted by the vendor. A variety of options are available. In the web-enabled model, an annual fee is paid to the vendor to maintain the application.

A detailed overview of the components of an EHR developed in 2006 by the National Institutes of Health National Center for Research Resources can be accessed at www.ncrr.nih.gov/publications/informatics/ehr.pdf.

A study by Thakkar and Davis (2006) on the reasons why the healthcare setting moved to an EHR cited that the motivating factors included the capturing of data and the ability to review and update information. Additionally, 75 % of the respondents indicate that the EHR:

- Improves clinical processes or workflow efficiency
- Improves quality of care
- Shares patient record information with healthcare practitioners and professionals
- Reduces medical errors

Although this study was conducted looking at a broader population of healthcare users, the results are applicable to the post acute settings.

Point-of-Care Technology

Many home health agencies have moved to using point of care (POC) technology to enable ease of documentation. Today the majority of agencies have their clinical staff using POC technology to collect data and document clinical care in the home. It is both more accurate and more efficient to collect information related to the patient at the time of the visit rather than at the end of day. The latter often involves visiting home care staff to make a written note of the visit that is entered into the computer at a later time. When using POC technology, the software is divided into two components. There is a server side application that is generally used by the in office staff and a POC application. In most cases the clinical staff member using the POC device will log into the server application and electronically download the files of the assigned patients. This is accomplished through a synchronization process. The process can be done using either a phone line (dial-up methodology, broadband, or cable) or an Internet connection which is a faster connection to data transfer. At the end of the care day, another synchronization is performed, and the data collected on each patient is uploaded to the server application. To improve the accuracy of data on the server side or to communicate new patient information to the end user, some agencies are now providing their staff with air cards so that data can be synchronized during the business day. There are several technologies used for POC devices. The most common is to use a lightweight personal computer (PC) or notebook. The average weight of these devices is about 2 pounds. The clinical staff easily transports them between visits. A standard PC is not generally used because of their weight. Other devices used are tablet PCs with a touch screen to allow for easier and faster data entry. These devices may also be used to capture patients' signatures for consents for care and other documents that required a written signature. Another popular option is the use of a handheld device such as a personal digital assistant (PDA). Because PDAs are lightweight and small, the clinical staff member can very easily transports them. The downside of the device, however, is the need to frequently change the screen due to the small screen size. As the clinical staff members get older, reading the small screen is a concern and font size may need to be enlarged. This further decreases the amount of data that can be shown on the screen.

One consideration that must be stressed with the use of any POC device is the need to protect the patients' information. Security of the data is of primary importance. Log-ons to both the POC device and the software application are required. Additionally, some agencies have taken to tracking POC devices electronically and have the ability to remotely destroy the contents of the device if it is lost or stolen.

Reporting capabilities are an integral part of having an EHR. Some vendors have built in a variety of report options. Others have limited reporting capabilities built into the software. This capability should be explored when selecting a clinical information system for any setting. For those agencies that require additional reports, most vendors will provide a customized report for a fee or the agency may have an internal report writer. Ad hoc reports can be generated using Crystal report writing software, SQL, or in some instances Microsoft Access. The software vendors themselves or external third parties also now offer the opportunity to purchase decision support software which gives the agency additional opportunities to obtain data and reports from the clinical information system.

Hospice

Caring for the terminally ill in a specific program or place has been an accepted method of healthcare delivery starting at the time of the Crusades. Some report hospice care beginning even earlier in the fourth century. It was not until payment methodologies were enacted by CMS in the mid-1980s that hospice care practices grew in the United States. Up until that time the hospice movement was limited to demonstration programs and small grass roots efforts that were supported by private funding and donations.

Under Medicare reimbursement, the hospice movement took hold with small but sustained growth in the United States. Many hospices were initially established as a part of home health agency. In some instances, staff provided care to both home health agencies and hospital patients. Over time there has been a growth in independent hospice companies. Currently, as with home health, there are several national companies that provide care nationwide. Hospice care, under Medicare guidelines, provides four levels of care. These levels of care are routine care, respite care, inpatient care (more acute services are provided), and continuous care. Generally, a hospice episode of care is measured in 90-day periods with a cap on services at 180 days. Payment is episodic and includes all care and services related to the terminal diagnosis. Each level of care has a different reimbursement. Patients may receive different levels of care within an episode. Tracking of the levels of care and the complex regulatory requirements of providing hospice care to Medicare and other insurance covered recipients has lead to the use of clinical information systems in hospice.

Hospice information systems are provided by many of the same vendors who offer home health system. In many instances this is an advantage to the agency that provides both services. Patient records for the patient who moves from home health to hospice can be maintained in the same system. Staff needing to look up information from the previous level of care can do so. In addition to the features and functions offered as part of the home health system, hospice software generally includes modules for interdisciplinary care, volunteer services and tracking, conferences, and bereavement. Expanded clinical assessments are also provided to include pastoral care services. In past years the ability to document the in-patient cares that is provided in a respite facility or an inpatient hospice setting has been problematic. Vendors who support both home health and hospice applications were slow to make program changes to include these levels of care provisions.

More recently, software companies have developed niche markets that are separate from home healthcare and provide EHR exclusively for the hospice market. These products are enhanced and meet more of the needs of the hospice providers. Some incorporate a pharmacy and a durable medical equipment module as part of the software. This enables the hospice to accurately account and bill for these services that are part of Medicare reimbursement. Additionally, these programs are set up to accommodate the billing of physician services provided for hospice patients. One minor disadvantage with using the hospice stand-alone system is the inability to monitor patients along the home care continuum from home health to hospice. Using two separate vendors requires an interface to link the records. Often the interface is costly and cumbersome.

New hospice regulations now require hospices to track and trend quality data and outcomes (OBQI). Unlike home health, however, there is no mandated data set to report outcomes of care.

Home Infusion

Home Infusion is a smaller home care market than either home health or hospice. As a result, there are more limited choices of software vendors. At the current time there are no vendors that provide an option that gives the end user the option of selecting all three home care components within one software application.

The home infusions software application focuses more on the pharmacy, inventory, delivery and billing modules than on clinical documentation. This is not surprising since up until recently, nursing care costs were bundled into the drug charges. Changes in reimbursement, however, now separate nursing costs, and as a result infusion software vendors are enhancing clinical modules.

Similar to home care and hospice, software application can be Web-based or hosted by the infusion company. POC devices are used by the delivery staff to track supplies and medication provided to a patient and the clinical staff for the assessment and documentation of clinical care and teaching.

Home Medical Equipment

Home Medical Equipment (HME) companies also provide durable goods and services to the home care population. Although these companies provide some professional care (nurses who provide wound care management and respiratory therapists to work with ventilator dependent patients), payment is generally bundled. Clinical documentation is limited and POC devices are not generally employed to document care. Drivers to tract and record inventory and deliveries made to patients may employ POC technology. The focus of the HME software is inventory control and billing.

Private Duty and Aide Services

Private duty companies for the most part have utilized internally developed or proprietary billing systems to track services and bill clients and insurance companies. Because of the minimal amount of mandated requirements, handwritten records are used to document clinical care. This has been the norm in this segment of the home care industry. Recently, national firms are expanding; they are requiring more complex billing systems. Often these companies are billing for several different services some of which may be reimbursed by managed care companies or Medicaid. Also in recent years there is more public scrutiny of the industry, especially, those companies that serve the Medicaid population. Increased demand is being placed on software vendors for clinical information systems that will support this business line. Home health systems, geared towards Medicare recipients, are often not suited for use with this population of chronically ill patients.

Currently several vendors are developing new platforms that support care across the continuum of post acute services.

Use of Standard Formats

The Health Insurance Portability and Accountability Act of 1996 (HIPAA) Privacy and Security Rules has three sections. The first part of the Act dealt with administrative simplification. It provided for the adoption of national standards for electronic healthcare transactions and code sets, unique health identifiers, and security. The remaining part of the Act deals with the privacy and security of the electronic record. It is the latter two parts of the Act that receive more attention in the literature.

For purposes of this discussion it is the standardization of code sets that played a major role in the infrastructure of all home care records and billing practices. Up until the implementation of HIPAA, software vendors and insurance companies were free to use their own internally developed code sets and billing formats. This prevented bills from being processed electronically and for data to be compared. As of October 2003, home care vendors, companies, and insurance companies all need to utilize the same standard formats. CMS adopted the use of Healthcare Common Procedure Coding System (HCPCS) to standardize and streamline billing. According to the CMS Website: The HCPCS Level II Code Set is one of the standard code sets used for this purpose. The HCPCS is divided into two principal subsystems, referred to as level I and level II of the HCPCS. Level I of the HCPCS is comprised of CPT (Current Procedural Terminology), a numeric coding system maintained by the American Medical Association (AMA). The CPT is a uniform coding system consisting of descriptive terms and identifying codes that are used primarily to identify medical services and procedures furnished by physicians and other healthcare professionals. These healthcare professionals use the CPT to identify services and procedures for which they bill public or private health insurance programs. The AMA makes decisions regarding the addition, deletion, or revision of CPT codes. The CPT codes are republished and updated annually by the AMA. (CMS, 2010)

Also adopted was the use of Current Procedural Terminology (CPT) that uses standard terms for medical procedures. Other standards were related to mandated claim formats. Another standard set by the technology industry is referred to as Health Level 7 language (HL-7) interface requirements. This requirement that has been adapted as an industry standard allows for the interfacing of two unrelated software programs by establishing common formatting of data elements. HL7 specifies a number of flexible standards, guidelines, and methodologies by which various healthcare systems can communicate with each other. Such guidelines or data standards are a set of rules that allow information to be shared and processed in a uniform and consistent manner. These data standards are meant to allow healthcare organizations to easily share clinical information. Theoretically, this ability to exchange information should help to minimize the tendency for medical care to be geographically isolated and highly variable (www. HL-7.org.).

A subsequent requirement of Medicare related to the use of standardized codes was enacted in 2003. It established a common language and coding guidelines for all prescription drugs. This required standardization with the pharmaceutical industry of which home infusion companies are a subset.

The Use of ANA-approved Nursing Languages in Home Care Applications

There are several approved nursing languages that are used in home care software. The major software vendors have been slow to adopt the use of standard nursing terminologies with their systems. The reasons for not including a nursing language are varied. One consideration that needs to be stated is that the industry is not requesting that these languages be imbedded in the software. Nursing leaders may not be aware of the value of using a standard language and clinical staffs have not been exposed to these languages as part of their undergraduate curriculum. Once in practice, the expense of teaching staff a new language falls on the agency. This is a sizable expense when one takes it into consideration the costs associated with the roll out of a new technology. An article by Canham and colleagues (2008) provides the steps necessary to implement the Omaha system into an academic Nurse-managed center. These steps are also of interest for introducing not only this system but any system into nursing practice.

There are two notable exceptions that have been identified and included in several post acute software applications. They are the Clinical Care Classification System and the Omaha System. Other classification systems such as Nursing Intervention Classification (NIC), Nursing Outcome Classification (NOC), and North American Nursing Diagnosis Association (NANDA) have also been used in part within software application that supports the home care industry. These languages may be added as part of an agency's customization of the software.

The Clinical Care Classification (CCC) system was developed as part of a research study conducted by Dr. Virginia Saba and her colleagues at Georgetown University, School of Nursing. The research consisted of a national sample of 646 health agencies, randomly stratified by staff size, type of ownership, and geographic location. They collected data on 8961 newly discharged Medicare cases representing each patient's entire episode of home healthcare from admission to discharge (www.sabacare.com) (Saba, 2010). According to information posted on the Sabacare Website, CCC is formally recognized by the American Nurses Association (ANA) as a recognized language. Further, "The Clinical Care Classification (CCC) System (version 2.0) provides a standardized framework and a unique coding structure for assessing, documenting, and classifying patient care by nurses and other clinical professionals in any healthcare setting." The CCC system consists of two interrelated terminologies "empirically developed from 40,000 problems and 80,000 patient statements from live patient records":

- CCC of Nursing Diagnoses consists of 182 (59 major & 123 subcategories)
- CCC of Nursing Interventions consists of 198 (72 major & 126 subcategories)

The two terminologies are both classified by 21 Care Components that represent the Functional, Health Behavioral, Physiological, and Psychological Patterns of patient. The CCC system is HL-7 compliant and it integrates with Logical Observation Identifiers, Names, and Codes (LOINC), and SNOMED CT.

Further, the Website states the software can be "used to track and measure patient/client care holistically over time, across settings, population groups, and geographic locations". It is suitable for use in an electronic medical record. CCC is beginning to build clinical care pathways. CCC is being implemented "in all types of healthcare facilities worldwide" (www.Sabacare.com, 2010).

Another ANA recognized standard language is the Omaha System. Like the CCC system, it has its roots in home health. In a telephone interview with Karen Martin, RN, MSN, FAAN, Ms. Martin stated that the Omaha system was initially developed by staff at the VNA of Omaha (Nebraska) under the direction of DeLanne Simmons, VNA of Omaha Chief Executive Officer. Subsequently the classification system was refined based on the finding of three research studies funded by the funded by the Division of Nursing, US DHHS between 1975 and 1986 (personal conversation, July 6, 2010).

According to the Omaha Website, the Problem Classification Scheme (within the Omaha System) provides a structure, terms, and system of cues and clues for a standardized assessment of individuals, families, and communities. It helps practitioners collect, sort, and document, classify, analyze, retrieve, and communicate health-related needs and strengths. It is a comprehensive, orderly, non-exhaustive, mutually exclusive taxonomy or hierarchy. The Problem Classification Scheme consists of four levels of abstraction. Four domains appear at the first or most general level. Forty-two client problems or areas of concern are at the second level; by definition, problems are neutral, not negative. The third level consists of two sets of problem modifiers: health promotion, potential and actual, as well as individual, family, and community. Clusters of signs and symptoms that describe actual problems are at the fourth or most specific level. Using the Problem Classification Scheme with the Intervention Scheme and Problem Rating Scale for Outcomes creates a comprehensive problem-solving model for practice, education, and research (www.omahasystem.org, 2010) (Martin, 2010).

In a commentary in the *Home Care Technology* (2009) the changes on culture one agency experienced after implementing the Omaha System as part of its EHR are described (Home Care Technology, p. 4–5).

As with the CCC system, Omaha is also recognized by the ANA as an official language. It has met the standards for interoperability for electronic health records after successfully passing the Healthcare Information Technology Standards Panel (HITSP), and it is compatible with LOINC and SNOMED CT, and is (recognized) by HL-7. According to the Website, www. omaha.com, "it is congruent with the reference terminology model for the International Organization for Standardization (ISO). It is being mapped to the International Classification of Nursing Practice (ICNP). It meets Medicare/Medicaid, Joint Commission, and CHAP guidelines and regulations". Currently, according to Martin, many national and international groups use the Omaha system as their accepted standard. Currently the Omaha system is being considered for inclusion by a major software vendor for their home care and hospice software product. Its major advantage for use in the post acute service area is the fact that it is designed for use by a multidisciplinary team.

2010 AND BEYOND

As the country moves into the new century, the focus of healthcare is again on reform and cost saving. The Obama plan calls for improving access to all Americans, while at the same time it also calls for reduced government spending. Under the Obama plan, funding to home care and hospice programs will be cut over the next few years. The initial impact of cost saving measures will go into effect in Fall 2011 and continue for at least the following 3 years.

The American Recovery and Reinvestment Act (ARRA) places more emphasis on spending in the form of grants to improve the use of technology in healthcare, especially in the area of interoperability. In an editorial comment, Lisa Remington (2010) notes that the ARRA will lead to new programs being initiated. Demonstration projects that support the use and or expand the use of EHR, smart phones, tele-health, wireless remote health EHRs, or systems that enable provider to provider communication, e-Health collaborative, such as Regional Health Information Organizations (RHIO), will be undertaken. Bush (2009), however, predicted "the final version of the stimulus package removed $600 million in grant funding specifically geared toward the adoption of EHRs for post-acute facilities. But nursing homes, home health agencies and hospices are eligible for general technology grants, and the law includes a study of "potential use of new aging services technology to assist seniors, individuals with disabilities and their caregivers throughout the process." The impact on software vendors will be to focus on technology that enhances the interoperability of the EHR across settings (Bush, 2009).

The trends indicate that CMS is continuing to focus on the models of care for the chronically ill and to improve quality outcomes. As healthcare spending for the chronically ill raises, CMS is planning to implement strategies to limit spending. It is estimated that 23% of Medicare recipients have five or more chronic diseases and account for 68% of Medicare spending. Two focuses of CMS will limit payment for patients who are readmitted to the hospital within 30 days of discharge and to evaluate new models or expanded use of post acute care delivery. Cost reduction related to re-admissions will take effect in Fall 2013 with data gathering related to the following diseases, heart attack, heart failure, and pneumonia as part of the quality reporting program beginning in fiscal year 2011. A concept that underlines both of these items is that of care transitions. Care transitions will be explored in the next section of this chapter. Also, the PPS Refinement Act of 2010 seeks to limit reimbursement to home care industry and sets additional standards for quality and increase access to care.

Expanding on the concepts in the previous chapters, there are three main themes that are relevant to the use of technology in the post acute service area. They are the focus of CMS on chronic care initiatives including Care Transitions and new models of care, increased importance of the interoperability of the EHR to provide the link between providers of care and the use of remote monitoring devices to support the management of the chronically ill population. Inherent in these themes are the requirements to demonstrate quality outcomes at a reduced cost. Simply stated, the home care industry will be moving towards a variety of approaches that will service the needs of the chronically ill. The focus will change from intermittent care to long term care for the chronically ill. These approaches will be supported and enhanced by the use of technology.

Care Transition Models

There are many articles that support the approach of improving care transitions. Ventura and colleagues (2010) state that one in five discharges are followed by readmission within 30 days. This is a major driver of healthcare costs. The article proves an excellent summary of the Care Transitions Themes that were funded by CMS through the auspices of the Quality Improvement Organizations. Of the 21 projects cited, seven projects focused on formal programs to improve care transitions, while the remainder focused on intervention strategies to improve care transitions. Notable are the works by Nayor (2006) which focus on the use of an advanced practice nurse to mentor and instruct the patient after hospital discharge to return to the community; the Best Practice Intervention Package: Transitional Care Coordination offers a tool kit for home health agencies to use to ease patients' transitions from hospital to home; and the Telemedicine project which uses remote electronic monitoring to link the patients' physiologic data to the provider. Remington (2010) elaborates on other CMS funding that is looking at the patient centered medical home. Bartelstone and Rackow (2010) state that the term medical home " has evolved over time and currently is thought of as the provision of service delivery that enables the provision of primary care in the community and takes into consideration the needs of the patient, the family and the environment including health, educational and social support system" (p.18). Four medical associations have developed standards for the term medical home and have enacted guidelines for medical home programs. "The guidelines focus on five areas: collaboration and leadership; practice recognition; practice support; reimbursement; and assessing and reporting results" according to Epperly (2009). Epperly further notes that the emphasis is on health information technology care coordination and improving clinical outcomes.

Interoperability of the EHR

With the move towards chronic care and coordination of care within the community, communication across setting and practitioners will be required. This will lead to

the development of EHRs that allow interoperability. In separate interviews (2010) with Dan Cobb, co-founder of HealthMEDX) and Chris Dollar (Vice President and General Manager of McKesson), both leading companies that provide software solutions to the post acute service industry, there was agreement that interoperability of EHR must be addressed by the technology industry. Cobb stated that the home care industry is currently working to set standards for interoperability (personal communication, April 23, 2010). Dollar states that there is a need to link all agencies providing care to the chronically ill population. His list includes not only all practice settings but also includes less thought of services like meals on wheels and community funded transportation companies (personal communication, April 12, 2010). The approach of their respective companies varies on how to achieve the goal; there is, however, overwhelming support for the interoperability of the EHR. Both men currently sit on a national panel of post acute software providers who are working together to set standards which will allow interoperability of different software programs. See Table 33.1 and Figures 33.1 and 33.2.

Hammond and colleagues state, "Interoperability of health information systems is a fundamental requirement to accomplish healthcare goals through the use of data and information. Interoperability means the ability to communicate and exchange data accurately among different IT system, software applications, and networks. An absolute necessity for achieving interoperability is the existence of agreed upon standards." (Hammond, Bailey, Boucher, et al., 2010) According to the authors the five priority areas for achieving interoperability in healthcare applications are: 1) patient identifier, 2) semantic interoperability, 3) data interchange standards, 4) core data sets, and 5) data quality. Currently as the work done with the IT industry, most

TABLE 33.1	Standards Adopted by Health Information Technology
Interface	Health Level 7 (HL-7)
Problem lists	ICD-9-CM (or 10) or SNOMED
Medication list	RxNorm
Allergies	UNII
Procedures	CPT-4 or ICD-9_CM (or 10)
Vital signs	CDA template
Lab orders and results	LOINC

http://healthit.hhs.gov/portal/server.pt/community/healthit_hhs_gov__health_it_standards_committee/1271

Why Standards and Exchanges ?

Without....

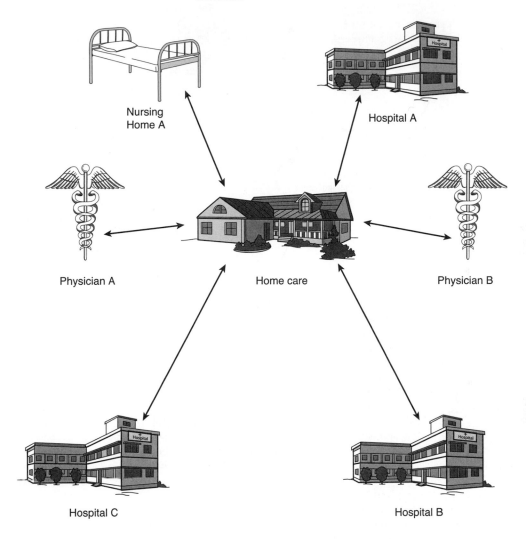

... multiple point-to-point inerfaces (if at all)

• **FIGURE 33.1.** Why Standards and Exchanges? Reprinted with permission from Dan Cobb, July 2010.

of the standards required to develop in interoperable health system exist today.

Bush (2009) quotes Majd Alwan, Director of the Center for Aging Services Technology, saying that the RRAA offers all providers a singular opportunity to connect with each other and achieve interoperability. According to a 2008 study conducted by Alwan's organization, 43 percent of U.S. nursing homes maintain

electronic health records (Bush, 2009). This is in comparison to a report from Hammond (2010) that stated that as of 2008, only 9.1% of hospitals have comprehensive health IT systems with a basic EHR. Hammond (2010) further states that this is true despite the fact that more than 90% of hospitals use computers for at least some purpose. Primary care offices are little better: Only 13% have a fully functional EHR system

Why Standards and Exchanges ?

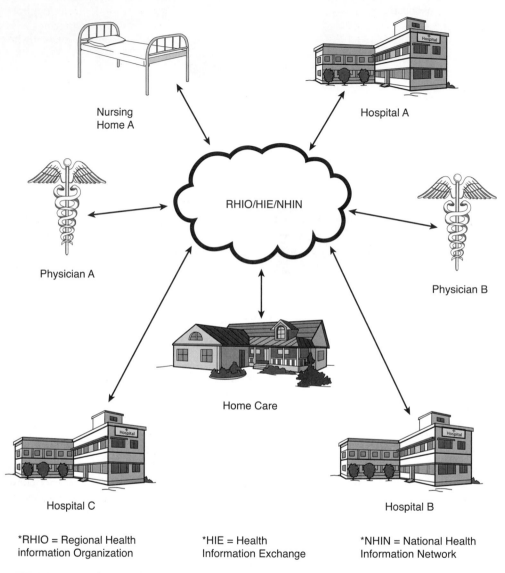

Nursing
Home A

Hospital A

RHIO/HIE/NHIN

Physician A

Physician B

Home Care

Hospital C

Hospital B

*RHIO = Regional Health
information Organization

*HIE = Health
Information Exchange

*NHIN = National Health
Information Network

• **FIGURE 33.2.** Why Standards and Exchanges? Reprinted with permission from Dan Cobb, July 2010.

(Hammond, 2010). Terry (2010) states, "65% of all home health agencies have electronic record, while 83% of hospital based home health agencies have an EHR."

Carol Raphael, President and CEO of the Visiting Nurse Service of New York comments in the *Remington Report* (Raphael, 2006) that through the use of federal stimulus funding under HITECH there is a project in New York City that is part of a state initiative which looks for interoperability and functionality to link between primary care practitioners, health centers, rural health clinics, hospitals, and home health agencies. Given the fact that nationally not all of these entities have an EHR, the task is formidable. It will be one, however, that will go forward over the next 10 years. Bush (2009) sums up the discussion on interoperability: "We hope to see a true partnership between the acute and long-term care settings." He goes on to state, "This is a once in-a-lifetime investment in the infrastructure, and we would be more than remiss if we miss this opportunity" (Bush, 2009). Post acute settings have much to gain from partnering in any and all opportunities to promote the interoperability of the EHR across the practice area.

Tele-Health and Remote Patient Monitoring

Remote patient monitoring through the use of tele-health devices has been used in home care industry for over 10 years. Much of the initial use of tele-health monitoring was a result of payment changes to Medicare recipients for home health services. The move to an episodic payment that included all supplies and services led the way for more efficient use of agency resources. Conducting visits electronically enabled home health agencies to monitor specific physiologic measures (pulse, blood pressure, blood glucose levels, and oxygen saturation) as a method of determining when an in-person visit needed to be made. Other forms of tele monitoring included the use of video conferencing and telephonic visits with patients. The latter two examples do not produce an electronic collection of physiologic measures.

Home Health News (2010) reported that one Dallas based agency had a significant reduction in the re-hospitalization rate of their tele-health monitored patients. Of the 11,000 completed episodes that yielded improved outcomes, only 5.98% of the Medicare tele-health monitored episodes vs. 14.89% of non tele-health monitored Medicare episodes were re-hospitalized. With re-hospitalization rates for Medicare patients being one of the quality measures for both home health agencies and hospitals, these results support the continued use of tele-health monitoring. Home Health News (http://www.homehealthnews.org/2010/06). Litan reports (2008), the use of remote monitoring translates into both saving and enhancing lives. In his article, he states that the use of remote monitoring can save millions of dollars in unnecessary costs resulting from needless re-hospitalizations. Today remote monitoring has moved beyond the monitoring of vital signs; it has become a tool to promote and educate chronically ill patients to care for themselves. During the 5-year period between 2006 and 2011, remote monitoring and other wellness monitoring services will expand over 50% (Medical Devices & Surgical Technology Week, 2006). While this prediction may not be realized, there is significant interest in the

use of remote monitoring devices to enhance communication between practitioners and their patients. Some of the applications now in remote tele-monitoring applications include the use of PDAs, video monitoring, Web applications, and e-mail. Smart phones may currently be enhanced with an app to monitor diabetes and other chronic diseases.

In the post acute setting, the most widely used form of tele-health has expanded from the collection and recording of vital signs and other physiologic measures to more as a tool used in the management of chronic disease. The devices used continue to monitor and record these measures. However, education modules and artificial intelligence are now built into complex algorithms that are designed to instruct the patient on techniques related to self-care. The most common tele-health programs established by home health agencies require the use of a portable tele-health monitor that is set up in the patient's home. The device is equipped with tools that are used to monitor the desired physiologic readings. The device can be either hard wired into the monitor or it can use airwave capabilities to transmit readings to the monitor. Many products have the capability to allow the patient to enter in the readings. This is especially useful for weight and blood glucose monitoring where the patient may have his or her own device. Recorded parameters are then transmitted to the base station and monitored by health professionals. Transmission may be done over phone lines, Internet or DSL lines or in some cases transmitted via air cards. The results are transmitted either to a Web-based host site or to a PC that is monitored by the agency. One of the advantages for the Web-based site is that not only the tele-monitoring staff can read the results but agency care givers and physicians can also see the data. New systems allow for agencies to provide the patient with disease specific information and videos. These can be purchased from the tele-monitoring vendor or they can be customized by the agency (Lorentz, 2008).

Use of Tele-Health by the Veterans Administration

Overall, the results from research studies of agencies using tele-health to improve patient outcomes or from anecdotal reporting of findings by home health agencies using tele-health indicate that one of the most significant results was demonstrated by the Veterans Administration (VA). In a study in the journal *Telemedicine and e-Health*, Dakins and colleagues reported the results of an in-depth study conducted by the VA. The study was conducted on veterans who were over the age of 65. Most of the subjects were men with chronic diseases. The subjects all received tele-health monitoring services in their homes. The study looked at health outcomes in a total of 17,025 VA home tele-health patients. The findings included a 25% reduction in the average number of days hospitalized and a 19% reduction in hospitalizations for patients using home tele-health. The data also show that for some patients the cost of tele-health services in their homes averaged $1600 a year—much lower than in-home clinician care costs. The key to the program's success is VA's computerized patient record system. Data obtained from the home such as blood pressure and blood glucose, along with other patient information in the electronic system, allows our healthcare teams to anticipate and prevent avoidable problems (Dakins, Ryan, Foster, Edmonson & Wakefield, 2008).

SUMMARY

From the 1990s and continuing through the current decade, the role of technology as an enabler of care in the post acute service area continues to expand. The initial impetuses for the earlier use of technology were compliance with regulations and financial reimbursement. This focus has shifted and the current drivers control of expenses related to chronic care, measuring and monitoring of quality outcomes, and providing regional access to the health records of an ever-mobile society and their providers. As technology applications continue to increase, the use of these technologies in the post acute service arena will also grow.

REFERENCES

Bartelstone, R., & Rackow, E. (2010). Intergraded Care Management Services for the Medical Home. *The Remington Report, May/June*, 18–20.

Bush, H. (2009). Post-acute providers see health IT money slip away. *Hospitals & Health Networks, 83*, 14.

Canham, D., Mao, C., Yoder, M., Connolly, P., & Dietz. D. (2008). The Omaha system and quality measurement in academic nurse-managed centers: Ten steps for implementation. Journal of Nursing Education, 47, 105–111.

Dakins, A., Ryan, P., Foster, L., Edmonson, E. and Wakefield, D. (2008). Care coordination/home telehealth: The systematic implementation of health informatics, home telehealth, and disease management to support the care of veteran patients with chronic disease. *Telemedicine and e-Health, 12*, 1118–1126.

Epperly, T. (2009). President's message. *Annals of Family Medicine, 7*, 279–280.

Hammond, WE, Bailey, C, Boucher, P, Spohr M, Whitaker P. *Connecting information to improve health*. Health Aff (Millwood). 2010 Feb; 29(2): 284–8.

Home Care Technology. (2009). Editorial. *Home Care Technology, Fall*, 4–5.

Home Health News. Retrieved on July 1, 2010 from http://www.homehealthnews.org/2010/06

Litan, R. (2008). Vital signs via broadband: Remote health monitoring transmits savings, enhances lives. Retrieved June 15, 2010 from www.betterhelthcaretogether.org

Lorentz, M. (2008). Telehealth and home healthcare. *Home Healthcare Nurse, 26*(4), 237.

Martin, K. (2010). Omaha Classification System. Retrieved May 10, 2010. http://www.omahasystem.org

Martin, K. 2010 retrieved from www.omahasystem.org/

Medical Devices & Surgical Technology Week. (2006). Editorial. Information technology; Revenues from digital home health services to top $2.1 billion by 2010. *Medical Devices & Surgical Technology Week*, 269.

Naylor, M. D. (2006). Transitional care: a critical dimension of the home healthcare quality agenda. *Journal for Healthcare Quality, 28(1)*, 48–54.

Raphael, C. (2006). Technical Presentation. Retrieve June 30, 2010 from http://www.academyhealth.org/Events/content.cfm?ItemNumber=1269

Remington, L. (2010). Emerging technology is re-connecting healthcare. *The Remington Report*, 1, 1, 20–24.

Retrieved from http://www.hl7.org/

Retrieved from http://www1.va.gov/opa/pressrel/pressrelease.cfm?id=1637, Jan 2009

Retrieved from http//www.hipaa.org

Retrieved from https://www.cms.gov/HomeHealth QualityInits/01_Overview.asp#TopOfPage/

Retrieved from www.cms.gov/medhcpcsgeninfo/

Retrieved from www.cms.gov/TransactionCodeSetsStands/02_TransactionsandCodeSetsRegulations.asp

Retrieved from www.ncrr.nih.gov/publications/informatics/ehr.pdf

Saba, V. (2010). Clinical Classifications Intervention. Retrieved June 2, 2010 from http://www.sabacare.com/interventions.

Stolle, P., Steeves, B., Glenny, C., & Filsinger, S. (2010). The use of electronic health system in home care. *Home Healthcare Nurse, 28*, 3.

Terry, K. (2010). Implementing an EHR. Preparing for launch. *Medical Economics, 84*(3), TCP2, TCP4, TCP6-8.

Thakkar, M., & Davis, C. (2006). Risks, Barriers, and benefits of EHR system: A comparative study based on size of hospital. *Perspectives in Health Information Management*, 3, 5.

Ventura, T., Brown, D., Archibald, T., & Brock, J. (2010). Improving care transitions and reducing hospitalizations. *The Remington Report, Jan-Feb*, 24–30.

34

Public Health Practice Applications

Judy D. Gibson / Janise Richards / Arunkumar Srinivasan / Derryl E. Block

• OBJECTIVES

1. Define public health informatics and the public health nurse informatician.
2. Describe the National Electronic Disease Surveillance System.
3. Describe two public health electronic information systems with implications for the public health nurse.
4. Discuss the public health informatician role and the emerging role of the public health nurse informatician in case studies.

• KEY WORDS

Public health informatics
Electronic public health surveillance
Electronic public health information systems
Interoperability standards
Office of National Coordinator for Health Information Technology
National Electronic Disease Surveillance System

OVERVIEW

For many years, public health practitioners stated the belief that if nobody thought about public health, then public health must be doing its job. The battles that health practitioners waged against infectious diseases (such as malaria, tuberculosis [TB], and leprosy), chronic diseases, and environmental health hazards were often not highlighted in the media. In recent years, after recent outbreaks of SARS and Influenza A virus (H1N1), dramatic large-scale foodborne disease outbreaks, and the explosion of chronic illnesses that are linked to multiple vectors such as obesity, public health is frequently in the media limelight. The continuing need to be alert to emerging public health problems, responsive in emergencies, and accountable to the public has intensified health departments' efforts to collect data and information from multiple sources.

Health departments are collecting and analyzing data on a scale that was inconceivable even 10 years ago (Figure 34.1). To be able to manage this overwhelming deluge of data and information, public health practitioners have tapped into information technology. During 2000–2010, information systems have become widely adapted to fit the special needs within public health. Recognizing the importance of linkages among clinical care (also known as direct care), clinical care information systems, laboratory information systems, and other data sources to better understand and improve the state of the nation's health, public health has helped to establish data and information exchange standards to support system interoperability.

This chapter provides an overview of the application of informatics to public health, describes legislation that has affected public health information systems, and provides examples of electronic data exchange between

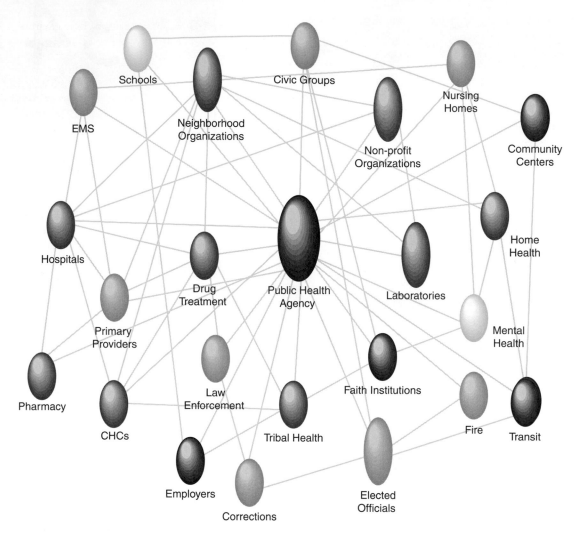

• **FIGURE 34.1.** Local public health information and data exchange entities (OSTLTS, 2009).

clinical care and public health. The chapter also introduces the emerging role of the Public Health Nurse Informatician (PHNI) and gives examples differentiating the public health nurse (PHN) and the PHNI.

PUBLIC HEALTH, PUBLIC HEALTH INFORMATICS, PUBLIC HEALTH NURSING, AND THE PUBLIC HEALTH NURSE INFORMATICIAN

In 1920, C.-E. A. Winslow defined public health as "the science and art of preventing disease, prolonging life and promoting health through the organized efforts and informed choices of society, organizations, public and private, communities and individuals (Winslow, 1920)." The roots of public health were established in the United States when the Public Health Service (PHS) was established in 1798 by the Marine Hospital Service Act. In 1944, with the passage of the Public Health Service Act [Title 42 U.S. Code], the PHS mission was broadened to protect and advance the nation's physical and mental health. To accomplish this mission, public health had to clearly define the activities that would lead to this desired outcome.

In a seminal study by the Institute of Medicine, *The Future of Public Health*, the functions of public health were described as assessment, policy development, and assurance (Institute of Medicine, 1988). Assessment

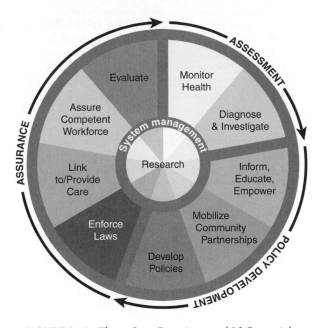

• **FIGURE 34.2.** Three Core Functions and 10 Essential Services of Public Health(ASTDN, 2000; Public Health Functions Steering Committee, 1994).

includes activities of surveillance, case finding, and monitoring trends, and is the basis for the decision making and policy development by public agencies. Policy development is the broad community involvement in formulating plans, setting priorities, mobilizing resources, convening constituents, and developing comprehensive public health policies. Assurance covers activities that verify the implementation of mandates or policies, and guarantees that the provision of necessary resources is provided to reach the public health goals. To further enhance the core public health functions, a committee of public health agencies and organizations convened by the U.S. Public Health Service described the 10 essential services of public health (Public Health Functions Steering Committee, 1994). Figure 34.2 describes the relationship between the core functions and essential services of public health.

The essential governmental role in public health is guided and implemented by a variety of federal, state/territorial, and local regulations and laws as well as federal, state/territorial, and local governmental public health agencies. At the local level, tens of thousands of governmental units at the county, municipality, town ship, school district, and other special jurisdiction levels must interact to provide public health services. This complex array of public health functions, services,

responsibilities, and interactions is not a static environment, but one that is constantly changing.

Information forms the basis of public health. To make informed decisions and policies, public health practitioners require timely, quality information. The 1996 World Health Report cites the continuing need to "disseminate health information widely, in the sharing of epidemiological and statistical data, reports, guidelines, training modules and periodicals (WHO, 1997)." Although there are numerous sources of public health data and information, the sources lack standardization in data organization, nomenclature, and electronic transmission. Innovative methods for storing, organizing, exchanging, and disseminating the millions of pieces of data gathered during public health activities have provided the foundation for the field of public health informatics.

Public health informatics has been defined as "the systematic application of information and computer science and technology to public health practice, research, and learning (Friede, Blum, & McDonald, 1995)." Public health informatics, like public health, focuses on populations. In public health informatics, population-level data and information are collected, analyzed, and disseminated with the ultimate goal of supporting preventive, as opposed to curative, interventions.

The demarcation between public health and clinical healthcare systems is frequently blurred, especially given legislation that has provided the funding and legal platforms to build the information systems needed to protect and advance the nation's physical and mental health. The provision in the 2004 Health Insurance Portability and Accountability Act (HIPAA) that generally prohibits disclosure of an individual's medical record and payment history without expressed authorization of the individual is known as the Privacy Rule. For public health purposes, the law provides for the disclosure of patient information to public health without authorization from the patient, for the purpose of preventing or controlling disease, injury, or disability, and for the purpose of conducting public health surveillance, public health investigations, and public health interventions (HIPAA, 2002). The 2010 Patient Protection and Affordable Care Act (PPACA) provides for the establishment of policies and technically interoperable and secure standards and protocols to facilitate the enrollment of individuals in federal and state health and human services programs (PPACA, 2010). As public health, clinical care, information science, computer science, and information technology continue to come together, the field of public health informatics will continue to expand to support the public health functions of assessment, policy development, and assurance to promote a healthy nation.

Public health nursing is the practice of promoting and protecting the health of populations using knowledge from nursing, and public health sciences. The practice is population focused with the goals of promoting health and preventing disease and disability for all people, through the creation of conditions in which people can be healthy. There are eight principles of public health nursing: the population is the unit of care; the primary obligation is to achieve the greatest good for the greatest number of people as a whole; PHNs work with the client as equal partner; primary prevention is the priority in selecting appropriate activities; focus is on strategies that create healthy environmental, social, and economic conditions in which populations may thrive; the PHN is obligated to actively identify and reach out to all who might benefit from a specific activity/service; the key element of practice is optimal use of available resources to assure best overall improvement in health of the population; and PHNs collaborate with a variety of other professions, populations, organizations, and stakeholder groups to promote and protect the health of the people (American Nurses Association, 2007).

The *Public Health Informatician (PHI)* is a "public health professional who works either in practice, research, or academia and whose primary work function is to use informatics to improve population health. The role requires more expertise than the multi-highly functional public health professional that assists with informatics-related challenges or supports personal productivity with information technology (CDC, 2009)."

The proposed role of the *Public Health Nurse Informatician (PHNI)* combines the competencies of PHI and nursing informatics (American Nurses Association, 2008). The PHNI systematically applies information, computer science and technology, and nursing science to PHN practice, research, and learning. A PHNI is a PHN who has specialized in nursing informatics and has skills in supporting the establishment of systems to improve public health surveillance through access to clinical care information. Further, the PHNI has advanced skills in supporting the use of nursing datasets for more effective clinical care in community surveillance programs. PHNIs ensure that data needs for population groups are adequate for knowledge models related to performance measures. These are just some examples of the differences between the PHN and the PHNI that will be described and explained in this chapter.

The Public Health Surveillance Landscape

The public health mission is to promote the health of the population rather than to treat individuals. In support of this mission, public health workers collect data on the determinants of health and health risks from factors in the pre-exposure environment, the presence of hazardous agents, behaviors, and exposures (CDC, 2010a; World Health Organization, 2010). Public health workers monitor the occurrence of health events, conditions, deaths, and the activities of the healthcare systems and their effects on health. Public health professionals use these data to inform decisions about the most effective mechanisms for interventions. Information from multiple, sometimes incompatible, systems or sources must be combined for an accurate depiction of problems (Figure 34.1). There is a need for rapid and comprehensive access to data across system boundaries, that is, the system at all levels as well as the healthcare industry systems (Koo, Morgan, & Broome, 2003).

Data collection and sharing in public health occurs at three levels: local, state/territorial, and federal (eg, Centers for Disease Control and Prevention [CDC]). Programs at each level have similar organization and management structures. Since most funding is based on programmatic need, many information systems have been built to support specific programs, thereby creating "silo"-like systems. To be productive, the program-oriented funding streams and information systems need to flow together.

Efforts are underway to assist healthcare providers in overcoming barriers to data collection and sharing through the implementation of regional, state/territorial, and local health information exchanges (HIEs) (Wild, Hastings, Gubernick, Ross, & Fehrenbach, 2004) and the National Electronic Disease Surveillance System (NEDSS) initiative. This comprehensive rather than disease-specific approach to data collection and sharing is the foundation of public health informatics and warrants further inspection.

Infectious Disease Electronic Surveillance

The three levels of the organizational structure of public health have distinct data collection and sharing roles in support of the electronic surveillance system (Figure 34.3). Each year, the Council of State and Territorial Epidemiologists (CSTE) and the CDC jointly update a list of reportable diseases and conditions. The CSTE recommends that all states and territories enact laws (statue or rule/regulation as appropriate) to make nationally reportable conditions reportable in their jurisdiction (CSTE, 2010). The local (city or county) health department—the frontline of public health—interacts most closely with clinicians and agencies in the community, gathers reports of communicable dis-

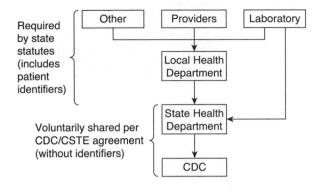

• **FIGURE 34.3.** Notifiable Disease Surveillance Data Flow to Public Health (Birkhead & Maylahn, 2000).

eases, tracks and monitors cases, conducts investigations, and often provides direct services (STD testing, vaccines, contact tracing, directly observed therapy, case management). The state health department uses legislation as well as regulations to require reporting by healthcare entities: to report certain illnesses, to require vaccinations for school entry, to coordinate statewide disease surveillance and to monitor incoming reports from counties, and then submit those reports, voluntarily and minus names, to the CDC. The state prioritizes problems and develops programs, runs the state public health laboratory, and serves as liaison between the CDC and local level. The CDC publishes national surveillance summaries and conducts research and program evaluations to produce public health recommendations. The CDC provides grants to states for specific programs, technical assistance, and, by invitation, outbreak response for state and local partners (Birkhead & Maylahn, 2000).

National Electronic Telecommunications System for Surveillance (NETSS)

In 1984, the CDC, in cooperation with the CSTE and epidemiologists in six states, began testing the Epidemiologic Surveillance Project. The project's goal was to demonstrate the effectiveness of computer transmission of public health surveillance case-based data between state health departments and the CDC. By 1989, all 50 states were participating in the reporting system. The Epidemiologic Surveillance Project was renamed the National Electronic Telecommunications System for Surveillance (NETSS) to reflect its national scope (CDC, 2010b). The NETSS system includes

22 core data elements for reportable disease conditions. The CDC analyzes these data and disseminates them in the *Morbidity and Mortality Weekly Report (MMWR)*. This overwhelming volume of data to be managed by health departments led to the National Electronic Disease Surveillance System (NEDSS) initiative, which provides guidance for the technical architecture and standards for nationally reportable condition reporting. When the CDC decided to transition from NETSS to NEDSS, it was determined that no further modification to NETSS would be made. NETSS differs from NEDSS in several ways. NETSS was case based; NEDSS is person-based. And, NETSS used proprietary codes, but NEDSS is based on standards so it can capture data already in electronic healthcare data streams. These differences precipitated the need to transition to NEDSS.

National Electronic Disease Surveillance System (NEDSS)

In 1999, the CDC, the CSTE, and state and local public health department staff began work on information system standards for the NEDSS initiative (NEDSS, 2001). The NEDSS initiative uses standards to advance the development of efficient, integrated, and interoperable surveillance systems at the state and local levels. This initiative facilitates the electronic transfer of information from clinical information systems in healthcare, reduces the provider's burden of providing data, and enhances the timeliness and quality of information provided.

Implementation of the NEDSS initiative was supported by the CDC. States were funded to assess their current systems and develop plans to implement criteria compatible with the NEDSS initiative. The criteria included (1) browser-based system data entry, (2) an Electronic Laboratory Results (ELR) system for laboratory staff to report results to health departments as authorized, and (3) a single repository for integrated databases from multiple health information systems. Also supported were system-wide electronic messaging upgrades for sharing the data. Finally, the CDC developed a platform called the NEDSS-Base System (NBS) for public health surveillance functions, processes, and data integration in a secure environment. States then had the option to choose this platform or another NEDSS-compatible system.

Some states developed systems using specified NEDSS standards, while other states used a CDC-developed system. To better understand how the NEDSS initiative meets its mission, we will examine the NBS role in supporting public health surveillance.

Healthcare Providers Role and the NBS

Healthcare providers are responsible for providing clinical care and reporting state-designated reportable conditions to public health departments. As a registered user of the NBS, a healthcare provider can directly enter data from case and laboratory reports into the state's electronic surveillance system at the point of care. In addition to the direct entry of data, healthcare providers can securely query the database, verify completeness of reporting using analysis tools, and ensure compliance with state public health laws. Healthcare providers can send electronic case reports using the Health Level Seven Clinical Document Architecture (HL7 CDA) format when their electronic health record (EHR) is equipped to report in the standard format.

Clinical Laboratories and the NBS

Staff members in public and private laboratories are required by law to notify public health departments of state reportable conditions. Timely reports are critical to public health surveillance because they prompt investigations of cases of reportable diseases or outbreaks. Registered laboratory users of the NBS system enter reports directly using the Web-based laboratory reporting function of the NBS. This report is then readily available to the public health NBS users to conduct the investigation (Levi, Vinter, & Segal, 2009).

Public Health Practitioner Role and the NBS

The local or state public health practitioner responds to incoming data on reportable conditions and implements appropriate public health case finding, tracking, and monitoring. Public health practitioners, who are registered users of the NBS, may review reports from laboratories and healthcare providers for patients residing within their jurisdictional boundaries. The public health practitioner may create an "alert" function for new data received in the NBS (such as for reports of meningococcal disease). Upon receipt of a new report, the public health practitioner may order a public health field investigation. Clinical, laboratory, epidemiologic, and follow-up data are entered at point of care and stored in the NBS. Stored data can be read, analyzed, and shared. The public health practitioner classifies the case, based on stored data and standard case definitions, and forwards the notification to CDC using the NEDSS messaging format, HL7, or NETSS (if no messaging guide exists). A data transfer function in the NBS allows users to notify another jurisdiction when a patient moves and to transfer records for follow-up.

Federal (CDC) Role and the NBS

A key part of the public health surveillance process is assessment of population health in the United States. The capabilities of the NBS support public health investigations and interventions at the state level and allow reporting of nationally notifiable diseases in a more complete and standardized manner and in near real-time for analysis by CDC program areas. This supports effective policy formation at the national level when events of public health significance happen. The data are disseminated through the *Morbidity and Mortality Weekly Reports (MMWR)*.

Privacy Protection and the NBS

In order to protect personally identifiable information, the NBS requires user authentication, authorization, and auditing protocols. To verify the identity of the user, the NBS supports custom authentication. Once authenticated, the NBS application authorizes access to data based on user role, geographical area(s), disease(s), public health event(s), and action(s). For example, a local public health practitioner may be assigned access to Foodborne and Diarrheal (FDD) investigations and laboratory reports for a public health jurisdiction. The supervisor can be assigned access to multiple public health jurisdictions across multiple families of diseases (eg, FDD and hepatitis). The NBS creates an audit file containing a fingerprint trail with a timestamp of the user's activities.

Value of Information Solutions to Surveillance Practice

NEDSS-compatible infectious disease electronic surveillance systems change how public health departments at all levels communicate to perform their mission. Access to data repositories is no longer limited to a central location. Rather, epidemiologists, registered as the NBS users, may have data access at all public health levels. These systems enhance the capacity of local and state public health agencies to react quickly to disease occurrences.

Future Directions for Infectious Disease Surveillance

State public health programs face major funding and infrastructure challenges in adopting the standards-driven information systems for electronic disease surveillance. The CDC encourages adequate and sustained funding by public health programs for the NEDSS initiative and encourages partners and clinical providers at the point of care to adopt standards and create a uniform, interoperable, and bi-directional process for electronic disease surveillance. Initiatives such as the CDC's Public Health Informatics Fellowship Program train professionals to apply information science and technology to the practice of public health (CDC, 2010c).

Because public health informatics requires the integration of computer science, information science, and information technology into the public health system and with clinical care, one method to better understand how public health information systems work is to examine their application in collecting, organizing, exchanging, and disseminating data and information. The following two cases illustrate public health information systems applied in the context of an immunization information system and a TB electronic surveillance system.

Using Informatics in an Immunization Information System

Public health has been an advocate for immunization to prevent disease for decades. Currently, vaccine-preventable diseases are at, or near, record lows (Roush, Murphy, & Vaccine-Preventable Disease Table Working Group, 2007). Some basic facts provided by the Every Child By Two organization regarding the need for immunization registries indicates that in the United States, there are around 4 million births each year (11,000/day); by age 2, a child will need to have up to 20 vaccinations; 2.1 million children are under-immunized; and 22% of American children see two immunization providers in their first 2 years (Every Child By Two, 2010).

Immunization records and registries began as paper forms that were completed by hand at the point of service. The immunization record was kept with the patient's file, and an official copy was given to the patient or patient's guardian. On a periodic basis, usually once a month, all the immunizations records were aggregated by hand (or calculator) with patient demographics and vaccine information written into a registry that was shared with the local health agency. This time-consuming process contained many vulnerable points where the data could be wrongly entered, incorrectly calculated, or not included in the overall tally.

Newer immunization registries are based on electronic Immunization Information Systems (IIS). These IIS are confidential, computerized information systems that allow for the collection of vaccination histories and provide immediate access by authorized users to a child's current immunization status. One impetus for IIS arose from the *Healthy People 2010* objective (14.26), which stated that 95% of children younger than 6 years of age would be registered in a fully operational IIS (U.S. Department of Health and Human Services, 2010). In 2008, 75% of U.S. children younger than 6 years of age (approximately 18 million children) participated in an IIS, compared to 65% in 2006 (Kelly, Heboyan, Rasulnia, & Urquhart, 2010).

Benefits of the implementation of an IIS for the public include having a private and secure place to safeguard important immunization information from multiple providers that will be used throughout a person's life; receiving timely immunization reminders; and eliminating duplicate immunizations. Benefits for healthcare providers include consolidating immunization records from different sources; automatically calculating the immunizations needed; easily providing official copies of immunization records; reducing chart pulls for coverage assessments and Healthcare Effectiveness Data and Information Set (HEDIS) reviews (NCQA, 2010); automating vaccine inventory and ordering procedures; allowing for vaccine tracking during vaccine shortages or manufacturer recalls; flagging high-risk patients for timely vaccination recalls; and assisting with vaccine safety and adverse event reporting. To accomplish these activities, the IIS must be able to exchange data and information.

Data, vocabulary, and transmission standards are critical to IIS success. A core IIS dataset has been defined, current procedural terminology (CPT) codes have been mapped to CVX (vaccine codes), and MVX (manufacturers of vaccines) codes have been developed to facilitate immunization data exchange between IIS, billing and administrative systems, inventory management systems, and other support systems. In addition, HL7 standards are used for codes as well as patient demographics, appointment scheduling, file synchronization, and other data management transactions produced and received by the systems.

The IIS has been successfully implemented in many states. Examples include the Michigan Care Improvement Registry (MCIR, 2010), the Oregon Immunization ALERT system (Oregon DHHS, 2010), the Wisconsin Immunization Registry (WIR) (Wisconsin Immunization Program, 2010), the Iowa Immunization Registry Information System (IRIS, 2010), and the Louisiana Immunization Network for Kids Statewide (LINKS) (AIRA, 2010).

Challenges to moving IIS forward include funding and human capacity to build and manage the system. The HITECH Act (ARRA, 2009) provides funding, and educational programs focusing on informatics will help nurses and others develop skills to refine and effectively use this important public health information system.

Using Informatics in a Tuberculosis Electronic Information System

Tuberculosis is a chronic bacterial infection caused by *Mycobacterium tuberculosis*. The most common site of infection is the lung, but other organs may be involved. Healthcare providers are required by laws in all 50 states to report patients with TB and other conditions on the state's list of notifiable conditions. Confirmed TB cases are reported by clinicians and laboratory staff to local health departments and then to statewide disease surveillance programs connected to state health departments. A confirmed case of TB is one that meets the clinical case definition or is laboratory confirmed. Reporting is also recommended for patients who have suspected respiratory TB, to expedite contact tracing and TB transmission control prior to laboratory confirmation.

Multiple systems are involved in electronic TB reporting. Data reporting systems include the National TB Surveillance System (Division of TB Elimination, 2010a), the TB Genotyping Information Management System (Division of TB Elimination, 2010b), and the Electronic Disease Notification System (Division of Global Migration and Quarantine, 2010).

The National TB Surveillance System is an electronic incidence surveillance system that collects 49 data items on newly diagnosed verified cases of TB in the United States. Data are held by the appropriate authority in the state or designated health jurisdiction and transmitted to CDC at three intervals: initially at the time of case verification, at receipt of initial drug susceptibility test results, and at treatment closure. Formats for reporting TB cases have evolved over decades from paper-based reporting beginning in 1952, to electronic reporting introduced in the mid-1980s, to a NEDSS-compatible, electronic surveillance system, using HL7 messaging, operational in 2010 for verified TB cases reported in 2009.

The TB Genotyping Information Management System (TB GIMS) builds upon the established infrastructure of the CDC's National TB Surveillance System and incorporates genotype data to create a centralized database and reporting system. State public health laboratories submit isolates from culture-confirmed cases to one of two designated genotyping laboratories for molecular characterization, which

helps with identifying recent transmission and potential outbreaks.

The Electronic Disease Notification System alerts state and local health department programs of the arrival of refugees and immigrants to their jurisdictions and provides overseas medical screening results and treatment follow-up information. Each refugee or immigrant with a TB classification is referred to the TB program for medical screening and treatment follow-up.

CDC uses data from these reporting systems to disseminate performance measurement reports for national TB-related performance indicators. CDC shares these reports electronically with health department programs receiving federal funding for TB prevention and control. The national reports are used by state programs to set performance targets, measure performance, and evaluate the program's capacity to control and prevent TB (Division of TB Elimination, 2010c).

Work continues on managing data quality to improve accuracy, completeness, consistency in collecting data, and timeliness of reporting in the National TB Surveillance System. Additionally, future applications are needed to automate data exchange between the TB reporting systems and to standardize laboratory data for direct reporting to the National TB Surveillance System.

The Public Health Informatician and the Emerging Roles for Public Health Nurse Informatician

The emerging role of the PHNI is illustrated in case studies to demonstrate the core public health functions of assessment and assurance performed by the PHNI and the PHI. In the first case study, the PHI ensured the retrieval of destroyed health records (immunization data) for displaced Hurricane Katrina communities by linking people with their records through informatics. By retrieving health records, the PHI enforced the rules regarding immunization record requirements while ensuring provision of needed immunizations. In the second case study, the PHI, while participating in assessment activities to monitor health status and health problems in displaced Hurricane Katrina communities, identified a norovirus outbreak. The PHI developed and used a simple data checklist of symptoms, and compiled daily information reports and environmental risk information to evaluate the ongoing effectiveness and quality of emergency public health services. In the third case study, the PHNI designed an assessment activity for barriers to adherence behaviors with TB treatment. The PHNI described a clinical nursing information system (CNIS) for a behavioral adherence model adapted to TB program literature. The resulting dataset can be used for data management and performance plan monitoring and to evaluate the effectiveness and quality of personal health services.

CASE STUDY 34.1. IMMUNIZATION REGISTRIES AND EMERGENCY RESPONSE AFTER HURRICANE KATRINA

Hurricane Katrina made landfall in Louisiana on August 29, 2005. To escape the storm, more than 200,000 residents of New Orleans and the surrounding area evacuated to shelters in Houston, Texas. In their hurry, they left behind most personal belongings, including immunization records or medical records. Since the hurricane landed as the fall school session was about to begin, state and local school boards in Texas agreed to accept the displaced children into schools without proof of immunization, but stated that proof of immunizations would be necessary to remain in school.

To assist families in finding their children's records, the Houston-Harris County (Texas) Immunization Registry (HHCIR) staff contacted their vendor, who was also the vendor for the Louisiana Immunization Network for Kids Statewide (LINKS), to investigate the possibility of linking the two IIS. In less than 24 hours the HHCIR, vendor, and LINKS personnel had developed a technological bridge built on HL7 standards connecting the two systems. Ten days later they had created a mechanism that allowed health authorities to acquire child and adolescent immunization histories from LINKS. This merged Web-based immunization registry was made available to public health officials and selected healthcare providers in temporary clinics in the Astrodome and George R. Brown Convention Center. Originally the new IIS was a "search and view" only system; the HL7 data exchanges capability was added to allow the LINKS- HHCIR connection to exchange patient data and information from one system to the other.

Over the next month, more than 20,000 records were searched and approximately 10,000 were successfully matched for displaced children in the greater Houston area. By September 2006, 1 year later, nearly 19,000 records had been successfully matched. The estimated cost savings of this on-the-fly, hybrid IIS, just in vaccines for these children, is slightly over $1.6 million. These costs do not factor in the savings in time, pain, and lost work time or missed school that would have occurred if the children had needed to be re-immunized. Nor do the costs reflect the societal costs that may have occurred if the children had not been allowed to attend school (Boom, Dragsbaek, & Nelson, 2007). The use of the IIS immunization registry post-Katrina empowered patients, parents, and healthcare providers to know immunization history.

CASE STUDY 34.2 . NOROVIRUS OUTBREAK IN PERSONS DISPLACED BY HURRICANE KATRINA

Collecting and sharing data and information is essential for public health practice. In September 2005, nearly 1000 evacuees from Hurricane Katrina and relief workers in numerous facilities had symptoms of acute gastroenteritis. A checklist of symptoms was used to collect data on an intake form in medical facilities set up to provide care on an outpatient basis. This information was gathered and entered into a database, and results were distributed each morning.

On September 2, staff observed an increase in adults and children with symptoms of acute gastroenteritis. On some days, nearly 21% of adults and 40% of children visiting one clinic had acute gastroenteritis. They conducted enhanced surveillance to improve identification of acute gastroenteritis, investigated the apparent outbreak, identified the infectious agent, and implemented control measures.

The reported epidemiologic and laboratory findings suggested that an outbreak of norovirus gastroenteritis had affected individuals in numerous facilities. These outbreaks are not associated with contaminated food or water, but spread through person-to-person contact or from fomites in crowded settings. This information was used to provide a health alert for epidemiologic features and clinical presentation, and to promote rehydration treatment and measures to prevent secondary transmission (CDC, 2005).

CASE STUDY 34.3 . USING INFORMATICS FOR PUBLIC HEALTH PROGRAM EVALUATION

A diagnosis of TB disease or latent TB infection in a child represents recent transmission of *M tuberculosis*; therefore trends in TB disease and latent TB infection in young children are important indicators to assess the effectiveness of TB prevention and control efforts. Investigations of persons having infectious pulmonary TB can avert TB in children who have been infected with *M tuberculosis* by finding and treating these children before they progress to TB disease (Lobato et al., 2008).

TABLE 34.1	Patient-Centered Care Model (PCC Model) for Barriers to Patient Adherence with Taking Medication and Keeping Appointments for Tuberculosis Treatment (Gibson, Boutotte, Wilce, & Field, 2010)	
Patient Diagnosis (NANDA-I)	**Nursing Interventions (NIC)**	**Patient Outcomes (NOC)**
Ineffective health maintenance	Sustenance support	Social support
Ineffective protection	Infection control	Immune status
Adjustment impaired/Risk-prone health behavior	Decision-making support	Well-being
Decisional conflict: whether to participate in treatment	Mutual goal setting	Participation in healthcare decisions
Defensive coping	Patient contracting	Coping
Fear (stigma)	Emotional support	Fear self-control
Powerlessness: perceived threat	Patient's rights protection	Health beliefs: perceived ability to perform
Ineffective therapeutic regimen management	Medication management	Medication response
Ineffective family therapeutic regimen management	Discharge planning	Family participation in professional care
Noncompliance	Health policy monitoring	Compliance
Knowledge deficit	Teaching	Knowledge of
• disease process	• disease process	• disease process
• treatment regimen	• treatment regimen	• treatment regimen
Communication impairment	Culture brokerage	Communication ability

NANDA-I, Nanda International; NIC, Nursing Interventions Classifications; NOC, Nursing Outcomes Classification (Johnson et al., 2006).

Monitoring standardized nursing activities can help identify missed opportunities for prevention. The main types of missed opportunities for preventing TB in young children include not screening the exposed child, perhaps because of incomplete identification of contacts (case interview/investigation adequacy); ensuring that the child starts TB treatment, but not ensuring treatment is completed (caregiver adherence issues); and the infected adult contact who is recommended for treatment either not starting treatment, or starting treatment but not completing it (adherence issues).

A clinical nursing information system (CNIS) dataset, constructed with standardized nursing terminology recognized by the American Nurses Association, is used by PHNs to account for nursing activities, to manage program outcomes, and to describe a planned approach to nursing care. Although the CNIS dataset is used to generate data on patient assessments and to characterize interactions with healthcare providers, it is not targeted to treatment barriers for the patient's adherence needs. In this case, the CNIS dataset would be adapted for the prevention efforts listed above.

Various CNIS datasets can be used. A vendor application of a CNIS is currently used in county and state public health programs in Maine and Minnesota. In Maine, the CNIS is a statewide PHN initiative within the state public health system. It is used to document clinical care and to inform program evaluation. Common tools are nursing care and education plans, flow sheets, and encounter forms for individual client services (TB, MCH, childhood lead poisoning) (Correll & Martin, 2009). In Minnesota, the Omaha system contributes to the outcomes management program in local public health departments by providing quantitative data and graphs for program planning, evaluation, and communication with administrators and local government officials (Monsen, Martin, Christensen, & Westra, 2009).

The standard clinical nursing information has been used to describe a planned approach to perceived barriers to adherence with TB treatment by describing the appropriate support needed to address the challenges of completing long-term TB treatment and perceived barriers to adherence (Table 34.1). Such support is characterized by productive interactions between persons with TB and their healthcare providers who are often TB nurse case managers. The Patient Centered Care (PCC) Model for Perceived Barriers to Adherence with TB Treatment (Table 34.1) helps the nurse identify and document multiple determinants of adherence behavior and useful interventions (Gibson, Boutotte, Wilce, & Field, 2010).

FUTURE DIRECTIONS IN PUBLIC HEALTH INFORMATION SYSTEMS

Although public health information systems have matured over the past decade, many challenges remain. In general, public health practitioners have not taken an active role in the development of health information systems within their jurisdictions. Since the bulk of public health activities occur within state/territorial level and local health departments, public health practitioners must provide support and leadership to local healthcare systems in the emerging concept of multiagency responsibility for health. Local agencies and institutions such as managed care organizations, hospitals, laboratories, environmental health agencies, nursing homes, police staff, community centers, pharmacies, civic groups, corrections staff, drug treatment centers, EMS staff, and home health agencies are partners in maintaining the public's health. Figure 34.1 illustrates entities involved in local data/information exchange. Additionally, public health practitioners have the expertise needed to inform health information system developers about specific data and information that are needed to make population-based analyses in order to recognize emergent issues in the community, to assist in diagnostic and treatment decisions, and to better understand methods to improve the health of the community. Federal agencies involved in public health can provide the leadership and expertise in developing consensus on data and health information technology standards that will allow for the exchange of public health data and information across public health jurisdictions creating a "network of networks" that function as a national public health information system.

Using data in innovative ways through the use of data visualization and decision support systems will increase public health's ability to understand disease trends, make decisions, and apply the appropriate resources where needed. The use of decision support based on clinical and prevention guidelines can integrate prevention messages into primary care.

As some health information technology stabilizes and other technology innovations occur, public health can be the beneficiary of the focus and funding that are driving healthcare reform. As clinical care and public health continue to integrate and support each other's goal of keeping people healthy, health information technology will provide the platform to improve the health of the nation.

The Future of the Public Health Nurse Informatician Role

The evolving role of the PHNI can contribute to public health practice and the Nation's health in several ways:

the PHNI can support the establishment of systems to improve electronic surveillance through access to clinical care information; describe data needs for knowledge models related to performance measures for community surveillance programs (eg, persons with infectious disease); and evaluate the effectiveness, accessibility, and quality of personal and population-based health services in support of electronic surveillance programs (American Nurses Association, 2008; ASTDN, 2003; CDC, 2009; Public Health Foundation, 2009; Public Health Functions Steering Committee, 1994).

SUMMARY

In summary, public health, public health informatics, public health information systems, and the ever-increasing integration of public health and healthcare present many opportunities to continually improve the Nation's health. Recent legislation has provided the guidance and funding platforms to create a seamless integration of health information systems to assist with better decision-making in patient care and in policy development. The development of individual data and information system standards is occurring less frequently as nationally recognized health information technology and data exchange standards are stabilizing. Efforts supporting the certification of the information technology used in health have an impact on the adoption and integration of these standards by information system vendors. Successful implementations of standards-based information systems have demonstrated enormous cost savings in time and money.

PHNs contribute data to the standards-based data exchange systems; use information to target care for individuals, families, groups, and populations; and then evaluate programs by means of the information systems. The PHNI seeks partners to understand variables of concern to nurses in clinical care, such as barriers to adherence behaviors, in the development of the standards-based data exchange systems. The PHNI provides leadership to the PHNs in the use of health information technology to improve the health of the nation.

REFERENCES

American Immunization Registry Association (AIRA). (2010). *State immunization information systems*. Public Health Solutions. http://www.immregistries.org/index. phtml. Accessed 11.06.2010.

American Nurses Association. (2007). *Public health nursing: Scope and standards of practice*. Silver Spring: Nursebooks.org.

American Nurses Association. (2008). *Nursing informatics: Scope and standards of practice*. Silver Spring: Nursebooks.org.

American Recovery and Reinvestment Act (ARRA). (2009). Department of Health Human Services, Pub. L. No. 111-5 (Feb. 17). http://frwebgate.access. gpo.gov/cgi-bin/getdoc.cgi?dbname=111_cong_ bills&docid=f:h1enr.pdf. Accessed 23.05.2010.

Association of State and Territorial Directors of Nursing (ASTDN). (2000). *Public health nursing: A partner for healthy populations: Linking nursing and public health core functions and essential services*. Washington, DC: American Nurses Association.

ASTDN. (2003). Quad Council of Public Health Nursing Organizations. *Public health nursing competencies— 2003*. Association of State and Territorial Directors of Nursing (ASTDN). http://www.astdn.org/publication_ quad_council_phn_competencies.htm. Accessed 7.06.2010.

Birkhead, G. S., & Maylahn, C. M. (2000). State and local public health surveillance. In S. M. Teutsch, & R. E. Churchill (Eds.), *Principles and practice of public health surveillance* (2nd ed., pp. 253–286). Oxford University Press.

Boom, J. A., Dragsbaek, A. C., & Nelson, C. S. (2007). The success of an immunization information system in the wake of hurricane Katrina. *Pediatrics, 119*(6), 1213–1217.

CDC. (2005). Norovirus outbreak among evacuees from hurricane Katrina—Houston, Texas, September 2005. *MMWR—Morbidity & Mortality Weekly Report, 54*(40), 1016–1018.

CDC. (2010a). *National environmental health data tracking network*. CDC. http://ephtracking.cdc.gov/showHome. action. Accessed 6.06.2010.

CDC. (2010b). *National Electronic Telecommunications System for Surveillance (NETSS)*. Centers for Disease Control and Prevention. http://www.cdc.gov/ncphi/ disss/nndss/netss.htm. Accessed 6.06.2010.

CDC. (2010c). *Public health informatics fellowship program*. CDC. http://www.cdc.gov/phifp/. Accessed 6.06.2010.

CDC and University of Washington's Center for Public Health Informatics. (2009). *Competencies for public health informaticians 2009*. U.S. Department of Health and Human Services, CDC. http://www. cdc.gov/InformaticsCompetencies/downloads/PHI_ Competencies.pdf.

Correll, P. J., & Martin, K. S. The Omaha System helps a public health nursing organization find its voice. *Computers, Informatics, Nursing, 27*(1), 12–16.

Council of State and Territorial Epidemiologists (CSTE). (2010). *Modification of the process for recommending conditions for national surveillance*. 10-SI-02. CSTE, 1–4. http://www.cste.org/ps2010/10-SI-02.pdf. Accessed 22.03.2010.

Division of Global Migration and Quarantine. (2010). *Electronic Disease Notification System (EDN)*. Centers for Disease Control and Prevention. http://www.cdc. gov/immigrantrefugeehealth/about-refugees.html. Accessed 11.06.2010.

Division of TB Elimination. (2010a). *Tuberculosis information management*. Centers for Disease Control and Prevention. http://www.cdc.gov/tb/programs/tims/ default.htm.

Division of TB Elimination. (2010b). *TB genotyping information management system (TB GIMS) fact sheet*. Centers for Disease Control and Prevention. http://www.cdc.gov/tb/programs/genotyping/ tbgims/implementation_statelab.htm. Accessed 11.06.2010.

Division of TB Elimination. (2010c). *National TB Indicators Project (NTIP)*. Centers for Disease Control and Prevention. http://www.cdc.gov/tb/publications/ factsheets/statistics/NTIP.htm. Accessed 11.06.2010.

Every Child By Two. (2010). *About registries (Immunization Information Systems)*. Every Child By Two. http://www.ecbt.org/registries/.

Friede, A., Blum, H. L., & McDonald, M. (1995). Public health informatics: how information-age technology can strengthen public health. [Review] [19 refs]. *Annual Review of Public Health, 16*, 239–252.

Gibson, J. D., Boutotte, J., Wilce, M., & Field, K. (2010). A patient-centered care model for perceived barriers to adherence with tuberculosis treatment. Ref Type: Unpublished Work.

Health Insurance Portability and Accountability Act (HIPAA) Privacy Rule. (2002). DHHS, *45*, CFR Parts 164. http://www.access.gpo.gov/nara/cfr/ waisidx_02/45cfr164_02.html.

Immunization Registry Information System (IRIS). (2010). Iowa Department of Public Health. http:// www.idph.state.ia.us/adper/iris.asp. Accessed 11.06.2010.

Institute of Medicine. (1988). *The future of public health*. Washington, DC: National Academy Press.

Johnson, M., Bulechek, G., Butcher, H., Dochterman, J. M., Maas, M., Moorhead, S., et al. (2006). *NANDA, NOC, and NIC Linkages: Nursing diagnoses, outcomes, and interventions* (2nd ed.). St. Louis: Mosby Elsevier.

Kelly, J., Heboyan, V., Rasulnia, B., & Urquhart, G. (2010). Progress in immunization information systems— United States, 2008. *MMWR—Morbidity and Mortality Weekly Report, 59*(5), 133–135. http://www.cdc.gov/ mmwr/preview/mmwrhtml/mm5905a3.htm. Accessed 11.06.2010.

Koo, D., Morgan, M., & Broome, C. V. (2003). New means of data collection. In P. W. O'Carroll, W. A. Yasnoff, M. E. Ward, L. H. Ripp, & E. L. Martin (Eds.), *Public health informatics and information systems* (pp. 379–536). New York City: Springer.

Levi, J., Vinter, S., & Segal, L. M. (2009). Ready or Not? Protecting the public's health from diseases, disasters, and bioterrorism 2009: Biosurveillance—NEDSS compatibility. Trust for America's Health, 24. Robert Wood Johnson Foundation. http://healthyamericans.org/reports/bioterror09/pdf/TFAHReadyorNot200906.pdf. Accessed 1.10.2010.

Lobato, M. N.; Sun, S. J.; Moonan, P. K.; Weis, S. E.; Saiman, L.; Reichard, A. A.; et al. (2008). Underuse of effective measures to prevent and manage pediatric tuberculosis in the United States. *Archives of Pediatrics & Adolescent Medicine, 162*(5), 426–431.

Michigan Care Improvement Registry (MCIR). (2010). *Michigan Care Improvement Registry*. http://www.mcir.org/. Accessed 23.05.2010.

Monsen, K. A., Martin, K. S., Christensen, J. R., & Westra, B. L. (2009). Omaha System data: methods for research and program evaluation. *Studies in Health Technology & Informatics, 146*, 783–784.

National Committee for Quality Assurance (NCQA). (2010). *2009 HEDIS performance measures*. NCQA. http://www.ncqa.org/tabid/855/Default.aspx. Accessed 23.05.2010.

National Electronic Disease Surveillance System Working Group. (2001). National Electronic Disease Surveillance System (NEDSS): a standards-based approach to connect public health and clinical medicine. *Journal of Public Health Management & Practice, 7*(6), 43–50.

Oregon DHHS. (2010). *Oregon immunization alert system*. Oregon DHHS. http://www.immalert.org/new/. Accessed 23.05.2010.

OSTLTS. (2009). National Public Health Standards Program. Centers for Disease Control and Prevention. http://www.cdc.gov/ostlts/.

Public Health Foundation. (2009). *Council on linkages between academia and public health practice. Core competencies for public health professionals*. Public Health Foundation. http://www.phf.org/link/prologue.htm#definitions. Accessed 3.06.2010.

Public Health Functions Steering Committee. (1994). *Public health in America*. DHHS. http://www.health.gov/phfunctions/public.htm . Accessed 11.06.2010.

Roush, S. W., Murphy, T. V., & Vaccine-Preventable Disease Table Working Group. (2007). Historical comparisons of morbidity and mortality for vaccine-preventable diseases in the United States. *JAMA, 298*(18), 2155–2163.

The Patient Protection and Affordable Care Act (PPACA). (2010). DHHS, Pub. L. No. 111–148 (March 23). http://frwebgate.access.gpo.gov/cgi-bin/getdoc.cgi?dbname=111_cong_bills&docid=f:h3590enr.txt.pdf.

U.S. Department of Health and Human Services. (2010). *Healthy people 2010: Understanding and improving health* (2nd ed.). U.S. Department of Health and Human Services.

Wild, E. L., Hastings, T. M., Gubernick, R., Ross, D. A., & Fehrenbach, S. N. (2004). Key elements for successful integrated health information systems: lessons from the states. *Journal of Public Health Management & Practice*, (Suppl.), S36–S47.

Winslow C.-E. A. (1920). The untilled fields of public health. *Science New Series, 51*(1306), 23–33.

Wisconsin Immunization Program. (2010). *Wisconsin Immunization Registry (WIR)*. Wisconsin Department of Health Services. http://dhs.wisconsin.gov/immunization/WIR.htm. Accessed 11.06.2010.

WHO. (1997). *The world health report 1996—Fighting disease, fostering development*. World Health Organization. http://www.who.int/whr/1996/en/index.html.

World Health Organization. (2010). *The determinants of health*. World Health Organization. http://www.who.int/hia/evidence/doh/en/.

Informatics Solutions for Emergency Planning and Response

Elizabeth (Betsy) Weiner / Capt. Lynn A. Slepski

• OBJECTIVES

1. Describe the contributions that informatics can provide to emergency planning and response.
2. Illustrate various ways that informatics tools can be designed and used to support decision making and knowledge base building in emergency planning and response efforts.
3. Utilize the 2009 H1N1 example as a case study in how informatics were used to plan and respond to this pandemic event.
4. Project areas of emergency management and response that would benefit from informatics assistance.

• KEY WORDS

Emergencies
Disasters
Public health informatics
Bioterrorism
Biosurveillance

INTRODUCTION

The first decade of the 21st century has proven to be an era with increased emphasis on emergency planning and response. There has been a documented rise in terrorism incidents, as well as natural disasters worldwide. Natural events have ranged from earthquakes, tsunamis, floods, hurricanes, typhoons, to pandemic disease events affecting billions. According to a World Health Organization (WHO) report, the number of natural disasters affecting urban populations has risen four-fold since 1975 (WHO, 2008a). In addition to natural disasters, political and social upheavals massively disrupt the lives and livelihoods of populations and result in the forced displacement of millions of people. Today, more than

40 countries with a combined population of more than 1.3 billion are faced with emergencies and humanitarian crises (WHO, 2008a). As a result, both planning and response efforts have taken on new importance in relation to emergencies and disasters. The purpose of this chapter is to explore the intersection between informatics and emergency planning and response in order to determine current and future informatics contributions. The United States is not immune from this increased emphasis on emergency preparedness. The events of September 11, 2001, catapulted the United States into the realization that the country was not adequately protected from terrorism. Then, within a short window of time, the anthrax outbreaks stressed the public health

infrastructure to the point that bioterrorism arose as an additional deadly threat. As a result of these two experiences, the government of the United States responded at an unprecedented pace to better prepare and manage terrorist events. Furthermore, the pandemic H1N1 incident in 2009 created data collection challenges that caused public health officials to creatively provide solutions for meaningful data acquisition in order to be able to effectively manage the event.

Early response by the informatics community focused on contributions toward surveillance of threat detection; however, a broader assessment of possible informatics contributions unveiled that in addition to biosurveillance and bioagent detection, informatics could also contribute to increasing the efficiency in disaster response as well as providing a telepresence for remote medical care-givers (Teich, Wagner, Mackenzie, & Schafer, 2002). Additional informatics contributions have since emerged.

The most consistent challenge for emergency and disaster response continues to be communication and information management. Effective response requires a moment-to-moment "situational analysis" and real-time information to assess needs and available resources that can change suddenly and unexpectedly (Chan, Killeen, Griswold, & Lenert, 2004). There is a critical interdependence between data collected in the field about a disaster incident, casualties, healthcare needs, triage, and treatment and the needed community resources such as ambulances, emergency departments, hospitals, and intensive care units. Concurrently, information from the various inpatient facilities and ambulance resources alters the management and disposition of victims at the scene of a disaster. Opportunities abound for new telecommunication technologies. Smart devices, wireless connectivity, and positioning technologies are all advances that have application during disaster events. These technologies are being used and evaluated to improve patient care and tracking, foster greater safety for patients and providers, enhance incident management at the scene, coordinate response efforts, and enhance informatics support at both the scene of the disaster and at the community resource levels.

The 2004 earthquake and tsunami that devastated parts of Southeast Asia illustrated the uncoordinated invasion of people and organizations that resulted in unnecessary duplication, competition, and failure to assist many of the victims in need (Birnbaum, 2010). Subsequently, the Interagency Standing Committee (IASC) of the United Nations Office for the Coordination of Humanitarian Affairs (UN-OCHA) initiated changes called the "humanitarian reform." This reform effort organized clusters whose principal mission was to assist the impacted government with coordination of all responses and with evaluations of the impact of interventions. The World Health Organization was appointed as the lead agency for health, which includes coordination and production of health information (WHO, 2009, p. 8). This organization at the global level was aimed at discouraging individual and organizational response efforts that were not part of this coordinated response. The United States has also organized their planning and response efforts for the same reasons, and informatics is increasingly taking on more important roles in these efforts.

THE FEDERAL SYSTEM FOR EMERGENCY PLANNING AND RESPONSE

Most disasters and emergencies are handled by local and state responders. The federal government provides supplemental assistance when the consequences of a disaster exceed local and state capabilities.

Under the Homeland Security Presidential Directive 5 (HSPD5) (White House, 2003), the Secretary of Homeland Security, as the principal Federal official for domestic incident management, coordinates Federal actions within the United States to prepare for, respond to, and recover from terrorist attacks, major disasters, and other emergencies. Coordination occurs if and when any one of the following four conditions applies: (1) a Federal department or agency acting under its own authority has requested the assistance of the Secretary; (2) the resources of State and local authorities are overwhelmed and Federal assistance has been requested by the appropriate State and local authorities; (3) more than one Federal department or agency has become substantially involved in responding to the incident; or (4) the Secretary has been directed to assume responsibility for managing the domestic incident by the President. Further, HSPD5 directs Federal department heads to provide their full and prompt cooperation, support and resources to the Secretary in protecting national security.

The National Response Framework, enacted in January 2008, established a comprehensive, national and all-hazards approach to respond to disasters and emergencies (Department of Homeland Security [DHS], 2008a). Built on its predecessor, the National Response Plan, it includes guiding principles that detail how federal, state, local, tribal and private sector partners, including the healthcare sector, prepare for and provide a unified domestic response, improving coordination and integration. The Framework emphasizes prepared-ness activities that include planning, organizing, training, equipping, exercising, and applying lessons learned and assigns lead federal agencies to each of 15 Emergency Support Functions (ESF) (DHS, 2008b).

The ESFs group functions are used to provide Federal support during a response (Table 35.1), and assigns leads for each functional area. The Department of Health and Human Services leads public health and medical responses, including biosurveillance.

TABLE 35.1	Emergency Support Functions by Lead Department and Scope	
Function	**Lead Department/ Agency**	**Scope**
ESF #1 – Transportation	Transportation	Aviation/airspace management and control Transportation safety Restoration/recovery of transportation infrastructure Movement restrictions Damage and impact assessment
ESF #2 – Communications	Homeland Security/Federal Emergency Management Agency	Coordination with telecommunications and information technology infrastructures. Restoration and repair of telecommunications infrastructure Protection, restoration, and sustainment of national cyber and information technology resources Oversight of communications within the Federal incident management and response structures
ESF #3 – Public Works and Engineering	Defense/ U.S. Army Corps of Engineers	Infrastructure protection and emergency repair Infrastructure restoration Engineering services and construction management Emergency contracting support for life-saving and life-sustaining services
ESF #4 – Firefighting	Agriculture/ Fire Service	Coordination of federal firefighting activities Support to wildland, rural and urban firefighting activities
ESF Scope ESF #5 – Emergency Management	Homeland Security/Federal Emergency Management Agency	Coordination of incident management and response efforts Issuance of mission assignments Resource and human capital Incident action planning Financial management
ESF #6 – Mass Care, Emergency Assistance, Housing, and Human Services	Homeland Security/Federal Emergency Management Agency	Mass care Emergency assistance Disaster housing Human services
ESF #7 – Logistics Management and Resource Support	Homeland Security/Federal Emergency Management Agency	Comprehensive, national incident logistics planning, management, and sustainment capability Resource support (facility space, office equipment and supplies, contracting services, etc.)
ESF #8 – Public Health and Medical Services	Health and Human Services	Public health Medical Mental health services Mass fatality management
ESF #9 – Search and Rescue	Defense Homeland Security/Federal Emergency Management Agency	Life-saving assistance Search and rescue operations

(continued)

TABLE 35.1	Emergency Support Functions by Lead Department and Scope *(continued)*	
Function	**Lead Department/ Agency**	**Scope**
ESF #10 – Oil and Hazardous Materials Response	Homeland Security/ U.S. Coast Guard	Oil and hazardous materials (chemical, biological, radiological, etc.) response Environmental short- and long-term cleanup
ESF #11 – Agriculture and Natural Resources	Agriculture Interior	Nutrition assistance Animal and plant disease and pest response Food safety and security Natural and cultural resources and historic properties protection and restoration Safety and well-being of household pets
ESF #12 – Energy	Energy	Energy infrastructure assessment, repair, and restoration Energy industry utilities coordination Energy forecast
ESF #13 – Public Safety and Security	Justice	Facility and resource security Security planning and technical resource assistance Public safety and security support Support to access, traffic, and crowd control
ESF #14 – Long-Term Community Recovery	Homeland Security/Federal Emergency Management Agency Urban Development Small Business Administration	Social and economic community impact assessment Long-term community recovery assistance to states, local governments, and the private sector Analysis and review of mitigation program implementation
ESF #15 – External Affairs	Homeland Security/Federal Emergency Management Agency	Emergency public information and protective action guidance Media and community relations Congressional and international affairs Tribal and insular affairs

Department of Homeland Security, 2008b.

CASE STUDY 35.1. INFORMATICS AND 2009 H1N1

The 2009 H1N1 influenza pandemic provides a recent illustration of how informatics can contribute to an emergency response. Initially concerned that a circulating H5N1 virus (Avian Influenza A) was mutating and could cause a human pandemic, global experts had focused efforts over the last several years on rapidly developing catastrophic plans even though a pandemic virus had not emerged. There were significant concerns, given that during the 20th century three flu pandemics were responsible for more than 50 million deaths worldwide and almost a million deaths in the United States (Department of Health and Human Services (DHHS), 2005) (Table 35.2).

Many governments believed that if a pandemic-capable virus emerged, there would be rapid world-wide spread as the 1918 Pandemic had spread across countries and continents in less than one year in a time without commercial air travel to facilitate the spread of disease (DHHS, 2005). It was understood that a world-wide influenza pandemic occurring in this century could have major effects on the global economy, especially travel, trade, tourism, food, consumption and eventually, investment and financial markets and could lead to widespread economic and social disruptions. As a result, many countries engaged in detailed pandemic planning and prepared to adopt draconian-like measures to delay but not stop the arrival of the virus, such as border closures and travel restrictions.

TABLE 35.2	History of Pandemics by Deaths, Causative Strain and At-Risk Population			
Pandemic	Estimated U.S. Deaths	Estimated Worldwide Deaths	Influenza A Strain	Populations at Greatest Risk
1918–1919	500,000	40 million	H1N1	Young, healthy adults
1957–1958	70,000	1–2 million	H2N2	Infants, elderly
1968–1969	34,000	700,000	H3N2	Infants, elderly

Department of Health and Human Services, 2005, p. B-7.

Here in the United States, modelers predicted catastrophic death estimates (Table 35.3). The 1918–1919 flu pandemic, to date the most severe, had caused the deaths of at least 675,000 Americans and affected about one-fifth of the world's population. Researchers believed that if a pandemic of similar severity occurred today, 90 million Americans could become ill, quickly exceeding available healthcare capacity and result in approximately 2 million Americans deaths (DHHS, 2005).

Preparedness planners assumed that all populations were at risk. They believed that disease would be widespread, affecting multiple areas of the United States and other countries at the same time preventing the redistribution of resources. The world would experience multiple waves of outbreaks potentially occurring for an extended period of time (over 18 months), affecting the entire United States for a period of 12 to 16 weeks with community waves each lasting 6 to 8 weeks (DHHS, 2005). One to three pandemic waves would occur (Occupational Safety and Health Administration [OSHA], 2007). Further, planners believed that a pandemic could affect as many as 40% of the workforce during periods of peak flu illness, predicting that employees could be absent because of their own illness, or would be caring for sick family members or for children if schools or daycare centers are closed. They also recognized that workers would be absent if public transportation was disrupted or if they were afraid to leave home (DHS, 2007).

Adopting a "worst case scenario," government experts rapidly developed a number of strategies to help local governments plan, stating that the Federal government would not likely be able to provide any assistance during the actual pandemic. For example, DHHS (2007) developed a Pandemic Severity Index (PSI) to characterize the severity of a pandemic. It was designed to predict the impact of a pandemic and provide local decision makers with standardized triggers that were matched to the severity of illness impacting a specific community (Table 35.4). The severity index was based on a case-fatality ratio to measure the proportion of deaths among clinically ill persons. Recommended actions were identified in advance, and communicated to the public in hopes of increasing their understanding and compliance. Using the PSI, a severe pandemic influenza, similar to the 1918 Pandemic, was defined as a category 4 or 5, with 20% to 40% of the population infected. For a severe pandemic, HHS recommended that localities be prepared to dismiss children from schools and close daycares for up to 12 weeks; as well as initiate adult social distancing, which included suspension of large public gatherings and modification of the work place schedules and practices (eg, telework and staggered shifts).

The Centers for Disease Control and Prevention, part of HHS, monitors influenza activity and trends and virus characteristics through a nationwide surveillance

TABLE 35.3	Estimates of Numbers of Episodes of Illness, Healthcare Utilization, and Death Associated with Moderate and Severe Pandemic Influenza Scenarios* in the United States	
Characteristic	Moderate (1958/68 -like)	Severe (1918 -like)
Illness	90,000,000 (30%)	90,000,000 (30%)
Outpatient Medical Care	45,000,000 (50%)	45,000,000 (50%)
Hospitalization	865,000	9,900,000
ICU Care	128,750	1,485,000
Mechanical Ventilation	64,875	742,500
Deaths	209,000	1,903,000

*Estimates based on extrapolation from past pandemics in the United States. Note that these estimates do not include the potential impact of interventions not available during the 20th-century pandemics.
Department of Health and Human Services Pandemic Plan, 2005, p. 18

TABLE 35.4   Matrix of Community Mitigation Strategies by Pandemic Severity Index

Interventions by Setting	Pandemic Severity Index		
	1	2 and 3	4 and 5
Home			
Voluntary isolation of ill at home (adults and children); combine with use of antiviral treatment as available and indicated	Recommend[b,c]	Recommend[b,c]	Recommend[b,c]
Voluntary quarantine of household members in homes with ill persons[d] (adults and children); consider combining with antiviral prophylaxis if effective, feasible, and quantities sufficient	Generally not recommended	Consider[e]	Recommend[e]
School			
Child social distancing			
• dismissal of students from schools and school-based activities, and closure of childcare programs	Generally not recommended	Consider: ≤ 4 weeks[f]	Recommend: ≤ 12 weeks[g]
• reduce out-of-school social contacts and community mxing	Generally not recommended	Consider: ≤ 4 weeks[f]	Recommend: ≤ 12 weeks[g]
Workplace / Community			
Adult social distancing			
• decrease number of social contacts (e.g., encourage teleconferences, alternatives to face-to-face meetings)	Generally not recommended	Consider	Recommend
• increase distance between persons (e.g., reduce density in public transit)	Generally not recommended	Consider	Recommend
• modify or cancel selected public gatherings to promote social distance (e.g., postpone indoor stadium events)	Generally not recommended	Consider	Recommend
• modify work place schedules and practices (e.g., telework, staggered shifts)	Generally not recommended	Consider	Recommend

Department of Health and Human Services, 2007, p. 12.

Generally Not Recommend = Unless there is a compelling rationale for specific populations or jurisdictions, measures are generally not recommended for entire populations as the consequences may outweigh the benefits;

Consider = Important to consider these alternatives as part of a prudent planning strategy, considering characteristics of the pandemic such as age-specific attack rate, geographic distribution, and the magnitude of adverse consequences. These factors may vary globally, nationally, and locally.

Recommened = generally recommended as an important component of planning strategy

[a]All these interventions should be used in combination with other infection control measures including hand hygiene, cough etiquette, and personal protection equipments such as face masks. Additional information on infection control measures is available at www.pandemicflu.gov (DHHS, 2007).

[b]This intervention may be combined with treatment of sick individuals using antiviral medications and vaccine campaigns, if supplies are available.

[c]Many sick individuals who are not critically ill may be managed safely at home.

[d]The contribution made by contact with asymptomatically infected individuals to disease transmission is unclear. Household members in home with ill member. These household members may have asymptomatic illness and may be able to shed influenza virus that promotes community disease transmission. Therefore, household members of homes with sick individuals would be advised to stay home.

[e]To facilate compliance and decrease risk of household transmission, this intervention may be combined with provision of antiviral medications to household contacts depending on drug availability, feasibility, and effectiveness; policy recommendations for antiviral prophylaxis are addressed in a separate guidance document.

[f]Consider short-term suspension of classes, that is, less than 4 weeks.

[g]Plan for prolonged suspension of classes, that is, 1 to 3 months; actual duration may vary depending on transmission in the community as the pandemic wave is expected to last 6-8 weeks.

system as well as estimates the burden of flu illness using statistical modeling (CDC, 2010a). On April, 29, 2009, the CDC began reporting cases of respiratory infection with swine-origin influenza A (H1N1) viruses transmitted through human-to-human contact (CDC, 2009a, 2009b). It established the case definition for 2009 H1N1 as an acute febrile respiratory illness in a person and laboratory-confirmed swine-origin influenza A (H1N1) virus infection at CDC by either of the following tests: real-time reverse transcription-polymerase chain reaction (rRT-PCR), or viral culture (CDC, 2009a). The CDC began tracking and reporting the number of cases, hospitalizations and deaths at state, local and national levels using standard state reporting mechanisms. It was soon apparent that using actual case counts resulted in dramatically underreported disease.

On July 24, 2009, CDC abandoned initial case counts, when it recognized that those numbers represented a significant undercount of the actual number of 2009 H1N1 cases. They found that 2009 H1N1 was less severe and caused fewer deaths than expected when compared to the pandemic planning assumptions. As a result, existing plans, which used case fatality numbers as the trigger for initiating response actions, were not effective.

Scientists turned to other means to begin to understand the effects of disease and predict its future course. For example, because trending indicated that children and young adults were at higher risk, the Department of Education began looking at school closures and school absenteeism, examining both teacher and student absences. Each of the critical infrastructure key resource sectors held weekly calls with private sector partners to elicit whether there were trends beginning to indicate business interruption problems, which might forecast social disruptions. The National Retail Data monitoring system tracked the real-time purchase of over-the-counter (OTC) medications, such as fever reducers and influenza treatments, in over 29,000 retail pharmacies, groceries, and mass merchandise stores. This University of Pittsburgh system (n.d.) is used to provide early detection of naturally occurring disease outbreaks as well as bioterrorism.

The CDC moved to using estimates. Using the influenza module from BioSense, CDC tracked flu with data from over 500 local and state health departments, hospital emergency rooms, Laboratory Response Network labs, Health Information Exchanges as well as the Departments of Defense and Veterans Affairs. A similar system, the Electronic Surveillance System for the Early Notification of Community-Based Epidemics (ESSENCE) was also used. ESSENCE is a Department of Defense tool that fuses syndromic information from multiple data sources that differ in their medical specificity, spatial organization, scale, and time-series behavior to provide early warning at the community level (Burkhom, Elbert, & Lin, 2004).The Real-time Outbreak Disease Surveillance (RODS) took chief complaint information from clinical encounters hospitals and classified it into one of seven syndrome categories using Bayesian classifiers. The data is stored in a relational database, used univariate and multivariate

statistical detection and alerted users of when the algorithms identify anomalous patterns in the syndrome count (Tsui, Espino, Data, et al., 2003). Interpreting these estimates, one study hypothesized that for every reported lab-confirmed case of H1N1 between April and July 2009, there were an estimated 79 total cases. The same study found that for every identified hospitalized case there were more likely 2.7 hospitalized people (Reed, Angulo, Swerdlow, et al., 2009) (Table 35.5).

Concerned that the limited capacity of the healthcare system would be overwhelmed and finite resources such as H1N1 test kits would be consumed, CDC published updated self-treatment guidance and told the public that H1N1 testing was no longer necessary. Instead, persons with minor flu-like illnesses were assumed to be infected and encouraged to utilize advice lines staffed by nurses to obtain answers to questions rather than to seek appointments with healthcare providers. For the first time the U.S. government established a one-stop federal Website (www.flu.gov) that housed information such as frequently asked questions as well as messaging aimed at individuals and families, businesses, and healthcare professionals from across the federal interagency. The Website contained tailored planning documents for schools and communities, and included targeted information for special populations. One particularly helpful site was a Flu Vaccine Locator, which contained a database that provided the general public with the locations of clinics that had vaccine supplies utilizing zip codes (DHHS, n.d.)

For the first time, HHS used social media to communicate with young people. Recognizing that large numbers of young adults were affected, they launched a Facebook application "I'm a Flu Fighter!" that allowed and encouraged users to spread information about H1N1, such as where they received the H1N1 vaccine, to their Facebook friends (Mitchell, 2010).

Healthcare Consumers Contribute to Surveillance Activities

In the H1N1 case study described above, healthcare consumer data became an important aspect of the disease surveillance model that augmented data collected by the CDC. Why was that the case? Now more than ever before consumers have the opportunity to contribute to surveillance activities. In some cases, the participation is a conscious decision, but in others consumers may be unknowingly contributing to this informatics process.

Part of the advantage of externally generated CDC surveillance mechanisms is that they shorten the typical lag time to publication for CDC's publicly reported data which is currently estimated to be from 10 to 14 days

TABLE 35.5	Technology and Informatics Contributions to Incident Management	
Functions	**Possible Technologies**	**Informatics Processing**
Data for Incident Command Center	Smart White Board Electronic Dashboards Resource Modeling Internet Access to Information Resources Staffing and Scheduling Records Electronic Logs to Capture Data and Decisions Resource Inventories Resource Distributor Database Online Disaster Manual with Job Action Sheets	Organize and detect patterns and trends in data Predict resource needs and safety zones Access additional data and information Record and process decisions for legal and financial purposes Analyze data to determine statistical significance Report and analyze internet surveillance systems Promote standardization of data collection and vocabulary
Communications	Landlines Radio Communications Cell Phones Satellite phones Amateur Radios Third and Fourth Generation Wireless Devices Electronic Mail Internet, Twitter, FaceBook Television and Radio announcements	Standardized vocabulary and roles Communication standards set in order to prioritize and determine accuracy of data transmission Data collection from the field is sent back to EOC Data collection and analysis contributes to situational awareness
Patient Tracking	Global Positioning systems (GPS) Bar code tracking Radio frequency identification	Data and Information processed for purposes of triage and transport Data collected to determine magnitude of disaster
Provider Safety	Radiation monitors and badges Radio communications GPS devices Cell phones	Data collection and Monitoring to determine safe radiation levels Cellular triangulation to determine location
Ambulance Tracking	GPS Cell phones Radio communication	Monitor for triage and admission purposes
Patient data acquisition and monitoring	Electronic PDA record Wireless monitoring; ED status system Pharmacy electronic records	Collect and analyze to determine trends across geographic area

(Ginsberg, Mohebbi, Patel, et al., 2009). Telephone triage data is now being used to help track influenza in a specified geographic location with the added advantage that the data is real-time in nature. In addition, patient demographics and disease symptoms can also be captured in a standard format. Another new mechanism for data capture about influenza is through physician group proprietary systems. In these systems, the healthcare providers enter the data for suspected or confirmed influenza patients. By far, the most talked about trend in influenza surveillance for the 2009 H1N1 outbreak was Google's Flu Trends. The assumption made with this system was that there was a relationship between how many people search the internet for flu-related topics and how many people have flu-like symptoms.

In studies conducted by Google.org comparing Google Flu Trends to CDC published data, they found that the search-based flu estimates had a consistently strong correlation with real CDC surveillance data (Ginsberg et al., 2009).

COMPETENCY-BASED LEARNING AND INFORMATICS NEEDS

In order to provide a successful nursing response effort, nurses must be appropriately and consistently educated to provide the right response. Competency-based education provides an international infrastructure for nurses to learn about emergency preparedness and response (Weiner,

2006). Yet, currently there are no accepted, standardized requirements for disaster nursing training or continuing education (Slepski & Littleton-Kearney, 2010).

There have been, however, a number of competency development efforts geared to different nursing audiences. In collaboration with the CDC, researchers from the Columbia University School of Nursing identified nine objectively measurable skills for public health workers and seven competencies for leaders, followed by an additional three competencies for public health professionals (Columbia University School of Nursing Center for Health Policy, 2002). There were also two competencies identified for public health technical and support staff relating to (1) demonstration of equipment and skills associated with his/her functional role in emergency preparedness during regular drills and (2) description of at least one resource for backup support in key areas of responsibility. In 2003, the International Nursing Coalition for Mass Casualty Education (later renamed the Nursing Emergency Preparedness Coalition, or NEPEC) generated a list of 104 competency statements for all nurses responding to disasters using domains developed by the American Association of Colleges of Nursing (Weiner, 2006). Additional competencies were developed by the University of Hyogo and the International Council of Nurses. All of the competency efforts were considered by a WHO group of nursing experts as they developed competency domains during the first consultation on nursing and midwifery in emergencies (WHO, 2007, p. 10).

Bakken (2002) noted that the detection of and response to the threat of bioterrorism requires an informatics infrastructure that includes: (1) continuous monitoring of a variety of data; (2) standards for combining data from different sources and coordination of such efforts; (3) computer-based processing and analysis that help detect unusual and statistically significant patterns; (4) centralized diagnostic and therapeutic tools such as computer-based algorithms and protocols for treating conditions caused by infectious agents; and (5) communication technology. Furthermore, she selected four general informatics competencies and provided examples of their use in biodefense (Bakken, 2002, p. 79).

Efforts to identify content to match competencies have also proven successful. An additional group of experts met following WHO's first consultation on nursing and midwifery contributions in emergencies to identify possible content that matched the identified competencies at the undergraduate nursing level (WHO, 2008b). Online modules produced by NEPEC (www.nepec.net) and the National Nursing Emergency Preparedness Initiative (NNEPI) (www.nnepi.org) both

received international awards from Sigma Theta Tau International for quality computer-based education programs.

The CDC currently sponsors a public health informatics fellowship program that is a two year paid fellowship in public health informatics (CDC, 2010b). The competency-based and hands-on training allows students to apply information and computer science and technology to solving real public health problems.

Informatics and Incident Management

Information technology staff members have long been familiar with emergency planning for disaster recovery related to their systems, but find themselves in a new role as part of a more comprehensive team approach to disasters and emergencies. The incident management system (IMS) was first used by firefighters to control disaster scenes in a multijurisdictional and interdepartmental manner. The IMS calls for a hierarchical chain of command led by the incident manager or commander. Each job assignment is consistently followed by assigned personnel who refer to a specific job action sheet. This system improves communication through a common language, allows staff to move between management locations, and facilitates all responders to understand the established chain of command. The IMS has been adapted for hospital use and is called the Hospital Incident Command System (HICS).

The Emergency Operations Center is the physical location where the Incident Management Team convenes to make decisions, communicate, and coordinate the various activities in response to an incident. Accurate, real-time data acquisition regarding patient needs, rescue personnel, and resources available is critical to overall coordination. Table 35.5 presents functions where technology can be used to capture and represent data for purposes of increasing situational awareness in the EOC for the purposes of making the most informed and efficient decisions. In addition, the informatics processing efforts that contribute to the incident management system are also described.

Informatics and Volunteerism

Healthcare volunteers are a necessary component of mass casualty events but also create challenges. How do you count volunteers so that they are only entered once? How do you educate them so that they can perform effectively when needed? How are liability issues dealt with? Are there certain tasks that lend themselves to volunteer efforts? Some states offer their nurses the opportunity to volunteer when they renew their nursing licensure. It is then possible for state-wide volunteer databases to be built, but these are only shared within the state system. Some states require a set number of hours of continuing education in emergency preparedness in order to renew licensure.

The federal government does have a system for organizing teams that are willing to travel to other regions of the country in the event of an emergency. These teams are called disaster medical assistance teams (DMATs). When DMATs are activated, members of the teams are federalized or made temporary workers of the federal government, which then assumes the liability for their services. Their licensure and certifications are then recognized by all states.

The Medical Reserve Corps (MRC) and the Emergency System for Advance Registration of Volunteer Health Professionals (ESAR-VHP) both represent initiatives of the Department of Health and Human Services to improve the nation's ability to prepare for and respond to public health emergencies. The MRC was founded after President Bush's 2002 State of the Union address, in which he asked all Americans to volunteer in support of their country (MRC, 2010). The MRC is a national network of community-based volunteer units that focus on improving the health, safety and resiliency of their local communities. MRC volunteers include medical and public health professionals such as physicians, nurses, pharmacists, dentists, veterinarians, and epidemiologists. Many community members—interpreters, chaplains, office workers, legal advisors, and others—can fill key support positions. For example, nurses trained in informatics are often used by MRC units to compile needed databases depending on the response effort at hand. At the time of this writing, there are 888 units composed of 208,979 volunteers, covering 70.4% of the United States (MRC, 2010).

The national ESAR-VHP program provides guidance and assistance for the development of standardized state-based programs for registering and verifying the credentials of volunteer health professionals in advance of an emergency or disaster. Each state program collects and verifies information on the identity, licensure status, privileges, and credentials of volunteers. These programs are built to a common set of national standards and give each state the ability to quickly identify and assist in the coordination of volunteer health professionals in an emergency. These registration systems include information about volunteers involved in organized efforts at the local level (such as MRC units) and the state level (DMAT and state medical response teams). In addition, individuals who prefer not to be part of an organized unit structure can also be entered into the registry in order to allow for a ready pool of volunteers. State ESAR-VHP programs provide a single, centralized source of information to facilitate the intrastate, interstate, and state-to-federal deployment or transfer of volunteer health professionals. Several collaboration suggestions have been generated in an effort to integrate both the MRC and ESAR-VHP initiatives, including having state coordinators for both initiatives (MRC, 2008).

Most volunteer opportunities require education prior to responding to the event. MRC units have competency based education requirements. The American Red Cross has a long history of volunteerism during disasters, and has education requirements for nurses depending on what roles they will play in disaster relief. Regardless of the group, nurses are urged to be a part of an organized group rather than simply showing up on the scene of a disaster and contributing to the confusion. All of these initiatives require informatics solutions in order to function effectively. Organizing the results of these efforts into a standardized registry allows for more informed decisions and increased efficiency of services during times of response and relief efforts.

Future Advances

While the recent pandemic fortunately was far less severe than the "Armageddon-like" event that planners forecasted, it served to highlight many opportunities for the use of informatics to assist in emergency preparedness and response. Health information technology investments are a necessary foundation in healthcare reform, linking potentially valuable information such as vaccination records and subsequent use of healthcare services to provide information about adverse events as well as vaccine effectiveness (Lurie, 2010).

Using "grids" to connect multiple computers across the country will allow data sources to share and view large amounts of health information. Grid participants will be able to analyze data in other jurisdictions without moving the actual data, which is an important step forward in overcoming policy barriers to moving data out of a jurisdiction to protect individual privacy.

Expanding the use of the electronic health record should help both patients and their healthcare providers during times of emergencies and disasters. Accessing clinical data for displaced patients should improve tremendously with interoperable data and the sharing of clinical information. A pilot project called KatrinaHealth illustrates such potential with the pooling of information resources across federal and private sectors. KatrinaHealth.org is a free and secure online service that provides Katrina evacuees, their authorized healthcare providers and pharmacists with a list of the prescription medications evacuees were taking before they were forced to leave their homes, lost their medications, and the medical records (KatrinaHealth, 2010).

SUMMARY

In conclusion, the 2009 H1N1 outbreak was a recent example of emergency preparedness and response. It reinforced the fact that estimating the number of actual flu cases is very challenging as current case counting relies on encounter information, which is prone to underreporting. Informatics is an emerging field that has the potential to immediately support the early identification of a communicable disease such as pandemic influenza, reducing loss of life and the consumption of limited resources. Use of automated case specific disease monitoring applications such as BioSense, ESSENCE and RODS and tracking retail data such as OTC medication purchases allows researchers to collect, analyze and present real-time disease information which allows users to have immediate access to information that previously would have taken days to assemble. Technological developments will further enhance the ability to use informatics to detect the first warning signs during an emergency.

Consumers themselves have assumed surveillance roles in their quest to seek data and information resources. The increase use of social media provides a new mechanism for data collection and trending.

Coordinated response efforts require excellent communication based on efficient decision making. Informatics can contribute to this agenda, particularly in an era when healthcare resources are dwindling. As a result, informatics solutions need to remain central to emergency planning and response efforts.

REFERENCES

Bakken, S. (2002). Biodefense and nursing informatics: The skills and technology nurses need. *American Journal of Nursing, 102*(9), 79–80.

Birnbaum, M. L. (2010). Stop!!!!!. *Prehospital and Disaster Medicine, 25*(2), 97–98.

Burkhom, H. S., Elbert, Y. and Lin, J. (2004, September 24). Role of data aggregation in biosurveillance detection strategies with applications from ESSENCE. *Morbidity and Mortality Weekly Report, 53*(Suppl), 67–73.

Centers for Disease Control and Prevention. (2009a). *Update: Swine Influenza A (H1N1) infections— California and Texas,* April 2009. Retrieved on April 12, 2011 from http://www.cdc.gov/mmwr/preview/mmwrhtml/mm5816a7.htm

Centers for Disease Control and Prevention. (2009b). *Update: Infections with a swine-origin Influenza A (H1N1) virus—United States and other countries, April 28, 2009.* Retrieved on April 12, 2011 from http://www.cdc.gov/mmwr/preview/mmwrhtml/mm5816a5.htm

Centers for Disease Control and Prevention. (2010a). *CDC estimates of 2009 H1N1 influenza cases, hospitalizations and deaths in the United States, April 2009- April 10, 2010.* Retrieved on April 12, 2011 from http://www.cdc.gov/h1n1flu/estimates_2009_h1n1.htm

Centers for Disease Control and Prevention. (2010b). *Public health informatics fellowship program.* Retrieved on April 12, 2011 from http://www.cdc.gov/PHIFP/More.html

Chan, R. C., Killeen, J., Griswold, W., & Lenert, L. (2004). Information technology and emergency medical care during disasters. Academic *Emergency Medicine, 11*(11), 1229–1236. doi:10.1197/j.aem.2004.08009

Columbia University School of Nursing Center for Health Policy. (2002, November). *Bioterrorism and emergency readiness competencies for all public health workers.* Retrieved on April 12, 2011 from http://www.cumc.columbia.edu/dept/nursing/chp/pdfArchive/btcomps.pdf

Department of Health and Human Services. (n.d.). *Know what to do about the flu.* Retrieved on April 12, 2011 from www.flu.gov

Department of Health and Human Services. (2005). *HHS pandemic influenza plan.* Retrieved on April 12, 2011 from http://www.hhs.gov/pandemicflu/plan/pdf/HHSPandemicInfluenzaPlan.pdf

Department of Health and Human Services. (2007). *Interim pre-pandemic planning guidance: Community strategy for pandemic influenza mitigation in the United States.* Retrieved on April 12, 2011 from www.pandemicflu.gov/plan/community/community_mitigation.pdf

Department of Homeland Security. (2008a). *Introducing the National Response Framework.* Retrieved on April 12, 2011 from http://www.fema.gov/pdf/emergency/nrf/about_nrf.pdf

Department of Homeland Security. (2008b). *National Response Framework. Emergency Support Annexes: Introduction.* Retrieved on April 12, 2011 from http://www.fema.gov/pdf/emergency/nrf/nrf-esf-intro.pdf

Department of Homeland Security. (2007). *Pandemic influenza preparedness, response, and recovery guide for critical infrastructure and key resources.* Retrieved on April 12, 2011 from http://www.flu.gov/professional/pdf/cikrpandemicinfluenzaguide.pdf

Ginsberg, J., Mohebbi, M., Patel, R., Brammer, L., Smolinski, M. & Brillant, L. (2009). Detecting influenza epidemics using search engine query data. *Nature, 457*, 1012–1015. Doi:10.1038/nature07634

KatrinaHealth. (2010). Retrieved on April 12, 2011 from http://www.katrinahealth.org/

Lombardo, J. *Public health informatics and the H1N1 pandemic*. Retrieved on April 12, 2011 from http://firstmonday.org/htbin/cgiwrap/bin/ojs/index.php/ojphi/article/viewFile/2778/2425

Lurie, N. (2009). H1N1 influenza, public health preparedness, and healthcare reform. *New England Journal of Medicine, 361*(9), 843–845. Retrieved on April 12, 2011 from http://content.nejm.org/cgi/content/short/361/9/843

Medical Reserve Corps. (April, 2008). *Integration of the Medical Reserve Corps and the Emergency System for Advance Registration of Volunteer Health Professionals*. Retrieved on April 12, 2011 from http://www.medicalreservecorps.gov/file/esar_vhp/esar-vhpmrcintegrationfactsheet.pdf

Medical Reserve Corps. (2010). *About MRC*. Retrieved on April 12, 2011 from http://www.medicalreservecorps.gov/About

Mitchell, D. (2010). *Facebook application "I'm a Flu Fighter" announced by Sebelius*. Retrieved on April 12, 2011 from http://www.emaxhealth.com/1275/90/35120/facebook-application-im-flu-fighter-announced-sebelius.html

Occupational Safety and Health Administration. (2007). *Pandemic influenza preparedness and response guidance for healthcare workers and healthcare employers*. Retrieved on April 12, 2011 from http://www.osha.gov/Publications/OSHA_pandemic_health.pdf

Reed, C., Angulo, F. J., Swerdlow, D. L., Lipsitch, M., Melter, M. I., Jernigan, D., et al. (2009, December). Estimates of the prevalence of pandemic (H1N1) 2009, United States, April-July 2009. *Emerging Infectious Disease*. Retrieved on April 12, 2011 from http://www.cdc.gov/eid/content/15/12/pdfs/09-1413.pdf. doi: 10.3201/eid1512.091413

Slepski, L., & Littleton-Kearney, M. T. (2010). Disaster nursing educational competencies (pp. 549–559). In R. Powers, & E. Daily(Eds.), *International disaster nursing*. New York: Cambridge University Press.

Teich, J. M., Wagner, M. M., Mackenzie, D. F., & Schafer, K. O. (2002). The informatics response in disaster, terrorism, and war. *Journal of American Medical Informatics Association, 9*(2), 97–104. doi:10.1197/jamia.M1055

Tsui, F., Espino, J. U., Data, V. M., Gesteland, P. H., Hutman, J., and Wagner, M. M. (2003). Technical description of RODS: A real-time public health surveillance system. *Journal of the American Medical Informatics Association; 10*(5), 399–408. doi:10.1197/jamia.M1345

University of Pittsburgh. (n.d.). About the National Retail Data Monitor. Retrieved on April 12, 2011 from https://www.rods.pitt.edu/site/content/blogsection/4/42/

Weiner, E. (2006, September 30). Preparing nurses internationally for emergency planning and response. *OJIN: The Online Journal of Issues in Nursing, 11*(3), Manuscript 3. Retrieved on April 12, 2011 from www.nursingworld.org/MainMenuCategories/ANAMarketplace/ANAPeriodicals/OJIN/TableofContents/Volume112006/No3Sept06/PreparingNurses.aspx

White House. (2003, February 28). *Homeland Security Presidential Directive 5: Management of domestic incidents*. Retrieved on April 12, 2011 from http://www.fws.gov/Contaminants/FWS_OSCP_05/fwscontingencyappendices/A-NCP-NRP/HSPD-5.pdf

World Health Organization. (2007). T*he contribution of nursing and midwifery in emergencies: Report of a WHO consultation*. WHO Headquarters, Geneva, November 22-24. Retrieved on April 12, 2011 from http://www.who.int/hac/events/2006/nursing_consultation_report_sept07.pdf

World Health Organization. (2008a). *WHO humanitarian action 2008-2009: Biennial work plan to support WHO's capacity for work in emergencies and crises*. Retrieved on April 12, 2011 from http://www.who.int/hac/about/workplan.pdf

World Health Organization. (2008b). *Integrating emergency preparedness and response into undergraduate nursing curriculum*. Retrieved on April 12, 2011 from http://whqlibdoc.who.int/hq/2008/WHO_HAC_BRO_08.7_eng.pdf

World Health Organization. (2009, December). *Strengthening WHO's institutional capacity for humanitarian health action: A five-year programme progress report*. Retrieved on April 12, 2011 from http://www.who.int/hac/events/5years_progress_report_brochure.pdf

PART 6

Educational Applications

Diane J. Skiba

36

Web 2.0 and Its Impact on Healthcare Education and Practice

Diane J. Skiba / Paul D. Guillory / Kay Lynn Olmsted

• OBJECTIVES

1. Describe the evolution of the Internet and the movement toward Web 2.0.
2. Describe the use of Web 2.0 tools in healthcare education and practice.
3. Discuss the impact of consumer-generated content and collaboration on the Web.
4. Identify the challenges and issues related to the use of social media in healthcare education and practice.

• KEY WORDS

Web 2.0
Health 2.0
Social Networking
Social Media
Virtual Worlds
Internet

INTRODUCTION

The Internet has revolutionized the computer and communications world like nothing before. The Internet is at once a world-wide broadcasting capability, a mechanism for information dissemination, and a medium for collaboration and interaction between individuals and their computers without regard for geographic location (Leiner, Cerf, Clark, Kahn, Kleinrock, et al., 1997, p. 102).

There is no doubt the Internet provided the necessary infrastructure to revolutionize the way scientists and researchers from the worlds of academia, business, and government could share data, interact, and collaborate with each other. But it was not until the introduction of the World Wide Web that "everyday people" with-

out computer programming skills were enabled to reap the benefits of this revolution. The Web not only changed how governments and businesses operate, it has impacted every facet of society—how we work, learn, play, and now, even how we manage our health.

In this chapter, there is a brief history of the evolution of the Web and its growing use in healthcare. There is a specific focus on the use of Web 2.0 tools and the growing movement of Health 2.0. Web 2.0, especially social media tools, are dramatically changing the way consumers seek health information, interact with their healthcare providers, and ultimately how healthcare will be delivered in the future. As Sarasohn-Kahn (2008, p. 2) noted, "the use of social media on the Internet are empowering, engaging and educating consumers and providers in healthcare." This chapter presents current examples of Web 2.0 tools such as social networking and virtual worlds in healthcare. The challenges related to the growing use of these tools are also discussed.

HISTORICAL PERSPECTIVE

As early as the 1960s, computer scientists began to write about the creation of a network of interconnected computers where scientists could share and analyze data by interacting across the network (Leiner, et al., 1997). According to Cerf (1995), "the name 'Internet' refers to the global seamless interconnection of networks made possible by the protocols devised in the 1970s through DARPA-sponsored research." The Internet is defined as "a computer network consisting of a worldwide network of computer networks that use the TCP/IP network protocols to facilitate data transmission and exchange" (http://wordnetweb.princeton. edu/perl/webwn). Several underlying technical principles facilitated the development of the Internet. The first was the idea of open architecture networking and a set of operating principles set forth by Robert Kahn at Defense Advanced Research Projects Agency (DARPA) (Leiner, et al., 1997). The second was the development of the Transmission Control Protocol/Internet Protocol (TCP/IP) by Kahn and Cerf. In 1972, ARPANET, predecessor of the Internet, had its first public demonstration. According to Leiner and colleagues (1997), a basic message (send and read) software designed by Ray Tomlinson was introduced and started the evolution of electronic mail as an application. "From there, email took off as the most popular network application and as a harbinger of the kind of people-to-people communication activity we see on the World-Wide Web today" (Leiner, et al., 1997 p. 103). Over the next decade, various government agencies and companies conducted considerable research to support the advancement of the Internet. It was not until 1985 that a broader community, in particular the academic community beyond the computer scientists, was given access to the Internet. At this time, the National Science Foundation (NSF) sanctioned the use of the Internet to serve the total higher education community. NSF funding for the Internet continued for almost a decade before the Internet was redistributed to regional networks with the eventual move toward interconnecting networks across the globe.

As the Internet came to expand, Tim Berners-Lee wrote his seminal paper *Information Management: A proposal* that circulated throughout the European Council for Nuclear Research (CERN) organization.

The paper explicated his ideas that using a hypertext system that would allow for storage and retrieval of information in a "web of notes with links (like references) between them is far more useful than a fixed hierarchical system" (Berners-Lee, 1989). The paper built upon the ideas set forth by Vannevar Bush in 1945 and Doug Engelbart, Ted Nelson, and Andrew van Dam in the 1960s (Cailliau & Connolly, 2010). In 1990, Berners-Lee's paper was recirculated and he began development of a global hypertext system that would eventually become the World Wide Web (WWW). As the WWW concept evolved, Marc Andreessen and Eric Bina at the University of Illinois developed a browser called Mosaic that provided a graphical interface for users. This browser is credited with popularizing the Web. The development of other browsers and online services that expand consumer access to the Web still continues today.

It is important to note that although many use the terms *Internet* and *Web* synonymously, there are differences between them. Whereas the Internet is the network of interconnected computers across globe, the Web is an application that supports a system of interlinked, hypertexted documents. One uses the Internet to connect to the Web. A Web browser allows the user to view Web pages that contain text, images, and other multimedia.

The Web in its first iteration (Web 1.0) allowed users to access information and knowledge housed on Web pages complete with text, images, and even some multimedia. It was considered a dissemination vehicle that democratized access to information and knowledge. Consumers could access information and knowledge that was now being made publically available. Information and knowledge was not bound by geography or time. The Web consisted of individual Web pages. To create a Web page, one needed to understand how to create hypertext mark up language (HTML) documents. Although information and knowledge was being shared, static Web pages were only changeable by the owner of the document.

Many in the field designate the time period between 1991 and 2004 as Web 1.0. This was an important era and, as noted by Friedman (2005), the world suddenly became flat—his metaphor for the leveling of the global playing field. The convergence of the personal computer with the world of the Internet and all its services facilitated the flattening. The flattening was particularly powerful in the world of commerce but also exploded in higher education, making it easier for students to access knowledge beyond their own academic campus. For healthcare, it was a time where consumers could now have access to health information and knowledge that was not locked in an academic library or in a distant place.

O'Reilly and Doughtery introduced the term *Web 2.0* at a 2004 conference brainstorming session about the failures of the dot-com industry. It was apparent that despite the demise of the dot-com industry, "the web was more important than ever, with exciting new applications and sites popping up with surprising regularity" (O'Reilly, 2005). There were several key concepts that formed the definition of Web 2.0. First, the Web is viewed as a platform rather than an application. Second, the power of the Web is achieved by harnessing the collective intelligence of the users. A third important principle was that the Web provided rich user experiences. According to O'Reily (2005), "the core competencies of Web 2.0 companies include:

1. Services, not packaged software, with cost-effective scalability
2. Control over unique, hard-to-recreate data sources that get richer as more people use them
3. Trusting users as co-developers
4. Harnessing collective intelligence
5. Leveraging the long tail through customer self-service
6. Software above the level of a single device
7. Lightweight user interfaces, development models, and business models"

The introduction of Web 2.0 embodies the long history of community spirit of the Internet conceived by its originators. As Leiner and colleagues (1997, p. 206) noted, "the Internet is as much a collection of communities as a collection of technologies, and its success is largely attributable to satisfying basic community needs as well as utilizing the community effectively to push the infrastructure forward."

The transition from an information dissemination platform to an engaging, customizable, social and media-rich environment epitomizes this next generation of the Web. As Downes (2005) stated, "the Web was shifting from being a medium, in which information was transmitted and consumed, into being a platform, in which content was created, shared, remixed, repurposed, and passed along." Another important feature was the idea of users interacting and sharing information, ideas, and content. Owen, Grant, Sayers, and Facer (2006) aptly described the transition of the Web, "we have witnessed a renaissance of this idea in the emergence of tools, resources and practices that are seen by many as returning the web to its early potential to facilitate collaboration and social interaction."

To set the context for the description of Web 2.0 tools and their uses in healthcare, it is important to understand the environmental context. The Internet Web Stats Web site, www.internetworldstats.com/stats,htm, collects information about Internet usage. In 2000, the number of people worldwide using the Internet was 360,985,492 and the current usage as of June 2010 is 1,966,514,816. The current usage represents a 28.7% penetration of the total global population. This represents a growth of 444.8% over the last decade. The largest penetration of Internet users is North America at 77.4%, followed by Oceania/Australia at 61.3%, and Europe with a 52.4% penetration. Although their penetration is only 21.5%, Asia represents 42% of all Internet users as of June 2010.

WEB 2.0 TOOLS IN EDUCATION AND PRACTICE

The growth of Web 2.0 tools in the healthcare delivery system has served as a catalyst for the Health 2.0 movement (Hughes, Joshi, & Wareham, 2008). Although, there is no single accepted definition of Health 2.0, most definitions include the idea of Web 2.0 tools applied to health (Van De Belt, Engelen, Berben, & Schoonhovenm, 2010). The Health 2.0 movement is, in essence, the overall umbrella to categorize the various uses of Web 2.0 tools in healthcare.

Web 2.0 applications can be categorized in several different ways. Some authors break down these tools into communications, social writing, social bookmarking, social networking, and social media. Some authors equate Web 2.0 tools with the term *social software*. Shirky (2002) simply defined this term as "software that supports group interactions." He goes on to explicate that social software has the ability to connect people together on an intellectual level to share and evolve ideas. Boyd (2003) further suggested that "social software have three defining characteristics: (1) Support for conversational interaction between individuals or groups ranging from real-time instant messaging to asynchronous collaborative teamwork spaces; (2) Support for social feedback which allows a group to rate the contributions of others, perhaps implicitly, leading to the creation of digital reputation, and (3) Support for social networks to explicitly create and manage a digital expression of people's personal relationships, and to help them build new relationships."

In some cases, social media is used as the broad category that encompasses all of the Web 2.0 tools. For example, the Web site *SearchEngineWatch* (searchengine watch.com/define) defines social media as "a category of sites that is based on user participation and user-generated content. They include social networking (e.g., LinkedIn, Facebook) social bookmarking (e.g., Del.icio.us), social news (e.g., Digg, Reddit), and other sites that are centered on user interaction. Anthony Bradley (2010) in his blog (blogs.gartner.com/anthony_bradley/2010/01/07/ a-new-definition-of-social-media) offers a new definition, "social media is a set of technologies and channels targeted at forming and enabling a potentially massive community of participants to productively collaborate.... enable collaboration on a much grander scale and support tapping the power of the collective in ways previously unachievable." According to Bradley (2010), there are 6 defining characteristics that distinguish social media from other collaboration and communication IT tools. These characteristics are: Participation, Collective, Transparency, Independence, Persistence, and Emergence. Participation echoes the "wisdom of the crowds" concept, but note that there is no wisdom if the crowd does not participate. The term *collective* refers to the idea that people collect or congregate around content to contribute, rather than the way individuals create and distribute content in the Web 1. 0 world. Transparency refers to the fact that everyone can see who is contributing and what contributions are made. Independence refers to the anytime, anyplace concept; people can participate regardless of geography or time. Persistence refers to the notion that information or content being exchanged is captured and not lost as in a synchronous chat room. Lastly, "the emergence principle embodies the recognition that you can't predict, model, design and control all human collaborative interactions and optimize them as you would a fixed business process" (Bradley, 2010). Taken together these characteristics define the new world of social media.

Given our understanding of Web 2.0 tools and some of the definitions associated with them, what follows are examples of these tools and their uses in healthcare education and practice. The examples are grouped into 2 categories: Communications and Social Writing and Social Media. Within social media, both social networking and virtual world examples are included.

COMMUNICATION AND SOCIAL WRITING

Social writing is another online phenomenon that can take many forms. These include, but are not limited to, wikis, blogs, and microblogging. Wikis are coined after the

Hawaiian work for fast, and are a means to establish an easily and quickly accessed consumer-driven knowledge base (Meister, 2008); they are essentially collaborative tools that are "based on social regulation rather than technical safeguards" (Digital Library Federation, 2008). Blogs, short for Web logs, are considered to be personal Web sites where content is displayed for visitors to review and comment upon (Adams, 2008).

Wikis, as a form of social writing, are also prevalent in healthcare. CliniWiki (www.informatics-review.com/ wiki/index.php/Main_Page) is a popular wiki targeted toward clinical informatics topics. This wiki contains information on a variety of topics in such areas as clinical decision support systems, unintended consequences of technology, federal initiatives, and usability. Many universities also maintain wikis to house pertinent information for their students and colleagues such as the University of Utah's Biomedical Informatics Wiki. For consumers, there is a host of wikis available and David Rothman maintains a current list of these resources (davidroth man.net/list-of-medical-wikis). Here are some examples: Medipedia (www.medipedia.com), Flu wiki (www. newfluwiki2.com), Aids Wiki (www.reviewingaids.com/ awiki/index.php/Main_Page) and Wiki Cancer (www. wikicancer.org).

Wikio, an information portal with a news search engine, searches for blogs and press sites. According to their recent August 2010 listing, some of the top blogs include: Booster Shots from the *Los Angles Times*, Well from the *New York Times* and KevinMD. In informatics, blogs can be associated with magazines such as *Healthcare Informatics* and individual professionals such as Ted Eytan, MD (www.tedeytan.com) that focuses on Health 2.0, John Halamka (geekdoctor.blogspot.com) that focuses on life as a CIO, and professional blogs such as the North Carolina Nursing Informatics blog (http:// informatics.toolshed.com).

According to Bennett (2010), of the current 762 hospitals using social media tools, there are 99 hospitals with blogs. One such example is the Mayo Clinic that maintains numerous blogs targeted toward consumers, such as Alzheimer's, Living with Cancer, and the Mayo Clinic Diet. The Children's Hospital in Boston, has a pediatric blog called *Thrive* that presents a host of pediatric news, cutting edge research, and videos about amazing patients and their families. In addition, there are many blogs that are generated by consumers. Examples of consumer-generated blogs include: Diabetes Mine (www.diabetesmine.com) and Assertive Cancer patient (www.assertivepatient.com).

Another Web 2.0 application, combining texting and blogging, adds a new dimension to communication and social writing. Historically, electronic mail (e-mail), instant messaging, and text messaging, have been less public forms of communication than the aforementioned Web 2.0 applications. E-mail, along with instant and text messaging, requires knowing a recipient's address before the communication can be sent—not unlike mailing a letter through the postal service. Recent Web 2.0 applications, however, have put a twist on such messaging by creating the microblog (Hawn, 2009). Sites like Twitter now allow consumers to post content to a Web site, which then automatically distributes the content to others who have "subscribed" to the individual's site; this creates short bursts of communication among any number of individuals (Hawn, 2009). These microblogging sites allow social communication to come directly to consumers, rather than requiring that consumers go and seek it out themselves.

According to Bennett (2010), of the current 762 hospitals using social media tools, there are 583 that use Twitter. Again, Mayo Clinic leads the way with over 66,000 followers on their Twitter account. The remaining 4 hospitals in the top 5 include: St. Jude's Research Hospital (over 8,000 followers), Aurora St. Luke Medical Center (7,600 followers), Children's National Medical Center (6,762 followers), and Emory Johns Creek Hospital (5,963 followers).

Another tool worth mentioning is the concept of social bookmarking. This tool allows users to save, organize, and share bookmarks. This tool allows one to use Web-based services for saving, organizing through tagging, and sharing with others on the network. Social bookmarking can be described as saving links from other Web sites to a public site so that they may be shared with others (Educause, 2005). Skiba (2006) provided some good examples of how universities are using social bookmarking in their courses and as a method of sharing resources across the campus. She mentions the use of Deli.cio.us as one tool to use with students. Healthcare professionals, students, and even consumers can use this particular social bookmarking tool. In addition, Skiba (2006) described a professional bookmarking tool, Connotea, provided by the publishers of the journal *Nature*, that is used primarily by the scientific community. This particular tool allows one to share not only Web sites but also journal articles in a collaborative manner. For example, a research team might share research articles and Web sites pertinent to their particular study. A recent addition to the marketplace is Health Mine (www.healthmine.com), which is targeted toward healthcare Web sites.

Barton (2009) highlighted the following advantages of social bookmarking: accessibility, tagging as a method

of organization, and the collaborative aspect. Some downsides of tagging are lack of standardization due to the personal nature of the tags, mis-tagging (typos, spelling errors, singular versus plural formats), and the inability to hierarchically associated terms. Chu, Young, Zamora, Kurup, and Marcario (2010) caution users that free sites, in particular, may be vulnerable as they are dependent upon their popularity. Using social bookmarking tools allows the ability to guide other users to relevant content on the Internet (Eysenbach, 2008) and engenders a new level of information sharing.

Keeping track of all of these new applications can be a daunting task. How can professionals and consumers stay updated on their favorite blogs, wikis, and other social media sites? The answer is via an RSS newsreader. Blogs, podcasts, and other Web 2.0 sites can be actively sought out or subscribed to via an RSS feed (Meng, 2005). RSS, or real simple syndication, is a label that is attached to a Web object, such as a Web page, which can then be targeted for subscription (Meng, 2005). A consumer can select any number of these Web objects to be delivered, or automatically uploaded, to an RSS news reader that can be embedded in a Web page or exist as an independent Web site in and of itself, such as Google Reader. The consumer can then go to a single location, the RSS newsreader, to view summaries of compiled Web sites or social media sites.

SOCIAL MEDIA

Social media, as the second category of tools, embraces many of the defining characteristics of the Web 2.0 and, consequently, the Health 2.0 movement. First, participation and collaboration are two of the principle themes in Web 2.0 (Eysenbach, 2008) and are the driving forces behind the social media movement. The ability for people to connect with others and become part of a network with like-minded people is a pervasive concept, not only in healthcare but also in society. This is definitively exemplified in the phenomenal growth of social networks such as Facebook and MySpace. According to statistics on Facebook, the site has more than 500 million users. Many in the social media industry tout that if Facebook was a county it would be the third largest county in the world. According to Eysenbach (2008), "Social networking is central to many Web 2.0 and Medicine 2.0 applications and involves the explicit modeling of connections between people, forming a complex network of relations, which in turn enables and facilitates collaboration and collaborative filtering processes."

Second, is the concept of user-generated content. Whether their motivation is peer support, knowledge acquisition, or expressive writing, patients are now consumers and codevelopers of the content being created (O'Reilly, 2005). Social media aims at sharing personal information. Unlike social networking, however, social media Web sites focus on a particular media format as its genesis for public interaction. Web sites such as YouTube, Flickr, and Podbean all allow consumers to add videos, photos, music, podcasts, and other types of media. The term *Podcast* is a composite of the name iPod™, which is the popular media player produced by Apple, Inc and the word broadcast, meaning to send forth (Sarasohn-Kahn, 2008). Meng (2005) defines it further as the capture of an audio occurrence, whether it is a speech or a song, posted on a Web site. Consumers only need to follow a few simple steps in order to create an account, and then they are able to upload, or contribute, content right away. In addition to adding and viewing content, consumers can also post comments to media someone else has contributed thus adding another level of communication to these sites (Skiba, 2007). Depending on their location and distribution, social media sites may be subject to state and federal laws and may have certain constraints that limit the size or content of the media. For example, YouTube limits content by not permitting its users to add copyright protected or overly explicit content (YouTube, n.d.).

Third, is the idea that interactions and collaboration can occur in rich immersive virtual environments. In the past, these rich virtual environments were only accessible through virtual reality tools in a physical space. By definition, virtual reality (VR) is a computer-simulated reality that projects the user into a 3-dimensional (3D) experience "in which users can navigate in a world and interact with it while being immersed in another environment in real time" (Koerner, 2003, p. 12). 3D virtual environments (VEs) afford a variable immersive experience (Deucher & Nodder, 2003). The fully immersive VEs require the use of multimedia peripherals such as haptic devices, stereoscopic goggles or helmets, data gloves, handheld devices, and body suits, which monitor the user and modify the simulation (Dalgarno & Lee, 2010; Koerner, 2003; Simpson, 2002). But more recently, it is the multiuser virtual environments (MUVEs) accessed through the personal computer and high-speed Internet connectivity that have gained recognition and popularity across the landscapes of entertainment, business, education, and healthcare.

Of the available Web 2.0 tools, social networking offers the most opportunity for peer support and consumer engagement. The term social network is not new and can be described as a system where individuals from all backgrounds can be regarded as relative equals and engage in cooperative efforts (Barnes, 1954). In recent times, the social network has come to describe a Web-based service that allows consumers to create profiles that can attract other users who share similar interests. Users can make connections with people that they already know in person or may connect with others through associations that they create (Boyd & Ellison, 2007). Through social networks, consumers are able to build personal profiles, create a community of friends or colleagues, and share personal information (Eysenbach, 2008; Wink, 2010). Once created, the personal site turns into a dynamic interface between the site "owner," his or her friends, and possibly even strangers. The individual can share content with others in the form of images, text, and even video. Depending on the individual's preferences, other consumers can be allowed to add content to the individual's site as well, in either text or other formats. Essentially, the social networking site serves as a powerful tool to engage and motivate consumers to share personal information, establish relationships, and communicate with others. Examples of social networking Internet sites are Facebook, MySpace, Yammer, and Ning (List of social networking websites, Wikipedia).

Higher education, including healthcare professional education, is taking full advantage of the collaborative features of Web 2.0 tools that provide a context for mobile learning, ubiquitous learning, and social presence that is unprecedented. The dynamic nature of collaboration via the Internet offers learners the opportunities to share working knowledge, provide professional support, and create communities of learning. Social media compliments and supports e-learning opportunities where students are able to have more control over the pace, sequence, and timing of their learning experience (Ruiz, Mintzer, & Leipzig, 2006). Pedagogical implications for social media extend beyond lectures and assignments being presented or submitted in such formats (Meng, 2005); students can access a library of necessary audio or video resources, such as heart and lung sounds, within a podcast site (Meng, 2005) or, possibly, via YouTube (Agazio & Buckley, 2009). These new digital learning environments aim at deepening the level of engagement for the student experience (Boulos, Maramba, & Wheeler, 2006).

Learners can also network and blog as a way to connect with others who are involved in similar programs (Downes, 2004). The primary benefit of utilizing Web 2.0

applications is to improve the quality and access to these education resources and programs. Social networking sites in particular, like Facebook, are demonstrating their utility in education by fostering interpersonal relationships through communication, sharing, collaboration, and ease of use (Mazman & Usluel, 2010). By effectively connecting students and academic institutions, these tools can provide a means to expand the reach of academic courses, allow for establishing a faculty of qualified instructors, and aid in increasing the nursing informatics workforce (Murray, 2007). Social networking tools can also be used in recruitment and retention of students in online programs (Skiba & Barton, 2009).

Various educational programs are already implementing Web 2.0 applications in order to enhance the educational experience and provide more opportunities. Programs that focus on particular areas of specialty, such as anesthesia (Chu, Young, Zamora, Kurup, & Macario, 2010) and dermatology (Kaliyadan, Manoj, Dharmaratnam, & Sreekanth, 2010), highlight the benefits of Web 2.0 tools. In the field of informatics, Skiba & Barton (2009) described the use of social networking tools at the University of Colorado College of Nursing. In this graduate program, they have embraced the use of social media to engage and retain online learners but also to attract potential students to the program. The program incorporates various social media, such as social networking and virtual worlds, as part of the online learning environment. Another example is the University of Oregon Biomedical Informatics program that includes the use of blogs to connect students and faculty within their programs. There are two specific blogs related to informatics. Students and faculty manage the first blog, OnInformatics (oninformatics. com). Another example is Informatics Professor, written by the Chair of the department, Dr. William Hersh (informaticsprofessor.blogspot.com). Duke University School of Nursing has a YouTube video created by students to describe nursing informatics (www.youtube. com/watch?v=Eq4n8u6H-WM). Children's Hospital in Boston also created a YouTube video to describe the role of an informatics nurse specialist (www.youtube.com/ watch?v=S2Rj4nz0zmc).

Clinicians are also using Web 2.0 tools to connect with others in their profession, thus sharing ideas and experiences across multiple facilities (Barton, 2010). Medical and nursing practices both can utilize Web 2.0 tools to collaborate in ways never before possible (Allison, 2009; Anderson, 2009). The prospect of seeing other nurses' best practices not only impacts quality of care delivery but can also save organizations

valuable time when trying to create a process that has already been developed elsewhere. Such outcomes can improve the individual organizations where the nurses are working and can even benefit the nursing profession as a whole (Barton, 2010). Perhaps one of the largest social networks for physicians is Sermo (www.sermo. com) with over 115,000 members.

Healthcare institutions and consumers have already begun to capitalize on the limitless utility of Web 2.0 applications. Numerous hospitals and healthcare–related organizations have social networking sites where patients and visitors can explore details about the facility, learn more about available services, and find information about diseases and/or treatments (Sarasohn-Kahn, 2008). Of the available social networking sites, Facebook stands out as one of the more popular, as it has proven useful for resource sharing, communication, and collaboration (Mazman & Usluel, 2010).

According to Bennett (2010), of the 762 hospitals using social media, there are 551 hospitals with Facebook pages and 348 hospitals with YouTube channels. According to recent statistics, the 5 healthcare institutions with the highest numbers of Facebook members are: St. Jude Research Hospital (249,000), Children's Hospital Boston (>151,000), Arkansas Children's Hospital (59,000), Mayo Clinic (>21,000), and the Veterans Health Administration (20,000). The Veterans Health Administration's (VHA) Facebook network provides a family-friendly open environment to encourage patients and family to learn and interact with the VHA. The Mayo Clinic's Facebook network has 137 videos, numerous discussions, as well as a wall of photos and news events. On it, consumers can request an appointment, look at job openings, or get involved in a discussion (Mayo Clinic, 2010). Consumers can also post comments, questions, and view informational videos regarding specific disease conditions or health topics. At the time of this writing, over 17,000 individuals have signed in to May Clinic's Facebook network and voted in favor of it. The Children's Hospital in Colorado has an active Facebook presence with over 5,900 friends. The network includes a wall full of events, promotions, and breakthroughs posted by both the hospital and others. There are photos, a blog, and a RSS news feed.

In terms of YouTube channels, Bennett (2010) lists the top 5 hospitals in terms of subscribers: University of Southern California (2,168), Mayo Clinic (1,717), Veterans Health Administration (1,658), University of Maryland Medical Center (1,415), and St. Jude Children's Research Hospital (661). At the University of Maryland's YouTube site (www.youtube.com/user/ummcvideos), there are well over a hundred videos showcasing health-care professional profiles, patient success stories, tips for a healthy pregnancy, and surgical Webcasts.

From a consumers' perspective, Sarasohn-Kahn's (2008) report, *Wisdom of Patients: Healthcare Meets Social Media*, provided an excellent synopsis of the current usage by consumers. Since that report, there have been several studies examining the area of social networking in healthcare. Fox and Jones (2009) examined the social life of health information and described the e-patient. The e-patient is engaged and uses a variety of resources to seek health information particularly on the Internet. Fox and Jones (2009, p. 3) reported "the majority of e-patients access user-generated health information." In this study, 39% of the e-patients used social networks like Facebook or MySpace. In a recent study conducted by the Pew Internet and American Life with the California Health Foundation, the researchers found some interesting results on the use of the Internet by those with chronic diseases. Fox and Purcell (2010) found that a disproportionate number of adults with chronic disease have access to the Internet (62%) in comparison with healthy adults with access to the Internet (81%). "However the social life of chronic disease is robust" (Fox & Purcell, 2010, p. 3). Once online, these patients were more likely to participate in blogs or online discussions. As Fox and Purcell (2010) noted, once on the Internet they were more likely to use user-generated information and use the Internet for communication as well as for seeking information.

One of the first social networks in healthcare was Matthew Zackery's i2y social network (I am too young for this Cancer Foundation; i2y.com). At one of the first Health 2.0 conferences, Zackery presented his experiences in creating the social network targeted for young adults with cancer. The history of his network and how he wanted people to find not only information but to connect with each other about their cancer is provided on a YouTube video (www.youtube.com/watch?v=6nkSieQ2aFw).

WebMD Exchange allows users to join a number of health communities either created by WebMD or by members of the community. One can join the Pregnancy First Trimester Community created by a member and now 8,000 members strong. Or, one can join the WebMD Cholesterol Management Control Community. Another social network is Inspire (www.inspire.com), which connects patients, families, friends, caregivers, and healthcare professionals with each other through various support groups. There are groups related to specific diseases or health and wellness. They

have a vast array of partners like the Asthma and Allergy Foundation of America and Discovery Health Channel. Their tag line says it all: "together we are better."

The Center for Disease Control (CDC) has embraced the use of social media and was used extensively in their H1N1 campaign. The CDC site (www.cdc.gov/h1n1flu) not only connects people to the CDC, but also to other social networks such as Facebook, My Space, and Daily Strength. It provides videos, podcasts, e-cards, widgets, RSS feeds, and the ability to get text messages and join their Twitter subscription. Another network associated with the CDC site is Daily Strength (www.dailystrength.org), which contains over 500 health support groups.

Perhaps one of the most interesting social networking sites is PatientsLikeMe (www.patientslikeme.com). Through this social networking application, patients from all over the world convene and share their experience,s while dealing with chronic conditions such as Multiple Sclerosis (Sarasohn-Kahn, 2008). The creators' brother, who was living with amyotrophic lateral sclerosis (ALS), was the inspiration for the network. Two brothers and a friend, all Massachusetts Institute of Technology engineers, created this network with the following goals in mind: (1) share health data, (2) find patients with similar conditions, and (3) learn from each other. Patients are asked to share data in the hope of improving the lives of all diagnosed with that particular disease.

The site does not have any fees and is kept free from advertising through revenues stemming from research awareness programs, market surveys, and the sale of processed anonymized data (Brownstein, Brownstein, Williams, Wicks, & Heywood, 2009). Members use aliases rather than real names and can openly share details about their healthcare experiences, drug regimens, and treatment side effects (Hansen, Neal, Frost, & Massagli, 2008; Sarasohn-Kahn, 2008). The primary motives behind such sharing are to ask or offer advice and to build a relationship with others in similar situations (Hansen, Neal, Frost, & Massagli, 2008). "Rather than disseminating medical advice, PatientslikeMe serves as a platform for peers to interact with one another in a data-driven context" (Brownstein et al., 2009, p. 889). Patients have actually taken information they have learned from PatientsLikeMe to their own healthcare providers to request to be put on specific treatments (Goetz, 2008). There is a detailed privacy policy provided for all interested members (www.patientslikeme.com/about/privacy).

Although PatientsLikeMe is similar to other social networks like Daily Strength and Inspire, it is different in its collection and aggregation of patient data in an open environment (Nature Biotechnology Editorial, 2008). The editorial raises questions about user-generated data, but also speaks to the use of this community to recruit potential patients for clinical trials. In fact, many companies and research institutions are leveraging the use of social networks to accelerate patient recruitment and decrease recruitment costs. Allison (2009) noted that many researchers are using social networking sites to help recruit participants and collect data for clinical trials. This usage not only improves enrollment, but also is reshaping the way research protocols are conducted. There are numerous examples of companies and their corresponding social networks that inform patients of clinical trials. Diabetic Connect (www.diabetic connect.com), operated by Alliance Health Network, both provides a community for diabetic patients and helps recruit patients for clinical trials. TrialX (trialx.com) is a search service that allows patients to search for a clinical trial or be matched up using their personal data from a Microsoft Health Vault or Google Health Personal Health Record. Susan Love's Army of Women's goal is to recruit 1 million healthy women to participate in research related to breast cancer. Allison (2009) acknowledged there is a flurry of activity using social networks, and although there are bumps in the road, it is hoped these "new products will help advance research and accelerate the development of improved treatments" (p. 902).

In addition to social networks, the popularity of virtual worlds is increasing. One of the better known MUVEs is the virtual world known as Second Life (SL). Launched in 2003 by developer Philip Rosedale from Linden Lab, SL is an online community imagined, created, and owned by its residents (Schmidt & Stewart, 2010). Second Life has both free and subscription modes, allows residents to own land, and to develop open or closed societies with both public and private spaces. To use SL, one downloads the application, creates an avatar, and signs a user agreement. With millions of residents globally and a virtual land mass 4 times the size of New York City, SL exists in both time and space (Schmidt & Stewart, 2010). Welcome Island in SL teaches the user the basics of navigation through the VE, including walking, chatting, standing, sitting, flying, and teleporting. The residents of SL are portrayed through avatars, the digital representation of the user, and may be humanoid or creature in appearance. Avatars allow users to interact, obtain a sense of presence, communicate, collaborate, and develop relationships in the virtual world (deFreitas, Rebolledo-Mendex, Liarokapis, Magoulas & Poulovassilis, 2010).

Second Life and other VEs share 3 key properties, as identified by Dalgarno and Lee (2010): presence, representational fidelity, and immediacy of control. Although the terms are sometimes used interchangeably, a distinction should be made between *presence* and *immersion*. Dalgarno and Lee (2010) note that immersion is the "objective and measurable properties of the system or environment", which leads to a sense of presence, "the subjective sense of being in a place" (p. 13). Representational fidelity is achieved through the lifelike appearance of the environment, smooth view changes, motion of objects, sensory experience within the environment, and user representation through an avatar. Representational fidelity, combined with the interactivity and immediacy of control found in real time, is what leads "to a high degree of immersion and consequently, a strong sense of presence" (Dalgarno & Lee, 2010, p. 13).

Avatars are at the heart of the interactions in virtual worlds. The word avatar is derived from the Sanskrit word *avatara*, which means incarnation (Messinger et al., 2009). Whereas "First life" selves are limited by body habitus, gravity, and aging, "Second Life" selves are not. One's avatar may be physically and emotionally like the user, or may present itself as an alter ego, with differing gender, physical characteristics, and mannerisms. For some, the anonymity afforded through an avatar permits the user an expressiveness and confidence not usually achieved in the real world (Falloon, 2010). The sense that the avatar is a portrayal of the user lends itself to the sense of psychological immersion in the virtual world (Dalgarno & Lee, 2010). It is through the avatar that interaction in the virtual world occurs, representational fidelity developed, and copresence, or the sense of being there together, is experienced. It takes a modicum of skill and experience for the avatar to navigate in the virtual world, to avoid bumping into other avatars or otherwise behave strangely.

Higher education, including for the health professions, has begun to use SL as a teaching and learning tool. Boulos, Hetherington, & Wheeler (2007) highlighted the various potential and current uses of virtual worlds in medical and health education. Skiba (2007b, 2009a) provided a snapshot of SL usage by several schools of nursing. Chapter 41 provides an excellent description of how the University of Kansas is using SL to teach nursing informatics as well as other clinical practice areas.

SL is also a venue for individuals, nonprofit organizations, corporations, hospitals, and government agencies and serves as a tool for socialization, training, and business (Schmidt & Stewart, 2010). Second Life can transport an individual to real and imagined places, give legs to the wheelchair-bound, and give hearing and voice to the deaf. As noted by Schmidt and Stewart, "Second Life is not a game; instead it is the next evolutionary step of the Internet. It merges many qualities of the Web, online games, social networking, user generated content, creativity applications, and telecommunication technologies" (p. 74).

For consumers, there are a number of recognized healthcare entities within SL, such as the Centers for Disease Control (CDC), the American Cancer Society, and Britain's National Health Services (Bruck, 2008). An early adopter in SL was the CDC, which maintains 2 islands in SL (www.cdc.gov/SocialMedia/Tools/VirtualWorlds.html). The first island, CDC in SL, features streaming video, historical public health posters, and numerous links to information on CDC.gov. It also contains a virtual lab and a conference center. The second island, called Whyville, is targeted to "tweens" and the importance of seasonal flu vaccinations. This community allows tweens to experience the benefits of being vaccinated and engages them in 6 weeks of exercises.

Second Life is host to an exceptional and dynamic group: Virtual Ability is a nonprofit organization whose mission is to "enable people with a wide range of disabilities by providing a supporting environment for them to enter and thrive in online virtual worlds like Second Life" (Virtual Ability, n.d.). One of the founders, Alice Krueger, has a YouTube video (www.youtube.com/watch?v=UV52WRXm1Cg) that explains the creation of the Heron Sanctuary in SL in 2007. This sanctuary was expanded and renamed Virtual Ability in 2008. On their Web site, one can learn about the many projects and components of Virtual Ability Island. For example, an excellent resident orientation has been developed according to adult learning principles and to accommodate challenges of one's disability (Babiss, 2009). Cape Able Island provides a haven for the hearing impaired, and the AVESS project is a VE amputee support space for military amputees and their families. The virtual world can assist military amputees through peer support, the opportunity to practice the skills needed to proceed with rehabilitation in real life, promote reintegration into society, and in general, improve physical and mental wellness. There is also a Virtual Ability Research Group whose goals are to encourage, promote, support, and disseminate sound research activities within disabilities communities in SL.

Virtual Ability is also committed to connecting SL with Real Life (RL). For example, an SL and RL connection took place when RL nursing students from Tacoma Community College met with SL Virtual Ability Island residents with disabilities to garner firsthand perspec-tives on life with a disability. Not only were the students able to meet with many at one time, the barrier of RL travel was overcome in the virtual world.

Another consumer-generated example in SL is Healing in Community Online (HICO), a virtual world that provides support for families whose children have been diagnosed with life-threatening diseases. A YouTube video (www.youtube.com/watch?v=FlwjONYfahs) explains the potential of using a virtual world like SL to create a supportive environment for families. Their Web site (www.sophiasgarden.org/index.html) provides more detail about this concept and the Web-based resources available.

These are two of many examples of how virtual worlds are being used not only to gather information about health, wellness, and diseases, but about how one can begin to use virtual worlds as a treatment modality for the social support of patients and their families.

IMPACT ON CONSUMERS

"When technology changes enough, it doesn't just change how we do things, but what we do." (Wulf, 1997)

As new tools are introduced in healthcare, it is not only changing how we deliver care but it is changing the dynamics of healthcare and the interactions between consumers and their providers. This is particularly true as one explores the growing use of Web 2.0 tools in healthcare. It is important to note that many of the advances in the use of Web 2.0 tools and the creation of the Health 2.0 movement are generated by the consumer and not necessarily from healthcare providers. The Pew Internet and American Life studies have been focused on consumer engagement in healthcare and use of the Web 2.0 tools on the Internet. For the past decade, there has been a steady rise in the number of people seeking health information on the Internet, with an increasing number of e-patients that are seeking and sharing their experiences on the Web.

Web 2.0 applications provide numerous benefits for healthcare consumers. As the primary stakeholder in their health, consumers are quickly learning that they are the custodians of their own care. They can seek out information and support from any number of online applications (Eysenbach, 2008). Though each tool offers its own perspective on the patient experience, consumers are not likely to rely on just one source (Sarasohn-Kahn, 2008). Hence, there is a collective and symbiotic value that each Web 2.0 tool brings to the consumers' pursuit of health information and understanding of the health experience. Blogs, wikis, and social media provide educational information to help consumers make informed decisions (Sarasohn-Kahn, 2008). Capitalizing on their ability to improve health outcomes (Sarasohn-Kahn, 2008), social networking sites are likely to have the largest impact on the shape of healthcare.

Blogs and wikis allow patients to transform from information consumers to information producers (Adams, 2008). Patients can keep a running diary of their thoughts and experiences when dealing with a particular disease or treatment (Adams, 2008). Social media offers an avenue for patients to listen or watch informative content that they feel pertains to them or is of significant interest. In addition to gathering such information for themselves, patients are bringing what they learn to their providers in order to seek validation or clarification about what they find (Powel, Darvell, & Gray, 2003).

Social networks offer support through positive social relations, stress adaptations, lay person explanations, experience sharing, and healthy behaviors encouragement (Sluzki, 2010). Consumers can receive positive affirmations, thus improving their self-esteem, and can also receive encouragement to stay on track with certain wellness behaviors (Sluzki, 2010). Smoking cessation programs, for example, are employing Web 2.0 modalities to further their campaigns (Freeman & Chapman, 2009) and some have demonstrated that participants who used Web forums showed a higher rate of abstinence than participants who did not (Severson, Gordon, Danaher, & Akers, 2008).

As with social networking, virtual worlds also provide numerous opportunities for nursing in the realms of education, healthcare treatment, and research (Davis, Khazanchi, Murphy, Zigurs, & Owens 2009). Virtual worlds allow for simulations that provide visual and sensory feedback, foster spatial knowledge, and afford the opportunity to master skills that are impossible or difficult to do in the clinical setting without compromising patient safety or that may be cost prohibitive. The globalization of virtual worlds makes it possible to collaborate with nurses from various parts of the United States and other countries. Virtual conferencing, networking, development of support systems, education, and knowledge exchange are possible. Second Life or other virtual worlds can provide the venue for trial and error or working out problems or issues, before taking something to the real world. It can also make it possible to enrich the knowledge base from which one draws conclusions, explores solutions, or develops skills in a safe and unique environment. These worlds can also provide valuable environments for consumers to learn about healthcare, engage in communities to support a

patient or family during an illness, or provide enhanced quality of life for those consumers with disabilities. Imagine in the future prescribing active involvement in the Virtual Ability Island as a method to increase quality of life. As healthcare clinicians examine and study the benefits of virtual worlds, they could become a future therapeutic intervention.

Challenges

Despite their prospects, Web 2.0 applications do not come without certain limitations and risks. Like any element of the Internet, they pose concerns for privacy, security, and legal issues. Healthcare organizations and clinicians are already entrenched in regulations governing the protection and transmission of health information and, thus, must proceed with caution when venturing into the realm of the social Web. The ramifications of poorly managed information on the Internet threaten the practical application of Web 2.0 tools for healthcare use, and potentially put consumers at greater risk for abuses that have yet to be fully realized.

Healthcare organizations and clinicians are required to abide by standards set forth in the Healthcare Insurance Portability and Accountability Act (HIPAA), which was passed in 1996 (Centers for Medicare and Medicaid Services, 2007). It defines the appropriate handling of protected health information, or individually identifiable information that is related to delivery of healthcare (DHHS, 2003). It further delineates that persons and entities, which participate in a network for the purpose of electronic exchange of protected health information, have a responsibility to ensure it is used for its intended purposes (DHHS, 2008). The law mandates that the exchange of protected health information be restricted to certain transactions, involve the transmission of the least amount of information needed to provide care, and abide by the rules governing disclosure (DHHS, 2003). Healthcare institutions and clinicians may only disclose, or share, protected health information if the patient authorizes the exchange (DHHS, 2003).

The Web 2.0 environment places unique circumstances around the sharing of protected health information, as it is generally patient or consumer-driven. That is, the consumer voluntarily divulges his or her information. In such cases the HIPAA regulations do not apply, however, healthcare institutions' attempts to abide by the law may hinder their adoption of Web 2.0 applications (Hawn, 2009). The scenario could change, however, if the healthcare provider were to openly solicit information from consumers or provide the avenue that encourages unprotected exchange of protected health information; legislation governing such uses of protected health information by healthcare institutions is nascent at this time (Tang & Lee, 2009). Certainly, sites such as the Mayo Clinic's Facebook page are operating within the scope of the law since they do not encourage patients to openly discuss their specific health issues, nor are they the caretakers of the Web site storing the information being shared. If, on the other hand, a healthcare institution were to sponsor a site like PatientsLikeMe, where patients are encouraged to divulge personal information, such an organization is acting outside the realm of protecting the privacy of their patients. Further investigation is needed to define the responsibilities of healthcare providers who engage in Web 2.0 activities that specifically place protected health information at risk.

The hesitation surrounding the use of Web 2.0 applications is not limited to healthcare institutions and providers. Although statistics show growing levels of adoption, consumers are also concerned about their privacy (Sarasohn-Kahn, 2008). Their concerns are not unfounded since the rates of identity theft are on the rise and Internet security cannot ever be fully ensured (Acoca, 2008; LaRose & Rifon, 2006). Web 2.0 applications promote information sharing and the open display of personal information, such as age, gender, and location. Posting this and other content creates digital footprints, or lingering information that can be connected back to the consumer who provided it (Madden, Fox, Smith, & Vitak, 2007); these bits of information can then be found and coalesced to form a more complete picture of the individual, thus negating the apparent transparency supposed by Web 2.0 applications (Madden, Fox, Smith, & Vitak, 2007). Whenever such information is made available on the Internet there is always a chance that it could be used for purposes other than what the consumer intended (Lee, Im, & Taylor, 2008; Marx, 1998). Not only are the risks related to the information being displayed on Web 2.0 sites (Fogel & Nehmad, 2009), there are also threats present in the exchange of online media and from others who try to coax private information from others, known as phishing (Acoca, 2008). Through these avenues consumers may end up downloading malicious software, also called malware, on their computers or mobile devices. These harmful applications can operate in the background unknown to the consumer and steal passwords, account data, and other person information (Acoca, 2008).

In addition to identity theft, consumers using Web 2.0 applications are at risk for social threats as well (Nosko, Wood, & Molema, 2010). Characterized as stigmatizing and bullying, social threats can pose significant dangers to consumers and those with whom they are affiliated (Nosko, Wood, & Molema, 2010). Stigmatizing can take the form of prejudice toward religious affiliation, sexual orientation, political views, or group association (Nosko, Wood, & Molema, 2010). Bullying, referred to as cyber-bullying or digital abuse when related to the internet, can involve online threats or aggression toward individuals or groups with the intent to intimidate or coerce someone who is perceived to be unable to retaliate (Dooley, Pyzalski, & Cross, 2009; Spears, Slee, Owens, & Johnson, 2009). Although Web 2.0 applications have propagated this phenomenon in the Internet environment (Spears, Slee, Owens, & Johnson, 2009), they are part of the solution to address it (Valentino-DeVries, 2010).

These issues are well known to Web 2.0 developers, and most applications delineate their terms in privacy policies when consumers register or enroll as a user of the applications. Facebook, for example, outlines details of how they protect and share consumer information; included is how Facebook uses its member information for targeted advertising, and how it declines responsibility for the misuse of a member's personal information by another member (Facebook, 2010). Sites operating in the United States are required to abide by regulations set forth by the Federal Trade Commission, but there is concern that these regulations are not sufficient (LaRose & Rifon, 2006). Some Web sites have adopted additional privacy and security assurances by participating in privacy seal programs (LaRose & Rifon, 2006). These programs claim that participating Web sites comply with practices regarding the access, disclosure, safe keeping, and choices surrounding the use of consumers' personal information (LaRose & Rifon, 2006); the individual Web site's actual compliance with these practices, however, can be brought to question in some cases (LaRose & Rifon, 2006). It is important to note that many organizations have not created social media policies to address these challenges. To learn more about these policies, Bennett (2010) has a listing of social media policies (ebennett.org/hsnl/hsmp).

Where the laws and regulations fall short, ethics must prevail (Marx, 1998). As the Web 2.0 environment evolves and consumers become more active and aware of the risks and benefits, they will be better able to make informed decisions on how they chose to use these applications. Awareness is increasing and users are being more cautious, however, more needs to be done to help users decide when it is acceptable to share personal information and just how much (Nosko Wood, & Molema, 2010). Risks encountered by consumers also impact healthcare organizations that have employees who engage in Web 2.0 use and may access the applications on computers at work; security measures must be implemented to ensure the integrity and security of the protected health information the organization stores and uses (Miles, 2010). Healthcare organizations and clinicians will have to be cognizant of the risks to their patients and the legal ramifications should they pursue applications that encourage consumers to share their personal health information.

In addition, there may be legal issues related to risk management and liabilities. It has long been known that Internet content is not regulated and may be unreliable (Eysenbach & Diepgen, 1998; Powel, Darvell, & Gray, 2003). The primary reason for the variance of information is the fact that virtually anyone can enter, edit, alter, and even vandalize Web 2.0 applications (Boulos, Maramba, & Wheeler, 2006). Hence, it is up to the individual and the involved organizations to self-regulate and process all information found online (Eysenbach & Diepgen, 1998). Consumers have already moved toward self-regulation by sharing opinions in the realm of "wisdom of the crowd" (Sarasohn-Kahn, 2008), but also feel healthcare providers should offer guidance (Hollander & Lanier, 2001). Healthcare organizations and clinicians will also find themselves serving as interpreters or mediators as patients visit and bring Web-based information to their office visits (Keelan, Pavri-Garcia, Tomlinson, & Wilson, 2007; Rodriques, 2000).

As healthcare organizations and clinicians move toward hosting Web 2.0 applications, they must also be cognizant of the legal implications. Not only will they have to monitor the content being shared on their site for appropriateness and reliability, they will also need to be sure there are no copyright infringements (Lawry, 2001). Clinicians will also need to be careful of the potential for fraud and abuse since some information exchanges on the internet could be construed as kickbacks or inappropriate in the medical-legal world (Lawry, 2001). Medical practice licenses will be in question as well since they are provided according to each state's policies, limiting how clinicians utilize Web 2.0 tools that cross all borders (Hawn, 2009).

The advent of virtual worlds such as Second Life has created unique legal issues. The informaticist must be cognizant of the developing laws and legal stances pertinent to virtual worlds. Virtual property is digital, existing only in the virtual world. It has value, however, to the many real-world users that access the property through their avatars. Hunt (2007) defines virtual property as persistent (it does not go away when the computer is turned off) and interconnected (other people can interact with it). Hunt (2007) also describes, "millions of people worldwide interact with virtual property on a daily basis and millions of dollars of transactions have been based upon virtual property sales and transfers. The trouble is that neither the public nor the legal community is entirely sure what it means to 'own' virtual property" (pp. 145–146). Extending legal protection to virtual property offers security for the investment in time and resources by the users and fosters innovative applications for the future. In addition to property disputes, other crimes in the virtual world are piracy (copying of others' characters, objects, and buildings), harassment or "griefing," and theft. In response to the perceived need, a community called the Second Life Bar Association, comprised of real-world legal experts and scholars, was founded for the express purpose of addressing technology and legal issues (Talbot, 2008).

Web 2.0 and virtual worlds provide the foundation for information-age healthcare. Affordances to the provider or patient include ease of collaboration, knowledge sharing or development, skill acquisition, socialization, and support. The future requires a new technological paradigm for both provider and patient to embrace and promote the capabilities of Web 2.0 and virtual worlds.

Web 2.0 applications are altering the patient-provider relationship in ways never before imagined. More and more patients are seeking health information online (Powel, Darvell, & Gray, 2003). Consequently, interpersonal communications have reached such heights of interactivity that healthcare organizations may not have a choice but to utilize Web 2.0 tools if they want to keep up with their patients (Hawn, 2009). Through the Internet, patients are in more contact with each other and their providers (Downes, 2005). Many healthcare providers are starting to recognize how these tools offer ease of use, sharing capabilities, and timely updates (Ajjan & Hartshorne, 2008; Mejias, 2005). While consumers are finding the health information and support they need on the Internet (Sarasohn-Kahn, 2008), organizations are finding economical means to educate patients, market their resources (Boulos, Maramba, & Wheeler, 2006), and build client loyalty (Chaiken, 2009).

As healthcare organizations and clinicians move toward adopting Web 2.0 applications as means for outreach, education, and solicitation, they must be cognizant about consumers who may not be able to access such resources or may be particularly vulnerable. A digital divide, or gap in usability, exists for some consumers who either lack physical access to the Internet or do not have knowledge or skills to navigate the myriad information on the Internet safely and effectively (Baur, 2006; Cashen, Dykes, & Gerber, 2004). Physical access limitations can be described as lack of resources to obtain the hardware or software to utilize these tools (Baur, 2006; Cashen, Dykes, & Gerber, 2004). Lack of experience describes the knowledge and skill deficit that hinders a consumer's ability to navigate the Web 2.0 tools effectively and safely. Some have also found that ethnic disparities do exist in regard to Internet access but, surprisingly, not in regard to social media use (Chou, Hunt, Beckjord, Moser, & Hesse, 2009).

The proliferation of mobile technology offers a means to address the challenges of Internet access. Whether it is through laptop computers or smart phones, more and more consumers are gaining Internet access from such devices (Horrigan, 2009; Sarasohn-Kahn, 2008). More than half of consumers use the Internet to find health information, and growing numbers of consumers are demanding mobile access to health information (Deloitte Center for Health Solutions, 2010). The industry is responding to such demands by lowering the cost of Internet-capable mobile phones, or smart phones (Reuters, 2010), and increasing Internet use by healthcare providers (Bennett, 2010).

Healthcare organizations are taking on roles as both consumers and developers of Web 2.0 applications (Nordqvist, Hanberger, Timpka, & Nordfeldt, 2009) and must incorporate cultural and ethnic issues in their pursuits (Institute of Medicine, 2002). Along with using the appropriate vocabularies (Smith & Wicks, 2008), they will need to consider age groups (Chou, Hunt, Beckjord, Moser, & Hesse, 2009), and accommodate those with visual, hearing, and other disabilities (Baur, 2006; Cashen, Dykes, & Gerber, 2004). Ultimately, healthcare organizations who operate Web 2.0 applications should strive to educate and empower consumers, support their decision making, and reduce the inequalities in health (Powel, Darvell, & Gray, 2003). To help with the further implementation of social media tools in healthcare, the Mayo Clinic recently announced the formation of their Center for Social Media (socialmedia.mayoclinic.org).

Capitalizing on the "wisdom of the crowds" (Sarasohn-Kahn, 2008; Skiba, 2009), patients are utilizing the Internet more and more to guide their decision making and are gaining increasingly more control over their own healthcare (Hawn, 2009; Powel, Darvell, & Gray, 2003). Rather than seeking advice solely from their healthcare providers, patients are now providing it to each other (Hansen, Neal, Frost, & Massagli, 2008; Sarasohn-Kahn, 2008; Skiba, 2009) and may even feel their peers are more reliable sources of such information (Sarasohn-Kahn, 2008). In addition to seeking support, consumers are searching for advice about treatment decisions and disease management (Sarasohn-Kahn, 2008). Soon patients will be looking to the Internet for health ratings to find the best doctors, hospitals, and treatments (Sarasohn-Kahn, 2008).

Although the long-term implications of such behavior have yet to be actualized, at the least clinicians are seeing more patients bringing Internet content to their appointments (Keelan, Pavri-Garcia, Tomlinson, & Wilson, 2007; Rodriques, 2000). A decentralization of healthcare may also occur (Sarasohn-Kahn, 2008), along with more consumer-driven expectations and standards.

As with most innovations, these challenges can be partially addressed through the development and implementation of social media policies by organizations, including user-generated networks. This is particularly important given that most healthcare agencies are risk adverse regarding patient care.

SUMMARY

There is no doubt that the world has been transformed by the Internet. By providing Web 2.0 tools to students, healthcare professionals and consumers, we are transforming healthcare education and practice. Web 2.0 tools provide users with the ability to generate their own content (text, images, and multimedia) and share this content on the Web. Web 2.0 tools allow people to engage, collaborate, share, and communicate. They are empowering and encourage interactivity. The Health 2.0 movement, built upon the Web 2.0 framework and tools, will ultimately change the way healthcare is delivered and the relationships between healthcare professionals and consumers. Although there are challenges related to each of the Web 2.0 tools, the movement to engage consumers in their healthcare is unstoppable. Person-centered care is becoming the norm, and Web 2.0 tools are fostering the participatory health movement. Giustini (2006) perhaps summarized the impact of the Web in his statement, "The web is a reflection of who we are as human beings—but it also reflects who we aspire to be."

REFERENCES

Acoca, B. (2008). *Scoping paper on online identity theft.* Retrieved from http://www.oecd.org/dataoecd/35/24/40644196.pdf.

Adams, S. A. (2008). Blog-based applications and health information: Two case studies that illustrate important questions for Consumer Health Informatics (CHI) research. *International Journal of Medical Informatics,* 79(6), e89–e96.

Agazio, J., & Buckley, K. M. (2009) An untapped resource: Using YouTube in nursing education. *Nurse Educator, 34*(1), 23–28.

Ajjan, H., & Hartshorne, R. (2008). Investigating faculty decisions to adopt Web 2.0 technologies: Theory and empirical tests. *The Internet and Higher Education, 11*(2), 71–80.

Allison, M. (2009). Can web 2.0 reboot clinical trials? *Nature Biotechnology, 27*(10), 897–902.

Anderson, C. (2009, September). How does social networking enhance the nursing narrative? *Nursing Management*, 16–20.

Babiss, F. (2009). Heron sanctuary. *Occupational Therapy in Mental Health, 25* (1), 1–3.

Barnes, J.A. (1954). Class and committees in a Norwegian island parish. *Human Relations, 7*(1), 39–58.

Barton, A. J. (2009). Social Bookmarking: What every clinical nurse specialist should know. *Clinical Nurse Specialist, 23*(5), 236–237.

Barton, A. J. (2010). Using technology to enhance the effectiveness of social networks to promote quality patient care. *Clinical Nurse Specialist, 24*(1), 6–7.

Baur, C., & Kanaan, S. (2006, June). *Expanding the Reach and Impact of Consumer e-Health Tools*. Washington DC: US Department of Health and Human Services Office of Disease Prevention and Health Promotion Health Communication Activities. Retrieved from http://www.health.gov/communication/ehealth/ehealthTools/default.htm.

Bennett, E. (2010, July 24). Hospital Social Media List. Found in cache Web site. Retrieved from http://ebennett.org/hsnl.

Berners-Lee , T. (1989). *Information Management: A Proposal*. CERN. Retrieved from http://www.w3.org/History/1989/proposal.html.

Boulos, M. N. K., Maramba, I., & Wheeler, S. (2006). Wikis, blogs and podcasts: A new generation of Web-virtual collaborative clinical practice and education. *BMC Medical Education, 6*, 41.

Boulos, M., Hetherington, L., & Wheeler, S. (2007). Second Life: An overview of the potential of 3-D virtual worlds in medical and health education. *Health Information and Libraries Journal.* 24(4), 233–245.

Boyd, S (2003). Are You Ready for Social Software? *Darwin Magazine.* Available at http://www.darwinmag.com/read/050103/social.html.

Boyd, D. M., & Ellison, N. B. (2007). Social network sites: Definition, history, and scholarship. *Journal of Computer-Mediated Communication, 13*(1), Article 11. Retrieved from http://jcmc.indiana.edu/vol13/issue1/boyd.ellison.html.

Bradley, A. (2010, January 7). A new definition of social media. *Gartner Blog.* Retrieved from http://blogs.gartner.com/anthony_bradley/2010/01/07/a-new-definition-of-social-media.

Brownstein, C. A., Brownstein, J. S., Williams, D. S., Wick, P., & Heywood, J. A. (2009). The power of social networking in medicine. *Nature Biotechnology, 27*(10), 888–890.

Bruck, L. (2008). Second life: Test-driving real-world innovations. *Hospitals & Health Networks, 82*(10), 50, 52, 54.

Cailliau R., & Connolly, D. (2010, July 26). A little history of the World Wide Web. *World Wide Web Consortium.* Retrieved from http://www.w3.org/History.html.

Cashen, M. S., Dykes, P., & Gerber, B. (2004). eHealth technology and internet resources: Barriers for vulnerable populations. *Journal of Cardiovascular Nursing, 19*(3), 209–214.

Centers for Medicare & Medicaid Services. (2009). *HIPAA Security Series.* Retrieved from http://www.hhs.gov/ocr/privacy/hipaa/administrative/securityrule/securityruleguidance.html.

Cerf, V. (1995). Computer networking: Global Infrastructure for the 21st Century. *Computer Research Association.* Retrieved from http://www.cs.washington.edu/homes/lazowska/cra/networks.html.

Chaiken, B. P. (2009). Social networking: A new tool to engage the clinical community. *Patient Safety and Quality Healthcare.* 6(2), 6–7.

Chou, W. S., Hunt, Y. M., Beckjord, E.B., Moser, R.P., & Hesse, B.W. (2009). Social media use in the United States: Implications for health communication. *Journal of Medical Internet Research, 11*(4), e48. Retrieve from http://www.jmir.org/2009/4/e48.

Chu, L. F., Young, C., Zamora, A., Kurup, V., & Macario, A. (2010). Anesthesia 2.0: Internet-based information resources and Web 2.0 applications in anesthesia education. *Current Opinions in Anesthesiology, 23*, 218–227.

Dalgarno, B., & Lee, M. (2010). What are the learning affordances of 3-D virtual environments? *British Journal of Educational Technology, 41*(1), 10–32.

Davis, A., Khazanchi, D., Murphy, J., Zigurs, I, & Owens, D. (2009). Avatars, people, and virtual worlds: Foundations for research in metaverses. *Journal of the Association for Information Systems, 10*(2), 90–117.

Deliotte Center for Health Solutions (2010). *Social Networks in Healthcare: Communication, collaboration and insights.* Retrieved from http://www.deloitte.com/view/en_US/us/industries/US-federal-government/center-for-health-solutions/research/2fbc755f3c1b9210VgnVCM100000ba42f00aRCRD.htm.

DeFreitas, S., Rebolledo-Mendex, G., Liarokapis, F., Magoulas, G. & Poulovassilis, A. (2010). Learning as immersive experiences: Using the four-dimensional framework for designing and evaluating immersive learning experiences in a virtual world. *British Journal of Educational Technology, 41*(1), 69–85.

Department of Health and Human Services, Office for Civil Rights. (2003, May). *OCR privacy brief: Summary of the HIPAA privacy rule*. Retrieved from http://www.hhs.gov/ocr/privacy/hipaa/understanding/summary/privacy.html.

Department of Health and Human Services, Office of the National Coordination for Health Information Technology. (2008, June 3). *Synopsis: The ONC-Coordinated Federal Health Information Technology Strategic Plan: 2008–2012*. Retrieved from http://healthit.hhs.gov/portal/server.pt/gateway/PTARGS_0_10731_848084_0_0_18/HITStrategicPlanSummary508.pdf.

Deucher, S., & Nodder, C. (2003). The impact of avatars and 3D virtual world creation on learning. *Proceedings of the 16th Annual NACCQ*, 255–258. doi 10.1.1.60.6787.

Digital Library Federation. (2008). *A quick guide to wiki*. Retrieved from http://www.diglib.org/pubs/execsumm/wikiexecsumm.htm.

Dooley, J. J., Pyzalski, J., & Cross, D. (2009). Cyberbullying versus face-to-face bullying. *Journal of Psychology, 217*(4), 182–188.

Downes, S. (2005, October 17). E-learning 2.0. *eLearn Magazine*. Retrieved from http://www.elearnmag.org/subpage.cfm?section=articles&article=29-1.

Educause. (2005, May). *7 things you should know about … social bookmarking*. Retrieved from http://net.educause.edu/ir/library/pdf/ELI7001.pdf.

Eysenbach G. (2008). Medicine 2.0: Social networking, collaboration, participation, apomediation, and openness. *Journal of Medical Internet Research. 10*(3), e22.

Eysenbach, G., & Diepgen, T. L. (1998). Towards quality management of medical information on the internet: Evaluation, labeling, and filtering of information. *British Medical Journal, 317*, 1496–1502.

Facebook. (2010). *Facebook's privacy policy*. Retrieved from http://www.facebook.com/policy.php.

Fairfield, J. (2008). Anti-social contracts: The contractual governance of virtual worlds. *McGill Law Journal, 53*(3), 427–476.

Falloon, G. (2010). Using avatars and virtual environments in learning: What do they have to offer? *British Journal of Educational Technology, 41*(1), 108–122.

Fogel, J., & Nehmad, E. (2009). Internet social network communities: Risk taking, trust, and privacy concerns. *Computers in Human Behavior, 25*, 153–160.

Fox, S., & Jones, S. (2009). The Social Life of Health Information. California Health Foundation and Pew Internet and American Life Project. Retrieved from http://www.pewinternet.org/Reports/2009/8-The-Social-Life-of-Health-Information.aspx.

Fox, S., & Purcell, k. (2010, March). Chronic Disease and the Internet. California Health Foundation and Pew Internet and American Life Project. Retrieved from http://www.pewinternet.org/Reports/2010/Chronic-Disease.aspx.

Freeman, B., & Chapman, S. (2009). Open source marketing: Camel cigarette brand marketing in the "Web 2.0" world. *Tobacco Control, 18*, 212–217.

Freidman, T. (2005). *The World is Flat: A Brief History of the 21st Century*. New York: Farrar, Straus & Giroux Publishers.

Giustini, D. (2006). How Web 2.0 is changing medicine. [Editorial]. *British Medical Journal, 333*, 1283–1284.

Goetz, T. (2008, March 23). Practicing patients. *New York Times*. Retrieved from http://www.nytimes.com/2008/03/23/magazine/23patientst.html.

Hansen, D., Neal, L., Frost, J. H. & Massagli, M. P. (2008). Social uses of personal health information within Patientslikeme, an online patient community: What can happen when patients have access to one another's data. *Journal of Medical Internet Research, 10*(3), e15. Retrieved from http://www.ncbi.nlm.nih.gov/pmc/articles/PMC2553248.

Hawn, C. (2009). Take two aspirin and Tweet me in the morning: How Twitter, Facebook, and other social media are reshaping healthcare. *Health Affairs, 28*(2), 361–368.

Hollander, S., & Lanier, D. (2001). The physician-patient relationship in an electronic environment: A regional snapshot. *Bulletin of the American Library Association, 89*(4), 397–399. Retrieved from http://www.pubmedcentral.nih.gov/articlerender.fcgi?artid=57970.

Horrigan, J. (2009). *Wireless internet use*. Washington, DC: Pew Internet & American Life Project. Retrieved from http://pewinternet.org/Reports/2009/12-Wireless-Internet-Use.aspx.

Hughes, B., Joshi, I., and Wareham, J. (2008). Health 2.0 and Medicine 2.0: Tensions and controversaries in the field. *Journal of Medical Internet Research. 10*(3), e23.

Hunt, K. (2007). This land is not your land: Second Life, CopyBot, and the looming question of virtual property rights. *Texas Review of Entertainment and Sports Law, 9*(1), 141–173.

Institute of Medicine. (2002). *Speaking of health: Assessing health communication strategies for diverse populations*. National Academies Press; Washington D.C.

Kaliyadan, F., Manoj, J., Dharmaratnam, A. D., & Sreekanth, G. (2010). Self-learning digital modules in Dermatology: A pilot study. *Journal of the European Academy of Dermatology & Venereology, 24*, 655–660.

Keelan, J., Pavri-Garcia, V., Tomlinson, G., & Wilson, K. (2007). Youtube as a source of information on immunization: A content analysis. *Journal of the American Medical Association, 298*(21), 2482–2484.

Koerner, J. (2003). The virtues of the virtual world: Enhancing the technology/knowledge professional interface for life-long learning. *Nursing Administration Quarterly, 27*(1), 9–17.

LaRose, R., & Rifon, N. (2006). Your privacy is assured—of being invaded: Websites with and without privacy seals. *New Media and Society, 8*, 1009–1029.

Lawry, T. C. (2001). Recognizing and managing website risks. *Health Progress, 82*(6), 12–13, 74.

Lee, D. H., Im, S., & Taylor, C. R. (2008). Voluntary self-disclosure of information on the internet: A multi-method study of the motivations and consequences of disclosing information on blogs. *Psychology & Marketing*. Special Issue: New Developments in E-commerce, *25*, 692–710.

Leiner, B., Cerf, V., Clark, D., Kahn, R., Kleinrock, L., Lynch, D., et al. (1997). The past and future history of the Internet. *Communications of the Association of Computing Machinery, 40*(2), 102–108.

Linden Lab. (n.d.). Retrieved from http://lindenlab.com/lindenprize/finalists/virtualability.

List of social networking websites. (2010, May 8). In *Wikipedia*. Retrieved from http://en.wikipedia.org/wiki/List_of_social_networking_websites.

Madden, M., Fox, S., Smith, A., & Vitak, J. (2007). *Digital footprints: Online identity management and search in the age of transparency*. Washington, D. C.: Pew Internet and American Life Project.

Marx. G. (1998). Ethics for the new surveillance. *The Information Society, 14*, 171–185.

Mayo Clinic. (2010). *Mayo Clinic is on Facebook*. Retrieved from http://www.facebook.com/MayoClinic.

Mazman, S. G., & Usluel, Y. K. (2010). Modeling educational usage of Facebook. *Computers & Education, 55*(2010), 444–453.

Meister, J. C. (2008, February). Wikis at work: Benefits and practices. *Chief Learning Officer*. Retrieved from http://www.clomedia.com/in-conclusion/jeanne-c-meister/2008/February/2064/index.php.

Mejias, U. (2005). *Nomad's guide to learning and social software*. Retrieved from http://knowledgetree.flexiblelearning.net.au/edition07/download/la_mejias.pdf.

Meng, P. (2005). Podcasting and vodcasting, a white paper. Columbia, MO: University of Missouri IAT Services. Retrieved from http://www.tfaoi.com/cm/3cm/3cm310.pdf.

Miles, S. (2010, February 26). New policy authorizes social media access, with caveats. *Armed Forces Press Service*. Retrieved from http://www.defense.gov/news/newsarticle.aspx?id=58117.

Messinger, P., Stroulia, E., Lyons, K., Bone, M., Niu, R., Smirnov, K., Perelgut, S. (2009). Virtual worlds—past, present, and future: New directions in social computing. *Decision Support Systems, 47*, 204–228.

Nature Biotechnology Editorial. (September 2008). Calling all Patients. *Nature Biotechnology, 26*(9), 953.

Nordqvist, C., Hanberger., L., Timpka, T., & Nordfeldt, S. (2009). Health professionals' attitudes towards using a web 2.0 portal for child and adolescent diabetes care: Qualitative study. *Journal of Medical Internet Research, 11*(2), e12. Retrieved from http://www.jmir.org/2009/2/e12.

Nosko, A., Wood, E., & Molema, S. (2010). All about me: Disclosure in online social networking profiles: The case of FACEBOOK. *Computers in Human Behavior, 26*, 406–418.

O'Reilly, T. (2005, September 30). What is Web 2.0? O'Reilly Media, Inc: Sebastopol, CA. Retrieved from http://oreilly.com/web2/archive/what-is-web-20.html.

Owen, M., Grant, L., Sayers. S., and Facer, K.(2006). Social software and learning. Bristol, United Kingdom: FutureLabs. Retrieved from http://www.futurelab.org.uk/research/opening_education.htm.

Powel, J. A., Darvell, M., & Gray, J. A. (2003). The doctor, the patient and the world-wide web: How the internet is changing healthcare. *Journal of the Royal Society of Medicine, 96*, 74–76.

Reuters. (2010). *Smartphone competition to bite in 2010 after Q4 boom*. Retrieved from http://www.reuters.com/article/idUSTRE61012O20100201.

Rodrigues, R. J. (2000). Ethical and legal issues in interactive health communication: A call for international cooperation. *Journal of Medical Internet Research, 2*(1), e8. Retrieved fro http://www.jmir.org/2000/1/e8.

Ruiz, J. G., Mintzer, M. J., & Leipzig, R. M. (2006). The impact of e-learning in medical education. *Academic Medicine, 81*(3), 207–212.

Sarasohn-Kahn, J. (2008, April). *The wisdom of patients: Healthcare meets online social media*. Oakland, California: California HealthCare Foundation. Retrieved from http://www.chcf.org/topics/chronicdisease/index.cfm?itemID=133631.

Schmidt, B., & Stewart, S. (2010). Implementing the virtual world of second life in community nursing theory and clinical courses. *Nurse Educator, 35*(2), 74–78.

Severson, H. H., Gordon, J. S., Danaher, B. G., & Akers, L. (2008). ChewFree.com: Evaluation of a web-based cessation program for smokeless tobacco users. *Nicotine & Tobacco Research, 10*(2), 381–391.

Shirky, C. (2002). Social Software and the Politics of Groups. *Writing About the Internet*. Retrieved from http://www.shirky.com/writings/group_politics.html.

Simpson, R. L. (2002). The virtual reality revolution: Technology changes nursing education. *Nursing Management, 33*(9), 14–15.

Skiba, D. (2006). Web 2.0: Next Great Thing or Just a Marketing Hype? *Nursing Education Perspectives, 27*(4), 212–213.

Skiba, D. (2007a). Nursing education 2.0: YouTube. *Nursing Education Perspectives, 28*(2), 100–102.

Skiba, D. (2007b). Nursing Education 2.0: Second Life. *Nursing Education Perspectives, 28*(3), 156–157.

Skiba, D. (2009a). Nursing Education 2.0:A Second Look at Second Life. *Nursing Education Perspectives, 30*(2), 129–131.

Skiba, D. (2009b). Nursing practice 2.0: The wisdom of the crowds. *Nursing Education Perspectives, 30*(3), 191–192.

Skiba, D., & Barton, A. (2009). Using social software to transform informatics education. In K. Saranto, P. Brennan, H. Park, M. Tallberg & A. Ensio. (Eds.), *Connecting Health & Humans: Proceedings of NI2009.*

The 10th International Congress of Nursing Informatics (pp. 608–612). Amsterdam: IOS Press.

Sluzki, C. E. (2010). Personal social networks and health: Conceptual and clinical implications of their reciprocal impact. *Families, Systems, & Health, 28*(1), 1–18.

Smith, C. A., & Wicks, P. J. (2008). PatientsLikeMe: Consumer health vocabulary as a folksonomy. *AMIA 2008 Symposium Proceedings*, pp. 682–686.

Spears, B., Slee, P., Owens, L., & Johnson, B. (2009). Behind the scenes and screens insights into the human dimension of covert and cyberbullying. *Journal of Psychology, 217*(4), 189–196.

Talbot, D. (2008). The fleecing of the avatars. *Technology Review, 111*(1), 58–62.

Tang, P. C., & Lee, T. H. (2009). Your doctor's office or the internet? Two paths to personal health records. *New England Journal of Medicine, 360*(15), 1276–1278.

Valentino-DeVries, J. (2010, March 16). Tool aims to help kids avoid 'digital abuse'. *Wall Street Journal*. Retrieved from http://pewinternet.org/Media-Mentions/2010/Tool-Aims-to-Help-Kids-Avoid-Digital-Abuse.aspx.

Van De Belt, T. H., Engelen, L. J., Berben, S. A. A., Schoonhoven, L. (2010). Definition of Health 2.0 and Medicine 2.0: A systematic review. *Journal of Medical Internet Research. 12*(2), e18.

Virtual Ability. (n.d.). Retrieved from http://virtualability.org/default.aspx.

Warren, J., Connors, H., & Trangenstein, T. (2011). A paradigm shift in simulation: Experiential learning in Second Life. In V. Saba and K. McCormick (Eds). *Essentials of Nursing Informatics*. Fifth Edition. New York: McGraw Hill.

Wink, D. M. (2010). Technology corner: Social networking sites. *Nurse Educator, 35*(2), 49–51.

Wulf, W. (1997). Look in the spaces for tomorrow's innovations. *Communications of the Association of Computing Machinery, 40*(2), 109–111.

YouTube. (n.d.). *Terms of service*. Retrieved from http://www.youtube.com/t/terms.

37

Initiation and Management of Accessible, Effective Online Learning

Patricia E. Allen / Khadija Bakrim / Darlene Lacy / Enola Boyd / Myrna L. Armstrong

• OBJECTIVES

1. Explore the past and present perspectives of distance education.
2. Compare and contrast important interactive electronic tools that support online learning.
3. Examine essential strategies and types of support required for the online learner and faculty.
4. Recognize future trends in online education.

• KEY WORDS

distance education
faculty workload
online learning
faculty development

DEFINITIONS

The literature still tends to use a variety of terms such as distance education, Web-based or online learning, and online education to reflect this type of nontraditional education, which in educational reality is becoming a mainstream approach to learning. Some definitions include "institution-based, formal education where the learning group is separated, and where interactive telecommunications systems are used to connect learners, resources, and instructors" (Simonson, Smaldino, Albright & Zvacek, 2009, p. 12). The concept is now associated with learner accessibility, since online learning is experienced locally or globally, at home, a dormitory, or in the work place, regardless of a rural or urban setting, across state lines, and even internationally. The American Association of Colleges of Nursing (AACN) continues to use Reinert and Fryback's (1997) and

Russell's (1998) definitions to further clarify this type of learning as "a set of teaching/learning strategies to meet the learning needs of students that are separate from the traditional classroom setting and the traditional role of faculty." Today with the use of the internet, the terms *online education* and *online learning* (which will be used interchangeably in this chapter) are being used to reflect the broader view of these educational experiences.

EFFECTIVENESS OF ONLINE EDUCATION

Online learning for nursing courses is exploding. Advertisements about "new online education for working professionals" certainly have appeal, capturing the attention of many people seeking to fit further education into their busy schedules. Yet, there are still some traditional students who do not pay attention to online education, there are still some faculty who avoid the concept by raising questions of quality rather than exploring the educational principles used in online learning, and there are still some who believe the only "gold standard" of education continues to be the traditional classroom setting (Allen, Arnold, & Armstrong, 2006). Additionally, questions emerge concerning the validity of the courses: Is it really possible to earn a degree while at home or in the work setting without driving long distances and sitting in tedious lecture classes? Is the interaction with the faculty equal to the same interaction that occurs in the classroom? Is this really applicable to clinical nursing?

Overall, market-driven demands of educational reform and creative, visionary faculty have moved online learning, transforming both academic and continuing nursing education, by capturing new types of educational experiences and innovative kinds of pedagogy (Allen & Seaman, 2010; Allen et al., 2006). The outcomes have been an empowerment of the nursing student and working professional to have numerous important educational choices. Now, in addition to quality, the educational decisions are often based on accessibility and the amount of time needed to complete the course or program.

Online learning offers more alternatives to accommodate individual circumstances and educational needs. Now, it is becoming a commonly accepted instructional method in higher education institutions, and the numbers of online courses are constantly increasing to accommodate the large number of students enrolling. For the past 6 years, online enrollment has grown at a greater rate than the total higher education enrollment (Allen & Seaman, 2010). According to the Sloan Consortium Report (2008), overall online enrollment increased from 1.98 million in 2002 to 4.6 million in 2008, with the majority of doctoral-granting universities (80%) offering online courses or programs.

In order to purport quality, educational outcomes must be similar for both the on-campus and online learning students; countless studies over at least 3 decades have documented this (Dede, 1990; Mahan & Armstrong, 2003; Schlosser & Anderson, 1994). Findings reflect that regardless of the delivery method, online learning students receive the same grades or do better than those students receiving traditional instruction. Overall, student evaluations are good to very good following online education activities. One factor commonly identified by students as a tremendous value in online learning is a collection of learners at a location, which promotes the sharing of ideas, partners to debate

the issues, and educational camaraderie (Armstrong, 2003). In essence, good online education theory and good education theory are actually the same; the education just transcends the barriers of time and space.

Yet, online learning is not a magic bullet, and an examination of the cost and benefits continues to be important. Benefits include increased access, increased interaction, speed, ease of use, novelty, revenue, and improved learning (Bart, 2010). While it can be viewed as an inexpensive way to provide education because there are neither classroom enrollment restrictions, nor costs for students coming to campus, often only the initial, fixed costs are considered. Additional costs that need to be considered include technology and production support (24%), administrative support (18%), academic and student support services (17%), marketing (5%), and research and development (4%) (para 2).

GOALS FOR THIS CHAPTER

Following a brief historic review of distance education, this chapter focuses on today's high-quality, cost-effective, learner-centered approach to online education, examining it from both the student and faculty perspectives. This includes the importance of applicable educational principles needed to promote interactivity; legal, ethical, and copyright issues; active learning; and effective learner and student support, as well as some of the major academic and pedagogic issues impacting faculty developing creative courses.

THE HISTORICAL EVOLUTION

This type of education has always experienced bumps and surges of acceptance. Even the term *distance* education denotes remoteness or isolation to call attention to the differences from the traditional classroom education. While distance education has been available in the United States since before the turn of the nineteenth century, schools and educators have often required a reason to develop and conduct education for students beyond the traditional classroom setting. Initial development centered primarily on vocational training.

Historically, educational regulatory agencies have not been very supportive; approval for off-campus or extension sites were needed when the sites were separated from the originating school or when geographical barriers existed, even when the same faculty were teaching both types of courses. Some states even defined the number of miles for approval. Another approach to distance education, depending on the school's technological resources, could also mean that the faculty drove "the distance" to the off-campus sites, then provided face-to-face (F2F) instruction.

Use of Technology

The advent of print, audio, television, and the computer have assisted distance education strategies, and eventually led to online learning. In the United States, the distance education movement began with the Boston-based Society to Encourage Studies at Home in 1873, followed in 1885 by the University of Wisconsin developing "short courses" and Farmer's Institutes. By 1920, a Pennsylvania commercial school for correspondence studies had enrollments of more than 2,000,000. Unfortunately, dropout rates averaged around 65%. In 1919 radio was the first technology used for distance education, later followed by telephone service. Wisconsin again became a pioneer by using audio conferencing equipment with telephone handsets, speaker phones, and an audio bridge to connect multiple phone lines for the first 2-way interactive distance education for physicians and nurses (Armstrong, 2003; Schlosser & Anderson, 1994). Next came television, so that complex and abstract concepts could be illustrated through motion and visual simulation. Satellite technology for distance education in the United States was implemented in the early 1980s. As these methodologies grew in sophistication and complexity, distance education students began to experience greater transparency of the technology, which enhanced the educational experience. Computer technology came slowly to the forefront of distance education with computer-based education (CBE), computer-assisted instruction (CAI), and computer-managed instruction, and then its use exploded. Yet, it has been the combination of the various interactive Web-based technologies that have really provided the force for creative educational strategies, as well as innovative ideas from faculty that have provided the momentum and impact of online education.

ACADEMIC VERSUS "CORPORATE" OR "E-LEARNING" MODELS

The significant growth of online learning includes not only the technical development of more devices but also the professional development of instructional designers, instructors, and learners. Academic online learning programs differ from "corporate" or "e-learning models" of education in several ways. The academic learning model places the emphasis and responsibility for designing,

developing, and assessing courses on the faculty who teach the courses. While developing an effective and efficient course requires content knowledge, instructional design skills, and technology requirement, it is the school that employs the developmental team personnel. These academic programs deliver a total program with standards established by state, regional, and national accreditation agencies.

In contrast, e-learning models exist when an educational organization contracts to develop online courses from corporate institutions; the corporate organization creates them and the educational organization has its faculty teach them. These types of courses are designed and developed by a specific team that includes a content expert, instructional designer, technology expert, and graphic designer, but they are employed by the corporate group. Advantages of using outsourced online learning courses include standardizing content delivery as well as saving faculty time for other scholarly activities.

STANDARDS FOR QUALITY IN ONLINE EDUCATION

To ensure the quality of online education, various accreditation agencies and organizations have recently developed standards for this type of education. The main purpose of these standards is to guide the development and evaluation of online learning programs offered through colleges and universities. Accreditation agencies require that each facet of the online program be critically and logically appraised to reflect the quality of the programmatic goals and outcomes designated within the program.

ORGANIZATIONAL ACCREDITATION STANDARDS

There is no one type of accreditation applied to online education. In fact, there are several types of accreditations for different institutional statuses, and they are categorized into regional, national, and professional accreditations. Each organization has a particular emphasis, and sometimes they have specific geographical areas that they cover (Koenig, Lofstad, & Staab, 2004), although all accrediting agencies ensure standards of quality have been met.

Regional Accreditation organizations

There are 6 regional accreditations: Middle States Association of Colleges and Schools, New England Association of Schools and Colleges, North Central Association of Colleges and Schools, Northwest Commission on Colleges and Universities, Southern Association of Colleges and Schools, and the Western Association of Schools and Colleges. These agencies accredit both public and private schools, and 2-year or 4-year institutions by reviewing their program and delivery methods based on established standards and requirements. The online programs are expected to meet the general institution standards as well as other criteria specific to online setting such as faculty support, faculty qualification, student support, and the necessary infrastructure to develop and deliver effective online education. For more information, see www.neasc.org.

National Accrediting Organizations

The Council of Higher Education Accreditation (CHEA) is a national nonprofit organization of higher education. This organization relies on peer review rather than governmental regulation. The members of this accreditation define standards of good practice and evaluate the institutions as to whether they meet these standards. Its purposes are to promote academic quality and diversity and provide relevant information on accreditation through research, publications, services, and recognition to colleges and institutions.

Professional Accreditation

Professional accreditation varies by discipline and is a key to defining a quality unit or discipline within a community college, college, and/or university. For nursing, two widely sought professional accrediting agencies are the National League for Nursing Accrediting Council (NLNAC) and Commission on Collegiate Nursing Education (CCNE). Both NLNAC and CCNE are recognized by the U.S. Department of Education. The CCNE agency accredits only baccalaureate and higher degree programs in nursing. NLNAC offers accreditation to vocational and practical nursing programs, associate's, diploma, bachelor's, master's, and doctoral programs within nursing schools and/or departments. Both require online education offerings to be equivalent to site-based offerings and may have specific standards to be addressed by the school in the accreditation process. These additional standards require institutions to ensure online education programs are complemented by resources and structures that allow for student success for online learning.

EXAMINING TECHNOLOGIES USED IN ONLINE LEARNING

A number of technologies are employed in the delivery of online learning, yet not all online programs use all of the technologies described.

Learning Management Systems

A Learning Management System (LMS) is a software product that was first designed for corporate and government training divisions as a tool to assess workers' skills for job positions, and then provide specific training, either individually or in groups. Learning management systems are also commonly used for K–12 education and the higher education level to track student achievement in outcomes-based educational programs (Waterhouse, 2005). LMS software includes the following functions:

- Distribution of course content
- Communication among the users
- Interaction with course resources
- Testing, grading, and tracking records

Another term for LMS that is used more frequently in academic settings is Course Management System (e.g., Blackboard and Desire2Learn). They provide the same functionality as an LMS. For more information visit this site: www.edutools.info/item_list.jsp?pj=4.

Content Management Systems

A content management system is a database of learning objects, which may include many items developed for instructional use. A content management system allows course developers to develop learning objects such as videos, modules, assessments, or any other materials used for online learning. It provides version tracking so that changes to these learning objects can be implemented without losing previous versions of the items. Another benefit to such systems is the ability of developers to share learning objects. They can be used as previously developed or modified to fit the need of the current course. Finally, content management systems are designed to integrate with course management systems. This allows the development of materials to take place outside the course itself. Then, building the course becomes as simple as selecting learning objects and placing them into the course. Course management systems such as *Blackboard* offer a content management system that is designed to fully integrate with their system.

WEB-BASED TOOLS

There are a number of technologies that are currently used or that are under consideration for future use in online learning. No single technology is considered the best technology. The focus today in online learning has been mostly on Web- and video-based delivery via the course management systems described previously. Newer technologies such as mobile computing and Web-based conferencing are beginning to be used as they become more accessible.

Web Conferencing

Interacting and communicating through Web conferencing applications have made online learning a much more engaging and interactive experience. Web conferencing allows a participant to communicate with a personal computer, Internet access, microphone, and Web camera (Webcam). With a Web-conferencing format, students and instructors ask questions in real time, build relationships, and experiment with different learning techniques in order to gain a better understanding of the course material. While there are free programs that allow the user to share and meet online, there are also some full-featured online meeting software programs such as GoToMeeting and WebEx. Full-featured means they can accommodate many more people and provide some great interactive tools.

Tools for Collaborative Projects Development

The Web offers a variety of tools (software) that allow users to share documents online and work on them in real time. The most common Web-based collaborative tools are Google Docs, Zoho, and ThinkFree. These tools are used to participate and collaborate in projects. Other Web 2.0 applications that offer the opportunity for powerful information sharing and ease of collaboration, particularly wikis, blogs, and podcasts, have been increasingly adopted by many online health-related professional and educational services. Wikis are Web sites that can be edited by anyone who has access to them. The word *blog* is a contraction of Web Log—an online Web journal that can accommodate a rich multimedia environment.

Pageburst by Elsevier is an Internet application allowing students to go beyond searching in the textbook to accessing and integrating over 500 references, multimedia resources, and collaborative tools for specific topics. This is an example of an Internet application focused on combining health science content with interactive media, collaborative tools, and class management functions, allowing educators to create an active and engaging, learning experience for students (pageburst.elsevier.com). Consequently, content can "come to life" for the student by tapping into real-time discussions and accessing visual images, video clips, and audio files for topic-specific learning reinforcement.

Social Networking

Social networking can enhance distance education programs by providing more interactive communication and informational sites. Facebook, Twitter, and Linkedin are social networking sites that provide distinct platforms for communication. Facebook, the most frequently used social networking site today, allows the student to link to peers and/or the instructor for messaging, connecting with social groups with similar knowledge interests, and updates on university activities through university-sponsored Facebook pages. Twitter is a social networking site for sharing thoughts, activities, and events occurring as they unfold through messages known as *tweets*. Linkedin began as a business networking site and continues to encourage the exchange of ideas and knowledge among professional associates. Resume suggestion updates, maintaining reference contacts, and exploring professional opportunities are just a few of the features Linkedin might be used for distance learning today.

MOBILE COMPUTING

A broad definition of *mobile computing* is, a technology that allows transmission of data via a limited computer, without having to be connected to a fixed physical link (Seppala & Alamaki, 2003; University of Miami, 2008). There are many different mobile devices including personal digital assistants (PDAs) smart phones, tablet PCs, and laptop computers. Use of portable computational devices is an increasingly compelling choice of technology for higher education. Many universities and colleges are now requiring students to have a mobile computing device, such as a laptop or tablet PC, to access information at any time from any place. Although the integration of functional mobile computing devices is no longer the real challenge, the focus becomes mainly on how this technology should be used to fulfill the core mission of learning (Cain, Bird, & Jones, 2008). Swan, Hooft and Kratcoski (2005) found that the use of the mobile device increases the quality and quantity of student work.

Applications for Mobile Computing

Mobile devices, such as smart phones and touch-screen computers, are beginning to be introduced into the educational setting (Abilene Christian University, 2009). Applications of mobile technology in education can provide benefits to both students and educators. Students can use the mobile device to access information including searching, reading, and organizing. In addition, they can use mobile devices to facilitate collaborative activities, support group work on projects, and communicate with their peers within the course management system, as well as using the other collaborative systems previously mentioned (Yousuf, 2007).

Recently, a highly anticipated tablet computer, Apple's iPad, has been introduced. It offers an increased number of features for communication, interaction, and engagement. Smart phones, iPhones, and iPads all allow mobile computing applications, enabling at-your-fingertips information access. *Apps*, as they are called in the world of technology, can bring information to the point of care at the bedside for information about how to perform nursing procedures as well as updates on vaccines, immunizations, the latest drug interactions, and CDC warnings just to name a few. A recent newspaper article (Gallaga, 2010) describes a physician reviewing her Labor and Delivery patients' fetal monitor recordings while away from the hospital; the app had been developed by another physician.

Apps are free or can be purchased for minimal fees. Apps are listed by current usage and recommendations from other healthcare providers, and smart phone users are alerted to the latest apps in their fields. A quick Google search can determine the top 25 apps for healthcare team members.

FACULTY SUPPORT

With the number of online courses increasing, the American Association of State Colleges and Universities emphasizes the critical need for faculty well experienced in teaching online (Orr, Williams, & Pennington, 2009). In order to assist in successful online education, faculty must receive appropriate support, technical expertise, and online infrastructure.

Faculty Development

Faculty development is a critical component to the success of any online education, especially as colleges and universities are using numerous Adjunct Faculty to assist with the increased student enrollments and teaching responsibilities (Allen et al, 2006). Academic institutions are taking a proactive approach to faculty support. Numerous workshops and one-to-one support in course development and technical issues are the most common types of training faculty receive. The faculty development activities are designed to assist and improve faculty teaching at all levels of the educational programs. Workshops, seminars, Webinars, and peer coaching are among services available for faculty development. The focus of these services should not be limited to technical skills development, but must include pedagogical issues. For example, strategies to create active learning activities, engage online learners, or motivate online students are topics that, if explored in depth, would help faculty be more effective online teachers (Lahaie, 2007).

Support for Course Development

Developing and delivering an effective online course requires pedagogical and technological expertise. Instructors new to online teaching are not likely to have such skills. An example used at our university is the Jumpstart Program. Hixon (2007) defined Jumpstart as a series of workshops that may take more than a week. These workshops include a team of support professionals, including instructional designers, librarians, and media production specialists, who help faculty increase their knowledge, productivity, and teaching experience with technology. Evaluation findings document that this Jumpstart program significantly influences the faculty members in their online course development process.

Moller, Foshay, and Huett (2008) note that online course development requires a team involving instructional designers, technical support staff, and content experts. The content expert offers an outline of topics that should be covered. The instructional designer provides help in course structure organization and functionality, and the technical support provides assistance with integration of technology tools. This model of team course development is common in most nonacademic settings and has been adopted by a number of academic organizations. However, course development carried out by the instructors who will be teaching the course is still a common practice in many colleges and universities that offer online learning.

Technological tools for online learning are constantly being developed and improved, with the aim to make online learning more interesting and more effective (Maor, 2003). Regardless of faculty teaching experience, technology support is critical in online teaching. Appropriate training on using new technologies, routine technical support, and instructional guidance are the common support that faculty receive (Gopalakrishnan, 2006).

Pedagogy and Role Change

The instructor's role in the online environment becomes a significant element in creating quality learning (Maor, 2003). The role of the online instructor has developed into that of a facilitator rather than a knowledge distributor. This is achieved by monitoring and guiding students to learn critical concepts, principles, and to develop skills, rather than just lecture material (Easton, 2003). The technical component of the instructor's role often requires assistance when using technology such as software and hardware interfaces, systems access, and passwords.

Faculty Workload

Faculty workload refers to the number of courses taught by an instructor (Boyer, Butner, & Smith, 2007). The allocation of faculty time in Higher Education usually includes teaching, scholarship activities, and community service. Because teaching online is thought to require more time and effort compared with traditional face-to-face teaching, workload adjustment is usually used by institutions to promote faculty involvement in non-teaching activities.

Actual research into the assumption of increased development time has been limited. Freeman's (2008) research findings suggest that the time spent with online course development seems to be proportional to classroom teaching. As with traditional classroom development, usually the extra time devoted to making the course effective and applicable then produces a significant reduction of faculty time after first-time delivery. Freeman (2008) offers four Lessons for Distance Education Administration:

1. "Make sure faculty understand that they are starting something new."

2. "Teach your faculty to think about their course in a different way, to be ready to do things differently."

3. "Use your instructional designers. As the faculty member is developing the course with the instructional designer, the designer should be on the lookout for time-consuming approaches."

4. "The more an administrator knows about the process of course development, the better he/she can manage [the faculty workload issue]." (para. 9)

COURSE DEVELOPMENT

The use of the Web for courses can be divided into three categories: hybrid courses, Web-enhanced face-to-face courses, and fully online courses. The selection of approach depends on the needs of the organization, the nature of the content, and the faculty.

Hybrid Courses

A hybrid, or blended course, is defined as any course combining elements of face-to-face instruction and activities with elements of Internet instruction. Research conducted by Buzzetto & Sweat-Guy (2006) indicated that the main advantage of this approach is to make use of the best features of both approaches in promoting active learning and reducing class seat time. According to Singh (2003), the benefit of this approach is that the two different platforms provide different types of learning activities and promote students-to-students and students-to-instructor interactions.

Web-Enhanced F2F Courses

Face-to-face courses can use Web-based technology to facilitate self-studying. This type of course usually uses a course management system or Web pages to post the syllabus, readings, and assignments. The course management system may also be used for testing or other assessments.

Fully Online Courses

A fully online course refers to a course where most or all of the content is delivered online, and has no face-to-face meetings. Due to the increasing student enrollment, more and more colleges and universities are offering fully online courses.

Learner Assessment in Online Courses

Assessment is an important aspect in the learning process. *Assessment* is defined as a means to test and evaluate student performance and ensure that students meet the outcomes designed for the course (Waterhouse, 2005). The assessment may take different forms, such as:

- Online quizzes and exams.
- Self-assessment: Students assess their own learning as they progress through the course.
- Online discussion: Students respond to questions, reply to peers messages, and discuss course materials.
- Papers: Students submit research papers, or essays. Posting papers to the online discussion forum can spark discussion. Rubrics provide guidelines and a method for self-evaluation.
- Individual or collaborative projects: Students develop a project individually or as members of a group by using clear directions and guidelines.
- Presentations: Synchronous communication systems can be used to make presentations or even have debates. A student can use a whiteboard or show a Web site they would like everyone to view while holding a live discussion.

STUDENT SUPPORT

One of the most critical factors in a student's success with online learning is student support. Moore and Kearsley (2005) noted that the absence of student support could drastically affect student retention, and tends to increase student frustration and feelings of inadequacy, which in turn leads to the student dropping out of the program. Several investigators have proposed a wide range of student support services that should help students be successful. These services include precourse orientation (Nash, 2005), free tutoring services (Raphael, 2006), and online technical support (Moore & Kearsley, 2002). These academic services allow students to be familiar with the technology and improve student-to-instructor and student-to-student communication. The main goal is to increase students' ease with the cyber environment and encourage constant connection with their peers. In addition to academic support, services that focus on students' affairs are also important to success and retention. Services such as online library resources (Gaide, 2004; Raphael, 2006), online advising (Herbert, 2006; Osika, 2006), and a common course management system (Osika, 2006) could be part of an integrated student support system aimed at making online learning exciting and successful.

Orientation to the Online Environment

Orientation programs designed to introduce new students to the online environment are crucial to assure a smooth transition, especially for students without prior experience in online learning. The goals of orientations and tutorials are to ensure that students are familiar with the online environment and are aware of expectations. Free tutorials are also helpful, especially with difficult or challenging tasks such as navigating the Web course space, using new software packages and/or equipment, or performing technical procedures (e.g., uploading a file to a Web site).

Communication and Flexibility

There are two basic types of Web-based communication:

- Asynchronous communication tools such as e-mail, discussion boards, and blogs. Course participants use these tools when they are online; however, the person to whom they communicate may not be online. They serve as a messaging interface between communicators.

- Synchronous communication tools require participants to be online to communicate at the same time. These tools include chat, whiteboard, desktop conferencing, and video conferencing such as Skype.

To ensure effective communication, instructors must select the most appropriate tool for their class. This will depend on accessibility to the technology and the levels of students' skills. Communication is strongly affected by course flexibility (due dates and/or assignment submission). Building flexibility in the course structure allows the faculty to compensate for unexpected technological problems, as well as provides opportunities to respond to student feedback.

LEGAL, ETHICAL, AND COPYRIGHT ISSUES

The faculty is accountable for educational content they teach. However, accountability is even more at the forefront of education at this time. According to Shupe (2008), as educators have more educational delivery choices available, the standard for accountability for educational results rise. Billings and Halstead (2009) reminds us that higher education largely depends on governmental funding and, thus, is accountable to the public for academic productivity and fiscal prudence. With this in mind, there is a meshing of legal and ethical issues for faculty to take into consideration when presenting educational content.

Legal concerns relate to established laws associated with telecommunication technologies, whereas ethical concerns relate to the rights and wrongs stemming from the values and beliefs of the various users of the distance education system. Three major areas that are of concern regarding legal issues include copyright protection, interstate commerce, and intellectual property. Privacy, confidentiality, censorship, freedom of speech, and concern for control of personal information continues to be as relevant today as in 1998 when Bachman and Panzarine (1998) identified these cyber ethical issues.

Copyright Protection

Copyright is a category of intellectual property and refers to creations of the mind (World Intellectual Property Organization, n.d.). This protection for Copyright is based on the Copyright Act of 1976, a federal law that went into effect January 1978 (Radcliff & Brinson, 1999). Copyright law protects "works of authorship," giving developers and publishers the right to control unauthorized exploitation of their work (Radcliff & Brinson, 1999). Although there have been no new federal laws since 1976 to address educational multimedia concerns, the Consortium of College and University Media Centers has published the Fair Use Guidelines for Educational Multimedia (Dalziel, 1996). When combining content such as text, music, graphics, illustrations, photographs, and software it is important to avoid copyright infringement (Radcliff & Brinson, 1999). Additionally, the Digital Millennium Copyright Act was passed in October 1998. The UCLA Online Institute for Cyberspace Law and Policy list the highlights of the Digital Millennium Copyright Act at gseis.ucla.edu/iclp/dmca1.htm and the United States Copyright Office Summary can be located at www.copyright.gov/legislation/dmca.pdf. As noted by the dates of citations here, regulations and legislative guidance seem to lag from the technological changes incorporated within the online educational arena.

Intellectual Property

A common question by faculty is, "Who owns the course?" According to Kranch (2008) there is a great deal of controversy over who owns academic coursework materials. United States copyright law is intended to provide ownership and control of what an individual has produced. However, its relationship to faculty-produced work is not as clear. Although faculty may own the materials they have developed for use in their online courses, it is always good to have a memo of understanding documenting the specific use of the materials as well as the accrued benefits (Billings, 1996).

The issue of "work made for hire" is the point of controversy. According to the 2003 U.S. Copyright Office document, as indicated by Kranch (2008), a "work made for hire" is defined in the following ways:

1. A work prepared by an employee within the scope of his or her employment

2. A work specially ordered or commissioned for use as a contribution to a collective work

The bottom line of this section is that faculty should know their employer's policy pertaining to intellectual property rights. Over the last several years, universities, government, and private organizations have noted the need to clearly delineate their policies in this area. For example, our school has an established university-wide committee providing advisory opinions to the Provost on matters related to patentable discoveries and inventions, and/or copyrightable material, which had been developed by University employees.

Open Courseware (2010) is a free and open digital publication of educational material (www.ocwconsortium.org/about-us/about-us.html). However, there are specific guidelines and requirements for the use of Open Courseware. Although Open Courseware is available to anyone, material used in education from any Open Courseware participant is consistent with materials from any university and or faculty. Additional information on Open Courseware can be found at ocw.mit.edu/OcwWeb/web/help/faq3.

Extensive resources on intellectual property law and rights can be found at the following sites:

- Indiana University Information Policy Office (informationpolicy.iu.edu)

- Office of Technology Transfer and Intellectual Property at Texas Tech University Copyright (www.ttuhsc.edu/HSC/OP/OP57/op5702.pdf); Intellectual Property (www.ttuhsc.edu/hsc/op/op52/op5206.pdf)

- Legislative initiatives regulating intellectual property and copyright are found in the Technology, Education and Copyright (TEACH) Act (www.arl.org/pp/ppcopyright/index.shtml)

- The Berkeley Digital Library at Sunsite is an excellent resource for national perspectives on intellectual property (sunsite.berkeley.edu/Copyright)
- The Creative Commons Web site (creativecommons.org/about/what-is-cc) is a nonprofit organization that works to increase the amount of creativity in the body of work available to the public for free and legal sharing, use, repurposing, and remixing.

Ethical behaviour in the nursing profession has been established by groups such as the American Nurses Association (ANA) in the Code of Ethics (2001) and the American Association of Colleges of Nursing's (AACN) (2008) competencies for baccalaureate nursing education. These nursing values and ethics are fundamental in practice decisions and are just as applicable in nursing education, whether education be face-to-face or online. Mpofu (n.d.) regards ethical considerations in online teaching as performing your work within the context of professional practice and the confines of institutional regulations. However, over and above professional and institutional ethics, nurse educators must contend with legal and ethical issues that take on a new dimension when applied to online education. While issues such as copyright, privacy, licensing, fair and acceptable use, and plagiarism are certainly not unique to online education, they assume new dimensions and different proportions. Another source for consideration with ethics issues can be found in *Best Practice Strategies to Promote Academic Integrity in Online Education*, (Version 2.0, June 2009) (wiche.edu/attachment_library/Student_Authentication/BestPractices.pdf).

PROGRAM EVALUATION

Program evaluation is an ongoing process in online education and requires a framework for evaluation to be adopted by the faculty, standards and outcomes to be defined, as well as a timeline for measurement of outcomes. Program evaluation focuses on review and improvement. The need for curriculum revision, resources, and faculty and staff may become apparent during this ongoing review process. Program evaluation allows educators to facilitate meaningful change, while providing feedback. Whether a framework is selected for an evaluation focused on attainment of objectives or a management-oriented framework, all program evaluation gathers evidence for measurement against

predetermined outcomes. The framework will provide the steps to outcome attainment. All program evaluation should be systematic and ongoing to be effective. With systematic program evaluation, revision decisions are based on the evidence from findings rather than assumptions. To obtain this evaluative data, program surveys by faculty, students, and administrators should be completed and analyzed annually. Additionally, course surveys should be completed by students at the end of each course.

Regional accreditation agencies assist in guiding programs for maintaining standards in program delivery, and regional credentials are sought after by major colleges and universities. Regional accreditation is a continuous improvement process involving the entire university or college. Many of the regional accrediting agencies, such as the Southern Association of Colleges and Schools (SACS), engage the college or university to pursue a continuous improvement process of self-evaluation, reflection, and improvement for not only face-to-face learning but distance learning as well (Southern Association of Colleges and Schools, 2010). Other regional accrediting agencies providing excellent resources for online program assessment and evaluation include Western Interstate Commission on Higher Education (WICHE) and WICHE Cooperative for Educational Technologies (WCET), a division of WICHE, providing good practices and policies to ensure the effective adoption and appropriate use of technologies in teaching and learning online (wcet.wiche.edu/advance).

Quality Matters

Quality Matters (QM) is another evaluative process that employs a set of standards based on best practices in instructional design developed to verify the quality of online or hybrid courses. It is based on faculty-oriented peer review and provides tools for the review process while focusing on course design more than content or delivery method. The standards of the QM consist of 8 elements: Course Overview and Introduction, Learning Objectives, Assessment and Measurement, Resources and Materials, Learner Engagement, Course Technology, Learner Support, and Accessibility (Pollacia & McCallister, 2009). For more information visit www.qualitymatters.org.

Sloan Consortium

Additional resources for the evaluation of online education that promote quality can be found at the Sloan Consortium Web site (www.sloan-c.org). The Sloan Consortium (2008) is dedicated to making online learning a mainstream higher education delivery methodology, and this international consortium provides tools, best practices, and directions for educators. The Sloan Consortium addresses effective best practices with an excellent model for quality education. This model features the concepts of scale, access, faculty and student satisfaction, and learning effectiveness overlapping in the quest for distance learning effectiveness (www.sloan-c.org/effective).

Teaching, Learning, and Technology Group

The Teaching, Learning, and Technology Group (TLT) is an important not-for-profit group providing excellent resources related to online learning and the effective evaluation and assessment of online programs. The group provides technology updates to help college and university faculty improve online learning methodologies through the use of the latest technology. Many resources for educators can be found on the TLT Group's Web site (www.tltgroup.org/about.htm).

A major project of interest by the TLT Group has been the Flashlight Program. This program is an inexpensive Web 2.0 tool for program evaluation and evaluation research opportunities. This rich online resource for educators provides evaluation measures, validated surveys, rubrics, model questions and survey matrices for use by institutions. Institutions from across the country contribute to the database of evidence-based resources, and the system is interactive and secure. Visit their Web site for additional information about this helpful evaluation and assessment tool (www.tltgroup.org/Flashlight/flashlightonline.htm).

FUTURE TRENDS

The future trends in online learning will be defined by student empowerment and technological advancements. The population and student enrollments have grown extensively during the last 6 years (Allen & Seaman, 2010) and it is anticipated that the field of online education will witness a tremendous growth both in terms of quantity as well as quality. For example, Hodgins (2007) predicts that learning content will be customized for each learner, rather than mass-produced. This approach is called adaptive Web-based instruction, where the learning environment is created to meet the individual student's needs (Inan & Grant, 2008).

The other most apparent trend changing online learning is the advancement of technologies. The Internet is becoming more interactive and visual, and soon high-speed network connections will be the standard. In addition, the capabilities of computers and mobile devices are significantly improving in speed while decreasing in cost. These changes along with others are boosting online education. By 2018, computers will be able to "routinely translate languages in real-time with the accuracy and speed necessary for effective communications" (Cetron & Daview, 2003). There will be more technologies that offer live interactive instruction. With all the growth in online education, the need for effective course management systems will be ever more crucial. Furthermore, technological advancements will also increase the need for developing effective teaching strategies that exploit the capabilities of technology.

Futurists have been predicting the rise of the *ubiquitous computing device* for years (Bull & Garofalo, 2006; Swan, Van 'T Hooft, Kratcoski, & Schenker, 2007; Weiser, 1991). A ubiquitous device is one to which users have become so accustomed, they no longer notice the device itself when they are using it. Instead, users tend to focus on what they get from the device. One example of this in our life is the refrigerator. We may open the door of the refrigerator, but often are thinking of the food we get from the device, rather than the device itself. Some authors go even farther, defining the ubiquitous device as a single device or service that takes care of all of our computing needs (Pendyala & Shim, 2009). These computing devices will continue to be part of an exciting new world for online learning opportunities.

The 2010 Horizon Report by the New Media Consortium described 6 technologies that universities will likely mainstream within the next 5 years. One of these technologies is gesture-based computing, which is also called Gesture Recognition. This refers to technology that recognizes and interprets the motions and movements of its users. Instead of using the mouse or keyboard, the users employ natural body movements to control the device, such as shaking, rotating, tilting, touching, or moving the device in space. It is expected that in 4 to 5 years this type of technology will emerge in educational settings and have a considerable impact on teaching and learning (www.nmc.org/horizon).

REFERENCES

Abilene Christian University. (2009, October 30). *ACU connected: Mobile learning innovation* Retrieved from http://www.acu.edu/technology/mobilelearning/index.html.

Allen, I. E., & Seaman, J. (2010). *Learning on demand: Online education in the United States, 2009.* Retrieved from http://www.sloanconsortium.org/publications/survey/pdf/learningondemand.pdf.

Allen, P. E., Arnold, J., & Armstrong, M. L. (2006). Accessible, effective distance education, anytime, anyplace. In V. K. Saba and K. A. McCormick (Eds.), *Essentials of nursing informatics*, (4th ed., pp. 533–548). New York: McGraw-Hill.

American Association of College of Nursing. (2008). *The essentials of baccalaureate education for professional nursing practice.* Washington, DC: Author.

American Nurses Association. (2001). *Code of ethics for nurses with interpretive statements.* Washington, DC: Author.

Armstrong, M. L. (2003). Distance education: Using technology to learn. In V. K. Saba and K. A. McCormick (Eds.), *Essentials of computers for nurses: Informatics for the new millennium* (3rd ed., pp. 413–425). New York: McGraw-Hill.

Bachman, J. A., & Panzarine, S. (1998). Enabling student nurses to use the information superhighway. *Journal of Nursing Education, 37*(4), 155–161.

Bart, M. (2010). *Distance education—Measuring the benefits and costs.* Retrieved from http://www.facultyfocus.com/articles/distance-learning.

Billings, D. M. (1996). Distance education in nursing: Adapting courses for distance education. *Computers in Nursing, 14*(5), 262, 263, 266.

Billings, D. M., & Halstead, J. A. (2009). *Teaching in nursing: A guide for faculty.* St.Louis, MO: Saunders Elsevier.

Boyer, P. G., Butner, B. K., & Smith, D. (2007). A portrait of remedial instruction: Faculty workload and assessment techniques. *Higher Education, 54,* 605–613.

Bull, G., & Garofalo, J. (2006). Commentary: Ubiquitous computing revisited—A new perspective. *Contemporary Issues in Technology & Teacher Education.* 271–274.

Buzzetto, N., & Sweat-Guy, R. (2006). Hybrid learning defined. *Journal of Information Technology Education, 5,* 153-156 Retrieved from http://www.umes.edu/webct/pdf%20files/Hybrid%20Course%20Handout.pdf.

Cain, J., Bird, E. R., & Jones, M. (2008). Mobile computing initiatives within pharmacy education. *American Journal of Pharmaceutical Education, 72*(4), 1–7.

Cetron, M. J., & Daview, O. (2003). *50 trends shaping the future.* Special report published by the World Future Society. Retrieved from http://www.eric.ed.gov/ERICDocs/data/ericdocs2sql/content_storage_01/0000019b/80/1b/28/40.pdf.

Dalziel, C. (1996). *Fair use guidelines for educational multimedia.* Retrieved from http://www.libraries.psu.edu/mtss.fairuse/dalziel.html.

Dede, C. J. (1990). The evolution of distance learning: Technology-mediated interactive learning. *Journal of Research in Computing in Education, 22*(3), 247–264.

Easton, S. S. (2003). Clarifying the instructor's role in online distance learning. *Communication Education, 52*(2), 87–105.

Freeman, L. (2008, February 1). Time requirements for teaching online: Beyond the myths. *Distance Education Report.* Retrieved from Permalink:http://www.facultyfocus.com?p=11460.

Gallaga, O. L. (2010, April, 4). Dr. technology. *Austin American-Statesman,* Section H, 1–3.

Gaide, S. (2004). Best practices for helping students complete online degree programs. *Communication Education, 52*(2), 87–105.

Gopalakrishnan, A. (2006). Supporting technology integration in adult education. Critical issues and models of basic education. *Adult Basic Education, 16(1),* 39–56.

Herbert, M. (2006). Staying the course: A study in online student satisfaction and retention. *Online Journal of Distance Learning Administration.* Retrieved from http://www.westga.edu/~distance/ojdla/winter94/herbert94.htm.

Hixon, E. (2007). *Working as a team: Collaborative online course development.* 23rd Annual Conference on Distance Teaching & Learning. Retrieved from http://www.uwex.edu/disted/conference/Resource_library/proceedings/07_5084.pdf.

Hodgins, W. (2007). Distance education but beyond: "meLearning"—What if the impossible isn't? *Journal of Veterinary Medical Education, 34*(3), 325–329.

Inan, F., & Grant, M. (2008). *Individualized web-based instructional design.* Hershey, New York: Information Science Reference. DOI: 10.4018/978-1-59904-865-9.

Koening, A. M., Lofstad, R., & Staab, E. (2004). *Higher education accreditation in the United States.* Higher Education Accreditation in the United States. EAIE Conference.Retrieved from http://www.eaie.org/pdf/torino/205.pdf. 4/7/2010.

Kranch, D. A. (2008). Who owns online course intellectual property?*Quarterly Review of Distance Education Research That Guides Practice, 9*(4), 349–356.

Lahaie, U. (2007). Web-based instruction: Getting faculty onboard. *Journal of Professional Nursing, 23(6),* 335–342.

Mahan, K., & Armstrong, M. L. (2003). Distance education: What was, what's here, and preparation for the future. In M. Armstrong and S. Fuchs (Eds.), *Providing successful distance education and telehealth* (pp. 19–37). New York: Springer.

Maor, D. (2003). The teacher's role in developing interaction and reflection in an online learning community. *Education Media International, 40,* 127–138.

Moller, L., Foshay,W. R., & Huett, J. (2008). The evolution of distance education: Implications for instructional design on the potential of the Web. *TechTrends, 52*(4), 66–70.

Moore, M. G., & Kearsley, G. (2005). *Distance education: A systems view* (2nd ed.). Belmont, CA: Wadsworth.

Mpofu, S. (n.d.). *Ethics and legal issues in online teaching.* Retrieved from http://www.col.org/pcf2/papers/mpofu.pdf.

Nash, R. (2005). Course completion rates among distance learners: Identifying possible methods to improve retention. *Online Journal of Distance Education Learning Administration, 8(4).* Retrieved from http://www.westga.edu/~distance/ojdla/winter84/nash84.htm.

Open Courseware Consortium. (2010). *Information about the consortium.* Retrieved from http://www.ocwconsortium.org/about-us/about-us.html.

Orr, R., Williams, M., & Pennington, K. (2009). Institutional efforts to support faculty in online teaching. *Innovation Higher Education, 34,* 257–268.

Osika, E. (2006). The concentric support model: How administrators can plan and support effective distance learning programs. *Distance Education Report, 10*(21), 1–6.

Pendyala, V. S., & Shim, S. S. Y. (2009). The Web as the ubiquitous computer. *Computer, 42*(9), 90–92.

Pollacia, L., & McCallter, T. (2009). Using Web 2.0 technologies to meet Quality Matters™ (QM) requirements. *Journal of Information Systems Education, 20*(2), 155–164.

Radcliff, C. F., & Brinson, R. P. (1999). *Copyright Law* (1999). Retrieved from http://library.findlaw.com/1999/Jan/1/241476.html.

Raphael, A. (2006). Need assessment: A study of perceived need for student services by distance learners. *Online Journal of Distance Education Learning Administration.* Retrieved from http://www.westga.edu/~distance/ojdla/summer92/raphael92.htm.

Reinert, B., & Fryback, P. (1997). Distance learning and nursing education. *Journal of Nursing Education, 36*(9), 421.

Russell, T. L. (1998). *The no significant difference phenomenon.* Retrieved from http://cuda.teleeducation.nb.ca/nosignificantdifference.

Schlosser, C. A., & Anderson, M. L. (1994). *Distance education: Review of the literature.* Washington DC: Association for Educational Communications & Technology.

Seppala, P,. & Alamaki, H. (2003). Mobile learning in teacher training. *Journal of Computer Assisted Learning, 19,* 330–335.

Shupe, D. (2008). Toward a higher standard: The changing organizational context of accountability for educational results. *On The Horizon, 14*(2), 72–96.

Simonson, M., Smaldino, S., Albright, M., & Zvacek, S. (2009). *Teaching and learning at a distance: Foundations of distance education* (4th ed.). Boston, MA: Allyn & Bacon & Pearson.

Singh, H. (2003). Building effective blended learning programs. *Issues of Educational Technology, 43*(6), 51–54.

Sloan Consortium Report (2008). *Staying the course—Online education in the United States 2008.* Retrieved from http://sloanconsortium.org/publications/survey/pdf/staying_the_course.pdf.

Southern Association of Colleges and Schools (SACS). (2010). *Standards and accreditation process for schools.* Retrieved from http://www.advance-ed.org/accreditation/schools_accreditation/accreditation_process.

Swan, K., Hooft, M., & Kratcoshi, A. (2005). Uses and effects of mobile computing devices in K–8 classrooms. *Journal of Research on Technology in Education, 38(1),* 99–112.

Swan, K., Van 'T Hooft, M., Kratcoski, A., & Schenker, J. (2007). Ubiquitous computing and changing pedagogical possibilities: Representations, conceptualizations and uses of knowledge. *Journal of Educational Computing Research, 36*(4), 481–515.

University of Miami Leonard C. Miller School of Medicine. (2008). *Information and Technology: Terms and definitions* Retrieved from http://it.med.miami.edu/x2224.xml.

Waterhouse, S. (2005). The power of eLearning: The essential guide for teaching in the digital age. Boston, MA: Pearson Education, Inc.

Weiser, M. (1991). The computer for the 21st century. *Scientific American, 265*(3), 94.

World Intellectual Property Organization (n.d.). *What is intellectual property?* Retrieved from http://www.wipo.int/about-ip/en.

Yousuf, M. (2007). Effectiveness of mobile learning in distance education. *Turkish Online Journal of Distance Education, 8*(4), 114–124.

38

Innovations in E-Health

Marilyn M. Nielsen / Amy J. Barton

• OBJECTIVES

1. Define concepts of e-Health, telehealth, and m-health.
2. Explore applications of e-Health for healthcare, education, and research.
3. Examine evidence on the impact of e-Health in health promotion and health maintenance.
4. Analyze challenges and issues surrounding these applications.
5. Discuss telehealth case study.

• KEY WORDS

Telemedicine
Telehealth
e-Health
m-health

A renewed emphasis on patient-centered care is enabling more complete participation in the healthcare environment by patients and their families.

E-Health, the use of health information and communication technologies, is slowly being replaced by fundamental structural changes in healthcare, such as the advent of new care and communication patterns. The goals of such new communication patterns and systems are (1) making the scientific body of medicine available to clinicians in a decision-supporting format, (2) facilitating communication between patients and clinicians outside of the traditional visit, and (3) enabling new communication among clinicians (medical networking) (Waegemann, 2010, p. 24).

This chapter highlights the transformations in healthcare and education within the context of advances in computing and communications technologies. The goals of this chapter are twofold: to explore how e-Health innovations will transform healthcare, education, and research and to present the challenges and issues as a result of these potential transformations. The chapter covers the progression of e-Health applications; e-Health and other associated concepts; future innovations in advanced practice, education, and research; and the challenges and issues arising as a consequence of these transformations.

HISTORICAL CONTEXT OF E-HEALTH

The rudimentary roots of telemedicine extend back to ancient times where simple forms of distance communication, such as the use of light reflections and smoke signals, were used to relay messages about external threats, famines, and disease. Long-distance communication evolved from these modest beginnings to systems such as the telegraph, radio, and onward to advanced digital communication and communication systems (Bashshur & Shannon, 2009).

In the early 1900s, the Netherlands became the site of the earliest modern telemedicine application, which was the transmission of heart rhythms over telephone lines. Radio consultations followed patients aboard ships at sea and on remote islands (Bashshur & Shannon, 2009). Universal phone service was established as a public policy goal in the 1930s. Telephone use became wide spread due to its advantages: relatively low cost for installation, low cost per use, minimal training for use, and ubiquity (Witherspoon, et al., 1994). Beginning in the 1950s the transmission of radiographic images began and the first telemedicine programs were started in the United States (Bashshur & Shannon, 2009). By the early 1960s the practice of medicine through telecommunications was being refined by the National Aeronautics and Space Administration (NASA) with efforts to put men in space. Physiologic measurements of astronauts were monitored from the spacecraft, and space suits were telemonitored during space flights (Welsh, 1999).

The development of satellite technology further advanced the development of telemedicine. Projects such as STARPAHC (Space Technology Applied to Rural Papago Advanced Healthcare), which ran from 1972 to 1975, utilized a van staffed by paramedics carrying a variety of medical instruments to link, via 2-way microwave transmission, to the Public Health Service Hospital, thus providing care to the remote Papago Reservation. The first international telemedicine project was conducted in 1989 following a devastating earthquake in Soviet Armenia. Telemedicine consultations were conducted by the U.S./U.S.S.R. Joint Working Group on Space Biology, with several medical centers in the United States and a medical center in Armenia. In 1997, the project was extended to Russia to aid burn victims following a railroad accident (Welsh, 1999).

Telehealth applications have evolved from simple communications to sophisticated, pervasive, and widespread systems in the home that make use of wireless, wearable, robotic, and multisensorial technologies. In the past, trends in telehealth applications were grouped according to the various media: voice, data, and video. But with the convergence of these technologies, newer technologies merge across these media. Despite these newer technologies, voice applications remain a mainstay of telehealth applications. The tools of telemedicine offer effective and efficient solutions for remote monitoring of the chronically ill, as well as an avenue to allow for diagnosis and treatment of individuals who have no access to healthcare because of geographic limitations (Bashshur & Shannon, 2009).

THE CONCEPT OF E-HEALTH

E-Health is a relatively new term, barely used before 1999. In the literature, e-Health might be referred to as e-medicine, telehealth, or telemedicine. There is no single agreed upon definition of e-Health. Initially, the term was an attempt to encompass all the possibilities and excitement the Web had to offer for healthcare and to include the concepts of health, technology, and commerce. It was created as other areas such as e-commerce and e-business were being developed. Because the Web created new opportunities, as well as challenges, the use of a new term seemed appropriate; it provided a new perspective on healthcare where technology is viewed as the tool that enables a process, function, and service. E-Health includes the capability of consumers to interact with their providers online; improves possibilities for institution-to-institution transmissions of data; and presents exciting new possibilities for peer-to-peer communication among consumers (Eysenbach, 2001; Oh, Rizo, Enkin, & Jadad, 2005).

E-Health is an emerging field of medical informatics, referring to the organization and delivery of health services and information using the Web and related technologies. In a broader sense, the term characterizes not only technical development, but also a new way of working, an attitude, and a commitment for networked, global thinking to improve healthcare locally, regionally, and worldwide by using information and communication technology. E-Health represents optimism, allowing patients and professionals to do what was previously impossible (Eysenbach, 2001; Pagliari, et al., 2005; Oh, Rizo, Enkin, & Jadad, 2005).

The term e-Health is now in widespread use, which suggests that it is an important concept (Oh et al., 2005). E-Health technologies provide opportunities for customized and meaningful communication, enabling patients to receive individually tailored information that can be viewed and responded to at their convenience. Patients can also post their comments and advice to virtual communities (Neuhauser & Kreps, 2010).

E-Health can empower consumers and patients, and it opens doors for new types of relationships, such as shared decision making between a patient and his healthcare provider. "E-Health is the single-most important revolution in healthcare since the advent of modern medicine, vaccines, or even public health measures like sanitation and clean water" (Silber, 2003, p. 7).

The Concepts of Telemedicine and Telehealth

To examine the concept of telehealth, it is important to define the term *telecommunications*. According to the Institute of Medicine (IOM, 1996), "it is the use of wire, radio, optical or other electromagnetic channels to transmit and receive signals for voice, data, and video communications." The American Nurses Association (ANA) defined telecommunications as, "the transmission, emission, or reception of data or information, in the form of signs, signals, writings, images and sounds or any other form, via wire, radio, visual or other electromagnetic systems" (ANA, 1997).

Media that can be used for telecommunications include the telephone, video, and computer systems that now provide for interactive live video conferencing. Data, images, and video are transmitted through a variety of methods including phone lines, fiber-optic cables, satellites, and microwave systems. Today, store-and-forward connections allow audio clips, video clips, still images, or data to be held and transmitted when the user chooses. Recipients can choose to view the media in real time or at a later time (Whitten & Sypher, 2006).

Over the past several years the Internet has given rise to newer methods of communication such as Voice over Internet Protocol (VoIP). This function allows a voice to be converted into a digital signal that can then travel over the Internet, allowing users to make a call directly from a computer (Federal Communications Commission, 2010). There is Internet Protocol Television (IPTV), where Internet television services are delivered using the methods of the Internet protocol over a network infrastructure, such as the Internet and broadband Internet networks, rather than through traditional radio-frequency broadcast, satellite signal, or cable television formats. The advantage of IPTV is that it allows real-time participation from people watching, and one can receive Web service notifications for things such as incoming e-mail and instant messages (IPTV, 2008).

> Today, telemedicine is again at the frontier of the forward march in medical care. Its purpose is not only to increase access to healthcare but also to promote the efficiency, effectiveness, and quality of mainstream clinical care and to enable the integration of complex health systems. It is also at the frontier of the pursuit of a health lifestyle, patient empowerment, as well as preparedness and response to natural and man-made threats (Bashshur & Shannon, 2009, p. 8).

Early definitions of telemedicine included the use of interactive, or 2-way, television to provide healthcare. This was later expanded to include the concept of diagnosing or treating a patient who was in a different location (Whitten & Sypher, 2006). According to the IOM (1996, p. 16) telemedicine is broadly defined as "the use of electronic information and communication technologies to provide and support healthcare when distance separates the participants."

The American Telemedicine Association (ATA) uses the terms *telemedicine* and *telehealth* interchangeably. "Telemedicine is the use of information exchanged from one site to another via electronic communications to improve patients' health status. Closely associated with telemedicine is the term *telehealth*, which is often used to encompass a broader definition of remote healthcare that does not always involve clinical services" (ATA, 2010b).

Telehealth can be considered another component of the e-Health concept, with the difference being around the delivery mechanisms, which can include live video conferencing; store-and-forward systems, such as those used to store digital images; telephone conferencing; and remote patient monitoring and e-visits via a secure Web Portal. Teleconferencing and digital networking systems are now merging, giving rise to "group consultation" opportunities (Waegemann, 2010; Doty, 2008).

Focusing on nursing, the American Nurses Association (ANA, 1997) wanted a more inclusive term and proceeded to define telehealth as, "delivery of healthcare services or activities with time and distance barriers removed and using technologies such as telephones, computers, or interactive video transmissions." This organization considers telehealth an umbrella term that encompasses telemedicine, telenursing, teleradiology, and telepsychiatry.

Loane and Wootten (2002) suggested that telehealth is not a technology, but rather a technique for the remote delivery of healthcare. In the *2001 Report to the Congress on Telemedicine*, Thompson and Fox (2001) defined telehealth as "the use of electronic information and telecommunications technologies to support long-distance clinical healthcare, patient and professional health-related education, public health, and health administration." Brantley, Laney-Cummings, and Spivack (2004, p. 9–10) expanded the definition to include "a comprehensive system for integrating various applications—clinical healthcare delivery, management of medical information, education, and administrative service—within a common infrastructure." This report (Brantley et al., 2004) stated that "any examination of the nation's healthcare system should also acknowledge the convergence that combines such healthcare technologies as medical devices, healthcare informatics, IT for healthcare, telehealth, and healthcare over the Internet (e-Health)" (p. 10).

While variations in the definitions of telemedicine and telehealth exist, there is agreement on the broad conception of this field as, "the delivery of personal and non-personal health services and of consumer and provider education as well as a means for safeguarding the living environment via information and communication technology" (Bashshur & Shannon, 2009, p. 601). Using the broadest definition of telehealth as a foundation, this chapter will explore the past, present, and future innovations as they apply to healthcare delivery, education, and research.

E-HEALTH APPLICATIONS

Telehealth has both clinical and nonclinical uses. Nonclinical applications include professional education; healthcare administrative duties; research; and the aggregation of health data, excluding patient-specific medical treatments and decisions. Clinical uses include medical decisions involving patient care, diagnostics, and treatments. However, these two categories are somewhat blurred, as patients and providers exchange e-mail communications that are being stored in the patient's computerized record (Bauer, 2009).

Clinical applications for telemedicine can be provided at the point of service or at another location (e.g., in the home for patients who may be home-bound, who reside in rural communities, or who are living in correctional facilities). Telemedicine applications can be specialized, such as with telepathology, telepsychology, or remote patient monitoring services for ICUs in acute care facilities. Telemedicine is forging new relationships between patients and all types of practitioners; it is moving care out the physician-centric perspective into the 21st century model of healthcare that will see more consumer empowerment (ACNP, 2006).

Impact of the Web

With the introduction of the World Wide Web (WWW), electronic support groups expanded to offer other healthcare services such as e-mail communication with providers, decision support tools, and customized discharge planning. Consumer demand for e-mail continued to place demands on healthcare professionals. Early e-mail practices (Widman & Tong, 1997; Borowitz & Wyatt, 1998; Diepgen & Eysenbach, 1998) and corresponding

guidelines (Kane & Sands, 1998; Spielberg, 1998) provided a solid foundation for the increasing demand for electronic communication between consumers and providers.

Today, 74% of American adults (ages 18 and older) are using the Web; 60% of them access via broadband connections at home, and 55% connect wirelessly to the Web via their laptops or handheld device such as smart phones (Raine, 2010). A 2010 Pew Internet and American Life Project study indicates 81% of adults with no chronic diseases go online, while only 62% of adults living with chronic disease are likely to access to the Web (Fox & Purcell, 2010). These findings are in line with trends in public health and technology adoption. Chronic disease is typically associated with being older, African American, less educated, and living in a lower-income household. While Internet use is associated with being younger, white, college educated, and living in a higher-income household (Fox & Purcell).

People living with chronic disease have complicated health issues and are disproportionately offline. Those who are online, however, have additional support; they have each other. Two online activities that are common among people living with chronic diseases are blogging and online health discussions. Having a chronic disease significantly increases the likelihood that the user will use the Web to read and share information. "Nuggets" of information are discovered via these online discussion groups; individuals in the groups connect and they "just keep going" (Fox & Purcell, 2010).

The Concept of M-Health

One component of e-Health is mobile-health (m-Health), which can be considered a delivery mechanism for e-Health. M-Health typically refers to the use of a wireless communication device that supports public health and clinical practices (Eytan, 2010; TBHome, 2010). M-Health is seen as a valuable tool as the digitization of health and wellness data increases. It is postulated that many tools will be required, as no single tool will serve all people. As a result, there is a need to stop focusing on the technological components separately and work toward aggregating these communication technologies in an integrated system. Once this is accomplished, an ecosystem for integrated broad-scale deployment of e-Health tools can be achieved (Eytan, 2010; TBHome, 2010).

Ted Eytan, MD, Medical Director for Delivery Systems Operations Improvement for the Permanente Federation, offers 6 distinctions between the concepts of e-Health and m-Health:

1. Access to mobile devices: Discussions regarding Web access often are directed toward the 26% of adults who are not online. This compares with 91% of the U.S. population who subscribe to cell phone service (Eytan, 2010; Rainie, 2010).

2. Digital divide: When considering disparities, 9 out of 10 (92%) adults in the United States access information in multiple formats, on multiple platforms, and on a variety of devices (Purcell, Rainie, Mitchell, Rosenstiel, & Olmstead, 2010). Desktop usage favors more educated and affluent people, with the highest usage among Caucasians (75%) and the lowest usage among Hispanics (64%). Interestingly, there is an inverse relationship when one looks at wireless usage: the highest usage (62%) is among Hispanics (English- and Spanish-speaking); followed by African Americans (59%); and the lowest usage is by Caucasians (52%) (Eytan, 2010; Rainie, 2010).

3. Application development: Developers of mobile devices face more challenges and difficulties, while applications for the desktop computer are much easier to build.

4. Interoperability: When discussing m-Health, telecommunications companies must be included, which is not the case when developing code for a Web page.

5. Public health: Much of the innovation around m-Health is coming from resource-poor countries utilizing m-Health innovations to meet the public and primary healthcare needs of populations within those countries.

6. Personal versus public: Finally, m-Health often is viewed as more personal when compared with a Web site accessed via a desktop computer (Eytan, 2010).

Waegemann (2010) views m-Health as the new generation of telemedicine that is laying the foundation for a new generation of healthcare. He describes e-Health as having a focus on using electronic medical records and other technologies, while m-Health focuses on behavioral and structural changes. The current idea that telemedicine requires dedicated connections does not fit the new world view of m-Health. The m-Health revolution is introducing patient-centered, communication-based care in a system that includes wellness and healthcare providers (Bloch, 2010). The healthcare model itself is moving from a provider-driven one to a largely participatory model including all stakeholders such as long-term caregivers, dentists, insurance companies, hospitals, public health officials, primary care providers, consumers, and health systems involved in wellness (Bloch, 2010).

It is crucial to note that these changes will be global in distribution. M-Health is going to allow basic care to be provided that might not otherwise be available in regions of African, Asia, and South America. In developing countries, mobile phones far outnumber personal computers, and they offer support services on both health and technology fronts. As United Nations Foundation President Timothy E. Wirth emphasizes, the power of these technologies to improve health and the human condition cannot be underestimated: "Modern telecommunications, and the creative use of it, has the power to change lives and help…. solve some of the world's biggest challenges" (United Nations Foundation, Vodafone Group Foundation, & Telemedicine Society of India, 2008). For most of the world this will be the only computer they will own; it is on the Web and they can carry it everywhere. The impact on healthcare could be great (The doctor in your pocket, 2005).

For example, in Zimbabwe, villagers have been trained to easily key data into phones, such as the number of cases of malaria and number of infant and maternal deaths from remote locations. Analyzing this information, national health ministries can mobilize care to select villages. Most importantly, data that formerly required years to collect can now be viewed in a timely fashion. Determinations concerning interventions, such as providing mosquito nets to villagers, have consequently been timelier and more effective (Dambita, 2010). Another example comes from SIMPill, a firm in South Africa that has developed a small device that can be placed inside the lid of a medicine bottle. Whenever the lid is opened a message is sent to a central server, if no message is received the patient or caregiver receives a text message reminder. This technology has improved medication compliance, which is of vital importance for the management of conditions such as HIV (The doctor in your pocket, 2005).

Mobile phone teledensity (number of phones per 100 people) has been estimated to exceed 100% within the next 10 years, meaning everyone in the world who wants a mobile telephone will likely have one. South Africa passed 100% and Ghana reached 98% in January of 2009. Kenya and Tanzania are expected to be at 100% by 2013 (Finishing the Job, 2009).

As m-Health continues to progress, nursing care will need to evolve. Traditionally, nurses have been hands-on caregivers; now, nurses are challenged with developing new models for nursing care that address "care at a distance" using innovations such as mobile phones and text messaging. Communication is at the core of nursing care, and the methods of communication are rapidly changing and growing. Nurses will be able to utilize text messaging over a secure network to send automated appointment reminders, health tips, and messages about available resources in the area. Nurses will need to consider their standards of care and the impact these new modalities will have on care delivery.

Transforming the Practice of Healthcare

Wearable and Portable Monitoring Systems. Remote patient monitoring, considered experimental a few years ago, is now maturing, with a number of applications available. Employers and insurance companies are all interested in disease management programs and the abilities to measure physiologic responses and communicate in real time with patients at a distance, as these activities have the potential to change health behaviors. Everyone is seeking quality outcomes, ease of delivery, as well as cost savings. Remote monitoring fits this bill (Blanchett, 2008). The VitalJacket is one example that utilizes microelectronics in a wearable T-shirt that continuously monitors electrocardiogram waves and heart rate. The shirt can be used for patients or for healthy subjects involved in fitness activities or sports (Biodevices, 2009; Blanchett, 2008).

Wireless body area networks (WBAN) are now in development. Utilizing low-powered embedded systems along with developing cellular phone technologies, work is ongoing to develop smart systems that continuously monitor an individual's health. The concept involves multiple sensors communicating wirelessly with each other and with a centralized node, called a *personal server*. The choice for this type of server is the modern cell phone, which has the processing power to handle the demands of physiologic monitoring along with the ability to connect with any other computer anywhere in the world. Designers of these systems are challenged with keeping products light and unobtrusive, much like a wristwatch, as well as keeping costs down. Utilizing a personal server, information can be integrated to form a big picture, and some of the data from sensors will be able to create new information not available from individual sensors (Terry, 2010).

This type of mobile, patient-centric, personal monitoring will greatly enhance health awareness for all healthcare providers and for the patient. A system available today from BodyMedia is a wearable monitoring system that focuses on weight loss, health, and fitness. The armband has sensors that collect heat flux, galvanic skin response, skin temperature, as well as an accelerom-

eter. Utilizing a USB cable, one can sync the data with Activity Management software where it is stored and can be tracked by the user (Terry, 2010).

The Health Buddy System is a remote monitoring platform that provides a daily interface between care coordinators and patients with chronic illnesses; this system has a proven track record over the past decade. The appliance can also connect glucose meters, weight scales, blood pressure cuffs, and other medical devices so additional patient data are sent to the healthcare professionals. Health Buddy has been used with a variety of patients including coronary artery bypass graft (Zimmerman, Barason, Nieveen, & Schmaderer, 2004), chronic heart failure (LaFramboise, Todero, Zimmerman, & Agrawat, 2003), diabetes (Cherry, Moffat, Rodriguez, & Dryden, 2002), and asthma (Guendelman, Meade, Benson, Chen, & Samuels, 2002). Care providers access data that can provide an early alert of warning signs that the patient is deteriorating; it addresses gaps in care before the patient becomes critical.

A Veterans Health Administration (VHA) study examined 4 years of data from their telehealth program. Results showed a 19% reduction in hospitalizations and a 25% reduction in bed days of care for patients using Health Buddy (Darkins, et al., 2008; Ratan, 2010). A new Health Buddy messaging feature allows customized notifications to specific patients or to a clinic's entire population. Examples of messages include a reminder to patients with heart failure to limit their salt intake if a slight increase in their blood pressure was seen that week, or encouragement to a diabetes patient struggling with managing their blood glucose levels (Ratan, 2010).

Telemedicine and Telecare Web-Based Services. New industries are now entering the healthcare arena. At Intel, research is underway to find in-home technologies to help people with illness and injury prevention, early detection, caregiver support, and independent living. In-home sensors are being considered to detect visits and phone calls, and combined with online tools will summarize social activity to help support changing social lives and engagement with patients suffering from cognitive decline. The Sensing Health with Intelligence, Modularity, Mobility and Experimental Reusability (SHIMMER) project is investigating development of a small sensing device for long-term wear that will capture physiologic and behavioral data (Blanchett, 2008).

Cisco Healthcare is working on a pilot project to launch a telemedicine platform that will link Long Beach physicians with underserved residents in San

Diego, CA, and nearby communities. This public-private partnership will allow physicians to use audio, video, and data-sharing services to create an experience for patients similar to visiting their own healthcare providers. This represents another step toward bringing about new models of healthcare delivery (Wicklund, 2010).

Google Health now offers telehealth services through its online platform, in partnership with MDLiveCare. Users with MDLiveCare log into secure video, phone, or e-mail telehealth consultations with a board-certified physician or mental health therapist. Medical records can be shared prior to an appointment and can be accessed after the appointment, thus allowing for portability and continuity of care (Merrill, 2009).

Telemedicine is actively being considered as an aid for such things as fall-risk detection in telerehabilitation. For the stroke patient, remotely assessing fall risk has been a major problem. A novel wearable device is being investigated that utilizes a data collection tool integrated into a global positioning system (GPS) to assign a fall risk (Giansanti, Morelli, Maccioni, & Constantini, 2009).

Advanced ICU Care offers a staffing solution where board-certified critical care physicians and CCRN-certified nurses monitor ICU patients 24 × 7. Utilizing telemedicine technology that combines clinical management software and patient data with real-time video feeds, patients can be monitored remotely leading to improved care and safety in the ICU setting (Advanced ICU Care, 2009).

Robotics. Robotics is the frontier for telemedicine. The RP-7 Remote Presence Robot allows providers to project themselves anywhere and anytime to another location to move, see, hear, and talk as if they were actually there. Under direct control of a remote physician seated in a control station, the robot moves allowing the caregiver to observe the patient, check bedside monitors and ventilator settings, listen to heart and lung sounds, and interact with staff and family members (InTouch Health, 2010).

Telenursing and Decision Support Tools. Nurses have always been the link between the patient and the physician. Telenursing is broadening the role of nurses and advancing their value in the chain of healthcare delivery to consumers in remote regions or to homebound patients. These nurses are the first to observe, evaluate, and initiate action by facilitating collaboration with the physician engaged via telecommunication technology.

Nurses who practice telenursing perform tasks such as providing advice via phone triage services and staffing remote walk-in clinics where the closest physician may be 150 miles away. They conduct physical assessments, utilize a "smart stethoscope" to hear lung and heart sounds, and examine skin lesions with a high-intensity camera. If necessary, physicians at a regional medical center can be consulted via teleconference. These nurses prevent the chain of care delivery from being broken, delayed, or totally neglected (Naditz, 2009).

Home health nursing via visual communication is a technique that provides accessible care and reduces both travel time and expense. Using videophones, the nurse and patient can establish a more personal relationship. Images can be transmitted interactively from the patient's home directly to attending physicians improving follow up and treatment for things such as leg wounds. This technology can be used to plan care interventions and to train patients and their caregivers. Utilizing field notes, photos, and video-recorded dialogues, all care providers can easily follow any changes in leg wounds (Jönsson & Willman, 2008).

Teletriage is a component of telenursing. Decision support tools have been developed as a guide for the teletriage nurse assessing a patient. These tools provide the nurse with structure around the teletriage processes. Utilizing these decision support tools, along with nursing judgment and critical thinking skills, helps to minimize risk when providing telephone assistance. For example, the Medicare Quality Improvement Community (MedQIC) Web site has a free online teletriage resource toolkit to support consistent and appropriate teletriage assessments for many conditions including adverse drug reaction; breathing difficulty; depression; feeding tube problems; nausea, vomiting, and fluid loss; wound drainage; and pain management (QualityNet, 2007).

Possibility of Virtual Worlds. Web-based 3D virtual worlds are currently being investigated as a potential tool to engage a variety of audiences in healthy behavior and lifestyle choices regardless of location. These tools are also being used as a new educational method for the healthcare professions that will help facilitate learning through interactive, collaborative learning environments (Skiba, 2007).

The 3D worlds are created online using a virtual persona, or avatar, which interacts with other avatars in the online world. The Centers for Disease Control and Prevention (CDC) has established a Second Life island where users can see streaming videos and access links to information on CDC.gov. The island has a virtual lab and conference center (CDC, 2009). The Second Life platform is being investigated as a tool to train hospital staff in a mass casualty incident, or discuss how to design and evaluate an evacuation plan for a fire emergency scenario. These virtual worlds take up no space and can be accessed at a distance. Well designed training environments immerse the player—a key factor when evaluating training effectiveness. The popularity of this training method continues to grow, with possibilities not only for nursing education but also for patient and telehealth applications and for surgical training (Boulos, Ramloll, Jones, & Toth-Cohn, 2008; Wilson, Stevenson & Cregan, 2010).

Health Portals and Web 2.0. Web access is increasing, and more people are online using a desktop or laptop computer or mobile phones. Web 2.0 social networking sites such as Facebook, Twitter, YouTube, and MySpace are proliferating. People are going to these sites to communicate, learn, and become active participants on the Web. Internet users are creating forums for discussion and learning to be more engaged and informed. Health consumers feel empowered and now want to participate in decisions about their healthcare. Support groups are using the Web as a new platform to organize, share experiences, seek online counseling, and simply connect with others. Web sites are now being utilized by healthcare providers as a place to engage with colleagues on clinical and nonclinical issues.

Hospital portals are being developed where patients can make appointments, renew prescriptions, and review test results and their medical records online. An example is My Health*e*vet, which offers veterans, active duty service members, their dependents, and caregivers access anytime to VA healthcare information and services that include tracking tools and journals to help the user track their health activities (My Health*e*vet, 2010).

Google Health is a Web-based personal health record where patients can store and manage all of their health information and access it anywhere at anytime. Users can build health profiles, import records from hospitals and pharmacies, share their records, and explore online health services (Google Health, 2010).

WebMD is a consumer portal that is a leader in providing online health information. It provides the ability to browse condition-specific and wellness-related topics. Individuals have the ability to participate in moderated exchanges where they can get expert feedback on a variety of topics such as osteoporosis, skin problems, and gynecology problems. There are also member-created exchanges where users discuss parenting issues or participate in a diet club (WebMD, 2010).

PatientsLikeMe is a popular social networking site. This site contains communities that have been developed to allow patients to become proactive. The community forums include patients, doctors, and organizations. Users learn about treatments and symptoms, and can participate in the forum or have one-on-one discussions. The site was developed for individuals with life-changing diseases such as Amyotrophic Lateral Sclerosis (ALS), Parkinson disease, and epilepsy (PatientsLikeMe, 2010).

The impact that social networking sites will have on not only patient education but also nursing education in the future remains to be seen. These sites have the potential to distribute health information to millions in a matter of seconds. Web users are no longer just consumers of information, they are generating information and content.

M-Health Applications. The rapid and pervasive worldwide adoption of mobile cell phones is going to drive tremendous growth in handheld healthcare over the next decade. Wireless communication technologies are forcing a transformation in how and where healthcare is delivered. The abilities to collaborate, share high-resolution images, and even have live broadcasting of surgeries are all enabled by new technologies.

Applications areas for m-Health include consumer education, emergency response systems, professional and patient communications (e.g., text messaging, e-mail, social networking), health promotion and community mobilization, and public and population health to name a few (Waegemann, 2010).

One example of the value of m-Health technology was seen immediately following the disastrous Haiti earthquake in January, 2010. Cell phones were the only technology available for communication. They were used by relief workers to stay connected to each other and to the outside world; workers were able to gather information from Twitter, and they used Google maps to access routes to the airport and hospital (Inside Haiti's makeshift hospitals, 2010).

M-health growth has been around the world with significant demand from "bottom-of-the-pyramid" consumers located in rural areas. Pilot projects are ongoing in countries such as Indonesia, Brazil, Sudan, and Uganda. In Africa, health personnel use mobile phones to provide emergency medical care; their phones use solar charges. A toll-free mobile service is being launched in remote areas of Tanzania, Kenya, and Uganda. In developing economies, m-Health will be a major part of e-Health. M-Health will need to be integrated into the training of healthcare workers, so professionals have the knowledge and skills required to use the technology safely and effectively (Ganapathy & Ravindra, 2008).

IMPACT OF E-HEALTH APPLICATIONS

Transforming the Way We Learn

Web-based educational programs are changing the way consumers and healthcare providers learn. These programs continue to proliferate, providing the opportunity for interactive learning and simulations with the ability to have multiuser discussions and presentations in a collaborative learning environment. Faced with limited funds, nursing schools now have the ability to form partnerships and share their resources via the virtual classroom. The Web allows nurses and students the ability to access the most up-to-date research and knowledge facilitating evidence-based practice. Technological innovations, such as video streaming and virtual reality 3D displays, are providing more sophisticated formats in which to deliver educational materials. Web-based educational programs can reach remote students who otherwise would be unable to attend class (Sakraida & Draus, 2003; Smith-Stoner, 2003, Simpson, 2003; Brantley, Laney-Cummings & Spivack, 2004).

The role of the nurse as a patient and consumer educator in the digital age is evolving as well. Computer-based education programs are becoming an effective method to present information and improve outcomes. Online educational materials can be tailored to an individual's literacy level and presented in a bilingual format (Lewis, 2003). Remote interactive telehealth networks have been shown to be effective in providing preoperative patient education to rural locations and are increasingly being used for disease management (Thomas, Burton, Withrow, & Adkisson, 2004; Roupe, 2004).

Research Opportunities

The changes around e-Health applications are occurring at a rapid pace. More and more consumers want to become active participants in the management of their healthcare and will be looking at a variety of technologies to facilitate this. Today the Web is the preferred platform for young people to share ideas and opinions on issues. This is also the direction in which the world of e-Health is heading. There will be an increasing need for interactions with healthcare professionals via the Web on a variety of platforms (Nugyen, 2010; Grady & Tschirch, 2006).

Much is written on how e-Health applications may help provide care for an aging population, improve care in rural areas, and decrease healthcare disparities in the United States and increasingly around the world. While the potential for telehealth and m-Health is great, costs to convert to such applications and to train and change current medical practice remains underfunded. There is an increasingly important need to look at the impact of e-Health applications on the care provider–patient relationship and how these applications affect outcomes (Merrell & Doarn, 2010; McGowan, 2008).

Specific to telehealth nursing, there is a need to study symptom management and effectiveness of "distant" clinical assessments to identify standardized best practices. The Web can be the avenue for education and support for patients with chronic conditions. Communication can be synchronous via video Web conferencing applications, traditional telephone landlines, or cell phone. On the other hand, communication may be asynchronous via e-mail and the variety of social networking sites and Web portals. Also, the future may see more communication via avatars or "virtual agents." The effectiveness of all these communication methods as avenues to provide healthcare will need to be researched. Cell phones and the Web were not originally intended to provide healthcare; it is only fairly recently that these technologies have been adopted by healthcare providers and consumers. Nursing research will need to adapt to this ever-evolving landscape of technologies (McGowan, 2008).

Nugyen (2010) identifies unique methodologic research issues and challenges for nursing around the use of information and communication technologies (ICT). Research efforts should not focus on the effectiveness of healthcare delivered through different modes; rather, the focus needs to be on "understanding what intervention component, through what mechanism, for whom, and under what conditions will produce the most optimal health outcome" (p. 31).

When looking at Internet-based health management programs, concentrate on determining which active components of a multicomponent intervention will be involved in the study design, instead of trying to investigate all possible combinations of components. This narrowing of the research focus will facilitate more refinement of individual ICT components that appear to be effective (Nugyen, 2010). Gibbons and colleagues (2009) found 3 factors in consumer health applications that had a significant effect on health outcomes: (1) individual tailoring, (2) personalization, and (3) behavioral feedback. In essence, build the intervention based on actual characteristics of the individual, and deliver personal messages in an appealing format as the consumer progresses through the intervention.

While randomized controlled trials provide evidence for effectiveness of an intervention relative to a control, there is difficulty in finding consistency of control groups when studying ICT applications. It is often difficult to recruit the desired sample size; there is little consistency in how to design or select the control group. In addition, there are competing applications and resources all easily accessible via multiple modalities to anyone with Web access. These are just a few of the challenges to traditional research methodologies when looking at ICT applications. With the increasing pervasiveness of e-Health, nurse researchers will have to evolve their scientific approaches in order to produce the practice-based evidence that is going to be needed (Nugyen, 2010).

With the advent of social networks and the willingness of consumers to share information about themselves and their conditions, there are increasingly complex ethical, social, and legal issues to face regarding how to collect this data. Patients with few or no options for new treatments are not willing to wait for the conventional scientific process to take place. These patients are now using Web 2.0 platforms to log their own data. There are, however, unintended consequences from consumers participating in this "knowledge generation" including misinformation, user-generated data quality and credibility, and natural biases. Today with consumers managing, storing, and obtaining health records and information from diverse sources, this information can now be shared with care providers or researchers. Work needs to be done on how to best connect with individual health consumers on large Web platforms for powering the epidemiologic studies of the future (Nugyen, 2010; Grady & Tschirch, 2009, Randeree, 2009).

Another gap in current research is on the use of telehealth applications for emergency and disaster preparedness and response. There is a need for larger studies to explore the potential uses of these tools to facilitate the national public health agenda and research initiatives such as the Public Health Information Network (PHIN) initiative from the Center for Disease Control and Prevention (CDC). There are opportunities for interdisciplinary research on public health surveillance networks to determine pattern recognition algorithms that address threats to public health including flu outbreaks, environmental disasters and man-made threats such as terrorist attacks (Alverson et al., 2009).

Transforming Emergency Preparedness and Response

Over the years, there has been a shift from "closed system" technologies used by police and fire departments to "open systems" such as Twitter and FaceBook where families and neighbors communicate and offer help. We need to leverage these systems, including social media and mobile technologies, as delivery mechanisms to communicate with affected populations where to find emergency services (Bloch, 2010; Ackerman, 2010).

During a disaster situation, healthcare personnel are often affected as well. The use of telehealth technology would allow physicians to provide healthcare services remotely. M-Health technologies allow physicians to contact and have remote consultations with peers. It has been proposed that in the future, it would be advantageous to have a provision that would allow for telehealth cross-state consults in cases of disasters. There is a need as well for a wide-grid, fault-tolerant network capable of continuous operations despite disruptions in parts of the system, similar to what exists now in electrical systems and natural gas systems (Ackerman, 2010).

A locally based network of physicians linked via modern communication would help reduce major disruptions in healthcare. Protocols need to be developed for mobile communication devices before disasters so they can be rapidly deployed to provide routine care, triage, and shelter-in-place medical care (Bloch, 2010; Ackerman, 2010).

Advanced wireless electronic technologies are the quickest vehicles to communicate needs during emergency situations. State, federal, and international emergency efforts have not evolved as rapidly as these new technologies. However, some communities are turning to subscription services to notify residents of threats related to severe weather (Media Weather Innovations, LLC, 2010). There needs to be more collaboration to develop redundancy networks partnerships with commercial providers to ensure well planned disaster preparations (Bloch, 2010; Ackerman, 2010).

E-Health Challenges and Issues

Innovations in e-Health do not come without challenges and issues that healthcare professions must address. As the transformation of healthcare moves toward patient-centric models, the healthcare professionals must resolve some key challenges and issues.

These issues center on the legal, ethical, and public policy arenas.

Licensure

The lack of infrastructure for interstate licensure was a key impediment to the growth of telehealth. Each state has established practice acts for medical, nursing, and allied health professionals that dictate the procedures for obtaining and renewing a license to practice within that state. In April 1996, the Federation of State Medical Boards proposed creation of a limited interstate license for teleconsulting physicians, which was rejected by the American Medical Association in June 1996. The issues contributing to the defeat of the measure included a concern that rural patients would leave their rural primary care provider for a specialist, the cost of telehealth equipment, and payment for provision of telehealth services (Telemedicine Editorial, 1997).

The U.S. Congress contracted with the Center for Telemedicine Law for a background paper concerning telehealth licensure issues in early 1997(Telemedicine Report to Congress). Alternative approaches to licensure outlined in that report include consulting exceptions, endorsement, mutual recognition, reciprocity, registration, limited licensure, national licensure, and federal licensure. Much progress has been made to date, allowing physicians to obtain a license to diagnose and treat patients using electronic communication tools, despite the patient's location. Additionally, in 2010, the Centers for Medicare and Medicaid Services (CMS) proposed a rule that would allow a streamlined credentialing and privileging process for physicians and practitioners providing telemedicine services (Telehealth Law Center, 2010b).

The National Council of State Boards of Nursing (NCSBN), in 1998, developed a mutual recognition model of licensure. This allows nurses licensed in their home state to practice in other states under their respective state's Nurse Practice Act, when that state is part of the interstate compact. Over the past 10 years, many states have concluded that they could benefit from more coordination around multistate licensure. In 2006, the NCSBN received a grant to work with states to reduce licensure barriers impacting telehealth and interstate nursing practice. As of May 2010, 22 states have enacted the nurse licensure compact, with an additional state having proposed legislation (Telehealth Law Center, 2010a). Nurses remain accountable to their home state board of nursing, but the nurse does not have to get a new license for temporary practice in a party state, and can start practice when needed.

Ethical Issues

The predominant ethical issues concerning telehealth are privacy, confidentiality, and security. The following definitions have been set forth by the American Society for Testing and Materials Committee E31 on Healthcare Informatics, Subcommittee E31.17 on Privacy, Confidentiality, and Access (1997):

Privacy. "The right of individuals to be left alone and to be protected against physical or psychological invasion or the misuse of their property. It includes freedom from intrusion or observation into one's private affairs, the right to maintain control over certain personal information, and the freedom to act without outside interference." The Health Insurance Portability and accountability Act (HIPAA) was enacted in 1996, with the privacy rule taking effect in 2003. This rule regulates the use and disclosure of protected health information and applies to e-Health applications. Encryption is the best option when providing any videoconferencing services or when transferring video or digital images to other sites. Patients may release their health information via e-mail, but once received the provider is responsible for protecting it (Telehealth Law Center, 2010b).

Confidentiality. The "status accorded to data or information indicating that it is sensitive for some reason, and therefore it needs to be protected against theft, disclosure, or improper use, or both, and must be disseminated only to authorized individuals or organizations with a need to know."

Data Security. "The result of effective data protection measures; the sum of measures that safeguard data and computer programs from undesired occurrences and exposure to accidental or intentional access or disclosure to unauthorized persons, or a combination thereof; accidental or malicious alteration; unauthorized copying; or loss by theft or destruction by hardware failures, software deficiencies; operating mistakes; physical damage by fire, water, smoke, excessive temperature, electrical failure or sabotage; or a combination thereof. Data security exists when data are protected from accidental or intentional disclosure to unauthorized persons and from unauthorized or accidental alteration."

System Security. "The totality of safeguards including hardware, software, personnel policies, information practice policies, disaster preparedness; and oversight of these components. Security protects both the system and the information contained within from unauthorized access from without and from misuse from within. Security enables the entity or system to protect the confidential information it stores from unauthorized access, disclosure, or misuse, thereby protecting the privacy of the individuals who are the subjects of the stored information."

It is imperative that providers and healthcare systems establish policies concerning privacy, confidentiality, and security as they create systems to facilitate patient-centered care through the provision of e-Health. In addition to these issues, Khoja, Durrani, and Fahim (2008) identified the additional issues of consent for care in e-Health and the patient's right to access information as important considerations going forward.

Public Policy. The American Telemedicine Association (2010a) outlined policy initiatives concerning rule-making within the Centers for Medicaid and Medicare services to facilitate reimbursement for telemedicine care. Their agenda includes the following:

- Medical Staff Credentialing and Privileging for Telehealth Networks
- Expand Medicare coverage for telehealth
  - Remove Medicare barriers
  - Encourage remote monitoring, home telehealth, and chronic disease care
- Expand Medicaid coverage for telehealth
- National broadband deployment and upgrade
  - Streamline and expand the rural health program
  - Encourage Interconnections of Remote Healthcare Networks
  - Expand support for universal services
- Support Federal Programs and Initiatives that Deploy Telemedicine Technology and Services
- Resolve Barriers to Telemedicine
  - State Physician Licensure
  - Interstate Compacts
  - Internet Practice Issues (most notably concerning e-mail consultations, prescribing medications, and facilitating meeting consumer demand)
  - Malpractice Coverage
  - Use Telemedicine for Emergency Preparedness and Response

Emerging Issues and Challenges

Patients are the only constant across the care continuum. Patients need to ensure the accuracy of their information including demographics, allergies, and medication lists, thus placing accountability in their hands and likely having a significant impact on the quality of care delivered. There is a progressive movement toward patients becoming true partners with their care providers by co-managing their care. Those in the business of healthcare information technology need to look at clinical changes and patient impact enabled, supported, and facilitated by the technology (Murphy, 2009).

There is a growing movement to ensure that all consumers not only have access to healthcare, but are provided with all the information needed to prevent disease and improve health. This might include details on how to lose weight and quit smoking, the importance of complying with medication regimens, learning about personal health needs, and the importance of participating in routine health screening exams.

Healthcare professionals and healthcare institutions have been actively creating Web-based applications for the direct delivery of healthcare. Pioneering work by Brennan and colleagues (1991a,b) served as a catalyst for the development of computer-mediated systems to provide healthcare for persons living with AIDS and caretakers of Alzheimer disease patients. In both instances, Brennan and colleagues used a community-computing network, ComputerLink, to provide support services (e.g., contact with a nurse, informational resources, electronic support groups, and access to a decision-making tool) in the homes of patients and their caretakers. Results of these experiments (Brennan & Ripich, 1994; Brennan, Moore, & Smyth, 1995) demonstrated the value and effectiveness of computer-mediated support systems. As a continuation of this work, Brennan and colleagues (2001) designed HeartCare, which creates individual Web pages for cardiac artery bypass graft patients upon discharge.

For all the possibilities it presents, e-Health does come with challenges including privacy concerns, equity across populations, and the need to define a new type of relationship between the patient and healthcare provider (Eysenbach, 2001). Other issues include integration and networking interoperability, and usability. Nurse educators are challenged with preparing students for work in an electronic environment, and how to educate on the use of innovative technologies that can facilitate effective and efficient communication with patients. Finally, there is the challenge to determine what impact these new technologies will ultimately have on patient outcomes.

Disparities in healthcare and access to care still persist and a true solution eludes us. Telehealth and m-Health technologies can provide high-quality connections with public and nonprofit providers in rural and urban locations by bridging these geographic areas, redistributing medical expertise, and creating new avenues for education. Underserved communities can benefit from improved access to clinical expertise in specialties such as oncology, radiology, infectious disease, and psychiatry. Telehealth applications can provide greater access and help reduce healthcare costs (Merrill, 2010). The tools of telemedicine are useful for administrators and managers of health systems, as they continue to operate in more complex and restrictive regulatory environments that demand more efficiency, increased productivity, and greater assurance of patient safety and autonomy (Bashshur & Shannon, 2009).

With all its promise, telehealth is an equipment-intensive program, and it is expensive to get started. Unfortunately, many health providers have not shown interest in making capital investments, paying monthly fees, and training staff. A solid business case is a prerequisite for successful implementation. Further, reimbursement for telehealth interventions and a positive cost-benefit ratio are necessary before providers can consider adopting technological innovation into their practice environments. Health systems may want to fund programs if telemedicine visits prevent trips to congested emergency departments. As the healthcare industry is forced to deliver more with less, flexible telemedicine will need to come to the mainstream (Enrado, 2009).

Looking specifically at m-Health technology, there is the potential to save billions of dollars. M-health applications can be simple and low cost. There are now new communication possibilities with patients, including easy access to Web resources, phone-based personal health records and education programs, point-of-care documentation, and communication-based disease management. An individual can network with other professionals and use administrative and financial applications. There are emergency medical, public health, and research applications available, and there is the potential to have body area networks where implanted and wearable devices capture and send data to mobile phones (Wagermann, 2010; Bloch, 2010). As 78 million baby boomers enter

their 60s, the ability to continuously monitor data such as vital signs, calorie usage, and activity levels may help reduce healthcare costs and will play a role in improving lifestyle choices (Terry, 2010). Additional challenges include limited and fluctuating bandwidth; the need to configure application-specific uplink and downlink speeds; and the need for operating protocols to coordinate, integrate, and compress media streams.

A 2009 Price Waterhouse Coopers Research Institute report notes, one of the top issues for healthcare is the need for alternative care models outside of physician offices and hospitals. Needed changes are beginning to occur in the healthcare industry; expect to see an increase in home health services, work-site clinics, and programs for telehealth and remote patient monitoring (Doarn, 2010; PricewaterhouseCoopers, 2009). Telehealth and m-Health applications stand at the forefront of these needed changes for cost-effective care.

Challenges to address include information accuracy and quality, privacy and security issues, data portability, information literacy including patient literacy levels, Web site literacy levels, and technology access skills. The benefits of Healthcare 2.0 remain to be seen; it is in the early stages, and the adoption of these tools by healthcare providers and small physician groups is still less than 20%. These new services come at a cost, and the case needs to be made that they can improve quality of care and lower costs before private insurers can be expected to invest in these systems (Randeree, 2009).

CONCLUSION

Without a doubt, e-Health applications will proliferate in the future. Healthcare professionals need to seize the opportunities made possible by advanced technologies and create powerful and human-centered applications to facilitate consumers' full participation in health and wellness. To evolve this process, healthcare professional need to be actively involved in resolving challenges, shaping public policy, and evaluating health outcomes.

TELEHEALTH CASE STUDY

FG, is a 67-year-old African American who has been living with diabetes for several years. She lives alone in a rural community that is 100 miles from the nearest hospital. In addition to her diabetes, FG suffers from hypertension.

FG had missed a routine check up with her family physician because she did not have transportation to his office in a neighboring town. She rescheduled the visit 3 weeks later and was found to have a blood pressure of 185/100, and a fasting blood sugar of 285. The family physician chose to admit her to the hospital in order to bring her blood sugar and blood pressure under control. FG is able to monitor her blood glucose, but she has neither consistently monitored her blood glucose or her diet. FG has been experiencing increasing difficulty with her eyesight and while in the hospital has been given a new prescription for glasses.

Upon discharge, FG was approved for telehealth services and monitoring. Her family does not live nearby and she tends to become depressed; it was felt that the regular counseling and communication she would have with the home health nurse would be beneficial in helping her with ongoing long-term management of her conditions.

The telehealth workstation being considered for FG's home includes a blood pressure cuff, glucose meter, and an automated weight scale connected to FG's home phone line that will transmit the number directly to the home telehealth agency.

- There is a need for an involved patient assessment when looking at whether the patient is a candidate for telehealth services—what skills and behaviors and physical capabilities would need to be evaluated for limitations when determining if FG is a candidate for telehealth monitoring?

- An important consideration when looking at telehealth candidates is whether telehealth equipment could be set up in the patient's existing residence. In looking at the home environment and the telehealth system to be used, what are some user interface considerations to address when determining if the patient and their home setting would be appropriate for telehealth nursing care?

- When setting up questions for the telehealth station, why is it important to design easy-to-understand and easy-to-answer customizable questions?

- FG is a Medicaid patient. Research whether Medicaid reimbursement of services is available in your state.

- Discuss some of the issues of privacy, informed consent, equal access, and patient-provider communication that need to be addressed when utilizing a telehealth application in a patient's home.

REFERENCES

Ackerman, K. (2010, April 22). New toolkit for disaster response: Social media, mobile tools & telehealth. *iHealthBeat*. Retrieved from http://www.ihealthbeat. org/features/2010/new-toolkit-for-disaster-response-social-media-mobile-tools--telehealth.aspx.

Advanced ICU Care. (2009). *Together, we can realize and new level of care in the ICU*. Retrieved from http://www.icumedicine.com.

Alverson, D. C., Edison, K., Flournoy, B. A., Korte, B., Magruder, C., & Miller, C. (2010, January/February). Telehealth tools for public health, emergency, or disaster preparedness, and response: A summary report. *Telemedicine and e-Health, 16*(1), 112–114. Retrieved from http://www.liebertonline.com/doi/pdf/10.1089/tmj.2009.0149.

American College of Nurse Practitioners (ANCP). (2006, June 12). *What is telehealth?* Retrieved from http://www.acnpweb.org/i4a/pages/index.cfm?pageid=3470.

American Society for Testing and Materials Committee E-31 on Healthcare Informatics, Subcommittee E-31.17 on Privacy, Confidentiality, and Access. (1997). *Standard Guide for Confidentiality, Privacy, Access, and Data Security Principles for Health Information Including Computer-based Patient Records*. Philadelphia, PA: ASTM (Designation E-1869-97).

American Nurses Association (ANA). (1997). Telehealth: A tool for nursing practice. In *Nursing Trends & Issues, ANA Policy Series*. Washington, DC: ANA.

American Telemedicine Association (ATA). (2010a). *Telemedicine Policy Priorities: 2010*. Retrieved from http://www.americantelemed.org/files/public/policy/2010%20Policy%20Priorities.pdf.

American Telemedicine Association (ATA). (2010b). *ATA Defining Telemedicine*. Retrieved from http://www.atmeda.org/news/definition.html.

Bashshur, R., & Shannon, G.W. (2009). *History of telemedicine: Evolution, context, and transformation*. New Rochelle, NY: Mary Ann Liebert, Inc.

Bauer, K. (2009) Healthcare ethics in the information age. In R. Juppicini & R. Adell (Eds.), *Handbook of research on technoethics: Vol.1.* (pp. 171–172). Pennsylvania: IGI Global.

Biodevices. (2009). *Vital Jacket® knowing your heart*. Retrieved from http://www.vitaljacket.com.

Blanchett, K. (2008, March). Remote patient monitoring. *Telemedicine and e-Health, 14*(2), 127–130. Retrieved from http://www.acnpweb.org/i4a/pages/index.cfm?pageid=3470.

Bloch, C. (2010, April 21). UTMB responds to disasters. *Federal Telemedicine News*. Retrieved from http://telemedicnenews.blogspot.com/2010/04/utmb-respons-to-disasters.html.

Blumenthal, D. (2010, February 4). Launching HITECH. *New England Journal of Medicine, 362*(5), 382–385.

Boulos, M., Ramloll, R., Jones, R., & Toth-Cohen, S. (2008). Web 3D for public, environmental and occupational health: Early examples from second life. *International Journal of Environmental Research and Public Health, 5*(4), 290–317. doi:10.3390/ijerph5040290.

Borowitz, S. M., & Wyatt, J. C. (1998). The origin, content, and workload of e-mail consultations. *The Journal of the American Medical Association, 280*(15), 1321–1324.

Brantley, D., Laney-Cummings, K., & Spivack, R. (2004). *Innovation, demand and investment in telehealth*. U.S. Dept. of Commerce: Office of Technology Policy. Retrieved from http://www.technology.gov/reports/TechPolicy/Telehealth/2004Report.pdf.

Brennan, P., Moore, S., Bjornsdottir, G., Jones, J., Visovsky, C., & Rogers, M. (2001). HeartCare: An Internet-based information and support system for patient home recovery after coronary artery bypass graft (CABG) surgery. *Journal of Advanced Nursing, 35*(5), 699–708.

Brennan, P., Moore, S., & Smyth, K. (1995). The effects of a special computer network on caregivers of persons with Alzheimer's disease. *Nursing Research, 44*, 166–172.

Brennan, P., & Ripich, S. (1994). Use of home-care computer network by persons with AIDS. *International Journal of Technology Assessment in Healthcare, 10*, 258–272.

Brennan, P., Ripich, S., & Moore, S. (1991). The use of home-based computers to support persons living with AIDS/ARC. *Journal of Community Health Nursing, 8*, 3–14.

Brennan, P., Moore, S., & Smyth, K. (1991). ComputerLink: Electronic support for the home caregiver. *Advances in Nursing Science, 13*(4), 14–27.

CDC Home. (2009, August 10). *Social media at CDC—Virtual worlds*. Retrieved from http://www.cdc.gov/SocialMedia/Tools/VirtualWorlds.html.

Cherry, J. C., Moffat, T. P., Rodriguez, C., & Dryden, K. (2002). Diabetes disease management program for an indigent population empowered by telemedicine technology. *Diabetes Technology & Therapeutics, 4*(6), 783–791.

Dambita, N. (2010, May). *Leveraging IT to deliver healthcare in low resource settings: Lessons given, lessons taken*. Paper presented at the meeting of the Colorado Health Information Management and Systems Society, Denver, CO.

Bloch, C. (2010, February 8). Status of mobile health. *Federal Telemedicine News*. Retrieved from http://telemedicinenews.blogsspot.com/2010/02/status-of-mobile-health.html.

Darkins, A., Ryan, P., Kobb, R., Foster, L., Edmonson, E., Wakefield, B., & Lancaster, A. E. (2008). Care coordination/home telehealth: The systematic implementation of health informatics, home telehealth, and disease management to support the care of veteran patients with chronic conditions. *Telemedicine and e-Health, 14*, 1118–1126. Retrieved from http://www.liebertonline.com/doi/pdfplus/10.1089/tmj.2008.0021.

Diepgen, G., & Eysenbach, T. (1998). Responses to unsolicited patient e-mail request for medical advice on the World Wide Web. *The Journal of the American Medical Association, 280*(15), 1333–1335.

Doty, C. A. (2008, November) Delivering care anytime, anywhere: Telehealth alters the medical ecosystem. *California Healthcare Foundation*. Retrieved from http://www.chcf.org/publications/2008/11/delivering-care-anytime-anywhere-telehealth-alters-the-medical-ecosystem.

Eysenbach, G. (2001). What is e-Health? *Journal of Medical Internet Research, 3*(2), e20.

Enrado, P. (2009, August 19). California telemedicine shortage aims to alleviate nurse shortage. *Healthcare IT News*. Retrieved from http://www.healthcareitnews.com/news/california-telemedicine-program-aims-alleviate-nurse-shortage.

Eytan, T. (2010, February 18). Six Reasons Why mHealth Is Different Than eHealth [Web log post]. Retrieved from http://www.tedeytan.com/2010/02/18/4731.

Federal Communications Commission (FCC). (2010, February 1). *Voice Over Internet Protocol (VoIP)*. Retrieved from http://www.fcc.gov/voip.

Finishing the Job. (2009, September 24). *Economist* Retrieved from http;//www.economist.com/specialreports/printerfriendly.cfm?story_id=14483856.

Fox, S., & Purcell, K. (2010, March). Chronic disease and the Internet. *Pew Internet & American Life Project*. Retrieved from http://www.pewinternet.org/Reports/2010/Chronic-Disease/Summary-of-Findings.aspx?r=1.

Ganapathy, K., & Ravindra, A. (2008, July 13–August 8). mHealth: A potential tool for healthcare delivery in India. *Making the eHealth Connection*. Retrieved from http://www.ehealth-connection.org/files/conf-materials/mHealth_A%20potential%20tool%20in%20India_0.pdf.

Giansanti, D., Morelli, S., Maccioni, G., & Constantini, G. (2009, April). Toward the design of a wearable system for fall-risk detection in telerehabilitation. *Telemedicine and e-Health, 15*(3), 296–299. Retrieved from http://www.liebertonline.com/doi/pdfplus/10.1089/tmj.2008.0106.

Gibbons M. C., Wilson, R. F., Samal, L., Lehmann, C. U., Dickersin, K., Lehmann, H. P., & Bass, E. B. (2009, October). *Impact of Consumer Health Informatics Applications*. Evidence Report/Technology Assessment No. 188. (Prepared by Johns Hopkins University Evidence-based Practice Center under contract No. HHSA 290-2007-10061-I) AHRQ Publication No. 09(10)-E019. Retrieved from http://www.ahrq.gov/downloads/pub/evidence/pdf/chiapp/impactchia.pdf.

Google Health. (2010). *About Google Health*. Retrieved from http://www.google.com/intl/en-US/health/about.

Grady, J., & Tschirch, P. (2006, May 9). Creating a national telehealth nursing research agenda. *American Telehealth Association 11th Annual Meeting.* Retrieved from http://www.acnpweb.org/files/public/ProposedTelenursingResearchAgenda.pdf.

Guendelman, S., Meade, K., Benson, M., Chen, Y. Q., & Samuels, S. (2002). Improving asthma outcomes and self-management behaviors of inner-city children: A randomized trial of the Health Buddy interactive device and an asthma diary. *Archives of Pediatric and Adolescent Medicine, 156*(2), 114–120.

HHS names David Blumenthal as National Coordinator for Health Information Technology. (2009, March 20). *U.S. Department of Health & Human Services, News Release.* Retrieved from http://www.hhs.gov/news/press/2009pres/03/20090320b.html.

Inside Haiti's makeshift hospitals. (2010, May 3). *GovernmentHealthIT.* Retrieved from http://govhealthit.com/newsitem.aspx?nid=73658.

Institute of Medicine. (1996). *Telemedicine: A guide to assessing telecommunications in healthcare.* Washington, DC: National Academy Press.

Internet Protocol Television. (2008) *What is Internet protocol television.* Retrieved from http://internetprotocoltelevision.com.

InTouch Health. (2010). RP endpoint devices. Retrieved from http://www.intouch-health.com/products_remote_presence_endpoint_devices.html.

Jönsson, A., & Willman, A. (2008, December). Implementation of telenursing within home healthcare. *Telemedicine and e-Health, 14*(10), 1057–1062.

Kane, B., & Sands, D. Z. (1998). AMIA Internet Working Group, Task Force on Guidelines for the Use of Clinic-Patient Electronic Mail: Guidelines for the clinical use of electronic mail with patients. *Journal of the American Medical Informatics Association, 5*(1), 104–111.

Khoja, S., Durrani, H. & Fahim, A. (2008, July). *Scope of policy issues for eHealth: Results from a structured review.* Paper presented at Making the eHealth Connection Global Partnerships, Local Solutions—The Rockefeller Foundation, Bellagio, Italy. Retrieved from http://www.ehealth-connection.org/files/conf-materials/Scope%20of%20Policy%20Issues%20for%20eHealth_0.pdf.

LaFramboise, L. M., Todero, C. M., Zimmerman, L., & Agrawat, S. (2003). Comparison of Health Buddy with traditional approached to heart failure management. *Family and Community, 26*(4), 275–288.

Lewis, D. (2003). Computers in patient education. *Computers, Informatics, Nursing, 21*(2), 88–96.

McGowan, J. (2008). The pervasiveness of telemedicine: Adoption with or without a research base. *Journal of General Internal Medicine, 23*(4), 505–507.

Media Weather Innovations, LLC (2010). *WeatherCall.* Retrieved from http://www.weathercall.net/wc_home.html.

Merrell, R. C., & Doarn, C. R. (2010, March). Where is the proof? *Telemedicine and e-Health, 16*(2), 125–126. Retrieved from http://www.liebertonline.com/doi/abs/10.1089/tmj.2010.9995.

Merrill, M. (2009, October 8). Google Health adds telehealth services to the mix. *Healthcare IT News.* Retrieved from http://www.healthcareitnews.com/news/google-health-adds-telehealth-services-mix

Merrill, M. (2010, April 14). California embarks on "future of medicine" with telehealth project. *Healthcare IT News.* Retrieved from http://www.healthcareitnews.com/news/california-embarks-future-medicine-telehealth-project.

My HealtheVet. (2010). My HealtheVet home page. *United States Department of Veterans Affairs.* Retrieved from http://www.myhealth.va.gov.

Naditz, A. (2009, December). Telenursing: Front-line applications of telehealthcare delivery. *Telemedicine and e-Health, 15*(9), 825–829. Retrieved from http://www.liebertonline.com/doi/pdfplus/10.1089/tmj.2009.9938.

Neuhauser, L., & Krepts, G.L. (2010, February). eHealth communication and behavior change: Promise and performance. *Social Semiotics, 20*(1), 9–27.

Nguyen, H. (2010, April). *Digital health consumers: Transforming the clinical research landscape.* Paper presented at the Western Institute of Nursing Annual Communicating Nursing Research Conference, Phoenix, AZ.

Oh, H., Rizo, C., Enkin, M., & Jadad, A. (2005, February 24). What is eHealth?: A systematic review of published definitions. *Journal of Medical Internet Research, 7*(1), e1. Retrieved from http://www.jmir.org/2005/1/e1.

PatientsLikeMe. (2010). *PatientsLikeMe home page.* Retrieved from http://www.patientslikeme.com.

Pagliari C., Sloan D., Gregor P., Sullivan, F., Detmer, D., Kahan, J. P., & MacGillivray, S. (2005) What is eHealth? A scoping exercise to map the field. *Journal of Medical Internet Research, 7*(1), e9.

PricewaterhouseCoopers' Health Research Institute (2009, December). *Top 10 health industry issues in 2010: Squeezing the juice out of healthcare.* Retrieved from http://pwchealth.com/cgi-local/hregister.cgi?link=reg/top-ten-health-industry-issues-in-2010.pdf.

Purcell, K., Rainie, L., Mitchell, A., Rosenstiel, T., & Olmstead, K. (2010, March). New news landscape: Rise of the Internet, understanding the participatory news consumer. *Pew Research Center Publications,* Retrieved from http://pewresearch.org/pubs/1508/internet-cell-phone-users-news-social-experience.

QualityNet. (2006/2007). Tools: Home telehealth reference 2006/2007. Retrieved from http://www.qualitynet.org/dcs/ContentServer?c=MQTools&pagename=Medqic%2FMQTools%2FToolTemplate&cid=1157485199575.

Rainie, L. (2010, January). Internet, broadband, cell phone statistics. *Pew Internet and American Life*

Project. Retrieved from http://www.pewinternet.org/Reports/2010/Internet-broadband-and-cell-phone-statistics.aspx?r=1.

Randeree, E. (2009, April). Exploring technology impacts of healthcare 2.0 initiatives. *Telemedicine and e-Health, 15*(3), 255–260. Retrieved from http://www.liebertonline.com/doi/pdfplus/10.1089/tmj.2008.0093.

Ratan, S. (2010, May 10). Highlights at ATA Conference 2010. *Bosch Healthcare introduces new telehealth solutions and presents outcomes. Technology for Better Quality of Life*. Retrieved from http://www.marketwire.com/press-release/Highlights-ATA-Conference-2010-Bosch-Healthcare-Introduces-New-Telehealth-Solutions-1259369.htm.

Roupe, M. (2004). Interactive home telehealth: A vital component of disease management programs. *Case Management, 9*(1), 47–49.

Sakraida, T. & Draus, P. (2003). Transition to a Web-supported curriculum. *Computers, Informatics, Nursing, 21*(6), 309–315.

Silber D. (2003, May). *The case for eHealth*. Paper presented at the European Commission's First High-Level Conference on eHealth - European Institute of Public Administration. Retrieved from http://www.epractice.eu/files/download/awards/D10_Award1_ResearchReport.pdf.

Simpson, R. (2003). Welcome to the virtual classroom: How technology is transforming nursing education in the 21st century. *Nursing Administration Quarterly, 27*(1), 83–86.

Skiba, D. (2007). Emerging Technology Center: Nursing Education 2.0: Second Life. *Nursing Education Perspectives, 28*(3), 156–157.

Smith-Stoner, M. & Willer, A. (2003). Video streaming in nursing education: Bringing life to online education. *Nurse Educator, 28*(2), 66–70.

Spielberg, A. R. (1998). On call and online, sociohistorical, legal, and ethical implications of e-mail for the patient-physician relationship. *Journal of the American Medical Association, 280*(15), 1353–1359.

TBHome. (2010, February 21). *Re: 6 Reasons Why mHealth is different than eHealth* [Web log comment]. Retrieved from http://tedeytan.com/2010/02/18/4731.

Telehealth Law Center. (2010a). Licensure main page. Retrieved from http://www.telehealthlawcenter.org/?c=143&a=1388.

Telehealth Law Center. (2010b). *Major changes in HIPAA and privacy regulations: What telehealth providers need to know*. Retrieved from http://www.telehealthlawcenter.org/?c=125&a=2187.

Telemedicine Editorial. (1997). Obstacles to tele-medicine's growth. *Medical Economics, 74*(23), 69.

Telemedicine Report to Congress. (1997). *Legal Issues—Licensure and Telemedicine*. Retrieved from http://www.ntia.doc.gov/reports/telemed/legal.htm.

Terry, M. (2010, March). Wearable health monitors: Real-time, patient-friendly data collection. *Telemedicine and e-Health, 16*(2), 1–5. Retrieved from http://www.liebertonline.com/doi/pdfplus/10.1089/tmj.2010.9994.

The doctor in your pocket. (2005, September 15). *Economist*. Retrieved from http://www.economist.com/displaystory.cfm?story_id=E1_QPGRTQD.

Thomas, K., Burton, D., Withrow, L., & Adkisson, B. (2004). Impact of a preoperative education program via interactive telehealth network for rural patients having total joint replacement. *Orthopaedic Nursing, 23*(1), 39–44.

Thompson, T. G., & Fox, C. E. (2001). *2001 Report to Congress on Telemedicine*. Retrieved from http://www.hrsa.gov/telehealth/pubs/report2001.htm.

United Nations Foundation, Vodafone Group Foundation, & Telemedicine Society of India. (2008, July/August). mHealth and mobile telemedicine—An overview. *Making the eHealth Connection*. Retrieved from http://www.ehealth-connection.org/content/mhealth-and-mobile-telemedicine-an-overview.

Waegemann, C. P. (2010, January/February). mHealth: Next generation of telemedicine. *Telemedicine and e-Health, 16*, 23–25. Retrieved from http://www.liebertonline.com/doi/pdfplus/10.1089/tmj.2010.9990.

Welsh, T. S. (1999, June 20). Telemedicine. *UT Telemedicine Network*. Retrieved from http://ocean.st.usm.edu/~w146169/teleweb/telemed.htm.

WebMD. (2010). WebMD Better Information. Better Health. Retrieved from http://www.webmd.com.

Whitten, P. & Sypher, D. (2006, November 6). Evolution of telemedicine from an applied communication perspective in the United States. *Telemedicine and e-Health, 12*, 590–600.

Wicklund, E. (2010, February). Cisco launches telemedicine pilot. *Healthcare IT News*, pp. 32–33.

Widman, L. E., & Tong, D. A. (1997). Requests for medical advice from patients and families to healthcare providers who publish on the World Wide Web. *Archives of Internal Medicine, 157*(2), 209–212.

Wilson, L., Stevenson, D., & Cregan, P. (2010, January/February). Telehealth on advanced networks. *Telemedicine and eHealth, 16*(1), 69–79. Retrieved from http://www.liebertonline.com/doi/pdf/10.1089/tmj.2009.0153.

Witherspoon, J., Johnston, S., & Wasem, C. (1994). *Rural telehealth, telemedicine, distance education and informatics for rural healthcare*. Boulder, CO: Western Interstate Commission of Higher Education Publications.

Zimmerman, L., Barason, S. Nieveen, J., & Schmaderer, M. (2004). Symptom management intervention in elderly coronary artery bypass graft patients. *Outcomes Management, 8*(1), 5–12.

39

Consumer and Patient Use of Computers for Health

Rita D. Zielstorff / Barbara B. Frink

- OBJECTIVES

  1. Review the types of technology applications used by patients and consumers related to health.
  2. Discuss several issues related to patient and consumer applications in health, and promising developments for dealing with these issues.
  3. Explain the nurse informaticist's role in patient and consumer computing.
  4. List some areas for research related to patient and consumer computing.
  5. Provide a list of resources for further learning.

- KEY WORDS

  consumer computing
  patient computing
  Internet-based health applications
  computer information systems
  consumer health informatics
  nursing informatics
  healthcare consumerism
  e-patients

INTRODUCTION

Consumerism has seen a dramatic rise in the United States over the past decades. Not surprisingly, this movement has expanded into the arena of health. Consumers of health services (patients, families, and family caregivers) are educating themselves on all aspects of health, wellness, and disease; they are seeking out comparative information on insurance plans, physicians, hospitals, and other health-related services (Binder, 2008; Keckley & Eselius, 2009). Armed with more information, they are exercising a greater say in decisions that affect them and the persons they care about. The traditional role of the patient as the object of care, acquiescent to decisions made by the experts, is changing (Binder, 2008; Keckley & Eselius, 2009; Miller, 2010). Today, patients and families expect to be partners in care, evaluating with their caregivers the implications of diagnostic tests and the ramifications of treatment modalities, including cost and effectiveness (Fox & Jones, 2009). Indeed, a new voluntary organization, the Society for Participatory Medicine, has been formed to bring about a world "in which networked patients shift from being mere passengers to responsible drivers of their health, and in which providers encourage and value them as full partners" (Society for Participatory Medicine, 2010).

The movement is sanctioned by government policy as well. A new developmental goal proposed for Healthy People 2020 is to "Increase the proportion of persons who report that their healthcare providers always involved them in decisions about their healthcare as much as they wanted" (U.S. Department of Health and Human Services, 2009). As part of the American Recovery and Reinvestment Act of 2009 (ARRA, 2009), one of the recommendations for Meaningful Use of health information technology (HIT) is the principle to "include patients and families as primary participants in health information sharing," with the objective to "…engage patients and caregivers in shared decision making…" (Office of the National Coordinator for Health Information Technology, 2010).

The Health Insurance Portability and Accountability Act (HIPAA) Privacy Rule grants specific rights to patients and family members regarding their health information. For example, patients must be made aware when their record is shared outside of prespecified boundaries, and patients must be granted the ability to view their medical record and to correct information if that is warranted (U. S Department of Health and Human Services, 2003). Consumer-friendly guides to the HIPAA Privacy Rule and the rights granted under the rule have been published by the Office for Civil Rights (Office for Civil Rights, n.d.).

The Internet has been a boon to healthcare consumerism. A Google search on any health topic will typically return thousands of pages, varying greatly in relevance and quality, but nonetheless usually useful to the health information seeker (Fox & Jones, 2009). Caregivers routinely report the phenomenon of patients arriving for a visit with a stack of printouts related to their diagnosis or treatment, asking the physician or nurse to comment on the material's relevance to their particular case.

Static content pages are only one type of health-related resources on the Web. Links to diagnosis-specific support groups, the ability to communicate with family, friends, and healthcare providers about one's health, and a variety of interactive resources for record keeping, monitoring, and decision making are also available. A movement that is at the intersection of consumerism and technology is Health 2.0 (Shreeve, 2008). Evolved from Web 2.0, with its emphasis on user-generated content, community, and personalized computing, Health 2.0 has been defined as "The use of social software and light tools to promote collaboration between patients, their caregivers, medical professionals, and other stakeholders in health" (Sarasohn-Kahn, 2008, p. 2.).

This chapter provides an overview of applications, discusses several issues related to consumer use of technology for health, and reviews current developments for dealing with these issues. In addition, it provides a rationale for nurses' involvement in this arena, lists special considerations in designing computer applications for patients and consumers, and discusses some areas for research related to patient and consumer computing for health.

APPLICATION AREAS: CONSUMER USE OF COMPUTERS FOR HEALTH

Information Seeking

Information seeking about health matters is a common use of computers by patients and consumers. According to a 2008 Harris Interactive survey, approximately 81% of the adult U.S. population has access to the Internet (Harris Interactive, 2008, November 17); of these, 4 out of 5, or 150 million people, had used the internet recently for health-related matters, and about a quarter of them did so often (Harris Interactive, 2008, July 29). Just as many people now consult the internet for health information as they do physicians (Sarasohn-Kahn, 2008).

In a different survey, the Pew Internet & American Life project found that 61% of all American adults, and 8 in 10 Internet users, went online to access health information (Fox & Jones, 2009). About 60% of these said the information they found online influenced their decision making related to health, and that they or someone they knew were helped by the information they found. This is twice the number of respondents who said that in 2006 (Fox & Jones, 2009, p. 4). The topics most frequently searched on, according to the report, are diseases, treatments, and exercise and fitness information. A new finding is that wireless devices are "changing the behavior of healthcare consumers," and that the "mobile internet draws people into conversations about health as much as online tools enable research" (Fox & Jones, 2009, p. 6).

Sponsorship of static content sites varies widely. Healthcare organizations may offer their communities a public Web site that includes health articles developed by their own professional experts, or licensed from vendors. A well known example is the Mayo Clinic, whose public site (www.mayoclinic.com) provides a wealth of health information and tools. For-profit entities such as pharmaceutical firms, drugstore chains, and durable medical equipment vendors frequently sponsor public sites. An example is www.diabetes.com sponsored by GlaxoSmithKline. Professional societies and foundations frequently sponsor public sites devoted to educating consumers about health matters that are their particular focus. Examples are www.american-heart.org sponsored by the American Heart Association, and www.lungusa.org sponsored by the American Lung Association. Some vendors develop health Web site applications and license them to other entities, allowing branding or co-branding by the licensing organization.

The U.S. government has developed several resources for consumers seeking health information. These include www.healthfinder.gov, a collection of vetted links to health-related Web sites that is sponsored by the Office of Disease Prevention and Health Promotion of the U.S. Department of Health and Human Services; www.medlineplus.gov, a consumer-friendly site developed by the National Library of Medicine and the National Institutes of Health; and www.medicare.gov, devoted to information specific to the Medicare program and to health topics for seniors, sponsored by the Centers for Medicare and Medicaid Services (CMS) of the U.S. Department of Health and Human Services.

With respect to purchasing decisions, several sites are now available to help consumers compare costs and quality for hospitals, nursing homes, home health agencies, insurance plans, and physicians. Two examples are the Leapfrog Group (www.leapfroggroup.org) and the Centers for Medicare and Medicaid Services (www.cms.gov). Consumers can research the background of individual physicians, including patient reviews, on such sites as www.PhysicianReports.com, and www.Vitals.com.

For the tech-savvy, static content may not be enough. Exposed to social networks that provide interactive access to dynamic user-generated content, these users instead seek the collective wisdom of "patients like me" (Frost, Massagli, Wicks, & Heywood, 2008; Sarasohn-Kahn, 2008). They may anonymously browse a site, seeking content relevant to their particular situation, or become an active, contributing member, forming online relationships based on common experience (Fox & Jones, 2009). In a 2009 survey, Manhattan Research found that about 35% of American adults used social media for health-related purposes (Manhattan Research, 2010).

Communication and Support

Electronic mail continues to be the pervasive application of the Internet. Many e-mail users find it particularly useful for health-related matters. They may communicate informally with friends and family about health. They may use e-mail to keep family informed about the health status of one of the family. They may engage in online support groups and social networks whose focus is on a particular disease or condition. Or they may communicate directly with their healthcare providers about their own or a family member's condition (Fox & Jones, 2009).

Online support groups and topic-specific social networks can provide an indispensable, even life-saving resource to patients and families. Interested persons can find an online support group for almost any condition, ranging from Alzheimer disease to Zellweger syndrome. Again, the sponsorship varies, from healthcare organizations providing local groups for their patients, to national organizations and foundations, to privately sponsored groups, to grant-funded research projects. Participation in the group can also vary. Some groups are monitored by health professionals such as medical social workers, nurses, or physicians. Others are unmonitored. For suffering patients and families, the knowledge that others are facing similar situations, and have found ways to cope, can be a source of hope and consolation (Civan & Pratt, 2007; Civan, Skeels, Stolyar, & Pratt, 2006; Durant, Safran, & McCray, 2010; Fox, 2007; Fox & Jones, 2009). These participants in Health 2.0 often share information about latest research, treatments, and clinical trials that may not be common knowledge, developing what Weiss and Lorenzi call "community wisdom" (Weiss & Lorenzi, 2008). Some communities have generated new information about side effects of drugs (Fox, 2008a; Sarasohn-Kahn, 2008), and in one instance, an online community collaborated in the generation of new knowledge regarding the use of lithium for Amyotrophic Lateral Sclerosis (ALS) (Frost, et al., 2008). Examples of social networking sites include PatientsLikeMe (www.patientslikeme.com) (Frost et al., 2008), WEGO Health (www.wegohealth.com), Diabetic Connect (www.diabeticconnect.com, the Association of Cancer Online Resources (www.ACOR.org), Quitnet (www.quitnet.com) aimed at those who want to quit smoking, and Disaboom (www.disaboom.com) for persons with disabilities. For those who are homebound or living with chronic conditions, the online group may be a lifeline (Fox & Purcell, 2010; Miller, 2008; Sarasohn-Kahn, 2008). Assistive devices such as screen readers, screen magnifiers, alternative keyboards, and foot mice can even assist those who have physical disabilities to use the computer for online support (World Wide Web Consortium, 2010).

Direct communication with one's healthcare provider is high on the list of desired resources for most patients and families. A survey by the California Healthcare Foundation found that about three-fourths of Internet users would like to be able to communicate with their doctor or doctor's staff (Seidman & Eytan, 2008). About a quarter of these would even be willing to pay extra for it. A separate survey of healthcare consumers conducted by Deloitte Center for Health Solutions found similar results (Copeland, Keckley, Eselius, Greene, & Underwood, 2008). The functions most requested in these surveys include online appointment requests, access to online medical records and test results, and direct e-mail to physicians.

The number of providers offering this type of service, though increasing, is still much less than the demand. In both the CHCF and Deloitte surveys, fewer than 10% of respondents had access to the applications they wanted. However, a recent survey by Manhattan Research (2010) found that about 39% of physicians currently offer online communication with their patients, up from 30% in 2008. Slow uptake by physicians is generally linked to concerns about liability, reimbursement, confidentiality and security, and impact on office workflow (Brooks & Menachemi, 2006; Byrne, Elliott, & Firek, 2009; Manhattan Research, 2010). Byrne and colleagues noted a "clinical adoption inertia" in a Veterans Administration setting that was already highly automated (Byrne et al., 2009). Yet those who do offer secure messaging have reported increased patient satisfaction as well as increased efficiency and quality of communication (Byrne et al., 2009; Ralston et al., 2009; Tang et al., 2003).

In some arrangements, patients communicate with staff for issues such as appointment requests and prescription renewal requests. In others, patients are able to send nonurgent clinical questions to nursing staff or directly to the physician. Generally, the practice absorbs the cost of the technology supporting the service, although some health plans may charge a subscription fee for clinical messaging.

The technology for providing the service ranges from simply giving patients the provider's e-mail address, to registering them with a username and password to use a secure Web site. The Web site may be administered by the practice, or by the provider group, payer, or network, or the clinician may subscribe to a vendor-provided service. Often the messaging application is embedded in a patient portal that has other functions such as a personal health record, access to vetted health information, and administrative functions such as bill pay. Examples of portals that include patient-clinician messaging are Patient Site at Beth Israel Deaconess Medical Center in Boston (www.patientsite.org), PAMFOnline at Palo Alto Medical Foundation (www.pamfonline.org), and My Health Manager at Kaiser Permanente

(www.kaiserpermanente.org). Commercial systems available to physician practices, payers, and health delivery organizations include MedFusion, now owned by Intuit (see www.medfusion.com) and Relay Health, now owned by McKesson (www.relayhealth.com).

Further along the spectrum are "e-visits," or structured interactions that enable patients to describe a problem in some detail (usually with the help of a topic-specific questionnaire), and receive advice from the healthcare provider, thus avoiding the time and expense of an in-person visit. Even more than with e-mail, providers are cautious about adopting the technology, citing concerns about liability, privacy, reimbursement, and impact on their own and their staff's productivity (Byrne et al., 2009; Liederman, Lee, Baquero, & Seites, 2005a; Painter, 2007; Stone, 2007; Tang et al., 2003); Gradually, these concerns are being mitigated. A number of organizations have published guidelines for the use of patient-provider electronic communication that are aimed at reducing risk. These include the American Medical Association (Bovi, 2003), the American Nurses Association (Hutcherson, 2001), the American Academy of Pediatrics (Gerstle and the Task Force on Medical Informatics, 2004), the American Medical Informatics Association (Kane & Sands, 1998), the eRisk Working Group for Healthcare (Troxel, 2009), and the Federation of State Medical Boards (2002). The advent of secure, Web-based messaging requiring password access from known patients has reduced the fears associated with open Internet e-mail. Reimbursement for online visits has also improved, with several national insurers and health plans now paying physicians $25 to $50 per visit, some with a patient co-pay, some not (Marte, 2009; Robeznieks, 2007a, 2007b; Schneider, 2010). Some employers, seeing the evidence of lessened absenteeism due to doctors' visits for minor acute problems, are requiring that their contracts with insurers include reimbursement for e-visits (Gearon, 2008). Even when insurance won't pay, many patients with access to the service are willing to pay for the convenience from their own pockets (Copeland et al., 2008; Marte, 2009; Schneider, 2010).

The fear that the physician's practice will be inundated with messages and inappropriate demands has proven unfounded. It appears that while a majority of consumers want the ability to communicate with their providers and their staff, and will even switch providers to get it (Copeland et al., 2008), those who do have it use the function sparingly (Adamson & Bachman, 2010; Halamka, Mandl, & Tang, 2008; Liederman et al., 2005a; Painter, 2007; Ralston et al., 2007; Zhou, Garrido, Chin, Wiesenthal, & Liang, 2007). Lastly, with respect to impact on productivity, we are beginning to see reports from larger-scale evaluations that show promise. One very large integrated delivery system found that patient access to a secure messaging system that included online visits was associated with decreased rates of primary care office visits and telephone contacts (Zhou et al., 2007). Although this may be a negative incentive in a fee-for-service environment, the authors note that this leaves more time to care for more seriously ill patients, whose visits may be reimbursed at a higher rate. In another one-year study in a large academic medical system, where physicians were compensated based on Relative Value Units (RVUs), those who offered online visits averaged 10% more RVUs per day than a control group who did not, and the increase was not due to "intensity" of visits, but to practice efficiencies that led to 11% more visits per day (Liederman, Lee, Baquero, & Seites, 2005b).

More than just positive impacts on productivity, some are now reporting the potential for improved quality of care at lower cost, particularly in monitoring chronic conditions like diabetes, hypertension, congestive heart failure, and other conditions that depend on patient reports of symptoms and findings (Adamson & Bachman, 2010; Bredfeldt, Compton-Phillips & Snyder, 2009; Matthews, 2009). Rohrer and colleagues (2010), in a 6-month study conducted in a conventional medical office setting, found that patients who received secure online visits were less likely to be cost outliers in the subsequent 6 months than patients who received standard care. This may be another reason that health plans are seeing value in reimbursing providers for online visits.

Personal Health Records

Even though patients' medical records are more available to them now, thanks to the HIPAA Privacy Rule, many consumers are daunted by the size, complexity, illegibility, and sheer number of institutionally-based medical records that accumulate over a person's lifetime. As an alternative, many keep their own personal health records, both for themselves and for their family members. The structure of computer-based personal health records varies widely, from those that simply collect text under major headings such as allergies, problems, drugs, procedures, and so forth, to those that encode users' entries with ICD9 and CPT codes, or even with the broad range of terms found in the National Library of Medicine's Unified Medical Language System (UMLS) (National Library of Medicine, 2006).

Although the concept of a personal health record has been evolving, one commonly accepted definition is this one from the American Health Information Management Association (AHIMA) (AHIMA e-HIM Personal Health Record Work Group, 2005):

> The personal health record (PHR) is an electronic lifelong resource of health information needed by individuals to make health decisions. Individuals own and manage the information in the PHR, which comes from healthcare providers and the individual. The PHR is maintained in a secure and private environment, with the individual determining rights of access. The PHR is separate from and does not replace the legal record of any provider. (p. 24)

There are many ways to acquire a PHR. Consumers can create a *stand-alone* PHR by buying personal health record software for a reasonable cost (typically $30 to $75), downloading the program, then entering and storing their information on their own computer. One example is Health-Minder (www.health-minder.com); another is CheckUp (www.checkupsoftware.com). Some, like MyMedicalCD (www.MyMedicalCD.com), Minerva (www.myminerva.com), and VitalKey (www.VitalKey.com), store the data on portable media like small CDs and USB drives than can be carried with the person and accessed on any computer whose user has the appropriate password. Another option for those looking for ubiquitous access is to download an application to their smart phone or personal digital assistant (PDA) that allows for entry of personal health information including health conditions, medications, allergies and health monitoring data (see, for example, the Capzule PHR at www.capzule.com/phr and ProfileMD at www.e-medtools.com/profilemd.html).

Alternatively, consumers can subscribe to a Web site where their record will be held securely. Many healthcare organizations offer the service free of charge on their community Web sites, as do many health insurers. A number of these applications include interactive health management tools such as health risk assessments, smoking cessation programs, fitness trackers, pregnancy centers, calorie intake monitors, and any number of calculators. WebMD's Personal Health Manager, available through individual registration (www.webmd.com) or through sponsoring organizations that offer it on their Web site, even includes the ability for the user to subscribe to a wireless messaging service. Reminders can be sent to the user's Web-enabled phone to take medication, record blood pressure, and so forth. Built-in alerts can advise the user to call the physician if recorded values are outside the acceptable range. Other free, Web-based PHRs include Google Health Records (www.google.com), and Microsoft HealthVault (www.myhealthvault.com).

A number of issues arise when the PHR is stored in a place other than the user's own computer. Security of access to the data must be assured as well as privacy. Will the data be shared with anyone other than the user? Are policies for data sharing clearly described and accessible to the user? Can the user opt out of data sharing or e-marketing of goods and services based on the data entered in the record? If the user terminates his or her relationship with the vendor, can a paper or electronic version of the accumulated record be provided, and will the data subsequently be purged from the server? If the vendor goes out of business, will the user be notified, and what will happen with the information that is stored on the vendor's servers? The American Health Information Management Association (AHIMA) provides a comprehensive Web site (MyPHR.com) with multiple pages informing consumers of the benefits of PHRs, what information should be included in a PHR, and criteria for selecting one, along with a nonbiased listing of dozens of available products. AHIMA has also provided a guide for professionals to help them educate consumers on evaluating the various types of products and selecting an appropriate PHR product for their needs (AHIMA Personal Health Record Practice Council, 2006). The individual products listed on MyPHR.com have been evaluated along a number of dimensions by Heinold and colleagues (2009a,b) as part of a larger government initiative regarding health information security and privacy. A collaborative of groups including insurers and professional organizations created two reference guides, one for consumers and one for professionals, on PHRs—what they are and the value of using them (the guides are available at www.bcbs.com/cp/phr_guide) (American College of Physicians, 2010).

Several organizations have developed standards and guidelines relating to the consumer's relationship with vendors who supply PHR systems and health information over the Internet. They include URAC (www.urac.org), ASTM International (Standard E2211.02, available at www.astm.org), Health on the Net Foundation (www.hon.ch), and TRUST-e (www.truste.com).

A major drawback to stand-alone PHRs is the fact that consumers are entirely responsible for entering their data. The burden of doing this with data that are often incomprehensible to the average lay person discourages most people from keeping their records up to date, thus defeating the purpose when an emergency arises.

Different from the stand-alone PHR that is created and maintained by an individual, a *tethered* PHR is one that is originated by a provider organization or insurer. Data in the PHR is populated by the owning organization. This may be information about billed services, or, in the case of provider organizations, it may be clinical information such as laboratory test results, current active medications, past and future scheduled visits, and even visit summaries. In some cases, the consumer can add information in designated sections of the record. There are many examples, but here are a few:

- Caregroup's PatientSite is a Web-based application that permits patients to view their medical record, and to record information online in a separate section of the record (www.caregroup.org/patientsite.asp) (Weingart, Rind, Tofias, & Zands, 2006).

- Palo Alto Medical Foundation provides a patient portal called PAMFOnline where patients can view components of their medical record, obtain their health summary, and make notes on the record for their own personal use (www.pamfonline.org). Tang and colleagues reported that the PAMFOnline portal (which includes secure messaging) improves patient access to health information, improves communication with physicians and staff, promotes patient satisfaction, and improves office efficiency (Tang et al., 2003).

- Group Health Cooperative, a large mixed-model healthcare system, provides a patient portal called MyGroupHealth that includes a shared medical record and secure messaging. Components of the record that can be viewed by the patient include test results, after-visit summaries, medical conditions, allergies, and immunization history (Ralston et al., 2007). Patients can enter information in a designated section of the record, which becomes part of the medical record and viewable by clinicians. A survey of 900 users of the portal revealed that 94% were satisfied or very satisfied with the portal overall, with the highest feature ratings for medication refills (96%), patient-provider messaging (93%), and medical test results (86%) (Ralston et al., 2007).

- Other large organizations that offer a shared medical record to their members and patients include Kaiser Permanente, which offers My Health Manager (www.kp.org), and the U.S. Veterans Administration, which offers My HealtheVet (www.myhealth.va.gov) (Nazi et al., 2010).

While tethered PHRs relieve the consumer of entering large amounts of data, and have the potential to improve communication with one's care providers, they have a disadvantage in that they are not interoperable, and they are not portable (Detmer, Bloomrosen, Raymond, & Tang, 2008; Halamka et al., 2008; Kahn, Aulakh, & Bosworth, 2009; Pringle & Lippitt, 2009; Tang, Ash, Bates, Overhage, & Sands, 2006). When the patient severs ties with the insurer, health plan or provider, the record stays with that organization. And if the patient is being seen by multiple providers who offer separate shared records, they are likely to exist as "siloed" records. Recognizing that the issue of interoperability is a major deterrent to greater adoption of PHRs combined with EHRs, a number of governmental, quasigovernmental, and private organizations are working on standards for interoperability. These are being harmonized by the Health Information Technology Standards Panel (www. HITSP.org). In addition, America's Health Insurance Plans (AHIP), has developed standards for data architecture so that consumers who wish to do so can port their records from one insurer to another when they switch coverage (Edlin, 2007). The Centers for Medicare and Medicaid Services (CMS) and the Veterans Affairs Department are developing the ability for users of their PHRs to download information into their own PHR or any electronic medium (Mosquera, 2010a).

One currently available solution to the dilemma of multiple siloed records is the *aggregated* PHR. In this model, information entered by the consumer is supplemented with professionally sourced reports that can be faxed, scanned, mailed or uploaded to the vendor. The vendor maintains the secure, centralized record on its own servers. In some cases, the consumer can authorize direct data import from medical devices and other information sources. Examples of aggregated records are Google Health Record (www.google.com/health) and Microsoft HealthVault (www.healthvault.com). Alternatively, the consumer can subscribe to a service that queries all entities that provide service to the subscriber, and aggregates the information into one record that is accessible to the subscriber and to whomever the subscriber designates (for example, see www.peoplechart.com). Google Health and MS HealthVault are free as of this writing. Other services charge a monthly or annual fee (Heinold et al., 2009b). In addition to completeness, the advantage is that when information is shared with professionals, it has much more credibility, since the actual reports, not the consumer's interpretation, are included. The services are not without their issues, though, and consumers should be aware that third party reports, especially those based on claims data, can contain misleading and even erroneous information (Wangsness, 2009a). Because of this, at least one provider organization has stopped sending claims data as patient summaries to Google Health (Wangsness, 2009b).

Even further along the spectrum toward an ideal solution is the *integrated* personal health record, where all entities that provide service to a consumer automatically populate a centrally stored record, to which the consumer can add information as appropriate. The consumer could not alter professionally sourced information, but, consistent with the ideal of a PHR, would control access to the centralized record. There are many barriers to this solution, including legal issues such as ownership of information, technical issues surrounding interoperability, privacy and security, and ethical issues regarding governance and use and distribution of personal data (Garvin, Odom-Wesley, Rudman, & Stewart, 2009; Lobach et al., 2009; Mosquera, 2010b). Detmer and colleagues (2008) provide an in-depth exploration of the current state of PHRs and the transformative potential of truly integrated PHR systems for facilitating consumer-centric care.

Many believe that the concept of a PHR as just a repository of information is too narrow, and that instead, the PHR should be conceptualized as a "PHR system," a "suite of personal tools that recommend healthy actions based on data from many sources" (Brennan, 2007, p. 8.). Project HealthDesign, sponsored by the Robert Wood Johnson Foundation, is an initiative that promotes the development of next-generation PHRs, using new technologies based on user-centered design and a focus on functionalities that support personal health management, all built independently to operate on a common platform (Brennan, Downs, Casper & Kenron, 2007; Brennan, Casper, Downs, & Aulahk, 2009; Robert Wood Johnson Foundation, 2007, May).

A group of nurses from around the world convened in Finland in 2009 to examine the topic of Personal Health Information Management Systems (PHIMS), including definitions, user requirements, policies regarding confidentiality and safety, current applications, and considerations for educating nurses to practice "in a wired world." (Saranto, Brennan and Casey, 2009, p. 1). The proceedings demonstrate the breadth of the topic, and the variety of applications currently available and in development. The document is freely available at www.uku.fi/vaitokset/2009/isbn978-951-27 1321-9.pdf.

Despite the number of products and tethered PHRs now available to the public, the uptake of PHRs is low. In a large survey, Deloitte found that only 9% of consumers used a PHR (Keckley & Eselius, 2009). California Healthcare Foundation found a similar result (Undem, 2010). The Markle Foundation's Connecting for Health survey of 2008 shows a much lower percentage, less than 3% (Connecting for Health, 2008). While surveys show that people who use PHRs tend to like them (Nazi & Woods, 2008; Ralston et al., 2007; Tang et al., 2003), there are many reasons for the slow uptake in the general population. The major concerns are usually about privacy and security, but others include cost, lack of awareness, lack of incentives, lack of computer skills, lack of perceived value, cultural barriers, and lack of access to computer resources (Brennan, 2007; Garvin et al., 2009; Lobach et al., 2009; Mosquera, 2010b; Tang et al., 2006). Although use of PHRs is very slowly rising, a critical mass will likely not accrue until these concerns are resolved, and resolving them will require a combination of technical, legislative, policy, social, and ethical advances (Bernstein, Murchinson, Dutton, Keville, & Belfort, 2008; Brennan et al., 2009; Detmer et al., 2008; Gearon, 2007; Kahn et al., 2009; Reti, Feldman, Ross, & Safran, 2010; Reti, Feldman, & Safran, 2009; Tang et al., 2006; Connecting for Health, 2008; Lecker et al., 2007; National Center on Vital and Health Statistics, 2006). Weaver and Zielstorff (2011) provide a fuller discussion of consumer empowerment and PHRs as part of the Technology Informatics Guiding Education Reform (TIGER) initiative (www.tigersummit.com/Home_Page.php). A synthesis of knowledge and compendium of resources on current and future prospects for personal health records can be found on the Robert Wood Johnson Web site entitled "Feature: The Power and Potential of Personal Health Records" (www.rwjf.org/pr/product.jsp?id=49988).

Decision Support

A broad range of decision-support applications is available to the interested consumer. Some incorporate multimedia presentations of patients who have the condition that is the subject of the search (for example, www.healthcentral.com has videos on several cancer subjects as well as heart conditions, epilepsy, and many others). EverydayHealth.com (www.everydayhealth.com) has a multimedia "Symptom Checker" feature where an interactive video of a physician elicits answers for a specific topic (such as back pain) and provides basic advice on how to follow up with the problem. Usually these features are based on straightforward decision trees. The more comprehensive sites may offer the user the ability to log on to speak directly with a

physician, or to join disease-specific forums and blogs. A comprehensive site dealing with drugs is Drugs.com which offers not only static content from a choice of databases, but also a drug interaction checker and an interactive pill identifier (www.drugs.com). Registered users of the site can sign up to keep a personal drug profile that provides alerts about drug-drug interactions, recalls, and so on.

Some sites provide sophisticated risk assessment tools that use the consumer's input to summarize health risks, then suggest individualized changes in lifestyle that may influence these risks. For example, the Personal Health Manager tools available to registered users of WebMD (www.WebMD.com) provide a variety of health risk assessments, both general and topic-specific. One popular tool is the Readiness to Quit Smoking quiz that elicits responses about the user's intent to quit, then offers action steps appropriate to the user (WebMD.com, Health.com and many other sites offer this tool). Kukafka and colleagues described an evidence-based decision aid that helped users to prioritize behavior changes after receiving estimates of risk (Kukafka, Kahn, Kaufman, & Mark, 2009). The authors believe the application can form the basis for more informed behavioral counseling with clinicians.

Holbrook and colleagues (2009) describe a Web-based diabetes tracker application that provides advice based on monitored clinical parameters. The application was shared by 46 physicians and their patients in a primary care practice. A randomized trial demonstrated that patients who used the system showed greater satisfaction with care, as well as improvements in process of care and in some clinical parameters, such as decline in blood pressure and glycated hemoglobin.

More sophisticated multimedia applications have been developed that incorporate statistics-based models of risk and alternatives on topics such as heart disease prevention, PSA testing, early-stage prostate cancer treatment, breast cancer surgery, genetic testing and others (Stacey, Samant, & Bennett, 2008; Volk et al., 2007). These decision aids are often used to support shared decision making between clinicians and patients, especially in cases where patient preferences play a large role, and there are trade-offs in testing, treatments, or outcomes (Stacey et al., 2008). There is a large amount of literature on the subject, including a recent Cochrane review on effectiveness of the technology (O'Connor et al., 2009). This review found that based on the evidence, these aids "increase people's involvement and are more likely to lead to informed values-based decisions" and that they "reduce the use of discretionary surgery without apparent adverse effects on health outcomes or satisfaction" (O'Connor et al., 2009, p. 2).

A technology that is newly making its way into the health arena is the "recommender system." Consumers who have used Amazon.com or Netflix.com have seen the output of a recommender system. Briefly, the software proposes that "if you chose this, you will probably like this" (the content-based approach), or "people who are like you, or who chose what you chose, also chose this" (the collaborative filtering approach); some systems combine both approaches (Felfernig, Friedrich, & Schmidt-Thieme, 2007). It seems simple, but the software engines are complex and often highly proprietary, although some are open-source. Witteman and colleagues (2008) describe the development of a recommender system to assist men who are searching the Web for prostate cancer information that is relevant to their personal situation. Based on user characteristics that include clinical parameters, health status, sociodemographic factors, e-Health literacy and others, the system's goal is to direct the user to the Web sites that are predicted to be most useful to them. The technology seems highly relevant in the Health 2.0 world, where community is all, and collaboration is the predominant force. The caution is that if there is no transparency in the algorithms, the user may not trust the recommendations, especially in high-stakes decisions (Sinha and Swearingen, 2002). Various solutions have been proposed, including an "explanation interface," where the system provides the user with an explanation of how the system arrived at the recommended results (Pu & Chen, 2007). This principle has long been established in user acceptance by professionals of medical decision support systems.

Use of the computer for decision support among patients and consumers is covered in depth in another chapter 28.

Disease Management

Technological support for joint patient-provider collaboration in disease management is a promising application area. Patients or family caregivers are enrolled in a program and participate using one of a number of technologies. They may log on to an Internet portal or use their mobile phone to record parameters such as blood pressure, blood sugar, or peak flow. They may periodically complete a disease-focused questionnaire that captures broader data about mental and physical function or use a device that captures physical parameters such as weight or blood sugar and connect it to a telephone or computer, causing the information to be relayed to nurses whose responsibility is to monitor

the incoming data. Interactive voice response systems have been used successfully to monitor patients with conditions such as obsessive-compulsive disease, hypertension, asthma, and others. Values outside the desired range may prompt a phone call requesting the patient to alter their regimen or come in for a visit. Paré and colleagues (Paré, Moqadem, Pineau, & St-Hilaire, 2010) conducted a systematic review of home telemonitoring for 4 diseases, and found that clinical parameters for diabetes, asthma, and hypertension were improved with the home monitoring, but that congestive heart failure needed further, larger studies.

Some studies report reduced hospitalizations and reduced use of emergency rooms by employing these technologies (Paré, Jaana, & Sicotte, 2007). In one pilot study at the Cleveland Clinic, patients using medical devices at home that interfaced directly with their shared medical record showed longer times between office visits for diabetes and hypertension, but shorter times for heart failure (Theiss, 2010). Investigators believed that necessary treatment for heart failure was delivered in a timelier manner, possibly averting more serious consequences. Brennan and colleagues have reported on Heart Care II, a Web-based resource supporting home care of patients with chronic heart disease (Brennan, Casper, Kossman & Burke, 2007; Johnson et al., 2008). One important contribution of the study is its examination of the dynamics of introducing technology into the home, with subsequent impacts on both patients and nurses. For nurses, there were challenges in learning to do tasks differently—incorporating technology that was supposed to help, but that was sometimes seen as interference. For patients, there were challenges in finding space for equipment in homes that may already have been cramped for space, resentments in having to move belongings to accommodate the technology, and fears that the equipment would be damaged or stolen. For both groups, there were sometimes feelings that technology didn't belong in the home. There were some in both groups who were not computer literate, and had difficulties learning to use the technology (Johnson et al., 2008).

In a large government-funded randomized controlled trial at Columbia University named IDEATel (Informatics for Diabetes Education and Telemedicine), researchers assessed the effects of a comprehensive home-based telemedicine program with underserved rural and inner-city patients with diabetes (Shea et al., 2009). Live videoconferencing with nurses, use of devices to record and electronically transmit fingerstick glucose and blood pressure, and access to a project Web site were the technologies used with the intervention group. Evaluation showed that some clinical parameters (hemoglobin A1c, LDL cholesterol, and blood pressure) showed net improvements, but Medicare claims costs were not reduced (Palmas et al., 2010).

In a more consumer-driven, provider-independent mode, some Web sites offer the user a disease self-management program, providing educational materials, tools, links to additional resources, recipes and nutritional information, and the ability to record disease-specific parameters. One provider of such a site for diabetics is the American Diabetes Association (www.diabetes.org).

ISSUES IN CONSUMER COMPUTING FOR HEALTH

Variability in Quality of Information Available to Consumers

Because there are no quality controls on the content of health information available on the Internet, health professionals have been concerned about the influence of unreliable information on consumer and patient behavior. Research shows, however, that the fears may be unfounded. One survey reported that only 3% of e-patients said they or someone they knew had been seriously harmed by information they found on the internet (Fox & Jones, 2009). Consumers have developed a number of strategies for determining the veracity of information they find on the Web. They include recommendation of a site from their nurse or physician; determining the sponsor of the site (academic, non-profit organization, commercial, or vendor-sponsored); the credentials of the writer of the content (healthcare professional or not); and whether the same information appears in more than one site. HarrisInteractive (2008, July 29) found that almost half of those who searched for information online discussed the results of their searches with their physician.

A number of organizations have developed guidelines for health information seekers to use when evaluating the quality of materials they read. For example, The Consumer and Patient Health Information Section of the Medical Library Association evaluates Web sites based on the following criteria: credibility, sponsorship/authorship, content, audience, currency, disclosure, purpose, links, design, interactivity, and disclaimers. Its list of top 10 health Web sites is at www.mlanet.org/resources/medspeak/topten.html. Links to sites that offer guidelines for evaluating health materials are gathered in a special section of the National Library of Medicine's MedlinePlus site: www.nlm.nih.gov/medlineplus/evaluatinghealthinformation.html.

The Health On the Net Foundation (HON) has developed a set of principles and corresponding guidelines for developers of health information published on the Web. The 8 principles are authority, complementarity, confidentiality, attribution, justifiability, transparency of authorship, transparency of sponsorship, and honesty in advertising and editorial policy. They can be found at www.hon.ch/HONcode/Pro/Conduct.html (Boyer, Gaudinat, Baujard, & Geissbühler, 2007). Developers who follow the guidelines are encouraged to apply for certification, which grants them the right to place the HON Code seal on their site.

URAC, another certification body, applies a rigorous set of 50 standards when evaluating a site. The standards cover such areas as privacy and security, disclosure, how content is developed and revised, and how the site chooses to link to other sites. There are also standards about policies, procedures, and quality oversight processes. The URAC seal on a Web site assures the user of the site's compliance with these standards. Further information can be found atwww.urac.org/consumers/resources/accreditation.aspx.

The increasing popularity of health-related social networks has revived fears among healthcare professionals about the quality of user-generated information on the Internet (Adams, 2010; Fox, 2008b; Miller, 2008; Sarasohn-Kahn, 2008). Unlike Web 1.0, where attribution and provenance may be more easily determined, consumers who engage in Health 2.0 look for "just-in-time just-like-me" information whose authorship may be anonymous (Fox & Jones, 2009). Researchers find, however, that as with most communities, "opinion leaders" and "expert patients" emerge who become trusted peers, and that the sites tend to be self-correcting. Furthermore, the collective wisdom of the group becomes greater than the knowledge of any one individual (Civan & Pratt, 2007; Sarasohn-Kahn, 2008; Weiss & Lorenzi, 2008). Manhattan Research found that editorial content on the Web had more influence on consumers than information they found in social media, and that both are superseded by the influence of healthcare professionals (Manhattan Research, 2010). Surveys are consistent in finding that the patient's physician is ultimately the most trusted source of health information (Copeland et al., 2008; Hesse, Moser, & Rutten, 2010).

Privacy and Security of Data on the Internet

Surveys consistently show that privacy and security are major concerns among consumers who are asked about personal health records and health communication over the Internet (Keckley & Eselius, 2009; Undem,

2010; Dhopeshwarkar et al., 2009). The advent of Web portals secured with passwords has helped, but even as consumers want interoperability of health records, they worry about who has access to their information and how that access is controlled (Lobach et al., 2006; Connecting for Health, 2008; Wynia and Dunn, 2010). One government-sponsored study found that one-third of 92 PHR products reviewed made no statement about privacy or security, and that most of the 92 did not mention secondary uses of the data they store (Heinold et al., 2009a). Since independent PHR vendors are not considered covered entities under HIPAA regulations, consumers are on their own to determine what the policies are of the product or service they use (Heinold et al., 2009; Kahn et al., 2009). Another study sponsored by the Office of the National Coordinator for Health Information Technology (ONC) examined the privacy policies of 30 PHR vendors, and found significant gaps in all of them (Lecker et al., 2007). The researchers concluded that a model PHR privacy policy should be developed for the industry. The Department of Health and Human Services is currently engaged in the process of developing such a model policy.

The federal government recognizes that the National Health Information Infrastructure and health information exchange cannot be achieved without robust structures in place to assure privacy, confidentiality, and security of data. As of this writing, several committees are in place to review, recommend, and implement privacy and security policies. The interested reader can visit www.healthit.hhs.gov and click on the "Privacy and Security" link to see the many initiatives in place.

The Digital Divide

From the time that statistics were first gathered about Internet usage, it was apparent that Internet users were not representative of the population at large. Surveys consistently showed that Internet users were better educated, wealthier, younger, urban, and largely white (Rainie et al., 2003; Fox, 2005). According to more recent surveys, the demographics of internet users are slowly coming to reflect those of the entire country (HarrisInteractive, 2008, November 17). A major barrier to timely Internet access is lack of broadband in the home. Despite the fact that home broadband access has grown substantially in the past few years (from 47% in 2007 to 65% in 2010), there still are disparities among the elderly, the less educated, and the poor (Horrigan, 2010; Horrigan & Smith, 2007). In other words, the Digital Divide still exists. This is a matter of concern to health providers and public health officials, because poorer, minority, and older populations have more health problems, and are the very ones who could benefit most from Internet-based healthcare applications.

Healthy People 2020, the U.S. government's agenda for population health in the current decade, has as one of its overarching goals the elimination of health disparities among different segments of the population (www.healthypeople.gov/hp2020). In the focus area of health communication and health IT, one specific proposed objective is to "Increase individuals' access to the Internet." The U.S. Congress agrees. Recognizing that unequal access to technology has a number of social, economic, civic, public safety, and health consequences, Congress in 2009 mandated that the Federal Communications Commission create a National Broadband Plan that would "ensure that all people have access to broadband capability" (ARRA, 2009). The Plan has been created, and contains numerous initiatives and recommendations to achieve the goal (to see the plan and the funded initiatives, visit www.broadband. gov). The effort is seen as parallel to the government's initiatives in the 1930s to ensure that all Americans had access to radio and telephone services (Federal Communications Commission, 2010, Chapter 1).

Educational, Ethnic and Cultural Barriers

Even among those who have access to the Internet, factors such as literacy, language preference, and cultural background can be barriers to use of the Internet for health. Surveys continue to show that among Internet users, Latinos and blacks are underrepresented (Fox & Livingston, 2007). Language explains some of this: among Latinos, a recent survey finds that only 32% of those who are Spanish-dominant use the Internet, compared with 78% who are English-dominant and 76% who are bilingual. With respect to education, the same survey finds that regardless of ethnicity, those with a college degree are 3 to 4 times more likely to go online than those without a high school diploma (Fox & Livingston, 2007).

Literacy in the population remains a major barrier to use of the Internet for health. The 2003 National Assessment of Adult Literacy survey (the most recent one performed) found that 14% of adults had below-basic proficiency in prose literacy, 12% had below-basic proficiency in document literacy, and 22% had below-basic proficiency in quantitative literacy (National Center for Education Statistics, 2003). African Americans, Hispanics, those over the age of 65 and those with multiple disabilities were disproportionately represented in below-basic proficiency in all 3 categories.

For the first time, health literacy was measured in the survey, using the definition quoted by the Institute of Medicine as "the degree to which individuals have the capacity to obtain, process, and understand basic health information and services needed to make appropriate health decisions" (Institute of Medicine, 2004, p. 2). The assessment found that 14% of adults had below-basic health literacy, with a greater percentage of minorities (black, Hispanic, American Indian/Alaska Native) in that category (Kutner, Greenberg, Jin, Paulsen, & White, 2006). The Hispanic population had the greatest proportion of below-basic health literacy at 41%.

A new concept, e-Health literacy, has been added to the lexicon. Norman and Skinner (2006a) provide this definition: "the ability to seek, find, understand, and appraise health information from electronic sources and apply the knowledge gained to addressing or solving a health problem" (p. 1). The authors describe a model that encompasses the skills required to leverage technology for health. Its components are traditional literacy, information literacy, media literacy, health literacy, computer literacy and scientific literacy. They have also developed an 8-item instrument to measure e-Health literacy, named eHEALS (Norman & Skinner, 2006b).

Internet users on the wrong side of the Digital Divide face daunting challenges in trying to use the Internet for health. Research consistently shows that most Web content is written at high school level or above (Badarudeen & Sabharwal, 2010; Friedman, Hoffman-Goetz, & Arocha, 2006; Kaphingst, Zanfini, & Emmons, 2006; Lachance, Erby, Ford, Allen, & Kaphingst, 2010). It is generally agreed that to be accessible to those with limited literacy (about 20% of the population), material should not be written above sixth-grade level (Eichner and Dullabh, 2007). There are many resources for those who would develop content for Web-based health materials. Two excellent resources are *Clear and Simple* from the National Cancer Institute (2003), and *Accessible Health Information Technology (IT) for Populations with Limited Literacy* from the Agency for Healthcare Research and Quality (AHRQ) (Eichner & Dullabh, 2007).

Medical terminology, by its nature, is difficult to comprehend for even highly literate consumers. Some vendors have developed proprietary consumer-friendly terminologies that map to medical terminologies to assist consumers with finding, understanding, and recording health-related material. A government-sponsored initiative to develop and maintain a public-domain consumer health vocabulary is ongoing (www.consumerhealthvocabulary.org) (Zeng & Tse, 2006).

In another effort, a large healthcare system has developed a consumer-friendly vocabulary to assist consumers to enter coded family health histories (Hulse, Wood, Haug, & Williams, 2010, April 9). With the advent of shared medical records, and with ever-greater consumer access to medical literature, several efforts are underway to develop tools that "translate" medical documents into material that is more accessible to consumers (for example, see Miller, Leroy, & Wood, 2006; Zeng-Treitler, Goryachev, Kim, Keselman, & Rosendale, 2007; Zeng-Treitler, Goryachev, Tse, Keselman, & Boxwala, 2008).

On the opposite side of the coin, the rising use of social networks for health is leading to large databases of consumer- and patient-generated expressions of symptoms, findings, diagnoses, and health impacts. Smith and Wicks (2008) found that on PatientsLikeMe.com, 43% of terms used by consumers had exact or synonymous matches in the Unified Medical Language System. They described difficulties in classifying the rest, leading to problems with coding, and therefore, difficulties in matching members appropriately. The authors describe the database as a "folksonomy," the opposite of a taxonomy. They argue that imposing a rigid terminology on the users of the site would be a mistake, while acknowledging that "a deficiency in knowledge representation affects not only the professionals, but the consumers as well."

Physical and Cognitive Disabilities

A recent survey showed that adults with disabilities were less likely to have access to the Internet than persons without disabilities (62% versus 81%), and if they had more than one disability, even less likely (52%) (Fox & Purcell, 2010). Persons with disabilities are more likely to turn to health professionals, family, or print materials than the Internet, unlike persons with no disabilities. Those with disabilities who do use the Internet for health, however, are more likely to engage in blogs, social networks, and support groups, to consume and contribute user-generated content, and to feel that these resources are helpful to them in their everyday lives (Fox & Purcell, 2010). Zeng and Parmanto (2004) found that of 103 consumer health information Web sites, none complied completely with Web accessibility guidelines. For example, text equivalents for all nontext objects on a page should be embedded in the code, so that it is accessible to automated screen readers that are used by the blind (to access the W3C Web Accessibility Guidelines, visit www.w3.org/WAI/intro/wcag). In a more recent study, Luchtenberg and colleagues (Lüchtenberg, Kuhli-Hattenbach, Sinangin,

Ohrloff, & Schalnus, 2008) found only 18% of 139 Web sites they examined complied with Web accessibility guidelines at the lowest level (A), only 1% complied at the next highest level (AA), and none complied at the highest level.

Elderly users are even more specialized in their needs. In a review of design considerations for elderly users, Good and colleagues point out that diminished visual acuity and color discrimination, memory deficits, and increased need for processing time impose specific requirements on the design of applications (Good, Stokes, & Jerrams-Smith, 2007 Summer). Lober and colleagues (Lober et al., 2006) cite similar deficits, as well as high incidence of decreased upper limb mobility. In addition, a large proportion of the elderly are inexperienced using computers, so the applications must be especially easy to use.

Impact on Relationship with Healthcare Providers

Just as computers have revolutionized consumers' and patients' abilities to care for themselves, so have they affected patient-clinician relationships. The knowledgeable patient is no longer so dependent on the clinician's advice, and, in fact, may challenge it. The empowered patient wishes to collaborate in the clinician's care, and wants to be treated respectfully as a full-fledged partner in achieving mutually agreed-on goals (Fox & Jones, 2009). Some clinicians welcome the new partnership, believing that better-quality, lower-cost care will result (Disch, 2009; Slack, 2007; Lundberg 2009). Others have a more difficult time adjusting to the power shift, and would rather not deal with patients who will not accept their recommendations at face value (described in Bylund et al., 2007). Disch (2009) maintains that nurses have always seen patients as partners in care, that they "inherently value the concept of partnership, of complementary expertise, of collaboration."

Another area that threatens many healthcare professionals is the notion of patients as independent co-practitioners. Online support groups provide consolation, comfort, hope, and empathetic human contact—hallmarks of the care that any good nurse would provide. Furthermore, these are available 24 hours a day and on demand, something that no individual professional could do. In addition, support groups and social networks may provide cutting-edge knowledge of disease processes, treatments, and clinical trials of which even the patients' providers may not be aware. Patients within the group may bring their background expertise to the knowledge that is shared, helping to evaluate it for validity (Fox & Jones, 2009; Sarasohn-Kahn, 2008).

Kaplan and Brennan (2001) advocate for a 3-way partnership among patient, provider, and technology. This partnership should be centered on the patient and consumer, not on the provider or institution. Wald and colleagues (Wald, Dube, & Anthony, 2007) have a similar outlook, describing a "triangulation" of patient-Web-provider, and providing guidelines to help the clinician to integrate patients' use of the Web into practice.

The Nurse Informaticist's Role in Consumer and Patient Computing

It seems obvious that a technology that so impacts patients' and consumers' health decisions should be a central focus of nurse informaticists. The most recent edition of the American Nurses Association Scope and Practice of Nursing Informatics Practice (ANA, 2008) makes this explicit. The new definition of the field states that:

> NI [Nursing Informatics] supports consumers, patients, nurses, and other providers in their decision-making in all roles and settings. (p. 1)

In addition, the revised Scope and Standards makes several references to patients' use of technology for managing their health, and the role of nursing informatics specialists in supporting that function. For example, the patient is now included as a focus of education about effective and ethical uses of technology, and the patient's use of information tools and resources for health information is included as a focus for nursing informatics research. Collaboration with patients, clients, and families in informatics activities is also one of the standards of nursing informatics practice.

Areas of Nursing Expertise that can be Applied to Consumer and Patient Computing. Informaticists who are nurses bring unique skills to the arena of consumer informatics by virtue of their professional education in nursing. Among these skills:

- *Deep expertise in patient education:* A core competency of nursing professionals is patient education. Nurse informaticists can combine their expertise in patient education with their informatics skills to design content and applications that are effective for imparting knowledge and skills needed to maintain health and manage acute and chronic conditions. It is well within the nursing informatics skill set to design content that is interactive, effective, and sensitive to patients' literacy, language, and cultural needs. Nurse informaticists may need additional education in adapting or developing content for the Web, which has unique requirements and capabilities. Good resources are Nielsen's *Writing Style for the Web* (Nielsen & Loranger, 2006), and Nielsen's *Writing for the Web*, a collection of essays summarizing research on how users read Web pages as opposed to print. This is available at www.useit.com/papers/webwriting.

- *Cultural diversity in the workforce and a strong ethic of cultural sensitivity:* The nursing workforce itself is more ethnically and culturally diverse than most professions. Cultural sensitivity is highly valued in nursing education and practice. This background serves nurse informaticists well in producing applications and materials that are culturally appropriate.

- *Strong background in both patient- and community-focused research:* Nurses have a long tradition of patient-focused research, a strength that can be applied to the many areas of consumer and patient computing that are begging for research. At the same time, nurses are very comfortable in the areas of implementing and evaluating interventions targeted at populations, by virtue of their expertise in community health.

- *Strong heritage of patient advocacy and patient empowerment:* While nurses are not immune to feeling threatened by the empowered patient, it is also true that nurses have always had as a central goal to assist each patient to achieve as much self-sufficiency as possible (ANA, 2010). Encouraging and enabling the patient to use technology to achieve that self-sufficiency is a natural extension of nursing care.

Special Considerations in Designing Applications for Patients and Consumers. Nurse informaticists who have designed or implemented applications for health professionals to use should be aware of the special considerations required in applications for consumers and patients. They may need to seek further education to gain the skills and knowledge needed to design, implement, and evaluate these systems (PC Tang et al., 2006). These special considerations include:

- *Lay versus professional nomenclature:* Professional nomenclature is so ingrained in most clinicians

that they often are not even aware that they are using language that is foreign to the patient or consumer. Interactive applications, forms, and static content designed for patients and consumers must be scoured for professional terms. Lay terms must be substituted whenever possible. When professional terms must be used, a definition or an equivalent lay term in parentheses should be supplied. Though it does not incorporate a formal consumer nomenclature, the UMLS has many consumer-friendly synonyms for medical terms. The UMLS Metathesaurus can be browsed online by applying for a free license at umlsks.nlm.nih.gov/kss/servlet/Turbine/template/admin,user,KSS_login.vm. The online, open-source Consumer Health Vocabulary Initiative is another good source of consumer-friendly terms (www.consumerhealthvocabulary.org). The Harvard School of Public Health's Health Literacy Studies Web site (www.hsph.harvard.edu/healthliteracy) has a set of Plain Language Glossaries aimed at improving communication about specific diseases such as asthma, arthritis, and others.

- *General literacy and health literacy*: It is a myth that materials written at a sixth-grade level will not be appropriate for more highly educated people. All readers, no matter what their educational level, appreciate material that is written clearly and in plain language (National Cancer Institute, 2003). There are many books, courses, and other resources to assist the health educator or system designer to develop materials that are accessible and understandable to most readers. Comprehensive bibliographies and references on this topic are available in the Institute of Medicine's Health Literacy: A Prescription to End Confusion (www.nap.edu/openbook.php?isbn=0309091179). The Harvard School of Public Health's Health Literacy Studies Web site (www.hsph.hardard.edu/healthliteracy) has a wealth of resources, including links to a number of literature reviews and research findings. The Agency for Healthcare Research and Quality (AHRQ) has developed a guide for developers and purchasers for Accessible HIT for Populations with Limited Literacy (Eichner & Dullabh, 2007). It is full of practical, research-based guidelines for all technical media, with a list of additional resources. The federal government sponsors a site named Plain

Language (www.plainlanguage.gov) that is a rich compendium of resources, including guidelines, checklists, and training programs. There is also content specific to writing for the Web, with links to additional resources on that topic.

- *Computer literacy and the digital divide*: Using a computer for a health-related application (such as participating in a support network or recording physiologic parameters from home) may be a person's introduction to the use of the technology. Nurses who have implemented health-related systems to persons who are not computer literate realize the importance of system design that emphasizes ease of use and easily available help functions. Evaluations of consumer health applications universally cite usability as a determining factor in patient acceptance and use (for example, see Klein, 2007; Or & Karsh, 2009). Web site usability poses a different set of requirements than desktop applications, so the nurse who is expert in one may not necessarily be expert in the other. There are many books available on user-interface design, Web design, usability principles, and methods of testing. Popular ones are (Brinck & Gergle, 2002; Garrett, 2002; Krug, 2005; Nielsen & Loranger, 2006). Shneiderman and colleagues (Shneiderman, Jacobs, Plaisant, & Cohen, 2009) advocate for "universal usability," with principles that foster a better user experience for all persons, regardless of age, educational status, or physical impairments. Those interested in periodic newsletters delivered online can subscribe for free to Jakob Nielsen's Alertbox by visiting www.useit.com and to Jared Spool's usability articles by signing up at www.uie.com/uietips.htm. One of the collaboratives of TIGER dealt with Usability and Application Design. Its report offers a wealth of information for system designers, as well as case studies and references (www.tigersummit.com/Usability_New.html). The U.S. Department of Health and Human Services sponsors a highly useful site named Usability.gov that lists, among other things, research-based guidelines for usability and Web design (www.usability.gov). While some designers think that usability is largely a matter of taste and opinion, the guidelines compiled on this site are rated for relative importance in overall success of the Web site, and for strength of evidence. With respect to lesser access to broadband for

some segments of the population, nurses should remember that cell phones are used by many in these groups to access the internet (Horrigan, 2009). In fact, mobile technology may be the preferred medium for some types of applications, like recording of physical findings, on-the-spot decision aids such as calorie counts, and reminders to take medications.

- *Special needs of the elderly:* Addressing the special needs of the elderly is a priority in healthcare and in e-Health. The National Institute on Aging and the National Library of Medicine have jointly published "Making Your Website Senior Friendly," a checklist with research-based guidelines (www.nia.nih.gov/HealthInformation/Publications/website.htm). Good and colleagues (2007) offer many practical suggestions for designing Web sites that take into account the limitations of older users.

- *Accessibility to persons with disabilities:* The World Wide Web Consortium's Web Accessibility Initiative (W3C/WAI) is an international effort to establish guidelines and promote technologies to increase accessibility of the World Wide Web to persons with physical and cognitive impairments. To see the guidelines and a prioritized checklist for assessing compliance with the guidelines, visit www.w3.org/WAI. The federal government has mandated accessibility for all government-sponsored Web sites under Section 508 of the Rehabilitation Act Amendments of 1998. The standards are available at www.section508.gov/index.cfm?FuseAction=content&ID=12. Designers wishing to use an automated tool to assess compliance of their Web pages with W3C/WAI guidelines and Section 508 standards can visit the W3C/WAI Web site (www.w3.org/WAI/ER/tools) to see a list of available tools, many of which are free.

- *User-centered design:* While nurse informaticists undoubtedly learn the importance of user-centered design during their education, nowhere is this more important than in designing applications for patients and consumers. The patient's and consumer's view of the world will be highly influenced by age, by health and computer literacy, by health status, by socioeconomic status, by environment, by language and culture, and even by situational circumstances. Focus groups, iterative testing and validation with target users, and a multidisciplinary approach that includes representatives of the target population are central to the process (for example, see Brennan, Casper, Kossman and Burke, 2007; and Dabbs et al., "2009)".

SOME RESEARCH AREAS RELATED TO CONSUMER AND PATIENT COMPUTING

It is difficult to read any article, report, or book about consumers' use of computers for health without finding the phrase "more research is needed." The e-Health revolution is a relatively new phenomenon, and every area described in this chapter could be a focus for in-depth research. While much good work has been accomplished and is in progress, the surface has barely been scratched. Several evidence reports and systematic reviews are available. A few examples are: the effect of decision aids (O'Connor et al., 2009); the use of health information technology by the elderly, chronically ill, and underserved (Jimison et al., 2008); a survey of literacy and health literacy in the United States (National Center for Education Statistics, 2003; Kutner et al., 2006); the impact of interactive consumer health applications on health outcomes (Gibbons et al., 2009); patient acceptance of consumer health information technology (Or & Karsh, 2009); and evaluation frameworks for collaborative, adaptive, and interactive technologies (O'Grady et al., 2009). Each review includes recommendations for further research.

Keselman and colleagues provide an overview of the consumer health informatics field, including its theoretical underpinnings and challenges. Among the research directions they propose are these: (1) development of methods to assess the quality of user-generated content and how to "gently moderate" such content as needed; (2) development of consumer health vocabularies that map to medical terminologies to facilitate "horizontal" communication between consumers and healthcare professionals, and among peers; (3) how to apply existing knowledge in the communication, marketing, and social science fields to health communication technologies; (4) how to dynamically tailor the presentation of information to the characteristics of the user, taking into account literacy, health literacy, and computer literacy; and (5) paying greater attention to the needs of caregivers and families (Keselman et al., 2008).

How to evaluate consumer health applications is itself a topic for research. Nazi and colleagues (2010)

advocate for a health services research perspective, particularly for personal health records. O'Grady and colleagues (2009), after doing a systematic review of evaluation frameworks for consumer health information technologies, propose a new one for evaluating Web 2.0 applications. Gustafson and Wyatt (2004) advocate for various levels of evaluation studies of e-Health systems based on the type of service offered. Services for patients who are in serious crisis situations demand higher standards of acceptability, usability, and veracity, and should be evaluated for such before implementation. Cost evaluations are infrequently carried out, but claims of replacing traditional forms of service with less expensive alternatives must be substantiated. Systems developed for underserved populations must be evaluated for usability, effectiveness, and impact (one good example is the evaluation of IDEATel by Shea and colleagues (2009)).

User-centered design and participatory design are important strategies for developing systems that meet the needs of the target population, leading to a greater chance of success. There are many examples in the literature. Brennan and colleagues at University of Wisconsin, Madison, have published extensively on their research into home-based systems, all developed after intensive investigation on how patients manage health information in the home (Brennan, Casper, Kossman, & Burke, 2007; Casper, Brennan, Burke, & Nicolalde, 2009; Johnson et al., 2008; Marquard, Moen, & Brennan, 2006; Moen & Brennan, 2005). Their work is foundational for future efforts to establish the Healthcare Home (often called the medical home). Many view the Healthcare Home as essential to achieving healthcare reform (Stange et al., 2010).

As nurses, we often respond to innovative technologies that are developed by others, using them or adapting them to create systems for consumers. We sometimes forget that we can drive technological innovations, contributing our insights and knowledge and inspiring multidisciplinary teams to stretch what is into what could be to meet the needs of our patients. Project HealthDesign, funded by the Robert Wood Johnson Foundation is one example (Brennan, Downs, Casper & Kenron, 2007; Brennan et al., 2009; Robert Wood Johnson Foundation, 2007). A new, multidisciplinary Living Environments Laboratory (LEL) has been established in the Institute of Discovery at University of Wisconsin, Madison to "enhance personal health through rapid-cycle design and deployment of personal care technologies... tested in a simulated living environment instead of an isolated laboratory" (P. Brennan, personal communication, 2010, June 23; also see the

LEL home page at discovery.wisc.edu/home/wisconsin/research/Living%20Environments%20Lab.cmsx).

Additional areas for research (among many more that could be mentioned) include:

- Development and evaluation of technologies to automatically translate health content and medical record data to meet the user's native language and educational level
- Contribution of personal health records to patient-provider communication, and to patient self-management and clinical outcomes
- Contribution of shared medical records to patient-provider communication, and to accuracy and completeness of the medical record
- Effect of the empowered patient on patient-nurse dynamics
- Effectiveness of various technologies to reach less educated, lower-income, and more culturally diverse populations
- Needs of underserved, less literate populations with respect to computer applications for health
- Contribution of automatic push of health-related materials based on user's expressed interests and recorded health problems to patient behavior and outcomes
- Contribution of consumer-friendly terminology to retrieval of health information online, and to recording of data in personal health records
- Unmet needs of patients and consumers with respect to online services
- Effects of highly tailored prognostic information based on user's individual profile on patient decision making
- Influence of e-Health technology on educational interventions in patient care
- Ethical considerations in all aspects of e-Health, including disclosure, informed consent, and providing full access to the medical record
- Influence of e-Health technology on educational interventions in patient care
- How to ethically mine the user-generated content of social networks both for new knowledge and to inform us of consumer needs in particular disease states
- How to reconcile consumers' concerns about privacy and confidentiality of data with their willingness to share large amounts of personal data on social networks

- Differences in effects of synchronous versus asynchronous communication with patient (e.g., videocalls versus secure messages)
- Impact of social networks on consumer health behavior and clinical outcomes

CONCLUSION

E-Health technologies for consumers and patients are widely viewed as transformative for consumer empowerment, healthcare reform, and in fostering healthy lifestyles. Clearly, the field of consumer health informatics, though young, is broad and multifaceted. It does not belong to any one discipline, but draws on the expertise of a variety of health, science, social, and technical fields. Armed with the additional knowledge of the special considerations in designing, implementing, and evaluating applications for use by patients and consumers, nurse informaticists have much to contribute to the field.

RECOMMENDED READINGS AND RESOURCES

Reports and Surveys

California HealthCare Foundation newsletter—iHealthBeat: www.ihealthbeat.org

California HealthCare Foundation—reports and surveys: www.chcf.org

HarrisInteractive: www.harrisinteractive.com

Pew Internet and American Life Project—Health: www.pewinternet.org/topics/Health.aspx

Principles, Guidelines, and Standards

Health On the Net (HON) Foundation: www.hon.ch

URAC Health Web Site Accreditation Program: Webapps.urac.org/Websiteaccreditation/default.htm

World Wide Web Consortium Web Accessibility Initiative (W3C WAI): www.w3c.org/wai

Usability.gov—Your Guide to Developing Useful and Usable Web Sites: www.usability.gov

Tools for Consumers to Evaluate Health Information on the Web

Health on the Net Foundation: www.hon.ch

MedlinePlus—Guide to Health Web Surfing: www.nlm.nih.gov/medlineplus/healthywebsurfing.html

National Cancer Institute: Evaluating Health Information on the Internet: www.cancer.gov/cancertopics/factsheet/information/internet

National Center for Complementary and Alternative Medicine: Evaluating Web-Based Health Resources: nccam.nih.gov/health/webresources

National Network of Libraries of Medicine: Evaluating Health Web Sites: nlm.gov/outreach/consumer/evalsite.html

Writing for the Web and for Accessibility

Nielsen, J. (2008, June 9). *Writing Style for Print vs. Web*. Retrieved from http://www.useit.com/alertbox/print-vs-online-content.html.

Niesen, J. (2005, March 14). *Lower Literacy Users*. Retrieved from http://www.useit.com/alertbox/20050314.html.

National Institute on Aging. (2003). *Making Your Website Senior-Friendly*. Retrieved from http://www.nia.nih.gov/HealthInformation/Publications/website.htm.

Plain Language.gov (n.d.). *Improving Communication from the Federal Government to the Public*. Retrieved from www.plainlanguage.gov.

Harvard School of Public Health. (n.d.). *Health Literacy Studies Web Site*. Retrieved from http://www.hsph.harvard.edu/healthliteracy.

REFERENCES

Adams, S. A. (2010). Revisiting the online health information reliability debate in the wake of "web 2.0": An inter-disciplinary literature and website review. *International Journal of Medical Informatics*, 79(6), 391–400. doi: 10.1016/j.ijmedinf.2010.01.006.

Adamson, S. C., & Bachman, J. W. (2010). Pilot study of providing online care in a primary care setting. *Mayo Clinic Proceedings*, (June 1). Retrieved from http://www.mayoclinicproceedings.com/content/early/2010/06/01/mcp.2010.0145.abstract. doi:10.4065/mcp.2010.0145.

AHIMA e-HIM Personal Health Record Work Group. (2005). The role of the personal health record in the EHR. *Journal of AHIMA* 76(7), 64A–D. Retrieved from http://library.ahima.org/xpedio/groups/public/documents/ahima/bok1_027539.hcsp?dDocName=bok1_027539.

AHIMA Personal Health Record Practice Council. (2006). Helping consumers select PHRs: Questions and considerations for navigating an emerging market. *Journal of AHIMA*, 77(10), 50–56. Retrieved from http://library.ahima.org/xpedio/groups/public/documents/ahima/bok1_032260.hcsp?dDocName=bok1_032260

American College of Physicians. (2010, April 5). Healthcare groups collaborate on new reference guides for personal health records.. Retrieved from http://www.acponline.org/pressroom/phr_guides.htm.

American Nurses Association. (2008). *Scope and standards of nursing informatics practice*. Washington, DC: American Nurses Publishing.

American Nurses Association. (2010). *Nursing's social policy statement: The essence of the profession* Washington, DC: American Nurses' Association.

ARRA. (2009). American Recovery and Reinvestment Act of 2009, Pub. L. No. 111-5, § 6001(k)(2)(D), 123 Stat. 115, 516 (2009) (Recovery Act).

Badarudeen, S., & Sabharwal, S. (2010). Assessing readability of patient education materials: Current role in orthopaedics. *Clinical Orthopedics and Related Research*. (May 22). doi: 10.1007/s11999-010-1380-y.

Bernstein, W. S., Murchinson, J. V., Dutton, M. J., Keville, T. D., & Belfort, R. D. (2008, February). Whose data is it anyway? Expanding consumer control over personal health information Retrieved from http://www.chcf.org/~/media/Files/PDF/W/WhoseDataIsItAnywayIB.pdf.

Binder, L. (2008). The power of consumerism. *Modern Healthcare*, 38(45), 28–29. Retrieved from http://www.modernhealthcare.com/article/20081110/REG/811079988&Template=printpicart.

Bovi, A. M. (2003). Ethical guidelines for use of electronic mail between patients and physicians. *The American Journal of Bioethics*, 3(3), 43–47.

Boyer, C., Gaudinat, A., Baujard, V., & Geissbühler, A. (2007). Health on the Net Foundation: assessing the quality of health web pages all over the world. *Stud Health Technol Inform.*, 129(Pt 2), 1017–1021.

Bredfeldt, C., Compton-Phillips, A., & Snyder, M. (2009). *Secure messaging effect on health outcomes for diabetic patients*. Proceedings of the 2009 AMIA Annual Symposium 2009, p. 781.

Brennan P. F. (2007). The big-picture perspective. In C. J. Gearon, *Perspectives on the future of personal health records* (pp. 6–10). California Healthcare Foundation. Retrieved from http://www.chcf.org/~/media/Files/PDF/P/PHRPerspectives.pdf.

Brennan, P., Downs, S., Casper, A., & Kenron, D. (2007). *Project HealthDesign. Stimulating the next generation of personal health records*. Proceedings of the 2007 AMIA Annual Symposium, pp. 70–74.

Brennan, P. F., Casper, G., Downs, S., & Aulahk, V. (2009). Project HealthDesign: enhancing action through information. *Stud Health Technol Inform*, 146, 214–218.

Brennan, P. F., Casper, G., Kossman, S., & Burke, L. (2007). HeartCareII: Home care support for patients with chronic cardiac disease. *Stud Health Technol Inform.*, *129*(Pt 2), 988–992.

Brinck, T., & Gergle, D. (2002). *Usability for the web: Designing web sites that work.* San Francisco, CA: Morgan Kaufman Publishers.

Brooks, G. R., & Menachemi, N. (2006). Physicians' use of email with patients: Factors influencing electronic communication and adherence to best practices. *Journal of Medical Internet Research, 8*(1), e2.

Bylund, C., Gueguen, J., Sabee, C., Imes, R., Li, Y., & Sanford, A. (2007). Provider-patient dialogue about Internet health information: An exploration of strategies to improve the provider-patient relationship. *Patient Education and Counseling, 66*(3), 346–352.

Byrne, J. M., Elliott, S., & Firek, A. (2009). Initial experience with patient-clinician secure messaging at a VA medical center. *Journal Of The American Medical Informatics Association, 16*, 267–270.

Casper, G., Brennan, P., Burke, L., & Nicolalde, D. (2009). HeartCareII: Patients' use of a home care web resource. *Studies in Health Technology and Informatics, 146*, 139–143.

Civan, A., & Pratt, W. (2007). *Threading together patient expertise.* Proceedings of the 2007 AMIA Annual Symposium, pp. 140–144. Retrieved from http://www.ncbi.nlm.nih.gov/pmc/articles/PMC2655889/?tool=pubmed.

Civan, A., Skeels, M., Stolyar, A., & Pratt, W. (2006). *Personal health information management: Consumers' perspectives.* Proceedings of the 2006 AMIA Annual Symposium, pp. 156–160. Retrieved from http://www.ncbi.nlm.nih.gov/pmc/articles/PMC1839450/?tool=pubmed.

Connecting for Health. (2008). *Americans overwhelmingly believe electronic personal health records could improve their health.* Markle Foundation. Retrieved from http://www.connectingforhealth.org/resources/ResearchBrief-200806.pdf.

Copeland, W. J., Keckley, P. H., Eselius, L. L., Greene, J. B., & Underwood, H. R. (2008). 2008 survey of healthcare consumers. Executive summary. (pp. 1-24). Washington, DC: Deloitte Center for Health Solutions. Retrieved from http://www.deloitte.com/assets/Dcom-UnitedStates/Local%20Assets/Documents/us_chs_ConsumerSurveyExecutiveSummary_200208.pdf.

Dabbs, A. D. V., Myers, B. A., Mc Curry, K. R., Dunbar-Jacob, J., Hawkins, R. P., Begey, A., & Dew, M. A. (2009). User-centered design and interactive health technologies for patients. *Computers Informatics Nursing, 27*(3), 175. doi: 10.1097/NCN.0b013e31819f7c7c.

Dhopeshwarkar, R., O'Donnell, H., Patel, V., Kern, L, Barron, Y., Teixeira, P., Kaushal, R. (2009). Consumers' privacy and security preferences for electronic health information. Proceedings of 2009 AMIA Symposium, p. 818.

Detmer, D., Bloomrosen, M., Raymond, B., & Tang, P. (2008). Integrated personal health records: Transformative tools for consumer-centric care. *BMC Medical Informatics and Decision Making, 8*(1), 45. Retrieved from http://www.ncbi.nlm.nih.gov/pmc/articles/PMC2596104/pdf/1472-6947-8-45.pdf.

Disch, J. (2009). Participatory healthcare: Perspective from a nurse leader. *Journal of Participatory Med., 1*(1), e4. Retrieved from http://www.jopm.org/opinion/commentary/2009/10/21/participatory-health-care-perspective-from-a-nurse-leader-2/.

Durant, K., Safran, C., & McCray, A. (2010). *Social network analysis of an online melanoma discussion group.* Paper presented at the 2010 AMIA Clinical Research Informatics Summit.

Edlin, M. (2007, March-April). You can take it with you. *AHIP Coverage* Retrieved from http://www.ahip.org/content/default.aspx?bc=31|130|136|19318|19319.

Eichner, J., & Dullabh, P. (2007). *Accessible health information technology (HIT) for populations with limited literacy: A guide for developers and purchasers of health IT.* (Prepared by the National Opinion Research Center for the National Resource Center for Health IT). AHRQ Publication No. 08-0010-EF. Rockville, MD: Agency for Healthcare Research and Quality. Retrieved from http://healthit.ahrq.gov/images/literacy_guide102507/literacy_guide.html?fbr=1193341303546.

Federal Communications Commission. (2010). The national broadband plan: Connecting America. Retrieved from http://www.broadband.gov.

Federation of State Medical Boards. (2002). *Model guidelines for the appropriate use of the internet in medical practice.* Dallas, TX: Author. Retrieved from http://www.fsmb.org/pdf/2002_grpol_use_of_internet.pdf.

Felfernig, A., Friedrich, G., & Schmidt-Thieme, L. (2007). Recommender Systems. *IEEE Intelligent Systems,* May/June 2007, 18–21.

Fox, S. (2005) *Digital divisions.* Pew Internet & American Life Project. Retrieved from http://www.pewinternet.org/~/media//Files/Reports/2005/PIP_Digital_Divisions_Oct_5_2005.pdf.pdf.

Fox, S. (2007, October 8). *E-patients with a disability or chronic disease.* Pew Internet & American Life Project. Retrieved from http://www.pewinternet.org/~/media//Files/Reports/2007/EPatients_Chronic_Conditions_2007.pdf.pdf.

Fox, S. (2008a). *The engaged e-patient population. People turn to the internet for health information when the stakes are high and the connection fast.* Pew Internet & American Life Project . Retrieved from http://www.pewinternet.org/Reports/2008/The-Engaged-Epatient-Population.aspx?r=1.

Fox, S. (2008b). *Recruit doctors. Let e-patients lead. Go mobile.* Paper presented at the Health 2.0 Conference, San Diego, CA. Retrieved from http://www.

pewinternet.org/~/media//Files/Reports/2008/Fox_
Health_March_2008.pdf.pdf.

Fox, S., & Jones, S. (2009). *The social life of heath
information*. Pew Internet and American Life
Project. Retrieved from http://www.pewinternet.
org/Reports/2009/8-The-Social-Life-of-Health-
Information.aspx.

Fox, S., & Livingston, G. (2007). *Latinos Online.*
Pew Internet & American Life Project. Retrieved
from http://www.pewinternet.org/~/media//Files/
Reports/2007/Latinos_Online_March_14_2007.pdf.
pdf.

Fox, S., & Purcell, K. (2010, March 24). *Chronic disease
and the Internet*. Pew Internet and American Life
Project. Retrieved from http://www.pewinternet.org/
Reports/2010/Chronic-Disease.aspx.

Friedman, D. B., Hoffman-Goetz, L., & Arocha, J. F.
(2006). Health literacy and the World Wide Web:
Comparing the readability of leading incident cancers
on the Internet. *Informatics for Health and Social Care,
31*(1), 67-87. doi: 10.1080/14639230600628427.

Frost, J. H., Massagli, M. P., Wicks, P., & Heywood,
J. (2008). *How the social web supports patient
experimentation with a new therapy: The demand for
patient-controlled and patient-centered informatics.*
Proceedings of the 2008 AMIA Annual Symposium,
pp. 217-221. Retrieved from https://www.ncbi.nlm.
nih.gov/pmc/articles/PMC2656086.

Garrett, J. J. (2002). *The elements of user experience:
User-centered design for the web*. New York: American
Institute of Graphic Arts.

Garvin, J., Odom-Wesley, B., Rudman, W. J., & Stewart,
R. S. (2009). Healthcare disparities and the role of
personal health records. *Journal of AHIMA*, (June
web exclusive). Retrieved from http://library.
ahima.org/xpedio/groups/public/documents/ahima/
bok1_043826.hcsp?dDocName=bok1_043826.

Gearon, C. J. (2007). *Perspectives on the future of personal
health records*. Prepared for California HealthCare
Foundation. Retrieved from http://www.chcf.org/
publications/2007/06/perspectives-on-the-future-of-
personal-health-records.

Gearon, C. J. (2008, July/August). Take two and
email me at your convenience. *AHIP Coverage*.
Retrieved from http://www.ahip.org/content/default.
aspx?bc=31|130|136|24075|24077.

Gerstle R. S. & the Task Force on Medical Informatics.
(2004). E-mail communication between pediatricians
and their patients. *Pediatrics*, 114, 317–321. Retrieved
from http://pediatrics.aappublications.org/cgi/
reprint/114/1/317.

Gibbons, M. C., Wilson, R. F., Samal, L., Lehmann,
C. U., Dickersin, K., Lehmann, H. P., Aboumatar,
H.,...Bass, E. B. (2009). *Impact of consumer health
informatics applications*. Evidence Report/Technology
Assessment No. 188. AHRQ Publication No. 09(10)-
E019. Rockville, MD: Agency for Healthcare Research

and Quality. Retrieved from http://www.ahrq.gov/
downloads/pub/evidence/pdf/chiapp/impactchia.pdf.

Good, A., Stokes, S., & Jerrams-Smith, J. (2007, Summer).
Elderly, novice users and health information web
sites: Issues of accessibility and usability. *Journal of
Healthcare Information Management, 21*(3), 72–79.

Gustafson, D. H., & Wyatt, J. C. (2004). Evaluation of
ehealth systems and services. *BMJ, 328*(7449), 1150.
Retrieved from http://www.ncbi.nlm.nih.gov/pmc/
articles/PMC411080/?tool=pubmed. doi: 10.1136/
bmj.328.7449.1150.

Halamka, J. D., Mandl, K. D., & Tang, P. C. (2008). Early
experiences with personal health records. *Journal of
the American Medical Informatics Association*, 15, 1–7.
doi:10.1197/jamia.M2562.

HarrisInteractive. (2007, March 26). Many U.S. adults are
satisfied with use of their personal health information.
The Harris Poll. Retrieved from http://www.
harrisinteractive.com/vault/Harris-Interactive-Poll-
Research-Health-Privacy-2007-03.pdf.

HarrisInteractive (2008, July 29). Number of
"cyberchondriacs" – adults going online for health
information – has plateaued or declined. *The Harris
Poll*. Retrieved from http://www.harrisinteractive.com/
vault/Harris-Interactive-Poll-Research-Number-of-
Cyberchondriacs-Adults-Going-Online-for-2008-07.pdf.

HarrisInteractive (2008, November 17). Four out of
five adults now use the internet. *The Harris Poll*.
Retrieved from http://www.harrisinteractive.com/
vault/Harris-Interactive-Poll-Research-Internet-
Penetration-2008-11.pdf.

Heinold, J. W., Stone, D., & MacClary, M. (2009a).
*Health information security and privacy collaboration.
personal health record (PHR) website inventory,
analyses, and findings*. (Contract Number HHSP 233-
200804100EC). Washington, DC.

Heinold, J. W., Stone, D., & MacClary, M. (2009b).
Inventory matrix for personal health records. (Contract
Number HHSP 233-200804100EC). Washington,
DC.

Hesse, B. W., Moser, R. P., & Rutten, L. J. (2010). Surveys
of physicians and electronic health information. *New
England Journal of Medicine, 362*(9), 859–860. doi:
10.1056/NEJMc0909595.

Holbrook, A., Thabane, L., Keshavjee, K., Dolovich,
L., Bernstein, B., Chan, D., . . . Gerstein, H. (2009).
Individualized electronic decision support and
reminders to improve diabetes care in the community:
COMPETE II randomized trial. *CMAJ: Canadian
Medical Association Journal, 181(1–2)*(July 7), 37–44.
doi: 10.1503/cmaj.081272.

Horrigan, J. (2009, July). *Wireless Internet use*. Pew
Internet & American Life Project. Retrieved from
http://www.pewinternet.org/~/media//Files/
Reports/2009/Wireless-Internet-Use.pdf.

Horrigan, J. B. (2010). *Obama's online opportunities II. If
you build it, will they log on?* Pew Internet & American

Life Project. Retrieved from http://www.pewinternet. org/Reports/2008/Obamas-Online-Opportunities.aspx

Horrigan, J. B., & Smith, A. (2007, June). *Home broadband adoption 2007*. Pew Internet & American Life Project. Retrieved from http://www.pewinternet.org/~/media// Files/Reports/2007/PIP_Broadband%202007.pdf.pdf.

Hulse, N. C., Wood, G. M., Haug, P. J., & Williams, M. S. (April 9, 2010). Deriving consumer-facing disease concepts for family health histories using multi-source sampling. *Journal of Biomedical Informatics, 43*(2), 1-9. doi: 10.1016/j.jbi.2010.04.003

Hutcherson, C. M. (2001). Legal Considerations for Nurses Practicing in a Telehealth Setting. *Online Journal of Issues in Nursing, 6*(3). Retrieved from http://www.nursingworld.org/MainMenuCategories/ ANAMarketplace/ANAPeriodicals/OJIN/ TableofContents/Volume62001/No3Sept01/ LegalConsiderations.aspx

Institute of Medicine. (2004). *Health literacy: a prescription to end the confusion*. Washington DC: Institute of Medicine Board on Neuroscience and Behavioral Health, Committee on Health Literacy.

Jimison, H., Gorman, P., Woods, S., Nygren, P., Walker, M., Norris, S., & Hersh, W. (2008). Barriers and Drivers of Health Information Technology Use for the Elderly, Chronically Ill, and Underserved. *Evidence Report/ Technology Assessment No. 175 (Prepared by the Oregon Evidence-based Practice Center under Contract No. 290- 02-0024)*. AHRQ Publication No. 09-E004. Rockville, MD: Agency for Healthcare Research and Quality. November 2008. Retrieved from http://www.ahrq.gov/ downloads/pub/evidence/pdf/hitbarriers/hitbar.pdf

Johnson, K. A., Valdez, R. S., Casper, G. R., Kossman, S. P., Carayon, P., Or, C. K. L., … Brennan, P. F. (2008). Experiences of technology integration in home care nursing. Proceedings of 2008 AMIA Annual Symposium, pp. 389-393. Retrieved from http://www.ncbi.nlm.nih.gov/pmc/articles/ PMC2656057/?tool=pubmed.

Kahn, J. S., Aulakh, V., & Bosworth, A. (2009). What it takes: Characteristics of the ideal personal health record. *Health Affairs (Project Hope), 28*(2), 369–376.

Kane, B., & Sands, D. Z. (1998). Guidelines for the clinical use of electronic mail with patients. *Journal of the American Medical Informatics Association, 5*, 104–111. Retrieved from http://www.ncbi.nlm.nih.gov/pmc/ articles/PMC61279/?tool=pubmed. doi: 10.1136/ jamia.1998.0050104.

Kaphingst, K. A., Zanfini, C. J., & Emmons, K. M. (2006). Accessibility of web sites containing colorectal cancer information to adults with limited literacy (United States). *Cancer Causes and Control, 17*(2), 147–151.

Kaplan, B., & Brennan, P. (2001). Consumer informatics supporting patients as co-producers of quality. *Journal of the American Medical Informatics Association, 8*(4), 309–316. Retrieved from http://www.ncbi.nlm.nih. gov/pmc/articles/PMC130075/?tool=pubmed.

Keckley, P. H., & Eselius, L. L. (2009). *2009 Survey of healthcare consumers:Key findings, strategic implications*. Washington, DC: Deloitte Center for Health Solutions. Retrieved from http://www.deloitte. com/assets/Dcom-UnitedStates/Local%20Assets/ Documents/us_chs_2009SurveyHealthConsumers_ March2009.pdf.

Keselman, A., Logan, R., Smith, C. A., Leroy, G., Zeng-Treitler, Q. (2008). Developing informatics tools and strategies for consumer-centered health communication. *Journal of the American Medical Informatics Association*, 15, 473–483. Retrieved from http://www.ncbi.nlm.nih.gov/pmc/articles/ PMC2442255/?tool=pubmed. doi: 10.1197/jamia. M2744.

Klein, R. (2007). Internet-based patient-physician electronic communication applications: Patient acceptance and trust. *E-Service Journal. 5*(2), 27–52. Retrieved from http://inscribe.iupress.org/doi/ abs/10.2979/ESJ.2007.5.2.27?journalCode=esj.

Krug, S. (2005). *Don't make me think: A common sense approach to web usability*. Berkeley, CA: New Riders.

Kukafka, R., Kahn, S. A., Kaufman, D., & Mark, J. (2009). *An evidence-based decision aid to help patients set priorities for selecting among multiple health behaviors*. Proceedings of the 2009 AMIA Annual Symposium, pp. 343–347.

Kutner, M., Greenberg, E., Jin, Y., & Paulsen, C. (2006). *The health literacy of America's adults: Results from the 2003 National Assessment of Adult Literacy*. U.S. Department of Education. (NCES 2006–483). Washington, DC: National Center for Education Statistics. Retrieved from http://nces.ed.gov/ pubs2006/2006483.pdf.

Lachance, C., Erby, L. A. H., Ford, B. M., Allen, V. C. J., & Kaphingst, K. A. (2010). Informational content, literacy demands, and usability of websites offering health- related genetic tests directly to consumers. *Genetics in Medicine, 12*(5), 304–312.

Lecker, R., Armijo, D., Chin, S., Christensen, J., Desper, J., Hong, A., & Kneale, L. (2007). *Review of the personal health record (PHR) service provider market: Privacy and security*. Prepared for the Office of the National Coordinator for Health Information Technology (ONC) by Altarum Institute. Retrieved from http:// www.hhs.gov/healthit/ahic/materials/01_07/ce/ PrivacyReview.pdf.

Liederman, E., Lee, J., Baquero, V., & Seites, P. (2005a). Patient-physician web messaging. *Journal of General Internal Medicine, 20*(1), 52–57. Retrieved from http://www.ncbi.nlm.nih.gov/pmc/articles/ PMC1490042/?tool=pubmed.

Liederman, E. M., Lee, J. C., Baquero, V. H., & Seites, P. G. (2005b). The impact of patient-physician Web messaging on provider productivity. *Journal of Healthcare Information Management, 19*(2), 81–86.

Lobach, D. F., Waters, A., Silvey, G. M., Clark, S. J., Kalyanaraman, S., Kawamoto, K., & Lipkus, I. (2009). *Facilitating consumer clinical information seeking by maintaining referential context: evaluation of a prototypic approach*. Proceedings of the 2009 AMIA Annual Symposium, pp. 380–384. Retrieved from http://www.ncbi.nlm.nih.gov/pmc/articles/PMC2815459/?tool=pubmed.

Lobach, D. F., Willis, J. M., Macri, J. M., Simo, J., & Anstrom, K. J. (2006). Perceptions of Medicaid beneficiaries regarding the usefulness of accessing personal health information and services through a patient internet portal. Proceedings of 2006 AMIA Annual Symposium, pp. 509–513. Retrieved from http://www.ncbi.nlm.nih.gov/pmc/articles/PMC1839688/?tool=pubmed.

Lober, W., Zierler, B., Herbaugh, A., Shinstrom, S., Stolyar, A., Kim, E., & Kim, Y. (2006). *Barriers to the use of a personal health record by an elderly population*. Proceedings of the 2006 AMIA Annual Symposium, pp. 514–518. Retrieved from http://www.ncbi.nlm.nih.gov/pmc/articles/PMC1839577/?tool=pubmed.

Lüchtenberg, M., Kuhli-Hattenbach, C., Sinangin, Y., Ohrloff, C., & Schalnus, R. (2008). Accessibility of health information on the internet to the visually impaired user. *Ophthalmologica, 222*(3), 187–193.

Lundberg, G.D. (2009, October). Why healthcare professionals should practice participatory medicine: Perspective of a long-time medical editor. *Journal of Participatory Med.*, 1(1), e3. Retrieved from http://www.jopm.org/opinion/commentary/2009/10/21/why-health-care-professionals-should-practice-participatory-medicine-perspective-of-a-long-time-medical-editor-2/

Manhattan Research. (2010, February 9). *New report: The Internet has more influence over consumer health actions than traditional DTC channels.* Retrieved from http://www.manhattanresearch.com/newsroom/Press_Releases/internet-influence-consumer-health-actions.aspx.

Marquard, J., Moen, A., & Brennan, P. (2006). Photographic data—An untapped resource to explore complex phenomena such as health information management in the household (HIMH). *Studies in Health Technology and Informatics, 122*, 58–62.

Marte, J. (2009, August 9). Doctor is in—Online. *The Wall Street Journal*. Retrieved from http://online.wsj.com/article/SB124977187174117097.html.

Matthews, A. W. (2009, July 9). The doctor will text you now. *The Wall Street Journal*. Retrieved from http://online.wsj.com/article/SB10001424052970203872404574257900513900382.html.

Miller, C. C. (2008, July 24). Social networking for patients. *The New York Times*. Retrieved from http://bits.blogs.nytimes.com/2008/10/24/social-networking-for-patients.

Miller, C. C. (2010, March 24). Social networks a lifeline for the chronically Ill. *The New York Times*. Retrieved from http://alliancehealth.com/media/ah-news-032410.pdf.

Miller, T., Leroy, G., & Wood, E. (2006). *Dynamic generation of a table of contents with consumer-friendly labels.* Proceedings of the 2006 AMIA Annual Symposium, pp. 559–63. Retrieved from http://www.ncbi.nlm.nih.gov/pmc/articles/PMC1839557/?tool=pubmed.

Moen, A., & Brennan, P. F. (2005). Health@Home: The work of health information management in the household (HIMH): Implications for consumer health informatics (CHI) innovations. *Journal of the American Medical Informatics Association, 12*, 648–656. Retrieved from http://www.ncbi.nlm.nih.gov/pmc/articles/PMC1294036/?tool=pubmed. doi: 10.1197/jamia.M1758.

Mosquera, M. (2010a, June 8). HHS, VA will add download feature to patient portals. *Government Health IT*. Retrieved from http://www.govhealthit.com/newsitem.aspx?nid=73961.

Mosquera, M. (2010b, February 8). Most fed health plans offer PHRs, but few use them. *Government Health IT*. Retrieved from http://www.govhealthit.com/newsitem.aspx?tid=10&nid=73104.

National Cancer Institute. (2003). *Clear and simple: Developing effective print materials for low-literate readers*. Retrieved from http://www.cancer.gov/cancertopics/cancerlibrary/clear-and-simple.

National Center for Education Statistics. (2003). *National assessment of adult literacy (NAAL)*. Retrieved from http://nces.ed.gov/naal/kf_demographics.asp.

National Center on Vital and Health Statistics. (2006) *Personal health records and personal health record systems: A report and recommendations from the National Committee on Vital and Health Statistics*. Retrieved from http://www.ncvhs.hhs.gov/0602nhiirpt.pdf.

National Library of Medicine (2006). *Fact sheet: Unified medical language system*. Retrieved from http://www.nlm.nih.gov/pubs/factsheets/umls.html.

Nazi, K., Hogan, T., Wagner, T., McInnes, D., Smith, B., Haggstrom, D., . . . Weaver, F. (2010). Embracing a health services research perspective on personal health records: Lessons learned from the VA My HealtheVet system. *Journal of General Internal Medicine* .(Jan;25 Suppl 1), 62–67.

Nazi, K. M., & Woods, S. S. (2008). *MyHealtheVet PHR: A description of users and patient portal use.* Proceedings of the 2008 AMIA Annual Symposium, p. 1182.

Nielsen, J., & Loranger, H. (2006). *Prioritizing web usability*. Berkeley, CA: New Riders.

Norman, C. D., & Skinner, H. A. (2006a). eHealth literacy: Essential skills for consumer health in a networked world. *Journal of Medical Internet Research, 8*(2), e9. Retrieved from http://www.ncbi.nlm.nih.gov/pmc/articles/PMC1550701/?tool=pubmed.

Norman, C. D., & Skinner, H. A. (2006b). eHEALS: The eHealth literacy scale. *Journal of Medical Internet Research* , 8(4), e27. Retrieved from http://www.ncbi.nlm.nih.gov/pmc/articles/PMC1794004/?tool=pubmed.

O'Connor A. M., Bennett, C. L., Stacey D., Barry, M., Col, N. F., Eden, K. B.,...Rovner, D. (2009). Decision aids for people facing health treatment or screening decisions. *Cochrane Database of Systematic Reviews 2009, Issue 3.* doi: 10.1002/14651858.CD001431.pub2.

O'Grady, L., Witteman, H., Bender, J.L., Urowitz, S., Wiljer, D., & Jada, A. R. (2009, April–June). Measuring the impact of a moving target: Towards a dynamic framework for evaluating collaborative adaptive interactive technologies. *Journal of Medical Internet Research.* Retrieved from http://www.ncbi.nlm.nih.gov/pmc/articles/PMC2762807/?tool=pubmed. doi: 10.2196/jmir.1058.

Office for Civil Rights (n.d.). *Privacy and your health information.* Retrieved from http://www.hhs.gov/ocr/privacy/hipaa/understanding/consumers/consumer_summary.pdf. and *Your Health Information Privacy Rights.* Retrieved from http://www.hhs.gov/ocr/privacy/hipaa/understanding/consumers/consumer_rights.pdf.

Office of the National Coordinator for Health Information Technology. (2010). *Health IT strategic framework: Strategic goals, principles, objectives, and strategies.* Retrieved from http://healthit.hhs.gov/portal/server.pt/gateway/PTARGS_0_11673_911844_0_0_18/HIT_Strategic_Framework051010.pdf.

Or, C. K. L., & Karsh, B. T. (2009). A systematic review of patient acceptance of consumer health information technology. *Journal Of The American Medical Informatics Association: JAMIA,* 16(4), 550–560. Retrieved from http://www.ncbi.nlm.nih.gov/pmc/articles/PMC2705259/?tool=pubmed.

Painter, K. (2007, February 6). Few doctors are Web M.D.s, *USA Today.* Retrieved from http://www.usatoday.com/news/health/yourhealth/2007-02-04-web-mds_x.htm.

Palmas, W., Shea, S., Starren, J., Teresi, J. A., Ganz, M. L., Burton, T. M., . . . Weinstock, R. S. (2010). Medicare payments, healthcare service use, and telemedicine implementation costs in a randomized trial comparing telemedicine case management with usual care in medically underserved participants with diabetes mellitus (IDEATel). *Journal of the American Medical Informatics Association,* 17:, 196–202. doi: 10.1136/jamia.2009.002592.

Paré, G., Jaana, M., & Sicotte, C. (2007). Systematic Review of Home Telemonitoring for Chronic Diseases: The Evidence Base. *Journal of the American Medical Informatics Association,* 14., 269–277. Retrieved from http://www.ncbi.nlm.nih.gov/pmc/articles/PMC2244878/?tool=pubmed. doi: 10.1197/jamia.M2270.

Paré, G., Moqadem, K., Pineau, G., & St-Hilaire, C. (2010). Clinical effects of home telemonitoring in the context of diabetes, asthma, heart failure and hypertension: A systematic review. *Journal of Medical Internet Research,* 12(2), 1–15. Retrieved from http://www.jmir.org/2010/2/e21.

Pringle, S., & Lippitt, A. (2009). Interoperability of electronic health records and personal health records: Key interoperability issues associated with information exchange. *Journal of Healthcare Information Management,* 23(3), 31–37.

Pu, P., & Chen, L. (2007). Trust-inspiring explanation interfaces for recommender systems. *Knowledge-Based Systems,* 20(6), 542–556. doi: 10.1016/j.knosys.2007.04.004

Rainie, L., Madden, M., Boyce, A., Lenhart, A., Horrigan, J., Allen, K., O'Grady, E. (2003, April 16).*The ever-shifting internet population: A new look at internet access and the digital divide.* Pew Internet & American Life Project. Retrieved from http://www.pewinternet.org/Reports/2003/The-EverShifting-Internet-Population-A-new-look-at-Internet-access-and-the-digital-divide.aspx.

Ralston, J., Rutter, C., Carrell, D., Hecht, J., Rubanowice, D., & Simon, G. (2009). Patient use of secure electronic messaging within a shared medical record: A cross-sectional study. *Journal of General Internal Medicine,* 24(3), 349-355. Retrieved from http://www.ncbi.nlm.nih.gov/pmc/articles/PMC2642567/?tool=pubmed. doi: 10.1007/s11606-008-0899-z.

Ralston, J. D., Carrell, D., Reid, R., Anderson, M., Moran, M., & Hereford, J. (2007). Patient Web services integrated with a shared medical record: Patient use and satisfaction. *Journal of the American Medical Informatics Association,* 14, 798–806. Retrieved from http://www.ncbi.nlm.nih.gov/pmc/articles/PMC2213480/?tool=pubmed. doi: 10.1197/jamia.M2302.

Reti, S. R., Feldman, H. J., Ross, S. E., & Safran, C. (2010). Improving personal health records for patient-centered care. *Journal Of The American Medical Informatics Association,* 17(2), 192–195.

Reti, S. R., Feldman, H. J., & Safran, C. (2009). Governance for personal health records. *Journal of The American Medical Informatics Association,* 16(1), 14–17. Retrieved from http://www.ncbi.nlm.nih.gov/pmc/articles/PMC2605603/?tool=pubmed. doi: 10.1197/jamia.M2854.

Robert Wood Johnson Foundation. (2007, May). Project health design. Rethinking the power and potential of personal health records. Retrieved from http://www.rwjf.org/files/publications/other/HealthDesignMay07.pdf.

Robeznicks, A. (2007a, October 17). A virtual reality. *Modern Healthcare.* Retrieved from http://www.modernhealthcare.com/article/20071017/FREE/310170003.

Robeznieks, A. (2007b, October 18). Virtual visits: The new ATMs? *Modern Healthcare*. Retrieved from http://www.modernhealthcare.com/article/20071018/FREE/310180002.

Rohrer, J. E., Angstman, K. B., Adamson, S. C., Bernard, M. E., Bachman, J. W., & Morgan, M. E. (2010). Impact of online primary care visits on standard costs: a pilot study. *Population Health Management*, 13(2), 59–63. doi: 10.1089/pop.2009.0018.

Saranto, K. Brennan, P. F., Casey, A. (2009). *Personal health information management: Tools and strategies for citizens' engagement*. Proceedings of the Post-Congress Workshop of the 10th International Nursing Informatics Congress - NI 2009. Retrieved from http://www.uku.fi/vaitokset/2009/isbn978-951-27-1321-9.pdf.

Sarasohn-Kahn, J. (2008). *The wisdom of patients: Healthcare meets online social media*. California HealthCare Foundation. Retrieved from http://www.chcf.org/publications/2008/04/the-wisdom-of-patients-health-care-meets-online-social-media.

Schneider, M. E. (2010, January 1). Practice trends. Insurers, patients willing to pay for online visits. *Skin & Allergy News*. Retrieved from http://www.skinandallergynews.com/news/practice-trends/single-article/insurers-patients-willing-to-pay-for-online-visits/54da187e85.html.

Seidman, J., & Eytan, T. (2008). *Helping people plug in: Lessons in the adoption of online consumer tools*. California Healthcare Foundation. Retrieved from http://www.chcf.org/publications/2008/06/helping-patients-plug-in-lessons-in-the-adoption-of-online-consumer-tools.

Shea, S., Weinstock, R. S., Teresi, J. A., Palmas, W., Starren, J., Cimino, J. J., . . . Eimicke, J. P. (2009). A randomized trial comparing telemedicine case management with usual care in older, ethnically diverse, medically underserved patients with diabetes mellitus: 5 year results of the IDEATel study. *Journal of the American Medical Informatics Association*, 16, 446–456. Retrieved from http://www.ncbi.nlm.nih.gov/pmc/articles/PMC2705246/?tool=pubmed. doi: 10.1197/jamia.M3157.

Sinha, R. & Swearingen, K. (2002). The Role of Transparency in Recommender Systems. In Proceedings of the ACM Conference on Human Factors in Computing Systems (CHI'02) (pp. 830–831). Minneapolis, MN: ACM Press

Shneiderman, B., Jacobs, S., Plaisant, C., & Cohen, M. (2009). *Designing the user interface: Strategies for effective human-computer interaction*. Reading, MA: Addison Wesley.

Shreeve, S. (2008). What is Health 2.0: The enabling technologies and reform initiatives for next generation healthcare. Retrieved from http://health20.org/wiki/Shreeve_Health_2.0_Whitepaper.

Slack, W. V. (2007). Cybermedicine for the patient. *American Journal of Preventive Medicine*, 32(5, Supplement 1), S135–S136. doi: DOI: 10.1016/j.amepre.2007.01.024.

Smith, C. A., & Wicks, P. J. (2008). *PatientsLikeMe: Consumer health vocabulary as a folksonomy*. Proceedings of the 2008 AMIA Annual Symposium, pp. 682–686. Retrieved from http://www.ncbi.nlm.nih.gov/pmc/articles/PMC2656083/?tool=pubmed.

Society for Participatory Medicine. (2010, May 24). *It takes guts to be a neuroendocrine patient: A story of participatory medicine*. Retrieved from http://e-patients.net/index.php?s=%22networked+patients+shift%27.

Stacey, D., Samant, R., & Bennett, C. (2008). Decision making in oncology: A review of patient decision aids to support patient participation. *CA: A Cancer Journal for Clinicians*, 58(5), 293–304. Retrieved from http://caonline.amcancersoc.org/cgi/content/abstract/58/5/293. doi: 10.3322/ca.2008.0006.

Stange, K., Nutting, P., Miller, W., Jaén, C., Crabtree, B., Flocke, S., & Gill, J. (2010). Defining and measuring the patient-centered medical home. *Journal of General Internal Medicine*, 25(6), 601–612. Retrieved from http://www.ncbi.nlm.nih.gov/pmc/articles/PMC2869425/?tool=pubmed. doi: 10.1007/s11606-010-1291-3.

Stone, J. H. (2007). Communication between physicians and patients in the era of E-medicine. *The New England Journal Of Medicine*, 356(24), 2451–2454.

Tang, P., Ash, J., Bates, D., Overhage, J., & Sands, D. (2006). Personal health records: Definition, benefits, and strategies for overcoming barriers to adoption. *Journal of the American Medical Informatics Association*, 13(2), 121–126. Retrieved from http://www.ncbi.nlm.nih.gov/pmc/articles/PMC1447551/?tool=pubmed doi: 10.1197/jamia.M2025.

Tang, P., Black, W., Buchanan, J., Young, C., Hooper, D., Lane, S., . . . Turnbull, J. (2003). *PAMFOnline: Integrating ehealth with an electronic medical record system*. Proceedings of the 2003 AMIA Annual Symposium, pp. 121–126.

Theiss, E. (2010, March 16). Cleveland Clinic program linking chronic-disease patients directly to doctors online shows success. *The Plain Dealer*. Retrieved from http://www.cleveland.com/healthfit/index.ssf/2010/03/cleveland_clinic_program_linki.html.

Troxel, D. B. (2009). eRisk guidelines for online communication. *The Doctors Company*. Retrieved from http://www.thedoctors.com/KnowledgeCenter/PatientSafety/CON_ID_003167.

Undem, T. (2010). *Consumers and health information technology: A national survey*. California HealthCare Foundation. Retrieved from http://www.chcf.org/~/media/Files/PDF/C/althInfoTechnologyNationalSurvey.pdf.

U.S. Department of Health and Human Services. (2003, May). Summary of the HIPAA Privacy Rule. Retrieved from http://www.hhs.gov/ocr/privacy/hipaa/understanding/summary/privacysummary.pdf.

U.S. Department of Health and Human Services. (2009). Healthy People 2020: The road ahead. Retrieved from http://www.healthypeople.gov/HP2020/default.asp.

Volk, R. J., Hawley, S. T., Kneuper, S., Holden, E. W., Stroud, L. A., Cooper, C. P., . . . Pavlik, V. N. (2007). Trials of decision aids for prostate cancer screening: A systematic review. *American Journal of Preventive Medicine, 33*(5), 428–434.e411. doi: 10.1016/j.amepre.2007.07.030.

Wald, H., Dube, C., & Anthony, D. (2007). Untangling the Web—the impact of Internet use on healthcare and the physician-patient relationship. *Patient Education and Counseling, 68*(3), 218–224.

Wangsness, L. (2009a , April 13). Electronic health records raise doubt *Boston Globe*. Retrieved from http://www.boston.com/news/nation/washington/articles/2009/04/13/electronic_health_records_raise_doubt.

Wangsness, L. (2009b, April 18). Beth Israel halts sending insurance data to Google. Hospital admits 'mistake' as flaws in practice found. *The Boston Globe*. Retrieved from http://www.boston.com/news/nation/washington/articles/2009/04/18/beth_israel_halts_sending_insurance_data_to_google.

Weaver, C., Zielstorff, R. D. (2011). Personal Health Record: Managing Personal Health. In M. J. Ball, J. V. Douglas, P. H. Walker, D. DuLong, B. Gugerty, K. J. Hannah, J. M. Kiel, S. K. Newbold, JU. Sensmeier, D. J. Skiba, & M. R. Troseth (Eds.), Nursing Informatics: Where Technology and Caring Meet (4th ed.) (pp. 265–289). New York, New York: Springer.

Weingart, S. N., Rind, D., Tofias, Z., & Sands, D. Z. (2006). Who uses the patient internet portal? The PatientSite experience. *Journal of the American Medical Informatics Association, 13*, 13–91. Retrieved from http://www.ncbi.nlm.nih.gov/pmc/articles/PMC1380201/?tool=pubmed. doi:10.1197/jamia.M1833.

Weiss, J. B., & Lorenzi, N. M. (2008). *Synthesizing community wisdom: A model for sharing cancer-related resources through social networking and collaborative partnerships.* Proceedings of the 2008 AMIA Annual Symposium, pp. 793–797. Retrieved from http://www.ncbi.nlm.nih.gov/pmc/articles/PMC2656050/?tool=pubmed.

Witteman, H., Chignell, M., & Krahn, M. (2008). A recommender system for prostate cancer websites. Proceedings of the 2008 AMIA Annual Symposium, p. 1177.

World Wide Web Consortium (W3C). (2010, May 21). *Introduction to "how people with disabilities use the web."* Retrieved from http://www.w3.org/WAI/intro/people-use-web#ref.

Wynia, M., & Dunn, K. (2010). Dreams and nightmares: practical and ethical issues for patients and physicians using personal health records. *Journal of Law and Medical Ethics, 38*(1), 64–73.

Zeng-Treitler, Q., Goryachev, S., Kim, H., Keselman, A., & Rosendale, D. (2007). *Making texts in electronic health records comprehensible to consumers: a prototype translator.* Proceedings of the 2007 AMIA Annual Symposium, pp. 846–850. Retrieved from http://www.ncbi.nlm.nih.gov/pmc/articles/PMC2655860/?tool=pubmed.

Zeng-Treitler, Q., Goryachev, S., Tse, T., Keselman, A., & Boxwala, A. (2008). Estimating consumer familiarity with health terminology: A context-based approach. *Journal of the American Medical Informatics Association, 15*, 349–356. Retrieved from http://www.ncbi.nlm.nih.gov/pmc/articles/PMC2409994/?tool=pubmed. doi: 10.1197/jamia.M2592.

Zeng, Q. T., & Tse, T. (2006). Exploring and developing consumer health vocabularies. *Journal of the American Medical Informatics Association, 13*, 24–29. Retrieved from http://www.ncbi.nlm.nih.gov/pmc/articles/PMC1380193/?tool=pubmed. doi: 10.1197/jamia.M1761.

Zeng, X., & Parmanto, B. (2004). Web content accessibility of consumer health information web sites for people with disabilities: a cross sectional evaluation. *Journal of Medical Internet Research, 6*(2), e19. Retrieved from http://www.ncbi.nlm.nih.gov/pmc/articles/PMC1550595/?tool=pubmed. doi: 10.2196/jmir.6.2.e19.

Zhou, Y. Y., Garrido, T., Chin, H. L., Wiesenthal, A. M., & Liang, L. L. (2007). Patient access to an electronic health record with secure messaging: Impact on primary care utilization. *American Journal of Managed Care, 13*(7), 418–424.

40

Nursing Curriculum Reform and Healthcare Information Technology

Eun-Shim Nahm / Marisa L. Wilson

• OBJECTIVES

1. Describe the background of and needs for curriculum reform in nursing education in the 21st century.
2. Discuss prior academic and other professional organizational efforts to transform nursing education with an emphasis on healthcare information technology.
3. List information technology competencies required by nurses with different levels of education.
4. Identify current national trends in nursing education and the resources needed by nursing schools.

• KEY WORDS

American Association of Colleges of Nursing (AACN) Essentials for Nursing
Electronic health record (EHR)
Healthcare information technology (HIT)
HITECH Act
Informatics competency
Knowledge, skills, and attitudes (KSA)
Nursing education curriculum
Nursing informatics (NI)
Patient safety
Quality and Safety Education for Nurses (QSEN)
Technology Informatics Guiding Educational Reform (TIGER)

BACKGROUND: TRANSFORMATION OF HEALTHCARE USING INFORMATION TECHNOLOGY

Nursing care directly influences individuals' health and recovery from illnesses. Research and evidence-based practice have always been vital components to nursing (Grypma, 2005; Kudzma, 2006). For instance, Florence Nightingale eloquently demonstrated how nursing care lowered the mortality rate of British soldiers during the Crimean War by applying statistics (Grypma, 2005; Kudzma, 2006). Rapid advancement in healthcare information technology (HIT) in the 21st century offers nurses a great opportunity to augment their ability to manage patient information and provide quality care.

Since the Institute of Medicine's (IOM's) report *To Err is Human* was released, a great deal of effort has been made to transform healthcare using information technology (IT) (Committee on Quality of Healthcare in America & IOM, 2001; Newhouse, Dearholt, Poe, Pugh, & White, 2007). In fact, in the current digital era, hospitals cannot be sustained without HIT, which allows healthcare providers to deliver safer and efficient care. Aided by HIT, clinicians manage a large volume of clinical data and access the most up-to-date evidence-based health information. HIT also allows secure data exchange between care providers and organizations. The importance of HIT in healthcare organizations has also been recognized by credentialing organizations. In nursing, Magnet status recognition by the American Nurses Credentialing Center (ANCC) represents a healthcare organization's quality patient care, nursing excellence, and innovations in practice (ANCCenter, 2010). Hospitals can earn the recognition by meeting a set of standards for quality indicators and standards of nursing practice. A strong presence and effective utilization of HIT is an essential component in the Magnet recognition process.

Migration of paper-based health records to an electronic format was a national priority for the Bush administration, and remains an important priority for the current Obama administration. The American Recovery and Reinvestment Act (ARRA) plans to award nearly $1 billion to make HIT available to over 100,000 healthcare providers by 2014 (U.S. Department of Health & Human Services [DHHS], 2010a). Furthermore, Title XIII of the ARRA, the Health Information Technology for Economic and Clinical Health (HITECH) Act, authorized incentive payments through Centers for Medicare and Medicaid Services (CMS) to clinicians and hospitals when they used electronic health records (EHRs) privately and securely to achieve specified improvements in care delivery (Blumenthal, 2009; Blumenthal & Tavenner, 2010; Health Information Technology, 2010). The one caveat of the HITECH Act is that it emphasizes the "meaningful use" of EHRs and not just a simple adoption of EHRs. "Meaningful EHR users" must demonstrate the "meaningful use of a certified EHR, the electronic exchange of health information to improve the quality of healthcare, and reporting on clinical quality and other measures using certified EHR technology"(Centers for Medicare & Medicaid Services [CMS], 2007).

In order to provide optimal care in this rapidly changing and technology-laden healthcare environment, nurses must have a full understanding of the changes in healthcare and be properly prepared to use the available resources. This chapter will discuss:

1. The impact of HIT on the current state of healthcare.

2. Major efforts in nursing curriculum revisions.

3. Nursing education reform in the current technology-rich environment.

4. Major domains and attributes of HIT competencies needed for nursing students and practicing nurses in the current healthcare environment.

5. Current trends in nursing education and informatics competency for faculty members.

THE IMPACT OF HEALTHCARE INFORMATION TECHNOLOGY ON THE CURRENT STATE OF HEALTHCARE

Recent advancements of HIT revolutionized and impacted every aspect of healthcare delivery. For instance, currently most patients gather a significant amount of information about their health online even before they meet with healthcare providers. When patients go to a clinic or hospital, they are admitted to a system before the care provider sees them. Eventually, the data in those systems are forwarded to various clinical systems including EHRs, laboratory and pharmacy systems, as well as other ancillary systems. Eventually the health data in those systems are forwarded to finance systems and then sent to the appropriate insurance companies and other regulatory organizations (Saba & McCormick, 2006). In addition, a recent emphasis on personal healthcare records (PHR) demonstrates the ever-growing use of HIT (Ball, Smith, & Bakalar, 2007; CMS.gov, 2010; The HIMSS Personal Health Record Steering Committee, 2007).

Many years ago, healthcare teams used to bring a cart full of paper-based patient medical records during rounds. Physicians and nurses often furiously documented to-do lists on their notebooks. A clinician in the current era makes rounds with a portable workstation on wheels (WOW) (also called computers on wheels [COWS]), which is connected to the hospital's main EHR system using a wireless connection. They look for the most up-to-date evidence-based clinical information needed for the patient right at the bedside, using various portable systems (e.g., personal digital assistant [PDA] devices, iPad, tablet computers).

The nation has clearly recognized the importance of HIT in improving patient safety and the efficiency of healthcare delivery. The Obama administration called for a $10 billion-a-year investment in HIT over the next 5 years (Change.gov, 2007). This national agenda has significant implications for healthcare providers, and the use of HIT systems in healthcare settings will continue to increase at a rapid pace. Current HIT has already reconceptualized various aspects of healthcare delivery, including regulations related to healthcare data and information. For instance, previously, healthcare providers were concerned about the privacy and security of patients' data in the paper-based charts. However, they now have to establish mechanisms to secure the data stored in the server as well as during transmission to the other healthcare parties. The Health Insurance Portability and Accountability Act (HIPAA) addresses these privacy and security concerns for patient data, and most healthcare providers have been trained for these regulations (Centers for Medicare and Medicaid Services, 2010; U.S. Department of Health & Human Services, 2010b). At the systems level, healthcare providers must ensure the accuracy and completeness of data, as well as appropriate interoperability between the systems. Implementation and maintenance of HIT are a complex and dynamic process and increasing numbers of HIT experts and clinicians are being involved in this process. Preparation of a sufficient number of competent healthcare informaticists and the education of clinicians to be competent users of HIT have become an enormous challenge for healthcare organizations and educators.

Compared to the speed of recent advancements in HIT, both the adoption of these technologies by clinicians and the education of healthcare providers in HIT have been slow. It has been only a few years since the number of schools that offer healthcare informatics programs has increased. The recent support from the ARRA and Section 3016 of the HITECH Act significantly facilitated this effort. The act authorized the creation of a program to assist in the establishment and/or expansion of educational programs designed to train HIT professionals (U.S. Department of Health & Human Services, 2010a). The Office of the National Coordinator for Health Information Technology (ONC) awarded $84 million in funding to schools to train HIT professionals.

With the successful adoption of HIT in healthcare, it is also critical to ensure clinicians' competency to use HIT. Nurses' competency for using HIT is particularly important because they are the largest group of direct healthcare providers in the U.S., accounting for 19.6% of all healthcare workers in 2008 (approximately 3 million) (U.S. Bureau of Labor Statistics, 2010; U.S. DHHS Health Resources and Services Administration, 2010). In fact, nursing as a healthcare discipline has been ahead in terms of educating healthcare professionals who are specialized in HIT. For instance, nursing informatics (NI) was created as an area of graduate specialization at the University of Maryland School of Nursing in 1988, and NI was officially recognized as a specialty practice area by the American Nurses Association (ANA) in 1992 (Gassert, 2000). Since then, informatics has become a core course for many baccalaureate programs, and many nursing schools have offered graduate degree programs focusing on nursing and healthcare informatics.

The advancement of available information communication technologies has also changed nursing education drastically. Nursing schools teach their students using innovative technologies emphasizing evidence-based practice and problem-solving abilities. Many nursing schools have high-fidelity simulation labs that are incorporating the use of EHRs as a critical component of simulation cases. Stakeholders expect nursing students to be competent in using HIT when they arrive in practice settings. Nursing as a profession has recognized the major reform of nursing education, and significant efforts are being made in many areas of the nursing domain (AACN, 2008a; Cronenwett et al., 2007).

EFFORTS IN NURSING CURRICULUM REVISIONS

Background

An increased awareness of patient safety and the use of HIT in healthcare called for changes in the nursing curriculum. The IOM report *Health Professions Education: A Bridge to Quality* is a result of a 2002 summit that followed the IOM's report *Crossing the Quality Chasm*

(Committee on Quality of Healthcare in America & IOM, 2001). This interdisciplinary summit was held to discuss reforming education for health professionals to enhance quality and patient safety (IOM Committee on Health Education Profession Summit, 2002). The report proposed 5 core competencies for healthcare professionals (Committee on Quality of Healthcare in America & IOM, 2001; IOM Committee on Health Education Profession Summit, 2002):

- *Provide patient-centered care:* Identify, respect, and care about patients' differences, values, preferences, and expressed needs....and continuously advocate disease prevention, wellness, and promotion of healthy lifestyles, including a focus on population health.

- *Work in interdisciplinary teams:* Cooperate, collaborate, communicate, and integrate care in teams.

- *Employ evidence-based practice:* Integrate best research with clinical expertise and patient values for optimum care, and participate in learning and research activities to the extent feasible.

- *Apply quality improvement:* Identify errors and hazards in care; understand and implement basic safety design principles ... design and test interventions to change processes and systems of care, with the objective of improving quality.

- *Utilize informatics:* Communicate, manage knowledge, mitigate error, and support decision making using information technology.

Since then, many efforts have been made by nursing professional organizations and the AACN to revise the nursing curriculum to be aligned with the IOM competencies.

Quality and Safety Education for Nurses

The overarching goal of the 3 phases of the Quality and Safety Education for Nurses (QSEN) project, which was supported by the Robert Wood Johnson Foundation (RWJF), is to address the competencies necessary to continuously improve the quality and safety of the healthcare systems in which they work (Cronenwett et al., 2007; Quality and Safety Education for Nurses (QSEN), 2010). Phase I of the project identified 6 competencies that needed to be developed during prelicensure nursing education (Table 40.1). The group also proposed clarified competencies in the areas of knowledge, skills, and attitudes (KSAs).

Phase II work of QSEN was focused on competencies for advanced practice nurses (APNs). The QSEN faculty members collaborated with advanced practice nurses (APNs) who practiced in direct patient care and worked on the development of standards of practice, accreditation of educational programs, and certification (Cronenwett, Sherwood, Pohl et al., 2009). The workgroups that participated in Phase II generated KSAs for graduate-level education.

In summary, the IOM and QSEN competencies are embedded in the new AACN Essentials of Baccalaureate Education. In addition, many graduate

TABLE 40.1	QSEN Competencies
Patient-centered Care	Recognize the patient or designee as the source of control and full partner in providing compassionate and coordinated care based on respect for a patient's preferences, values, and needs.
Teamwork and Collaboration	Function effectively within nursing and interprofessional teams, fostering open communication, mutual respect, and shared decision making to achieve quality patient care.
Evidence-based Practice (EBP)	Integrate best current evidence with clinical expertise and patient and family preferences and values for the delivery of optimal healthcare.
Quality Improvement (QI)	Use data to monitor the outcomes of care processes and use improvement methods to design and test changes to continuously improve the quality and safety of healthcare systems.
Safety	Minimize the risk of harm to patients and providers through both system effectiveness and individual performance.
Informatics	Use information and technology to communicate, manage knowledge, mitigate error, and support decision making.

QSEN competencies in KSAs are embedded in AACN's *Essentials of Doctoral Education for Advanced Nursing Practice* (Cronenwett, Sherwood, & Gelmon, 2009; Cronenwett, Sherwood, Pohl et al., 2009; Dycus & McKeon, 2009).

The American Association of Colleges of Nursing Essentials for Nursing

In response to the urgent calls to transform healthcare delivery and to better prepare today's nurses for professional practice, the AACN convened a task force on essential patient safety competencies in 2006 (AACN, 2006b). The taskforce recommended specific competencies that should be achieved by professional nurses to ensure high-quality and safe patient care. Those competencies were identified under the following areas: (1) critical thinking, (2) healthcare systems and policy, (3) communication, (4) illness and disease management, (5) ethics, and (6) information and healthcare technologies. Since then, the AACN revised the *Essentials of Baccalaureate Education for Professional Nursing Practice* in 2008 (AACN, 2008a).

In regard to the essentials for graduate programs, the AACN made a decision to migrate advanced practice nursing programs from the master's level to the doctorate level (doctor of nursing practice [DNP] program) by the year 2015 (AACN, 2010a). Under this decision, all master's programs that prepare advanced practice registered nurses (APRNs) must transition to the DNP programs (currently some graduate specialty programs, such as nursing administration, community health nursing, and informatics, are not categorized as APRN programs). The *Essentials of Doctoral Education for Advanced Nursing Practice* were developed in 2006 (American Association of Colleges of Nursing, 2006a), and the informatics competency is one of the essentials for this education program. This has a major impact on education at the graduate level. Considering the migration of advanced practice nursing programs to the DNP level, the current *Essentials of Master's Education for Advanced Practice Nursing*, which was developed in 1994, was also revised as the *Essentials of Master's Education in Nursing* (AACN, 2011). The 1994 version of the *Essentials of Master's Nursing Education* does not clearly address an informatics competency as a separate essential (AACN, 1994). Management of information is only addressed as part of a research component. The new revision includes an essential concerning informatics and healthcare technologies (AACN, 2011).

Among various changes regarding essentials in nursing education since 2001, major emphasis has been on patient safety and HIT. The major focus of this chapter is to discuss nursing curriculum from the context of HIT, and Table 40.2 focuses on AACN essentials in the area of information management and technology.

Technology Informatics Guiding Educational Reform Initiative

The recent Technology Informatics Guiding Educational Reform (TIGER) Initiative epitomizes nurses' efforts to translate high-level initiatives on nursing education reform to a practice level (Hebda & Calderone, 2010; D. Skiba & Dulong, 2008; Technology Informatics Guiding Educational Reform (TIGER), 2010; Technology Informatics Guiding Educational Reform (TIGER) Informatics Competencies Collaborative, 2009). TIGER's aim is to fully engage practicing nurses and nursing students in the electronic era of healthcare. TIGER's goal is to create and disseminate action plans that can be duplicated within nursing and other multidisciplinary healthcare training and workplace settings. In Phase I of the TIGER summit, stakeholders from various fields, including nursing practice, education, vendors, and government agencies, participated in the discussions, and the TIGER team developed a 10-year vision and 3-year action plan for transforming nursing practice and education (TIGER, 2010). In Phase II, TIGER formalized cross-organizational activities and action steps into 9 collaborative TIGER teams (TIGER, 2009):

1. Standards and Interoperability
2. Healthcare IT National Agenda/HIT Policy
3. Informatics Competencies
4. Education and Faculty Development
5. Staff Development/Continuing Education
6. Usability/Clinical Application Design
7. Virtual Demonstration Center
8. Leadership Development
9. Consumer Empowerment/Personal Health Record

The National League for Nursing's Call for Reform

In 2006, with the heightened importance of using EHRs in the clinical setting, the National League for Nursing (NLN) Informatics Competencies Task Group of the Educational Technology and Information Management Council (ETIMAC) conducted a survey to assess the next generation of nurses' preparedness to work in a technology-rich informatics environment (National League for Nursing, 2008; Skiba, Connors, & Honey, 2010). The

TABLE 40.2	Information Management and Technology-Related Essentials for Nursing Education	
Baccalaureate Education. (2008). Retrieved from www.aacn.nche.edu/education/pdf/BaccEssentials08.pdf. (American Association of Colleges of Nursing, 2008a)	Essential IV: Information Management and Application of Patient Care Technology: • Knowledge and skills in information management and patient care technology are critical in the delivery of quality patient care.	The baccalaureate program prepares the graduate to: 1. Demonstrate skills in using patient care technologies, information systems, and communication devices that support safe nursing practice. 2. Use telecommunication technologies to assist in effective communication in a variety of healthcare settings. 3. Apply safeguards and decision-making support tools embedded in patient care technologies and information systems to support a safe practice environment for both patients and healthcare workers. 4. Understand the use of clinical information systems to document interventions related to achieving nurse sensitive outcomes. 5. Use standardized terminology in a care environment that reflects nursing's unique contribution to patient outcomes. 6. Evaluate data from all relevant sources, including technology, to inform the delivery of care. 7. Recognize the role of information technology in improving patient care outcomes and creating a safe care environment. 8. Uphold ethical standards related to data security, regulatory requirements, confidentiality, and clients' right to privacy. 9. Apply patient care technologies as appropriate to address the needs of a diverse patient population. 10. Advocate for the use of new patient care technologies for safe, quality care. 11. Recognize that redesign of workflow and care processes should precede implementation of care technology to facilitate nursing practice. 12. Participate in the evaluation of information systems in practice settings through policy and procedure development.
Master's Education (2011). *Retrieved from http://www.aacn.nche.edu/Education/pdf/Master%27sEssentials11.pdf. (American Association of Colleges of Nursing, 2011)*	Essential V: Informatics and Healthcare Technologies	The master's-degree program prepares the graduate to: 1. Analyze current and emerging technologies to support safe practice environments, and to optimize patient safety, cost-effectiveness, and health outcomes. 2. Evaluate outcome data using current communication technologies, information systems, and statistical principles to develop strategies to reduce risks and improve health outcomes. 3. Promote policies that incorporate ethical principles and standards for the use of health and information technologies. 4. Provide oversight and guidance in the integration of technologies to document patient care and improve patient outcomes. 5. Use information and communication technologies, resources, and principles of learning to teach patients and others. 6. Use current and emerging technologies in the care environment to support lifelong learning for self and others.

TABLE 40.2	Information Management and Technology-Related Essentials for Nursing Education *(continued)*	
Doctoral Education for Advanced Nursing Practice. (2006). www.aacn.nche.edu/ DNP/pdf/Essentials.pdf. (American Association of Colleges of Nursing, 2006a)	Essential IV. Information Systems/Technology and Patient Care Technology for the Improvement and Transformation of Healthcare	The DNP program prepares the graduate to: 1. Design, select, use, and evaluate programs that evaluate and monitor outcomes of care, care systems, and quality improvement including consumer use of healthcare information systems. 2. Analyze and communicate critical elements necessary to the selection, use, and evaluation of healthcare information systems and patient care technology. 3. Demonstrate the conceptual ability and technical skills to develop and execute an evaluation plan involving data extraction from practice information systems and databases. 4. Provide leadership in the evaluation and resolution of ethical and legal issues within healthcare systems relating to the use of information, information technology, communication networks, and patient care technology. 5. Evaluate consumer health information sources for accuracy, timeliness, and appropriateness.

American Association of Colleges of Nursing (2011). The Essentials of Master's Education in Nursing Retrieved April 11, 2011, from http://www.aacn. nche.edu/Education/pdf/Master%27sEssentials11.pdf

respondents included 545 school administrators and 1,557 faculty members. Only 50% to 60% of participants reported that informatics was integrated into the curriculum. Furthermore, many respondents equated online learning with informatics. More than 80% of faculty reported that their informatics knowledge was self-taught. In response, NLN issued the position statement *Preparing the Next Generation of Nurses to Practice in a Technology-rich Environment: An Informatics Agenda*, which called for nursing educators and administrators to advocate that all students graduate with competency in the following areas: computer literacy, information literacy, and informatics (NLN Board of Governors, 2008).

The NLN's recommendations are as follows (*Preparing the Next Generation of Nurses to Practice in a Technology-rich Environment: An Informatics Agenda (NLN Board of Governors, 2008)*:

For nurse faculty:

- Participate in faculty development programs to achieve competency in informatics.
- Designate an informatics champion in every school of nursing to: (a) help faculty distinguish between using instructional technologies to teach vs. using informatics to guide, document, analyze, and inform nursing practice, and (b) translate state-of-the-art practices in technology and informatics that need to be integrated into the curriculum.
- Incorporate informatics into the curriculum.

- Incorporate ANA-recognized standard nursing language and terminology into content.
- Identify clinical informatics exemplars, those drawn from clinical agencies and the community or from other nursing education programs, to serve as examples for the integration of informatics into the curriculum.
- Achieve competency through participation in faculty development programs.
- Partner with clinicians and informatics people at clinical agencies to help faculty and students develop competence in informatics.
- Collaborate with clinical agencies to ensure that students have hands-on experience with informatics tools.
- Collaborate with clinical agencies to demonstrate transformations in clinical practice produced by informatics.
- Establish criteria to evaluate informatics goals for faculty.

For Deans, Directors, and Chairs:

- Provide leadership in planning for necessary IT infrastructure that will ensure education that prepares graduates for 21st-century practice roles and responsibilities.
- Allocate sufficient resources to support IT initiatives.

- Ensure that all faculty members have competence in computer literacy, information literacy, and informatics.
- Provide opportunities for faculty development in informatics.
- Urge clinical agencies to provide hands-on informatics experiences for students.
- Encourage nurse-managed clinics to incorporate clinical informatics exemplars that have transformed nursing practice to provide safe quality care.
- Advocate that all students graduate with up-to-date knowledge and skills in each of the 3 critical areas: computer literacy, information literacy, and informatics.
- Establish criteria to evaluate outcomes related to achieving informatics goals.

For the National League for Nursing:

- Disseminate this position statement widely.
- Seek external funding and allocate internal resources to convene a think tank to reach consensus on definitions of informatics, competencies for faculty and students, and program outcomes that include informatics.
- Participate actively in organizations that focus on education in nursing informatics to ensure that recommendations from those organizations are congruent with the NLN's positions on curriculum.
- Use ETIMAC and its task groups to: (a) develop programs for faculty, showcasing exemplar programs, and (b) disseminate outcomes from the think tank.
- Encourage and facilitate accrediting bodies, regulatory agencies, and certifying bodies to reach consensus on definitions related to informatics and minimal informatics competencies for practice in the 21st century.

COMPETENCIES IN HEALTH INFORMATICS TECHNOLOGY

The essentials and competencies recommended by the IOM, AACN, and QSEN address essential competencies that need to be addressed across educational programs. A great deal of effort also has been made in developing more executable competency lists that can be used in practice settings.

American Nurses Association

Nursing Informatics: The Scope and Standard of Practice (American Nurses Association, 2008) addressed an NI-specific domain. As discussed earlier, NI is an essential component for any nurse. The competencies contained in the *NI Scope and Standard of Practice* matrix were categorized into 3 overall areas: (1) computer literacy, (2) information literacy, and (3) professional development and leadership (American Nurses Association, 2008). Computer literacy addresses competencies in the area of the psychomotor use of computers and other technological equipment. Information literacy competencies are related to the ability to identify a need for information as well as the ability to find, evaluate, organize, and use the information effectively. Professional development and leadership competencies address ethical, procedural, safety, and management issues for informatics solutions in nursing practice, education, research, and administration. The competency framework includes nurses with different levels of NI education (e.g., nurses with and without graduate-level NI specialty education) and different NI functional areas (e.g., analysis, consultation). The categories of educational and functional roles within the competency matrix include:

- Beginning Nurse
- Experienced Nurse
- Informatics Specialist/Informatics Innovator
- Administration Analysis
- Compliance and Integrity Management
- Consultation
- Coordination
- Facilitation and Integration
- Development
- Educational and Professional Development
- Policy Development and Advocacy
- Research and Evaluation
- Integrated Areas

TIGER Informatics Competencies Collaborative Recommendations

Upon extensive review of the literature, the TIGER Informatics Competency Collaborative (TICC) recommends specific informatics competencies for all practicing nurses and graduating nursing students (TICC, 2009). The TIGER NI competencies model consists of 3 areas: (1) basic computer competencies, (2) information literacy, and (3) information management.

For the basic computer competencies, the TICC adopted the European Computer Driving License (ECDL) competencies and recommends the following:

- All practicing nurses and graduating nursing students gain or demonstrate proficiency in ECDL modules 1, 2, and 7, as well as ECDL Category 3.1: Using the Application
- All practicing nurses and graduating nursing students become ECDL certified or hold a substantially equivalent certification.

The European Computer Driving License (ECDL)/ International Computer Driving License (ICDL) is an internationally recognized information and communication technology and digital literacy certification. (The ECDL Foundation Ltd., 2010) The ECDL certification program was developed through a task force of the Council of European Professional Informatics Societies in 1995. The current ECDL/ICDL Syllabus 5.0 includes 7 modules that define the competencies necessary to be a proficient user of a computer and common computer applications (The ECDL Foundation Ltd., 2007):

- Module 1: Concepts of Information and Communication Technology
- Module 2: Using the Computer and Managing files
- Module 3: Word Processing
- Module 4: Spreadsheets
- Module 5: Using Databases
- Module 6: Presentation
- Module 7: Web Browsing and Communication

The TICC's Information Literacy competency was adapted from the American Library Association's information literacy competency standards (TICC, 2009). Information literacy was defined as the ability to identify information needed for a specific purpose, locate pertinent information, evaluate the information, and apply it correctly.

All practicing nurses and graduating nursing students will have the ability to:

1. Determine the nature and extent of the information needed.
2. Access needed information effectively and efficiently.
3. Evaluate information and its sources critically and incorporate selected information into his or her knowledge base and value system.
4. Individually or as a member of a group, use information effectively to accomplish a specific purpose.
5. Evaluate outcomes of the use of information.

The TICC developed the information management competencies following the processes of data collection, data processing, and presenting and communicating the processed data as information or knowledge. The TICC conceptualized that this process can be well reflected in the EHR and recommends a set of competencies based on the application of the Health Level Seven (HL7) EHR System Functional Model and the ECDL.

E-Health Literacy

One area that needs further discussion in the competencies addressed by the AACN (ANA, 2008) and the TICC (TICC, 2009) is e-Health literacy. Norman and Skinner (2006) defined *eHealth literacy* as "the ability to seek, find, understand, and appraise health information from electronic sources and apply the knowledge gained to addressing or solving a health problem" (Norman & Skinner, 2006). E-Health, therefore, requires combined literacy skills in several domains. Norman and Skinner suggest 6 domains of e-Health literacy: traditional literacy, information literacy, media literacy, health literacy, computer literacy, and scientific literacy.

E-Health literacy is often discussed at the consumers level because consumers in the current age can access a large amount of health information online, and many of them may not be prepared to locate the information they need or evaluate the quality of the information found from different sources (Nguyen, Carrieri-Kohlman, Rankin, Slaughter, & Stulbarg, 2004). Although nurses have much more knowledge about general health than the public, e-Health literacy is also a concern for them. Unlike many younger generations, nurses who did not grow up with technology may spend less time exploring online health information and may be less familiar with search functions. Considering the nurse's role as an educator for consumers and the heightened emphasis on evidence-based practice, nurses must be properly prepared to be e-Health literate.

USE OF THE EHR IN NURSING EDUCATION

Informatics is now a core competency for nurses at all educational levels, and nursing students must be properly prepared to use EHRs at their clinical setting. During their course work, nursing students have the opportunity to rotate through various clinical settings that use different types of EHRs (Fauchald, 2008; Vestal, Krautwurst, & Hack, 2008). It would be ideal for students to learn to use EHRs from a simulation lab while they practice clinical skills before they enter clinical settings. Although some schools now have academic versions of EHRs in their simulation lab, many schools do not have the resources to support such technology. Thus, nursing schools have used a few different approaches to teach their students to use EHRs.

Collaboration Between the Nursing School and the Vendor

Implementing the EHR in simulation labs allows students to have an opportunity to develop competencies in using HIT before they go into clinical settings. In addition, most EHRs have decision support systems that could significantly augment students' learning. Using an academic version of the EHR, nursing educators can expand the nursing component (e.g., nursing documentation) of the EHR, which may not be highlighted in some hospital EHRs. Currently, several schools of nursing have an academic version of an EHR in their simulation lab (AllBusiness.com, 2009; Borycki et al., 2009; Fauchald, 2008; Joe et al., 2009; Otto & Kushniruk, 2009). In addition, some major HIT vendors (e.g., Cerner, Eclipsys) market academic versions of clinical information systems. When schools implement these academic EHR systems, they must have a thorough plan and a multitude of resources. For instance, the school must have funding to purchase the program, along with network infrastructures that can support it, and a designated project manger who is familiar with system deployment. There will be a great deal of work in developing use cases and building tables in the system, which also requires the clinical faculty members' participation. It will be necessary to educate faculty members about the system since they must be competent in order to teach classes using the EHR.

Collaboration among the Nursing School, Hospital, and the Vendor

An exemplary pedagogical model of teaching nursing students about EHRs would be the use of a collaborative approach among the nursing school, the hospital, and the vendor (Melo & Carlton, 2008). Using this approach, students can learn to use the hospital's EHR system from the simulation lab in their schools, so that when they arrive at their clinical settings, they are already familiar with the system.

Melo and Carton (2008) reported an exemplary case where Ball State University School of Nursing, Ball Memorial Hospital (BMH), and McKesson, Inc. all collaborated to educate students about the use of an EHR. In their project, the EHR simulation model was set up in the school's learning resource center. The vendor donated PCs equipped with the hospital's EHR and the licenses for the software. All 3 parties collaborated in building the infrastructure of the simulation model and the hospital's infrastructure for the students' access. Furthermore, the school of nursing's resource center became a hub for other nursing schools' students who rotate through clinicals at BMH.

Collaboration between the School of Nursing and the Hospital

Many hospitals face various levels (e.g., junior and senior) of nursing students who are not familiar with their clinical information systems. The hospitals, nursing instructors, and students may have difficulties in using the EHR in a safe manner that meets the hospital's policies and procedures (Fauchald, 2008; Vestal et al., 2008). Some hospitals use a creative approach to minimize this difficulty. For instance, Vestal, Krautwurst, and Hack (2008) reported their successful use of a designated liaison in the Department of Nursing Clinical Systems. The liaison identified the learning needs of the instructors and students who rotate through the hospital and developed educational materials that could be efficiently delivered to all nursing students and instructors. The person also enhanced some components of the EHR, which could be effectively used by the nursing instructors for the supervision of their students' practice.

Another important component of educating nurses about the use of an EHR is the inclusion of an interdisciplinary collaborative approach. When a nurse uses a system, her/his use affects many professionals in other departments because the data flows between different systems, and healthcare providers and staff from other departments must rely on their colleague's data entry in real time. In addition, when an HIT system is implemented in a hospital setting, various professionals (e.g., IT professionals, clinicians, administrators, vendors, lawyers) have to work together as a team for a prolonged period, and the system often affects many departments and professionals concurrently. Upon the completion of system deployment, the systems will continue to require management and upgrades. Learning about interdisciplinary collaboration is critical in nursing education, and is becoming more important as technology becomes more advanced and as healthcare becomes more complex.

NURSING INFORMATICS AS A SPECIALTY PROGRAM AT THE GRADUATE LEVEL

The ANA defines *Nursing Informatics* as (ANA, 2008):

"[A] specialty that integrates nursing science, computer science, and information science to manage and communicate data, information, knowledge and wisdom in nursing practice. NI supports consumers, patients, nurses, and other providers in their decision-making in all roles and settings. This support is accomplished through the use of information structures, information processes, and information technology."

The *NI Scope and Standards of Practice* clearly differentiates between informatics nurse specialists (INSs) and informatics nurses (INs). The INSs are those formally prepared at the graduate level in informatics, whereas INs are generalists who have gained on-the-job training in the field but do not have the educational preparation at the graduate level in an informatics-related area (ANA, 2008).

With the national emphasis on HIT education, various types of informatics-related educational programs are available at the graduate level, such as nursing informatics, healthcare informatics, biomedical informatics, and so on. Most informatics educational programs are moving toward online programs and/or hybrid (mainly online with some face-to-face classes) programs. The curriculum and credits vary a great deal depending on the program. The NI field also has unique characteristics. For instance, unlike other clinical nurses, the majority of colleagues of the INSs are from other disciplines, such as computer science, information management, business (vendors), or administrators (Ozbolt, Nahm, & Wilson, 2007). The roles that the INSs assume also vary (Sensmeier, 2007). In a 2009 Informatics Nurse Impact Survey (N = 432) conducted by the Healthcare Information and Management Systems Society (HIMSS), participants were asked to indicate the roles that nurses play with regard to IT (HIMSS, 2009).The findings showed the following results: user education (93%), system implementation (89%), user support (86%), workflow analysis (84%), getting buy-in from end users (80%), system design (79%), selection and placement of devices (70%), quality initiatives (69%), system optimization (62%), system selection (62%), database management and reporting (53%) (Note: only includes roles with greater than a 50% response rate).

Considering these varying roles and areas of practice, it is logical that each program may have a different emphasis or strength. Assurance of quality standards of each program, however, is particularly concerning considering that there is no regulatory body or speciality organization that could set standards for educational programs in NI.

HITECH HEALTHCARE IT ROLES

The current HITECH Act has a significant impact on the roles and competencies of HIT professionals. The ONC for Health IT has defined 12 key roles necessary to support the rollout of EHRs and the Health Information Exchange as part of the HITECH initiative to fund schools to train these professionals (U.S. DHHS, 2010a). In fact, nurses can assume most of these roles with proper preparation. The roles and educational levels delineated by the ONC would need to be considered in educating nurses in informatics.

Specific HIT professional roles requiring community college–level training:

- Practice workflow and information management redesign specialist
- Clinician/practitioner consultants
- Implementation support specialists
- Implementation managers
- Technical/software support staff and trainers
- Trainers

Specific HIT professional roles requiring university-level training:

- Clinical/public health leader
- Health information management and exchange specialist
- Health information privacy and security specialist
- Research and development scientist
- Programmer and software engineer
- Health IT subspecialist

INFORMATICS COMPETENCIES FOR FACULTY MEMBERS

Innovative technologies in teaching and learning can produce optimal outcomes only when the learners and instructors are competent in using those technologies. Previously we discussed the essential educational components needed to ensure nursing students' and practicing nurses' competencies in using HIT and managing information. Current students who grew up with technologies often outpace their faculty members in using technologies (Barton & Skiba, 2009; Skiba, 2009. Curran, Sheets, Kirkpatrick, & Bauldoff, 2007). Some faculty members struggle with not only HIT, but also emerging new technologies used in education (Barton & Skiba, 2009; Skiba, 2009). Faculty members must be properly supported to fully adopt the newest technologies (Griffin-Sobel et al., 2010).

The NLN's position paper *Preparing the Next Generation of Nurses to Practice in a Technology-rich Environment: An Informatics Agenda* specifically addresses the issue of faculty members' informatics competencies (NLM Board of Governors, 2008). It recommended that faculty members achieve informatics competencies through participation in faculty development programs and establish criteria to evaluate informatics goals for themselves. In addition, it also recommended that the school's administrative personnel ensure the faculty members' competence in computer literacy, information literacy, and informatics. Some continuing education modalities to support faculty members include half-day workshops, short refresher courses before the beginning of each semester, and online self-learning modules. If the school offers many online classes, a sufficient number of instructional design specialists should be part of the staff.

Faculty members who teach informatics must have a specific expertise in the field. With the heightened awareness of IT in healthcare and the revised essentials for the baccalaureate and DNP curriculums, increasing numbers of informatics classes are being required as core courses in nursing programs. The AACN's decision to migrate the ANP programs to the DNP level further accelerates this need. However, there is a significant shortage of faculty members who have an expertise in healthcare informatics and who can teach students (AACN, 2010b). More doctorally prepared informatics faculty members with proper education and preparation are needed in NI education.

INFORMATION TECHNOLOGY INFRASTRUCTURE OF THE SCHOOL

In the current information age, the IT infrastructure of the nursing school is critical for the success of the program and for the students' satisfaction. Current students are familiar with a high-tech environment and expect that type of environment in school as well. For instance, based on the 2009 Pew Internet survey, 63% of adult Americans now have a broadband Internet connection (Horrigan, 2009). Many public places and shops have a wireless connection. Students may expect to have a wireless connection at school and be able to connect to the EHR simulation from home for homework. Many online courses that use a video-conferencing platform for classes are often offered in the evening, requiring support staff during off-hour shifts. To maintain a supportive infrastructure, the schools must have strategic plans and establish a sufficient budget, staff, and policies and procedures. In addition, the schools must maintain clear communication with the students about their expectations of the students' individual IT requirements and the technologies available at school. It is advisable for the school to have a high-level administrative person who has expertise in IT to oversee the tasks related to the IT infrastructure of the school.

CONCLUSION

Information technology has revolutionized the current state of healthcare. Consumers now can access enormous amounts of health information online, even before they come to the hospital. Healthcare providers and students can access evidence-based health information right at the bedside. However, adoption of EHRs in healthcare has been slow, resulting in missed opportunities to provide safer and better-quality care. Recently, there has been heightened awareness of the importance of HIT in reducing medical errors and improving the efficiency of healthcare delivery. The government started to fund healthcare organizations to implement and use EHRs. This is an exciting time of change for nursing education. Face-to-face classes are being replaced by online classes, and high-tech and high-fidelity simulation-based nursing education has become a standard. New generations of nursing students are expected to be informatics competent. This chapter reviewed major HIT-related changes in our current healthcare system and efforts made by nursing organizations to reform the nursing curriculum. In the past decade, the nursing profession has made great advancements in transforming nursing practice, education, and research. Recent emphasis on interdisciplinary collaboration will further accelerate its progress.

REFERENCES

AllBusiness.com. (2009). *University of Pennsylvania School of Nursing and Eclipsys form academic partnership to bring HIT*. Retrieved from http://www.allbusiness. com/technology/software-services-applications-information/11749157-1.html.

American Association of Colleges of Nursing. (1994). *The essentials of master's education for advanced practice nursing*. Retrieved from http://www.aacn.nche.edu/education/mastessn.htm.

American Association of Colleges of Nursing. (2006a). *the essentials of doctoral education for advanced nursing practice*. Retrieved from http://www.aacn.nche.edu/DNP/pdf/Essentials.pdf.

American Association of Colleges of Nursing. (2006b). Hallmarks of quality and patient safety: Recommended baccalaureate competencies and curricular guidelines to ensure high-quality and safe patient care. *Journal of Professional Nursing, 22*(6), 329–330.

American Association of Colleges of Nursing. (2008a). *The essentials of baccalaureate education for professional nursing practice*. Retrieved from http://www.aacn.nche.edu/education/pdf/BaccEssentials08.pdf.

American Association of Colleges of Nursing. (2008b). *Task force on the essentials of master's education in nursing*. Retrieved from http://www.aacn.nche.edu/contactus/MastersEssentialsTF.htm.

American Association of Colleges of Nursing. (2010a). *The doctor of nursing practice (DNP)*. Retrieved from http://www.aacn.nche.edu/dnp.

American Association of Colleges of Nursing. (2010b). *Nursing faculty shortage: Fact sheet*. Retrieved from http://www.aacn.nche.edu/Media/Factsheets/facultyshortage.htm.

American Nurses Association. (2008). *Nursing informatics: Scope and standards of practice*. Silver Spring, MD: American Nurses Association.

American Nurses Credentialing Center. (2010). *The Magnet Recognition Program® overview*. Retrieved from http://www.nursecredentialing.org/Magnet/ProgramOverview.aspx.

Ball, M. J., Smith, C., & Bakalar, R. S. (2007). Personal health records: Empowering consumers. *Journal of Healthcare Information Management, 21*, 76–86.

Barton, A., & Skiba, D. (2009). Informatics curriculum integration for quality and safety in nursing education. In K. Saranto, P. Brennan, H. Park, M. Tallberg & A. Ensio (Eds.), *Connecting health and humans - Proceedings of NI2009 - The 10th International Congress on Nursing Informatics* (pp. 593–597). Amsterdam: IOS Press.

Blumenthal, D. (2009). Stimulating the adoption of health information technology. *The New England Journal of Medicine, 360*(15), 1477–1479.

Blumenthal, D., & Tavenner, M. (2010, August 5). The "meaningful use" regulation for electronic health records. *The New England Journal of Medicine. 363*, 501–504.

Borycki, E. M., Kushniruk, A. W., Joe, R., Armstrong, B., Otto, T., Ho, K., et al. (2009). The University of Victoria interdisciplinary electronic health record educational portal. *Studies in Health Technology and Informatics, 143*, 49–54.

Centers for Medicare & Medicaid Services. (2007). *Fact sheet: Details for Medicare and Medicaid health information technology: Title IV of the American Recovery and Reinvestment Act*. Retrieved from http://healthit.hhs.gov/portal/server.pt?open=512&objID=1325&parentname=CommunityPage&parentid=1&mode=2.

Centers for Medicare and Medicaid Services. (2010). *HIPAA - General information: Overview*. Retrieved from http://www.cms.hhs.gov/HIPAAGenInfo/01_Overview.asp.

Change.gov. (2007). *Barack Obama Presidential Announcement Speech in Springfield, IL*. Retrieved from http://change.gov/agenda/technology_agenda.

CMS.gov. (2010). *Medicare PHR choice*. Retrieved from http://www.medicare.gov/navigation/manage-your-health/personal-health-records/medicare-phr-choice.aspx.

Committee on Quality of Healthcare in America, & Institute of Medicine. (2001). *Crossing the quality chasm: A new health system for the 21st century*. Washington, DC: National Academy Press.

Cronenwett, L., Sherwood, G., Barnsteiner, J., Disch, J., Johnson, J., Mitchell, P., et al. (2007). Quality and Safety Education for Nurses. *Nursing Outlook, 55*(3), 122–131.

Cronenwett, L., Sherwood, G., & Gelmon, S. B. (2009). Improving quality and safety education: The QSEN learning collaborative. *Nursing Outlook, 57*(6), 304–312.

Cronenwett, L., Sherwood, G., Pohl, J., Barnsteiner, J., Moore, S., Sullivan, D. T., et al. (2009). Quality and safety education for advanced nursing practice. *Nursing Outlook, 57*(6), 338–348.

Curran, C., Sheets, D., Kirkpatrick, B., & Bauldoff, G. S. (2007). Virtual patients support point-of-care nursing education. *Nursing Management, 38*(12), 27–33.

Dycus, P., & McKeon, L. (2009). Using QSEN to measure quality and safety knowledge, skills, and attitudes of experienced pediatric oncology nurses: An international study. *Quality Management in Healthcare, 18*(3), 202–208.

Fauchald, S. K. (2008). An academic-industry partnership for advancing technology in health science education. *CIN: Computers, Informatics, Nursing, 26*(1), 4–8.

Gassert, C. (2000). Academic preparation in nursing informatics. . In M. J. Ball, K. J. Hannah, S. K. Newbold & J. V. Douglas (Eds.), *Nursing informatics: Where caring and technology meet* (pp. 15–32). New York, NY: Springer.

Griffin-Sobel, J. P., Acee, A., Sharoff, L., Cobus-Kuo, L., Woodstock-Wallace, A., & Dornbaum, M. (2010). A transdisciplinary approach to faculty development in nursing education technology. *Nursing Education Perspectives, 31*(1), 41–43.

Grypma, S. (2005). Florence Nightingale's changing image? Part I: Nightingale the feminist, statistician and nurse. *Journal of Christian Nursing: A Quarterly Publication of Nurses Christian Fellowship, 22*(3), 22–28.

Health Information Technology. (2010). *Meaningful use.* Retrieved from http://healthit.hhs.gov/portal/server.pt?open=512&objID=1325&parentname=CommunityPage&parentid=1&mode=2.

Healthcare Information and Management Systems Society (HIMSS). (2009). *HIMSS 2009 Informatics Nurse Impact Survey.* Retrieved from http://www.himss.org/content/files/MSS2009NursingInformaticsImpactSurveyFullResults.pdf.

Hebda, T., & Calderone, T. L. (2010). What nurse educators need to know about the TIGER Initiative. Technology Informatics Guiding Education Reform. *Nurse Educator, 35*(2), 56–60.

Horrigan, J. B. (2009). *Home broadband adoption 2009.* Retrieved from http://www.pewinternet.org/Reports/2009/10-Home-Broadband-Adoption-2009.aspx.

Institute of Medicine Committee on Health Education Profession Summit. (2002). *Health professions education: A bridge to quality.* Washington, DC: National Academy Press.

Joe, R. S., Kushniruk, A. W., Borycki, E. M., Armstrong, B., Otto, T., & Ho, K. (2009). Bringing electronic patient records into health professional education: software architecture and implementation. *Studies in Health Technology and Informatics, 150,* 888–892.

Kudzma, E. C. (2006). Florence Nightingale and healthcare reform. *Nursing Science Quarterly, 19*(1), 61–64.

Melo, D., & Carlton, K. H. (2008). A collaborative model to ensure graduating nurses are ready to use electronic health records. *CIN: Computers, Informatics, Nursing, 26*(1), 8–12.

National League for Nursing. (2008). *National League for Nursing issues call for faculty development and curricular initiatives in informatics.* Retrieved from http://www.nln.org/newsreleases/informatics_release_052908.htm.

National League for Nursing Board of Governors. (2008). *Preparing the next generation of nurses to practice in a technology-rich environment: An informatics.* Retrieved from http://www.nln.org/aboutnln/PositionStatements/informatics_052808.pdf.

Newhouse, R. P., Dearholt, S. L., Poe, S. S., Pugh, L. C., & White, K. M. (2007). *Johns Hopkins Nursing - evidence-based practice model and guidelines.* Indianapolis, Indiana: Sigma Theta Tau International.

Nguyen, H. Q., Carrieri-Kohlman, V., Rankin, S. H., Slaughter, R., & Stulbarg, M. S. (2004). Supporting cardiac recovery through eHealth technology. *Journal of Cardiovascular Nursing, 19*(3), 200–208.

Norman, C. D., & Skinner, H. A. (2006). eHEALS: The eHealth literacy scale. *Journal of Medical Internet Research, 8*(4), e27.

Otto, A., & Kushniruk, A. (2009). Incorporation of medical informatics and information technology as core components of undergraduate medical education - time for change! *Studies in Health Technology and Informatics, 143,* 62–67.

Ozbolt, J., Nahm, E.-S., Wilson, M., & Roberts, D. (2007). Careers in nursing informatics: The future is now! American Nurses Today, 2(9), 35–36.

Quality and Safety Education for Nurses (QSEN). (2010). *Quality and safety education for nurses.* Retrieved from http://www.qsen.org.

Saba, V., & McCormick, K. (2006). *Essentials of nursing informatics* (4th ed.). New York, NY: McGraw-Hill.

Sensmeier, J. (2007). Survey demonstrates importance of nurse informaticist role in health information technology design and implementation. *CIN: Computers, Informatics, Nursing, 25,* 180–182.

Skiba, D., Connors, H., & Honey, M. (2010). Growth in nursing informatics educational programs to meet demands. In C. A. Weaver, C. W. Delaney, P. Weber, & R. L. Carr (Eds.), *Nursing and informatics for the 21st century: An international look at practice, trends and the future* (2nd ed.).

Skiba, D., & Dulong, D. (2008). Using TIGER vision to move your agenda forward. *Nursing Management, 39*(3), 14–16.

Skiba, D. J. (2009). Teaching with and about technology: Providing resources for nurse educators worldwide. *Nursing Education Perspectives, 30*(4), 255–256.

Technology Informatics Guiding Education Reform. (2009). *Collaborating to integrate evidence and informatics into nursing practice and education: An executive summary.* Retrieved http://www.tigersummit.com/uploads/TIGER_Collaborative_Exec_Summary_040509.pdf.

Technology Informatics Guiding Educational Reform (TIGER). (2010). *About TIGER.* Retrieved from http://www.tigersummit.com/About_Us.html.

Technology Informatics Guiding Educational Reform (TIGER) Informatics Competencies Collaborative. (2009). *Technology Informatics Guiding Educational Reform (TIGER) Informatics Competencies Collaborative (TICC): Final report.* Retrieved from http://tigercompetencies.pbworks.com/f/TICC_Final.pdf.

The European Computer Driving Licence Foundation Ltd. (2007). *European Computer Driving License (ECDL)/International Computer Driving License (ICDL) syllabus version 5.0.* Retrieved from http://ecdl.com/programmes/files/2009/programmes/docs/20090507100415_ECDL_ICDL_Syllabus_Version_5.p.pdf.

The European Computer Driving Licence Foundation Ltd. (2010). *ECDL / ICDL: What is it?* Retrieved from http://ecdl.com/programmes/files/2009/programmes/docs/20090507100415_ECDL_ICDL_Syllabus_Version_5.p.pdf.

The HIMSS Personal Health Record Steering Committee. (2007). *HIMSS personal health records definition and position statement.* Retrieved from http://www.himss.org/content/files/PHRDefinition071707.pdf.

U.S. Bureau of Labor Statistics. (2010). *Employment projections: Labor force (demographic) data.* Retrieved from http://www.bls.gov/emp/ep_data_labor_force.htm.

U.S. Department of Health & Human Services. (2010a). *HITECH priority grants program: Health IT workforce development program.* Retrieved from http://healthit.hhs.gov/portal/server.pt?open=512&objID=1487&parentname=CommunityPage&parentid=9&mode=2&in_hi_userid=10741&cached=true.

U.S. Department of Health & Human Services. (2010b). *Privacy and security standard.* Retrieved from http://www.cms.gov/HIPAAGenInfo/04_PrivacyandSecurityStandards.asp.

U.S. DHHS Health Resources and Services Administration. (2010). *The registered nurse population: Initial findings from the 2008 National Sample Survey of Registered Nurses.* Retrieved from http://bhpr.hrsa.gov/healthworkforce/rnsurvey.

Vestal, V. R., Krautwurst, N., & Hack, R. R. (2008). A model for incorporating technology into student nurse clinical. *CIN: Computers, Informatics, Nursing, 26*(1), 2–4.

A Paradigm Shift in Simulation: Experiential Learning in Second Life

Judith J. Warren / Helen R. Connors / Patricia A. Trangenstein

• OBJECTIVES

1. Describe the use of Second Life in simulations.
2. Discuss the pedagogy of using simulations and Second Life in health professional education.
3. Compare and contrast simulation strategies for educating students in Second Life.
4. Design a simulation in Second Life.
5. Identify the administrative, faculty, and student support needed to use Second Life.

• KEY WORDS

Second Life
simulation
online education
informatics education
health professional education
virtual worlds
user computer interface

INTRODUCTION

Hundreds of leading schools and universities across the globe use Second Life (SL) as an innovative part of their educational courses and programs. Second Life is a 3-dimensional (3D) virtual world developed by Linden Lab and uniquely imagined and created by its residents. The online virtual world Second Life (www.secondlife.com) has multiple uses for teaching and learning. It enhances student engagement with course content and develops a sense of community among and between students and faculty. This virtual environment creates a powerful platform for interactive experiences that brings new dimensions to support best practices for learning. In this virtual environment, students and faculty can work together from anywhere in the world giving education a global perspective and an expanded reach.

The major challenge for online education is student engagement and the evaluation of skill attainment. Second life provides an online, virtual laboratory that solves most of this challenge. Faculty and student avatars can interact with each other, physically and verbally, in real time, thus facilitating simulations where students engage in demonstrating skill acquisition. Faculty are able to coach the skill development, as they now control the environment and can see what the student is doing. This type of evaluation in a real or simulated environment was previously unattainable in an online course. Furthermore, the environment provides a forum for student presentations and interactions with an audience. Field trips to other SL environments create opportunities to hone skills in information searching and observation of activities and settings that can be viewed by the faculty and other students. Second Life provides a virtual learning environment that only is limited by one's imagination.

Some of the advantages of student engagement in SL are active interaction, role-playing professional skills, and increased competency in learning a new skill (Hansen, 2008). The degree of immersion and interactivity available in SL allows for a greater sense of presence, which is believed to contribute to meaningful learning, especially when the course is online (Johnson, 2009; Richardson & Swan, 2003). Second Life facilitates real-time interaction between faculty and students when they are geographically apart. Furthermore, the environment can be controlled or simulated to create a learning environment desired by the faculty member to achieve pedagogical goals. These planned learning environments previously had to be in one physical place (e.g., learning laboratories, clinical facilities). Second Life supports online education by moving the geography to a virtual space, thus creating a sense of presence for the faculty and students.

The sense of presence is important while engaging in learning, regardless of whether the experience is real or virtual. *Presence* is defined as "the subjective experience of being in one place or environment, even when one is physically situated in another" (Witmer & Singer, 1998). The students feel as if they are actually in the virtual environment. A sense of immersion is also necessary for learning. *Immersion* is the sense of being enveloped by and interacting with the environment. While *involvement* is "a psychological state experienced as a consequence of focusing one's energies and attention on a coherent set of stimuli or meaningfully related activities and events" (Witmer & Singer, 1998). Second Life activities and simulations create presence and immersion for faculty and students, whether they are in traditional classes or online classes. The lack of a sense of presence has always been a major critique of online education. Now there is a tool that minimizes the sense of aloneness and distance.

Second Life, developed by Linden Lab, has been available over the Internet since 2003. Currently, there are over 16 million registered users with over 300 universities teaching courses or conducting research in SL (Michels, 2008). There are active educational special interest groups and listservs enabling faculty to share pedagogical strategies, ideas, and simulations. Within the nursing education community, there are 18 schools that have an active presence and/or own land in SL (Table 41.1).

LEARNING THEORIES THAT SUPPORT VIRTUAL WORLDS

Although it is not the purpose of this chapter to discuss learning theory in detail, it is important to know there are several learning theories that support teaching and learning in SL. To begin with, learners in SL are adults and, therefore, Malcom Knowles' (1984) theory of androgogy provides an overarching framework for designing learning activities for adult learners. Androgogy is based on the following assumptions about adult learners: (1) adults are self-directed, goal oriented, and need to know why they are required to learn something; (2) they approach learning as problem-centered rather than content-centered; (3) they need to recognize the value of learning and how to incorporate that learning into their jobs or personal lives; and (4) they learn best through experiential learning that incorporates their diverse life experiences in the development of new knowledge. Since adult learners take a great deal of responsibility for their own learning, this greatly alters the role of the faculty in learning environments in general but especially in virtual worlds such as SL. It also should be noted that environments like SL are well suited to applying the assumptions of adult learning theory; however, teachers and learners must adapt to this paradigm shift and to this new environment.

Other learning theories utilizing the principles of androgogy that educators most frequently apply to SL are experiential learning theory, social learning theory, constructivism, connectivism, and collaborative learning theory (Kolb, Boyatzis, & Mainemelis, 2000; Bandura, 1977; Bruner, 1966; Bruner, 1996; Siemens, 2004; Smith & MacGregor, 2010). Many of these theories have overlapping principles that can be mixed and matched to enhance best practices in education (Chickering & Gamson, 1987). Technology advancement and social networking tools such as SL provide rich learning environments for developing and facilitating learning activities that promote the use of these theories. In the authors' opinions, no one model fits best as it will depend upon the goals of the course as well as the teaching and learning style of the faculty and students. Also, some components of a particular theory may not be satisfied in a virtual world like SL. Today, although explosive, only the tip of the iceberg is being seen by colleges, universities, and training programs using SL. As the trend continues to grow in popularity, educators and researchers will realize the expansion of current

TABLE 41.1	University Developers of Nursing Sites	
Site	**Region**	**Slurl**
1. University of Wisconsin—Green Bay	UWGB	http://maps.secondlife.com/secondlife/UWGB Nursing Complex/112/104/21
2. Ball State	Ball State University	http://maps.Secondlife.com/secondlife/ BallStateUniversity/136/135/22
3. Boise State	EdTech	http://maps.Secondlife.com/secondlife/ EdTech.130.124.24
4. Duke	DUSON	
5. Kansas University Medical Center (KUMC)	KUMC Isle	
6. Ohio University	Ohio University	http://maps.Secondlife.com/secondlife/ OhioUniversity/50/50/26
7. University of Arizona	Arizona Island	<http://maps.Secondlife.com/secondlife/ Universityof Arizona/128/128/21>
8. Vanderbilt University School of Nursing and the University of Kentucky College of Nursing	NurSIM4U	
9. Washington State Board for Community and Technical Colleges (Tacoma Community College)	Evergreen Island	http://maps.Secondlife.com/secondlife/ EvergreenIsland/76/165/28
10. Wisconsin TECHE(University of Wisconsin Oshkosh; U of Wisconsin, Milwaukee)	Wisconsin Techne	http://maps.Secondlife.com/secondlife/ WisconsinTechne/84/80/29
11. Caledonian University Saltire Centre, Glasgow Scotland	Glasgow Caledonian	http://maps.Secondlife.com/secondlife/ GlascowCaledonian/107/106/23
12. HealthLink New York	HealthLink New York	http://maps.Secondlife.com/secondlife/ HealthLinkNewYork/188/187/25
13. Learning Commons for Nurses	Teaching 10	http://maps.Secondlife.com/secondlife/ Teaching10/152/141/37
14. Second Health Imperial College of London (University of Nottingham, U. K.)	UK Virtual Hospital	http://maps.Secondlife.com/secondlife/ ImperialCollegeLondon/150/86/27
15. SLENZ, New Zealand Tertiary Education Commission (University of Auckland)	Kowhai	http://maps.Secondlife.com/secondlife/ Kowhai/148/164/32
16. Texas State Tech. College	TSTC Commons	http://maps.Secondlife.com/secondlife/ TSTCommons/130/125/31
17. University of Michigan	Wolverine Island	
18. University of Texas Medical Branch at Galveston	UTMB Alpha, Main Campus	

theories as well as new theories and patterns of learning will be developed.

EXEMPLARS OF LEARNING IN SECOND LIFE

Orienting Faculty and Students to Second Life

Orienting faculty and students to SL should follow the precepts of experiential learning. The SL Web site has very clear directions for downloading the portal to the environment and then leads the individual through creating an avatar. Encourage students to engage in this experience of downloading software and creating an avatar by letting them know they are developing health informatics competencies. An orientation to participating is SL also is needed. Within directions for this exercise, a possible statement to achieve this purpose may be:

"Second Life is an immersive virtual environment. An avatar is a user's self-representation in the form of a 3-dimensional model. In Second Life, creating your avatar is part of how you will interact with

TABLE 41.2	Resources for Orienting New Second Life Userst
Resources for orienting new SL users	**Urls and Slurls**
Virtual Ability, virtualability.org/default.aspx	If you have an SL account, teleport to slurl.com/secondlife/Virtual%20 Ability/170/99/22
YouTube videos created by Virtual Ability	Part One: www.youtube.com/watch?v=XAjG4Tv6LvU
	Part Two: www.youtube.com/watch?v=AVzyi0MOsJM&feature=related
	Part Three: www.youtube.com/watch?v=Cnyt6rASfo0&feature=related
New Media Consortium (NMC) Virtual World, virtualworlds.nmc.org	If you have an SL account, teleport to slurl.com/secondlife/NMC%20 Orientation/106/113/39
Getting Started in Second Life by Savin-Bade, Tombs, White, Poulton, Kavia, and Woodham	www.jisc.ac.uk/publications/generalpublications/2009/ gettingstartedsecondlife.aspx

other residents. Some people design their avatar as a life-like representation of self. As the popularity of Second Life grows, many professional meetings occur in this virtual world; please dress you avatar in casual or professional clothes. The user controls the avatar through the use of the mouse or keyboard to walk, fly, and sit. An avatar can interact with other avatars through instant messages or the audio function (using a headset)."

Once the avatar is created there are several video tutorials to teach students how to navigate their avatars in SL, see Table 41.2 for suggestions. Upon completion of the tutorials, the faculty and student avatars should be ready to enter SL. During the first SL activity, a support person, knowledgeable in SL technology, should be available to trouble shoot problems with software and microphone use. After the first SL experience, students are ready to engage in more activities and openly share their enthusiasm for this type of interaction. As faculty begin to envision more activities, they will need additional support to make these happen without having to take time to become experts in using and building in SL.

The University of Kansas School of Nursing Experience

For the University of Kansas School of Nursing (KUSON), since a teaching, learning, and technology (TLT) infrastructure was already in place with 4 instructional designers and 3 technology specialists for the campus, the first step was to discuss the desire to use SL in the graduate health informatics program. The Director of our TLT support group was very familiar with the educational potential of virtual worlds. He had a presence in SL and knew of other faculty in the physical therapy and nurse anesthesia programs who

were ready to move to an "inworld" with their educational programs. Involving the TLT support group from the beginning assured faculty that the technology infrastructure was in place to support the teaching and learning needs. Faculty worked closely with TLT to established some goals and objectives for teaching in SL and to get started by purchasing the necessary land to build the program. Virtual land in SL is space where one can build your learning environment to support learning events and activities. For KUSON's purposes, it was decided to purchase an island or private region and call the space KUMC (University of Kansas Medical Center) Isle (Figure 41.1). An island or private region allows for restricted access and other levels of control not available on the virtual mainland. This was important for the academic mission. The cost of the KUMC Island was $700.00 for initial setup and $147.50 per month for monthly maintenance. These costs are shared by the School of Nursing and the School of Allied Health. Other costs include the cost for materials to build the various learning environments. As in real life, these costs can vary according to your needs and desires. Collaboration among the campus academic programs helps to set standards and create academic environments that are efficient and effective as well as model the real world academic environment. After the success experienced in health informatics, physical therapy, and nurse anesthesia, the undergraduate nursing program began to use SL to broaden the experience of students and as a strategy for teaching informatics competencies.

Graduate Health Informatics Program

Learning to be a health informaticist requires developing skills identifying use cases and workflows in clinical environments. These are experiential skills multiple states and time zones. Virtual reality environments, like SL, provided the online platform for simulations to experience and practice informatics skills. Second Life was selected as the simulation environment for our online health informatics graduate program. These simulations facilitate the development of informatics competencies for future work environments.

The curriculum, among other skills, teaches information system design and database development. An SL simulation was constructed to facilitate learning these skills. The faculty designed the Jayhawk Community Living Center (JCLC), an assisted living facility, for the simulation. The JCLC was designed to include rooms for 6 residents, a day room, dining room, clinic room, nurses' station, medical records room, medication room, director's office, and conference room. Landscaping, including a deck over the water surrounding our island, was also provided to enhance the reality of the simulation (Figure 41.2). Cues concerning information system requirements were placed in various locations within the center so that students practiced observing the environment. Some of these cues were multiple telephones for residents, computer locations for staff, and floor plans for workflows. Faculty played the roles of Director of Nursing and staff nurse.

The purpose of the simulation is to design a fall-risk management information system for the JCLC. This would be the first electronic health record for the JCLC. Students are given a Request for Proposal and information about falls: evidence-based protocols, workflows and policies for the management of fall risk, and resident

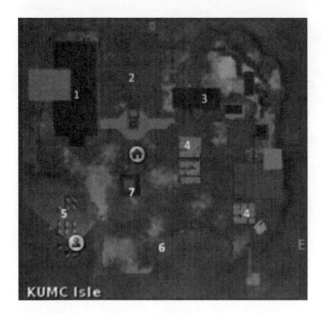

• **FIGURE 41.1.** KUMC Isle with the designed learning areas: (1) Jayhawk Community Living Center, (2) Virtual KU Center for Health Informatics and Nurse Anesthesia Suite, (3) Row Houses and Wellness Center buildings, (4) Poster Pavilions, (5) Amphitheater, (6) The Beach, and (7) Orientation Pavilion.

and are difficult to master in an online environment. Simulations and clinical experiences are the traditional approaches for teaching these skills, yet are not feasible in online courses where students reside in

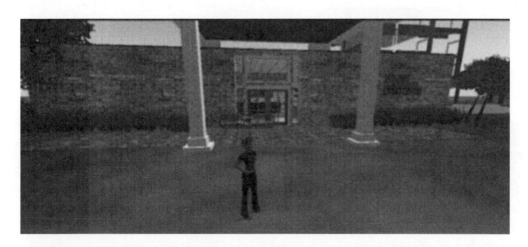

• **FIGURE 41.2.** The Jayhawk Community Living Center.

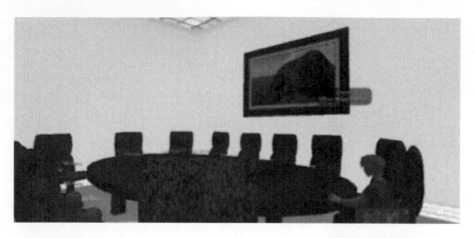

• **FIGURE 41.3** Conference room of the Director of Nursing with Director Ellipse Wrigglesworth seated.

data concerning fall risk. Their first task is to meet with the Director of Nursing in her conference room to clarify the requirements for the information system. This meeting is conducted through text messaging within SL so that a transcript of the meeting is available for analysis (Figure 41.3).

Next the students are taken on a tour of the JCLC, as they would be in real life, to observe and ask questions to clarify the requirements for the fall-risk information system. Students must design the entire system—architecture, software, Internet access, security and confidentiality constraints, and other relevant system functions. The deliverables for the design are storyboards,

use cases, use-case diagrams, workflow diagrams, and activity diagrams for both current and future states.

In the database theory course, the students return to the JCLC to design and build an access database for the fall-risk management assessments. They must work with the staff again to determine database table structures (conceptual, logical, and physical data models), data entry forms, standard data queries, required reports, and training needs. This time the cues are very important, as the students must realize that each resident has 2 telephones that must be in the database as well as other physical cues regarding data collection and input (Figure 41.4). This is a common problem in

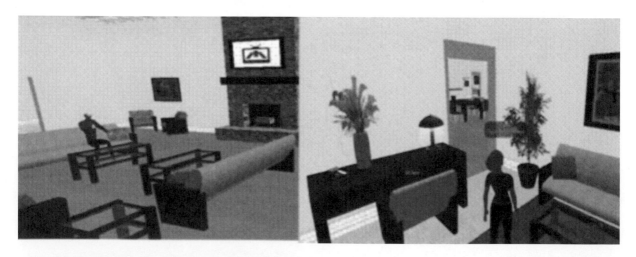

• **FIGURE 41.4.** Resident in the lounge talking on a cell phone and a resident sitting room with phone on the desk.

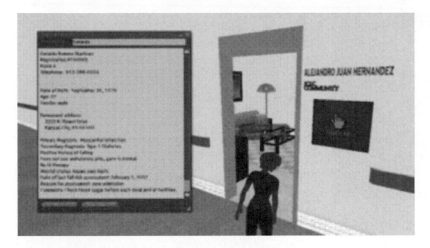

• **FIGURE 41.5.** "Touch Me" cards with resident information to be placed in the database.

database design. Information concerning each resident is posted on a "Touch Me" card outside the resident's room (Figure 41.5). The database produced by the students must contain all the information and address each design challenge embedded in the simulation.

Students enjoy the experience, request more class time in SL, and successfully develop informatics projects. SL is a great way to simulate a facility so students can learn to elicit user requirements for information systems. The challenges are scheduling meeting times, managing group interactions, practicing etiquette in group interactions, and learning to use the technology of SL.

Students present posters in SL as a way to demonstrate learning. Many of the presentations are about usability and design issues, system security approaches, federal regulations impacting the discipline of informatics, database management systems, and so forth. The simulation helps them to learn to put together a poster and answer questions of attendees at the poster session. A poster pavilion module was created with 6 poster boards (Figure 41.6). This module can be recreated to host as many presenters as is required. Figure 41.1 shows that the Isle is currently set up with 3 pavilions.

Course Evaluations

A serendipitous finding in using SL was using The Beach on KUMC Isle as a place to celebrate the end of a course and for students to share with faculty what worked and what didn't work. Early on, students suggested adjourning to the beach after the last

class. Faculty facilitated the meeting and engaged the students in informal discussions about the use of SL. Students shared their enthusiasm for SL and then began to share perspectives on the course. The informal environment, outside the course, encouraged very productive discussions that lead faculty to change several course strategies. Now after every course, a Beach Party is conducted to debrief the course. Students continue to be very professional in their desire to help the courses evolve into highly successful experiences. The Beach is shown in Figure 41.7.

Use of Second Life in Undergraduate Nursing Courses

The undergraduate nursing courses use SL in 3 major ways. First, by having students download the portal to

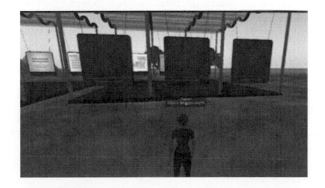

• **FIGURE 41.6.** Poster Pavilions.

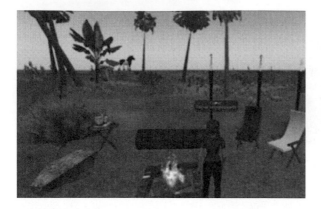

• **FIGURE 41.7.** The Beach, complete with palm trees, fire pit, places to sit, and tiki torches.

TABLE 41.3	SLURLs for Health-Related Places to Visit)
1. Centers for Disease Control Island, slurl.com/secondlife/CDC%20Island/191/86/22	
2. HealthInfo Island, slurl.com/secondlife/Healthinfo%20 Island/127/154/22	
3. Agoraphobia Support Headquarters, slurl.com/secondlife/Neptune/125/108/27	
4. Breast Cancer Network of Strength, slurl.com/secondlife/Association%20Works/236/155/27	
5. National Health Service, slurl.com/secondlife/National%20Health%20Service/167/27/27	
6. Ohio State University Health Island, slurl.com/secondlife/OSU%20Medicine/100/92/26	
7. Virtual Hallucinations, slurl.com/secondlife/Sedig/26/43/22	
8. Second Life Medical Library, slurl.com/secondlife/Healthinfo+Island/171/204/26	
9. Second Health London, slurl.com/secondlife/UK%20Virtual%20Hospital/144/115/24	
10. Second Health Hospital, slurl.com/secondlife/Second%20Health%20London/127/220/25	
11. Polomar West Hospital, slurl.com/secondlife/PalomarWest%20Hospital/120/134/35	
12. Biomedical Research Island, slurl.com/secondlife/Biomedicine%20Research%20Labs/53/169/22	
13. TLC Babies Maternity Pediatric Clinic New Orleans, slurl.com/secondlife/New%20Orleans/60/62/23	
14. PJ Maternity, slurl.com/secondlife/Paradise/163/179/602	
15. Virtual Cancer Institute, slurl.com/secondlife/ISN%20VISIONS/184/110/26	
16. Autistic Liberation Front, slurl.com/secondlife/Porcupine/29/177/107	
17. Cystic Fibrosis, slurl.com/secondlife/BOOMER%20ISLAND/95/143/27	
18. Center for Hope (Grief and Loss), slurl.com/secondlife/Topaz%20Square/85/20/25	
19. Lyme Disease, slurl.com/secondlife/Bella%20Isola/249/235/21	

SL and create avatars, they demonstrate computer and informatics competencies. Second, scavenger hunts are created as a way to teach health information literacy skills. (See Table 41.3 for health-related SL sites.) The students are given slurls (locations in SL) of these sites and asked to teleport there and to locate information relating to the assignment. KUSON guides the student to appropriate locations to decrease the stress of interacting in a new environment. Third, students present their findings in the Poster Pavilion, demonstrating presentation skills. An advantage of presenting in SL is that faculty do not have to find the physical space or the poster boards to host this session, plus students find this to be a fun activity.

Use of Second Life in Doctoral Nursing Courses

During the first semester, all doctoral students enroll in a technology and informatics course. This course is designed to assist the student in developing skills to complete an online doctoral program. Second Life is one of several Web 2.0 programs introduced to the students. Formal presentations of team projects are required. Students use instant messaging and SL to meet as a team to organize the work of their projects, thus enhancing their informatics skills. The presentations are conducted in the amphitheater, using microphones and speakers. Students are able to see the audience, pace the presentation, and answer questions just as they would in the real world. These students also enjoy the Beach Party at the end of the course and have helped to make this course very popular (Figures 41.8, 41.9, and 41.10).

Use of Second Life in Physical Therapy and Nurse Anesthesia Courses

Physical therapy students go into SL to evaluate the home of a disabled client. There are a series of 3 homes with different hazards to be identified. Students are given a patient record with information concerning the patient's abilities and disabilities. They then conduct a walk through and make recommendations for creating a safer home environment. Faculty control the visual cues and hazards, and so know when the students make

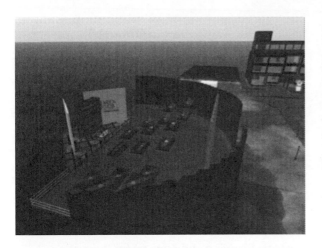

• **FIGURE 41.8.** The Amphitheater used for formal presentations.

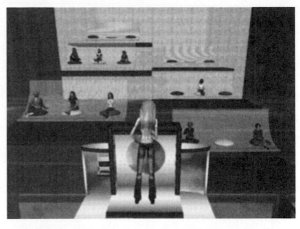

• **FIGURE 41.10.** Students interacting with the audience.

accurate assessments and are ready to make real home evaluations (Figures 41.11 and 41.12).

The nurse anesthesia faculty use SL to teach the students how an operating room is organized. Students learn how to move through the operating room and practice organizational skills for the anesthesia role. Some of the equipment is designed to be interactive so the students can manipulate them and gain confidence prior to participating in a real operating room environment.

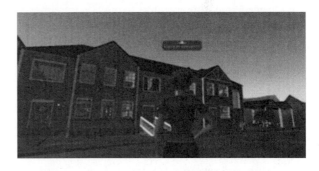

• **FIGURE 41.11.** The Row houses for home evaluations.

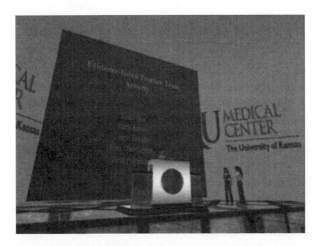

• **FIGURE 41.9.** Students giving the presentation and using slides.

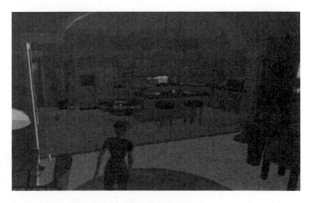

• **FIGURE 41.12.** Living room and kitchen of one of the row houses, showing safety hazards.

Administrative Considerations: Creating a Supportive Environment

Educational innovation is a process of bringing new teaching strategies to satisfied learners and future knowledge workers. It is a conversion of new knowledge into value-added outcomes enhanced by novel teaching strategies. Innovation in education involves not only technological advances, but also pedagogical approaches.

Most innovative educators are beginning to recognize and experiment with the educational possibilities of virtual worlds. Also, student enthusiasm for these learning formats is strong, creating uniquely powerful interactive and compelling educational possibilities. At the same time, for many faculty members, teaching in SL can be daunting. Learning the new technology, meeting the needs of the technologically diverse students, understanding virtual reality pedagogy, and managing workload and time are some of the challenges. It is up to academic administrators to provide the support and resources to encourage faculty to use new technologies such as Second life and to continue to use these emerging technologies. The goal is to minimize organizational barriers to student and faculty success. Challenges at the organizational level need to be anticipated and policies, procedures, and guidelines should be in place to help mitigate their impact on faculty and students. Faculty who desire to use SL need to be heard, to feel supported, and to have an infrastructure in place that not only supports the present, but allows for growth and rewards faculty's efforts. Creating a supportive environment for successful adaptation of innovative teaching strategies requires resources, but, more importantly, it requires a cultural shift for many academic institutions.

A Culture of Innovation. As technology advances, today's learning environment needs to convey a culture of innovation and strategically plan to meet the challenge of change. Every academic organization has a culture; the issue is whether and how that organization supports innovation. A culture of innovation gives you a competitive edge because it makes you more nimble with an increased ability to respond to change. To be successful, a culture of innovation should reflect a balance between an openness to allow ideas to flow, and the creation of controls and supports around those ideas.

Academia is steeped in a tradition of hierarchical beliefs where research and scholarship is rewarded and educational innovation is not. To fully integrate a culture of innovation within the organization, key concepts of innovation need to be reflected in the organization's mission, vision, leadership, core values, hiring practices, metrics, rewards, and compensation. The concepts call for new interactions and partnerships involving a team approach to teaching and learning. Also, success requires clear communication from leadership that describes how the institution understands educational innovation and that understanding should be built into the organizational behavior and modeled by the leader. Faculty and staff in this environment should feel comfortable and supported to take risks without fear of failure or retribution. As Melnyk and Davidson (2009) point out, "success in an innovative culture is viewed as going from one failure to the next with enthusiasm" (p. 2).

Strategic Planning and Support for Innovation

In the early 1990s, the University of Kansas Medical Center (KUMC) Division of Information Resources, in collaboration with the Schools of Medicine, Nursing and Allied Health, and the Division of Continuing Education, embarked on a strategic planning process to position the academic environment for the new wave of technology-based education. This planning process resulted in the formation of a re-envisioned academic support department—the Department of Teaching and Learning Technologies (TLT). The department is housed within the KUMC Information Resource Division. Central to it's mission, the department has evolved over time to support new and diverse technologies. The mission of the TLT department is: "working collaboratively with the schools and campus support units, the Teaching & Learning Technologies department provides KUMC faculty, staff, students, and community with leadership and support for the successful integration of new and existing educational technology into KUMC learning environments." The vision is for KUMC to be "a recognized leader in using technology to enrich and transform the teaching and learning experience. KUMC faculty, staff, students, and community have dependable access to core teaching and learning technologies as well as the knowledge, skills, and support to be successful with those tools. They are also aware of promising new technologies, and they have both the technical and pedagogical support to explore and evaluate the educational possibilities of these tools. As these technologies mature, those with the greatest potential to enhance teaching and learning are integrated into our core technologies, establishing a pattern of innovation and success." This infrastructure, which includes 4 instructional designers and 3 technology specialists, has served the Medical Center campus well over the ensuing years as educational technologies advanced and became more affordable and acceptable. Key to our success is the partnership between faculty and the TLT staff to design, develop, and implement courses using enhanced technologies and to work collaboratively across KUMC academic programs to develop a community of technology educators who share ideas and challenge each other. One of these newer technologies is SL, which KUMC uses for communication, presentations, and learning activities.

School of Nursing Administrative Support

The School of Nursing (SON) administration fully supports teaching in SL and serves as a liaison between the faculty and the TLT administrator to assure academic innovation and maintain quality and integrity of academic programs. Clear communication about faculty's pedagogical needs is essential to good outcomes and assures faculty the support they need. Faculty who are champions in this new learning environment need to be encouraged to take risks and should be rewarded for their efforts. By late in the 1990s, the SON revised its appointment, promotion, and tenure criteria, using Boyer's model of scholarship, to reflect the value of innovation in education, practice, and research. Boyer (1997) proposed an expanded definition of *scholarship* within the professorate based on 4 functions: discovery, integration, application, and teaching. He argues that all forms of scholarship should be recognized and rewarded, and that this will lead to more personalized and flexible criteria for gaining tenure. Boyer proposes using "creativity contracts" that emphasize quality and innovation in teaching, while fostering professional growth that supports individuals and their passions. A balanced focus on all forms of scholarship is critical to meet the challenges in creating and sustaining innovative academic programs. Using this model, faculty are encouraged, supported, and rewarded for risk taking, pilot testing, and design thinking in their teaching practices.

Searching for nursing sites in SL is a challenge, as the search engine does not distinguish between nursing and breastfeeding. For scholarly work to be recognized in SL, it is incumbent on the faculty to create profiles that support accurate search strategies. A barrier to identifying nursing education's immersion in SL is the lack of any standardized template as to what to include in descriptions of regions or groups or in individual profiles. A consensus within nursing users of SL as to a standardized approach to listing information would vastly improve search capabilities. A template similar to the one used by the SLHealthy

wiki (2009) could be adopted and might contain the following information: group or SIM name, purpose, contact information, educational activities provided, target audience, open to all or closed (except to members), special or unique features, related blogs, wikis and other outworld content, tags and keywords, and additional comments. In addition, many simulations could be observed by other users if YouTube videos were posted that describe and provide greater insight into select simulations.

The technology service support in the SON is another example of administration's support for the use of SL and other technology-supported practices. These services include an advanced technology environment for all faculty and staff, coordinated with all of the services at the KUMC campus level. The SON supports 2 dedicated professionals who exclusively serve the technology needs of the school. The lead person is a network engineer who manages the school's file servers and other advanced technologies and is assisted by a person who provides local desktop assistance, database programming, and video-conferencing assistance to assist faculty teaching with a wide variety of technologies. The school's support staff also provides services such as notebook computer support for faculty and staff, assistance in purchasing hardware and software to support research and educational innovation, and assistance with handheld computing devices. Teaching in SL requires a computer with hefty specs to run properly. Through these technology services and futuristic planning, the SON assures that faculty have what it takes to successfully teach in SL (see Table 41.4 for resources).

Faculty are the most important factor in the overall success of using SL and other innovative teaching strategies. If faculty feel well supported (technology, design, administrative) and have a voice in determining policies and procedures for fostering innovative environments, they will be more willing to move "in-world" with SL. Specifically, faculty need training, professional development, and release time for initial increased workload and design issues. Since faculty work collaboratively with instructional design and technology specialists, recognize that training needs shift from training faculty on software to training them on new teaching approaches, instructional design strategies, and workload management topics. Keep in mind that virtual worlds may not be for everyone; work with your champions and let them be the driver and set the standard. Celebrate your successes by having your champions showcase their work at faculty meetings and professional development sessions.

TABLE 41.4	Faculty Resources for Learning More About Second Life
Articles	Innovate (innovateonline.info/?view=issue) contains several articles on Second Life and the use of virtual worlds in education. Check out the June/July 2009 and the August/September 2009 issues.
	Boulos, M, Hetherington, L., & Wheeler, S. (2007). Second Life: An overview of the potential of 3-D virtual worlds in medical and health education. *Health Information and Libraries Journal, 24*(4), 233–245.
	Davis, A., Khazanchi, D., Murphy, J., Zigurs, I, & Owens, D. (2009). Avatars, people, and virtual worlds: Foundations for research in metaverses. *Journal of the Association for Information Systems, 10*(2) 90–117.
	Harrison, D. (2009, February 18). Real-life teaching in a virtual world. *Campus Technology.* Retrieved from http://campustechnology.com/Articles/2009/02/18/Real-Life-Teaching-in-a-Virtual-World.aspx.
	Ongley, J. (2009, October). Education by avatar at the University of Hawaii. Retrieved from http://www.hawaii.edu/malamalama/2009/10/second-life.
	Skiba, D. (2007). Emerging Technology Center: Nursing education 2.0: Second Life. *Nursing Education Perspectives, 28*(3), 156–157.
	Skiba, D. (2009). Nursing education 2.0: A second look at Second Life. *Nursing Education Perspectives, 30*(2), 129–131.
	Woodford, P. (2007, March 30). Medicine's not-so-secret Second Life: Public health education thrives in so-called virtual worlds. *National Review of Medicine, 4*(6). Retrieved from http://www.nationalreviewofmedicine.com/issue/2007/03_30/4_advances_medicine_6.htmlChapter41 Warren_Final_Chapter_SecondLife_8-6-10.DOCX.
	Journal of Virtual Worlds Research. Available at http://jvwresearch.org/index.php?_cms=default,3,0.
Books	Boellstorff, T. (2008). *Coming of age in second life: An anthropologist explores the virtually human.* Princeton, NJ: Princeton University Press.
	Krotoski, A., Cezanne, P., Rymaszewski, M., Rossignol, J., Wagner, & Au, J. (2008). *Second Life: The official guide* (2nd ed.). New York: John Wiley & Sons.
	Bell, M., & Robbins, S. (2008). *Second life For dummies.* New York: John Wiley & Sons.
	Bruns, A. (2008). *Blogs, Wikipedia, Second Life, and beyond: From production to produsage.* New York: Peter Lang Pub Inc.
	Weber, A, Rufer-Bach, K, Platel, R. (2007). *Creating your world: The official guide to advanced content creation for Second Life.* New York: John Wiley & Sons.
	Percival, S. (2007). *Second Life: In-world travel guide.* Indianapolis, IN: Que Publishing.

CONCLUSIONS

Second Life is an environment that can provide valuable educational experiences in nursing. The degree of immersion and interactivity available provides a greater sense of presence, contributing to better learning outcomes in both in-person and online courses. Faculty and staff are able to engage their creativity to provide dynamic simulations for students in a novel, virtual world. The outcomes are well worth the effort and resources required to produce high-quality learning experiences.

REFERENCES

Boyer, E. L. (1997). *Scholarship reconsidered: Priorities of the professoriate.* San Francisco: Jossey-Bass.

Bandura, A.(1977). *Social learning theory.* New York: General Learning Press.

Bruner, J. (1966). *Towards a theory of instruction.* Cambridge, MA: Harvard University Press.

Bruner, J. (1996). *The culture of education.* Cambridge, MA: Harvard University Press.

Chickering, A.E., & Gamson, Z. F. (1987). Seven principles for good practice in undergraduate education. *AAHE Bulletin, 39*(7), 3–6.

Hansen, M. M. (2008). Versatile, immersive, creative and dynamic virtual 3-D healthcare learning environments: A review of the literature. *Journal of Medical Internet Research, 10*(3), 26.

Johnson, C. M. (2009). Virtual worlds in healthcare higher education. *Journal of Virtual Worlds Research. 2*(2), 3–12.

Knowles, M. (1984). *The adult learner: A neglected species* (3rd ed.). Houston, TX: Gulf Publishing.

Kolb, D., Boyatzis, R., & Mainemelis, C. (2000). Experiential learning theory: Previous research and new directions. In R. J. Sternberg, & L.F. Zhang (Eds.), *Perspectives on cognitive, learning and thinking styles*. NJ: Lawrence Erlbaum.

Melnyk, B. M., & Davidson, S. (2009). Creating a culture of innovation in nursing education through shared vision, leadership, interdisciplinary partnerships, and positive deviance. *Nursing Administration Quarterly, 33*(4), 288–295.

Michels, P. (2008, February 26).Universities use Second Life to teach complex concepts. *Government Technologies*, Retrieved from http://www.govtech.com/gt/252550?topic=118264.

Richardson, J.C., & Swan, K. (2003). Examining social presence in online courses in relation to students' perceived learning and satisfaction. *Journal of Asynchronous Learning: 7*(1), 68–88.

Siemens,G. (2004, December 12). Connectivism: A learning theory for the digital age. *Elearnspace*. Retrieved from http://www.elearnspace.org/Articles/connectivism.htm.

SLHealthy. (n.d.) Retrieved from the SLHealthy Wiki: http://slhealthy.wetpaint.com.

Smith, B. L. & MacGergor, J. T. (1992). *What is collaborative learning?* Retrieved from http://learningcommons.evergreen.edu/pdf/collab.pdf.

Whitmer, B. G., & Singer, M.J. (1998). Measuring presence in virtual environments: A presence questionnaire. *Presence. 7*(3): 229–240.

42

The TIGER Initiative

Michelle R. Troseth

- OBJECTIVES
  1. Discuss the TIGER Initiative agenda.
  2. Describe the different phases of the TIGER Initiative.
  3. Describe examples of how TIGER Initiative efforts have created changes that impact the future of nursing.

- KEY WORDS

  Decade of Healthcare Technology
  Sense of Urgency
  Grassroots Effort
  Technology Informatics Guiding Education Reform
  Invitational Summit
  Collaborative Workgroups
  Virtual Learning Environment

INTRODUCTION

This chapter describes a wonderful story about what can occur when individuals committed to a common cause come together and take action. The best part is that this story has no end; the roots of the Technology Informatics Guiding Education Reform (TIGER) Initiative are already deeply embedded and causing significant effects across the healthcare industry. The work that is being accomplished through TIGER is now being cited as a significant catalyst in addressing the Institute of Medicine's (IOM's) calls for healthcare transformation, which came in the form of their landmark reports *Crossing the Quality Chasm* (2001) and *Health Professional Education: A Bridge to Quality* (2003). These reports addressed major changes needed for both practicing clinicians and educators. Addressing practicing clinicians, the 2001 report notes that, "The use of tools to organize and deliver care has lagged far

behind biomedical and clinical knowledge. Carefully designed, evidence-based care processes, supported by automated clinical information and decision support systems, offer the greatest promise of achieving the best outcomes from care for chronic conditions. Systems must facilitate the application of scientific knowledge to practice, and provide clinicians with the tools and supports necessary to deliver evidence-based care consistently and safely" (Institute of Medicine [IOM], 2001, p. 12). Addressing educators, the 2003 report called for new ways for health professions to be educated and identified 5 core competencies for all healthcare professionals: (1) provide patient-centered care, (2) work in interdisciplinary teams, (3) employ evidence-based practice, (4) apply quality improvement, and (5) utilize informatics (IOM, 2003, p. 3). Both of these reports, along with the federal efforts described below to address the need for widespread health information technology (HIT) adoption, were the catalysts for the beginning of the TIGER Initiative and its continued evolution.

THE DECADE OF HEALTHCARE TECHNOLOGY (2004)

National HIT Agenda

In early 2004, U.S. President George W. Bush declared the "Decade for Health Information Technology" and created the Office of the National Coordinator of Health Information Technology (ONC). In May 2004, Secretary of Health and Human Services, Tommy Thompson, appointed Dr. David Brailer as the first National Health Information Technology Coordinator. This was an exciting time for health professionals committed to the transformational role health information could play in improving in safety, efficiency, and other health reform efforts. In July 2004, Brailer convened the first National Health Information Technology Summit in Washington, DC and launched a strategy to provide U.S. citizens with the benefits of an electronic health record within 10 years.

Where is Nursing?

A very important observation was made at this first ONC event. The nation's 3 million nurses, who comprise up to 55% of the healthcare workforce, were not represented and/or clearly identified as an integral part of achieving the ONC's vision and implementing it's strategy. It left many begging the question, "Where is nursing?" There was keen awareness that without nursing engagement, the National HIT Agenda would be at risk and nursing would miss the wonderful opportunity to significantly advance the plan to transform healthcare practice and education with evidence and informatics. Kotter, in his books *Leading Change* (1996) and *A Sense of Urgency* (2008), describes the impact that a true sense of urgency can have on large-scale, effective change. When the sense of urgency is as high as possible and among as many people as possible, the greater the successes of leading transformational change efforts will be. Leaders in nursing realized the sense of urgency to begin a grassroots effort following this initial HIT summit and moved to birth a movement that would assure nursing was at the table as key stakeholders and advocates while HIT was integrated into the nation's healthcare delivery systems and academic programs.

THE BIRTH OF THE TIGER INITIATIVE (2005)

Challenges and Opportunities Facing Nursing

The grassroots leadership efforts began to take action, networking with others to determine first steps and gathering key individuals to attend the first TIGER meeting. The first official TIGER gathering was held on January 14, 2005, hosted by Johns Hopkins University School of Nursing. A diverse group of nursing leaders across the country engaged in conversation about the skills and knowledge needed by healthcare providers and nurses in the 21st century. Trends and patterns on topics such as basic skills, critical thinking, change management, evidence-based practice, knowledge workers, curriculum integration, professional practice, interdisciplinary collaborative practice, leadership, global military systems, national standards, clinical documentation, public policy, and more emerged as current challenges and opportunities facing nurses during this informatics revolution. These nurses realized that the opportunity was more than just tackling informatics; the focus also needed to be on high-quality and evidence-based care. TIGER presented a unique window of opportunity to build on the successes of informatics and connect more key stakeholders in an effort to make large strides in guiding true transformation. Lastly, finding ways to engage the power of the 3 million nurses in the healthcare workforce was crucial for moving the TIGER agenda forward. It was decided to hold an invitational summit in an effort to bring together a diverse group of stakeholders (e.g., professional organizations, governmental organizations, technology vendors, informatics specialists) to further advance the sense of urgency and actions needed to ensure that nurses were able to provide safe, efficient, and patient-centered care to all. At that time, questions were raised concerning whether the summit should include all disciplines to help meet the IOM aims and competencies. While this was recognized as being very important, there was consensus that it was critical to begin with moving the nursing workforce forward first, and then to expand out as recommendations were made from the summit.

Setting the Vision for TIGER

The following vision statement and expected outcomes were developed to guide the TIGER Initiative:

TIGER Vision

- Allow informatics tools, principles, theories, and practices to be used by nurses to make healthcare safer, effective, efficient, patient-centered, timely, and equitable.
- Interweave enabling technologies transparently into nursing practice and education, making information technology the stethoscope for the 21st century.

TIGER Expected Outcomes

- Publish a summit report, including summit findings and exemplars of excellence.
- Establish guidelines for organizations to follow as they integrate informatics knowledge, skills, and abilities into academic and practice settings.
- Set an agenda whereby the nursing organizations specify what they plan to do to bridge the quality chasm via information technology strategies.

THE TIGER SUMMIT (2005)

See Figure 42.1.

The Invitational Summit

To prepare for the invitational summit, a program committee was formed over a year in advance to plan the event. A fundraising committee was also formed to secure funds to support the TIGER Summit and expected outcomes. Over 25 diverse sponsors made contributions to the summit, including grants received from the Agency for Healthcare Research and Quality (AHRQ), Robert Wood Johnson Foundation (RWJF), and the National Library of Medicine (NLM).

The invitational summit was held at the end of October in 2006 and was hosted by the Uniformed Services University of the Health Sciences in Bethesda, MD. Over 100 leaders from the nation's nursing administration, practice, education, and informatics; technology organizations; governmental agencies; and other key stakeholders participated in the very interactive 2-day summit. External facilitators from Bonfire Communications created an open-space experience that included small and large group dialogues; unique graphic art to capture the vision, outcomes of the dialogues, and action plans; and the use of an audience response system (ARS) to capture current realities as well as gain consensus. To stimulate imagination and thinking, the first included a Gallery Walk experience in which participants were able to walk through and review cutting-edge technology and clinical decision support systems being utilized in healthcare environments today.

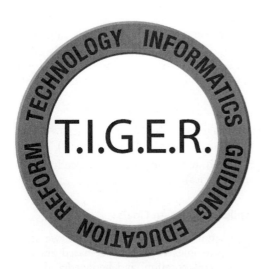

• **FIGURE 42.1. TIGER SUMMIT LOGO**

National Exemplars

The TIGER Executive and Program Committee felt it was important to build on some national exemplars in practice and education today. A total of 7 national exemplars were shared, with time for questions and answers from participants. For example, two chief nursing officers representing different health systems (Holmes Regional Medical Center, Palm Bay Community Hosptial and Cape Canaveral Hospitals of the HealthFirst system in Florida and Rush-Copley Medical Center of Illinois) presented one of the best practice exemplars. Their presentation highlighted the successes of multiple settings implementing a common professional practice framework as part of a large international healthcare consortium that is integrated into HIT vendor applications to support professional workflow, evidence-based practice, interdisciplinary integration, and patient-centered care. Demonstrated outcomes such as decreased patient falls, decreased pressure ulcers, decreased ventilator-associated pneumonia, and increased nursing satisfaction were shared.

The Informatics for Advanced Nursing program at Columbia University stands out as a best practice exemplar in education. The program merges curriculum and informatics tools to foster competency development and, ultimately, safe, evidence-based care. Their presentation at the summit covered various generations of applications that support nurse practitioners, including handheld devices, decision support, hazard and near-miss reporting, and tobacco cessation, along with key information resources. Some of the valuable lessons learned include the importance of organizational buy-in, user support, evolving technologies, funding, and expertise.

Developing a 10-Year Vision and 3-Year Action Plan

The entire summit was focused on creating movement toward consensus on a 10-year vision and 3-year action plan. First, the group did collective work around 7 defined pillars. From there, the significant patterns and most salient points were extracted through content streaming. This process helped to clearly evolve the 10-year vision. With the 7 pillars of nursing and rich content as its framework, the participants identified a 3-year action plan to achieve the 10-year vision of evidence and informatics transforming practice and education. This required intense group work and collaboration among the participants.

The last call for action before participants left the summit was for each leader of a participating organization to identify definable action plan goals that they could take back to their organizations. Each participant signed the TIGER Commitment Wall to show their commitment to the TIGER vision and action plans, as well as to continue to promote and engage others in the TIGER Initiative.

Following the TIGER Summit, a Web site was established (www.tigersummit.com) to record the several events and actions that arose as well as to post new information. In addition, the summit report *Evidence and Informatics Transforming Nursing: 3-Year Action Steps toward a 10-Year Vision* (TIGER, 2007) was developed and widely distributed as both a published report and a pdf download from the TIGER Summit Web site. The report provided a summary of the summit as well as recommendations for specific stakeholder groups: Professional Nursing Organizations, Academic Institutions, Information Technology, Government and Policy Makers, Healthcare Delivery Organizations, Health Information Management Professionals, and Health Science Libraries. Leaders from the American Colleges of Nursing, American Nurses Association, American Organization of Nurse Executives, National League for Nursing, and Sigma Theta Tau International affirmed their commitment and the need for the profession to continue to support the TIGER Initiative.

THE TIGER COLLABORATIVE WORKGROUPS (2007–2008)

Several months after the summit and after numerous follow-up meetings with the TIGER Executive Steering Committee, it was decided to move into phase II of TIGER. Building off the summit's vision and action plans, 9 key collaboratives were formed to dig more deeply into the recommendations made at the summit and more broadly engage the nursing community. Each collaborative was assigned coleaders to facilitate the workgroup and write a final report of findings and recommendations. A TIGER wiki site was established for each workgroup to have a virtual workspace in which to store working documents. A summary of the purpose, outcomes, and reference sites of each of the collaborative workgroups can be found in Table 42.1.

The Usability and Clinical Application Design Collaborative is an example of how these collaborative efforts produced a report that continues to be shared with diverse audiences. It is important to note that this collaborative was ranked as being the highest priority, and it also had the greatest number of volunteers (53.5%) of all the TIGER Collaborative workgroups. This demonstrates the significance of the topic for practicing nurses and faculty today. Some of the nurses who actively led and contributed to this collaborative cited the following reasons for their involvement: "A good design can make the system easier to use and enhance clinical practice." "Usability is a make or break part of a clinical informatics solution." And, "Many lessons are learned from end users as Design is translated into Practice."

The collaborative established their goals and design principles:

Usability Goals

1. An early and consistent focus on users
2. Iterative design processes (multiple versions matched to users, tasks, and environments)
3. Systematic product evaluations (with product users and metrics)

Clinical Application Design Goals

Clinical Application Design addresses how we integrate usability principles with evidence-based practice, interdisciplinary collaboration, and knowledge discovery within a systems-thinking design. In essence, we are applying usability and other intentional design factors

TABLE 42.1	TIGER Phase II Collaborative Workgroups	
TIGER Collaborative	**Purpose**	**Outcome Summary**
Standards & Interoperability	To accelerate the following action steps identified at the summit: • Integrate industry standards for health information technology (HIT) Interoperability with clinical standards for practice and education • Educate practice and education communities on health IT standards • Establish use of standards and set hard deadlines for adoption	Provides definitions and rationale for standardization and interoperability. Developed Nursing Health IT Standards catalogue and provided Web-based tutorials on benefits of interoperable systems and standards harmonization. For more detailed information: www.tigersummit.com/Standards_New and tigerstandards.pbworks.com
National Health IT Agenda	To identify the most relevant HIT agenda and policies that are important to the TIGER and nursing profession's mission and to assist in closing any representation gaps on policy issues.	Identified major national HIT organizations that need nursing engagement and participation. Developed tutorials to educate and encourage nurses to participate in HIT-related policy development, healthcare reform, and accelerate widespread HIT adoption. For more detailed information: www.tigersummit.com/HIT_Agenda_New and tigerhitagenda.pbworks.com
Informatics Competencies	To establish the minimum set of informatics competencies for all practicing nurses and graduating nursing students.	Collected over 1,000 informatics competencies, then narrowed focus to describe the minimum set of competencies around: 1. Basic computer competencies 2. Information literacy 3. Information management (including use of an electronic health record [EHR]) Several educational resources for each type were identified and provided. For more detailed information: www.tigersummit.com/Competencies_New_B949 and tigercompetencies.pbworks.com
Education & Faculty Development	To engage key stakeholders to integrate informatics into curriculums and create resources and programs to implement and sustain changes. Collaborate with industry and service partners to support faculty creativity in the adoption of informatics tools within the curriculum.	Formed 7 workgroups to engage key stakeholders. Effective in influencing the accrediting agencies to include informatics education in nursing curriculum. NLN position statement titled *Preparing the Next Generation of Nurses to Practice in a Technology-Rich Environment: An Informatics Agenda*. AACN took the lead in incorporating informatics as an essential element of baccalaureate and doctoral nursing programs. Participation in surveys for ADN and state boards related to informatics were done. HRSA collaboration that resulted in the Integrated Technology into Nursing Education and Practice Initiative (ITNEP). Webinars for educators on how schools can integrate informatics into curriculum and partnership examples to teach about the electronic health record and clinical documentation. For more detailed information: www.tigersummit.com/Education_New and tigereducation.pbworks.com Links to position statements available at: www.nln.org/aboutn;n/PostionsStatements/index and www.aacn.edu/Education/essential

(continued)

TABLE 42.1	TIGER Phase II Collaborative Workgroups *(Continued)*	
TIGER Collaborative	**Purpose**	**Outcome Summary**
Staff Development	To identify educational needs and resources in practice environments for the successful adoption of new technology and improving patient safety.	Conducted an electronic survey of TIGER participants to evaluate how prepared their nurses were in using an EHR. Developed strategies how the TIGER Informatics Competencies could be adopted by staff development resources. Gathered case studies that could be replicated in multiple settings. For more detailed information: www.tigersummit.com/Staff_Development_New and tigerstaffdev.pbworks.com
Leadership Development	To engage nursing leadership to develop revolutionary leadership that drives, empowers, and executes the transformation of healthcare.	Evaluated current nursing leadership development programs for the inclusion of informatics competencies. Built upon the American Organization of Nurse Executives (AONE) and developed a survey to identify most urgent program development needs. The survey provided insight into leadership competencies required. Aligned with the Magnet Recognition program to highlight how nurse leaders use major HIT implementations as an integral part of their Magnet journey and meeting the 14 forces of magnetism. Identified criteria for leadership development related to informatics. For more detailed information: www.tigersummit.com/Leadership_New and tigerleadership.pbworks.com
Usability & Clinical Application Design	To further define key concepts, patterns, trends, and recommendations to HIT vendors and practitioners to assure usable clinical systems at the point of care.	Synthesized a comprehensive literature review from nursing and other disciplines and analyzed in the areas of determining clinical information requirements, safe and usable clinical design, usability evaluations, and human factor foundations. Collected case studies that illustrated usability and clinical application design, including good examples to follow and bad examples to avoid. Reviewed the AAN Technology Drill Down (TD2) Project findings. Developed recommendations for HIT vendors and practitioners to adopt sound principles of usability and clinical design for healthc are technology. For more detailed information: www.tigersummit.com/Usability_New and tigerusability. pbworks.com
Virtual Demonstration Center	To explore the creation of a virtual Gallery Walk for all nurses, nursing faculty, and nursing students via Web technology applications.	Provided visibility to the vision of IT-enabled practice and education. Demonstrated future IT resources. Demonstrated collaboration between industry, healthcare organizations, academic institutions, and professional organizations to create educational modules for nurses that are based upon informatics competencies. Used practice examples from different practice environments to demonstrate best practices, results of research, case studies, and lessons learned by partnering with professional nursing organizations. For more detailed information: www.tigersummit.com/Virtual_Demo_New and tigervirtualdemo.pbworks.com

TABLE 42.1	TIGER Phase II Collaborative Workgroups *(Continued)*	
TIGER Collaborative	**Purpose**	**Outcome Summary**
Consumer Empowerment & Personal Health Records (PHRs)	To make information available to nurses about PHRs and to encourage inclusion of this content into nursing curricula and practice.	Identified several ways that nurses can impact the adoption and use of consumer empowerment strategies such as PHRs. For more detailed information: www.tigersummit.com/PHR_New and tigerphr.pbworks.com

that are critical to making information technology the stethoscope of the 21st century.

The Collaborative collected case studies that illustrated usability and clinical application design in best-case and worst-case scenarios. Over 30 case studies were received and analyzed. Several key factors emerged. An example of one was the involvement of end-user engagement throughout the process:

- User acceptance and system adoption
- Accuracy and avoidance of duplication
- Patient safety due to synchronized and accurate information
- Timeliness of information collection, reporting, and use

Findings included uncovering usability as the common thread that binds system users, their work, and their environments. The workgroup determined the following imperatives: engage the point-of-care clinicians early in the process, understand their practice needs, and conduct usability testing and redesign prior to implementation. Findings also identified that clinical application design should employ systems thinking, including components that are critical to serving complex healthcare environments, cultivating accountability, and coordinating patient and family care needs. Contemporary designs include evidence-based practice, interdisciplinary collaboration, and knowledge-discovery.

One of the most important outcomes of this Collaborative was making clear and distinct recommendations for HIT vendors and healthcare practitioners. These valuable insights gained from the literature, case studies, and the many workgroup members were ultimately compiled into a final report. Later, leaders of this TIGER collaborative conducted a workshop at the NI2009 Conference in Helsinki, Finland, entitled "Crucial Conversation about the Design of Clinical Technology," which was based on their findings and resulting recommendations. The workshop was met with great affirmation; the universal frustration reported by the diverse body of international participants caused by living with poor usability and clinical application design was so resounding that a secondary paper is now being written as a follow-up. The collaborative is also exploring additional ways to engage HIT vendors in order to enhance their understand of these basic needs.

THE NEXT TIGER PHASES (2010 AND BEYOND)

The next phase is TIGER III. Some of the leaders involved in TIGER I and II continue to aid TIGER III, and there are some important new leaders involved. Every phase has gained momentum from the previous phase while keeping a focus on the TIGER vision. Also, as TIGER entered Phase III, it was decided to create a TIGER Champions group that includes important stakeholders and continues to reach out to the over 1,500 individuals that either want to join or stay engaged in this very important initiative.

TIGER III will focus on building a Virtual Learning Environment (VLE). Phases I and II of TIGER identified a great need for a Web site that would demonstrate successful adoption of Health IT as well as engage interdisciplinary team members (e.g., physicians, respiratory therapists, physical therapists, occupational therapists, pharmacy). There is also a need for basic educational materials and learning modules for faculty and practitioners to further advance the knowledge and dissemination of topics related to evidence and informatics. Collaborating partners, such as the National Library of Medicine, UPMC Center for Connected Medicine, and other public-private partnerships, will be key in supporting the VLE pilot and its continued expansion. TIGER III is intended to relate closely to the TIGER Collaboratives: Competencies, Staff Development, Education and Faculty Development, and Usability and Clinical Application Design.

At the time of this writing, plans for the VLE pilot include virtual communities focused on workforce development, future workforce development, and educational and faculty development. One community will be a TIGER OPEN DOOR, which will host free and available resources. The other communities will be developed through partnerships that share and/or help create content for learning modules. A governing committee will review and approve content. There is also a plan for a second VLE pilot phase, which would incorporate additional partner communities supporting the areas of leadership and management, toolkits and best practices, and science and technology. The ability to track the usage of classrooms and communities will be added so there is a database to measure utilization and outcome strategies. Future invitational summits are also being considered to further enhance interdisciplinary engagement as well as address healthcare disparity and rural healthcare needs as they relate to the role of technology and effective HIT adoption. A new Web site (www.thetigerinitiative.org) for the growing TIGER Initiative experience will be updated to reflect the current status of TIGER III efforts, as well as provide access to new and historical TIGER-related materials.

ONCE A TIGER ALWAYS A TIGER

Brief Summary and Conclusion

The sign of significant changes to come was palpable in 2004 as the United States began to address healthcare reform by announcing that this would be the decade for healthcare technology. A great sense of urgency to create a vision and course of action for nurses to lead, and, in turn, engage *all* nurses, set the stage for Technology Informatics Guiding Education Reform; the TIGER acronym fit perfectly as hundreds of nurses launched into action. The grass roots effort took root and merged into an innovative social disruption that continues to grow. Many TIGERS have shared that the sense of collaboration and teamwork has been an amazing experience. The number of volunteer hours has been simply astounding. The timing of TIGER is even more significant now with the passing of the 2009 American

Recovery and Reinvestment Act and the phased mandate for meaningful use of electronic health records. The TIGER I vision and action plans, TIGER II Collaborative Recommendations, and now the TIGER III Virtual Learning Environment, along with other outreaches, are all critical to meet the demands of the transforming healthcare environment. It is more important than ever to have clarity about what the best technology is to support practice and what is needed to prepare students for this new world. We need TIGERS everywhere! As the TIGER Initiative continues to evolve and grow in the United States, other countries are developing their own TIGER Initiatives. We are helping each other spread the vision and take the actions necessary to integrate evidence and technology informatics into our daily work to make healthcare safer, effective, efficient, patient-centered, timely, and equitable.

REFERENCES

Institute of Medicine. (2001). *Crossing the quality chasm: A new health system for the 21st century*. Washington, DC: The National Academy Press.

Institute of Medicine. (2003). *Health profession education: A bridge to quality*. Washington, DC: The National Academy Press.

Kotter, J. (1996). *Leading Change*. Boston, MA: Harvard Business Press.

Kotter, J. (2008). *A sense of urgency*. Boston, MA: Harvard Business Press.

Technology Informatics Guiding Education Reform. (2007). *The TIGER Initiative: Evidence and informatics transforming nursing: 3 year action steps toward a 10-year vision*. Retrieved from http://www.tigersummit.com/Summit.

Technology Informatics Guiding Education Reform. (2009). *The TIGER Initiative: Collaborating to integrate evidence and informatics into nursing practice and education: An executive summary*. Retrieved from http://www.tigersummit.com/9_Collaboratives.

Technology Informatics Guiding Education Reform (2009). *The TIGER Initiative: Designing usable clinical information systems: Recommendations from the TIGER Usability and Clinical Application Design Collaborative Team*. Retrieved from http://www.tigersummit.com/Usability_New.

PART 7

Research Applications

Virginia K. Saba

43

Computer Use in Nursing Research

Veronica D. Feeg / Theresa A. Rienzo

- ## OBJECTIVES
  1. Describe general data and computer applications related to proposal development and project implementation in both quantitative and qualitative research (computer use in research).
  2. Describe general categories of research focusing on computer use in clinical applications and informatics integration (nursing research on computer use).
  3. Summarize a range of computer-based applications that facilitate or support the steps of the research process, including data collection, data management and coding, data analysis, and results reporting.
  4. Compare and contrast select computer software applications that can be used in quantitative and qualitative research data analysis related to the steps of the research process.
  5. Describe specific research studies on computer use in nursing that exemplify quantitative and qualitative methodologies in the literature.
  6. Describe the context for nursing informatics research in the next decade.

- ## KEY WORDS

  nursing informatics research
  research process
  research methodology
  quantitative
  qualitative
  data collection
  data mining
  data management
  data analysis
  research applications
  computer applications

Nursing research today involves a plethora of tools and resources that researchers employ throughout the research process. From the individual or collaborative project initiation, through refinement of the idea, selection of approaches, development of methods, capturing the data, analyzing the results, and disseminating the findings, computer applications are an indispensible resource for the researcher. The investigators must be well prepared in a variety of computerized techniques for research activities as they are employed in the domain of knowledge that will be investigated. Without the power of technology, contemporary research would not reach the levels of sophistication required to discover and understand health and illness today. New opportunities to mine existing data for evaluation and discovery are forming a bridge between the process of conducting research and the products of discovery.

Additionally, the range and sophistication of research on computerized applications and informatics warrants attention in a discussion of computer use in nursing research. The context for nursing informatics research has proliferated since the National Institute of Nursing Research (NINR) published an agenda outlining the need for nursing informatics research in the Nursing Informatics Research Agenda (NINR, 1993). Other reports called for organizing priorities (Brennan, Zielstorff, Ozbolt, & Strombom, 1998) and constructing an organizing framework (Orem, 2001; Effken, 2003) to develop a context connecting nursing and informatics that would provide the basis for studying the practice of nursing informatics. In the rapidly changing world of Internet technologies, information management, and computer-enhanced therapies, nursing informatics research on the use of computers has produced a new body of science that will continue to grow. Blending the focus of computer use in research (tools and process) and research on computer use (informatics research) calls for an understanding of process and products. This chapter will provide an overview of the research process for two separate and fundamentally different research approaches—quantitative and qualitative—and discuss select computer applications and uses relative to these approaches. The discussion will be supplemented by examples and proposed future research on the impact of informatics, electronic records, treatments, and integrated technologies using the computer as a tool.

The computer has been a tool for researchers in various aspects of the research process and has gone beyond its historic application once limited to number crunching. Field-notes tablets and paper recordings have all but disappeared in the researchers' world. Personal computers, laptops, tablets, and even handheld PDAs (personal digital assistants) have become part of the researcher's necessary resources in mounting a research project or study. Wireless technologies are ubiquitous and connect people to people as well as researchers to devices. From word processing proposals and manuscripts to database management of subjects, contacts, or logistics, nurses have used a range of hardware and software applications that are generic to operations in addition to the tools and devices that are specific to research data collection, analysis, results reporting, and dissemination.

In today's electronic healthcare environment, numerous advances have been made with the sources of data collection relative to general clinical applications in nursing, health, and health services. System implementations for large clinical enterprises have also provided opportunities for nurses and health service researchers to identify and extract information from existing computer-based resources. In an era when the federal government is calling for comparative effectiveness research to address the rising costs of healthcare (Congressional Budget Office [CBO], 2007), the richness of capturing nursing data that can be managed and mined for advanced analyses should be recognized in the development of electronic health records (EHR) and other sources.

In addition, the era of Web-based applications has produced a plethora of innovative means of entering data and, subsequently, collecting data in ways that were not possible before. With the advancements in the implementation of clinical systems, acceptable terminology and vocabularies to support nursing assessment, interventions, and evaluation, computers are increasingly being used for clinical and patient care research. Although research is a complex cognitive process, certain aspects of carrying out research can be aided by software applications. For example, examination of nursing care patient outcomes and the effect of interventions would have been prohibitive in the past, but with the aid of computers and access to large data sets, many health outcomes can be analyzed quantitatively and qualitatively.

The objective of this chapter is threefold: (1) to provide an overview of general computer and software applications related to the stages of the research process; (2) to describe how computers facilitate the work of the researcher in both quantitative and qualitative aspects, and (3) to highlight research on computer use in healthcare in categories delineating nursing informatics research. These will serve as a snapshot of the research on computer use for the future with contextual influences.

To begin, the chapter will focus on some of the considerations related to the logistics and preparation of the research proposal, project planning, and budgeting, followed by the implementation of the proposal with data capture, data management, data analysis, and information presentation. The general steps of proposal development, preparation, and implementation are applicable to both quantitative and qualitative approaches. However, no discussion about research could begin without acknowledging the mountain of literature that must be organized. The use of literature search systems and online bibliographic retrieval and management applications are discussed in detail in the Chapter 44.

PROPOSAL DEVELOPMENT, PREPARATION, AND IMPLEMENTATION

All research begins with a good idea. The idea is typically based on the nurse researcher's identification of a problem that is amenable to study using a philosophical and theoretical orientation. The philosophical aspect sets the stage for selecting one's approach to investigating the problem or developing the idea. Good clinical ideas often come from personal experiences, based on the researcher's foundation of knowledge that aids in drawing inferences from real clinical situations. These unfold by way of iterative consideration of problem and process—leading the investigator to evolve an approach to the problem, and subsequently a theoretical paradigm to address the problem. Because the theoretical paradigm emerges from these iterative considerations, and because the theoretical perspective will subsequently drive the organization of the research study, it is important to distinguish between these two distinct approaches. Each theoretical paradigm directs how the problem for study will unfold. The researcher uses a selected theoretical approach and operationalizes each step of the research process that will become the research design and methodology, either qualitative, quantitative, or some combination of both. Each approach can be facilitated at different points along the proposal development process with select computer applications. These will be described as they relate to the theoretical approach.

Quantitative or Qualitative

The important distinction to be made between the quantitative and qualitative approaches is that for a quantitative study to be successful, the researcher is obliged to fully develop each aspect of the research proposal *before* collecting any data, whereas, for a qualitative study to be successful, the researcher is obligated to allow the data collected to determine the subsequent steps as it unfolds in the process and/or the analysis. Quantitative research is derived from the philosophical orientations of empiricism and logical positivism (Weiss, 1995), with multiple steps bound together by precision in quantification. The requirements of a hypothesis-driven or numerically descriptive approach are logical consequences of, or correspond to, a specific theory and its related tenets. The hypothesis can be tested statistically to support or refute the prediction selected a priori or in advance. Statistics packages are the mainstay of the quantitative methodologist.

The qualitative approaches are a collection of different research traditions (e.g., phenomenology, hermeneutics, ethnography, and grounded theory) that share a common view of reality, which consists of the meanings ascribed to the data such as a person's lived experiences (Creswell, 2009). With this view, theory is not tested, but rather, perspectives and meaning from the subject's point of view are described and analyzed. For nursing studies, knowledge development is generated from the patient's experiences and responses to health, illness, and treatments. The requirements of the qualitative approach are a function of the philosophical frames through which the data unfold and evolve into meaningful interpretations by the researcher. A variety of software applications assist the qualitative methodologist to enter, organize, frame, code, reorder and synthesize text, audio, video, and sometimes numeric data.

General Considerations in Proposal Preparation

Several computer applications have become indispensable in the development of the research proposal and generally in planning for the activities that will take place when implementing the study. These include broad categories of office programs including word processing, spreadsheet, and database management applications. According to Forrester Research, an independent research firm, Microsoft Office products currently capture 80% of users with 64% of enterprises using Office 2007 (Montalbano, 2009). Office 2010 is the new release, offering improved clerical tools to manage the text from numerous sources and assemble them in a cogent and organized package.

Microsoft Word (Microsoft Corporation, 2010b) and WordPerfect (Corel Corporation, 2010) provide capabilities and a platform into which other off-the-shelf applications can be integrated. Tables, charts, and figures can be inserted, edited, and moved as the proposal takes shape. Personal computer applications that allow inserting simple graphic designs give the researcher a powerful means of expressing concepts through art. Line art and scanned images with Adobe programs such as Illustrator CS5 (www.adobe.com) or Photoshop CS5 (www.photoshop.com) can be integrated into the document for clear visual effects. These offer the researcher and grants managers tools to generate proposals, reports, and manuscripts that can be submitted electronically directly or following conversion to portable document formats (pdf) using Adobe Acrobat or other available conversion products.

There are a variety of reference management software products available as add-ons to word processing, with ranging prices and functionalities. Common programs such as Reference Manager, Procite, and Endnote are products of the Thomson Corporation (2009) (www.refman.com/rmcopyright.asp), the industry standard software tools for publishing and managing bibliographies on the Windows and Macintosh desktops. RefWorks adds another option for reference management from a centrally hosted Web site (www.refworks.com). Searching online is one function of these applications, and then working between the reference database and the text of the proposal document is efficient and easy, calling out citations when needed with "cite as you write" capability into the finished document. Output style sheets can be selected to match publication or proposal guidelines.

Research applications and calls for proposals are often downloadable from the Internet into an interactive Adobe Acrobat form where individual fields are editable and the documents can be saved, printed, or submitted from the Web. The Web also allows the researcher to explore numerous opportunities for designing a proposal tailored to potential foundations for consideration of funding. Calls for proposals, contests, and competitive grants play a role in developing the idea in one direction or another, and the links from Web sites give the researcher a depth of understanding of what is expected in the proposal.

Research Study Implementation

A funded research study becomes a logistical challenge for most researchers in managing the steps of the process. Numerous demands for information management require the researcher to maintain the fidelity of the procedures, manage the subject information and paper flow, and keep the data confidential and secure. These processes mandate a system of database management

that are sometimes separate but essential to the research data. Several software applications exist and have evolved to assist the researcher in the overall process of study implementation. These applications are operations oriented, used in nonresearch programs and projects as well, but can assist the researcher in management of time, personnel, money, products, and ultimately dissemination.

The Microsoft Office suite includes programs that manage data (Microsoft Access) and number crunching (Microsoft Excel). General database applications including Microsoft Access, FileMaker Pro 11 (FileMaker, Inc., 2010), and more sophisticated, integrated, and proprietary database management applications from companies such as Oracle and Lotus provide the researcher with mechanisms to operationalize the personnel, subjects, forms, interviews, dates, times, and/or tracking systems over the course of the project. Most of these applications require specially designed screens that are unique to the project if the research warrants complicated connections such as reminders, but simple mailing lists and zip codes of subjects' addresses and contact information in a generic form can also be extremely useful for the researcher. Some of these applications are beginning to include add-ons such as FileMaker Go that provides application portability with devices such as the iPhone.

Several other generic computer programs can aid the researcher in daily operations and project management. Spreadsheet applications are invaluable for budgeting and budget planning, from proposal development through project completion. One multipurpose Microsoft Office application is Microsoft Excel. Universally understood and easy to use, Excel allows the researcher to manage costs and calculate expenses over the course of the project period, producing a self-documenting plan by categories to track actual spending and money left. Templates can be developed for repetitive tasks. Scheduling and project planning software is also available from Microsoft including Microsoft Project that allows the project director to organize the work efficiently and track schedules and deadlines using Gantt charts over the lifetime of the project.

In summary, the general considerations of developing and conducting a research study are based on philosophical approaches and will dictate which methodology the researcher will use to develop the study. Although this will subsequently influence the research and computer applications to be used in carrying out the project, the steps of proposal preparation are less specific, and the computer applications are useful in both quantitative and qualitative studies. After identifying the research problem, however, the researcher must proceed through the steps of the process, where computers play an important role that is unique to each of the methodologies.

THE QUANTITATIVE APPROACH

Data Capture and Data Collection

Data capture and data collection are processes that are viewed differently from the quantitative and qualitative perspectives. Nurses may already be familiar with data collection that is focused on the management of patient care. Patient monitoring, patient care documentation, and interview data are collected by nurses, although not always for research purposes. Data collection can take a number of forms depending on the type of research and variables of interest. Computers are used in data collection for paper-and-pencil surveys and questionnaires as well as to capture physiologic and clinical nursing information in quantitative or descriptive patient care research. There are also unique automated data capturing applications that have been developed recently that facilitate large group data capture in single contacts or allow paper versions of questionnaires to be scanned directly into a database ready for analysis.

Paper and Pencil Questionnaires. Surveys and questionnaires, traditionally administered in paper-and-pencil forms, can be programmed into a computer application either in a microcomputer or on a Web site accessed through the Internet. Computers are being used for direct data entry in studies where subjects enter their own responses via a computer, and simultaneous coding of response to questions and time "online" can be captured (Brennan & Ripich, 1994) or Web surveys can be distributed widely. These online survey tools can provide a wide range of applications, including paper or portable versions, and range in price and functionality.

The use of notebook microcomputers has gained popularity in recent years for allowing the user to enter the data directly into the computer program at the time of the interview with a subject, with innovations emerging in touch screens, light pens, and even wireless data entry with PDAs (Bakken et al., 2003). Responses to questions can be entered by the respondent or a surrogate directly into the computer or Web site through Internet access. Several research studies on patients with chronic conditions use a computer application or the Internet as the intervention as well as the data capture as the patients or caregivers respond to questions directly (Mullen, Berry, & Zierler, 2004; Wilkie et al., 2003). Individual devices such as the Medication Event

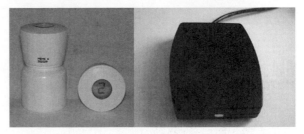

• **FIGURE 43.1.** MEMS (medication event monitoring system) SmartCap contains an LCD screen; MEMS Reader transfers encrypted data from the MEMS monitor to the Web portal. (Source: www.aardexgroup.com). Published with permission.

Monitoring System (MEMS) (Figure 43.1) capture data and can be downloaded for analysis in research such as patient adherence studies (Rolley et al., 2008).

A variety of online survey tools also provide researchers the power to collect data from a distance, without postage, using the Internet. These applications can present questionnaire data in graphically desirable formats, depending on the price and functionality of the software, to subjects delivered via e-mail, Web sites, blogs, and even social networking sites such as Facebook if desirable. Web surveys, although often criticized for yielding poorer response rates than traditional mail (Granello & Wheaton, 2004), are becoming increasingly popular for their cost and logistical benefits. The data from the Internet can be downloaded for analysis and several applications provide instant summary statistics that can be monitored over the data collection period. Several of these programs are available for free with limited use; others yield advanced products that can be incorporated into the research, giving mobility (e.g., PDAs) and flexibility (e.g., scanning or online entry) to the data capture procedures. Several of these applications include: (1) Survey Monkey (www.survey monkey.com); (2) E-Surveys Pro (www.esurveyspro. com); (3) Survey System (www.surveysystem.com); and (4) SNAP Survey software (www.snapsurveys.com/us). An example of screen flexibility and scanning output are in Figure 43.2.

Several special applications have been used in nursing research that can facilitate large group data capture. Group use applications in specially designed facilities have been developed to engage an audience in simultaneous activity, recording their impressions through electronic keypads located proximal to the users, and capturing that information for display or later analysis. One type of application, Expert Choice 11.5 (Expert

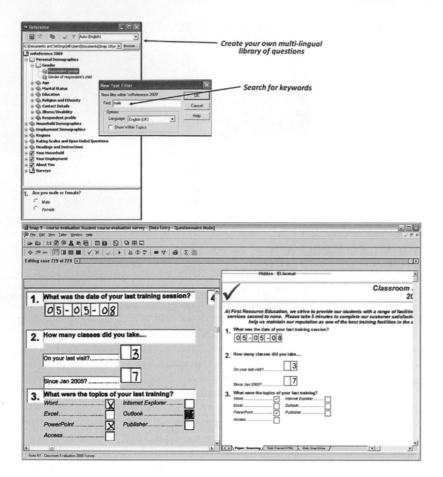

• **FIGURE 43.2.** Sample screens for SNAP Survey software (Source: Slideshow, www.snapsurveys.com/us)

Choice, 2009) uses the analytic hierarchy process, a mathematical technique, with handheld keypad technology to elicit group responses and automatically score, analyze, prioritize, and present information back to the group graphically. This kind of groupware for collaborative decision making can supplement data collection from a focus group to add a quantitative component to the subjective question as it elicits and captures opinion via pairwise comparisons (Feeg, 1999).

Software packages also exist that can be integrated with the researcher's scanner to optically scan a specially designed questionnaire and produce the subjects' responses in a database ready for analysis. OmniPage 17 (Nuance, 2010) is a top rated optical character recognition (OCR) program that converts a scanned page into plain text. Programs such as Remark Office OMR

(Gravic, 2010) can facilitate scanning large numbers of questionnaires with speed and accuracy. These products, enhanced even more with Web-based products such as Remark Web Survey (Gravic, 2010), increase the accuracy of data entry with very low risk of errors, thereby improving the efficiency of the data capture, collection, and entry processes.

Physiologic Data. The collection of patient physiologic parameters has long been used in physiologic research. Some of these parameters can be measured directly from patient devices such as cardiac monitoring of heart rhythm, rate, and fluid or electrolytes. For example, hospitals have developed mechanisms to use information from intensive care unit (ICU) data to calculate benchmarks for mortality and resource use resulting in the

APACHE Equations (Cerner Corporation, 2005). Now that many measurements taken from various types of imaging (e.g., neurologic, cardiovascular, and cellular) have become digitized, they can also be entered directly from the patient into a computer program for analysis. Each of these applications is unique to the measures, such as systems to capture cardiac functioning and/or pulmonary capacity, devices that can relay contractions, or monitors that pick up electronic signals remotely. Numerous measurements of intensity, amplitude, patterns, and shapes can be characterized by computer programs and used in research. Each of these measurement systems have evolved with the unfolding of research specific to their questions, and within each community of scholars, issues about the functionality, accuracy, and reliability of electronic data extracted from these physiologic devices are debated. For example, research on heart rate variability employs specialized recording and synthesizing devices. A longitudinal study on preterm infants' heart rate variability uses a physiologic monitoring device producing spectral analysis of heart rate variability (Krueger, van Oostrum, & Shuster, 2010).

Along with the proliferation of clinical diagnostic measurement systems, there has been a rapid expansion of unique computer applications that have emerged for the data analysis aspects of these clinical systems, physiologic and record sources. Millions of gigabytes of data are stored in machines that can be tapped for multiple studies on the existing data. Data mining is a powerful tool in the knowledge discovery process that can now be done with a number of commercial and open-source software packages (Berger & Berger, 2004). With increased attention to comparative effectiveness research, several government and private organizations are encouraging researchers to hone the techniques to extract valid and reliable information from large data sets. Data mining is a mechanism of exploration and analysis of large quantities of data in order to discover meaningful patterns and rules, applied to large physiologic data sets as well as clinical sources of data. The nature of the data and the research question determine the tool selection (i.e., data-mining algorithm or technique). Tools and consultants exist to help researchers unfamiliar with data mining algorithms to use data mining for analysis, prediction, and reporting purposes (MSDN Library, 2000). Many of the first commercial applications of data mining were in customer profiling and marketing analyses. Today, many special technologies can be applied, for example, to predict physiologic phenomena such as genetic patterns in tumors that might respond to therapy based on classification of primary tumor gene expression or tissue rejection post-heart transplantation from blood samples and biopsies (Berger & Berger, 2004).

Unique Nursing Care Data in Research. Scientists and technologists from a variety of disciplines are working hard to identify the domain of data and information that is transferable across situations, sites, or circumstances that can be captured electronically for a wide array of analyses to learn how the health system impacts the patients it serves. The American Nurses Association (ANA) has supported the need to standardize nursing care terms for computer-based patient care systems. The clinical and economic importance of structured recording to represent nursing care was recognized by the acceptance of the nursing minimum data set (Werley, Lang, & Westlake, 1986). The ANA has accepted 7 systems of terminology for the description of nursing practice: the North American Nursing Diagnosis Association (NANDA) taxonomy of nursing diagnosis, Georgetown Home Healthcare Classification (renamed Clinical Care Classification [CCC] System) (McCormick et al., 1994; Saba, 1997, 2007; Zielstorff et al., 1995), Nursing Interventions Classification (Bulechek & McCloskey, 1997), Nursing Outcomes Classification (Daly, Moss, & Johnson, 1997), patient care data set (Ozbolt, 1999), Omaha Home Healthcare (Martin & Norris, 1996), and the International Classification of Nursing Practice (Saba, 1997, 2007; Zielstorff et al., 1995). The Clinical Care Classification System (sabacare.com) nursing terminology has been accepted by the U.S. Department of Health and Human Services (HHS) Secretary Michael Leavitt as a named standard within the Healthcare Information Technology Standards Panel (HITSP) Interoperability Specification for Electronic Health Records, Biosurveillance and Consumer Empowerment as presented to a meeting of the American Health Information Community (AHIC), a federal advisory group on health information technology (DHHS, 2007, January). (See Chapter 14 for a full discussion of the CCC System.) Other terminology that may encompass issues of major interest to nursing is the minimum data set (MDS), which is part of the residence assessment inventory (RAI) used for the documentation of resident problems in nursing homes (Hansebo, Kihlgren, Ljunggren & Winbald, 1999; Zulkowski, 1999).

Although none of the above has emerged as a single standard, a structured coding system is needed for recording patient care problems that are amenable to nursing actions, the actual nursing actions implemented in the care of patients, and the evaluation of the effectiveness of these actions. Outcomes research and quality indicators extracted from health information systems (HIS) have become the data end-points that can justify healthcare services (Nahm, Vaydia, Ho, Scharf & Seagull, 2007). The use of structured terms across healthcare settings would provide for comparability of patient care using patient records. There is new emphasis in the federal government to produce electronic health records (EHRs) and cross-platform compatibility through the development of collaborative efforts across organizations in the government and the information technology industry (Thompson & Brailer, 2004). The American Recovery and Reinvestment Act (ARRA) of 2009 (Public Law 111-5) calls for increased development, certification, and wide-range meaningful use of EHRs across healthcare. Research on outcomes of care is the centerpiece of this stimulus legislation to catapult information technologies in healthcare. Nursing research on nursing practice captured from standardized terminology will be essential to document outcomes of nursing care.

Data Coding

In quantitative studies, the data for the variables of interest are collected in a numerical form. These numerical values are entered into designated fields in the process of coding. Coding may be inherent in software programs for the physiologic data and many of the electronic surveys. The coding may be generated by a computer program from measurements directly obtained through imaging or physiologic monitoring, or entered into a computer by a patient or researcher from a printout or a questionnaire or survey into a database program. Most statistical programs contain data editors that permit the entry of data by a researcher as part of the statistical application. In such a situation, fields are designated and numerical values can also be entered into the appropriate fields without the use of an extra program. For mechanisms that translate and transfer source data to prepare it for analysis, generic programs such as Microsoft Excel (Microsoft Office, 2010a) serve multiple needs. In addition to allowing simple transfers of data from source to a statistical analysis package, Excel has its own powerful, but simple, analysis capabilities and exceptionally easy to use graphic translators that can turn statistics into visual graphs and charts.

Coding data is a precise operation that needs careful consideration and presents the researcher with challenges that warrant technical or cognitive applications. Coding data is a combination of cognitive decisions and mechanical clerical recording of responses in a numerical form with numerous places for error to occur. There are several ways of reviewing and "cleaning" the data prior to analysis. Some computer programs allow for the same data to be entered twice (preferably by different people to check for errors), with the premise that if the double

entry does not match, one entry is wrong. One also must check for missing data and take them into consideration in the coding and analyses. Reviewing data for values outside of those allowable is another way of examining the data for errors. It can best be done by examining the multiple printouts produced by the statistical software packages or procedures invoked in the statistical application and by carefully perusing for outliers or artifacts. While coding data is a process activity in quantitative research to get results, it is a substantive activity for the qualitative researcher, as it becomes the essence of the interpretation of data collected.

Data Analysis

Data analysis in a quantitative study combines a variety of techniques that apply statistical procedures with the researcher's cognitive organization of research questions, results, and visual or textual information, translated into tables, charts, and graphs to make the data meaningful. It translates the numeric and conceptual elements of the inquiry into meaningful representations of information. In general, the statistical analyses are ordered by the conceptual arrangement of hypotheses, variables, measurements, and relationships, and ultimately answer the research questions. There are myriad ways to consider data analysis. The presentation below is organized around the broad types of research of interest in nursing and general research goals or questions. The researcher may use different types of analyses depending on the goal of research. These goals may require different statistical examinations: descriptive and/or exploratory analyses, hypothesis testing, estimation of confidence intervals, model building through multivariate analysis, and structural equation model building. Various types of nursing research may contain a number of these goals. For example, to test an intervention using an experimental or quasiexperimental design, one may first perform descriptive or exploratory analyses followed by tests of the hypotheses. Quality improvement, patient outcome, and survival analysis studies may likewise contain a number of different types of analyses depending on the specific research questions.

In general, the statistical analysis steps of the research process rely heavily on the functions specific to a variety of statistical software applications. Two of the most popular programs in use today are the IBM SPSS Statistics 18 (formerly Statistical Package for Social Sciences) (IBM SPSS Statistics 18, 2010) and Statistical Analysis Services (SAS Version 9.2) (SAS Institute, 2010), however a variety of other packages and programs exist, such as STATA (Statistical Software for Professionals,

2004), and are often supported by libraries or unique to particular scientific disciplines. Which package one selects depends on the user's personal preference, particular strengths, and limits of the applications including number of variables, options for analyses, and ease of use. These packages have given the user the power to manipulate large data sets with relative ease and test out statistical combinations that have exponentially improved the analyses possible in a fraction of time that it once took.

The different types of analyses required by goals of the research will be addressed further. This description will be followed by examples of types of nursing research that incorporate some of these types of analyses.

Descriptive and Exploratory Analysis. The researcher may first explore the data means, modes, distribution pattern, and standard deviations, and examine graphic representations such as scatter plots or bar graphs. Tests of association or significant differences may be explored through chi-squares, correlations, and various univariate, bivariate, and trivariate analyses, and an examination of quartiles. During this analysis process, the researcher may recode or transform data by mathematically multiplying or dividing scores by certain log or factor values. Combining several existing variables can also create new variables. These transformations or "reexpressions" allow the researcher to analyze the data in appropriate and interpretable scales. The researcher can then easily identify patterns with respect to variables as well as groups of study subjects of interest. Both commercial statistical packages provide the ability to calculate these tests and graphically display the results in a variety of ways.

IBM SPSS Statistics 18 (IBM SPSS, 2010) provides the user with a broad range of capabilities for the entire analytical process. SPSS is a modular, tightly integrated, and full-featured software comprised of the SPSS base and a range of add-on modules. With SPSS, the researcher can generate decision-making information quickly using a variety of powerful statistics, understand and effectively present the results with high-quality tabular and graphical output, and share the results with others using various reporting methods, including secure Web publishing. SAS 9.2 (SAS, 2010) provides the researcher with tools that can help code data in a reliable framework, extract data for quality assurance, exploration, or analysis, perform descriptive and inferential data analyses, maintain databases to track, and report on administrative activities like data collection, subject enrolment or grant payments, and deliver content for reports in the appropriate format. SAS allows for creating unique programming within the

variable manipulations. Stata 11 (SAS Institute, 2010) and SYSTAT 13 (SYSTAT 13, 2010) are also fully integrated statistical packages with full database management capabilities and a range of sophisticated statistical tests particularly useful for epidemiologists and physical scientists. All of these statistical packages have evolved to provide an integrated collection of tools that assist in aspects of research study management—from planning to dissemination—in addition to the reputable statistical analyses and data manipulation capabilities that they have provided for many years.

As part of exploratory analysis, simple and multiple regression analyses can be used to examine the relationships between selected variables and a dependent measure of interest. Certain models can be developed to determine which collection of variables provides the best prediction of the dependent measure. Printouts of correlation matrices and regression analysis tables provide the researcher with condensed, readable statistical information about the relationships in question.

Hypothesis Testing or Confirmatory Analyses. Hypothesis testing or confirmatory analyses are based on an interest in relationships and describing what would occur if a hypothesis were true. The analysis of data allows us to compare the actual outcomes with the hypothesized outcomes. Inherent in hypothesis testing is the probability (P value) of an event occurring given a certain relationship. These are conditional relationships based on the variables selected for study, and the typical mathematical tables and software for determining P values are accurate only insofar as the assumptions of the test are met (Polit, 2009). Certain statistical concepts such as statistical power, type II error, selecting alpha values to balance type II errors, and sampling distribution are decisions that the researcher must make regardless of the type of computer software. These concepts are covered in greater detail in research methodology courses and are outside the scope of the present discussion. Power and Precision (Version 2) is a computer program for statistical power analysis and confidence intervals (Biostat, 2000).

Model Building. An application used for a confirmatory hypothesis testing approach to multivariate analysis is structural equation modeling (SEM) (Byrne, 1984). Byrne describes this procedure as consisting of two aspects: (1) the causal processes under study are represented by a series of structural (i.e., regression) equations and (2) these structural relations can be modeled pictorially to enable a clearer conceptualization of the theory under study. The model can be tested statistically in a simultaneous analysis of the entire system of variables to determine the extent to which it is consistent with the data. If goodness of fit is adequate, the model argues for the plausibility of postulated relationships among variables (Byrne, 1984). Most researchers may wish to consult a statistician to discuss the underlying assumptions of the data and plans for testing the model. Different types of modeling programs, such as LISREL (Joreskog & Sorbom, 1978) (see www.ssicentral.com/index.html) or EQS (Byrne, 1984) (see Multivariate Software, www.mvsoft.com), are commercially available. The researcher will identify latent (unobservable) variables of interest (e.g., emotions) and link them to those that are observable (direct measurement) and plan with the statistician to specify and examine the impact of one latent construct on another in the modeling of causal direction.

IBM SPSS 18 (IBM SPSS Software Inc., 2010) offers Amos 4, a powerful SEM and path analysis add-on to create more realistic models than if using standard multivariate methods or regression alone. Amos is a program for visual SEM and path analysis. User-friendly features, such as drawing tools, configurable toolbars, and drag-and-drop capabilities, help the researcher build structural equation models. After fitting the model, the Amos path diagram shows the strength of the relationship between variables. Amos builds models that realistically reflect complex relationships because any variable, whether observed (such as survey data) or latent (such as satisfaction or loyalty) can be used to predict any other variable.

Meta-Analysis. Meta-analysis is a technique that allows researchers to combine data across studies to achieve more focused estimates of population parameters and examine effects of a phenomenon or intervention across multiple studies. It uses the effect size as a common metric of study effectiveness and deals with the statistical problems inherent in using individual significance tests in a number of different studies. It weights study outcomes in proportion to their sample size and focuses on the size of the outcomes rather than on whether they are significant.

Although the computations can be done with the aid of a reliable commercial statistical package such as Meta-Analysis (Biostat, 2000), the researcher needs to consider the following specific issues in performing the meta-analysis (Polit, 2009): (1) justify which studies are comparable and which are not, (2) rely on knowledge of the substantive area to identify relevant study characteristics, (3) evaluate and account for differences in study quality, and (4) assess the generalizability of the results from fields with little empirical data. Each

of these issues must be addressed with a critical review prior to performing the meta-analysis.

Meta-analysis offers a way to examine results of a number of quantitative research that meet meta-analysis researchers' criteria. Meta-analysis overcomes problems encountered in studies using different sample sizes and instruments. The software application Meta-Analysis (Biostat, 2006) provides the user with a variety of tools to examine these studies. It can create a database of studies, import the abstracts or the full text of the original papers, or enter the researcher's own notes. The meta-analysis is displayed using a schematic that may be modified extensively, as the user can specify which variables to display and in what sequence. The studies can be sorted by any variable including effect size, the year of publication, the weight assigned to the study, the sample size, or any user-defined variables to facilitate the critical review done by the researcher (Figure 43.3).

Graphical Data Analysis. There are occasions when data need to be displayed graphically as part of the analysis and interpretation of the information or for more fundamental communication of the results of computations and analyses. Most statistical packages including SPSS, SAS, and STATA, and even spreadsheets such as Excel, provide the user with tools for simple to complex graphical translations of numeric information, thus allowing the researcher to display, store, and communicate aggregated data in meaningful ways. Special tools for spatial representations exist, such as mapping and geographic displays, so that the researcher can visualize and interpret patterns inherent in the data. Geographic information system (GIS) technology is evolving beyond the traditional GIS community and becoming an integral part of the information infrastructure of visualization tools for researchers. For example, GIS can assist an epidemiologist with mapping data collected on disease outbreaks or help a health services researcher graphically communicate areas of nursing shortages. GIS technology illustrates relationships, connections, and patterns that are not necessarily obvious in any one data set, enabling the researcher to see overall relevant factors. ArcGIS 10 (ESRI, 2010) system is a GIS for management, analysis, and display of geographic knowledge, which is represented using a series of information sets. The information sets include maps and globes with 3-dimensional capabilities to describe networks, topologies, terrains, surveys, and attributes (Figure 43.4).

In summary, the major emphasis of this section has provided a brief discussion about the range of traditions, statistical considerations, and computer applications that aid the researcher in quantitative data analysis. As

```
Comprehensive meta analysis - [C:\Bristol\Magnesium.cma]                                    _ □ X

File  Edit  Format  View  Insert  Identify  Tools  Computational options  Analyses  Help

Run analyses  →  🔍 □ 🖿 🖻 🖫  🖨  ✂  🖹 🖻  🖫  '—'= '⦀  🔢 🔢 🗄  ▼  ↓ → + ✓ □  ↑↓ ↕ ⟲
```

	Study name	Treated Dead	Treated Total N	Control Dead	Control Total N	Odds ratio	Log odds ratio	Std Err	Year	J
1	Morton	1	40	2	36	0.436	-0.830	1.247	1984	
2	Rasmussen	9	135	23	135	0.348	-1.056	0.414	1986	
3	Smith	2	200	7	200	0.278	-1.278	0.808	1986	
4	Abraham	1	48	1	46	0.957	-0.043	1.430	1987	
5	Feldstedt	10	150	8	148	1.250	0.223	0.489	1988	
6	Schechter	1	59	9	56	0.090	-2.408	1.072	1989	
7	Ceremuzynski	1	25	3	23	0.278	-1.281	1.194	1989	
8	Bertschat	1	23	2	22	0.304	-1.192	1.661	1989	
9	Singh	6	76	11	75	0.499	-0.696	0.536	1990	
10	Pereira	1	27	7	27	0.110	-2.208	1.110	1990	
11	Schechter 1	2	89	12	80	0.130	-2.038	0.781	1991	
12	Golf	5	23	13	33	0.427	-0.850	0.618	1991	
13	Thogersen	4	130	8	122	0.452	-0.793	0.626	1991	
14	LIMIT-2	90	1159	118	1157	0.741	-0.299	0.147	1992	
15	Schechter 2	4	107	17	108	0.208	-1.571	0.574	1995	
16	ISIS-4	2216	29011	2103	29039	1.059	0.058	0.032	1995	

```
Cohort 2x2 (Events)
```

• **FIGURE 43.3.** Comprehensive meta-analysis (CMA) user interface. (Source: www.meta-analysis.com/pages/features/spreadsheet.html). Published with permission.

computers have continued to integrate data management functions with traditional statistical computational power, the researchers have been able to develop more extensive and sophisticated projects with data collected. Gone are the days of the calculator or punch cards, as the computing power now sits on the researchers' desktops or laptops, with speed and functionality at their fingertips.

THE QUALITATIVE APPROACH

Data Capture and Data Collection

The qualitative approach focuses on activities in the steps of the research process that differ greatly from the quantitative methods in fundamental sources of data, collection techniques, coding, analysis, and interpretation. Thus, the computer becomes a different kind of tool for the researcher in most aspects of the research beginning with the capture and recording of narrative or textual data.

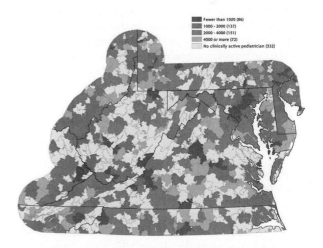

• **FIGURE 43.4.** ArcGIS map example: clinically active pediatricians. (Source: www.esri.com/what-is-gis/graphics/health_6b_lg.jpg)

In terms of qualitative research requiring narrative content analysis, the computer can be used to record the observations, narrative statements of subjects, and memos of the researcher in initial word processing applications for future coding. Software applications that aid researchers in transcription tasks include text scanners, such as OmniPage 17 (Nuance, 2010). Other devices include vocal recorders or speech recognition software such as Dragon Naturally Speaking 10 (Nuance, 2010), where the researcher can input the information into text documents by speaking into a microphone without typing. Some questions can elicit responses from subjects that can be captured directly. These narrative statements, like the quantitative surveys, can be either programmed for use in microcomputers or on the Internet's World Wide Web (WWW) so that subjects' responses can be entered directly into the computer.

Qualitative Data Collection. Simple electronic audio-taping is often used during interviews, whereby the content is entered into a word processing program by clerical assistants in preparation for analysis. The narrative statements entered into a word processor are stored for subsequent coding and sorting according to one's theoretical framework. Through analysis, categories from the data emerge as interpreted by the researcher. It is important to point out that for both quantitative and qualitative data, the computer application program is only a mechanical, clerical tool to aid the researcher in manipulating the data. Using the Internet for indirect and direct data collection in qualitative studies can also provide a vehicle for data analysis that yields a quantitative component as well as the qualitative analysis. Computers are not only able to record the subject's responses to the questions but also routinely record the number of minutes the subject was online and the number of times they logged in.

Data Coding and Data Analysis

Historically, qualitative researchers have relied on narrative notes, often first recorded as audio and later transcribed by a typist. Coding qualitative text data was a time-consuming task, often involving thousands of pages of typewritten notes and the use of scissors and tape for the development of coding and categories. With the advent of computer packages, the mechanical aspects of the coding and sorting have been reduced. The researcher must decide on which text may be of interest and use a word processing program to search for words, phrases, or other markers within a text file using any number of word processing software packages.

Some specific software packages developed for qualitative research coding and analysis interface directly with the most popular word processing software packages. The application program Ethnograph (Seidel & Clark, 1984; Seidel, Friese, & Lenard, 1994) was one of the first packages developed specifically for the purpose of managing some of the mechanical tasks of qualitative data analysis. The new version, Ethnograph 6.0 (Qualis Research, 2008), gives users a project management interface with functions to code, edit, and search data. The non-numerical unstructured data indexing, searching, and theorizing (NUD-IST) software was another qualitative package commonly used (Gahan & Hannibal, 1998; Richards & Richards, 1993). This program assisted the researcher to establish an index of data codes and seek relationships among the coding categories. The ease with which researchers can code and recode large amounts of data with the aid of computerized programs encourages the researcher to experiment with different ways of thinking about data and recategorizing them. Retrieval of categories or elements of data is facilitated by computer storage. Newer technologies have evolved from Ethnograph and NUD-IST with improved user interfaces, including the latest versions of NVivo 9, MAXQDA 10 (QSR, 2004), and ATLAS.ti 6 (ATLAS.ti 6, 2010).

Qualitative research, like quantitative research, is not a single entity, but a set of related yet individual traditions, aims, and methods. Some individual traditions within qualitative research are ethnography, grounded theory, phenomenology, and hermeneutics. The distinguishing feature of qualitative research is that the goal is to understand the qualities or essence of phenomena and/or focus on the meaning of these events to the participants or respondents in the study. The forms of data are usually the words of the respondents or informants rather than numbers. Computerization is especially helpful to the researcher in handling large amounts of data.

Computer Application Programs. A number of general-purpose or specific software packages can be used in qualitative analysis: one package is a free text retrieval program such as that available in a word processing program; another is any number of standard database management or indexing programs; third is a program specifically developed for the purpose of qualitative analysis. Table 43.1 presents side-by-side comparisons of 4 of the commonly used special-purpose programs for qualitative analysis.

General Purpose Software. Word processing programs in current use offer a number of features useful to the

TABLE 43.1 Comparison of Qualitative Data Analysis (QDA) Software

Software	Version	Web Source	Data Types	Length of Code Words/Node Titles	Display of Search Results	Platform(s)
ATLAS.ti	6	www.atlasti.com	Text (txt), graphic (jpeg, bmp, gif, png, pict), audio (wav, aif, mov, mp3), video (avi, mpeg, mov, swf, gif)	Not limited	Generates a hit list displaying a source tag and the first 30+ characters of coded segment. Report contains complete information about the source of the hit and the search function used.	PC, Mac, Sun Workstations
MAXqda	10	www.maxqda.com	Rich text	64 characters	Results are immediately displayed in a separate window. Source tags clearly identify the find. When running a search on selected codes, results can be displayed in table format.	PC
Ethnograph	6	www.qualisresearch.com	Plain text with special formatting rules, built-in editor	10 characters, longer definitions can be written in code book	Immediately displays the full results with detailed information. Search results can be displayed as text, count of hits, or percentages of hits within and across data files.	PC
NVivo	9	www.qsrinternational.com	Plain text and built-in editing of coded documents. Not including embedded objects. Video and audio links	Not limited	Results saved to a node in the Node Explorer. Results can be displayed in table format. Cells can display node addresses. Source tags clearly identify the find.	PC

qualitative researcher. The ability to search for certain key words allows the researcher to tag the categories of interest. In addition, such features as cut and paste; linking texts; insertion of pictures, tables, and charts; and the inclusion of video and audio data enhance the application. Add-on applications specific to integrating multiple elements help the researcher organize a range of data and materials for analysis. A comprehensive program is ATLAS.ti (Version 6.0) (ATLAS.ti 6, A2010), a powerful workbench for the qualitative analysis of large bodies of textual, graphical, audio, and video data. It offers a variety of tools for accomplishing the tasks associated with any systematic approach to "soft" data, such as material that cannot be analyzed by formal and statistical approaches in meaningful ways (ATLAS.ti 6,, 2010).

Data management programs (e.g., Excel) can be used to categorize data, link categories, and address a number of queries within categories, domains, or themes of interest. For example, the researcher can list all early adolescents who smoked more than one pack of cigarettes per day who gave birth to preterm babies. These programs work better for discrete rather than unstructured texts (Chang, 2001).

Special Purpose Software. Several software products have evolved and improved for the specific purpose of analyzing qualitative data. Ethnograph is one such program, which is used after the data have been entered with a word processing program and converted to an ASCII file. Each file can be designated by its context and identifying features using markers provided by the computer program. The researcher can have the program produce a file that numbers each line of the narrative data. From this line file, the researcher can begin to assign each line or paragraph a category. The researcher keeps track of the category definitions and is alert to dimensions that emerge. Recoding can be done to provide for inductive thinking and iterative comparisons. Through the use of a search command, the computer program can be made to search for data segments by categories throughout the typed document.

Ethnograph provides a column format, permitting numbered lines in the first column and categorical notations in the second column. Using a command entered by a researcher, it can selectively or globally delete or replace coding categories and produce an output file containing sorted, cross-referenced coded segments from the original text data sets entered via a word processing program. The split screen allows the researcher to view more than one file at a time, so is useful in constant comparison and contrasting of data. Researcher memos and theoretical notes written by the researcher

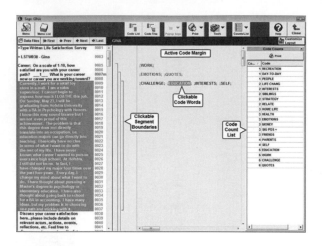

• **FIGURE 43.5.** Example of coding using Ethnograph. (Source: www.qualisresearch.com). Published with permission Qualis Research.

during analysis can also be stored and retrieved with Ethnograph. Figure 43.5 presents a sample screen of coding and data.

NVivo 9 and XSight from QSR (Qualitative Solutions & Research Pty. Ltd, 1999) provide a new generation of software tools with multiple advantages for researchers. Because qualitative research takes many forms, these two applications can be selected based on the user's specific methodologic goals, the nature and scale of the study, and the computer equipment. While NVivo 9 supports fluid, rich data, detailed text analysis, and theory building, it also can manage documents

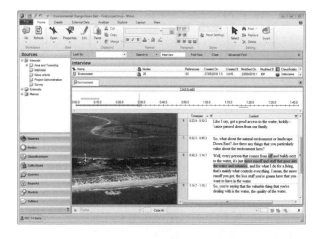

• **FIGURE 43.6.** Screenshot of NVivo9 main Window. (Source: www.qsrinternational.com). Published with permission from QSR International.

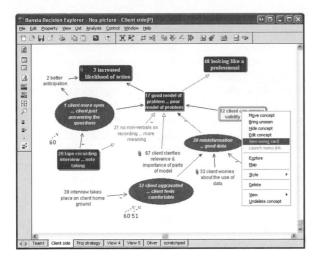

• **FIGURE 43.7.** Example of cognitive mapping analysis: (Source: www.banxia.com/dexplore/pictures.html). Published with permission.

or nodes in visual displays that show the structure and properties of the document (Figure 43.6).

Conceptual Network Systems. A system known as *concept diagrams, semantic nets, or conceptual networks* is one in which information is represented in a graphic manner. The objects in one's conceptual system (e.g., age and experiences) are coded and represented by a box diagram (node). The objects are linked (by arcs) to other objects to show relationships. Like rule-based systems, semantic nets have been widely used in artificial intelligence work. In order to view the relationships of an object in the system, the researcher examines the node in the graph and follows the arcs to and from it (Huberman & Miles, 1999). Semantic network applications may be useful in model building and providing a pictorial overview. Decision Explorer (Banxia, 2004) offers the user a powerful set of mapping tools to aid in the decision-making process for audience response activities. Ideas can be mapped and the resulting cognitive map can be further analyzed (Figure 43.7). The software has many practical uses, such as gathering and structuring interview data and as an aid in the strategy formulation process. The software is primarily described as being a recording and facilitation tool for the elicitation of ideas, as well as a tool to structure and communicate qualitative data. It allows the user to gather and analyze qualitative data and thus make sense of many pieces of qualitative data in order to achieve a coherent picture of a given issue or problem (Banxia, 2010).

Data Analysis for Qualitative Data. Qualitative data analyses often occur on an ongoing basis with data collection in a reflexive and iterative fashion. There is no clear demarcation of when data collection should end and analysis should begin. The process of obtaining observations, interviews, and other data over a period of time results in a vast body of data that may include hundreds or thousands of pages of field notes and researcher memos. Although computer applications can aid considerably in organizing and sorting this mass of data, the theoretical and analytical aspects of decision making about concepts and themes must be made by the researcher (Chang, 2001).

As an example, some of the tasks the computer can facilitate in data analysis using grounded theory (one approach to qualitative research) are as follows. Once a researcher has determined which parts of the interviews and observations can be tagged as categories, certain properties or dimensions can be determined and coded. The researcher may engage in "constant comparison," comparing the meanings of all incidents that have been similarly categorized. This process should continue until the researcher determines that the categories are internally consistent, fit with the data, and are saturated. Saturation is achieved when the researcher can find no more properties for a category and new data are redundant with the old (Cresswell, 2009).

Strauss and Corbin (1990) suggest that, in the later stages of research, the researcher may engage in axial coding. In this stage, the researcher elaborates and explains key categories, considering the conditions under which the event occurs, the processes that take place, and possible consequences. Glaser (1978) indicates that the researcher may engage in theoretical sampling, which is a deliberate search for episodes in incidents that enlarge the variances of properties and place boundaries around categories.

Uses and Caution. Software programs exist for qualitative research that save researcher time doing file management, reducing the manual labor of cutting, pasting, sorting, and manual filing. They may also encourage the researcher to examine the data from different perspectives, recoding and reorganizing the data in different frameworks.

One must be mindful that qualitative analysis is a cognitive process, not a mechanical one (Chang, 2001). The essence of qualitative research is the meaning and interpretation of the data within context. The ability of software enhancements to generate quasifrequency distributions and cross-tabulations tend to further increase the investigator's confidence in believing such findings and relationships, when in fact these may be an artifact of the way in which the data are manipulated. While computer programs facilitate coding, organization of data, and preparation of the data for interpretation, they cannot replace the thinking and decision making that is at the heart of qualitative analysis. As in all research, the burden of analysis and interpretation rests on the researchers (Chang, 2001).

Dissemination of Results

While dissemination of results continues to occur by traditional means such as presentations at professional meetings and publication in journals and monographs, online reporting is becoming increasingly common. Some Web sites frequented by nurses are peer review journals such as *Online Journal of Nursing Informatics* (www.cisnet.com) and selected nursing articles on various Web sites such as that of the ANA (www.nursing-world.org). Nursing forums sponsored by various professional nursing organizations (e.g., *American Journal of Nursing*, Sigma Theta Tau, and National League for Nursing) often allow participants to chat online with presenters or authors of certain articles on designated dates during scheduled times. Nearly all organizations have their own Web sites. Some examples are the Alzheimer's Disease Education and Referral Center (www.alzheimers.org), American Heart Association (www.americanheart.org), American Medical Informatics Association (www.amia.org), and RAND Corporation (www.rand.org). The Cochran Collection has numerous centers all over the world through the Cochrane Collaborative (www.cochrane.org). As with all publications, online as well as hardcopy, the information accessed must be evaluated by the users regarding appropriateness for the purpose for which it was retrieved.

Reports to most government and some nongovernment agencies require the researcher to submit a converted document online. Grant proposals submitted to the federal government currently require online submission with conversion to PDF. National Institutes of Health (NIH) applicants are directed to a page with downloadable programs to convert the documents before submitting them (www.grants.gov/help/download_software.jsp). In fact, there is a trend for all manuscript submissions to be accomplished online. Regardless of the method of submission and medium for publication, the published article may be incorporated into one or several online bibliographic retrieval systems.

This chapter has summarized the processes of quantitative and qualitative research and described select computerized tools that can assist the researcher in proposal preparation, data collection, data coding, data analysis, and dissemination for both types of research. The following section highlights examples for 3 categories of research on computer use and nursing informatics in: (1) electronic data such as data mining large electronic data sets and electronic nursing documentation; (2) Web-based interventions; and (3) specialized computer applications in clinical practice. The examples include both quantitative and qualitative studies in which the nurse researchers inevitably used a variety of software tools in the proposal development, data collection, measurement, analysis, and/or dissemination activities.

EXAMPLES OF RESEARCH STUDIES

Computers are inextricably tied to the process of conducting research, but there are also good examples of research on computer use in the nursing literature. Several of the following examples also describe computerized processes for conducting quantitative and qualitative research approaches. These examples provide focus on nursing research related to computer use and informatics as well as using computers in the process of doing the research.

Electronic Data and Electronic Documentation Research

There are several different studies that highlight using electronic data and electronic health records in data mining or care documentation.

Secondary Analysis of Large Data Sets. In a study by Atherton, Feeg, and El-Adham (2003), a secondary analysis was done on a publicly available data set from the federal government. The researchers hypothesized that race, ethnicity, and insurance coverage would be determinants of pregnant women receiving epidural anesthesia during delivery. They designed the study as an exploratory examination of data in the Agency for Healthcare Research and Quality (AHRQ) Medical Expenditure Panel Survey (MEPS) HC-046 (1996–2000 Pregnancy Files), a nationally representative survey of the U.S. civilian noninstitutionalized population (www.meps.ahrg.gov/mepsweb). This data set includes specific variables of interest collected by interviewers through a series of 5 rounds of interviews over a 2.5-year period. Using computer-assisted personal interviewing (CAPI) technology, data were collected from each household as part of the larger project cosponsored by AHRQ and the National Center for Health Statistics.

The sampling frame for the MEPS HC is drawn from respondents to the National Health Interview Survey (NHIS), which provides a nationally representative sample of the United States with over-sampling of Hispanics and blacks (MEPS HC-046, 2003). Based on predictions formed from the literature, the researchers predicted differences in race or ethnicity and health insurance coverage for use of epidural during normal, vaginal, uncomplicated delivery.

The data were downloaded from the Internet and imported into a spreadsheet data file using Microsoft Excel. After intensive cleaning and matching of the data with the panels containing full sets of demographic information available from the NHIS data on the subjects, the usable set of MEPS data was coded to control for extraneous variables that might have confounded the findings, including complications associated with childbirth. The clean data set was submitted to a logistic regression analysis to identify determinants of epidural use. With some patch coding between the files and logistic regression within the SAS options on the final data set, the researchers were able to determine that ethnicity and insurance coverage significantly influenced whether a woman received an epidural during childbirth.

Computerized Documentation of Nursing Care Plans.
In a randomized trial on electronic documentation of nursing care plans, Feeg, Saba, and Feeg (2008) tested the quality of nursing student care planning on a bedside personal computer (PC) using a standardized nursing terminology in a specially designed Microsoft Access database program (Clinical Care Classification System) compared with an open-text format type-in application with the same terminology. Students were randomly assigned to 1 of the 2 versions of electronic nursing documentation formats and interviewed 2 simulated patients who served for all of the participants. The simulated patients were interviewed about their symptoms: one presented with congestive heart failure, the other with pneumonia. Participants were instructed to document the care immediately following the interview on a laptop stationed at the patient's bedside. Measures were developed to assess the quality of the care plans and the participants' evaluation of using the system. Data were analyzed revealing a statistically significant difference ($p = .05$) for the Microsoft Access care plans completed by participants and a statistically significant difference in the students' reports on using the system ($p = .025$).

The results demonstrate that the data-based PC application is effective in recording nursing care planning information using the nursing process. It captures patient care information with a coded, standardized nursing language (CCC) ready for integration with other patient electronic medical record data and the participants preferred it over free-text entry.

Web-Based Tools and Interventions.
A significant body of research has been conducted on using the Internet as a tool for conducting research, as well as studies on Web-designed interventions for clinical problems. For example, Yen and Bakken (2009) tested the usability of a Web-based tool for managing open shifts on nursing units. Using observational and interview approaches, they evaluated a Web communication tool (BidShift) designed to allow managers to announce open work shifts to solicit staff to request their own work shifts. They used specialized software to capture screens and vocal utterances as participants were asked to think aloud as they completed 3 subtasks associated with the open-shift management process. After task completion, they were asked about the process and their responses were recorded. Their data were managed and coded using Morae, specialized software developed for usability testing (www.techsmith.com/morae.asp). This example of qualitative research reported participants' patterns of use and themes related to their perceptions of usability of the communication tool.

In another qualitative study on electronic encounters using Web-based videoconferencing, Nystrom and Ohrling (2007) created a series of e-meetings for new fathers of children under 1 year old to "meet" in parental support groups. The technology allowed both one-on-one and group encounters. The fathers were interviewed using a narrative approach and content analysis was applied to the interview data. The researchers identified 3 categories from the transcripts: (1) being unfamiliar and insecure talking about fatherhood, (2) sharing experiences and being confirmed, and (3) being supported and limited by the electronic encounters.

Andersen and Ruland (2009) studied an Internet-based online patient-nurse communication (OPNC) service to support patients with prostate and breast cancer. Using qualitative content analysis, they examined 276 messages in a tailored Internet support intervention over 15 months. Two main themes emerged: (1) concerns about physical symptoms and treatment side effects and (2) worries and questions about treatment and follow-up. They concluded that the OPNC service can meet patients' needs for advice and information, thus improving the quality of care.

In a meta-analysis on the effectiveness of Web-based and non–Web-based interventions on behavior change, Wantland, Portillo, Holzemer, Slaughter, and McGhee (2004) synthesized 22 articles identified from the

MEDLINE, CINAHL, Cochrane Library, EMBASE, ERIC, and PSYCHInfo databases that were appropriate for the analysis. They described a 12-fold increase in citations in a 7-year period without a substantial review on the use and effectiveness of Web-based interventions. Their meta-analysis of the 22 studies concluded that the effect-size comparisons in the use of Web-based interventions to achieve a specified knowledge and/or behavior change demonstrated significant changes: increase in exercise time, knowledge of nutritional status, knowledge of asthma treatment, and 18-month weight loss maintenance.

Specialized Computer Applications in Clinical Care. Computer based administration of assessment is a reliable means of collecting patient assessment data as demonstrated by the report by Wilkie and colleagues (2001) who evaluated the feasibility and acceptability of a computerized assessment of cancer-related symptoms in 41 patients. If information could be collected prior to encounters with physicians via a specially designed program on a laptop computer with touch screen, patients' reports on their perceived quality of life (QOL) and symptoms could be produced as a colorful graphic display and used in the patient-provider encounter. In a study conducted by Mullen, Berry, and Zierler (2004), 45 patients with cancer being evaluated for radiation therapy and 10 clinicians were asked to complete acceptability and usability survey questions. The patient acceptability survey indicated that 70% liked the computers; 79% thought the program was easy to use; 91% thought it was easy to understand; and 71% reported it was enjoyable. Of the clinicians, 83% found the graphic output helpful in promoting communication with patients, 75% found the computerized output to be helpful and 83% indicated that the output helped guide clinical interactions with patients. In this study, the specialized computer application served as an intervention and tool for data collection demonstrating that a computer-based QOL and symptom assessment tool was useful as a clinical intervention.

SUMMARY

This chapter has reviewed two research paradigms and philosophical orientations that specify different underlying approaches to research and the use of computers in various stages of the research process. It also highlighted examples of research on computer use with these quantitative and qualitative approaches. A variety of computer applications are available via commercialized packages that serve the nurse researcher in conducting research. In addition, research on computer applications and informatics is a growing body of science that will continue to proliferate in the literature.

According to Bakken, Stone, and Larson (2008), the context for nursing informatics research has changed significantly over the last 15 years. The emergence of genetic and genomic science promises to revolutionize healthcare. The rapid expansion of social (Web 2.0) technologies has unleashed new possibilities for patients and caregivers to share knowledge and decision making. The avalanche of information will bury us, and it mandates the refinement of technologies to organize, sort, synthesize, and evaluate data into meaningful knowledge for providers and consumers.

The contextual influences on nursing research are discussed by Bakken and colleagues (2008). The nursing informatics research agenda for the next 10 years must expand users of interest to include interdisciplinary researchers; build upon the knowledge gained in genomic and environmental data; guide the re-engineering of nursing practice; harness new technologies to empower patients and their caregivers in collaborative knowledge development, particularly related to the social network technologies; and evaluate innovative methodologies that recognize human-computer interface factors.

REFERENCES

Agency for Healthcare Research and Quality. (2003). Medical Expenditure Panel Survey. *1996–2000. Pregnancy Files*. Rockville, MD: Agency for Healthcare Research and Quality

Andersen, T., & Ruland, C. (2009). Cancer patients' questions and concerns expressed in an online nurse-delivered mail service: Preliminary results. In K. Saranto et al. (eds.), *Connecting Health and Humans*. Location: IOS Press, Fairfax, VA.

ATLAS.ti 6. (2010). Thousand Oaks, London: SAGE. Available at http://www.atlasti.com.

Atherton, M., Feeg, V., & El-Adham, A. (2003). Racial, ethnic and insurance determinants of epidural use in childbirth: Analysis of a national sample survey. *Nursing Economic, 22*(1), 6–13.

Bakken, S., Cook, S., Curtis, L., Soupios, M., & Curran, C. (2003). Informatics competencies pre- and post-implementation of a Palm-based student clinical log and informatics for evidence-based practice curriculum. In *Proceedings of the American Medical Informatics Association Symposium* (pp. 42–46).

Bakken, S., Stone, P. & Larson, E. (2008). A nursing informatics research agenda for 2008–2018: Contextual influences and key components. *Nursing Outlook, 56,* 206–214.

Berger, A. M., & Berger, C. R. (2004). Data mining as a tool for research and knowledge development in nursing. *Computers, Informatics, Nursing, 22*(3), 123–131.

Biostat. (2000). *Comprehensive MetaAnalysis*. Retrieved from http://www.meta-analysis.com/html/biostat.html.

Biostat (2000). *Power & precision version*. Englewood, NJ: Biostat.

Brennan, P. F., & Ripich, S. (1994). Use of a home-care computer network by persons with AIDS. *International Journal of Technology Assessment in Healthcare, 10,* 258–272.

Brennan, P. F., Zielstorff, R. D., Ozbolt, J. G., & Strombom, I. (1998). Setting a national research agenda in nursing informatics. *Medinfo, 9,* 1188–1191.

Bulechek, G. M., & McCloskey, J. (1997). All users of NIC encouraged to submit new interventions, suggest revisions. Iowa Intervention Project Research Team. *Image: The Journal of Nursing Scholarship, 1,* 10–20.

Byrne, B. M. (1984). *Structural equation modeling with EQS and EQS/Windows: Basic concepts, applications, and programming*. Thousand Oaks, CA: Sage.

Cerner Corporation (2005). White paper: *The APACHE® IV Equations: Benchmarks for mortality and resource use*. Kansas City: Cerner Corporation.

Congressional Budget Office (CBO). (2007, December). *Research on the comparative effectiveness of medical treatments: Issues and options for an expanded federal role*. Washington, DC: CBO Report.

Chang, B. L. (2001). Computer use in nursing research. In V. Saba & K. McCormick (Eds.), *Essentials of computers for nurses: Informatics for the new millennium*. New York: McGraw-Hill.

Corel Corporation. (2010). *Wordperfect X5*. Ottawa, ON.

Cresswell, J. W. (2009). *Research design: Qualitative, quantitative, and mixed methods approaches* (3rd ed.). Thousand Oaks, CA: Sage.

Daly, J. M., Maas, M. L., & Johnson, M. (1997). Nursing outcomes classification: An essential element in data sets for nursing and healthcare effectiveness. *Computers in Nursing 15,* S82–S86.

Department of Health and Human Services (DHHS). (2007, January). *Breaking news: Nationwide health information technology standard for nursing*. Washington, DC: Department of Health and Human Services.

Effken, J. A. (2003). An organizing framework for nursing informatics research. *Computers, Informatics, Nursing, 21,* 316–323.

Esri. (2004). *ArcGIS® 9*. Redlands, CA. Available at http://www.esri.com.

Expert Choice, Inc. (2009). *Expert Choice® 11.5*. Arlington, VA. Available at http://www.expertchoice.com.

Feeg, V. D. (1999). Using the analytic hierarchy process as an alternative weighting technique to magnitude estimation scaling. *Nursing Research, 48*(6), 207–214.

Feeg, V. D., Saba, V., & Feeg, A. (2008). Testing a bedside personal computer clinical care classification system for nursing students using Microsoft Access®. *Computers, Informatics, Nursing, 26*(6), 339–349.

FileMaker, Inc. (2004). *FileMaker Pro® 11*. Santa Clara, CA. Available at http://www.filemaker.com.

Gahan, C., & Hannibal, M. (1998). *Doing qualitative Research using QSR NUD.IST*. Thousand Oaks, CA: SCOLARI Sage Publications Software.

Glaser, B. G. (1978). *Theoretical sensitivity*. Mill Valley, CA: Sociological Press.

Granello, D., & Wheaton, J. (2004). Online data collection: Strategies for research. *Journal of Counseling and Development, 82,* 387–393.

Gravic, Inc. (2010). *Remark Office®, Remark Classic®, Remark Web Survey®*. Available at http://www.gravic.com/remark.

Hansebo, G., Kihlgren, M., Ljunggren, G., & Winbald, B. (1999). Staff views on the Resident Assessment Instrument, RAI/MDS, in nursing homes, and the use of the Cognitive Performance Scale, CPS, in different levels of care in Stockholm, Sweden. *Journal of Advanced Nursing, 3,* 642–653.

Huberman, A. M., & Miles, M. B. (1999). Data management and analysis methods. In N. K. Denzin and YSL (Ed.), *Handbook of qualitative research* (pp. 428–440). Thousand Oaks, CA: Sage.

IBM SPSS Statistics. (2010). *Statistical package for social sciences (SPSS)*. Chicago, IL. Available at http://www.spss.com/statistics.

Joreskog, K. G., & Sorbom, D. (1978). *LISREL IV's user's guide*. Chicago, IL: National Educational Resources.

Krueger, C., van Oostrum, J., & Shuster, J. (2010). A longitudinal description of heart rate variability in 28-34 week-old preterm infants. *Journal of Biological Nursing, 11*(30), 261–268.

Martin, K. S., & Norris, J. (1996). The Omaha system: A model for describing practice. *Holistic Nursing Practice, 11,* 75–83.

McCormick, K. A., Lang, N., Zielstorff, R., et al. (1994). Toward standard classification schemes for nursing language: Recommendations of the American Nurses Association Steering Committee on databases to support clinical nursing practice. *Journal of the American Medical Informatics Association, 1,* 421–427.

Microsoft Corporation. (2010a). *Excel®*. Redmond, WA.

Microsoft Corporation. (2010b). *Microsoft Word®*. Redmond, WA.

Montalbano, E. (2009, June 4). Forrester: Microsoft Office in no danger from competitors. *PC World*. Retrieved from http://www.pcworld.com/businesscenter/article/166123/forrester_microsoft_office_in_no_danger_from_competitors.html.

Mullen, K., Berry, D., & Zierler, B. (2004). Computerized symptom and quality-of-life assessment for patients with cancer. Part II: Acceptability and usability. *Oncology Nursing Forum, 31*(5), E84–E89.

MSDN Library. (2000). *Building and using data mining models.* Microsoft Corporation.. Retrievd from *http://msdn.microsoft.com/library/default.asp?url=/library/en-us/olapdmad/agdatamining_686r.asp.*

Nahm, E., Vaydia, V., Ho, D., Scharf, B., & Seagull, J. (2007). Outcomes assessment of clinical information system implementation: A practical guide. *Nursing Outlook, 55,* 282–288.

NINR Priority Expert Panel on Nursing Informatics. (1993). *Nursing informatics: Enhancing patient care.* Bethesda, MD: U.S. Department of Health and Human Services, U.S. Public Health Service, National Institutes of Health.

Nuance Dragon Solutions. (2010). *Dragon Naturally Speaking®10.* Burlington, MA. Available at *http://www.nuance.com/naturallyspeaking.*

Nuance Imaging. (2010). OmniPage *Pro® 17.* Burlington, MA. Available at http://www.nuance.com/imaging.

Nystrom, K., & Ohrling, K. (2008). Electronic encounters: Fathers' experiences of parental support. *Journal of Telemedicine and Telecare, 14,* 71–74.

Orem, D. E. (2001). *Nursing: Concepts of practice* (6th ed.). St. Louis, MO: C. V. Mosby.

Ozbolt, J. G. (1999). *Testimony to the NCVHS hearings on medical terminology and code development.* School of Nursing and Division of Biomedical Informatics, School of Medicine, Vanderbilt University.

Polit, D. (2009). *Statistics and data analysis for nursing research* (2nd ed.). Upper Saddle River, NJ: Prentice Hall.

Qualis Research. (2008). *Ethnograph 6.0.* Colorado Springs, CO. Available at http://www.qualisresearch.com/default.htm.

Qualitative Solutions & Research Pty. Ltd. (1999). *NVivo, NUD*IST, NUD*IST Vivo, NUDIST, & NUDIST VIVO.* Available at http://www.qsrinternational.com.

Richards, L., & Richards, T. J. (1993). *QSR NUD.IST.* Victoria, Australia: Qualitative Solutions and Research Pty. Ltd.

Rolley, J., Davidson, P., Dennison, C., Ong, A., Everett, B., & Salamonson, Y. (2008). Medication adherence self-report instruments: Implications for practice and research. *Journal of Cardiovascular Nursing, 23*(6), 497–505.

Saba, V. K. (1997). Why the home healthcare classification is a recognized nursing nomenclature. *Computers in Nursing, 15,* S69–S76.

Saba, V. K. (2007). *Clinical Care Classification (CCC) System Manual: A guide to nursing documentation.* New York: Springer Pub.

SAS Institute. (2010). *Statistical Analysis System.* Cary, NC: Scansoft, Inc. Available at http://www.sas.com/software/sas9.

SAS Institute. (2010). *Statistical Software for Professionals.* Cary, NC: Scansoft, Inc.

Seidel, J., & Clark, J. (1984). The Ethnograph: A computer program for the analysis of qualitative data. *Qualitative Sociology, 7*(12), 110–125.

Seidel, J., Friese, S., & Lenard, C. (1994). *Ethnograph* (Version 4.0). Amherst, MA: Qualis Research Associates.

Strauss, A , & Corbin, J.M. (1990). *Basics of qualitative research: Grounded theory procedures and techniques.* Newbury Park, CA: Sage.

SYSTAT 13. (2010). Systat Software Inc. Chicago, IL.

The Thomson Corporation. (2009). *Reference Manager* (Version 8). Carlsbad, CA: Thomson ISI ResearchSoft. Available at http://www.refman.com/pr-rm11.asp.

Thompson, T., & Brailer, D. (2004). *The decade of health information technology: Delivering consumer-centric and information rich healthcare.* Washington, DC: Department of Health and Human Services (DHHS).

Wantland, D., Portillo, C., Holzemer, W., Slaughter, R., & McGhee, E. (2004). The effectiveness of Web-based vs. non-Web-based interventions: A meta-analysis of behavioral change outcomes. 6(4), e40.

Weiss, S. J. (1995). Contemporary empiricism. In A. Omery, C. E. Kasper, & G. G.

Page (Eds.), In *Search of nursing science* (pp. 13–17). Thousand Oaks, CA: Sage.

Werley, H. H., Lang, N. M., & Westlake, S. K. (1986). The nursing minimum data set conference: Executive summary. *Journal of Professional Nursing, 2,* 217–224.

Wilkie, D., Huang, H., Berry, D., Schwartz, A., Lin, Y., Ko, N. et al. (2001). Cancer symptom control: Feasibility of a tailored, interactive computerized program for patients. *Family Community Health, 24*(3), 48–62.

Wilkie, D., Judge, M.K., Berry, D., Dell, J., Zhong, S. & Gilespie, R. (2003). Usability of a computerized PAIN ReportIt in the general public with pain and people with cancer pain. *Journal of Pain and Symptom Management, 25*(3), 213–224.

Yen, P., & Bakken, S. (2009). Usability testing of a Web-based tool for managing open shifts on nursing units. In K. Saranto et al., (Eds.), *Connecting health and humans.* Location: IOS Press, Fairfax, VA.

Zielstorff, R. D., Lang, N. M., Saba, V. K., et al. (1995). Toward a uniform language for nursing in the US: Work of the American Nurses Association Steering Committee on databases to support clinical practice. *Medinfo, 8*(2), 1362–1366.

Zulkowski, K. (1999). MDS + Items not contained in the pressure ulcer RAP associated with pressure ulcer, prevalence in newly institutionalized elderly. *Ostomy/Wound Management, 1,* 24–33.

Information Literacy and Computerized Information Resources

Diane S. Pravikoff / June Levy / Annelle Tanner

- OBJECTIVES
  1. Define information literacy.
  2. Identify steps in choosing appropriate databases.
  3. Identify steps in planning a computer search for information.
  4. Identify sources of information for practicing nurses.
  5. Identify the difference between essential and supportive computerized resources.

- KEY WORDS

  information literacy
  information retrieval
  MEDLINE/PubMed
  CINAHL
  Nursing Reference Center
  Mosby's Nursing Suite
  unified medical language system
  health reference databases
  electronic resources

INTRODUCTION

This chapter presents information about electronic resources that are easily available and accessible and can assist nurses in maintaining and enhancing their professional practices. These resources aid in keeping current with the published literature, in developing a list of sources for practice, research and/or education, and in collaborating with colleagues.

As is evidenced in earlier chapters, nurses use computers for many purposes. In the past, most of the focus has been on computerized patient records, acuity systems, and physician ordering systems. One of the major

purposes for which computers can be used, however, is searching for information. Many resources are available by computer, and the information retrieved can be used to accomplish different ends. Computers also are available in various sizes, improving portability and availability wherever a nurse is practicing. Many of the resources described in the following sections will be available via mobile devices.

To maintain professional credibility, nursing professionals must (1) keep current with the published literature, (2) develop and maintain a list of bibliographic and other sources on specific topics of interest for practice, research, and/or education, and (3) collaborate and network with colleagues regarding specifics of professional practice. Electronic resources are available to meet each of these needs. This chapter addresses each of these requirements for professional credibility and discusses both essential and supportive computerized resources available to meet them. *Essential* computerized resources are defined as those resources that are vital and necessary to the practitioner to accomplish the specific goal. In the case of maintaining currency, for example, these resources include bibliographic retrieval systems such as MEDLINE or the CINAHL database, current awareness services, review services, or point-of-care tools and may be accessible on the World Wide Web. *Supportive* computerized resources are those that are helpful and interesting and supply good information but are not necessarily essential for professional practice. In meeting the requirement of maintaining currency, supportive computerized resources include document delivery services, electronic publishers, and metasites on the World Wide Web. There are many resources available to meet each of the above requirements for professional credibility. For the purposes of this chapter, selective resources are identified and discussed as examples of the types of information available. Website URLs of the various resources are included as well. It is important that the nursing professional determine her or his exact requirements before beginning the search. Planning the search will be stressed throughout this chapter.

INFORMATION SEEKING BEHAVIOR OF REGISTERED NURSES

Multiple practice standards organizations [Institute of Medicine (IOM), Agency for Healthcare Research and Quality (AHRQ)], American Nurse Credentialing Center's Magnet Recognition Program, American Association of Colleges of Nursing, National League for Nursing, JCAHO) insist that nursing care be based on information derived from best practice evidence. To identify best evidence and apply it in the care of the patient, the nurse must apply the information literacy process (Association of College and Research Libraries, 2000):

1. Recognize the need for evidence
2. Know how to search and find relevant information
3. Access, utilize, and evaluate such information within the practice environment

Information literacy is identified as a competency for the basic nurse (American Nurses Association, 2008). The American Library Association describes the "information literate" person as one who can "recognize when information is needed and have the ability to locate, evaluate, and use effectively the needed information" and identifies it as a basic competency for higher education (American Library Association, 1989, p. 1).

While the importance of maintaining currency with published literature is stressed, research indicates that nurses often do not access the tools needed to do so. Neither do they have the ability to utilize these tools, if available within their work setting. A national study (Pravikoff, Pierce, & Tanner, 2005) of 3000 nurses licensed to practice in the United States was conducted in 2004 to better understand the readiness of nurses to utilize evidence-based nursing practice, based on their information literacy knowledge and competency. Results based on a 36.5% response rate indicated:

- 34.5% felt they needed information only seldom or occasionally
- Almost half were not even familiar with the term *evidence-based practice* (EBP)
- More than half had never identified a researchable problem
- Most did not search the most reliable sources for appropriate information (76% never searched Cinahl; 58% never searched Medline)
- Slightly over half had a medical or health sciences library where they work
- Almost half did not have access to print journals at their workplace
- Few had received training in the use of online bibliographic databases, the best tools for searching for evidence
- Even if tools were available in the workplace, 43% of the responding nurses considered them inadequate to meet their needs

This landmark study demonstrated that nurses were not aware that they needed information; once they recognized a need, online resources available for them to use were inadequate and respondents had not been taught how to use online databases to search for the information they needed. Additionally, they did not value research as a basis on which to formulate and implement patient care.

The rate of expansion in health information technology (electronic health records) is phenomenal; additionally, clinical knowledge is multiplying exponentially and dissemination methods are changing to include scholarly databases and social networking. Despite of the demands for EBP, nurses continue to have difficulty finding information they need for practice (Courey, Benson-Soros, Deemer, & Zeller, 2006; Dee, 2005).

Researchers at the University of Washington studied information seeking behavior of today's students and concluded, "Students conceptualize research, especially tasks associated with seeking information, as a competency learned by rote, rather than as an opportunity to learn, develop, or expand upon an *information-gathering strategy which leverages the wide range of resources available* to them in the digital age" (Head & Eisenberg, 2009, p. 1)

Nurses—students, clinicians, educators, and managers—must develop efficient and effective search strategies that embrace information literacy as a framework to search the myriad of information resources available for evidence. According to recent studies, education is embracing the change by imbedding well-designed courses that offer opportunities to develop these skills throughout program curricula (Schulte, 2008; Morgan, Fogel, Hicks, et. al., 2007; Skiba, 2005). Results indicate that such courses are indeed effective in improving the nurse's skills and confidence in searching for evidence (Bailey, Derbyshire, Harding, et al., 2007; Craig & Corrallt, 2007). Change in practice culture is needed to infuse information literacy throughout the workplace.

The resources and search strategy introduced in this chapter provide the reader with tools that will become the basis of life-long learning for the nurse—tools for evidence-based practice.

MAINTAINING CURRENCY WITH THE PUBLISHED LITERATURE

It is obvious that one of the most important obligations a nurse must meet is to maintain currency in her or his field of practice. With the extreme demands in the clinical environment—both in time and amount of work—nurses need easily accessible resources to answer practice-related questions and ensure that they are practicing with the latest and most evidence-based information. Information is needed about current treatments, trends, medications, safety issues, business practices, and new health issues, among other topics.

The purpose of the information retrieved from the sources listed below is to enable nurses to keep abreast of the latest and most evidence-based information in their selected field. Both quantity *and* quality must be considered. When using a resource, check that:

1. The resource covers the required specialty/field
2. The primary journals and peripheral material in the field are included

3. The resource is updated regularly and is current
4. The resource covers the appropriate period
5. The resource covers material published in different countries and languages
6. There is some form of peer review, reference checking, or other means of evaluation

Essential Computerized Resources

Essential computerized resources for maintaining currency include bibliographic retrieval systems for the journal literature, current awareness services, review services of the journal literature, point-of-care tools and currently published books. All of these assist the nurse in gathering the most current and reliable information.

Bibliographic Retrieval Systems

One of the most useful resources for accessing information about current practice is the journal literature. Although there may be a delay between the writing and publishing of an article, this time period is seldom more than a few months. The best way to peruse this literature is through a bibliographic retrieval system, since there is far too much literature published to read it all. Bibliographic retrieval systems also allow filtering and sorting of this vast amount of published material.

A bibliographic retrieval system database allows the nurse to retrieve a list of citations containing bibliographic details of the material indexed, subject headings, and author abstracts. The nurse can search these systems using specific subject headings or key words. Most bibliographic retrieval systems have a controlled vocabulary, also known as a thesaurus or subject heading list, to make electronic subject searching much easier. For this reason, the vocabulary is geared toward the specific content of the database. These controlled vocabularies are made available online as part of the database. Key word searching is necessary when there are no subject headings to cover the concepts being searched. The nurse can also search by specific fields including author, author affiliation, journal title, serial number (ISSN), grant name or number, or publication type. In bibliographic retrieval systems, most fields in the records are word-indexed and can be searched individually to retrieve specific information.

Previously available as print indexes, these systems are now available electronically through online services, or via the World Wide Web. To access them, a computer with a modem, and/or Internet access is required.

Since each of these bibliographic retrieval systems has its own specific content, a nurse may have to search several systems to retrieve a comprehensive list of citations on a particular topic. Directories of descriptions of bibliographic retrieval systems can be found on the World Wide Web, eg, DoCDat, directory of clinical databases in the U.K. (http://www.clingov.nscsha.nhs.uk/Default.aspx?aid=3303), Database Descriptions by Dykes Library (http://library.kumc.edu/), and the National Library of Medicine (NLM) databases (http://www.nlm.nih.gov/databases/).

The main bibliographic retrieval systems that should first be considered are MEDLINE, the CINAHL database, Mosby's Index, ERIC, PsycINFO, and the SocialSciences Citation Index.

MEDLINE/PubMed. The NLM provides free access to many online resources (Table 44.1). One of these, MEDLINE, covers 5,455 journals in 37 languages with over 20 million references from 1966 to the present in the fields of medicine, nursing, preclinical sciences, healthcare systems, veterinary medicine, and dentistry. The nursing subset in MEDLINE covers 189 nursing journals. The database is updated weekly on the World Wide Web (National Library of Medicine, 2010a, 2010b).

The NLM's databases use a controlled vocabulary (thesaurus), called MeSH (Medical Subject Headings) (MeSH: http://www.nlm.nih.gov/mesh/). These index terms facilitate subject searching within the databases.

TABLE 44.1	A List of Online Databases		
Database	**URL**	**Subject**	**Type**
	General Databases		
AIDSinfos	http://aidsinfo.nih.gov	HIV/AIDS clinical trials	Factual and referral
ClinicalTrials.gov	http://clinicaltrials.gov	Patient studies for drugs and treatment	Factual and referral
DIRLINE	http://dirline.nlm.nih.gov	Directory of organizations providing information services	Referral
HSRProj (health services research projects in progress)	http://gateway.nlm.nih.gov	Ongoing grants and contracts in health services research	Research project descriptions
HSRR Health Services and Sciences Research Resources	http://wwwcf.nlm.nih.gov/hsrr_search/home_search.cfm	Research datasets and instruments used in health services research	Factual
HSTAT Health Services Technology Assessment Texts	http://hstat.nlm.nih.gov	Clinical practice guidelines, technology assessments, and health information	Full text
Locator Plus	http://locatorplus.gov	Catalogs of books, audiovisuals, and journal articles held at National Library of Medicine	Bibliographic citations
MEDLINE/PubMed	http://www.ncbi.nlm.nih.gov/or http://gateway.nlm.nih.gov	Biomedicine. Includes the following databases/subsets: AIDS, BIOETHICSLINE, NURSING, HealthSTAR, HISTLINE, POPLINE, SPACELINE, CANCERLIT	Bibliographic citations
MedlinePlus	http://medlineplus.gov/Spanish: http://medlineplus.gov/esp/	Consumer health information	Factual, bibliographic citations
MeSH Vocabulary File	http://www.nlm.nih.gov/mesh	Thesaurus of biomedicine-related terms	Factual
OLDMEDLINE	http://gateway.nlm.nih.gov/or http://www.ncbi.nlm.nih.gov	Biomedicine	Bibliographic citations

TABLE 44.1	A List of Online Databases *(continued)*		
Database	**URL**	**Subject**	**Type**
TOXNET databases (NLM database and electronic resources): toxicology data network			
CCRIS (Chemical Carcinogenesis Research Information Systems)	http://toxnet/nlm.nih.gov	Chemical carcinogens, mutagens, tumor promoters, and tumor inhibitors	Factual
ChemIDplus	http://sis.nlm.nih.gov/chemidplus	Identification of chemical substances	Factual
DART (Developmental and Reproductive Toxicology Database	http://toxnet/nlm.nih.gov	Test results Developmental and reproductive toxicology	Bibliographic citations
GENE-TOX (genetic toxicology)	http://toxnet/nlm.nih.gov	Genetic toxicology test results on chemicals	Factual
Haz-Map	http://hazmap.nlm.nih.gov	Effects of exposure to chemicals. Links jobs and hazardous tasks with occupational diseases	Factual
HSDB (hazardous substances data bank)	http://toxnet/nlm.nih.gov	Hazardous chemical toxic effects, environmental fate, safety, and handling	Factual
IRIS (Integrated Risk Information Systems)	http://toxnet/nlm.nih.gov	Potentially toxic chemicals	Factual
ITER (international toxicity estimates for risk)	http://toxnet/nlm.nih.gov	Data of human health risk assessment	Factual
Tox Town	http://toxtown.nlm.nih.gov	Toxic chemicals and environmental health risks	Interactive guide
TOXLINE (toxicology information online)	http://toxnet/nlm.nih.gov	Toxicologic, pharmacologic, biochemical, and physiologic effects of drugs and other chemicals	Bibliographic citations
TRI (toxic release inventory)	http://toxnet/nlm.nih.gov	Annual estimated releases of toxic chemical to the environment, amounts transferred to waste sites, and source reduction and recycling data	Numeric

Source: National Library of Medicine. (2010a). *NLM Databases and Electronic Resources*. Retrieved May 21, 2010, from http://www.nlm.nih.gov/databases/

MEDLINE and the nursing subset are available free over the World Wide Web through the NLM's home page at http://www.nlm.nih.gov. There are two ways to search this database: PubMed and the NLM Gateway. The NLM Gateway is a Web-based system that allows users to search multiple NLM retrieval systems simultaneously. The database is also available through the commercial vendors mentioned below. All of these options allow the nurse to search by subject, key word, author, title, or a combination of these. An example of different searches with a display using the EBSCOhost interface is shown in Figures 44.1 and 44.2.

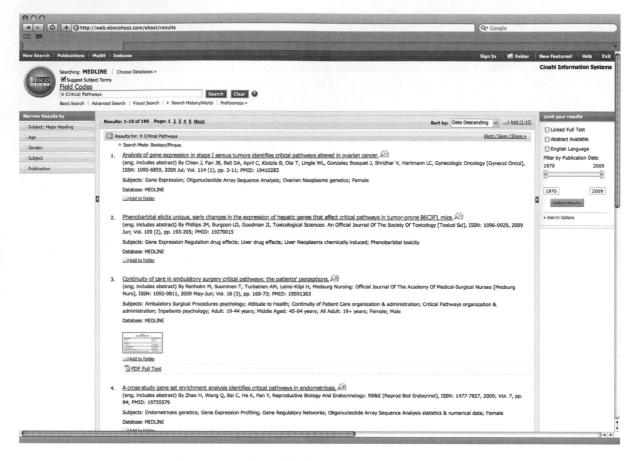

• **FIGURE 44.1.** MEDLINE search. (Courtesy of Cinahl Information Systems.)

Loansome Doc allows the nurse to place an order for a copy of an article from a medical library through PubMed or the NLM Gateway. The full text of articles for some journals is available via a link to the publisher's Website from the PubMed abstract or record display. Some of the full text is available free of charge. The links indicating free full-text display on the Loansome Doc order page prior to order placement and on the Loansome Doc Order Sent page immediately after the order is finalized. NLM has a fact sheet for Loansome doc users covering the registration process, how to place an order, order confirmation, check order status and updating account information (http://www.nlm.nih.gov/loansomedoc/loansome_home.html).

CINAHL. The CINAHL database, produced by Cinahl Information Systems, a division of EBSCO Publishing,

Inc., provides comprehensive coverage of the literature in nursing and allied health from 1982 to the present. CINAHL has expanded to offer four databases including two full-text versions. The database covers chiropractic, podiatry, health promotion and education, health services administration, biomedicine, optometry, women's health, consumer health, and alternative therapy (Cinahl Information Systems, 2010). More than 3,000 journals, as well as thousands of books, pamphlets, dissertations, audiovisuals, software, and proceedings are indexed. Some journals covered are published in other countries. Full text is available for some critical paths, research instruments, practice acts and standards of practice, patient education handouts, clinical innovation documents, and Website descriptions. It is updated weekly.

The CINAHL database also uses a controlled vocabulary for effective subject searching. The CINAHL

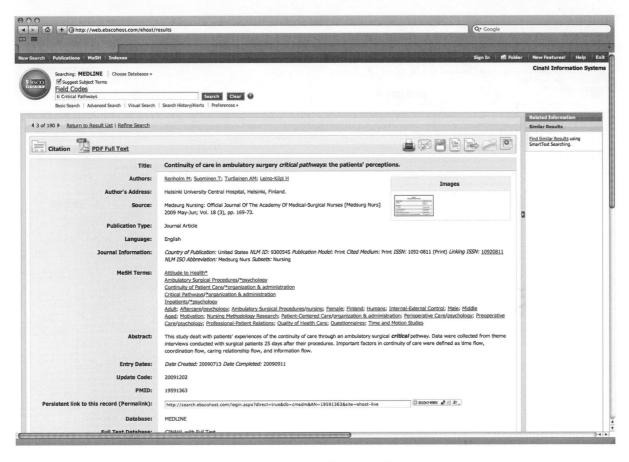

• **FIGURE 44.2.** MEDLINE search result. (Courtesy of Cinahl Information Systems.)

Subject Heading List uses the NLM's MeSH terms as the standard vocabulary for disease, drug, anatomic, and physiologic concepts (Cinahl Information Systems, 2010). There are approximately 5,360 unique CINAHL terms for nursing and the allied health disciplines. Specific field searching and quality filters are available in the CINAHL database and are similar to those found in MEDLINE. An example of different searches with a display using the EBSCOhost interface is shown in Figures 44.3 and 44.4.

An essential part of research papers is the list of references pointing to prior publications. Cited references for more than 1,290 nursing and allied health journals are searchable in the CINAHL database (EBSCO Publishing, 2010).

Mosby's Index. The database indexes content from over 2,800 peer-reviewed journals, trade publications, and electronic titles. It uses the EMTREE Thesaurus, a hierarchically structured, biomedical thesaurus, which has been enhanced for nursing. Both the thesaurus and the index are published by Elsevier B.V. (Elsevier, 2010b).

ERIC. The ERIC (Educational Resources Information Center) database is sponsored by the Institute of Education Sciences (IES) of the U.S. Department of Education and contains more than 1,300,000 citations covering education-related literature (Educational Resources Information Center, 2010a). It covers virtually all types of print materials, published and unpublished, from 1966 to the present day. It is updated monthly. This database gives the nurse a more comprehensive coverage of education than any other bibliographic retrieval system. The *Thesaurus of Eric Descriptors*, a controlled vocabulary, assists with computer searches of

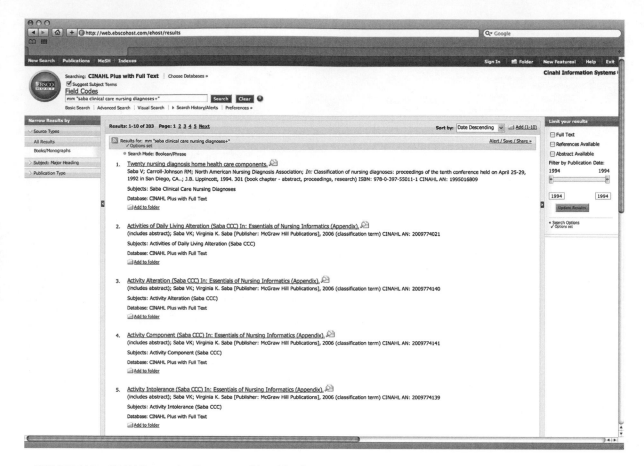

• **FIGURE 44.3.** CINAHL search. (Courtesy of Cinahl Information Systems.)

this database on the Internet through the World Wide Web (see the URLs mentioned previously) (Educational Resources Information Center, 2010b). As with the other two bibliographic databases mentioned, nurses are able to access all of the data in each record on ERIC by searching, using subject headings or key words or by searching for a word(s) in a specific field.

PsycINFO. The PsycINFO database, produced by the American Psychological Association, provides access to psychologically relevant literature from more than 2,450 journals, dissertations, reports, scholarly documents, books, and book chapters with more than 2.8 million references from the 1880s to the present. Updated weekly, most of the records have abstracts or content summaries from material published in over 49 countries. Using the *Thesaurus of Psychological Index Terms* of more than 8,400 controlled terms and cross references,

the nurse can search for specific concepts effectively. Key word and specific field searching are also available (American Psychological Association, 2010).

Social Sciences Citation Index. This database can be accessed via Web of Science for a fee. It was developed by the Institute for Scientific Information and is a multidisciplinary citation index which covers more than 1,700 journals in the social, behavioral, and related sciences. The nurse can search the cited references as in the citation index in the CINAHL database (Thomson ISI, 2010a).

A few other bibliographic retrieval systems to keep in mind are databases such as CHID online (Combined Health Information Database), produced by the federal government; the database AgeLine owned by EBSCO Publishing, Inc.; the Excerpta Medica database EMBASE; the National Technical Information

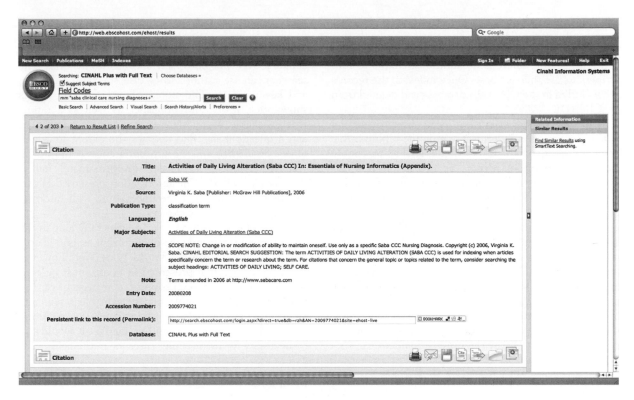

• **FIGURE 44.4.** CINAHL search result. (Courtesy of Cinahl Information Systems.)

Service NTIS database; and the UMI Proquest Digital Dissertations.

Current Awareness Services

Most bibliographic retrieval systems are updated weekly or monthly. In addition to the delay between the writing and publishing of the material that is indexed in the database, there is also a delay between the receipt of material, the indexing, and finally the inclusion of the citations for the indexed material in the database. To obtain access to more current material than that available in a bibliographic database, the nurse should use a current awareness service.

Current awareness services are helpful when used in addition to bibliographic retrieval systems. These services provide access to tables of contents of journals and allow individuals to request articles of interest. They may include not only journal articles but also proceedings from conferences, workshops, symposia, and other meetings. Often, hospital or university librarians may provide these services as well.

Unlike the bibliographic databases, where subject searching using controlled vocabulary is available, only key word searching for the subject, author, title, or journal is available in current awareness services or databases.

Some current awareness services or databases are Current Contents Connect, the in-process database for MEDLINE (formerly PREMEDLINE), and PreCINAHL on EBSCOHost.

Current Contents Connect from Thomson Reuters, provides a Web-friendly current awareness service to tables of content, abstracts and bibliographic information from the most recently published scholarly journals as well as from more than 7,000 relevant, evaluated websites (Thomson ISI, 2010b).

PubMed's in-process records (formerly PREMED-LINE) provide basic information and abstracts before the citations are indexed.

The current awareness service (PreCINAHL) offered by Cinahl Information Systems, a division of EBSCO Publishing, Inc., publishers of the CINAHL database, is available on EBSCOHost. This service is similar to that described above which contains citations of those articles received but not yet indexed with CINAHL subject headings from the CINAHL thesaurus. The fields that are key word searchable include the article title, author, and journal title. There is no additional charge to subscribers to use this database. Once indexed, the records are included in the CINAHL database and deleted from PreCINAHL.

The second type of current awareness provided by Cinahl Information Systems is within the bibliographic database itself, where the searcher is able to choose from a group of 34 specific or special interest categories, which actually function as "virtual" databases. Possibilities include such areas as advanced nursing practice, case management, home healthcare, or military/ uniformed services. By selecting one of these categories, documents are retrieved that are either in specific journals in the field or have been selected by indexers as being of interest to those in that field. The results can be limited by any of the available limits on the database, eg, publication type such as research, journal subset such as blind peer reviewed, and presence of full text. A nurse with limited time can peruse the latest literature in one of these fields in this way (Figures 44.5 and 44.6).

Review Services

Although the bibliographic retrieval systems and the current awareness services and databases act as filters to the ever-exploding volume of literature, sometimes the information retrieved needs to be evaluated to determine whether or not it is appropriate. For example, a monthly literature search might be done on a bibliographic and current awareness database and then a review service checked for commentaries on the sources retrieved. Supportive computerized resources that synthesize the literature include the Joanna Briggs Institute for Best Practice (http://joannabriggs.edu.au/), Clinical Evidence (BMJ Publishing at http://www.clinicalevidence.bmj. com) or the Cochrane Library Database of Systematic Reviews (http://www.cochrane.org/reviews). Review services such as Doody's Review Service or reviews noted in bibliographic databases or review journals, such as, *Evidence-Based Nursing*, *Evidence-Based Practice*, *Best Practice*, and *ACP Journal Club*, can also be used to evaluate sources. Review services provide information to searchers about recently published books, journal articles, audiovisuals, and software. These reviews may also include ratings, opinions, or commentaries about the material.

Doody's Review Service (www.doody.com/) is a service offered as a membership benefit to those belonging to Sigma Theta Tau and other nursing professional groups. Doody's Book Review Service develops a profile

on its members and sends a weekly electronic mail (e-mail) bulletin describing books and software that meet the parameters of the profile. The service currently contains over 110,000 print and electronic titles. The searcher can use author names, title, specialty, publisher, and key words to find books of interest. The results show price, ISBN, and publisher as well as a rating, when available. Materials are rated using a star system and a questionnaire that assesses the extent to which objectives are met and the appropriateness of the work's readability, among other criteria. (Approximately half of the titles are rated.) The information presented allows serious consideration of the book along with information to assist in making choices.

It is well known that books are generally long in the development stage and are not as current as journal articles or documents on the World Wide Web; however, the *depth* of material presented in books must be considered. An in-depth discussion of *all* aspects of cardiac rehabilitation, for example, may be valuable in planning care and would probably not be examined in a journal article where space is a consideration. Yet it would still be necessary for maintaining currency in the field.

Point-of-Care Resources

Point-of-care resources are resources that support patient care at the bedside. Lists of these resources are available from http://library.upstate.edu/evidence/ pointofcare, and from http://nnlm.gov/training/nursing/sampler.html#evid.

Mosby's Nursing Suite. Mosby's Nursing Suite from Elsevier includes Mosby's Nursing Consult, Mosby's Nursing skills and Mosby's Index. Mosby's Nursing Consult provides information to help nurses with patient care. The database includes evidence-based nursing monographs, over 38 nursing journals and clinics, over 38 nursing and medical reference texts, 350 practice guidelines, images, drug information, and 8,000 customizable patient handouts (Elsevier, 2010a). Mosby's Nursing Skills is an online skills reference and competency management resource from Elsevier. There are 940 nursing skills that use a learning management system (LMS) which allows nurse managers and educators to assign, track and manage skills and test hospital staff. It includes customizable patient handouts.

Nursing Reference Center. Nursing Reference Center (NRC), published by EBSCO Publishing, is a point-of-care tool designed to provide relevant clinical resources to nurses and other healthcare professionals. The database

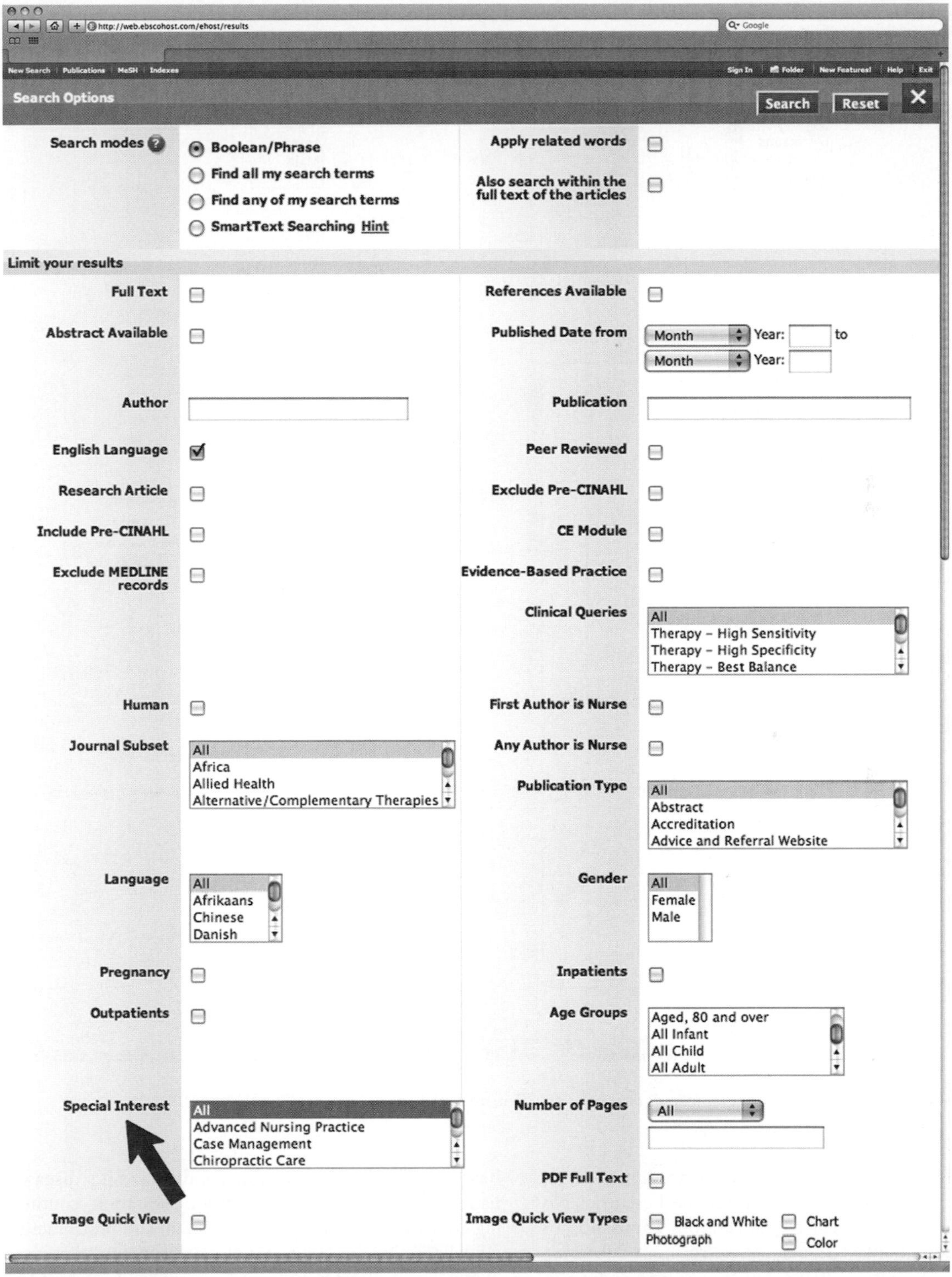

• **FIGURE 44.5.** Search for special interest categories. (Courtesy of Cinahl Information Systems.)

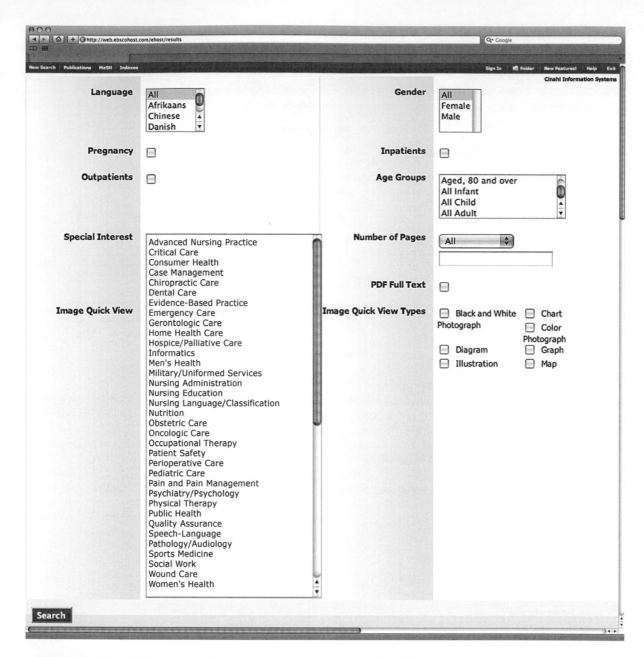

• **FIGURE 44.6.** Available 2010 special interest categories. (Courtesy of Cinahl Information Systems.)

offers staff nurses, nurse administrators, nursing students, nurse faculty, and hospital librarians the best available and most recent clinical evidence from thousands of full-text documents (University of Vermont Libraries, Dana Medical Library, 2010). Nursing Reference Center contains nearly 3,000 Quick Lessons and Evidence-

Based Care Sheets covering conditions and diseases, patient education resources, drug information, continuing education, lab and diagnosis detail, and best practice guidelines. Quick Lessons are clinically organized nursing overviews of diseases and conditions. They represent the best available evidence and are designed to match the nursing work flow. They provide nurses with information the nurses need about diseases, including a description of the disease; its signs and symptoms; typical tests the clinician will order to diagnose it, or measure progress in treating it; the interventions nurses will likely be involved in while the patient is in their care; and information necessary to share with the patient/patient's family.

Evidence-Based Care Sheets provide evidence about aspects of a disease or a condition in terms of what we know about it and what we can do about it. The evidence is coded as to its strength so the user can evaluate it and determine its applicability to their practice.

In the database, there are hundreds of nursing skills and procedures, providing access to clinical papers detailing the necessary steps to achieve proficiency in a specific nursing task. Skill Competency Checklists are provided with these documents. Many papers are also available that define key considerations to providing culturally competent care to specific population groups.

Point-of-care reference books include: *Davis's Comprehensive Handbook of Laboratory & Diagnostic Tests with Nursing Implications*; *Taber's Cyclopedic Medical Dictionary*; *Davis's Drug Guide for Nurses*; *AHFS Drug Essentials*; *Diseases and Disorders: A Nursing Therapeutics Manual*, and more.

There are more than 6,700 evidence-based customizable patient handouts (English and Spanish) together with thousands of detailed medical illustrations. More than 600 continuing education modules are also available. These modules are accredited through the American Nurses Credentialing Center (ANCC) and the International Association for Continuing Education and Training (IACET).

Users can search NRC by entering keywords in the **Find** field and then clicking on the **Search** button. NRC will display a Result List that is sorted by source type—for example, Quick Lessons, Skills, Evidence-Based Care Sheets, Drugs, etc. Users can search the database using the standard nursing process ADPIE (assessment, diagnosis, planning, implementation, evaluation). Nursing process limiters are used to clarify a search in NRC. Users can select one or multiple nursing process limiters to rapidly target applicable content.

Users can launch a *CINAHL*-type search, and limit searches by document types, full-text, publication date, or source. They can also browse CINAHL headings or indexes and other EBSCOhost databases that may be subscribed to by the institution.

Users can store search results, persistent links to articles, images, saved searches, alerts, and Web pages to pull in the latest information needed on the floor and to create department-specific patient education packets.

Supportive Computerized Resources

Supportive computerized resources that assist the nurse in maintaining currency provide additional information and enhance the value of the essential computerized resources described previously.

Document Delivery Services. Obtaining a bibliographic list of citations is only the first step in obtaining information on a particular topic. After carefully evaluating the citations, either from the title and/or the abstracts, or after using one of the review processes described previously, the nurse will need to get the full text of the sources retrieved. A local library would be the first place to go to locate the items retrieved in a search. Publishers of journals or books, database vendors and providers (NLM, American Psychological Association, Ovid Technologies, EBSCO Publishing, Proquest Information and Learning), and document delivery services are secondary sources through which full text of items can be obtained for a fee. Fees differ depending on the service, the urgency of the request, and the publisher's charges. Hard copy is usually sent via fax, mail, or electronic delivery.

Electronic Publishers. Another resource option is publications, such as electronic journals and *Morbidity and Mortality Weekly Report (MMWR)*, that are available on the World Wide Web. Sparks (1999) presents an excellent case for the importance of including electronically published information in a search for information. It offers several advantages over print material, including the speed of publishing, the comparatively small amount of space required for publishing, and the ease of availability of the documents. These advantages are important; however, because a document is published quickly it does not necessarily mean it is accurate. The credibility and accuracy of the source of electronically published material must always be considered. The criteria mentioned along with additional criteria discussed later can be useful in evaluating this material. Some of the main electronic-only nursing journals are the *Online Journal of Issues in Nursing*, published by the American Nurses Association; *On-Line Journal of Nursing Informatics*, published in Pennsylvania; and Worldviews on Evidence-Based Nursing, published by Wiley-Blackwell on behalf of the Honor Society of Nursing, Sigma Theta Tau International. Other journals such as *Nursing Standard Online* have print counterparts but may have portions that are only electronic.

Nursing publishers and organizations have their own Websites, which have details about new publications, sometimes full text of some of the latest journal articles, official position statements of organizations, and/or practice guidelines. To identify the Websites of nursing publishers and organizations, search Website indexes such as Yahoo (www.yahoo.com) or Google (www.google.com), or browse Website lists on Websites such as that of the University of Buffalo Library (http://ublib.buffalo.edu) or the Allnurses.com site (http://allnurses.com) have been provided. On a Website index such as Yahoo, do a general search for "nursing and publishers," "nursing and organizations," or "nursing and associations" or under the specific names of the publishers and organizations (eg, Delmar). Advanced searches are also available.

Lippincott Williams & Wilkins (www.nursingcenter.com) has placed over 60 journals including the *American Journal of Nursing, Nursing Research, CIN: Computers, Informatics, Nursing*, and *JONA: Journal of Nursing Administration*, among others, on their journals page with issues from January 1996 to the present. The site has search capability that allows key word searching of the contents of the journals on the site. Articles are available for a fee.

Many nursing organizations provide a significant amount of support to practicing nurses. Many publish journals and provide these as a member benefit. They also provide access to the full text of their position statements and/or practicing guidelines. Some of these publications are the American Nurses Association's Website NursingWorld (www.nursingworld.org) and the Websites of the American Academy of Nurse Practitioners (www.aanp.org), American College of Nurse Practitioners (www.acnpweb.org), the Association of Pediatric Hematology/Oncology Nursing (www.aphon.org), and many others. Details regarding new publications and ordering items can be found on the Websites of most publishers.

Metasites on the World Wide Web. Since there is so much information on the World Wide Web, identification and evaluation of Websites is very important to determine which provide valid information. One of the ways to identify Websites is to consult a metasite. There are several Websites that can be classified as metasites concerning the same specific topic. The Hardin Meta Directory of Internet Health Sources, sponsored by the Hardin Library for the Health Sciences at the University of Iowa (http://www.lib.uiowa.edu/hardin/md/) is one of these as is the National Information Center on Health Services Research & Healthcare Technology (NICHSR) (http://www.nlm.nih.gov/hsrinfo/index.html), a government site. These sites basically function as lists of lists that provide links to other subject-specific Websites.

Once the Websites have been identified, it is very important to evaluate them. At minimum, the nurse should ask the following questions (Schloman, 1999): (1) Who created the site? (2) Is the purpose and intention of the site clear? (3) Is the information accurate and current? (4) Is the site well designed and stable?

There are also Websites that can be used to evaluate other Websites. Intute (www.intute.ac.uk) is a free online service created by a consortium of seven universities in the UK that helps to identify, select, evaluate, describe, and provide access to biomedical network resources. HON (Health on the Net Foundation) (www.hon.ch) is an international initiative to promote effective Internet development and use in the areas of medicine and health. Other Websites that critically evaluate sites are National Council Against Health Fraud (www.ncahf.org), a voluntary health agency that focuses on health fraud; and Quack Watch (/www.quackwatch.org), a member of the Consumer Federation of America. Additionally, Websites providing information or discussions concerning specific diseases should be evaluated in this way (eg, the Websites of the American Diabetes Association [www.diabetes.org], American Heart Association [www.amhrt.org], and the Multiple Sclerosis Foundation [www.msfacts.org]).

DEVELOPING AND MAINTAINING A LIST OF SOURCES FOR RESEARCH/ PRACTICE/EDUCATION

Essential Computerized Resources

The purpose of the information retrieved from these information resources is to enable nurses to answer specific questions that relate to research, practice, and/or education. For example:

- A staff nurse needs to find information to share with her or his colleagues on oral care and the prevention of pneumonia.

- A nursing student has to finish a term paper and needs to find five nursing research studies on caring for a Hispanic patient with a myocardial infarction.

- A nurse manager needs to find research studies and anecdotal material showing the best way to prevent patient falls in her or his health facility.

Bibliographic Retrieval Systems. Resources essential in answering this type of question again include bibliographic databases as well as various Websites. Once again, the resources need to be carefully evaluated

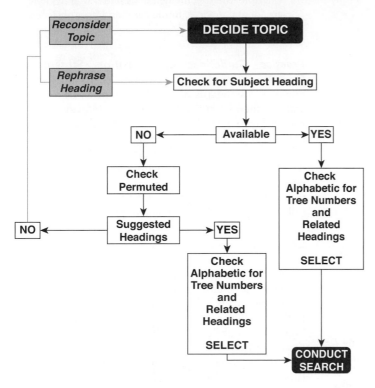

Strategy For A Successful Literature Search

Reconsider Topic → DECIDE TOPIC

Rephrase Heading → Check for Subject Heading

NO ← Available → YES

Check Permuted

Suggested Headings → YES → Check Alphabetic for Tree Numbers and Related Headings SELECT

NO ←

Check Alphabetic for Tree Numbers and Related Headings SELECT → CONDUCT SEARCH

• **FIGURE 44.7.** Strategy for a successful literature search. (Courtesy of Cinahl Information Systems.)

for coverage and currency. Once a resource has been selected, the nurse breaks down her or his needs into a search statement such as, "I need information on oral care and prevention of pneumonia." The information on this topic would best be found in a bibliographic database. On such a database, the best method of searching is to do a subject search using a controlled vocabulary (MeSH headings in MEDLINE, CINAHL subject headings in the CINAHL database, and so forth).

Search Strategies. One of the most important aspects of searching the literature is formulating the exact strategy to obtain the information from a resource, whether from a bibliographic retrieval system or a Website. There are six steps in planning the search strategy.

1. Plan the search strategy ahead of time.
2. Break down the search topic into components. To find information on oral care and the prevention of pneumonia, remember to include synonyms

or related terms. The components of the above search would be oral hygiene or mouth care and prevention of pneumonia. Sometimes the terms for the search will be subject headings in the database's subject heading list (often called a thesaurus); in other cases, they will not be (Figure 44.7).

3. Check for terms in a subject heading list, if available. If the concept is new and there are no subject headings, a text word or key word search is necessary. For example, before the term *critical paths* or *critical pathways* was added to MeSH or the CINAHL Subject Heading List, it was necessary to do a text word search for this concept. A search using the broad term *case management* would have retrieved many articles that would not necessarily discuss or include critical paths.

4. Select *operators*, which are words used to connect different or synonymous components of the

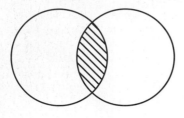

AND

Concept 1 "AND" Concept 2 = This means that only articles with both concept 1 and concept 2 are searched for.

• **FIGURE 44.8.** Venn diagram AND.

search. The AND operator, for example, makes the search narrower or more specific as the results of the search for two different terms will only result in records that include *both* terms as subject headings (Figure 44.8)

The OR operator can be used to connect synonymous or related terms, which broadens the search (Figure 44.9). An example combining subject headings using OR and AND operators is shown in Figure 44.10.

The NOT operator can be used to exclude terms (Figure 44.11).

5. Run the search. For the search on oral care and pneumonia, select the option *explode* for the subject headings oral hygiene and mouth care.

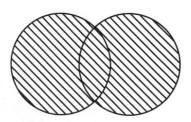

OR

Concept 1 "OR" Concept 2 = This means that articles with either concept 1 or concept 2 are searched for.

• **FIGURE 44.9.** Venn diagram OR.

This would ensure the retrieval of articles on the broad heading and the more specific headings. For example, the specific headings under oral hygiene are "dental devices, home care" and "toothbrushing."

6. View the results.

Practice Guidelines and Position Statements. Organization-specific practice guidelines, position statements, and standards of practice can often be accessed and obtained from the Website of an individual's professional organization. These are extremely useful documents that present information on the scope of practice, qualifications, and education among other important details. Additionally, Cinahl Information Systems currently includes nurse practice acts as one of its publication types in the CINAHL database. These appear in full text and can be read online or printed.

Continuing Education and Computer-Assisted Learning. Many nurses do not have the time or money to attend conferences and workshops to keep abreast of the latest information in their specialties or to complete the necessary units or credits for continuing education (CE) for relicensure or recertification. The World Wide Web is a wonderful source for nurses that can be used to satisfy their requirements for CE. To identify CE Websites visit the Nurse Friendly Nationwide Directory (http://www.nursefriendly.com/ceu/), or use one of several search engines (Alta Vista at www.altavista.com, Google at www.google.com, or Ask at www.ask.com) to obtain CE nursing sites. There are many nursing sites or point-of-care resources that offer online CE and CEU certificates, such as Nursing Reference Center, RnCeus.com at www.rnceus.com and the CE Connection at Lippincott Williams & Wilkins site at http://www.nursingcenter.com/prodev/ce_online.asp/. A directory of free online continuing education opportunities for nurses can be found at nurseceu.com (NurseCEU, 2010).

As mentioned at the beginning of this chapter, nurses use computers for many purposes. Computer-assisted instruction (CAI), computer-assisted learning (CAL), and interactive videodisc (IVD) provide easy learning experiences using a computer.

Supportive Computerized Resources

Supportive computerized resources that assist in practice, research, and education contain all types of health information including drug and treatment information, anatomy, and physiology. Specific products such

Subject headings using OR and AND operators

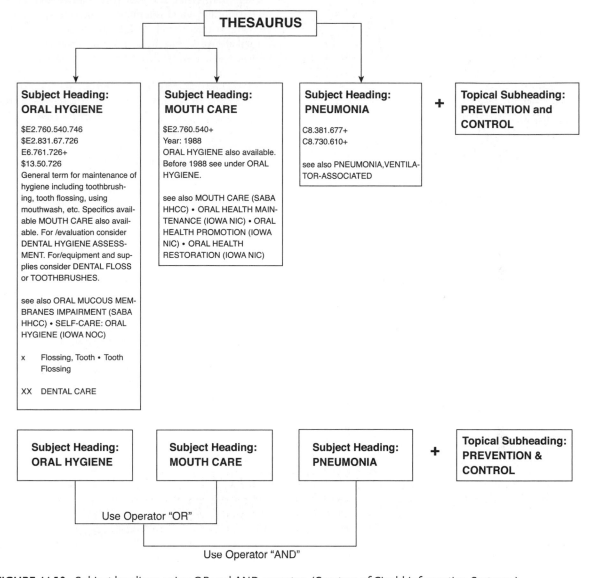

• **FIGURE 44.10.** Subject headings using OR and AND operator. (Courtesy of Cinahl Information Systems.)

as the *Merck Manual of Diagnosis and Therapy* (www. merck.com) or the *Physician's Desk Reference* available as *PDRhealth* (http://www.pdrhealth.com/drug_info/) are also available on the World Wide Web. The Visible Human Project includes complete, anatomically detailed, three-dimensional representations of the male and female human bodies. The National Library of Medicine itself claims the "largest collection of medical knowledge in the world." The Cochrane Library's Database of Systematic Reviews, available online, is another excellent source.

Websites of particular interest in this category include the Nursing Theory Page (http://www.sandiego.edu/academics/nursing/theory) and the Virginia Henderson International Library and Research Registry (http://www.stti.iupui.edu/library/) as well as the Interagency Council on Information Resources for Nursing (ICIRN) (http://icirn.org). ICIRN prepares "Essential Nursing

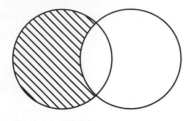

NOT

Concept 1 "NOT" Concept 2 = This means that articles with concept 1 that do not include concept 2 are searched for.

• **FIGURE 44.11.** Venn diagram NOT.

References" published biannually by the National League for Nursing in *Nursing Education Perspectives*.

COLLABORATION AND NETWORKING REGARDING ISSUES OF PROFESSIONAL PRACTICE

Nurses frequently gather information from their personal networks—either at the worksite or at professional meetings. The increased availability of computers makes contact with other professionals much easier, resulting in networking and collaboration possibilities heretofore impossible. Information retrieved by this method enables nurses to learn from their colleagues' experiences. When considering with whom to network, the specialty of the person should be evaluated along with experience, the material they have published in their field, and the research undertaken by the institution with which they are affiliated. Most of this information is not published and would be unavailable through traditional information resources.

Computerized resources for collaboration and networking vary in several technical details (eg, their focus, the presence or absence of a moderator to monitor messages, the number of participants, and their level of interactivity).

Essential Computerized Resources

Electronic Mail and Listservs. An important fundamental computerized resource for collaboration and networking is e-mail, which is at the core of almost any electronic communication. Necessary components for e-mail are access tp Internet services (often provided by cable television and local telephone companies) and e-mail viewing software, such as Internet Explorer or Firefox. E-mail allows one-to-one communication between individuals and can provide immediate response to practice-related questions.

A second essential computerized resource for collaboration is an electronic discussion group or "listserv." Listservs allow individuals to subscribe free of charge and to read and respond to messages via e-mail. Since the messages are posted to all of the members, the listserv allows sharing and dissemination of information with colleagues. Some listservs have a closed membership for a specific group (eg, librarians or specific nursing groups), and some are moderated. In a moderated group, an individual or group of individuals reads the messages prior to distribution to the group. Subject-specific listservs include NURSENET (general nursing), Nrsing-L (nursing informatics), NRSED (education issues/faculty), and NurseRes (research). Specialty listservs are very helpful in increasing dialogue between individuals within the same specialty.

Supportive Computerized Resources

Electronic Bulletin Boards, Forums, Newsgroups, and Chat Rooms. Bulletin boards, forums, newsgroups, and chat rooms are examples of supportive computerized resources. Similar to a traditional bulletin board, the electronic version has an administrator who sends the discussion to various Websites, where nurses visit to read and participate in the discussion. This format for electronic networking has almost entirely been replaced by forums and newsgroups, which have become more and more sophisticated in their interactivity and design. The premise behind each of them is similar. An individual posts a message concerning a topic (known as a thread) for others to read and respond to. Lippincott's Nursing Center (www.nursingcenter.com), for example, has many different forums under broad nursing categories such as roles, care settings, and areas of practice. Participants can respond to a previously posted thread or begin a new one in any of these broad areas or the subtopics within them. Newsgroups operate in much the same way but have a tendency to be less focused. All of these resources are interactive but on a delayed basis. An individual may respond to a message immediately or wait several days. Chat rooms, on the other hand, are interactive in real time. Conversations in chat rooms can be compared to telephone conversations—without the benefit of sound. Examples of chat rooms can be found at http://virtualnurse.com or www.nursechat.com.

Each of these methods of collaboration and networking provides an option for nurses to contact and build relationships with other professionals concerning issues important to them. New social networking sites such as Facebook and Twitter offer great potential for sharing experiences and ideas about practice issues.

SUMMARY

While these three categories of information needs have been discussed as if they were independent of one another, a nurse might often find that she or he has needs that transcend all three categories or that fall under a different category each time, depending on the task. For example, a staff nurse may need to investigate the best methods to assess and manage pain. The process of retrieving appropriate information would be to first search for research studies and anecdotal material on the topic of pain management and pain measurement. This would involve a search for pain measurement or pain with therapy, drug therapy, and diagnosis using essential computerized resources such as bibliographic retrieval systems like MEDLINE or the CINAHL database. The nurse would also consult a point-of-care tool such as Mosby's Nursing Consult or Nursing Reference Center to locate the latest evidence on a particular patient care topic.

Networking with other professionals facing the same task would be an additional step in this process. The nursing listservs mentioned under the "Collaboration and Networking Regarding Issues of Professional Practice" section would be an important and essential resource, while e-mailing or texting colleagues who are specialists in the field of pain would be a supportive resource. To locate specialists, a bibliographic retrieval system could be searched for research studies on pain measurement or management. The author affiliation field in the records retrieved would help track the institution with which the author is affiliated.

Making sure to keep current on any new material published on pain measurement and pain management, by using current awareness services or Websites, would also be vital in locating information on this topic. Bibliographic retrieval systems, already used as an essential resource, could be searched each month to assess what new material had been published on the topic. Supportive computerized resources might include a similar search for papers on the Cochrane Library's Database of Systematic Reviews, or consulting electronic publications such as *Worldviews on Evidence-Based Nursing*.

An important part of identifying and using these essential and supportive computerized resources is the evaluation of each of them to assess whether or not they contain the information needed. Therefore, the nurse must determine what she or he is looking for, identify the most appropriate resources to locate the information needed, and, using the criteria discussed throughout this chapter, evaluate the resources to assess if they are valid, current, and accurate.

Finally, it is important to realize that computerized information resources are like a "moving target," in that technology is changing so quickly that resources used today may be gone, unavailable, or outdated tomorrow. The use of bibliographic retrieval systems, search engines, and metasites encourages searching by *subject* or *concept*, which is the most reliable way to cope with the ever-changing nature of technology. This is vital to maintaining currency with the published literature, developing and maintaining a list of sources of topics of interest for practice, research, and/or education, and collaboration and networking with colleagues regarding issues of professional practice.

REFERENCES

American Library Association. (1989). *Presidential Committee on Information Literacy. Final Report*. Chicago, IL: American Library Association. Retrieved June 14, 2010 from http://www.ala.org/ala/mgrps/divs/acrl/publications/whitepapers/presidential.cfm

American Nurses Association. (2008). *Nursing informatics: Scope and standards of practice*. Silver Spring, MD: Nursebooks.org.

American Psychological Association. (2010). *PsycINFO*. Retrieved May 24, 2010, from http://www.apa.org/pubs/databases/psycinfo/index.aspx

Association of College and Research Libraries of the American Library Association. (2000, January 18). *Information literacy competency: Competencies for higher education*. Retrieved June 14, 2010 from http://www.ala.org/ala/mgrps/divs/acrl/standards/standards.pdf

Bailey, P., Derbyshire, J., Harding, A. et al. (2007). Assessing the impact of a study skills programme on the academic development of nursing diploma students at Northumbria University, UK. *Health and Information Libraries Journal, 24*(Suppl. 1), 77–85.

Cinahl Information Systems. (2010). *Subject Headings and Subject Coverage*. Retrieved May 24, 2010 from http://www.ebscohost.com/cinahl/default.php?id=8

Courey, T., Benson-Soros, J., Deemer, K., & Zeller, R. (2006, Nov–Dec). The missing link: Information literacy and evidence-based practice as a new challenge for nurse educators. *Nursing Education Perspectives, 27*(6), 320–323.

Dee, C. (2005, April). Information-seeking behavior of nursing students and clinical nurses: Implications for health sciences librarians. *Journal of the Medical Library Association, 93*(2), 213–222.

Craig, A., & Corrallt, S. (2007). Making a difference? Measuring the impact of an information literacy programme for pre-registration nursing students in the UK. *Health Information and Libraries Journal, 24*(2), 118–127.

EBSCO Publishing. (2010). The CINAHL database. Retrieved May 24, 2010 from http://www.ebscohost. com/thisTopic.php?.marketID=2&topicID=53

Educational Resources Information Center. (2010a). *About the ERIC program.* Retrieved May 24, 2010 from http://www.eric.ed.gov/ERICWebPortal/resources/ html/about/about_eric.html

Educational Resources Information Center. (2010b). *About the ERIC Thesaurus.* Retrieved May 24, 2010 from www.eric.ed.gov/ERICWebPortal/resources/ html/about/about_eric.html

Elsevier. (2010a). *Mosby's Nursing Consult.* Retrieved May 24, 2010 from http://www.elsevier.com.

Elsevier. (2010b). *Mosby's Index.* Retrieved June 14, 2010 from http://www.confidenceconnected.com/products/ mosbys_index/overview/

Head, A., & Eisenberg, M. (2009, December 1). *Lessons learned: How college students seek information in the digital age.* Seattle, WA: The Information School, University of Washington. Retrieved June 14, 2010 from http://projectinfolit.org/pdfs/PIL_Fall2009_ Year1Report_12_2009.pdf

Morgan, P. D., Fogel, J., Hicks, P., Wright, L., & Tyler, I. (2007, Spring). Strategic enhancement of nursing students information literacy skills: Interdisciplinary perspectives. *ABNF Journal, 18*(2), 40–45.

National Library of Medicine. (2010a). *NLM Databases and Electronic Resources.* Retrieved May 24, 2010, from http://www.nlm.nih.gov/databases/

National Library of Medicine. (2010b). *Number of titles currently indexed for Index Medicus and MEDLINE on PubMed.* Retrieved May 24, 2010 from http://www. nlm.nih.gov/bsd/num_titles.html

NurseCEU (2010). *Online CEUs: A Directory for Nurses.* Retrieved May 24, 2010 from http://www.nurseceu.com

Pravikoff, D. S., Pierce, S. T., & Tanner, A. B. (2005). Readiness of U.S. nurses for evidence-based practice. *American Journal of Nursing, 105*(9), 40–51.

Schloman, B. F. (1999). Whom do you trust? Evaluating Internet health resources. *Online Journal of Issues in Nursing.* Retrieved June 8, 2004 from http://www. nursingworld.org/ojin/infocol/info_1.htm

Schulte, S. (2008, Summer). Integrating information literacy into an online undergraduate nursing informatics course: The librarian's role in the design and teaching of the course. *Medical Reference Services Quarterly, 27*(2), 158–172.

Skiba, D. J. (2005). Preparing for evidence-based practice: Revisiting information literacy. *Nursing Education Perspectives, 26*(5), 310–311.

Sparks, S. M. (1999). Electronic publishing and nursing research. *Nursing Research, 48*, 50–54.

Thomson ISI. (2010a). *Social Sciences Citation Index.* Retrieved May 24, 2010 from http://thomsonreuters. com/products_services/science/science_products/a-z/ social_sciences_

Thomson ISI. (2010b). *Current Contents Connect®.* Retrieved May 24, 2010, from http://www thomsonreuters.com/products_services/science/ science_products/a-z/current_contents_connect. citation index._

University of Vermont Libraries. Dana Medical Library. (2010). Nursing Reference Center. Retrieved May 24, 2010 from http://library,uvm.edu/dana/help/featured_ resources/Nursing

RECOMMENDED READINGS

Beke-Harrigan, H., Hess, R., & Weinland, J. A. (2008). A survey of registered nurses' readiness for evidence-based practice: A multidisciplinary project. *Journal of Hospital Librarianship, 8*(4), 440–448.

Cleary, M., Hunt, G. E., & Horsfall, J. (2009). Conducting efficient literature searches: strategies for mental health nurses. *Journal of Psychosocial Nursing & Mental Health Services, 47*(11), 34–41.

Delwiche, F. A. (2008). Focus: information literacy. Searching MEDLINE via PubMed. *Clinical Laboratory Science, 21*(1), 35–41.

Evidence-based practice. Importance of nursing leadership in advancing evidence-based nursing practice. (2010). *Neonatal Network, 29*(2), 117–122.

Flemming, K., & Briggs, M. (2007). Electronic searching to locate qualitative research: evaluation of three strategies. *Journal of Advanced Nursing, 57*(1), 95–100.

Hoss, B., & Hanson, D. (2008). Evaluating the evidence: web sites. *AORN Journal, 87*(1), 124, 126–128, 130–132 passim.

Krom, Z. R., Batten, J., & Bautista, C. (2010). A unique collaborative nursing evidence-based practice initiative using the Iowa model: a clinical nurse specialist, a health science librarian, and a staff nurse's success story. *Clinical Nurse Specialist: The Journal for Advanced Nursing Practice, 24*(2), 54–59.

Lawrence, J. C. (2007). Techniques for searching the CINAHL database using the EBSCO interface. *AORN Journal, 85*(4), 779–780, 782–788, 790–791.

Markussen, K. (2007). Barriers to research utilization in clinical practice. *Vard I Norden, 27*(1), 47–49.

Milner, M., Estabrooks, C. A., & Myrick, F. (2006). Research utilization and clinical nurse educators: A systematic review. *Journal of Evaluation in Clinical Practice, 12*(6), 639–655.

Wong, S. S., Wilczynski, N. L., & Haynes, R. B. (2006). Optimal CINAHL search strategies for identifying therapy studies and review articles. *Journal of Nursing Scholarship, 38*(2), 194–199.

PART 8

International Perspectives

Susan K. Newbold

Nursing Informatics in Canada

Lynn M. Nagle / Kathryn J. Hannah / Nora Hammell

- OBJECTIVES
  1. Provide an overview of the status of nursing informatics in Canada.
  2. Describe the context of nurses' use of information and communications technologies in Canada.
  3. Describe the Canadian context of health information management systems.
  4. Describe obstacles and issues related to effective nursing management of information in Canada.
  5. Describe current Canadian nursing informatics initiatives and relevant national organizations.

- KEY WORDS
  health information
  nursing components
  outcomes
  information and knowledge management

INTRODUCTION

Registered nurses should advocate for and lead efforts toward the collection, storage, retrieval and use of nursing care data to generate information on nursing outcomes....These data are essential to expand knowledge, to evaluate the quality and impact of nursing care, to promote patient safety and to support integrated health human resources planning.

–Canadian Nurses Association, 2006a

Nursing's role in managing information in health service organizations and care facilities in Canada is similar to that in other developed countries. The Canadian Nurses Association (CNA) has taken the position that registered nurses and other stakeholders in healthcare delivery require information on nursing practice and its relationship to client outcomes. A coordinated system to collect, store, and retrieve nursing data in Canada is essential for health human resource planning, and to expand knowledge and research on determinants of quality nursing care. The CNA, the provincial and territorial nurses associations and nursing informatics interest groups across Canada, have been instrumental in supporting nurses' involvement with innovations in health informatics by disseminating information and promoting standards and ethics in the development of nursing informatics. Current applications of nursing informatics include many kinds of clinical, educational, administrative, research, and healthcare systems initiatives (e.g., telehealth, electronic health records, decision support systems, workload measurement tools, and online education).

Both internationally and nationally there has been a desire to put more emphasis on the delivery of primary healthcare. However, in Canada, the most substantial investments in information technology supporting healthcare delivery to date have been primarily directed toward systems supporting illness care. Likewise, the predominant focus of nursing informatics in Canada has been on supporting the work of nurses within health service organizations. Despite the prevailing focus on institutional care, primary care, public health, and community-based nursing are also experiencing the shift to clinical care and administrative activities supported by information and communication technology (ICT). In most health service organizations, nurses manage both client care and clinical operations. Usually nurse clinicians manage client care and nurse managers administer the clinical operations within organizations. For some time, nursing's role in the management of information has been considered to include both the information necessary to manage client care using the nursing process and the information necessary for managing clinical operations within an organization.

With regard to the nursing management of client care, nursing practice is information intensive. Nurses constantly handle enormous volumes of client care information. In fact, nurses constantly process information mentally, manually, and electronically. Nurses have long been recognized as the interface between clients and families, and health service organizations. Like nurses in other countries, Canadian nurses integrate information from many diverse sources to provide client care and coordinate client and family interactions with healthcare providers and services.

In recognition of the information-intensive nature of nursing practice and the significant emerging role of ICT, the CNA recently developed the *E-Nursing Strategy for Canada* to "promote and ensure changes that support quality nursing practice" (Canadian Nurses Association, 2006b). The strategy begins to elaborate on 3 key requirements for nurses to effectively use ICT in their practice: (1) access to user-friendly ICT that supports evidence-based care, (2) opportunities to acquire the requisite competencies to use these tools, and (3) active participation in the design, deployment, and evaluation of ICT solutions (2006a). Further, the strategy advocates that these activities will be most effectively accomplished through collaboration among nurses in practice, administrators, employers, health ministries, nursing organizations, educators, and researchers.

Nurses must be able to manage and process nursing data, information, and knowledge to support patient care delivery in diverse care delivery settings (Graves and Corcoran, 1989). For almost 40 years it has been widely recognized that nurses spend enormous amounts of time engaged in information handling; a seminal study, in 3 New York hospitals, found that registered nurses spend from 36% to 64% of their time on information handling, with those in administrative positions spending the most time (Jydstrup & Gross, 1966). Unfortunately, the continued preponderance of paper records in a majority of health service organizations suggests that the time nurses spend in the "care and feeding" of paper records has not significantly changed since this initial work.

There is an essential linkage between access to information and client outcomes and the delivery of safer care. Lang succinctly and aptly described the present situation: "If we cannot name it, we cannot control it, finance it, teach it, research it or put it into public policy" (Clark & Lang, 1992). Having access to information about their practice arms nurses with evidence to demonstrate the contribution of nursing to patient outcomes. Outcomes research is an essential foundation for evidence-based nursing practice. Evidence-based practice is a means of promoting and enhancing client safety.

In a 2006 statement on nursing information and knowledge management, the CNA articulated the following position (Canadian Nurses Association, 2006a):

- CNA believes that information management and communications technology are integral to nursing practice.

- Registered nurses should advocate for and lead efforts toward the collection, storage, retrieval, and use of nursing care data to generate information on nursing outcomes.

- CNA advocates data standards and supports the adoption in Canada of a single clinical care terminology with the capacity to represent client health data and the clinical practice of all healthcare providers.

- CNA advocates for a client-centred, pan-Canadian electronic health record.

The CNA's belief in the importance of information and knowledge management for nurses was underscored in the launch of NurseONE. In 2006, through a partnership between the CNA and the First Nations and Inuit Health Branch (FNIHB) of Health Canada, a nursing portal was made available to the Canadian nursing community. NurseONE is a national, bilingual Web-based health information service designed "to provide quick access to credible, up-to-date healthcare information to support nurses in Canada in delivering effective, evidence-based care, and to help them manage their careers and connect to colleagues, regardless of where or when they work" (NurseONE, 2010). The portal serves as a gateway to resources and information for healthcare professionals in all domains of practice—direct care, education, administration, research, and policy—to support and enhance their clinical and professional expertise. NurseONE offers all healthcare professionals access to healthcare news, bulletins, alerts, statistics, and more. While the secure, subscriber-only section provides nurses with access to a wide array of evidence-based tools and resources, from reference manuals and materials that support patient care and lifelong learning, to tools to build a portfolio and forums to connect with nursing peers (NurseONE, 2010).

At the time of this writing, Canada lacks a centralized system to collect, store, and retrieve information about nursing practice. However, it is becoming increasingly recognized within the nursing community that such information is essential "to expand knowledge, evaluate the quality and impact of nursing care, to promote patient safety and integrated health human resources planning" (Canadian Nurses Association, 2006a). Variations in decision making, clinical populations, documentation protocols, organizational governance, and nursing leadership all affect nursing's role in information management and the adoption of ICT solutions that support nursing practice. In particular, nursing leadership and participation in the decision making that will set the course for nursing representation in electronic health records for many years to come, is essential.

CONTEXTUAL FACTORS INFLUENCING THE DEVELOPMENT OF HEALTH INFORMATION IN CANADA

Canadians have a healthcare system that is the envy of many countries. One of the things that make the Canadian healthcare system unique is the belief in health as a right rather than a privilege or an economic commodity. This philosophy is reflected in the principles upon which the provincial and territorial health systems in Canada are based, and it is legislated through the *Canada Health Act* by which all Canadian jurisdictions abide. These principles include universality, portability, accessibility, comprehensiveness, and public administration. The publicly funded health system in Canada provides for about 70% of healthcare, the other 30% is paid for out of pocket or by health insurance companies. In addition, health is a provincial and territorial responsibility in Canada, not a federal one. Conformity on health matters between provinces, territories, and the federal government is by mutual consent and agreement, not legislation.

Unfortunately, like other healthcare systems, the provincial and territorial health systems in Canada are presently in a box analogous to the room in which Alice in Wonderland found herself when she began to grow. The system is under enormous pressures (Figure 45.1). These factors are well described and documented

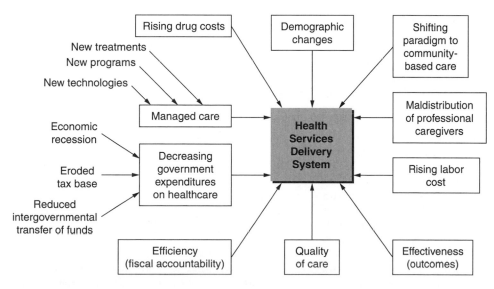

• **FIGURE 45.1.** Pressures on health services delivery systems.

elsewhere (Hannah, Ball, & Edwards, 1999; Hannah & Anderson, 1994).

The overall picture is one in which the expenses and costs associated with healthcare are rising and the resources needed to support healthcare delivery in Canada are being strained. We must identify strategies to provide enhanced information management and clinical decision making to optimize the use of our increasingly stretched health human resources. Hence, Canadian nurses are being engaged in efforts to find ways to be more efficient and effective through the use of ICT that will also reap the benefits of safer, quality care being provided to Canadians.

These are some of the factors that are influencing the drive toward identifying the essential data needs of nurses. In Canada, the information revolution has prompted initiatives by healthcare organizations to develop or acquire automated information systems focused on the utilization of data for the purposes of resource allocation, patient-specific costing, and health outcomes monitoring. The information revolution has also been a driving force in the evolution of national health information management as demonstrated by the formation of the Canadian Institute for Health Information (CIHI) in 1992.

New models of care delivery are also emerging, including *patient-focused care, hospitals without walls, and interprofessional practice.* These new models are directed at eliminating inefficiency in the structure and approaches to healthcare. There is also recognition that the ever-escalating costs associated with chronic disease management need to be contained. The use of ICT such as telemedicine is widely viewed as key to managing the issues and cost burden associated with the prevalence of chronic diseases in Canada. Deinstitutionalization of care and changes in the scope of medical and nursing practice are also occurring. There is an increasing trend toward consumerism in which self-help groups, disease-specific groups, and other special interest groups expect to be involved in their own care and the management of their health information. The power differential is equilibrating such that consumers have ubiquitous access to information about disease management, treatment options, and provider performance. Citizens are now utilizing ICT to communicate with clinicians and exchange information about their health. The face of healthcare delivery will be forever transformed through these changes and the Canadian nursing community is recognizing the need to respond.

In sum, a common outcome of health system reviews conducted by most provinces and territories throughout the first decade of the 21st century was the recognition

of information systems as a key enabler (and lack of quality information as a key barrier) to health sector reform. Across Canada, information management and supporting technologies have become increasingly important over the past 10 years. Canadian nursing must ensure that information related to nurses' contributions to patient care is available in local and national data sets. Thus, the data elements from which this information is derived must be collected and stored in a retrievable format.

NATIONAL HEALTH INFORMATION ORGANIZATIONS

Canadian Institute for Health Information

Created in 1992, the Canadian Institute for Health Information (CIHI) is an independent, pan-Canadian, not-for-profit organization, established jointly by federal, provincial, and territorial ministers of health that provides essential data and analysis on Canada's health system and the health of Canadians.

Information is derived from many sources including hospitals, regional health authorities, medical practitioners, and governments. This information is further supplemented from other sources to support CIHI's analysis and the generation of reports that focus on (Canadian Institute for Health Information, 2010):

- Healthcare services
- Health spending
- Health human resources
- Population health

CIHI has a mandate to:

- Coordinate the development and maintenance of a comprehensive and integrated approach to health information for Canada
- Provide and coordinate the provision of accurate and timely data and information required for:
  ◦ Establishing sound health policy
  ◦ Effectively managing the Canadian health system
  ◦ Generating public awareness about factors affecting good health

The core functions of CIHI are to (Canadian Institute for Health Information, 2010):

- Identify and promote national health indicators
- Coordinate and promote the development and maintenance of national health information standards

- Develop and manage health databases and registries
- Conduct analysis and special studies and participate in research
- Publish reports and disseminate health information
- Coordinate and conduct education sessions and conferences

In existence for nearly 2 decades, CIHI has become an acknowledged and trusted source of quality, reliable, and timely aggregated health information for use in understanding and improving the management of the Canadian health systems and the health of the population of Canada.

Canada Health Infoway

As CIHI and its various aggregated databases evolved and matured, the focus was on health indicators and population health as well as information to manage the healthcare system. The healthcare community came to realize that there was still limited information available to support decision making related to the clinical care of individuals and groups of patients or clients of the health systems. In October 2000, the federal government committed initial funding to support the development and coordination of pan-Canadian health information systems necessary to achieve an electronic health record (EHR). This funding was a recognition, by federal, provincial, and territorial governments, of the potential of ICT to improve the efficiency, cost-effectiveness, access, quality, and safety of health services in Canada. The Federal/Provincial/Territorial Advisory Committee on Health Infostructure (Advisory Committee on Health Infostructure, 2001) set its top priority as the development of EHR and telehealth. The committee identified an immediate need to begin putting building blocks in place for the next stages of EHR development.

Canada Health Infoway (Infoway) was incorporated in January 2001 and is an independent, not-for-profit organization funded by the federal government. Infoway jointly invests with every province and territory to accelerate the development and adoption of EHR projects in Canada. The Infoway mission is (Canada Health Infoway, 2002):

> To foster and accelerate the development and adoption of electronic health information systems with compatible standards and communication technologies on a pan-Canadian basis with tangible benefits to Canadians. The Corporation is building on existing

initiatives and pursuing collaborative relationships in the achievement of its mission.

Significant progress toward the EHR is being been made with federal investments of more than $2.1 billion to date (Canada Health Infoway, 2008).

The specific objectives of Infoway are to (Canada Health Infoway Inc., 2002):

- Accelerate the development and adoption of modern systems of health information and communication technologies (ICTs).
- Define and promote standards governing shared data to ensure the compatibility of health information networks.
- Support the adoption of such standards for health information and compatible communications technologies for the health sector in Canada.
- Enter into collaborative arrangements as required with the governments of Canada, the provinces and territories, corporations, not-for-profit organizations, and other public and private partners for the development and adoption of standards and technologies.
- Incorporate standards that protect personal privacy, confidentiality of individual records, and the security of health information.
- Carry out the work of Infoway in both official languages.

Infoway believes that investments in key aspects of "infostructure" will have direct benefits to Canadians by improving the quality, accessibility, portability, and efficiency of health services delivery across the continuum of care. Its mandate includes (1) strengthening and integrating health services through EHRs, (2) empowering the public by increasing health information access, (3) addressing issues of privacy, (4) developing and implementing standards, and (5) ensuring the adoption of emerging technologies through private and public sector collaboration (Canada Health Infoway, 2008). Strategic investments have been directed to each of the provinces and territories in support of initiatives that provide the foundation for an interoperable pan-Canadian EHR.

Most Canadian jurisdictions have the beginnings of a basic infrastructure in place to support an interoperable EHR including (1) client registries, (2) provider registries, (3) drug information systems, (4) laboratory information systems, (5) diagnostic imaging information systems, (6) telehealth systems, and (7) public health surveillance systems. These foundational systems are providing the basis for provincial and territorial EHRs. Beyond the data from the foundational systems, other key data elements to be included in the national and jurisdictional EHRs have yet to be confirmed. Canadian nurses have been working to ensure that jurisdictional EHRs include patient-centered information and clinical outcomes data. Presently, there is also substantial investment being directed to the deployment of primary care electronic medical records (EMR) to support physician practice and a growing nurse practitioner practice across the country (Canada Health Infoway, 2008).

Canada, through Infoway, was also a charter member of the International Health Information Standards Development Organization (IHTSDO) in 2006. The development and deployment of health data and technical standards are germane to the evolution of an interoperable EHR, and Infoway recognizes the centrality of this work in the achievement of their mission.

The emerging EHR will ultimately incorporate data related to patient assessment and interventions contributing to patient outcomes and providers' patterns of practice. As the single largest group of healthcare providers, is imperative that nursing's contributions to care included in the EHR.

OBSTACLES TO EFFECTIVE NURSING MANAGEMENT OF INFORMATION IN CANADA

In Canadian hospitals, like most U.S. or European hospitals, the major obstacles to more effective nursing management of information are the sheer volume of information, the lack of access to modern information handling techniques and equipment, and the inadequate information management infrastructure. The volume of information that nurses manage on a daily basis, either for patient care or organizational management purposes, is enormous and continuing to grow. Nurses continue to respond to this growth with incredible mental agility. However, human beings do have limits, and a major source of job dissatisfaction among Canadian nurses is information overload resulting in information-induced job stress.

Antiquated manual information systems and outdated information transfer facilities are information-redundant and labor-intensive processes, not to mention an inappropriate use of an expensive professional resource. Modern information transfer and electronic communication systems allow rapid and accurate transfer of information along electronic communication networks. Unfortunately, nursing clinical documentation has not typically been an early component of EHR deployments, but it will eventually have the most significant impact on nursing practice. Therefore, it is time for the profession to start building toward this eventuality and to take charge of directing the data elements and measures that nurses need to have included in the EHR.

Software and hardware for modern electronic communication networks are only two aspects of an information infrastructure. The other major aspect lacking in most hospitals and health services organizations, is appropriate infrastructure to facilitate information management. Infrastructure includes but is not limited to data management policies and procedures, methods for data stewardship and custodianship, user training, and information management support staff.

Even in instances where there are sufficiently functional information systems, a barrier that continues to be raised by nurses is the limited access to computing devices and online resources. While the provision of EHR functionality will derive many clinical care benefits, nurses should not be constrained by lack of access to information when and where it is needed. Having the capability to retrieve and enter information at the point of care needs to become a standard of practice in all health service organizations. Moreover, prohibiting nurses from having access to the Internet and the vast array on online knowledge resources is not acceptable. Nursing leaders need to advocate on behalf of nurses in all sectors to ensure that their practice is not encumbered or limited by inhibited information access.

ISSUES RELATED TO EFFECTIVE NURSING MANAGEMENT OF INFORMATION

Primary among the nursing issues related to information management in Canada is the lack of adequate educational programs in information management techniques and strategies for nurse clinicians and nursing managers. At the time of writing, there are only a few preservice nursing education programs in Canada offering a course in modern information management techniques and strategies related to nursing. At a minimum, such a program must include advanced study of information management techniques and strategies such as information flow analysis, the use of spreadsheets, databases, and word processing packages. Ideally such courses would also introduce concepts and provide hands-on experience related to the use of patient care information systems. In 2010, new entry-to-practice competencies related to collecting, using, and managing information were introduced in the newly revised Canadian Registered Nurse Examination. The expectation is that these competencies will have an impact on nursing curricula across Canada.

Another major issue is that nursing is frequently underrepresented in the selection and implementation of patient care information systems and financial management systems in Canada. Regrettably, many senior nurse managers fail to recognize the importance of this activity and opt out of the process. They then complain when the systems do not meet the needs of nursing. Canadian senior nursing executives must recognize the importance of allocating staff and money to participate in the strategic planning process for information systems in their organizations. Other senior management personnel must also recognize the importance of nursing input into the strategic planning process for information systems. In any hospital, nurses are the single largest group of professionals using a patient care system, and nursing represents the largest part of the budget requiring financial management. Nursing, therefore, represents the single largest stakeholder group in Canada related to either a patient care information system or a financial information system.

Nurses have been involved in the management of nursing information since the initial systems for gathering minimum uniform health data, which can be traced back to systems devised by Florence Nightingale over a century ago (Verley, 1970). This early role in the management of nursing information began to change dramatically with the introduction of computers into healthcare and nursing environments. The role evolved as nurses became more involved in the selection and utilization of information systems. These developments have been well documented elsewhere (Hannah, Ball, & Edwards, 1999) along with detailed information on the nursing responsibilities, roles, and contributions to the selection and implementation of information systems in healthcare organizations. The issues for nurses no longer relate to computers or management information systems but rather information and knowledge management. The computer and its associated software are merely tools to support nurses as they practice their profession. Far too much attention has been directed to the technology rather than its informational content. Current hospital information systems do little to assist nurses in their real role, which is providing nursing care. Canadian nurses must be able to manage and process nursing data, information, and knowledge to support patient care delivery in diverse care delivery settings. To accomplish this goal, Canadian nurses are increasingly focusing on the contents (the data) contained in information systems, instead of being distracted by the glamour and romance of the technology.

Nurses in Canada have been working toward achieving consensus on the minimum set of data elements essential to the practice of nursing and the coding of those elements. While there are presently efforts underway in a few Canadian jurisdictions, there is still only a limited set of nursing data being collected and stored for use in decision making related to health policy or resource allocation. Nurses in Canada who have developed a heightened awareness of the importance of collection, storage, and retrieval of nursing data have recognized these data gaps.

Thus, the salient issue in information management for nurses in Canada is that of identification of nursing data elements that are essential for collection and storage in a national health database. These data elements must reflect the data that nurses use to build information that is the foundation for clinical judgment and management decision making in any setting where nursing is practiced. The remainder of this chapter will focus on the issue of defining those data elements that are essential to the practice of nursing.

INITIATIVES DIRECTED AT THE DEVELOPMENT OF NURSING COMPONENTS OF HEALTH INFORMATION FOR USE IN CANADA

In Canada, nurses are in the fortunate position of recognizing the need for nursing data elements at a time when the status of national health information is under review. The challenge for nurses is to capitalize on this timing and define those data elements required by nurses in Canada. To prevent losing control of nursing data, Canadian nurses must take a proactive stance and mobilize resources to ensure the development and implementation of a national health database that is congruent with the needs of nurses in all practice settings in Canada. Some initiatives intended to promote the vision of a national health database becoming a reality in Canada are in progress.

- During the 1990s, the work of individual nurse leaders and the Canadian Nurses Association led to the 1997 consensus on 5 data elements. *Client status* is broadly defined as a label for the set of indicators that reflect the phenomena for which nurses provide care, relative to the health status of clients (McGee, 1993). Although client status is similar to nursing diagnosis, the term client status was preferred because it represents a broader spectrum of health and illness. The common label client status is inclusive of input from all disciplines. The summative statements referring to the phenomena for which nurses provide care (i.e., nursing diagnosis) are merely one aspect of client status at a point in time, in the same way as medical diagnosis.

- *Nursing interventions* refer to purposeful and deliberate health-affecting interventions (direct and indirect) based on assessment of client status, which are designed to bring about results that benefit clients (Alberta Association of Registered Nurses [AARN], 1994).

- *Client outcome* is defined as a "clients' status at a defined point(s) following healthcare [–affecting] intervention" (Marek & Lang, 1993). It is influenced to varying degrees by the interventions of all care providers.

- *Nursing intensity* "refers to the amount and type of nursing resource used to [provide] care" (O'Brien-Pallas & Giovannetti, 1993).

- *Primary nurse identifier* is a single unique lifetime identification number for each individual nurse. This identifier is independent of geographic location (province or territory), practice sector (e.g., acute care, community care, and public health), or employer.

Identifying those data elements that represent the most important aspects of nursing care is only the first step. Beyond their definition, there is the ongoing work of promoting and further developing the data elements and ensuring that they become integrated into an inter-professional, client-centred, pan-Canadian EHR. With every new government agency or initiative it is important to advocate for nursing data to be part of the inter-professional clinical data set.

In 2009, a nursing informatics think tank was hosted by the CNA and Infoway. It resulted in a renewed partnership with national nursing organizations representing nursing education, unions, nurse administrators, as well as professional colleges and associations that identified key strategies to advance nursing informatics in Canada (see National Nursing Reference Group later in this chapter). The first strategy area is the identification of nursing requirements for the pan-Canadian EHR, including both required functionality for nursing and the nursing core data. Just over a year later, another forum attended by an even larger group of nursing leaders had moved the issue of nursing data forward to a renewed 2010 consensus that nurses in Canada require data on: client assessment, nursing interventions, client outcomes, nursing intensity, and a unique nurse identifier. The forum also supported the position of the International Classification of Nursing Practice (ICNP), in line with the CNA, advocating (Canadian Nurses Association, 2006a):

> The adoption of a single clinical terminology that... facilitates communication across all health settings, spoken languages and geographic regions, that has the capacity to represent client health data and the clinical practice of all healthcare providers...For a clinical terminology to adequately represent the practice of registered nurses across all regions and settings it, must be developed in collaboration with the International Council of Nurses.... The International Classification of Nursing Practice (ICNP®) which is compliant with international standards in a manner consistent with other disciplines.

The Canadian Health Outcomes for Better Information and Care Project

Infoway has made an investment to support the early efforts to capture the "outcomes" dimension of nursing data. In the fall of 2006, the CNA partnered with the Ministries of Health in 3 Canadian provinces to undertake the inclusion of 8 nursing-sensitive patient outcomes in EHRs. Infoway provided funding for this work, launched as the Canadian Health Outcomes for Better Information and Care (C-HOBIC) project. This project supports the advancement and use of standardized patient assessments and related documentation. Further, these assessments enable the provision of feedback to nurses about patient outcomes and the ability to compare outcomes over time. Of additional value is that C-HOBIC provides an EHR adoption lever, providing information of use to nursing practice.

The C-HOBIC project builds upon a decade of work started in the province of Ontario in 1998. A detailed history of this work is chronicled elsewhere (Nagle, White, & Pringle, 2007; Nagle, White & Pringle, 2010; White & Pringle, 2005). The 8 C-HOBIC measures were derived from evidence in the nursing literature and include: (1) functional status, (2) pain, (3) dyspnea, (4) fatigue, (5) nausea, (6) falls, (7) pressure ulcers, and (8) readiness for discharge. The measures are constituted by 38 data elements of which 26 are being collected in 4 sectors of the healthcare system: (1) acute care, (2) long-term care, (3) home care, and (4) complex continuing care. The 8 measures each have a concept definition and an associated valid and reliable measurement instrument. As part of the C-HOBIC project, the concepts originally identified in Ontario were mapped to the International Classification of Nursing Practice. The specific details of this mapping are reported elsewhere (Kennedy, 2008). Hannah, White, Nagle, and Pringle (2009) have provided more details about the C-HOBIC initiative in another publication. Experience with C-HOBIC to date indicates that these outcome measures can be collected using standardized tools across the healthcare system. Moreover, the nurses using the measures are deriving value in addressing clinical care issues and quality improvement for their patients and clients.

In Canada, nurses have come to recognize the need to incorporate nursing data into the national health information infostructure (i.e., national databases and EHR) as federal, provincial, and territorial health information systems are being restructured. To ensure that nursing data are incorporated into the national health infostructure, nurses must participate in the design, standards development, and pilot studies to ensure the capture of data that are essential to reflect nursing's contribution to healthcare in Canada.

As nurses in Canada pursue the development of core nursing data for interprofessional clinical information systems, several issues are germane. The first need is to ensure that data are available, reliable, valid, and comparable (i.e., data standards are established). To this end, the CNA has endorsed the ICNP for use in Canada. It is also important to define the scope of the compiled data set to ensure that only those essential data elements are collected and to avoid proliferation of data. In addition, it is essential to promote the concept to ensure widespread use and educate the nurses to ensure the quality of the data that are collected.

IMPLICATIONS OF THE NURSING COMPONENTS OF HEALTH INFORMATION

In the absence of a national system for the collection, storage, and retrieval of nursing data elements, it is evident that a significant amount of valuable information is being lost. In Canada, as in other countries, this information is important to demonstrate the contribution nursing makes to the care of the patient and to demonstrate the cost effectiveness of nursing care (Werley & Zorn, 1988; Werley, Devine, Zorn, Ryan, & Westra, 1991). As we move away from nursing-oriented models of patient care delivery to models that focus on the patient, emphasizing collaboration of disciplines,

multiskilling of healthcare providers, standardization of care, and streamlining of documentation through charting by exception, it is imperative that nurses be able to articulate what the role of nursing entails, and what it does not entail. Nurses will be asked to demonstrate their contributions to patient care in terms of outcome measures that are objective and measurable. They will require nursing data to identify outcomes of nursing care, defend resource allocation to nursing, and justify new roles for nursing in the healthcare delivery system (Gallant, 1988; McPhillips, 1988; Werley et al., 1991). Similarly, nurses need to understand and value nursing data so that in the selection and implementation of information systems for their organizations, nurse administrators insist that they or their designee play a major role and that nursing data needs are incorporated into the selection and implementation criteria. (For greater detail on selection and implementation, refer to Hannah, Ball, & Edwards, 1999).

While on the one hand we must preserve our professional nursing identity, Canadian nurses must balance this against professional ghettoization. The collection and storage of essential nursing data elements that are not integrated as components of a national EHR and national patient care data sets will serve to ghettoize nursing especially in a socialized healthcare system such as Canada's. This is dangerous at a time when significant emphasis is being placed on multidisciplinary collaboration, patient-focused care, and patient outcomes. In Canada, contributions to the only national health database are voluntary rather than legislated, and the elements are established by consensus rather than by legislation. In view of priorities in Canadian healthcare as well as the culture of negotiation and consensus, the importance of nursing's participation in the determination of the integrated data elements could not be more apparent.

Nurses need to know what nursing elements are essential for archival purposes so that nursing documentation is inclusive of these elements. With the move toward standardization of care through the use of care maps, it is essential that outcomes of nursing care are determined and included in the care maps. As healthcare organizations embrace the concept of charting by exception in an effort to decrease the valuable hours spent by healthcare workers in documentation, nurses must be sure that those tools that outline the patient care delivered are not devoid of nursing's contributions to patient care. In the absence of data that reflect nursing activities, there is no archival record of what nurses do, what difference nursing care makes, or why nurses are required. At times of fiscal restraint, objective nursing data is required to substantiate the role of nurses and the nurse-patient ratios required in the clinical setting.

Nurse researchers need a database of essential data elements to facilitate the identification of trends related to the data elements for specific patient groups, institutions, or regions and to assess variables on multiple levels including institutional, local, regional, and national (Werley & Zorn, 1988). The collection and storage of essential nursing data elements will facilitate the advancement of nursing as a research-based discipline (Werley and Zorn, 1988). Nurse educators need these essential nursing data elements to develop nursing knowledge for use in educating nurses and to facilitate the definition of the scope of nursing practice (McCloskey, 1988).

Finally, defining the nursing components of health information is essential to influence health policy decision making. Historically health policy has been created in the absence of nursing data. At a time when we are in the midst of profound healthcare reform it is essential that nurses demonstrate the central role of nursing services in the restructuring of the healthcare delivery system.

MEETING THE CHALLENGE

Canadian Nursing Informatics Association

Although the cadre of Canadian nurses working in informatics roles has grown over the past decade, it is clear that efforts are needed to increase awareness among all nurses about the relevance of informatics to the profession. In particular, our nurse leaders in practice and education need to embrace and assist in advancing the health informatics agenda and assure that nurses are engaged. Throughout the 1990s, a few nursing informatics interest groups emerged in various parts of the country; some have endured while others have not.

In 2002, the Canadian Nursing Informatics Association (CNIA) was established with the goal of engaging nurses in all sectors and in all roles. In 2004, the scope and growth of the CNIA's national membership and compliance with the CNA criteria, afforded the CNIA "Associate Group" status. This status brings further credence to the CNIA along with opportunities to review and influence relevant national nursing policy and strategic planning.

The CNIA also has a formal alliance with Canada's Health Informatics Organization, COACH, which has facilitated the appointment of the Canadian nurse nominee to the International Medical Informatics Association—Nursing Informatics Working Group (IMIA-NI WG). The IMIA-NI WG provides an opportunity to engage with international nursing informatics colleagues and share our knowledge beyond national borders. Opportunities to further leverage respective expertise and experiences are already under discussion with colleagues in the United States, Europe, South America, and Australia.

The need to harness existing nursing informatics expertise, address the required informatics competencies of all nurses, and extend the profession's understanding of the significance of health informatics are key priorities for the CNIA. The overall objectives include the following:

- To provide nursing leadership for the development of nursing and health informatics in Canada
- To establish national networking opportunities for nurse informaticists
- To facilitate informatics educational opportunities for all nurses in Canada
- To engage in international nursing informatics initiatives
- To act as a nursing advisory group in matters of nursing and health informatics
- To expand awareness of nursing informatics to all nurses and the healthcare community

The achievement of these objectives is being operationalized through a number of initiatives including biannual national conferences, a Web site, and the online *Canadian Journal of Nursing Informatics*.

National Nursing Reference Group

In 2009, in partnership with the CNA, Canada Health Infoway established Clinical Adoption, a nursing reference group (NRG) that includes practicing nurses, national nursing associations, and other provincial nursing leaders and informatics experts. The purpose of the NRG is to provide national nursing leadership, engagement, expertise, and input to inform Infoway's nursing strategy and plans to accelerate nursing's adoption and realization of the benefits of EHRs. The objectives of the NRG are to:

- Provide strategic-level advice and input on policies, priorities, and strategic plans aligned with Infoway's Clinical Adoption business strategy and clinical engagement.
- Review and provide feedback on products, services, and projects under consideration, or being implemented where appropriate.

- Provide strategic input on the needs and engagement of nurses in practice, education, policy, administration, and research.
- Provide ongoing oversight and input into the established 6 key nursing strategic directions and tactical plans and associated working groups.
- Act as liaisons and promote a coordinated approach of activities and strategies within their organizations and across partners.

In May 2009, 6 strategic goals were developed and preliminary action plans were established to accelerate nursing engagement and EHR adoption:

1. Identification of nursing key business and functional requirements
2. Development of a structure and strategy for collaboration
3. Development of an education strategy
4. Development of a communications strategy
5. Advancing and leveraging the C-HOBIC implementation
6. Advancing and leveraging the NurseONE portal

In March 2010, the NRG met to review the previously identified nursing components of health information and to validate that these were still relevant and appropriate for inclusion in EHRs. The group overwhelmingly endorsed the elements as being relevant and worthy of continued development for capture within EHRs. Furthermore, the NRG supported the continued deployment and development of C-HOBIC and the need to secure additional funding to support this work.

CONCLUSION

It is clear that a continued priority for nursing in Canada is the deployment of solutions that support the capture and retrieval of essential nursing data. Further, Canadian nursing leaders are actively pursuing the vision to include these as core elements in a national health information database. There is no question that progress has been made during the last decade, but nursing leaders must continue to respond to the challenge to further advance this agenda. Early experience with the collection and use of the C-HOBIC measures demonstrates the great potential of a common clinical data set utilized across care settings. Establishing a standardized set of nursing components for health information has the potential to provide nurses with the data required to transform nurs-

ing into a profession prepared to respond to the health needs of Canadians in the 21st century; however, the window of opportunity to have nursing data elements included in a national data set is narrowing. We must continue our efforts to ensure that the vision of nursing components in our national health information system becomes a reality for nursing in Canada.

REFERENCES

Advisory Committee on Health Infostructure. (2001). *Tactical plan for a pan-canadian health infostructure: 2001 update*. Office of Health and the Information Highway, Health Canada, Ottawa.

Alberta Association of Registered Nurses (AARN). (1994). *Client status, nursing intervention and client outcome taxonomies: A background paper*. Edmonton: Author.

Canada Health Infoway Inc. (2002). *Annual report: Accelerating the development of electronic health information systems for Canadians*. Montreal: Author.

Canada Health Infoway. (2008). *Infoway's investment programs*. Retrieved from http://www.infoway-inforoute.ca/lang-en/about-infoway/approach/investment-programs.

Canadian Institute for Health Information. (2010). Retrieved from http://www.cihi.ca.

Canadian Nurses Association. (2006a). *Nursing information and knowledge management*. Ottawa: Author.

Canadian Nurses Association. (2006b). *E-nursing strategy for canada*. Ottawa: Author.

Clark, J., & Lang N. (1992). Nursing's next advance: An international classification for nursing practice. *International Journal of Nursing, 39*(4), 102–112, 128.

Graves, J. R., & Corcoran, S. (1989). The study of nursing informatics. *Image: Journal of Nursing Scholarshi,p 21*(4), 227–231.

Hannah, K. J., & Anderson, B. (1994). Management of nursing information. In J. Hibbert & M. Kyle (Eds.), *Canadian nursing management*. Toronto: W.B. Saunders.

Hannah, K. J., Ball, M. J., & Edwards,M. J. A. (1999). *Introduction to nursing informatics* (2nd ed.). New York: Springer-Verlag.

Hannah, K., White, P., Nagle, L. M., & Pringle, D. (2009). Standardizing nursing information for inclusion in electronic health records: C-HOBIC. *Journal of the American Medical Informatics Association, 16*, 524–530.

Jydstrup, R. A., & Gross, M. J. (1966). Cost of information handling in hospitals: Rochester region. *Health Services Research, 1*, 235–271.

Kennedy, M.A. (2008). *Mapping Canadian clinical outcomes in ICNP*. Retrievd from http://www.cna-aiic.ca/c-hobic/documents/pdf.

Marek, K., & Lang, N. (1993). Nursing sensitive outcomes. In *Papers from the Nursing Minimum Data Set*

Conference (pp. 100–120). Ottawa: Canadian Nurses Association.

McCloskey, J. C. (1988). The nursing minimum data set: Benefits and implications for nurse educators. In *National League for Nursing, perspectives in nursing 1987–1989* (pp. 119–126). New York: National League for Nursing.

McGee, M. (1993). Response to V. Saba's paper on Nursing Diagnostic Schemes. *Papers from the Nursing Minimum Data Set Conference* (pp. 64–67). Ottawa: Canadian Nurses Association.

McPhillips, R. (1988). Essential elements for the nursing minimum data set as seen by federal officials. In H. H. Werley & N. M. Lang (Eds.), *Identification of the nursing minimum data set* (pp. 233–238). New York: Springer.

Nagle, L. M., White, P., & Pringle, D. (2007). Collecting outcomes in spite of our systems. *Canadian Journal of Nursing Informatics, 2*(3), 4–8.

Nagle, L. M., White, P., & Pringle, D. (2010). Realizing the benefits of standardized measures of clinical outcomes. *Electronic Healthcare 9*(2), e3–e9.

NurseONE. (2010). About us. Rertieved from http://www.nurseone.ca.

O'Brien-Pallas, L., & Giovannetti, P. (1993). Nursing intensity. *Papers from the Nursing Minimum Data Set Conference* (pp. 68–76). Ottawa: Canadian Nurses Association.

Verley, H. (1970). *Florence Nightingale at Harley Street*. London: Dent & Sons.

Werley, H.H., Devine, E.C., Zorn, C.R., Ryan, P, and Westra, B.L. (1991). The nursing minimum data set: Abstraction tool for standardized, comparable, essential data. *American Journal of Public Health, 81,* 421–426.

Werley, H. H., & Zorn, C. R. (1988). The nursing minimum data set: Benefits and implications. In *National League for Nursing, Perspectives in Nursing—1987–1989* (pp. 105–114). New York: National League for Nursing.

White, P., & Pringle, D. (2005). Collecting patient outcomes for real: The Nursing and Health Outcomes Project. *Canadian Journal of Nursing Leadership, 18*(1), 26–33.

Nursing Informatics in Europe

Kaija Saranto / Virpi Jylhä / Kaarina Tanttu

• OBJECTIVES

1. Describe elements of the European Union e-Health initiatives.
2. Describe nursing terminology work in Europe.
3. Give examples of nursing informatics education in Europe.
4. Give examples of nursing informatics cooperation in Europe.
5. Describe possibilities of meaningful use of structured data.
6. Describe a national model for documenting nursing and implementing an electronic nursing care plan.
7. Give examples of future developments.

• KEY WORDS

Europe
education
e-Health
electronic health records
health and nursing informatics
nursing documentation
terminologies
standards

INTRODUCTION

The number of sovereign states in Europe is 50. This is not surprising for a continent, but when considering that the European Union has 27 member states and recognizes 23 official languages, the complexity of this geographical area becomes evident. The role of the European Union in both healthcare policy and practice has become increasingly important due to directives launched by the European Union Council. These initiatives, focused on specific developments and actions, have strengthened equality, quality, and safety among healthcare services for citizens in every country in the European Union.

The European Union plays an integral part in supporting research and development activities through various initiatives and programs that have created advances in both education and health. Concerning nursing, there are many formal and informal communities working toward joint efforts at the European level. Whether discussing education, practice, management, or research, the combining factor seems to be enthusiasm. This chapter focuses on the important subject of e-Health initiatives from the perspectives of nursing language, education, management, and practice. Finally, the national Finnish nursing documentation project is described as an example of implementing a standardized nursing terminology into an electronic health record (EHR) system.

NURSING INFORMATICS AS PART OF THE eHEALTH STRATEGIES

In 2005, Europe had 730 million inhabitants that constituted about 11% of the world's population (Eurostat, 2010). The European Union includes most of Europe, with 27 member countries and a population of nearly half a billion. This is over 50% larger than the population of the United States, although the European Union is less than half its geographic area (Europa, 2010). However, the European Union's population is not spread evenly across the continent; some countries are more densely populated than others. For example, Malta has about 1,300 inhabitants/km², whereas Finland has 15 inhabitants/km² (Eurostat 2010). This creates challenges for health services. National health services are delivered in different ways throughout the European Union. Thus, the numbers of registered

TABLE 46.1	Numbers of RNs and Physicians in European Union in 2008			
	RN (PP)	Physician (PP)	RN (PP) per 100,000	Physician (PP) per 100,000
Austria	62,657	38,313	752	460
Belgium	na	31,274	na	298
Bulgaria	32,314	27,480	424	360
Cyprus	3710	2276	468	287
Czech Republic	82,765	36,921	794	354
Denmark	na	na	na	na
Estonia	8,583	4,490	640	335
Finland	na	14,455	na	272
France	507,514	213,821	817	344
Germany	877,000	292,129	1,068	356
Greece	na	67,540	na	601
Hungary	61,783	31,024	615	309
Ireland	68,614	13,763	1,552	311
Italy	370,641	246,834	619	413
Latvia	12,090	7,040	534	311
Lithuania	23,884	12,413	711	370
Luxemburg	na	na	na	na
Malta	2,647	1257*	642	304*
Netherlands	na	na	na	na
Poland	197,929	82,397	519	216
Portugal	56,709	38,932	534	367
Romania	na	47,617	na	221
Slovakia	33,778	na	625	na
Slovenia	15,924	4,854	781	238
Spain	210,800	159,500	462	350
Sweden	na	na	na	na
United Kingdom	575,989	157,658	938	257

*2009
(WHO, 2010)

nurses (RNs) and physicians differ from country to country. Table 46.1 identifies the numbers of registered nurses and physicians in each member state. Some of the differences can be explained through skill-mix issues, in other words, the roles of nurses are varied from country to country.

Although the European Union includes many different cultures, and the ways that healthcare is organized differ substantially from country to country, the national health systems face similar sets of challenges. Population growth has decreased and life expectancy has increased within the European Union during recent years, causing a transition toward an older population. By 2050, almost one-third of the European Union's population will be over 65 years old (Eurostat, 2010). Due to the aging population, the demand for health and social services is increasing. Further, the demand for health professionals is increasing, and many countries have already reported shortages of skilled nursing personnel. In the future it will be a challenge to balance supply and demand of health professionals in the workforce. In addition to an aging population, higher income and educational level have some effect on the increased demand for services. Also, the expectations of citizens have increased; people are more conscious of their health and want the best care available (Commission of the European Communities, 2004). As use of the Internet has become more popular among citizens, it has also had an effect on the delivery of healthcare services. Thus, the traditional office visit model used in healthcare fails to meet citizens′ diverse needs. Consequently, new ways of accessing health services and information should be introduced. European countries have to be able to fulfill citizens' needs and, at the same time, cut the increasing costs of healthcare services.

eHealth in European Union Policy Frameworks

Health informatics can offer solutions for future challenges. To promote the use of information and communication technology, the European Commission has produced several strategy initiatives, including the use of e-Health tools, to improve healthcare services. According to the eHealth Action Plan published in 2004 (Commission of the European Communities 2004):

> e-Health is today's tool for substantial productivity gains, while providing tomorrow's instrument for restructured, citizen-centered healthcare systems and, at the same time, respecting the diversity of Europe's multi-cultural, multi-lingual healthcare traditions. There are many examples of successful e-Health developments including health information networks, electronic health records, telemedicine services, wearable and portable monitoring systems, and health portals. (p. 4)

More briefly, e-Health has been defined as health services and information delivered or enhanced through the Internet and related technologies (Eysenbach, 2001).

The European Commission introduced the eEurope initiative in 2000 (European Commission, 2000). The purpose of this policy framework was to enable an information society for all Europeans and to ensure that the European Union was ready for the development of the information society, with the aim of creating fully integrated, interoperable, and modernized health systems using digital technologies. To achieve this, the European Commission published the eEurope 2002 Action Plan in 2000 (Commission of the European Communities, 2000). The aims of this plan, namely extending Internet connectivity and helping the member states adopt an existing legal framework, were achieved by 2002. Later in 2002, the eEurope 2005 Action Plan was released, focusing on utilization of broadband technologies, electronic health services, and improvement of the quality and cost effectiveness of public services (Commission of the European Communities, 2002).

Europe's eHealth Action Plan

In tandem with the eEurope strategy initiatives, the European Commission introduced an Action Plan for a European eHealth Area in 2004 (Commission of the European Communities, 2004). The central points of the eHealth Action Plan were information transfer, health and patient information, patient identifiers, mobility of patients and health professionals, infrastructure and health information networks, as well as monitoring the effects of new interventions. According to the eHealth Action Plan three general targets were identified (Commission of the European Communities 2004, p. 16):

- Addressing common challenges and creating the right framework to support e-Health
- Setting up pilot actions to jump start e-Health delivery
- Sharing best practices and measuring progress

The eHealth Action Plan includes recommendations for disseminating best practices and experiences regarding e Health applications across the European Union. The progress of e-Health application implementation needs to be measured every two years during the period of 2004 to 2010. In addition, the Monitoring National eHealth Strategies study has analyzed the results obtained by European Union member states through 2009 (Empirica, 2009). The European commission has funded the eHealth Benchmarking study, which aimed to analyze existing benchmarking sources. Based on the results of this study, a European Union–level recommendation for e-Health benchmarking activities, including definition of indicators, data collection, and conclusions, was produced in 2009 (Meyer, Hüsing, Didero, & Korte 2009).

In 2008, the European Commission published a recommendation on cross-border interoperability of EHR systems to support the goals of the eHealth Action Plan (Commission of the European Communities, 2008). According to the recommendation, existing and future challenges of healthcare systems can be at least partly solved through implementation of e-Health applications. EHRs are a fundamental part of e-Health systems, and interoperability between information systems needs to be achieved in order to fully utilize the benefits of EHRs. The guidelines set minimum requirements for activities conducted by member states to ensure that EHR systems can work together across the European Union. In addition, the issues of evaluation and monitoring as well as education and awareness are introduced. The guidelines present the following objectives (Commission of the European Communities, 2008):

- Establish elements of EHRs that should be exchangeable between systems.

- Enable health data to be shared among different healthcare systems.

- Build appropriate networked systems and services covering all healthcare areas.

Interoperability between information systems is not only a technical issue. Health data is always sensitive, thus, patient confidentiality and data security are important issues. In addition, legal, ethical, economic, organizational, and cultural aspect needs to be considered.

National Roadmaps for eHealth

The eHealth Action Plan included a requirement for each member state to develop a national e-Health strategy in order to identify their current state and map a plan for future development (Commission of the European Communities, 2004). National strategies focused on implementing e-Health systems, interoperability, utilizing EHRs, reimbursing e-Health services, and other related issues. Evaluation of national strategies conducted in 2008 showed that 25 out of 27 member states had formulated a national e-Health strategy (Hämäläinen, Doupi, & Hyppönen, 2008). Many of these strategies had links to national information society programs as well as to eEurope and i2010 information society programs. The Monitoring National eHealth Strategies study, published in 2010, showed that almost all European Union member states have detailed documents concerning e-Health goals, implementation, and achievements (Stroetmann et al., 2011).

Finland introduced its e-Health strategy in 2007 (Ministry of Social Affairs and Health, 2007). It is based on the Finnish national information society strategy work started in the mid-1990s. The Finnish e-Health strategy has 2 main objectives: (1) to secure the access to information for those involved in care regardless of time or place, and (2) to enable the involvement of citizens and patients, increasing the citizens' access to information and offering a high-quality of health information. The interoperability of information systems in healthcare is the starting point for information accessibility, and national-level legislation, recommendations, and specifications have been produced. The first aim is to attain interoperability between public and private service providers and then later between health and social welfare systems (Ministry of Social Affairs and Health, 2007). Electronic patient records already have a nationally defined structure, and the specification has been implemented in the information systems. In addition, several classifications and codes, such as the Finnish Classification on Nursing Diagnosis and Interventions, have been agreed upon. Finnish legislation supports availability of health information for citizens and Finland has already conducted some implementation activities and plans. The core patient data will be stored in the national electronic archive. The e-archive will enable citizens to access their health data and e-prescriptions online in the near future. A national health information portal for citizens has been introduced for health promotion and guidance purposes. The portal includes evidence-based data published by public administrations, research institutes, and health organizations. Thus, it offers reliable information about health issues and supports citizens in decision making and self-care. In addition, some regional Internet-based health services were introduced in Finland. The Hyvis portal, for example, is a free service intended for inhabitants of the Etelä-Savo Hospital District that complements regional health services and promotes the welfare of inhabitants by offering information about health and healthcare services. The portal also includes the ability to make an appointment for a community nurse, enables communication with a nurse for diabetes patients, and offers an enquiry service for users to consult a healthcare professional. Questions for nurses can be presented either in the portal's public forum, allowing universal access to the information, or in a private forum, which is secure and can be accessed only by the person who asks the question. Citizens usually receive a personal response within 1 or 2 days.

The role of health informatics, and certainly nursing informatics, has become increasingly prominent within the United Kingdom over the course of 2010. The U.K. Government is investing billions of pounds in developing information and communications technology (ICT) within the National Health Services to ensure that modernization and utilization of e-Health becomes a reality. All 4 countries now have national programs for ICT. In England, it is called NHS Connecting for Health; the Wales program is Informing Healthcare; Scotland has the e-Health program; and Northern Ireland's program is called Health and Personal Social Services Information and Communications Technology Strategy (HPSS ICT). A comprehensive list of the activities of each of these programs is beyond the scope of this chapter; see the Web sites below for additional information:

England: www.connectingforhealth.nhs.uk

Wales: www.wales.nhs.uk/ihc

Scotland: www.ehealth.scot.nhs.uk

Northern Ireland: www.dhsspsni.gov.uk

i2010: European Information Society

i2010 was the European Union's strategic framework for the information society and media during the years of 2005 through 2009. It was aimed toward a single european information space focusing on the positive contribution of ICT on the economy, society, and personal quality of life (Commission of the European Communities, 2005). E-Health had an important role in i2010, which focused on accessible e-Health services and the participation and inclusion of Europe's citizens in healthcare provision through electronic tools (European Commission, 2010a). Concurrent with policy framework, a subgroup on e-Health was established (European Commission, 2010). The main objectives of the subgroup were to improve quality and accessibility of healthcare services, while supporting the cost effectiveness of e-Health systems and services. One of the main tasks of the subgroup was to facilitate and contribute the implementation of the previously mentioned eHealth Action Plan.

The i2010 framework was followed by a new policy framework, the Digital Agenda for Europe, which focused on the utilization of the economic and social potential of Internet technologies in all fields of society (European Commission, 2010b). In healthcare, the emphasis is on ambient assisted living (AAL) technologies, which makes ICT-based services accessible for all. To support these strategic plans, the European Union has launched the AAL Joint Program for conducting research on and development of e-Health applications. The program aims to enhance the quality of life of older people by extending the time people can live in their homes, supporting functional capability of the elderly, and increasing the efficiency and productivity of used resources (Ambient Assisted Living Joint Programme, 2010). From the viewpoint of nursing informatics, AAL technologies offer the means to care for older patients who remain in their own homes and enables health information management at the point of care. In addition to AAL activities, the following actions will be included in the Digital Agenda during the coming years: secure online access for Europeans to their medical health data, widespread deployment of telemedicine services, and definition of a common minimum set of patient data for interoperability of electronic patient records (European Commission, 2010b).

eHealth Applications

The Finnish National Institute for Health and Welfare (previously referred to as STAKES) in cooperation with the eHealth ERA project evaluated the implementation of e-Health policies and the deployment of e-Health applications in the European Union. According to the report (Hämäläinen et al., 2008), the main e-Health applications are EHRs, patient identifiers, health portals for informing patients and professionals on health issues and disease prevention, citizen card activities, and telemedicine. The Monitoring National eHealth Strategies study provided an update on the progress of e-Health activities in Europe. The results showed significant progress in eHealth activies among EU27 countries (Stroetmann et al., 2011). The analysis of progress published in 2008 combined with the total number of reported activities in 2010 is presented in Table 46.2. The table presents an overview of the situation, but is not conclusive due to differences in the features and functions of e-Health applications in different countries, and deployment can be present only in primary or secondary care. In addition, deployment can be partly national, regional, or local (Hämäläinen et al., 2008).

The 2008 report shows that Finland was the only country to report activities in all 14 areas. Additionally, 11 countries (Austria, Belgium, Denmark, Germany, Greece,

TABLE 46.2 Deployment Status of Various E-Health Applications

EHR	Austria	Belgium	Bulgaria	Cyprus	Czech Republic	Denmark	Estonia	Finland	France	Germany	Greece	Hungary	Ireland	Italy	Latvia	Lithuania	Luxembourg	Malta	Netherlands	Poland	Portugal	Romania	Slovakia	Slovenia	Spain	Sweden	United Kingdom	Total (n = 27)	Total 2010 Study*
Patient Summary		1	1			1	1	1			1			1					1			1				1	1	27	27
Data Definition/Coding	1	1		1	1	1	1	1			1	1		1					1	1		1				1	1	10	n/a
Standards	1	1			1	1	1	1	1	1	1	1			1	1		1	1	1		1		1	1	1	1	15	n/a
Semantic Interoperability		1	1		1		1	1	1	1	1	1		1		1			1	1				1	1	1	1	20	27
E-Prescription	1	1	2	1	1	1	1	1	1	1	1	1	1	1	2	1	1	1	1	1	1	1	1	1	1	1	1	14	n/a
Citizen Health Card	1	1	1	1	1	1	1	1	1	1	1	1		1		1	1			1	1	1	1	1	1		1	21	22
Professional Card																								1		1		22	25
Patient ID	1	1	1	1	1	1	1	1	1	1		1	1	1	1	1	1	1		1	1	1		1	1		1	7	18
Professional ID	1	1	1	1		1	1	1	1		1				1	1		1		1		1		1	1	1	1	24	26
Citizen Health Portals	1				1	1	1	1	1	1	1	1	1	1	1	1	1		1	1	1	1		1	1	1	1	16	22
Professional Health Portals	1	1	1		1		1	1	1	1	1	1	1	1		1	1	1		1	1	1		1	1	1		23	n/a
Telemedicine	1	1	1	1	1	1	1	1	1	1	1	1		1	1	1	1			1	1	1	1	1	1	1	1	16	n/a
Safety and Quality Activities	1	1	1		1			1		2	1				2								1	1	1	1	1	24	27
																												7	n/a

1: Reported activities (actual planning, development, use)
2: Reported no activities
Empty: No information
n/a: data not available
*(Hämäläinen et al., 2008, p. 44; (Stroetmann et al., 2011).

702

Hungary, Italy, Poland, Slovakia, Sweden, and the United Kingdom), have reported activities in more than 10 areas. All countries have reported activities on the EHR, but it is unknown whether these developments concern primary care, secondary, or both (Hämäläinen et al., 2008). More specific activities regarding the development of the EHR in 2008 are not conducted often: patient summary ($n = 10$), data definition/coding ($n = 15$), standards ($n = 20$), semantic interoperability ($n = 14$).

EHR deployment in the European Union has mainly progressed well, but there are interesting differences in the deployment status of other e-Health applications. In 2008, e-prescription activities were reported in 21 countries (22 countries in 2010), but it was in use in only 5 countries, while 9 countries were at the construction or piloting phase. In 2010, the citizen health card is used in almost all countries ($n = 25$), but activities regarding professional cards are reported by a smaller number of countries ($n = 18$). However, in 2008 only 7 countries reported professional card activities, so the progress has been good. Different functions are included in citizens' health cards in different countries; the most common were patient ID and national health insurance coverage (Hämäläinen et al., 2008). In many countries, health cards and identification issues are closely related to each other. Almost all countries ($n = 26$) reported patient ID activities in 2010, while 22 countries reported professional ID activities. The type of identification method differs between countries. In general, there are 2 methods: healthcare–specific identifiers and national identification numbers (Hämäläinen et al., 2008). Based on the 2008 report, health portals for citizens (23 countries) are introduced more often than health portals for professionals (16 countries). Typically, citizens' health portals include information about general health and service systems (Hämäläinen et al., 2008). In accordance with the European Union's strategic goals, telemedicine applications are reported in all countries. The most common types of applications were teleconsultation and teleradiology including picture archiving communication systems (Hämäläinen et al., 2008).

Improvements in patient safety and quality of care are identified as a major benefit of e-Health, and the European Union has included them in the eHealth Action Plan as part of the i2010 strategic framework. In addition, the European Commission introduced the eHealth for Safety study in 2006. These activities indicate the importance of patient safety issues in Europe, but surprisingly only 7 countries (Belgium, the Czech Republic, Finland, Greece, Slovakia, Sweden, and the United Kingdom) reported some activities in this field. Germany and Latvia reported no activities, and the data for the remaining 18 countries were missing.

NURSING TERMINOLOGY DEVELOPMENT IN EUROPE

In Europe, the first effort to have standardized nursing data took the form of a multinational study from 1976 through 1985 called People's Needs for Nursing Care, which included participation by 11 European countries and was sponsored by the World Health Organization (WHO, 1977). In this study, the nursing process model was used as a framework. Since then the model has served as a standard for nursing documentation in many countries; nurses have mainly adopted four of its phases: assessment of nursing needs, planning of care, implementation of nursing actions, and assessment of nursing outcomes. In the early 1980s, there was considerably discussion and debate about whether nurses should use the nursing diagnosis as the second phase of the process. However, in many European countries nurses decided not to use the term *nursing diagnosis* and instead named the important conclusion after the assessment phase *nursing needs* or *nursing problems*. Nowadays, the nursing process model with 4 or 6 phases is used as the basis for structuring nursing documentation in various electronic nursing information systems in Europe.

The European Union has played an important role in supporting research and development activities with various initiatives and programs since the 1980s. Although these activities did not include nursing practice in the beginning, with the inception of the third framework program the European Union launched the Concerted Action on Nursing and delegates from member countries were invited to present proposals. The Danish Institute for Health and Nursing Research was elected to coordinate the Concerted Action on Telematics for Nursing: European Classification on Nursing Practice with regard to patients problems, nursing interventions, and patient outcomes, including educational measures. The Concerted Action was later renamed the TELENURSING consortium and was funded by the European Union from 1991 through 1994. It brought together 15 member states.

At the same time, the International Council of Nursing (ICN) had started the development of the International Classification for Nursing Practice (ICNP), and since 1991 these two nursing classification projects worked together to support the development of the ICNP. Following the TELENURSING project, the consortium was successful in gaining further European Union funding to start the TELENURSE project (1995 to 1998) and 9 European countries were involved in the 3 phases of the project in 7 work packages. The central focus of the project was on clinical nursing's aim

TABLE 46.3	Use of Translated and Validated Terminologies in Some European Countries										
	ICNP	CCC	NANDA –I	NIC	NOC	PNDS	LOINC	SNO-MED	VIPS	OMAHA	Local/Other
Austria	U		UT		T						U
Belgium			T	UTV			U			T	U
Croatia	UTV		UTV								
Denmark								T	UT		U
England*								UV			U
Finland		UTV	T	T		UTV			UT		U
Germany	TV		UT	T	T						U
Iceland			UTV	UTV	T						
Ireland*	U			U	U						
Italia	UTV		UT	UT	UT						
Latvia									T		
Norway	UTV	UT	UTV	UTV	UT			UT	UTV	T	U
Poland	T										
Portugal	UT		U							T	
Sweden	T								UV		
Switzerland	UTV		UTV	UT	UT						U
Wales*											U

U, terminologies in use; T, translations of terminologies; V, validations of terminologies.
*English is the spoken and written first language; VIPS is developed and written in Swedish.
(Thoroddsen et al., 2009)

to offer advanced ways of handling both nursing classifications of problems, interventions, and results as part of the registration of clinical data and collecting the information necessary to enhance the quality of clinical practice in nursing (Clark, 2003; Danish Institute for Health and Nursing Research, 1995). The outcomes of these projects had a crucial impact on nursing terminology development; in 1999, the ICNP alpha version was launched by the ICN with joint international efforts. As is well know, the ICNP elements—nursing phenomena (nursing diagnoses), nursing actions, and nursing outcomes—are now published in the ICNP Version 2 launched in 2009

Use of Nursing Terminologies in Europe

Consisting of various countries with their own national languages, the use of nursing terminologies in Europe involves a considerable amount of translation and cultural validation, particularly regarding a terminology originally written in English. Based on the results of a 2008 survey, the use of nursing terminologies is not very common in European countries (Table 46.3). However, the results of the survey should be interpreted conditionally. Only 17 country members out of 38 countries replied to the electronic survey, and countries such as Italy, the Netherlands, and Spain are not included in the results (Thoroddsen, Saranto, Ehrenberg, & Sermeus 2009).

The NANDA International classification has been translated into many European languages, such as Dutch, French, German, Icelandic, Italian, Norwegian, Portuguese, and Spanish, but is still not in active use in nursing documentation. Seemingly, the countries that adopted the NANDA-I Classification have also translated the Nursing Interventions Classification (NIC) and Nursing Outcomes Classification (NOC). Some European countries have expressed a need to validate terminologies based on cultural differences in their healthcare service system.

Many European countries have followed the development work of the ICN and especially the ICNP terminology. Translations in French, German, Greek, Icelandic, Italian, Norwegian, Polish, Portuguese, Romanian, Spanish, Swedish, and Turkish are in process. Translation has often been supported by the national nursing organizations (ICNP, 2010). The active use of the ICNP in healthcare settings is still in its infancy in many European countries, mainly due to differences in nursing documentation legislation, policies, or electronic information systems. However, many nursing schools are using the terminology in teaching nursing documentation.

The VIPS model (acronym for the Swedish spelling wellbeing, integrity, personal, and safety) developed in Sweden by Professor Margareta Ehnfors and her associates is widely used in the Nordic countries. The VIPS model conceptualizes the essential elements of nursing care, clarifying and facilitating systems thinking and nursing recording. The focus of the model is on patients' functioning in daily life activities rather than on pathophysiologic problems (Ehnfors, Ehrenberg, & Thorell-Ekstrand, 2003; Ehrenberg, Ehnfors, & Thorell-Ekstrand, 1996.) A significant amount of research on the VIPS model has been conducted, showing that the model has good content validity in different areas of nursing care. The model has proven useful in different nursing specialties and is fully computerized in information systems (Saranto & Kinnunen, 2009).

Although not evident in Table 46.3, many European countries have also used the International Classification of Functions (ICF, formerly known as the ICIDH, or International Classification of Impairments, Disability, and Handicaps) launched by the WHO. The ICF puts the notions of health and disability in a new light. It acknowledges that every human being can experience a decrease in health, and thereby experience some degree of disability. The ICF has been used in nursing and rehabilitation contexts, and several countries have started the process of streamlining the ICF in their health and social information standards (e.g., Finland, Ireland, Italy, the Netherlands, and Sweden) (ICF, 2010).

The National Health Service in England and other countries of the United Kingdom decided in the early 2000s to use a single, multidisciplinary terminology across healthcare. This work evolved, combining with efforts in the United States and other countries, to become the Systematized Nomenclature of Medicine— Clinical Terms (SNOMED-CT). This terminology has maps to other classifications that have different but essential purposes. Nurses have been involved in the crucial task of ensuring that nursing content is adequately represented in this large, multidisciplinary terminology

(Casey, 2003). Since this terminology is of English language origin, there is a major translation challenge for European countries adopting and implement it into electronic information systems. At the moment, translations in European countries, such as Denmark and Sweden, are in process, but a Spanish version already exists.

Possibilities for Meaningful Use of Nursing Data

According to the study by Thoroddsen and colleagues (2009) the use of standardized nursing terminologies in Europe is still rare, which makes access to nursing data an obstacle. In more than 60% of the institutions in the countries that replied, nursing data were not stored and could, therefore, not be retrieved (Thoroddsen et al., 2009). Clinical patient data can answer a variety of questions presented by managers, researchers, or policy makers when it is collected and used appropriately. Documentation developments, such as the increased standardization of patient records and the use of classifications, make healthcare data more reliable and useful for practice development, management, and research.

There are various local terminologies in nursing practice in addition to the international nursing classifications (Table 46.3). This partly reflects the language differences, but also the differences in healthcare service systems. In many countries nurses have devoted their activities to making nursing visible. The nursing information reference model (NIRM) developed in the Netherlands by Goossen, Epping, and Dassen (1997) has also been used widely in other countries to accommodate both the information needs of nurses at the clinical level and for aggregating data at higher levels (Goossen, Epping, & Dassen, 1997). The model has also been exploited in Finland in the national nursing documentation project.

Along with the NIRM, nursing minimum data sets have been used to indicate nurses' contribution in healthcare from administrative and economic perspectives. The use of the Belgian nursing minimum data set (B-NMDS) was the first attempt among European nurses to show a nursing contribution since 1988. The B-NMDS consists of 23 nursing interventions, medical diagnoses, patient demographics, nurse variables, and institutional characteristics. The data were collected 4 times per year (Sermeus & Delesie, 1997; Sermeus, Delesie, Van Landuyt, Wuyts, Vandenboer, & Manna, 1994.) The B-NMDS has been revised into B-NMDS-II based on the Nursing Intervention Classification (Van den Heede, Michiels, Thonon, & Sermeus 2009; Sermeus et al., 2005).

In Ireland, the need to improve understanding of how to use nursing resources most effectively has also emerged

(MacNeela, Scott, Treacy, & Hyde 2006). The development of the Irish Nursing Minimum Data Set (I-NMDS) for general nursing and the I-NMDS for mental health nursing has advanced data collection for multiple purposes. There is a need to analyze and provide information on nursing trends; illustrate service provider trends and patterns in nursing and client care; inform hospital budgeting, nurse staffing levels, and consequently patient safety; as well as inform developments in nursing education. Further, there is a need for integrating the data used to forecast the supply and demand of nurses and midwives with specific knowledge, skills, and competencies into the electronic patient record to facilitate access to nursing information and decision-making (Morris et al., 2010; National Council, 2006). There have only been a few additional initiatives on NMDS in Europe (e.g., the Swiss CH-NMDS [Berthou & Junger, 2003] and FinNMDS, which is in its early phase).

Over the years, data collection and analysis has largely focused on indirect aspects of nursing service such as waiting times, length of stay, and operative procedures. Addressing the international challenge of expanding the nursing workforce with qualified nurses is of crucial importance and requires cooperation to accomplish. Researchers from 12 different European countries collaborated in one of the largest nursing workforce studies in Europe—the RN4CAST study (2009 to 2011). Through nurse, patient, and organizational surveys, the RN4CAST study aims to provide innovative forecasting methods by addressing not only volume, but also quality of nursing and patient care. Simultaneously to these research activities, the project entails dissemination and stakeholder activities aimed toward achieving the study's objectives. Strategic collaboration is maintained with a stakeholder panel consisting of 13 healthcare– and nursing administration–related organizations to raise awareness of the project. The ambition of the RN4CAST project is to produce a policy breakthrough commensurate with the scientific strength of the project's findings and the accumulated evidence in the sector. This includes producing both technical and scientific publications, as well as liaising with mass media. Thus, research findings will need to be refined through proactive stakeholder engagement (RN4CAST, 2010).

DEVELOPMENTS IN NURSING INFORMATICS EDUCATION

In 1999, the ministers responsible for higher education in European countries signed the Bologna Declaration (named after the city in Italy where the meeting was held). They agreed on objectives for the development of a coherent and cohesive European Higher Education Area by 2010. The Bologna Process aimed to increase competitiveness and strengthen social and gender cohesion and reduce social inequalities both at the national and European levels. The member countries will promote effective quality assurance systems, increase effective use of the system based on 2 cycles (first cycle degrees [bachelor level] should give access to second cycle programs, and second cycle degrees should give access to doctoral programs), and improve the recognition system of degrees and periods of studies. Further, the process includes the following important objectives: promotion of student and academic and administrative staff mobility, application of a system of easily readable and comparable degrees, active participation of all partners especially student involvement in the process, ensuring a substantial period of study abroad, developing scholarship programs for students from developing nations, and making lifelong learning a reality (Mantas, 2004).

Nursing informatics education has been a central topic among countries in the European Union. Parallel to the development of the Bologna Process within the fourth European Union framework program, the NIGHTINGALE project (1998 to 2002) aimed to create support for nursing informatics (NI) education and a means to describe state-of-the-art NI education, NI curriculum development, and educational material and validation of the products in the educators' group. Before NIGHTINGALE, there had already been active development work in health informatics education through the EDUCTRA (Education and Training in Health Informatics) project (1992 to 1994) and its successor, the IT-EDUCTRA project (1996 to 1998), both funded by the European Union, where the focus was not only on medical education but also on nursing IT competencies. Evident in the results of these projects, health and NI education varied greatly among and within the countries, providing a great challenge to develop course material for education. Since the NIGHTINGALE project, the structure and material for NI courses has been used as an example for enhancing NI curricula (Mantas, 1998).

During the 1990s, the European Union also funded the European Summer School in Nursing Informatics (ESSONI) consortium. Over the years, 8 summer schools were organized in various European countries by the consortium. Based on changes in the European Union funding mechanism, the consortium was not able to continue and the tradition of effective and enthusiastic collaboration ended. However, the networks built up during the ESSONI years have created an atmosphere of flexible cooperation among participants and have advanced the development of NI education and research. Based on the ESSONI model, German partners have still from time to time carried out the educational tradition successfully.

Since the implementation of the Bologna Process first cycle degrees (i.e., at the bachelor's level), various courses in NI have been integrated into the nursing curricula in many countries. The topics have focused on health information systems, confidentiality and data protection, aspects of information technology, and the organizational impact in healthcare. Some nursing schools offer a special track in nursing or health informatics.

European universities have mainly included health informatics education in their programs. In some universities, at the University of Eastern Finland for example, a Health Informatics program is offered as a specialty within the health and human services informatics master's degree program. However, the degree itself is multidisciplinary and students may have a bachelor's degree in nursing or other health sciences, computer science, or business sciences when entering the program (University of Eastern Finland, 2010).

In the United Kingdom, a master's degree in health informatics has existed since 1990, with programs open to nurses and other healthcare professionals. As a joint initiative of the University College London and the Whittington Hospital NHS Trust, health informatics courses are offered as multiprofessional education. The Lancashire School of Health and Post-Graduate Medicine at the University of Central Lancashire provides a wide range of relevant and effective educational courses. Undergraduate and postgraduate programs also include health informatics education. Glasgow Caledonian University has expanded its capacity to provide students with experiences and education in e-Health, and a Health Informatics master's program is under development (IMIA, 2010).

In Greece, the Health Informatics Laboratory, which is connected to the Faculty of Nursing of the University of Athens, serves the undergraduate and postgraduate studies of most of the Schools of Health Sciences of the university. In the Netherlands, the Institute of Health Policy and Management, as part of Erasmus Medical Center, offers 3 undergraduate English master's and 2 postgraduate English master's programs, which focus on different aspects of healthcare including health information management. In Denmark, Aalborg University offers a 3-year master's degree in health informatics attended by more than 120 midcareer students per year from Scandinavia, Iceland, and Greenland.

Beside the degree programs, ICT competencies can be achieved by obtaining a driving license for computer use, especially for nurses working in hospitals or other healthcare organizations. One example is the European Computer Driving License (ECDL), which is a relevant and internationally recognized qualification for all computer users, not only nurses in healthcare. The ECDL is designed to improve understanding and to render the use of computers more effective among employees. It is designed for both novice and intermediate computer users. To enhance computer literacy, several countries have adopted this model for their in-service training in hospitals (European Computer Driving License (ECDL), 2010).

NURSING INFORMATICS RELATED COOPERATION IN EUROPE

The NI cooperation in Europe is based on the national nurses associations (NNAs) and other nursing-related organizations, working groups, and networks. At the European level, NNAs have worked together toward development in quality assurance, nursing workforce, and competencies. In many countries, NNAs have nursing informatics working groups, as well as NI-track sessions during their annual seminars, which have been very popular. These regular events have been mainly informal, discussing meaning of the discipline. More specific and formal efforts are needed in many European countries concerning NI education and practice development, and especially for the recognition of NI as a specialty in nursing.

At a national level, the NNAs play a central role in bringing ICT use into nursing practice. The most recent initiative has been focused on e-Health, highlighting the European Commission's eHealth Action Plan. In this huge endeavor, cooperation with other member countries is crucial. The role of the European Federation of Nurses Associations (EFN), established in 1971, is integral for establishing this cooperation. The EFN is the independent voice of the profession in Europe and consists of NNAs from 32 European Union member states working for the benefit of 6 million nurses throughout Europe.

The mission of the EFN is to strengthen the status and practice of the nursing profession for the benefit of both citizens' health and the interests of nurses in the European Union and the rest of Europe. Concerning the e-Health initiatives in European Union member states, the EFN has encouraged nurses to focus on three targets: (1) the expected benefits of the e-Health movement such as optimization of services and continuity of care; (2) National e-nursing advancements like electronic documentation, patient and health professional cards, and telenursing; and (3) the barriers faced during implementation. According to the EFN, e-Health has enormous potential for enabling continuity of care, especially for individuals with long-term conditions, and improving the accessibility of health services leading to optimized and efficient care. Although the use of ICT in healthcare is highly advanced in Europe, there are still many developments, such as EHRs, e-prescribing, and patient and health professional cards, that urgently need to be implemented in various countries. Some countries like Finland, Ireland, Portugal, and Sweden already have successful examples of nurses' involvement in prescribing medicines. However, changes are needed, especially in legislation, to make advances in e-prescriptions. Thus, the primary obstacle to e-Health adoption is national legislation, which often needs to be developed or revised. In some countries like Austria, Finland, Germany, Slovenia, and Sweden, there are legal initiatives regarding the extent to which various professionals or citizens should have access to electronic patient information (EFN, 2010).

It is essential to developing effective indicators and measures that assess quality, performance, and cost regarding nursing's contribution to patient outcomes and public health on a national and international level. The Nordic Nurses Federation (SSN, acronym for the Swedish words Nurses Cooperation in Nordic countries) has focused on quality indicators and nursing terminology issues during recent years. Nurses from NNAs in Denmark, Finland, Iceland, Norway, and Sweden have worked together, aiming to define quality indicators for nutrition, pain, pressure ulcer sores, falls, and terminologies as well as workforce measures. This work reflects various development activities in the Nordic countries, and the results are shared in seminars and panels during annual meetings (SSN, 2010).

Consisting of numerous countries and their languages, Europe needs many forums to share and benchmark its developments in nursing. The Association for Common European Nursing Diagnoses, Interventions and Outcomes (ACENDIO) is a membership organization established in 1995 to promote the development of nursing's professional language and to provide a network across Europe for nurses interested in the development of a common language that describes the practice of nursing. The establishment of ACENDIO was heavily connected to the TELENURSING project (1992 to 1994). During that time and still today, there is a huge need for nurses throughout Europe to be able to share and compare information in order to research

and improve care, manage nursing resources effectively, and ensure that nursing is visible in local, national, and European policy.

Nurses in some European countries are developing their own terminologies to meet the need for a nursing language in their country. Others have adapted or translated terminologies and classifications developed in other countries or by other disciplines, but there is no overall coordination of these developments among countries. ACENDIO offers a discussion forum for European nurses, and also for nurses from outside Europe, to enable active participatation in the development work in their own countries. Through biannual meetings and national workshops the association tries to encourage its members to improve the status of nursing terminology, inform policy decisions, and strengthen or make visible the nursing contribution to health and patient care (ACENDIO, 2010).

The Association for Nomenclature, Taxonomy and Nursing Diagnoses (the Spanish acronym AENTDE stands for Asociación Española de Nomenclatura, Taxonomía y Diagnósticos de Enfermeros) was created in 1995 by a group of Spanish nurses envisioning the future of the profession. The aims of the association are: to contribute to the development of a nursing terminology able to identify the contribution of nursing care to the population's health and to improve and foster the knowledge and use of nursing terminologies among nurses in Spain. Further, to collaborate with National and International organizations in the promotion of research and sharing of knowledge and experiences on the use of nursing diagnoses and other nursing terminologies. The association welcomes the participation of all nurses working with standardized nursing languages in clinical nursing, education, research, or administration.

The main activities carried out by the AENTDE are a biennial international symposium on Nursing Diagnoses and Terminologies and a biennial workshop. Since 1996 when the first international symposium was held, 7 international symposia and 7 workshops have been organized by AENTDE, with the participation of both national and international nurses. The most recent symposium was held in Madrid in May 2010, together with NANDA-International. It was the first time that NANDA-International celebrated its congress outside the USA. Around 1,000 nurses from all over the world joined the event, demonstrating the interest and importance of the development of nursing languages for the future of the profession. The workshops are more local, where about 200 Spanish nurses meet every other year somewhere in Spain to share and advance knowledge in the use of nursing terminologies. The Spanish health system is quite advanced in the use of electronic systems, and this is one of the reasons why the use of standardized nursing languages is so common in Spain (AENTDE, 2010).

The European Federation of Medical Informatics (EFMI) was established in 1976, and the nursing working group, now known as NursIE, formed in in 1988. From the 32 member countries of EFMI, 18 country members and 10 associate members belong to the NursIE as of 2010. The first chair of the working group was Dr. Marianne Tallberg, an active nurse from Finland, although the EFMI working group rules stated that, "A working group consists of experts selected and assigned in a special area" not necessarily meaning nursing. From the beginning, the aims of the working group have been constant, focusing on support for nurses and nursing organizations in the European countries with information and contacts, and to offer nurses opportunities to build contact networks within the field of informatics. This has been accomplished by arranging sessions, workshops, and tutorials in connection with the Medical Informatics European (MIE) conferences. The working group aims to support the education of nurses with respect to informatics and computing as well as to support research and development work in the field and to promote publishing of achieved results (EFMI, 2010). Many NursIE members are also members of the International Medical Informatics Association's Special Interest Group for Nursing Informatics (SIGNI) (IMIA, 2010).

Another development that built on the TELENURSE initiative was the development of a European standard for nursing terminology. This brought together nurses across Europe with the objective of including nursing in the efforts of the health informatics committee of the European Standard Organisation (CEN). The work progressed well and was adopted by the International Standards Organisation (ISO) under a cooperation agreement between the two standards organisations (the Vienna agreement). The resulting international standard focused on the conceptual structures that are represented in a reference terminology model for nursing, supporting mapping among terminologies and harmonisation with terminology and information model standards outside the domain of nursing (ISO, 2003).

NURSING DOCUMENTATION IN FINLAND

The following paragraphs provide an example of how a standardized nursing terminology has been implemented in an EHR system. In Finland, the somewhat unified paper-based health record has been widely used for more than 30 years. Over the years, nursing documentation has been based on narrative text. Thus, it has been difficult to retrieve and reuse the information contained in care plans and nursing notes. Electronic information systems including some platforms for care documentation have been used for more than 10 years, but their structures have not been unified. This kind of development has not been given high priority in the nursing profession in the past. However, today nearly all public and private healthcare providers already employ electronic health records.

During the past decade in Finland, there has been considerable activity toward developing the EHR. In Finland, the Ministry of Social Affairs and Health launched a large project for improving health services from 2003 to 2007. The purpose of the project was to unify information systems, national data archives, and data security solutions. For the first time, nursing was recognized in the national project. As a part of the national project, the Nursing Documentation Project started in May 2005 and ended in October 2009.

In Finland, the ratio of nurses to physicians is 4 to 1. In clinical settings, this means that nurses, being the largest group of healthcare professionals, constitute the most active users of patient data in hospitals 24 hours per day, 7 days per week. This necessitates that tools and models adopted for daily practice support nursing from philosophical, ethical, and practical perspectives.

The Development of a National EHR System

The Council of State made a decision in principle in 2002, that Finland should have a nationally interoperable EHR by the end of the year 2007. Furthermore, the decree launched in 2007 requires public healthcare organizations to join the national patient record archive. The Ministry of Social Affairs and Health is in charge of the implementation of this decision and the specification of the EHR solution (Figure 46.1).

In 2004, the core data elements of the EHR were introduced as part of the national EHR project. A national consensus on the data elements was reached at 2 special consensus seminars and working group meetings of healthcare professionals and software developers from IT suppliers. The definitions were also publicly available for comment on the Internet. *Core data* means health-related information required for data exchange between health information systems in a standardized format. The core data are defined as the data that can be

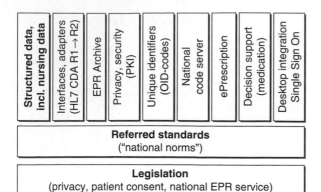

Niilo Saranummi, VTT Information Technology 2005

• **FIGURE 46.1.** The EHR solution in Finland.

standardized. Documentation of the core data requires the use of vocabulary, terminology, and classifications (Häyrinen, Saranto, & Nykänen, 2008).

The core data is the most significant information in the patient care process throughout different healthcare sectors, describing the patient's state of health or disease. The core information accumulates chronologically during patient care by different professionals. The aim of the core data is to give a holistic description of the patient's health and disease history, and of the care and guidance provided. The information is used in present and future care.

Development and Implementation of the Systematic Nursing Documentation Model

The national systematic nursing documentation model was adopted to describe nursing care in the EHR system. The systematic nursing documentation model was based on the nursing decision-making process introduced be the WHO in the late 1970s. The international model comprises 4 main phases:

• Assessment and naming the nursing needs (nursing diagnoses)

• Planning and describing the outcomes of care

• Description of interventions performed

• Assessment of nursing outcomes

The Nursing Minimum Data Set (NMDS) is a part of the core data elements. The NMDS includes information on the:

• Nursing diagnosis and needs

• Nursing interventions

• Nursing outcomes

• Nursing discharge summary

• Patient care intensity

The national nursing documentation model (Figure 46.2) and the Finnish Care Classification (FinCC) were developed in the National Nursing Documentation Project from 2005 to 2009. The aims in the nursing documentation project were to unify and standardize nursing documentation nationally and to connect it with the interdisciplinary core documentation of the patient history, national code server, and national data archive. The national NMDS and FinCC were integrated, between 2005 and 2007, into 8 health recording systems in 34 healthcare organizations. Piloting was carried out as an action research in 106 units or wards in 3 university hospitals, 11 district hospitals, 19 healthcare centers, and 1 private hospital. Integration, testing, and assessing in 8 EHRs was done in collaboration with 6 information technology suppliers. An education model and an e-education environment were also developed to support the implementation.(Ikonen, Tanttu, Hoffren, & Mäkilä, 2007).

The FinCC is a translation of the Clinical Care Classification (CCC) System (www.sabacare.com), and it was implemented after a cultural validation (Saba, 1992; Ensio, 2001). The CCC System is approved by the American Nurses Association (ANA) and is cross-mapped to the International Classification for Nursing Practice by the International Council of Nursing (ICN) and to the Unified Medical Language System (UMLS). The CCC System is also part of the international SNOMED-CT classification, and it can be used together with ICD-10. Clinical LOINC (Logical Observations, Identifiers, Names, and Codes) has integrated the CCC System of Nursing Diagnoses Outcomes in its clinical application. ABC Codes for Complimentary and Alternative Medicine (CAM) has adapted and selected the CCC System of Nursing Interventions for billing codes.

FinCC includes the Finnish Classification of Nursing Diagnosis (FiCND), Finnish Classification of Nursing Interventions (FiCNI), and Finnish Classification of Nursing Outcomes (FiCNO). The Finnish Classification of Nursing Diagnosis (FiCND) includes 19 care components, 88 main categories, and 179 subcategories defining care needs, and it is used to describe needs assessment and expected outcomes of patient care in various healthcare settings. The Nursing Interventions Classification (FiCNI) comprehends the

View: Patient care history

Interdiciplinary care process	Admission & Status						
		Planning			Action	Assessment	
Nursing process	Data collection and analysis*	Definition of patient needs / diagnosis	Aims	Planned nursing interventions	Nursing Interventions	Nursing Outcomes	Nursing discharge summary
FiCND 2.01 FiCNO 1.0	-	FiCND and assessment scales	FiCND	-	-	FiCND, FiCNO and assessment scales	Includes: Summary of the nursing process data exploiting the structured documentation and the patient care intensity grade.
FiCNI 2.01 FiCNO 1.0	-	-	-	FiCNI	FiCNI and assessment scales	FiCND, FiCNO and assessment scales - Measurement of patient care intensity (OPCq)	
Nursing core data	Inter-disciplinary core data	Nursing needs			Nursing interventions	Nursing outcomes	Nursing discharge summary	Patient care intensity

*Includes data of personal identification, risks, medication, medical diagnosis, examinations, operations and activity

060608 K.Tanttu

• **FIGURE 46.2.** The nursing documentation model in Finland.

same 19 care components, 164 main categories, and 266 subcategories defining planned and performed nursing actions. The care components represent the functional, health behavioral, physiologic, and psychologic patterns of a patient. FiCNO can be described using 3 qualifiers: improved, stabilized, or deteriorated. When comparing nursing diagnoses and outcomes of nursing care, it is possible to evaluate the care process and measure the care outcomes.

The components of FiCND and FiCNI are:

Activity	Metabolism
Coping	Circulation
Respiration	Role relationship
Elimination	Safety
Fluid volume	Self care
Health behaviour	Psychologic regulation
Health services	Sensory
Medication	Skin integrity
Nutrition	Life cycle
Continued treatment	

The Oulu Patient Classification (OPCq) is used to measure patient care intensity. The OPCq is based on the Roper, Logan, and Tierney model for nursing and the Oulu University Hospital's quality assurance program and value basis, which is characterized by a humanistic approach and current research results concerning patients' expectations of good care.

The OPCq is built on the following areas of need (Kaustinen, 1995; Onnela & Svenström, 1998):

1. Planning and coordination of care
2. Breathing, blood circulation, and symptoms of disease
3. Nutrition and medication
4. Personal hygiene and secretion
5. Activity/movement, sleep, and rest
6. Teaching and instruction in care/follow-up care and emotional support

In each of these areas, the nurse classifies from $A = 1$ point to $D = 4$ points once a day. The care intensity of a patient can be scored between 6 and 24 points. The higher the score, the higher is the care intensity of the patient (OHL, 2004).

The end product in the project was a cross-mapped classification material (FiCND, FiCNI, and OPCq) in the national code server. The databases enable evaluation, analysis, and utilization of data for administrative and research purposes.

Education Process

Nurses were educated on systematic nursing documentation. The education included theoretical education on the nursing process, nursing classification, and case studies. All nurses need a basic understanding of standardized terminology. It is imperative that nurses, who are expected to use the terminology accurately and consistently, receive a systematic introduction that is designed to meet their educational needs. Their learning needs were considered through well planned, comprehensive strategies. Learning a standardized terminology is similar to learning a new language; both require hard work. Learners need to understand the why, how, and when. Educators need to be sensitive to "just-in-time" opportunities, and match their presentations, materials, and schedules to diverse learning styles.

Case studies were one of the most important implementation strategies. The case study practice should be planned; it should proceed from simple to complex; it should be relevant to the daily experiences of the nurses; and it should be fun. Many wards do not have a tradition of a nursing care plan on paper, which is important when considering implementing a nursing care plan in the EHR. To these wards, the nursing care plan is a new approach. The key individuals should convince their colleagues why the patient should have a nursing care plan, engaging the discussion of useful content in the care plan and introducing the concept of functionality, which supports a new approach to documentation. The key individuals need to have expanded knowledge of and skills in the substance of nursing, including adequate supplementary training in addition to basic training in nursing, and be well prepared to teach and train their colleagues. Moreover, good cooperation between different interest groups is essential.

An education model and an e-education environment were also developed to support the implementation. Education was first launched to nurses in clinical settings, both in primary and specialized care. Education was built primarily on the content of classification and the theoretical assumptions of need theory. Surprisingly, having been in use for almost 30 years as a paper-based system, the nursing process model also required discussion and review.

Evaluation and Results

The model for systematic nursing documentation was assessed by continuous observations, questionnaires to nurses (N = 975), questionnaires to head nurses (N = 197), documentation cases, discussions, and by statistics of the classified documentation. Based on the experiences and evaluation results, the Finnish Care Classification can be implemented and used on all kinds of wards.

Overall, the quality of the nursing documentation has improved as a result of a unified model to describe nursing activities. They are more uniform, patient-centered, and based on guidelines accepted for care. This can be observed in the handovers between shifts. The length of oral reports has decreased during the project, giving more time for actual care. The use of systematic nursing documentation brings up the content of nursing care more clearly, allowing nurses to read patient information from the electronic records. In general, use of the EHR was routine after 3 months. Statistical information concerning use of FiCND and FiCNI were revealed between 2006 and 2009 in a nursing decision-making process. The statistical reports have been discussed in each ward. The discussion has been very meaningful. Statistical reports have also enabled more in-depth study of the care process and the interventions used in care.

The model based on the nursing decision-making process and FinCC is usable in all kinds of wards and units (e.g., primary care, special care, elderly care). FinCC can be used to:

- Document integrated patient care processes.
- Perform multiprofessional searches for information to aid the decision-making process.
- Analyze patient profiles and populations.
- Predict care needs, resources, and costs.
- Classify and track clinical care.
- Develop evidence-based practice models.
- Develop clinical plans of care, clinical pathways, and guidelines as well as for research and educational purposes.
- Develop reports for nursing management, planning, education, research, and quality assessment.

Among nurses, there is no desire to return to the old model of recording patient data. The users have begun to see the benefits of systematic nursing documentation and use of the EHR. The experiences of the systematic model of recording patient data are promising. Statistics and reports of nursing process by systematic documentation benefit nursing management, planning, education, research, and quality assessment.

It was important that all EHR suppliers in Finland were involved in the project to have equal core data structure in every EHR. Most important, the obstacles to be overcome were technical problems (e.g., failures and problems in new EHR versions), learning and accepting the new documentation model, which takes time approximately 3 months to become routine, and the maintaining organization-wide commitment.

The implementation process started in Finland in October 2007 and will end in 2011. A national network of mentors supported the adoption of the documentation model by using case studies developed for the implementation. All wards and units have named their own mentors who act as tutors in the beginning of the implementation.

FUTURE DEVELOPMENTS

European nurses have been eager to adopt a standardized nursing language. Activities have focused on translations, validations, and implementations of classifications and data sets into practice. In addition, the history of international cooperation in the development of the ICNP is promising. However, we need to have new beginnings, especially regarding the implementation of terminologies into electronic information systems, to be able to build databases for nursing. These databases will enable evaluation, analysis, and utilization of data for administrative and research purposes, in addition to clinical use of data.

The European Commission has stated in its recommendation (Commission of the European Communities, 2008), it is highly important that those systems implemented should be interoperable with other systems not only within organizations and nationally, but also internationally. This ensures that the health information of European Union citizens would be accessible safely and securely. Thus, data transfer will benefit patients' and professionals' mobility in the region of the European Union. This vision challenges nurses to guarantee that nursing data is transferable (i.e., standardized).

Concerns for the effects on the nurse-patient relationship are often important to those considering the advanced use of technology in healthcare. Although information and communication technology can enhance the nurse-patient relationship, it cannot entirely replace it. Based on studies, information gained through ICT applications empower users by encouraging active participation and increasing patient satisfaction. Thus, the use of ICT in nursing can be seen as a means to provide good quality care as well as to strengthen patient safety consistent with the aims in the European Commission's eHealth Action Plan.

Like in the United States, it may not be taken for granted that nurses have an informatics career pathway in Europe. Despite the active work among e-Health initiatives and IT capacity in healthcare settings, nurses often participate in development work in addition to their daily duties. A number of nursing professionals have already developed expertise or degrees in health or nursing informatics, yet, their knowledge and skills are not sufficiently recognized or used to deliver benefits to patients and colleagues. This deficiency reflects the lack of health or nursing informatics expert positions in healthcare organizations, partly due to the fact that NNAs are not recognized for IT expertise because most do not have nursing informatics as a recognized specialty in Europe.

National nursing development work is very demanding and cannot be regarded only as an implementation project. The Finnish nursing documentation model has now been introduced to nurses all over the country, and nurses have adopted the model mostly with satisfaction. An expert group has been established to take care of the updates to the FinCC, as well as to organize continuous assessments. There are also visions of how to implement clinical pathways and guidelines into the documentation model to be able to support evidence-based nursing. From the technological progress point of view, nurses would also like to have decision support actions including alarms added to the systems. As always, a considerably amount of development work is still needed to enhance usability of the information systems.

Information sharing from the databases is still in its infancy, and nurse managers mostly use frequencies from the databases. Thus, more sophisticated data acquisition, statistical analysis, and tools for reporting are in the development process to be used in benchmarking at the organizational, regional, and national levels (and hopefully at the European and international levels soon!).

ACKNOWLEDGMENTS

The authors would like to end this chapter with a very important reminder from their distinguished mentor, and a living legend, Dr. Virginia K. Saba: "Only coded data can be reused!" It is important to keep that in mind.

In addition, the authors want to acknowledge Adjunct Professor Dr. Marianne Tallberg, Information Standards Adviser Anne Casey, Associate Professor Carme Espinosa, and Professor Dr. Walter Sermeus for their important contributions to this chapter.

REFERENCES

ACENDIO. (2010). *Association for Common European Nursing Diagnoses, Interventions and Outcomes.* Retrieved from http://www.acendio.net.

AENTDE. (2010). *Asociación Española de Nomenclatura, Taxonomía y Diagnósticos de Enfermeros.* Retrieved from http://www.aentde.com.

Ambient Assisted Living Joint Programme. (2010). *Objectives.* Retrieved from http://www.aal-europe.eu/about-aal.

Berthou, A., & Junger, A. (2003). Nursing data-Developing a national nursing information system. In J. Clark (Ed.), *Naming nursing. Proceedings of the first ACENDIO Ireland/UK Conference* (pp. 197–207). Bern, Switzerland: Hans Huber.

Casey, A. (2003). Naming nursing in the UK. Goals and challenges. In J. Clark (Ed.), *Naming nursing. Proceedings of the first ACENDIO Ireland/UK Conference* (pp. 215–223). Bern, Switzerland: Hans Huber.

Commission of the European Communities. (2000). *eEurope2002. An information society for all. Action plan.* Retrieved from http://ec.europa.eu/information_society/eeurope/2002/documents/archiv_eEurope2002/actionplan_en.pdf.

Commission of the European Communities. (2002). *eEurope 2005: An information society for all.* Retrieved from http://ec.europa.eu/information_society/eeurope/2002/news_library/documents/eeurope2005/eeurope2005_en.pdf.

Commission of the European Communities. (2004). *e-Health – making healthcare better for European citizens: An action plan for a European e-Health Area.* Retrieved from http://eur-lex.europa.eu/LexUriServ/LexUriServ.do?uri=COM:2004:0356:FIN:EN:PDF.

Commission of the European Communities. (2005). *i2010 – A European Information Society for growth and employment.* Retrieved from http://eur-lex.europa.eu/LexUriServ/LexUriServ.do?uri=COM:2005:0229:FIN:EN:PDF.

Commission of the European Communities. (2008). *Commission recommendation of 2 July 2008 on cross-border interoperability of electronic health record systems.* Retrieved from http://eur-lex.europa.eu/LexUriServ/LexUriServ.do?uri=OJ:L:2008:190:0037:0043:EN:PDF.

Danish Institute for Health and Nursing Research (DIHNR). (1995). *The nursing research potential of electronic healthcare records and the role of nursing research centres in Europe.* Copenhagen: DIHNR.

EFN. (2010). *European Federation of Nurse Associations.* Retrieved from http:// http://www.efnweb.org/version1/EN/index.html.

EFMI. (2010). *European Federation of Medical Associations.* Retrieved from http://www.helmholtz-muenchen.de/ibmi/efmi.

Ehrenberg, A., Ehnfors, M., & Thorell-Ekstrand, I. (1996). Nursing documentation in patient records: Experience of the use of the VIPS-model. *Journal of Advanced Nursing, 24,* 853–867.

Ehnfors, M., Ehrenberg, A., & Thorell-Ekstrand, I. (2002). The development and use of the VIPS-model in Nordic countries. In N. Oud (Ed.), *ACENDIO 2002. Proceedings of the Special Conference of the Association of Common European Nursing Diagnoses, Interventions and Outcomes, in Vienna* (pp. 139–168). Bern, Switzerland: Hans Huber.

Empirica. (2009). *eHealth strategies.* Retrieved from http://www.ehealth-strategies.eu/index.htm.

Ensio, A., & Saranto, K. (2003). Finland: Finnish Classification of Nursing Interventions (FiCNI): Development and use in nursing documentation. In J. Clark (Ed.), *Naming Nursing. Proceedings of the first ACENDIO Ireland/UK Conference* (pp. 191–195). Bern, Switzerland: Hans Huber.

Europa. (2010). *Key facts and figures about Europe and the Europeans.* Retrieved from http://europa.eu/abc/keyfigures/index_en.htm.

European Commission. (2000). *eEurope. information society for all.* Retrieved from *http://ec.europa.eu/information_society/eeurope/2002/documents/archiv_eEurope2002/initiative_en.pdf.*

European Commission. (2010a). *i2010 subgroup on eHealth.* Retrieved from http://ec.europa.eu/information_society/activities/health/policy/i2010subgroup/index_en.htm.

European Commission. (2010b). *A digital agenda for Europe.* Retrieved from http://eur-lex.europa.eu/LexUriServ/LexUriServ.do?uri=COM:2010:0245:FIN:EN:PDF.

European Computer Driving License (ECDL) Foundation. (2010). Retrieved from http://ecdl.com.

Eurostat. (2010). *Europe in figures. Eurostat yearbook 2010.* Retrieved from http://epp.eurostat.ec.europa.eu/cache/ITY_OFFPUB/KS-CD-10-220/EN/KS-CD-10-220-EN.PDF.

Eysenbach, G. (2001). What is e-Health? *Journal of Medical Internet Research, 3*(2), e20.

Goossen, W. T. F., Epping, P. J. M. M., & Dassen, T. W. N. (1997a). Criteria for nursing information systems as a component of the electronic patient record: An international Delphi study. *Computers in Nursing, 15*(6),307–315.

Hämäläinen, P., Doupi, P., & Hyppönen, H. *eHealth policy and deployment in the European Union. Review and analysis of progress.* Stakes reports 26/2008. Retrieved from http://www.stakes.fi/verkkojulkaisut/raportit/R26-2008-VERKKO.pdf.

Häyrinen, K., Saranto, K., & Nykänen, P. (2008). Definition, structure, content, use and impacts of electronic health records: A review of the research literature. *International Journal of Medical Informatics, 77,* 291–304.

ICF. (2010). *International Classification of Functioning, Disability, and Health.* Retrieved from http://www.who.int/classifications/icf/en.

ICN. (2010). *International Council of Nurses.* Retrieved from http://www.icn.ch.

ICN. (2010). Retrieved on June 1, 2011. http://www.icn.ch/news/whats-new/a-new-multilingual-browser-for-the-international-classification-for-nursing-practice.html.

Ikonen, H., Tanttu, K., Hoffren, P., & Mäkilä, M. (2007). Implementing nursing diagnosis, interventions and outcomes in multidisciplinary practice: Experiences in Finland. In N. Oud, F. Sheerin, M. Ehnfors, & W. Sermeus (Eds.), *Proceedings of the 5th European Conference of ACENDIO* (pp. 183–187). Bern, Switzerland: Hans Huber.

IMIA. (2010). *International Medical Informatics Association.* Retrieved from http://www.imia.org.

International Standardization Organisation (ISO). (2003). *Health informatics—Integration of a reference terminology model for nursing.* ISO 18104:2003. Geneva: ISO

Kaustinen, T. (1995). *Development of the nursing intensity classification.* (In Finnish, Hoitoisuusluokituksen kehittäminen ja arviointi). (Licentiate thesis). University of Oulu, Department of Nursing. University of Oulu, Oulu.

Mantas, J. (1998). *Advances in health telematics education—A NIGHTINGALE perspective.* Amsterdam: IOS Press.

Mantas, J. (2004). Comparative educational systems. In E. J. S. Hovenga, & J. Mantas (Eds.), *Global health informatics education* (pp. 8–17). Amsterdam: IOS Press.

MacNeela, P., Scott, P. A., Treacy, M. P., & Hyde, A. (2006). Nursing minimum data sets: A conceptual analysis and review. *Nursing Inquiry, 13,* 44–51.

Meyer, I., Hüsing, T., Didero, M., & Korte, W. B. (2009). *eHealth benchmarking. Final report.* Retrieved from http://www.ehealth-benchmarking.eu/results/documents/eHealthBenchmarking_Final-Report_2009.pdf.

Ministry of Social Affairs and Health. (2007). *eHealth roadmap—Finland.* Reports of the Ministry of Social Affairs and Health (Vol. 15). Retrieved from http://pre20090115.stm.fi/pr1172737292558/passthru.pdf.

Morris, R., MacNeela, P., Scott, P.A., Treacy, P., Hyde, A., Morrisson, T., et al. (2010). The Irish nursing minimum data set for mental health: A valid tool for the collection of standardized nursing data? *Journal of Clinical Nursing, 19*(3–4), 359–367.

Müller-Staub, M., Lavin, M. A., Needham, I., & van Achterberg, T. (2006). Nursing diagnoses, interventions and outcomes: Application and impact on nursing practice: systematic review. *Journal of Advanced Nursing, 56*(5), 514–531.

National Council. (2006). *An evaluation of the extent of measurement of nursing and midwifery interventions in Ireland.* Retrieved from http://www.ncnm.ie.

Onnela, E., & Svenström, R. (1998). *Oulu-hoitoisuusluokituksen kehittäminen Oulun yliopistollisessa sairaalassa 1995–1997.* (In Finnish). Oulu: Loppuraportti.

OHL. (2004). *Oulu-hoitoisuusluokitus ohjekirja.* (In Finnish). Oulu: Pohjois-Pohjanmaan sairaanhoitopiiri.

RN4CAST. (2010). Retrieved from http://www.rn4cast.eu.

Saba, V. (1992). Home healthcare classification (HHCC) of nursing diagnoses and interventions. *Caring, 11,* 50–57.

Saranto, K., & Kinnunen, U-M. (2009). Evaluating nursing documentation—research designs and methods: Systematic review. *Journal of Advanced Nursing, 65*(3), 464–476.

Sermeus, W., van den Heede, K., Michiels, D., Delesie, L., Thonon, O., Van Boven, C., et al.. (2005). Revising the Belgian nursing minimum dataset: From concept to implementation. *International Journal of Medical Informatics, 74*(11–12), 946–951.

Sermeus, W., & Deleise, L. (1997). Development of a presentation tool for nursing data. In R. A. Mortensen (Ed.), *ICNP in Europe: Telenurse.* Amsterdam, The Netherlands: IOS Press.

Sermeus, W., Delesie, L., Van Landuyt, J., Wuyts, Y., Vandenboer, G., & Manna, M. (1994). *The nursing minimum data set in Belgium: A basic tool for tomorrow's healthcare management.* Leuven: Katholieke Universiteit Leuven.

SSN. (2010). *SSN—The Nordic Nurses Federation (NNF).* Retrieved from http://www.ssn-nnf.no/ikbViewer/page/ssn/english.

Stroetmann, KA., Artmann, J., Stroetmann VN. (2011). European countries on their journey towards national eHealth infrastructures. *Final European progress report.* Retrieved from http://www.ehealth-strategies.eu/report/report.html

Thoroddsen, A., Saranto, K., Ehrenberg, A., & Sermeus, W. (2009). Models, standards and structures of nursing documentation in European countries. In K. Saranto et al. (Eds.), *Connecting health and humans. Proceedings of NI2009* (pp. 146, 327–331). Amsterdam: IOS Press.

University of Eastern Finland. (2010). *Department of Health and Social Management.* Retrieved from http://www.uef.fi/stj.

Van den Heede, K., Michiels, D., Thonon, O., & Sermeus, W. (2009). Using nursing interventions classification as a framework to revise the Belgian nursing minimum data set. *International Journal of Nursing Terminologies and Classifications, 20*(3), 122–131.

WHO (1977). *Development of designs in and documentation of nursing process.* Report on a Technical Advisory Group. Copenhagen: WHO.

WHO. (2010). *European health for all database (HFA-DB).* Retrieved from http://data.euro.who.int/hfadb.

RECOMMENDED READINGS

Clark, J. (Ed.). (2003). *Naming nursing. Proceedings of the first ACENDIO Ireland/UK Conference.* Bern, Switzerland: Hans Huber.

Saranto, K., Brennan Flatney, P., & Casey, A. (Eds.). (2009). *Personal health information management tools and strategies for citizens' engagement.* University of Kuopio, Department of Health Policy and Management, Kuopio. Retrieved from http://www.uku.fi/vaitokset/2009/isbn978-951-27-1321-9.pdf.

47

Pacific Rim Perspectives

Evelyn J. S. Hovenga / Michelle Honey / Lucy A. Westbrooke / Robyn Carr

- ## OBJECTIVES
  1. Describe the development of nursing informatics in some Pacific Rim countries.
  2. Identify historical milestones, changes, and trends influencing nurses to embrace informatics.
  3. Discuss nursing informatics leadership, international links, education, and research, along with their impact upon the development of nursing informatics as a nursing discipline or specialty.

- ## KEY WORDS
  information systems
  standards
  hospital information systems
  public policy

The evolution of nursing informatics (NI) has varied in each of the Pacific Rim countries. The adoption of informatics usually began as a vision by one or more individuals. Such people used any number of opportunities plus their leadership skills to promote and disseminate the use of information technologies to support nurses in all areas of nursing practice. This occurred in healthcare, educational, and government organizations, as well as within the information technology (IT) industry and via any number of new and existing professional organizations. Events external to the nursing profession frequently became the catalyst stimulating some type of activity by nurses toward the adoption of informatics. International and multidisciplinary links have assisted these beginnings and its progression. Australia, New Zealand, and Hong Kong have made considerable progress since the early 1980s. Nurses in a number of other countries in the Pacific region have only just begun or have yet to learn about NI.

The Asia Pacific Medical Informatics Association (APAMI) was formed in 1993 as a regional group of the International Medical Informatics Association. APAMI has helped launch national healthcare informatics associations in Malaysia, Indonesia, and the Philippines and has generated awareness about the field in India, Pakistan, Sri Lanka, and Fiji. Other member nations are Australia, Hong Kong, Japan, Korea, New Zealand, the People's Republic of China, Singapore, Taiwan, and Thailand. Nurses in these countries who are interested in promoting informatics to their profession need to link up with this network.

Anecdotal evidence suggests that it continues to be a challenge for many nurses to obtain appropriate education in informatics both during their initial nurse education and as a component of post–nurse registration specialist courses. Notwithstanding these conditions, an increase in computer use by practicing nurses in Australia, New Zealand, and other Pacific countries is creating an awareness of the opportunities and gains to healthcare resulting from an increase in the use of computers, information, and telecommunication technologies. Thus, nurses in all health environments are becoming more dependent on electronic information.

This chapter aims to provide an overview of these historical events, primarily from Australia and New Zealand, relative to national health informatics, or e-Health, initiatives and trends, and to highlight critical success factors for the benefit of those who have yet to embark on such a journey. The chapter concludes by summarizing significant events and examining their impact on the evolution of nursing informatics in this region.

HEALTH AND NURSING INFORMATICS IN NEW ZEALAND

New Zealand's total population is reported as 4.4 million and approximately three-quarters of these people are found in urban areas, with the greater Auckland area having over a third of the total population (Statistics New Zealand, 2010). There are 40,616 registered nurses currently practising in New Zealand (Nursing Council of New Zealand, 2009). The nursing workforce in New Zealand is the single largest health professional group and is recognized as having enormous potential to advance health and disability outcomes (Nursing and Midwifery Workforce Strategy Group, 2006). With most of the nurses and midwives practicing in Auckland, Auckland by default becomes the focus of the drive for greater health informatics awareness.

Notable changes have occurred within New Zealand nursing legislation that impact the roles and future of nurses. Firstly, in line with international trends in nursing workforce development, the Nursing Council of New Zealand established the role of nurse practitioner, followed by the legislation enacting nurse prescribing that came into force in 2005. With nurse practitioners and prescribing being in place for less than a decade, in May 2010 there were 77 nurse practitioners and 50 nurses prescribing, but there is clearly a move toward further postgraduate education to attain these new nursing roles (District Health Boards New Zealand [DHBNZ], 2010). The impact of globalization has seen an increase in the movement of nurses into and out of New Zealand, which increases the challenges for the Nursing Council in terms of ensuring safety to practice at the level expected in New Zealand while not providing unnecessary barriers for overseas nurses. As part of ensuring standards of practice the Health Practitioners Competence Assurance Act (2003) requires each health

practitioner group to describe its profession in terms of scopes of practice. The purpose of scopes of practice is to ensure the safety of the public by defining the health services that health practitioners can perform.

Changes are continuous in the informatics arena and there are many sources and pressures for these. Figure 47.1 describes the major influences on informatics in New Zealand.

HEALTH AND NURSING INFORMATICS IN AUSTRALIA

Australia is a federation of 8 states and territories. It has a population of around 22 million. Around 9.1% of its gross domestic product (GDP) is spent on health services. Approximately 71% of its households are located in inner and outer urban and provincial areas, mostly near cities on the coast. There continues to be a workforce shortage across a number of health professions, including a need for around 10,000 nurses. In 2008, there were around 166,400 Full-Time Equivalent (35 hours per week) registered nurses and midwives of whom 18% were aged 55 or over (AIHW, 2010, p. 452). There were 776 registered nurses plus 112 enrolled nurses and 276 nursing and personal care assistants per 100,000 population (AIH&W, 2010, p. 454).

As a consequence of the globalization of the profession, Australia's contribution to international education, the resultant workforce mobility, economic growth, and changes in the healthcare industry resulting from technology and informatics advances, we are witnessing changes in the nursing workforce. Credentialing and accreditation of nursing specialties is now being promoted. Nursing specialty and other organizations have developed and adopted practice standards, competencies, guidelines for curricula development, and various professional development programs. Australia has more than 50 such specialty national nursing organizations (NNOs), where the Health Informatics Society Australia's nursing informatics special interest group (HISA NI Sig) is one of these. This group meets twice each year to discuss current issues impacting the nursing profession. Most have developed a set of specialty competencies and they provide credentialing services.

In 2003 the HISA NI Sig was funded to develop a strategic plan for nursing informatics capacity building, and a plan for the nursing profession's engagement with the Australian government and its informatics agenda. The plan has provided a lot of useful information for various bureaucrats, but there has not been a noticeable change in nurses' involvement at senior decision-making levels.

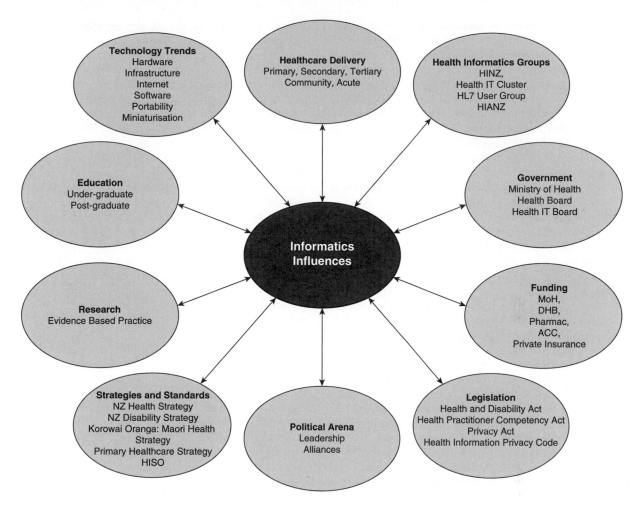

• **FIGURE 47.1.** Overview diagram: major influences in informatics in New Zealand.

Healthcare Funding Framework

In Australia, work began to develop patient classification systems to describe the case mix serviced by healthcare organizations in collaboration with Professor Fetter from Yale University during the 1980s. Since 1992, the Australian Refined Diagnosis Related Group (AR-DRG) standard has been in use first for the purpose of monitoring and comparison of hospital activity and later also for costing and funding purposes. This now forms the basis for a national approach to activity-based hospital funding. This Australian case-mix program relies on data obtained from individual patient records, including the ICD-10-AM codes. A number of case-mix systems

are in use to suit a variety of patient population types. Service weights to reflect the cost of providing various hospital-based services including nursing were developed and are currently in the process of being updated. These are included in various funding formulas adopted around the country. This same case-mix system has been adopted by a number of other countries. The 2009 review report on Australia's case-mix system states that, "this system reaps benefits to the community of around $4 billion per annum in savings (for bed days) against an estimated annual cost of $10 million" (Commonwealth of Australia, 2009). The government's Web site on case-mix is very informative.

Health spending continues to increase. In 2007–2008 this amounted to 9.1% of the GDP, compared with 7.8% ten years previously. All taxpayers contribute a 1.5% Medicare levy, and high-income earners who do not have private health insurance pay an additional 1%; this contributes around 18.2% to the health budget. The Australian government's contribution and the way all states and territories are funded to deliver health services changed significantly in 2009. This has been detailed in its 2010–2011 budget announcement available from the case-mix Web site. There has been major health reform policy that has hospital funding as its primary focus. It has its own Web site to explain these reforms to the population at large, as it does represent a very significant change. Starting on July 1, 2011, the Australian government will assume full funding and policy responsibility for GP and primary healthcare. In other words, from that date onward there will only be one level of government funding these services and, thus, the current common practice of "cost shifting" will be avoided (Commonwealth of Australia, 2010; www.yourhealth.gov.au). Information and technology, including e-Health, is a key foundational building block required to realize this vision. The Australian government is now actively promoting the use of electronic health records (EHRs) and new technologies to integrate care, better manage chronic conditions, and improve patient outcomes.

The management of cardiovascular disease constitutes the greatest health burden and accounts for the biggest percentage of health expenditures (AIH&W, 2010, p. 428). The Australian government also manages a Pharmaceutical Benefits Scheme (PBS) that is jointly funded by them and nongovernment sources; it accounts for 14% of recurrent health expenditures (AIH&W, 2010, p. 439).

Healthcare in New Zealand

New Zealand's healthcare system is primarily publicly funded by the government, through the Ministry of Health allocating funds based on population to 20 district health boards (DHB) who both purchase and provide healthcare services for their New Zealand resident population. DHBs need to ensure they work together for the most effective and efficient delivery of health services to meet national, regional, and local needs, and this is embodied in legislation.

The Accident Compensation Corporation (ACC) provides a range of health benefits and subsidies to assist individuals in the event of an accident. The establishment of the ACC has virtually eliminated suing for compensation in the event of an accident covered by the ACC. Funding for the ACC is provided through a levy on employers and employees.

The role of the private sector has increased significantly. Private insurance–funded healthcare is increasing, and given the aging population, improved options of health treatments, increased demands yet limited public budgets, and increased waiting times for elective surgery, this trend is likely to continue. The cost of private health insurance is growing, with premiums rising faster than the general cost of living, and consequently there is a widening gap between those who need and those who can afford private healthcare to supplement care provided through the public system.

All prescription-related medicines are regulated by the government through Pharmac. Subsidies are available on a range of medicines, although only a few options within each drug classification may be subsidized by Pharmac. The public can purchase an increasing number of over-the-counter remedies, and there is an increasing need for drug information for medical practitioners, nurses, and the public.

Information Governance

The Australian Institute for Health and Welfare (AIH&W) provides research and statistical support to the Australian, state, and territory governments. In 1993, all public health authorities, the Australian Bureau of Statistics, and the AIH&W signed an agreement to improve the quality of and cooperation in the development of national health information. This now provides the national infrastructure needed to provide high-quality health data. It includes Australia's repository for national metadata standards for health, METeOR, providing online access to a wide range of nationally endorsed data definitions and tools for creating new definitions based on existing already-endorsed components. Also available via METeOR are the National Data Dictionaries, national minimum data sets, and data set specifications.

A Community Nursing Minimum Data Set was developed during the early 1990s. This has been adopted and extended by the Department of Veteran Affairs (DVA) and is used by them to monitor the provision of community nursing services provided via DVA contracts. The DVA has also developed and adopted a Community Nursing Classification system consisting of 4 levels based on service type, client type, and clinical care, and technical care. A number of other minimum data sets (MDS) exist such as the palliative care MDS, the nurse practitioner MDS, the NSW State Spinal Cord Injury Service MDS, and health and community care (HACC) MDS. The Royal District Nursing Service (RDNS) in Melbourne makes use of a number of these in their information system via a data-mapping matrix. The RDNS also manages a data warehouse.

The University of Hong Kong is making good use of a number of standardized assessment instruments for older, frail, or disabled individuals. The assessment instruments were made available by interRAI, a collaborative network of researchers in over 30 countries, for their research. The interRAI minimum datasets for nursing home, home care, and mental health are now available in Chinese. Australia and New Zealand's interRAI coordinating center is located and managed by the Centre for Geriatric Medicine based at the University of Queensland in Brisbane. A nursing and midwifery MDS for human resources for health was developed by two Australian nurses (Jill While and Michele Rumsey) using data collected from 30 countries within the Western Pacific and Southeast Asia WHO Regions during 2006–2008 (WHO, 2008).

Australia's health sector governance is constantly changing. A 2004 review undertaken on behalf of the then newly established National Health Information Group (NHIG) and the Australian Health Information Council (AHIC) identified distributed governance over many jurisdictions as a significant impediment to the provision of better healthcare outcomes, safety, quality, and cost efficiencies. The NHIG became the National Health Information Management Principal Committee (NHIMPC), its role is to advise the Australian Health Ministers' Advisory Committee on planning and management requirements and to manage and allocate resources to health information projects and working groups. This committee produced a strategic workplan for 2007–2008 to 2012–2013 (NHIMPC, 2007), it's published model of the national governance structure for Information Management (IM) and Health Information Communication Technology (ICT) changed in 2008, following a change of government. NHIMPC became the National E-Health Principal Committee (NEHIPC) and was given a broader responsibility for national e-Health in addition to its existing focus on information management. A National Health Information Standards and Statistics Committee was established in 2008, its secretariat is at the Australian Institute of Health and Welfare.

The New Zealand Ministry of Health is interested in information collection and hosts 17 national collections and systems. New Zealand has been fortunate to have a National Health Index (NHI) database for registering all people who receive healthcare in New Zealand. Each person has a unique healthcare identifier, which is assigned at birth or on first contact with a healthcare provider, and this NHI number is designed to follow the individual through each healthcare event in her life allowing easier tracking of information through healthcare episodes.

The national data collections are developed in consultation with health sector representatives and provide valuable health information to support performance monitoring, decision making, policy formulation, funding, evaluation, and research (Ministry of Health, 2010a). Statutory requirements govern the reporting of certain mandatory items (e.g., cancer, tuberculosis, and other communicable diseases).

All information collection, storage, access, and retrieval in New Zealand is governed by the Privacy Act (1993), the Health Information Code (1994), and subsequent amendments. This act is one of the most comprehensive pieces of privacy legislation anywhere in the world.

Health Informatics Governance

The adoption of health informatics principles is seen as an enabler of coordination between the many stakeholders. The Boston Consulting Group (2004, p. 13) recommendations to the Australian Government Department of Health and Ageing included the establishment of a new entity with full-time staff to provide the necessary leadership and drive the IM & ICT agenda forward as well as promote the adoption of common standards to provide a national interoperability platform to maximize system connectivity, integrated decision support functionality, clinical information transfer, secure messaging, and broadband roll-out. The National eHealth Transition Authority (NEHTA) was established in 2004 as a not-for-profit company limited by guarantee and funded by all Australian governments. Its governance board represents these jurisdictions and is chaired by an independent businessperson. The release of the Australian government's National E-Health Strategy in December 2008 outlined 4 major strategic streams of activity: foundations, e-Health solutions, change and adoption, and governance. These formed the basis for the NEHTA's 2009–2012 strategic plan supporting the national vision for e-Health (NEHTA, 2009). A clinical leads group consisting of around 44 practicing clinicians has been assigned to various areas of the NEHTA's work program to provide an important sounding board for the development of its work in real-world contexts and to advise on likely issues and appropriate mechanisms for engaging with clinical stakeholders. Unfortunately, only one of these clinicians is a registered nurse.

Current National Initiatives in New Zealand

Healthcare in New Zealand is guided by a national health strategy, which has the goal of good health and well-being for all New Zealanders throughout their lives (Ministry of Health, 2000). Furthermore, the New Zealand Health Strategy (2000, p. 29) recognizes the importance of good information management and states: "The ability to exchange high-quality information between partners in healthcare processes will be vital for a health system focused on achieving better health outcomes". The overall vision for information management in New Zealand is set out in the Health Information Strategy (Health Information Strategy Steering Committee, 2005), as this document provides a direction and an impetus for the health and disability sector to improve information management and the sharing of information in order to underpin better health and disability outcomes for New Zealanders.

Following a Ministerial Review in 2009, changes to the health sector have been instigated with the overall objective of "better, sooner, more convenient health services." The implementation of these changes has been divided into 3 areas: organization change, implementation of the recommendations of the Ministerial Review Group (MRG) report, and review and amendments to legislation to support the changes.

One of the recommendations of the MRG was the establishment of the National Health Board and the formation of a subcommittee, the National Health IT Board. The MRG made a number of informatics-related recommendations that included strengthening health information technology and clinical leadership, prioritization of new technologies and medical devices, and addressing procurement from a national perspective. The National Health IT Board is seen as a health sector leadership group to support the delivery of high-quality healthcare by providing strategic leadership on health information investments and solutions and to lead a national health IT agenda. The Health IT Board has created a draft National Health IT Plan for consultation, which aims to "drive a culture of innovation, partnership and respect to support health sector leaders to make appropriate health IT investments in the context of the whole sector" (Ministry of Health, 2010b) and to work toward the e-Health vision: "To achieve high quality healthcare and improve patient safety, by 2014 New Zealanders will have a core set of personal health information available electronically to them and their treatment providers regardless of the setting as they access health services" (Ministry of Health, 2010b).

Although focused on person-centric health systems, there are generic principles that apply to other information systems. The first phase calls for reducing duplication by consolidation of systems in the health sector and leveraging the work already completed by other successful projects. With a more consolidated platform, shared care planning between providers can be enabled. The overall aim is to address New Zealand's most pressing health IT needs and significant issues that continue to form barriers to improving health outcomes and reducing delivery costs. The recent economic downturn is one of the drivers for this new initiative, with the Minister of Health hoping to achieve savings of $700 million over 5 years by having common back-office systems for the country's 20 district health boards. In addition, these strategies form the cornerstone of activity for a strong IT infrastructure to address longer-term issues such as electronic health records.

To date, the development of a national technology infrastructure has proved useful; however, securing appropriate access to relevant clinical and administrative information throughout the health sector remains the greatest challenge. Much progress has been made in primary healthcare. For example, in a comparative study of 11 countries, New Zealand was found to have 92% of community-based practices with advanced electronic health information capacity across functions, including electronic prescribing and ordering of tests; electronic access to test results, prescription alerts, and clinical notes; guidelines, preventive and follow-up care reminders; and computerized lists of patients by diagnosis, medications, due for tests, or preventive care (Schoen et al., 2009).

New Zealand's government health policy has been driving toward a population health management approach. Accordingly, the sector has been slowly moving away from a "bricks and mortar," hospital-centric approach toward integrated healthcare (Ministry of Health, 2001). Although significant gaps remain, the move has proved heavily reliant on collaboration between government, contracting agencies, and delivery units. The pressures New Zealand currently faces include:

- A growing older population, more people with long-term and complex health conditions (Davey & Gee, 2002), and a more informed consumer. As New Zealand has a history of free health service, there is an expectation that healthcare will continue to be freely available and that evidence-based best practice will determine the treatments with no consideration of cost.

- Workforce issues including an aging workforce, yet the nursing workforce is the single largest health professional group, and is recognized as having enormous potential to advance health and disability outcomes (Nursing and Midwifery Workforce Strategy Group, 2006).

- Health inequalities and the need to address Mâori (the indigenous people of New Zealand) health disparities because of their over-representation in morbidity and mortality data (Connolly et al., 2010; Ministry of Health, 2007, 2008; Statistics New Zealand, 2010).

These pressures exist now and can only be expected to intensify in the next decade. New Zealand has to target and prioritize where health IT investments are made, as judicious use of technology could be the key to the long-term sustainability of a free healthcare service and improving health outcomes.

National Initiatives in Australia

The national health information agreements and the establishment of the National Health Data Dictionary in 1993 laid the foundation for consistent health data sets in Australia. In 1999, the first national strategic information action plan, Health Online, was initiated. This was followed by a number of projects initiated by the Australian government: Health*Connect*, Medi*Connect*, the provision of quality health information for consumers known as Health*Insite*, and the national supply chain initiative along with more than 360 projects such as the integration of primary health and hospital care, several shared and coordinated care projects, and the establishment of health call centers. Since 2004, the Australian government has commissioned and received numerous reports with many recommendations. In addition, various state and jurisdiction reports were commissioned such as the NSW Health Garling Report on Acute Services. All such reports made reference to the need for widespread adoption of e-Health. The National Hospitals and Health Reform Commission's (NHHRC) report identified a number of gaps in safety and quality due to suboptimal information sharing, and proposed health informatics solutions that are expected to result in improvements (Australian Government, 2008).

The term *e-Health* only came into widespread usage a few years ago. There is no agreed-upon definition for *e-Health*; this term is widely used and has various meanings. Oh and colleagues (2005) undertook a systematic review of 1,209 abstracts and 430 citations and found

10 different definitions for the term *e-Health*, and from a Google search an additional 41 unique definitions were located ranging in length from 3 to 74 words. As a consequence, there is a lack of consistency in the population's understanding of and perceptions about the workforce's knowledge and skill requirements and the likely impact of successful e-Health strategy implementations.

In 2008, the Coalition of Australian Governments (COAG) made the decision to continue funding NEHTA's work, thus confirming a continuing government commitment to a national e-Health strategy. NEHTA has made a business case for the development of EHRs, but many argue that successful implementation is dependent upon an appropriately educated workforce. On April 30, 2009, the NHHRC published a supplementary paper to its 2008 Interim Report, outlining the commission's support for person-controlled EHRs for every Australian. The 2010 federal budget announced the governments intention to fund the adoption of personally held EHRs. Australia has also initiated a National Broadband Network roll-out, and more recently, the Healthcare Identifiers Bill was passed by the Australian Federal Parliament. One key national telecommunications infrastructure and service provider has just signed an agreement with the Royal Australian College of General Practitioners (RACGP) to deliver a Web-hosted service. This will have the capacity to host multiple healthcare applications including clinical software programs, decision support tools for diagnosis and management, care plans, referral tools, e-prescribing tools, and a range of online training and other administrative and clinical services.

Technology Trends

The healthcare environment is changing at an ever-increasing pace due to the proliferation of new and emerging technologies. Embracing the advances in technology enables us to deliver healthcare in new and innovative ways. Basic hardware has advanced into multiple components of input and output devices. Development of infrastructures has enabled this technology to be networked. The Internet provides a medium to transmit information nationally and internationally. The physical constraints and boundaries are now so blurred that healthcare delivery can occur and/or be supervised by experts located anywhere at any time.

Some Australian nurses are using personal digital assistants (PDAs) for point-of-care information and clinical documentation for community and acute hospital nursing, hospital-based infection control, and/or wound management. Many new monitoring devices are being connected to information systems for automated data entry. Improvements in portability are now enabling the use of technology in a greater range of settings. Both PDAs and tablets are being used or trialed in the clinical setting by students and healthcare professionals. One of the nursing schools has issued PDAs to its students and the success of this has been evidenced by the reluctance of the students to relinquish them.

Trends in New Zealand Healthcare

The changes in responsibility for healthcare provision in New Zealand have created a more collaborative approach, resulting in integrated care being seen as a priority. Integrated care is being supported by technology, enabling information to flow. Electronic health event summaries along with laboratory and radiology data are now being transmitted between providers and across primary and secondary sectors. In the pharmaceutical area, data will soon be available on prescriptions dispensed. The Internet and intranets are providing a wealth of information to health providers as well as consumers.

The Web environment and the use of powerful integration engines, is now providing contextual views of data that are browser-based and single log-on. Placed over multiple health information systems, this connection provides a single patient-centric view of data across all applications that can be used by the clinicians. There are tools available that enable ease of messaging and mapping along with products to support the clinical workflow process. Online technologies provide products and services that enhance patient care and improve clinical outcomes through evidence-based health information and decision support systems.

Although New Zealand is a small country, it has a surprising number of health IT companies producing software that is being used both locally and internationally. Information technology is New Zealand's third largest export behind dairy and tourism, and health IT applications are part of that (Heather, 2010).

Standards Development and Adoption in Australia

The national adoption of technical standards is a prerequisite to being able to optimize the use of IT by means of securing semantically interoperable clinical systems and contribute significantly to a sustainable national health system. Of particular importance is the design and architecture of any national health information and integration platform based on specific sets of technical standards.

Standards Australia (SA) was persuaded to establish a health informatics committee in 1992. The SA IT-14 Committee now has several active technical subcommittees and works closely with other similar groups such as HL7 International via HL7 Australia, the ISO Technical Committee 215, the Comite Europeen de Normalisation (CEN) Technical Committee 251, the Integrating the Healthcare Enterprise (IHE) international organisation, the International Health Terminology Standards Development (IHTSDO), and the openEHR Foundation. In Australia, nurses are represented via the Royal College of Nursing although other nurses also contribute from time to time.

The focus in Australia has been in the area of standards development to facilitate data interchange, initially designed to support all types of e-commerce and now expanded to support the interchange of clinical data. The Systematized Nomenclature of Medicine—Clinical Terms (SNOMED-CT) has been adopted as the national terminology standard. Australia is an active contributor to the development of international standards. This ensures that these standards are able to meet Australian and New Zealand industry needs. Once international standards have been completed and published, the SA IT-14 considers whether this can be adopted for Australia as is or if we need to develop an implementation guide that meets specific Australian needs. In some instances, Australian standards are being reviewed and modified via the ISO Technical Committee 215 to suit the international market. All Australian standards are freely available in pdf format via the SA's e-Health Web site (www.e-health.standards.org.au). This was made possible by Australian government funding, as IT industry standards compliance is highly valued.

The NEHTA now works closely with the SA IT-14 Committee to ensure that standards development priorities match its business priorities as detailed in its latest strategic plan. The NEHTA's role is to lead the uptake of e-Health systems of national significance and to coordinate the progression and accelerate the adoption of e-Health by delivering urgently needed integration infrastructure and standards for health information. Its vision is to enhance healthcare by enabling access to the right information, for the right person, at the right time and place. The NEHTA has adopted 4 strategic priorities that are guiding their work activities:

1. Urgently develop the essential foundations required to enable e-Health. This priority stresses the need to deliver essential e-Health services such as healthcare identifiers, secure messaging and authentication, and a clinical terminology and

information service. These will form the backbone of Australia's e-Health systems.

2. Coordinate the progression of the priority e-Health solutions and processes. Some e-Health solutions and processes provide the greatest opportunity to improve health practice and deliver benefit. Priorities include referrals and discharge, pathology and diagnostic imaging, and medications management.

3. Accelerate the adoption of e-Health. It is critical to increase the awareness and uptake of e-Health initiatives by the various stakeholder groups, through collaboration and communication programs, incentives, and implementation support.

4. Lead the progression of e-Health in Australia. This priority reflects that NEHTA has a significant role in leading the direction of the current and future state of e-Health in Australia, including future initiatives and the impacts on privacy and policy.

Standards Development and Adoption in New Zealand

Following the 2001 WAVE Report, the Minister of Health, directed that a WAVE working group, the Ministerial Committee on a Health Information Standards Organisation (HISO), be established to manage health information standards. HISO drew together hitherto disparate health-related groups with specific interest in producing IT standards for New Zealand. HISO's role included identifying, developing, publishing, and monitoring New Zealand's health information standards. HISO has been governed by different bodies over the years, but has been incorporated under the Health IT Board since 2009.

A key driver for HISO's role, the consistent use of standards, is aimed at acceptance throughout health and health-related industries of such standards. This requires enabling real-time access to information about the standards (i.e., Which standards are agreed upon? Which are being developed or proposed? What initiatives are taking place? What are the downstream implications?) including where the information may be freely accessed. The availability of detailed and clinically relevant data is essential for clinical care decisions and for oversight groups making decisions related to the quality of that care. Today, health information systems are expected to meet a variety of changing demands for data and information to support many purposes (e.g., automated alerts, decision support, quality monitoring, payment policy, and outcomes research).

Standardized terminology systems are essential to enable the use and exchange of clinical data across applications and IT systems. Given point-of-care documentation, technology is now available to build electronic health information systems that will efficiently meet a variety of needs. This includes providing immediate feedback to care providers by, for example, issuing alerts related to relevant best practice guidelines, generating data needed for internal and external quality monitoring, exchanging critical patient information in a timely manner across the healthcare continuum, and reducing provider burden associated with current documentation requirements.

National direction is provided for data collection and the use of standardized coding systems. Historically, primary care has used READ codes, the practice of which is continued by the New Zealand ACC. The ACC describes READ codes as "a hierarchical clinical coding system; each level provides a more specific diagnosis of an injury" (Accident Compensation Corporation [ACC], 2009). Secondary care used the International Statistical Classification of Diseases and Related Health Problems (10th revision), also known as ICD-10, originating from the World Health Organization as a coding of diseases and signs, symptoms, abnormal findings, complaints, social circumstances, and external causes of injury or diseases (World Health Organization, 2010). In addition, Logical Observation Identifiers, Names, and Codes (LOINC) is used for laboratory data and Health Level Seven (HL7) is the favored messaging standard. More recently, the government has introduced the use of the SNOMED-CT as a means to have a single coding system in place for the country (New Zealand Health Information Service, 2010).

Currently, one of the most significant challenges to implementing electronic health information systems is the lack of standards for electronic patient medical record information, especially standards for the terminology that expresses clinical documentation.

RESEARCH

Research in health informatics is supported through master's and doctoral programs in a number of the 8 government-funded universities in New Zealand. For example, Auckland University of Technology, Massey University, the University of Auckland, and the University of Otago offer postgraduate education that includes health informatics components. This also applies to a number of Australian Universities, especially those that have health or medical informatics research centers such as the University of Sydney, University of New South Wales, and the University of Melbourne.

Health-related information has a number of uses. Apart from the direct use of information in the care of clients, there is a growing awareness of the need for timely and accurate data for research. Three specific areas that are gaining more attention within nursing informatics are clinical pathways, evidence-based practice, and nursing service architecture.

One specific area of research that remains a focus for nursing informatics is evidence-based practice. In New Zealand, this is supported by The Centre for Evidence Based Healthcare Aotearoa. The Centre for Evidence Based Healthcare Aotearoa is a joint venture between the Auckland District Health Board and the University of Auckland and has strong links with other evidence-based practice organizations including the New Zealand branch of the Australasian Cochrane Centre, the New Zealand Guidelines Group, and the Effective Practice, Informatics & Quality Improvement Unit, based at the School of Population Health, University of Auckland. The New Zealand Guidelines Group (NZGG), while funded by the government through the Ministry of Health, remains an independent, not-for-profit organization that was established to promote effective delivery of health and disability services, based on evidence. It is overseen by an advisory board, which draws on leadership from nursing, Maori Health, Pacific Health, consumer representation, medicine, disability support, public health medicine, and general practice.

New Zealand also takes opportunities to participate in international research, such as the international survey regarding the role of health IT in acute care (Dykes et al., 2010). Despite the currently low use of nursing-specific health IT in acute care in New Zealand, this study was seen as an opportunity to benchmark the status and perceptions regarding the use of health IT, and as such a useful reference point for future initiatives. After a process of validation to ensure the survey tool, the Health Information Technology (I-HIT) Scale, was culturally appropriate and understandable by nurses in New Zealand (Dykes et al., 2009), dissemination of information about the survey and the link to the Web site to undertake the online survey was sent by e-mail using a snowball sampling technique where participants recruit other nurses from among their acquaintances. Only 124 nurses out of a targeted 300 finally completed the online survey. The results showed a regional disparity of responses, with the largest number of participants coming from the Auckland region (63%). Ninety two percent of the participants were female, with 56% aged from 41 to 50 years, and over 60% had 15 or more years

of nursing experience. Most nurses (73%) worked 36 or more hours per week, and 85% of the nurses were based in teaching hospitals (Dykes et al., 2010). An overview of the results indicated that the most experience nurses had with health IT was with their organization's systems, and the nurses reported that 94% of their organizations provided training. E-mail was used daily by 88% of nurses, word processing by 59%, and the World Wide Web by 66%. Overall, there was above average satisfaction with the health IT currently available. The findings from this survey confirm what was assumed about the state of health IT in New Zealand, including that many hospital systems are not nursing focused, and nurses use the systems mostly for accessing laboratory and x-ray results. This indicates that there is potential for further development and use of health IT that nurses will employ and benefit from (Dykes et al., 2010).

One of the main avenues for sharing health informatics research within New Zealand is through the Health Informatics New Zealand (HINZ) annual conference and quarterly seminars. In addition, *Healthcare and Informatics Review Online (HCIRO)* became the official journal of HINZ in 2007. *HCIRO* is dedicated to reviewing and interpreting significant developments in healthcare delivery with a particular focus on health informatics and is the only New Zealand–based journal focusing on health IT issues. The journal has a wide local and international readership, and is gaining credibility in business and academic circles. The focus of the journal is on knowledge gained through the practical experience of managing health issues. Its objectives are to facilitate the exchange of ideas among interested members of the health sector and to develop a widely accessible resource of experience in health delivery.

The Nursing Informatics Australia special interest group of HISA organizes an annual one day preconference to HISA's annual conference, known as HIC, where between 40 and 60 papers are presented each year. Papers presented at this conference are indexed in CINAHL and INFOMIT. They provide a good overview of progress in health informatics in Australia. In addition, ACHI and HISA sponsor the management of the free electronic *Journal of Health Informatics (eJHI)* that is becoming increasingly more popular among scholars and is attracting a good selection of fully refereed papers.

Health Informatics does not exist as a research category for the major government research funding organizations such as the Australian Research Council or the National Health & Medical Research Council, which makes it difficult to obtain research funds from these organizations. Despite this, some well established universty-based research centers have been more successful in attracting research funding for various health and nursing informatics projects.

HEALTH AND NURSING INFORMATICS EDUCATION IN AUSTRALIA

The first Australian experiences of nurses using computers were compiled into an edited text by Graham MacKay and Anita Griffin in 1989. The first Australian textbook on health informatics was published in 1996 (Hovenga et al., 1996), a second edition was published by IOS Press in 2010. Another popular Australian text was edited by the late Moya Conrick, a nurse who has made a significant contribution to nursing informatics in Australia over the years.

Much of nursing informatics education continues to be provided by nursing computer and informatics groups via study days, seminars, and conferences. The Lincoln Institute of Health Sciences (now Latrobe University) provided registered nurses undertaking postregistration degrees with opportunities to include computer studies in their coursework as early as 1979. Central Queensland University introduced nurses to computers in 1989 with a strong commitment to a computer-assisted and -managed learning project (Zelmer et al., 1991). A 1990 survey of all tertiary nursing programs in Australia found that 27% (10 out of 37 respondents) had more than 5 years of experience in teaching computing to nurses, and 73% (27) included computing within their nursing programs most frequently as a core unit (Hancock & Henderson, 1991). There has been little progress since then. Informatics education for nurses in Australia varies considerably from one university to another (Hovenga et al., 1999; Soar et al., 2003). Most have one person attempting the impossible, often in environments where fellow nurse academics have little or no knowledge of informatics. In some instances, there is active resistance to its introduction. This continues to be true in 2010.

Some schools of nursing integrate informatics into their undergraduate nursing program to some extent. Most universities offer one unit of study within their undergraduate nursing pre- and postregistration programs as an elective. Central Queensland University offered an undergraduate degree program in nursing informatics as a postregistration program, but it was discontinued in 2007. This enabled all registered nurses to either obtain a double degree or to convert their hospital-based certificate or university-based diploma into a bachelor's degree. A number of universities have recently commenced or continue to offer a certificate, postgraduate diploma, and master's degree in health informatics. Some of these graduates are now pursuing postdoctoral studies, others are actively engaged in promoting the use of IT in the workplace, and many work in hospital-based nursing informatics positions.

There continues to be a very significant skills shortage in this area, as was revealed in the numerous government reports commissioned in recent years. In an effort to address this, ACHI established an education committee in late 2008, which obtained Government funding in 2009 to establish what is now known as the Australian Health Informatics Education Council (AHIEC). The ACHI continues to provide the secretariat services for this group and it also communicates with a wide cross section of interested industry stakeholders. A strategic workplan was developed and published in late 2009. The AHIEC is now proceeding to implement this, but has yet to secure further funding. To fill this void, a private online e-Health education provider has been established by senior health informaics educators who had become disillusioned with the university system.

EDUCATION IN NEW ZEALAND

In New Zealand, nursing informatics has been recognized as significant by the Ministries of Health and Education since the early 1990s. The Nursing Council of New Zealand does not identify any specific computer skills within the competencies that registered nurses are required to attain; yet the competencies involve information management and communication that may be achieved using computer technology. Much of nursing informatics is integrated into undergraduate curriculum under the guise of other subjects (Honey & Baker, 2004). For example, law and ethics covers the Privacy Act (1993), which emphasizes the importance of the collection, storage, and use of client information, whether stored on paper or computer; evidence-based practice includes the discernment of evidence to ascertain its worthiness to base nursing practice on; and research includes literature searches, and therefore the use of the Internet and access to international nursing literature databases. Thus, undergraduate nurse education reflects the need for computer literacy. The new nursing student, most commonly from secondary school, enters with more computer skills than ever before. Rather than compulsory computer skills training, optional classes are available for those students that require additional assistance in this area.

Changes have taken place in undergraduate nursing education, including the computer literacy of entering students and the credentials with which new nurses qualify. Since the mid-1990s, nurses registering for practice in New Zealand also complete an undergraduate degree. The impact of these changes on undergraduate nursing education has a flow-on effect within postgraduate education. Furthermore, the changes in health service delivery in New Zealand and the establishment of new roles and career opportunities, such as the nurse practitioner, are drivers for the ongoing demand for postgraduate nursing education. These new advanced nursing roles require postgraduate qualifications, yet there have been barriers to nurses accessing postgraduate education, which is generally based in urban areas. Nurses are found throughout the country and the nature of nursing necessitates shift work. Nurses in New Zealand are predominantly women, and there are gender issues that make access to postgraduate education problematic. Learning that utilizes the benefits of technology is becoming increasingly common with flexible learning, e-learning, and online courses available for postgraduate nursing education (Honey, 2007).

The demand for health informatics education has increased over the last decade because of numerous international forces, to which New Zealand has also been subject. Two that particularly influence the role of health IT and the increasing demand for informatics are the increased prominence of patient safety and quality improvement in the healthcare arena and the increased importance of consumer-centric care and their use of the World Wide Web (Internet) to access health information, knowledge, and healthcare experts across the globe (Skiba, Connors, & Honey, 2010). As patients seek out information, become better informed, and request a range of options, nurses need to be able to assist patients in understanding their choices. Thus, information literacy is becoming an important competency for professional nursing practice.

Health informatics education in New Zealand has evolved in a different manner than other countries, such as the United States and Great Britain. Perhaps due to the smaller numbers of nurses, separate postgraduate courses in nursing informatics have not been viable. While nursing informatics as a postgraduate specialty has not been recognized in New Zealand, nurses are favoring health informatics options. A study that included an online survey and interviews with the major tertiary education providers within New Zealand offering postgraduate health informatics programs explored the potential for improving the health informatics workforce capability in New Zealand (Kerr et al., 2006). The study found that there is "clearly a role for graduates with a set of competencies that can provide a bridge between the IT specialist working in the health sector and the clinicians assisting with IT developments" (Kerr et al., 2006, p. 5). In New Zealand, 4 programs that provide postgraduate education in health informatics are slowly increasing enrolments, and are well regarded by students and graduates. These programs provide nurses with the opportunity to study informatics in a broad context alongside other health professionals. This study also suggests that national agreement on a postgraduate health informatics curriculum would improve the effectiveness and the marketability of programs (Kerr et al., 2006).

PROFESSIONAL ORGANIZATIONS AND GOVERNMENT ADVISORY GROUPS

Both New Zealand and Australia have many health informatics and related professional organizations and groups advising various government departments and specific projects. There tends to be a considerable overlap of members between these. Health Informatics New Zealand (HINZ) is working closely with the Australasian College of Health Informatics. Both organizations have many nurses as members and fellows.

NEW ZEALAND HEALTH INFORMATICS GROUPS

There are a number of informatics interest groups in New Zealand, each with a slightly different focus. Table 47.1 identifies and provides a high-level definition of these groups. HINZ is a national, not-for-profit organization whose focus is to facilitate improvements in business processes and patient care in the health sector through the application of appropriate information technologies (Health Informatics New Zealand, 2010). HINZ emerged in September 2000 from two health informatics organizations: Nursing Informatics New Zealand (NINZ) and New Zealand Health Informatics Foundation (NZHiF). HINZ does not compete with existing organizations or activities, but works to assist and network key influential partners to improve the effectiveness of health informatics in New Zealand.

HINZ acts as a single portal for the collection and dissemination of information about the New Zealand health informatics industry. Membership is for anyone who has an interest in health and informatics who wants

TABLE 47.1	New Zealand Health Informatics Groups
Group	**Description**
ACC www.acc.co.nz	The Accident Compensation Corporation (ACC) manages New Zealand's accident compensation scheme, which provides comprehensive no-fault personal accident insurance for all citizens. The ACC also works to prevent injury, and buy health and disability support services to treat, care for, and rehabilitate injured people.
DHBNZ www.dhbnz.org.nz	District Health Boards New Zealand (DHBNZ) is a national organization that has been set up by the 20 District Health Boards (DHB) to assist with representation, help coordinate joint DHB processes and activities, and undertake work that can be done more effectively and efficiently on a national basis.
Health Workforce NZ www.moh.govt.nz/ healthworkforcenz	Health Workforce New Zealand (previously known as the Clinical Training Agency Board) was formed to address the issues faced in health sector workforce development. It aims to provide a coordinated response to improving the ability to train, recruit, and retain the New Zealand health workforce.
HIANZ www.hianz.org.nz	Health Information Association of New Zealand (HIANZ) was founded in 1989 and is the networking and support organization for health information personnel, such as those involved in clinical coding, medical records, and health and medical libraries.
HINZ www.hinz.org.nz	Health Informatics New Zealand (HINZ) is a national, not-for-profit organization whose focus is to facilitate improvements in business processes and patient care in the health sector through the application of appropriate information technologies.
	HINZ has established working groups to mirror those within the International Medical Informatics Association Special Interest Group in Nursing Informatics (IMIA-NI). The HINZ Nursing Informatics Working Group is the most active of HINZ groups.
HISO www.ithealthboard. health.nz/hiso-2010	The purpose of the Health Information Standards Organisation (2010) is to support and promote the development, understanding, and use of fit-for-purpose health information standards to improve the New Zealand health system.
NZHITC www.healthit.org.nz	The New Zealand Health IT Cluster Inc. (NZHITC), established in 2002, sees itself as a neutral vehicle for dialogue between decision makers and industry through its consortium of over 80 organizations with a common interest in health information technology. The Cluster includes software and solution developers, consultants, health funders and healthcare providers who have agreed to work collaboratively to provide mutual support for local and international business development. The NZHITC mission statement is to "Collaborate to position New Zealand as a world leader in the supply and use of innovative health technology."
NZHUG www.hl7.org.nz	New Zealand Health Level 7 User Group (NZHUG) is the New Zealand arm of the international Health Level Seven (HL7) organization, which has a proven and widely used methodology for standards development that promotes information interoperability in healthcare. The organization is comprised of technical committees and special interest groups. The technical committees are directly responsible for the content of the standards. Special interest groups serve as a test bed for exploring new areas that may need coverage in HL7's published standards.
MoH www.moh.govt.nz	The Ministry of Health plays an important role in the formal intra- and intergovernment liaison work it undertakes, its influence on sector policy and strategy, and its funding capability. From 2008, the New Zealand Health Information Service (NZHIS) and HealthPAC have been merged into the Ministry of Health. HealthPAC, now known as Sector Services, are responsible for the administration and payment of government-funded core health services.
National Health IT Board www.ithealthboard.health. nz	The National Health Information Technology Board was established in 2009 and replaces Health Information Strategy Advisory Committee (HISAC). It works as a subcommittee of the National Health Board and aims to provide leadership across the health sector for IT investments in relation to patient safety and value for money, support for an improved health information model, and to set direction for the appropriate and effective use of personal health information.

(continued)

TABLE 47.1	New Zealand Health Informatics Groups (continued)
Group	Description
NIHI www.fmhs.auckland. ac.nz/soph/centres/nihi	The National Institute for Health Innovation (NIHI) is based at the University of Auckland and supports research through providing a Health Technology Laboratory for developing and testing ideas and products. This institute was established through partnership funding from the Tertiary Education Commission and founding partners.
Statistics New Zealand www.stats.govt.nz	Statistics New Zealand (Stats NZ) administers the Statistics Act (1975), producing the official statistics for the nation.

to be part of an organization that can provide relevant up-to-date information about health informatics. HINZ holds an annual conference in collaboration with other health IT organizations.

HEALTH INFORMATICS GROUPS IN AUSTRALIA

The history of the formation of medical, health, and nursing informatics groups reflects the difficulties experienced as a consequence of a federal system of government and vast distances between population centers.

Australia has had a representative to IMIA's Working Group 8 (WG8) (now NI sig) since 1984. Nurses were the second group of health professionals to organize themselves to promote health informatics in Australia. The general practitioners were first, beginning in the late 1970s. The Health Information Managers Association (HIMAA) has been in existance since 1949, but its integration of informatics is more recent. Nursing informatics is now a special interest group of the Health Informatics Society of Australia (HISA), which came into existence in 1993. It has been a long and torturous path to reach this position, as can be learned from the historical summary that follows.

Historical Developments

Nursing informatics in Australia began with the Royal Australian Nursing Federation (now ANF) in 1984. A year later, a small group of midwives in Victoria, including Joan Edgecumbe, who was the Executive Officer of HISA till 2009 the Executive Officer of the Health Informatics Society of Australia, decided to call a general meeting of nurses interested in computer use. About 70 nurses agreed to establish the Nursing Computer Group Victoria (NCGV). This group continued to flourish and hosted the Fourth International Symposium on Nursing Use of Computers and Information Science in Melbourne in 1991. The profits from this conference enabled the formation of the Health Informatics Society of Australia. These and other associated events are summarised in Table 47.2.

It has been a difficult path toward the recognition and professionalization of health (and nursing) informatics as a discipline. We have not yet managed to achieve a unity or consensus regarding how best to operate as one national professional organization to date, although increasingly joint activities are being organized.

NURSING INFORMATICS IN HONG KONG

Hong Kong nurses established NURSINFO (HK) Ltd. in 1991, and this organization has enjoyed a consistent increase in membership. They have as their motto, "Nursing Informatics for Excellence in Patient Care." They organize regular educational activities, use a communication network, produce a regular newsletter, and are actively involved with the Hong Kong Society of Medical Informatics and the Hong Kong Computer Society. Together, they participate in the organization of trade exhibits and regular conferences. The Hong Kong Hospital Authority is responsible for over 40 hospitals and over 50 specialist clinics that are part of a large multisite, multiprotocol intelligent data network to provide seamless data communications throughout Hong Kong. Implementation began in 1993. This included a clinical management system focusing on patient-oriented data sharing. This system provides longitudinal medical profiles for patients and can be accessed by healthcare professional on a need-to-know basis. Telemedicine and videoconferencing are in use, and multimedia enhancement in the clinical setting with voice recording and imaging now helps to speed up the work process and strengthens services in the clinical areas.

TABLE 47.2	History of Australian Health Informatics Professional Groups and the Promotion of the Discipline	
Year	**By Whom**	**Purpose**
1949	Health Information Managers Association (HIMAA)	Established. See www.himaa.org.au.
1984	Royal Australian Nurses Federation (RANF)	Adoption of position statement on "Computerisation in Health Services – Implications for Nursing" (RANF, 1984)
1985	RCNA	Seventh National Conference theme, "Information Processing—Challenges and Choices for Nurses," Melbourne. This inspired a small group of midwives.
1985	Midwives Association	General meeting of nurses interested in computer use; 70 nurses attended. The Nursing Computer Group Victoria (NCGV) was established.
1986	Royal Adelaide Hospital Nurses Education Fund	Sponsored a national nursing conference with the theme, "From Lamp to Light Pen – Computers in Nursing" to celebrate their 150th Jubilee. Nurses from Queensland and Western Australia computer groups established the previous year, networked.
1986	Health Commission of Victoria	Government funded the then senior nursing advisor to undertake a world tour to investigate the likely impact on nurses of computer use in the health industry.
1986	Royal Australian College of General Practitioners (RACGP)	National computer committee established following the formation of several state-based medical computing interest groups.
1986	Australian participants at Medinfo '86	Around 20 Australians met in Washington, DC, and decided to form a network with the aim of promoting health informatics among health professionals. This resulted in the formation of a number of computer groups in several states over the years that followed. Meanwhile, the Australian Computer Society (ACS) Inc. was the organization that represented Australia at IMIA.
1987	RACGP	Computer fellow position established in conjunction with Monash University's Department of Community Medicine.
1988	RACGP	Standards for computerized medical records systems released.
1989	Australian Medical Informatics Association (AMIA)	A Western Australia initiative to form AMIA with state-based branches. The inaugural meeting of AMIA (Victorian branch) was held in Melbourne in 1991. AMIA secured an affiliation with the Australian Computer Society (ACS) and became the ACS medical informatics special interest group.
1990	Australian Health Informatics Association SA	Sixteen health informatics enthusiasts met in South Australia and established AHIA SA. They published 6 issues of *Health Informatics News and Technology (HINT)* annually.
1991	Australian Computer Society (ACS) medical informatics special interest group	The ACS MI SIG organized a one-day health track at the ACS annual conference held in Adelaide that year. This was seen as an opportunity for members of the many disparate groups to meet and discuss the possibility of forming one national organization. Disagreement regarding the name (medical versus health) and the entry requirements remained unresolved.
1991	Australian Health Informatics Association Qld	A group of health professionals organized regular educational meetings in Brisbane and formed AHIA Qld.
1991	Health Informatics Association New South Wales (HIANSW)	HIANSW was established by 36 people representing a wide range of health and IT professionals including nurses. HIANSW produces a regular newsletter, *Computers in Health Information Processing (CHIP)*.

(continued)

TABLE 47.2	History of Australian Health Informatics Professional Groups and the Promotion of the Discipline *(continued)*	
Year	**By Whom**	**Purpose**
1991	Nursing Computer Group Victoria	International Nursing Informatics Symposium held in Melbourne hosted by the NCGV under the auspices of the IMIA Nursing Informatics working group.
1991	NI'91 Post Conference meeting	Nurses from all states and territories discussed the formation of a national nursing informatics group. Everyone agreed to work together, but the formalization of a new national organization was problematic due to differences between the state-based groups regarding affiliations with other professional nursing organizations. Subsequently, the Nursing Computer Group Victoria changed its name to Nursing Informatics Australia (NIA)
1992	Nursing Informatics Australia (NIA)	Postconference profits were used to establish a secretariat and launch a new look magazine.
1992	Australian Nursing Informatics Council (ANIC)	One representative from each state-based nursing informatics group was appointed to form ANIC.
1992	Standards Australia	Health Informatics Standards Committee IT-14 established.
1992	HIANSW Conference	Another attempt at uniting the 23 distinct groups was made at the first HIANSW conference held in Laura, New South Wales, to discuss how to best work together and how health (medical) informatics should be represented at IMIA. This resulted in a resolution to: 1. Form a national council of health informatics groups. 2. Combine 3 newsletters/journals—*CHIP, HINT,* and *Nursing Informatics Australia*—into a single national and multidisciplinary magazine with a national editorial board. The first issue of *Informatics in Healthcare Australia* came out in May 1992, funded by NIA.
1992	AMIA meeting, Melbourne	Discussion paper summarizing deliberations, and a scenario for the development of one new national organization to represent the field of health informatics in Australia was circulated widely.
1992	Australian Nursing Informatics Council (ANIC)	Initiated the idea to organize a national conference in 1993. Several groups supported this idea, and since NIA was the only organization with the necessary funds, this group managed the inaugural conference. This became an annual event known as HIC (Health Informatics Conference).
1993	Health Informatics Society of Australia (HISA)	A special meeting of representatives from interested groups, facilitated by Dr. Ian Graham, who was the Director of the Centre for Health Informatics at the Austin Hospital, was held in Sydney. This meeting produced a draft constitution for HISA, reflecting an agreed-upon set of principles. (See www.hisa.org.au.)
1993	HISA Victoria	NIA was reconstituted as the HISA Victoria branch.
1993	HISA Inaugural general meeting	The draft constitution was presented to potential HISA members at its inaugural general meeting held in conjunction with the inaugural Health Informatics Conference (HIC '93), and they voted for its adoption. Conference profits were then used to fund the further development of the constitution and incorporation.
1994	HISA Constituted	The NIA (now HISA Vic) secretariat became HISA's secretariat.
1994	HISA Standards SIG	HISA's representative to IT-14 informed the committee of the recommendation for the adoption of HL7 messaging standards, this was accepted.

TABLE 47.2	History of Australian Health Informatics Professional Groups and the Promotion of the Discipline *(continued)*	
Year	**By Whom**	**Purpose**
1995	HISA	HISA became the official group to represent Australia at IMIA
1996	HISA NI Sig	HISA Nursing Informatics special interest group established.
1997	General Practice Computing Group (GPCG)	Established by GPs, funded by the Australian Government Department of Health and Ageing to provide a strategic and cooperative approach to Australian GP informatics. (See www.gpcg.org.)
2000	HISA	A new constitution was adopted, making HISA a company limited by guarantee of its members.
2001	Australian College of Health Informatics (ACHI)	Meeting of 7 Health Informaticians funded by the Australian Department of Health and Aged Care resulted in the formation of ACHI in 2002, with 18 invited fellows selected via a peer review and consensus regarding the country's 20 top health informaticists to act as the peak reference body for health informatics in Australia. By 2004, there were 30 fellows and members. (See www.achi.org.au.)
2002	HL7 Australia	A Health Level Seven (HL7) user group established. An HL7 International Affiliates meeting held in Melbourne. (See www.hl7.org.au.)
2002	HISA	Hosted an international ISO TC215 meeting in Melbourne.
2003	HISA	A Pathology SIG established.
2004	HISA	An Aged Care SIG established.
2009	Australasian College of Health Informatics (ACHI)	The ACHI has increased its membership to suitably qualified candidates in New Zealand and Asia. There is an agreement between HINZ and ACHI to work together. ACHI initiated the establishment of the Australian Health Informatics Education Council (AHIEC), continues to provide a secretarial service for this Council, and prepared a strategic workplan for national health and nursing informatics education.
2010	ACHI	ACHI was accepted as a member of the Australian Council of Professions Ltd.

Hong Kong's Hospital Authority system has been widely accepted as part of the hospital infrastructure. It's Web site lists 75 local professional bodies but makes no mention of any health, medical, or nursing informatics professional organizations. Individual nurse informaticists do publish, however, there is no longer evidence of the existance of this nursing informatics group. Neither the College of Nursing in Hong Kong nor the Hong Kong Society of Medical Informatics makes any mention of nursing informatics.

raising, education, and dissemination of knowledge about the field of health and nursing informatics in the Pacific Rim. This is becoming increasingly complex with the proliferation of government initiatives spanning multiple government departments. This is also a reflection of the multidisciplinary nature of health informatics. Nurses, as the largest group of health professionals, have a major role to play. This requires sound knowledge about the numerous stakeholders so that nurses can benefit healthcare consumers—our patients, communities, and society as a whole.

SUMMARY

It is clearly evident that professional health, medical, and nursing organizations, along with educational providers and research centers play a major role in the awareness-

REFERENCES

Accident Compensation Corporation (ACC). (2009). *READ codes.* Retrieved from http://www.acc.co.nz/for-providers/lodge-and-manage-claims/prv00037.

Asia Pacific Medical Informatics Association (APAMI), an IMIA Regional Group. (n.d.). Retrieved from http://www.apami.org/ accessed 6 July 2010.

Australian Government. (n.d.). *Department of Health and Ageing eHealth initiatives*. (n.d.). Retrieved from http://www.health.gov.au/internet/main/publishing.nsf/Content/eHealth.

Australian Government. (n.d.). *National supply chain initiative*. Retrieved from http://www.nehta.gov.au/connecting-australia/e-health-procurement/healthcare-supply-chain-and-patient-safety.

Australian Government. (n.d.). *Health reform - GP (primary healthcare) and hospital care integration*. Retrieved from http://www.yourhealth.gov.au/internet/yourhealth/publishing.nsf/Content/Home.

Australian Government. (n.d.). *Aboriginal and Torris Strait Islander coordinated care trials*. Retrieved from http://www.health.gov.au/internet/main/publishing.nsf/Content/health-oatsih-pubs-coord.htm/$FILE/coord.pdf.

Australian Government. (n.d.). *Health call centres program*. Retrieved from http://www.health.gov.au/internet/main/publishing.nsf/Content/national-health-call-centre-network-team-overview.

Australian Government. (n.d.). *Department of Health and Ageing, towards a national primary healthcare strategy: A discussion paper from the Australian Government, Commonwealth of Australia, Canberra*. Retrieved from http://www.health.gov.au/internet/main/publishing.nsf/Content/PHS-DiscussionPaper.

Australian Government. (2008). National Health and Hospitals Reform Commission (NHHRC). *A healthier future for all australians—Interim report*. Retrieved from http://www.health.gov.au/internet/nhhrc/publishing.nsf/Content/interim-report-december-2008.

Australian Health Informatics Education Council (AHIEC). (2009–2010). *Strategic Workplan 2009-10 and beyond*. Retrieved from http://www.ahiec.org.au/Documents.htm.

Australian Healthcare Agreements. (n.d.). Retrieved from http://www.health.gov.au/ahca.

Australian Hospital Information. (n.d.). Casemix classifications. Retrieved from http://www.health.gov.au/internet/main/publishing.nsf/Content/Classificationshub.htm.

Australian Institute of Health and Welfare (AIHW). (2008). *Australia's health 2008*. Retrieved from http://www.aihw.gov.au/publications/index.cfm/title/10014.

Australian Institute of Health and Welfare (AIHW). (n.d.). *METeOR*. http://meteor.aihw.gov.au/content/index.phtml/itemId/181162.

Booz & Co E-Health. (2008 November). *Enabler for Australia's health reform, prepared for the NHHRC*. Retrieved from http://www.nhhrc.org.au/internet/nhhrc/publishing.nsf/Content/discussion-papers.

Chu, S., Mair, M., & Hobson, C. (2002). Developing the health event summary system. *Proceedings of Health Informatics New Zealand Congress 2002*. Auckland.

Commonwealth of Australia. (2009). *Casemix review report*. Retrieved from http://www.health.gov.au/casemix.

Commonwealth of Australia. (2010). *Building a 21st century primary healthcare system, Australia's first national primary healthcare strategy*. Retrieved from http://www.yourhealth.gov.au/internet/yourhealth/publishing.nsf/Content/Building-a-21st-Century-Primary-Health-Care-System-TOC.

Connolly, M., Boyd, M.-A., Kenealy, T., Moffitt, A., Sheridan, N., & Kolbe, J. (2010). *Alleviating the burden of chronic conditions in New Zealand: The ABCC NZ Study Workbook 2010*. Auckland: The University of Auckland and Freemason's Unit of Geriatric Medicine. Retrieved from http://dhbrf.hrc.govt.nz/media/documents_abcc/ABCC_Study_Workbook_Final.pdf.

Davey, J. A., & Gee, S. (2002). *Life at 85 plus: A statistical review*. Wellington, New Zealand: New Zealand Institute for Research on Ageing.

District Health Boards New Zealand (DHBNZ). (2010). *Future workforce: Nurse practitioner—A healthy future*. Retrieved from http://www.dhbnz.org.nz/Site/Future_Workforce/Nursing-Midwifery/Nursing-Projects/Nurse-Practitioner/Default.aspx.

Dykes, P. C., Brown, S., Collins, R., Cook, R., Docherty, C., Ensio, A., et al. (2010). *The impact of health information technology (I-HIT) survey: Results from an international research collaborative*. In C. A. Weaver, C. W. Delaney, P. Weber, & R. L. Carr (Eds.), *Nursing and informatics for the 21st century: An international look at practice, education and EHR trends* (2nd ed., pp. 69–88). Chicago: Healthcare Information and Management Systems Society.

Dykes, P. C., Hurley, A. C., Brown, S., Carr, R., Cashen, M., Collins, R., et al. (2009). Validation of the impact of health information technology (I-HIT) scale: An international collaborative. In K. Saranto, P. Flatley Brennan, H.-A. Park, M. Tallberg, & A. Ensio (Eds.), *Connecting health and humans: Proceedings of NI2009, The 10th International Congress on Nursing Informatics, Helsinki, Finland, 28 June–1 July* (pp. 618–622). Amsterdam: IOS Press.

Electronic Health Informatics Journal (eJHI). (n.d.). Retrieved from http://www.eJHI.net.

Enigma Publishing. (n.d.). Retrieved from http://enigma.co.nz.

Green, P. L. (1998). Improving clinical effectiveness in an integrated care delivery system. Online *Journal on Quality Improvement*. Retrieved from http://www.ncbi.nlm.nih.gov/pubmed/10351215.

Health Level Seven (HL7). (n.d.). *Electronic health record functional model and standard*. Retrieved from http://www.hl7.org/ehr.

Health Informatics New Zealand. (2010). *About health informatics New Zealand*. Retrieved from http://www.hinz.org.nz/page/about-hinz/about-hinz.

Health Information Strategy Steering Committee. (2005). *Health information strategy for New Zealand*. Wellington, New Zealand: Ministry of Health.

Heather, B. (2010, February 2). Technology third-biggest export. *Computerworld*. Retrieved from http://computerworld.co.nz/news.nsf/development/technology-third-biggest-export.

Ho, M. Y., & Hovenga, E. J. S. (1999). What do nurses have to say about information technology in their workplace? In J. Walker, S. Wheaton, M. Wise, & K. Stark (Eds.), *HIC 99 Handbook of Abstracts*. Full paper on CD-ROM of proceedings, HISA, Melbourne, Australia.

Ho, M. Y., & Hovenga, E. J. S. (2003). The study of Queensland nurses' attitude and behaviour towards computerisation at the workplace. In: H. de Fatima Marin, E. P. Marques, E. Hovenga, & W. Goossen (Eds.) *Proceedings of Nursing Informatics, Rio de Janeiro, June 2003*.

Honey, M. (2007). *Teaching and learning with technology as enabler: A case study on flexible learning for postgraduate nurses*. Unpublished doctoral thesis, University of Auckland, Auckland, New Zealand.

Honey, M., & Baker, H. (2004, July 27-29). *Integrated undergraduate curriculum for health informatics*. Paper presented at the HINZ 2004 Third National Health Informatics Conference: Towards a Healthy Nation, Wellington, New Zealand.

Hovenga, E. J. S., Kidd, M., & Cesnik, B. (1996). *Health Informatics, An overview*. South Melbourne: Churchill Livingstone.

Hovenga, E. J. S, Kidd, M., Garde, S., Hullin, C. (2010). *Health Informatics, An overview*. Amsterdam: IOS Press.

ICT Standards Committee. (2004). Foundations for the future: Priorities for health information standardisation in Australia, 2004–2008 unpublished working paper.

i-Health Ltd. (n.d.). Retrieved from http://www.i-healthviews.com/overview_profile.aspx.

InterRAI. (n.d.) Retrieved from http://www.interrai.org.

Karmel, T., & Li, J. (2002). *The nursing workforce 2010— national review of nursing education*. Retrieved from http://www.dest.gov.au/archive/highered/nursing/pubs/nursing_worfforce_2010/nursing_workforce_default.htm.

Kerr, K., Cullen, R., Duke, J., Holt, A., Kirk, R., Komisarczuk, P., et al. (2006). *Health informatics capability development in New Zealand: A report to the Tertiary Education Commission*. Wellington, New Zealand: National Steering Committee for Health Informatics Education in New Zealand. Retrieved from http://homepages.mcs.vuw.ac.nz/~peterk/healthinformatics/tec-hi-report-06.pdf.

MacKay, G., & Griffin, A. (1989). *Nurses using computers: Australian experiences*. Armidale, New South Wales: A.C.A.E Publications.

Microsoft Corporation. (2000). *NET for healthcare embraces new Internet standards to revolutionize healthcare*. Washington: Microsoft Corporation Presspass. Retrieved from http://www.microsoft.com/presspass/features/2000/Oct00/10-03healthcare.asp.

Ministry of Health. (2000). *The New Zealand health strategy*. Wellington, New Zealand: Ministry of Health.

Ministry of Health. (2001). *The health and independence report*. Wellington, New Zealand: Ministry of Health.

Ministry of Health. (2007). *Diabetes surveillance*. Wellington: New Zealand: Ministry of Health.

Ministry of Health. (2008). *The health and independence report 2008*. Wellington, New Zealand: Ministry of Health

Ministry of Health. (2010a). Data and statistics. Retrieved from http://www.moh.govt.nz/moh.nsf/indexmh/dataandstatistics-collections.

Ministry of Health. (2010b). *IT health board*. Retrieved from http://www.ithealthboard.health.nz/

National eHealth Transition Authority (NEHTA). (2009). *Strategic Plan 2009–2012*. Retrieved from http://www.nehta.gov.au/about-us/strategy.

National Nursing Organisations. (n.d.). Retrieved from http://www.conno.org.au.

New Zealand Health Information Service. (2010). *New Zealand SNOMED CT® National Release* Centre. Retrieved from http://www.nzhis.govt.nz/moh.nsf/pagesns/497.

Nursing and Midwifery Workforce Strategy Group. (2006). *Nursing workforce strategy*. Retrieved from http://www.dhbnz.org.nz/includes/download.aspx?ID=25740.

Nursing Council of New Zealand. (2009). *Annual report 2009*. Wellington, New Zealand: Nursing Council of New Zealand.

NHIMPC. (2007). *Strategic Workplan 2007–08 to 2012–13*. Retrieved from http://www.ahmac.gov.au/NHIMPC_Strategic_Work_Plan.pdf.

Oh, H., Rizo, C., Enkin, M., Jadad, A. (2005). What Is e-Health (3): A systematic review of published definitions. *Journal of Medical Internet Research*, 7(1), e1. Retrieved from http://www.jmir.org/2005/1/e1.

OpenEHR Community.(n.d.). Retrieved from http://www.openehr.org.

Parry, D., Holt, A., & Gillies, J. (2001). Using the internet to teach health informatics: A case study. *Journal of Medical Internet Research*, 3(3), e26. Retrieved from http://www.jmir.org/2001/3/e26.

Royal Australian Nurses Federation. (1984). *Computerised patient data and nursing information systems: Some considerations*. Melbourne, Australia: Royal Australian Nurses Federation.

Schoen, C., Osborn, R., Doty, M. M., Squires, D., Peugh, J., & Applebaum, S. (2009, November 5). A survey of primary care physicians in 11 countries, 2009: Perspectives on care, costs, and experiences Commonwealth Fund International Health Policy Survey of Primary Care Physicians. *Health Affairs Web Exclusive*, w1171–w1183.

Skiba, D. J., Connors, H. R., & Honey, M. L. L. (2010). Growth in nursing informatics educational programs to meet demands. In C. A. Weaver, C. W. Delaney, P. Weber, & R. L. Carr (Eds.), *Nursing and informatics for the 21st century: An international look at practice, education and EHR trends* (2nd ed., pp. 53–67). Chicago: Healthcare Information and Management Systems Society.

Standards Australia. (n.d.). *eHealth*. Retrieved from http://www.e-health.standards.org.au.

Statistics New Zealand. (2010). *QuickStats of 2006 census data*. Retrieved from http://www.stats.govt.nz/Census/2006CensusHomePage/QuickStats.aspx.

Soar, J., Marsault, A., Sara, T., Mount, C., Hardy, J., Swinkels, W., & Yearwoord, J. (2003). *Health informatics education, HISA, & Australian Department of Health and Ageing*. Retrieved from http://www.health.gov.au/internet/hconnect/publishing.nsf/content/7746B10691FA666CCA257128007B7EAF/$File/hiefrept.pdf.

University of Hong Kong. (n.d.). *interRAI coordinating centre*. Retrieved from http://ageing.hku.hk/interrai/index.html.

World Health Organization. (2010). *International Classification of Diseases*. Retrieved from http://www.who.int/classifications/icd/en.

World Health Organization. *2008 WHO human resources for health minimum data set*. Retrieved from http://www.who.int/hrh/documents/hrh_minimum_data_set.pdf.

Zelmer, A. C., Lynn, B., McLees, M. A., & Zelmer, A. E. (1991). A progress report on the use of CAL/CML in a three year pre-registration diploma program. In E. Hovenga, K. Hannah, K. McCormick, & J. Ronald (Eds.), *Nursing informatics '91; Proceedings of the fourth international conference on nursing use of computers and information science*. Melbourne: Springer-Verlag.

48

Asian Perspectives

Hyeoun-Ae Park

- **OBJECTIVES**
  1. Describe the development of nursing informatics (NI) in selected Asian countries.
  2. Identify historic milestones, changes, and trends influencing how nurses embrace informatics, such as government initiatives and international collaborations.
  3. Discuss NI practice, education, and research.

- **KEY WORDS**

  information systems
  standards
  health informatics
  government initiatives

INTRODUCTION

Since computers were first introduced into the healthcare sectors of Asian countries in the 1970s, there have been exciting developments in healthcare informatics associated with the rapid growth in information and communication technology. The first applications of information technology in healthcare in Asian countries were in administration, billing, and insurance; now these countries are moving toward implementing paperless electronic health records. This chapter provides an overview of the current status of the field of NI in South Korea, Japan, and Taiwan. It describes the history of NI, the use of informatics in clinical practice, informatics education, informatics research, and government initiatives and professional outreaches.

The short histories of NI have varied between the three countries, but all governments have played a very important role in introducing information technology into the healthcare sector by providing funds, developing infrastructure, and introducing policies to promote its use. Professional organizations have also played an important role. In most of these countries computers were first used in nursing during the early 1970s, although the terms health informatics and NI were not introduced until the 1980s or early 1990s following the establishment of professional organizations for health informatics.

The adoption of informatics in these three countries usually began as the vision of a group of individuals involved with the government or a professional organization, who promoted the use of information technology to support nurses in all areas of nursing. This occurred in nursing care practice, education, and research organizations, as well as within the information technology industry and via related government departments and exiting professional organizations.

As information technology has become indispensable to the daily activities of healthcare professionals, more and more nursing schools are beginning to realize the importance of providing informatics courses to nurses. Basic computer literacy education is now a part of nursing education in the three countries, and graduate programs majoring in NI are also available now in South Korea and Taiwan.

Reports of research into NI began to appear in the domestic nursing journals of the three countries in the 1990s. In the three countries, information technology first appeared as an educational tool, following by its use in clinical practice in applications such as expert systems and electronic nursing records. This use in clinical practice led to the development of standards becoming a favorite research topic. Current research topics include terminology and classification, decision support systems, mobile computing, and telemedicine.

Events external to the nursing profession frequently catalyzed the adoption of informatics by nurses. International multidisciplinary informatics links have assisted these beginnings and their progression. The progress in South Korea and Japan has been expedited by the hosting of the International Medical Informatics Association (IMIA) triannual conferences in 1980 and 1997. Moreover, the formation of the Asia Pacific Medical Informatics Association in 1993 helped promote national healthcare informatics association in the three countries due to the hosting of triannual conferences in the Pacific Rim. The China, Japan and Korea Medical Informatics Associations formed in 1999 helped nurses in these three countries to share and exchange experience and knowledge among both experts and users in these countries.

This chapter provides an overview of the historical events in South Korea, Japan, and Taiwan and highlights factors that are critical to success in healthcare informatics for the benefits of those who have yet to embark on such a journey. The chapter concludes by summarizing significant events and examining their impact on the evolution of NI in this region.

SOUTH KOREA

South Korea is located in the Far East of the Asian continent, and its territory consists of the Korean Peninsula extending southward with 4,410 islands around it. The area of South Korea is 99,392 km². Mountains account for almost 70% of the territory, and the cultivated area is only 21%. Currently, South Korea is the fourth largest economy in the Asia Pacific area and the 13th largest in the world. As of 2009, the population of Korea was about 50 million. The population predominantly lives in urban areas, with more than 41% living in 1 of the 5 major cities.

As of 2007, life expectancy in Korea was measured at 79.4, which exceeds the average life expectancy at birth (79.1) across countries measured by the Organisation for Econmic Co-operation and Development (OECD). The number of hospital beds was 7 per 1,000 individuals in 2007, ranking the second highest among OECD countries. With 1.7 physicians per 1,000 individuals, Korea ranked second lowest. Further, Korea had the lowest number of nurses among OECD countries in 2009, with 4.2 per 1,000 individuals (Statistics Portal, 2009).

South Korea introduced universal health insurance in 1989, covering hospital stays, physician visits, and prescription drugs for the whole population. The South Korean healthcare industry is on the growth track. Several new developments are contributing to the changing face of the South Korean healthcare industry. Biotechnology and health informatics are growing segments of the healthcare industry in Korea. In particular, health informatics in South Korea has grown considerably in recent years due to rapid growth of the information technology (IT) sector in Korea and with the help of the professional outreach activities of the Korean Society of Medical Informatics (KOSMI).

History of Nursing Informatics in Korea

The use of computers in South Korean healthcare began in the late 1970s in hospital finance and administration systems to expedite insurance reimbursements. Soon thereafter, the national health insurance system expanded to cover the whole population, and computers became necessary equipment to file reimbursement in healthcare organizations. The terms of *health informatics* and *nursing informatics* were first introduced in Korea when the KOSMI was founded in 1987.

A Nursing Informatics Special Interest Group was organized as 1 of the 5 special interest groups in the KOSMI in 1993. Since then, the Nursing Informatics Special Interest Group has held its own session at the biannual conference of the KOSMI. Nursing has been highly visible in the KOSMI through presenting and publishing papers on the use of computers in nursing at these conferences and in the *Journal of the KOSMI*. Currently, more than 200 of the KOSMI's active members are nurses.

Korean nurses have attended and participated in many international conferences promoted and organized by the International Medical Informatics Association (IMIA) and the International Medical Informatics Association Special Interest Group on Nursing Informatics (IMIA-NI) since the KOSMI was founded in 1987. Korean nurses represented the country at the IMIA-NI for the first time in 1995, since then Korea has sent a representative to the group and participated actively in developing and furthering nursing informatics within the country and outside of the country. The IMIA conference MEDINFO98 and the IMIA-NI conference NI2006 held in Seoul, provided excellent opportunities for Korean nurses to become acquainted with nursing informatics at the global level.

Further momentum for nursing informatics has been coming from funding for a nursing informatics study group provided by the Korean Science and Engineering Foundations since 1998. Activities of the study group include journal reviews and research activities such as survey studies of nursing informatics education and computer applications in nursing practice in Korean hospitals.

Use of Information Technology in Clinical Practice

According to a report published by the Korean Hospital Association in 2005, 100% of tertiary hospitals, 98.7% of community hospitals, and 95.4% of physician's offices have admission/discharge/transfer systems. Such a high implementation rate is believed to have been initially driven by financial factors associated with medical insurance claims. Eventually, the focus shifted to all areas of patient care as clinicians began to use computers in their practices. This report shows that almost 100% of tertiary hospitals, 84.2% of community hospitals, and 66.9% of physician's offices are using order communication systems, which enable physicians to communicate with other healthcare professionals for practice-related requisitions and the retrieval of data. In addition, about 90.5% of tertiary hospitals, 78.6% of community hospitals, and 22.6% of physician's offices are equipped with picture archiving and communication systems (PACSs). There has been a great deal of interest among healthcare organizations in acquiring these systems since the Korean government announced high reimbursement rates for diagnostic radiology examinations using PACS in early 2000. Hospitals are now beginning to implement paperless electronic medical record (EMR) systems. As of 2005, 21.4% of tertiary hospitals, 14.5% of community hospitals, and 21% of physician's offices have EMRs (Chae, 2005).

The use of computers in clinical nursing practice in Korea began first in medium-sized hospitals. These hospitals initially used computers mainly for administration and billing, as did most hospitals in other countries. These systems allow nurses to view their work list on screens or printouts so that they do not need to copy medica-

tion schedules or care activities onto the Kardex, or take notes on a piece of paper. Nursing information systems were proliferated when large hospitals with more than 1,000 beds began opening in the mid-1990s. These new hospitals were equipped with nursing information systems when they first opened. They included unique nursing activities such as nursing assessment, nursing care plans, and patient classifications in addition to nursing activities related to billing, managerial or coordinating activities, and physician-delegated tasks. Hospitals are now beginning to implement paperless electronic nursing record (ENR) systems. A standardized nursing terminology based on the International Classification for Nursing Practice was integrated into the ENR system and introduced at Seoul National University Hospital in Korea in 2003. Since then, nursing data collected with the system have been stored in a clinical data repository. Currently, data stored in the repository are being used for research and clinical practice.

Nursing Informatics Education

As IT has become indispensable in healthcare, and its impact on the daily activities of healthcare professionals has become significant, nursing schools are beginning to realize the importance of the health informatics education for clinicians. According to a survey on curriculums of Korean nursing schools posted in 2010, about 69% (78/135) of nursing schools with baccalaureate programs offer nursing informatics courses and 40.8% (29/71) of nursing schools with 3-year diploma programs offer nursing informatics courses (Lee, 2009). Nursing informatics courses were taught under different course titles, such as nursing informatics, nursing and informatics, nursing informatics and laboratory, medical and nursing informatics, nursing informatics and nursing process, nursing informatics and nursing management, nursing informatics science, and nursing informatics and evidence-based nursing. The course contents in these courses vary a great deal from school to school, and most of the instructors did not receive formal education on nursing informatics, rather they are self-taught instructors on the subject. This indicates that there is a need to identify content to cover in nursing informatics courses for 4-year programs and 3-year diploma programs, and standardize the programs based on the tasks of healthcare professionals.

Most nursing schools in Korea are adding informatics to the graduate-level curriculum so that students can take informatics courses as an elective. There is only one graduate program specializing in nursing informatics in Korea, which is at Seoul National University College of Nursing. This program started in 2003 and awards master's and doctoral degrees in nursing informatics. This program is playing a very important role in nursing informatics in Korea by producing not only nursing informatics practitioners, but also qualified nursing informatics educators.

Nursing Informatics Research

Since the introduction of the terms *medical informatics* and *nursing informatics* in 1987 in Korea, there have been many research studies on the use of information and technology in the healthcare field. We identified the trends of nursing informatics research since the introduction of medical informatics and nursing informatics in 1989 in Korea by reviewing nursing informatics–related literatures published in Korea (Lee, 2009). We reviewed the abstracts of oral and poster presentations at the KOSMI biannual conferences and papers published in the *Journal of Korean Academy of Nursing, Korean Journal of Nursing Query*, and *Journal of Korean Academy of Adult Nursing*. We included all of the abstracts and articles that were either authored by a nurse researcher or had relevance or application to nursing. A total of 192 papers were reviewed to examine the research trend of NI in Korea. We have grouped the NI research into the following 7 areas: clinical practice; teaching and learning; decision support; public and consumer health informatics; patient-centered healthcare such as telemedicine and ubiquitous healthcare; standardization activities; and use of IT for nursing research.

The number of NI-related papers published in Korea has increased dramatically over the past 20 years. Early studies on the use of computers for clinical nursing practice in the late 1980s and 1990s focused on attitudes toward or changes in workflow after computerized patient order entry (CPOE) implementation. In the mid-2000s, as terminology-based ENR systems were introduced, the outcomes of ENRs were studied in terms of direct and indirect care time and user satisfaction. Patient safety programs became part of the ENR. Quite a few papers have been published on the use of IT as a tool (e.g., CD-ROM, computer-assisted instruction, and Web-based learning) for learning and education in Korea. In the late 1990s and late 2000s, the popular research was in the area of decision support. With an aging population and increasing numbers of patients with aging-related diseases, there is a need for patient-centered healthcare such as telemedicine. Standardization activities in Korea are widely published and include work such as care plans, nursing practice guidelines and critical pathways, nursing document

forms, and the use of nursing terminology for ENR systems. Information technology has been used for research into nursing and for data analysis, including both qualitative and quantitative research.

The growing interest in IT has been reflected in nursing research in Korea. Over last 2 decades, the introduction of EMR and ENR systems, health informatics education, and health informatics research have either directly or indirectly influenced the development and expansion of NI research in Korea

Standardization Activities

There are current efforts to introduce various health informatics standards in healthcare information systems in South Korea. The primary motivation for this is compatibility of data, clinical documentation, and research outcomes across the country. Korean experts are actively involved in standards development activities in different international standards development organizations, such as the International Standards Organization (ISO) and Health Level Seven (HL7).

The Korean Ministry of Health introduced a Health Informatics Standards Committee in 2004 in an attempt to develop a single, integrated healthcare terminology in Korea as part of the National Health Information Infrastructure. This committee is in charge of developing, disseminating, and maintaining healthcare terminologies. There are 14 subcommittees working on healthcare terminologies in 14 different areas, such as medicine, dentistry, public health, and nursing. The Nursing Subcommittee translated the majority of existing nursing terminologies, such as the North American Nursing Diagnosis Association Taxonomy I and II, Nursing Interventions Classifications, Clinical Care Classifications, the Omaha System, and the International Classification for Nursing Practice (ICNP), into Korean. This committee also collected and standardized nursing statements documented in nursing records and mapped them to the ICNP. Outputs from this committee are available for Korean hospitals to access and use in their electronic patient record systems (Park, 2009).

Government Initiatives

The Korean government initiated information systems planning for the public health sector and the National Health Information Infrastructure in 2005. As part of these initiatives, the Korean government established the Center for Interoperable EHR (CiEHR) in 2005. The role of the CiEHR is to develop core technologies necessary to implement a lifetime electronic health record

(EHR), which enables the public to securely access and use their own medical record anytime and anywhere, as necessary, from the cradle to the grave.

Once the lifetime EHR is fully implemented, medical practitioners will be able to provide diagnoses and treatments with enhanced accuracy based upon sufficient patient data. The public benefits by receiving higher-quality medical care. In addition, the lifetime EHR will eventually reduce the costs and risks of medical care and eliminate redundancy in laboratory tests and prescriptions. Ultimately, the EHR promotes public health and chronic disease management, as it establishes the foundation for receiving systematic lifetime healthcare services.

In the first 2 years, CiEHR has established plans for a national healthcare information system. The center has been engaged in ongoing development of infrastructure for the next-generation EHR system by developing its necessary functions and standards including an integrated medical terminology and data model, administered service management system, and clinical decision support system. Research and development conducted by CiEHR is the outcome of collaboration with the 30 EHR-associated hospitals and 21 participating companies. This effort will be the cornerstone for utilizing health IT in the public healthcare sector and disseminating health IT to the private healthcare sector.

The research outcome of CiEHR creates a synergy effect through collaboration with national health IT projects, and public and private healthcare organizations. The ultimate goal of CiEHR is to enable the nation to conveniently receive healthcare at anytime and anywhere by practicing safe exchange of medical information between healthcare organizations. It aims to produce practical outcomes that can be applied by real users in real situations.

Professional Outreach

Since its inception in 1987, the KOSMI has played a key role in promoting and developing health informatics in Korea by holding biannual academic conferences, various seminars, workshops, and open forums, and by publishing journals. KOSMI has also offered educational programs for beginners in health informatics.

Professional organizations such as the Korean Medical Association and the Korean Nurses Association have also played significant roles by including health informatics in their continuing education programs. Another healthcare informatics expert group, the Health Informatics Standardization Committee, serving as the South Korean technical advisory group of the ISO Technical Committee 215, has held open forums and published health information standards.

The IMIA has contributed significantly to furthering the knowledge of South Korean healthcare professionals about worldwide trends in health informatics. South Korean experts in health informatics have attended and participated in many international conferences and meetings promoted or sponsored by the IMIA since 1989.

Technology Trends

The rapid growth in the number of mobile telephone users (currently estimated to be around 92% of the total population) and the advances in wireless local area network technology have lead to mobile computing in healthcare becoming a popular issue in South Korea, with many healthcare organizations testing its feasibility in special wards. The main users of mobile computing currently are nurses attending patients at bedsides, but this will soon be extended to other healthcare professionals. Although personal digital assistants (PDAs), tablet PCs, and notebooks are all suitable mobile computing platforms, users favor notebook computers with wireless LAN connections because of their large screen size and easier-to-use interface.

The need for telemedicine continues to grow in Korea with the increasing numbers of elderly patients, patients with chronic diseases, and patients who are discharged early. Many telemedicine systems have been tested over the past 10 years, one of which is a teleconsultation system initiated by the Korean government. Such systems allow, for example, a primary care physician at a health center in a remote area to have a telepathology or a teleradiology consultation with the specialists of a tertiary hospital. Another example of telemedicine is telecare at home, with the Telecare Center of Seoul National University Hospital and the Telemedicine Center of Gil Hospital being among the most active telecare-at-home clinics. Telepractioners at these centers maintain special schedules for their remote clients. They set aside 1 to 2 days per week to take care of their clients using virtual reality technology via the Internet. Currently, the teleconsultation fee is reimbursed by health insurance, but the use of telecare-at-home clinics is not covered. In July 2009, the Korean government began permitting telemedicine between healthcare professionals and clients.

Another technical trend in healthcare is called *ubiquitous computing in healthcare*. Ubiquitous healthcare can be defined as the environment where healthcare is available to everyone, everywhere without any dependence on time and location and where the technologies enabling ubiquitous healthcare will be assimilated flawlessly in our daily lives such that the technologies become invisible (Sneha and Varshney, 2006). It is being considered as an alternative to traditional face-to-face healthcare services in Korea. Since revision of medical laws to include e-prescriptions and telehealth was passed in 2002, several attempts were made to utilize ubiquitous computing in healthcare in both public and private sectors in Korea. For example, the Korean government initiated various pilot projects to promote ubiquitous computing in healthcare such as the Smart Digital Home, Health Management, and Health Promotion projects that use ubiquitous IT for underprivileged populations; the Ubiquitous Home Healthcare project for the elderly; and the u-City project. The local governments have also initiated various ubiquitous healthcare trials such as health center–based home healthcare, telemedicine in rural underserved regions, telemedicine for the elderly in nursing homes, and tele-emergency services.

The private sector has also made various attempts to utilize ubiquitous computing in healthcare. One example is the B2C ubiquitous healthcare model, which was developed to help manage chronic diseases (e.g., diabetes and hypertension), promote health in the general population (e.g., exercise, diet, and life style management), and support disease prevention in the private sector. Another example is the B2B model, where medical information solutions companies collaborate with healthcare organizations and insurance companies to provide ubiquitous healthcare services.

Recently, major healthcare organizations, leading telecommunication companies, universities and government research institutes, medical device and sensor companies, medical information solutions companies, and the safety and security industries are beginning to collaborate in ubiquitous healthcare in Korea. For example, a consortium of healthcare organizations with life insurance companies, medical information solutions companies, and local governments led by SK Telecom and LG Electronics, is developing ubiquitous healthcare models for private clinics and major healthcare organizations. About 8,000 patients with diseases such as diabetes, hypertension, cancer, chronic respiratory disease, and metabolic syndrome will participate in this pilot project.

Ubiquitous computing is being used in nursing too. Home care nurses send data measurements of their clients to doctors at health centers. Doctors monitor data measurements sent by the home care nurses and send recommendations to the nurses' PDAs. Nurses, in return, deliver nursing care to home care clients using short message service (SMS) systems or phones.

Another example is the use of ubiquitous computing by community health practitioners. Community health practitioners share bioinformation collected from clients with hypertensive and diabetic medications with doctors. Nurses prescribe and dispense medications for the patients based on doctors' orders delivered to them via wireless networks. Ubiquitous computing is also used in nursing homes; nurses working in nursing homes can consult with doctors at a hospital located remotely via teleconferencing technology. Nurses working in community settings and for vendors are actively involved in different types of ubiquitous healthcare activities as healthcare providers, business model planners, and developers.

JAPAN

The population of Japan is about 127 million, which is about twice that of the United Kingdom and half that of the United States. There are about 10,000 hospitals in Japan, of which about 430 have more than 400 beds. About 852,000 nurses work at these hospitals, including about 220,000 nurse aides (assistant nurses). There are about 278,000 medical doctors, 97,000 dentists, and 253,000 pharmacists (JPNA, 2010; Health and Welfare Statistics Association, 2009). The healthcare delivery system in Japan provides easy access to healthcare. All citizens can choose healthcare institutions and doctors freely, and their financial contribution to health insurance is proportional to their income. The insurance fee is deducted from the monthly salary and pooled by each insurance union. Insured individuals and families pay 20% and 30%, respectively, of all health expenditure, and the publicly funded health insurer pays the rest when a patient receives medical treatment in a hospital. The hospital receives reimbursement for the balance from the National Health Insurance system. The Japanese government will contribute a maximum of 70,000 yen to the medical treatment of a person during a 1-month hospital stay. Both the easy access to healthcare and low out-of-pocket cost in Japan help to provide the populace with a sense of security.

The total health expenditure of Japan remains lower than that in some other advanced nations, which is partially attributable to healthier dietary habits. The relatively small number of healthcare professionals working in Japan also helps to contain healthcare expenditures. The average length of hospital stays has recently been shortened, and thus many newly hospitalized patients are in the acute phase. This increases the probability of medical accidents, which can be offset by utilizing health informatics to improve medical safety.

Health informatics in Japan

Japan began to pay attention to the use of computers in healthcare during the late 1970s following the increased use of computers in other industries. Japan hosted MEDINFO80, the International Medical Informatics Association conference in 1980. The Japanese Association of Medical Informatics (JAMI) was founded at that time with the aim of supporting health informatics in Japan. Since then, JAMI has held 24 annual and biannual academic conferences, and these conferences have contributed considerably to the progress of health informatics in Japan (JAMI, 1996; Kamiitzumi, 2004). Initially, research was focused on computerized billing systems for medical fees, and the development of the use of personal computers at an individual level (JAMI, 2004). The focus then shifted to research and development of systems at the organizational level, such as hospital and regional information systems, and research into basic information technology for healthcare such as database design, network security, and data-switching technology. The current focuses are ethical issues in health informatics, medical finances, and quality assurance. This illustrates that the scope of health informatics has gradually expanded since it was first introduced into Japan during the 1980s.

Medical information departments in about 50 national university hospitals have made the largest contribution to the development of health informatics in Japan. Each organization has been developing its own hospital information systems for its own applications to clinical practice, education, and research (Japan Association of Medical Informatics, 1980–2003). This work helped Japan to determine the information, information technology, and mechanisms that were needed for healthcare applications, but the independence of these applications has hindered standardization in many healthcare fields. Standardization is one of the many problems in the use of healthcare information technology that needs to be resolved.

History of Nursing Informatics in Japan

The Third International Congress on Medical Informatics, MEDINFO80, organized by the International Medical Informatics Association, was held in Tokyo in 1980. This congress included a special interest group on nursing informatics, which represented the beginning of nursing informatics in Japan (JAMI, 1996; Kamiizumi, 2004). This did not result in immediate progress in Japanese nursing informatics education, due to schools being vocationally oriented. However, in the late 1990s nursing education in Japan rapidly shifted to a more academic orientation, and there are now more than 100 universities offering baccalaureate programs and 40 universities offering graduate programs. Some baccalaureate programs and graduate schools include nursing informatics courses in their curricula. Nursing informatics was applied more in clinical practice than in academic fields during the 1990s, with more nurses learning about utilizing computers in nursing practice through the activities of medical information departments in national university hospitals. It was also evident that clinical nurses presented more papers than academic researchers at the annual meetings of the JAMI. The Annual Meeting for Nursing Information Systems that was established as a task force of the JAMI also supports clinical practice, and most of its members are clinical nurses. The Nursing Division of the JAMI was established in 2000 and is managed by a team of clinical nurses and academic researchers. Several textbooks on nursing informatics have been published, but systematized nursing informatics education has not yet been implemented. The Japanese Nurses Association prepared a course on nursing information management as the first step toward a continuing education curriculum for ward managers. The standard textbook was published in March 2004 (Kamiizumi, 2004). The lecturers are researchers of health informatics and nursing informatics, and clinical nurses working at the hospitals where hospital information systems were introduced.

Nursing Informatics Education

As of April 2004, there were 505 professional schools, 33 junior colleges, 183 universities, and 125 graduate schools in Japan, compared with 461 professional schools, 74 junior colleges, and 30 universities in 1994 (JNAP, 2010). This comparison illustrates that nursing education in Japan has shifted from professional schools to universities and postgraduate education in the past 6 years. However, there are still very few universities with separate nursing informatics programs. The increasing development of hospital information systems in Japan has lead to discussions on the utilization of information technology in clinical nursing practice. Continuous education of nursing informatics is being emphasized, along with the promotion of electronic health records. However, it is difficult to conclude that the curricula of nursing schools have reflected the changes in society and clinical fields. Rather, it appears that clinical practice is now more advanced than nursing education.

Universities provided elementary computer literacy education during the first half of the 1990s, but this became unnecessary thereafter due to the introduction of computer education into elementary and junior high schools. Overall, the teaching of computer literacy on document retrieval, utilization of statistical processing, and Web utilization has increased, but barriers to the development of nursing informatics remain in Japan: (1) there are few researchers and educators in nursing informatics, (2) there is little development of educational tools, and (3) the cost of improving the network and computer environments is high. However, the importance of universities providing a satisfactory curriculum is being recognized due to the increasing importance of nursing informatics, with this being more so in graduate schools than in baccalaureate education.

Nursing Informatics Research

The amount of nursing informatics research is increasing in Japan, the two main purposes of which are improving the quality and standardization of nursing practice. Nursing informatics was one of the main subject areas of paper presentations at a recent annual meeting of the Japanese Academy of Nursing (Japan Academy for Nursing Science, 2003), indicating that it is becoming one of the major areas in nursing. There were many reports on research into the use of information technology as an educational tool during the 1990s (Ochiai, Sota, & Ezumi 1997; Kanai-Pak et al., 1997; Muranaka et al., 1997; Yamanouchi, Nakano, & Nojiri, 1997; Majima, 1997; Ezumi, Sota, & Ochiai, 1997), and on the use of information technology in clinical practice, especially on decision support systems for nursing in hospital information systems and electronic health records (JAMI, 2003). There has also been research into the use of information to prevent nursing-related accidents (Tsuru et al., 2004) and into telenursing (Kawaguchi, Azuma, & Ohta, 2004). Research into nursing-practice algorithms using thinking-aloud methods have begun in Japan (Tsuru, 2009, 2010).

Nursing Informatics Practice

Becoming a specialist in nursing informatics is useful when hospital information systems and electronic health records are introduced. However, the accreditation program of the Japan Nursing Association does not recognize the training for such specialists. Instead, the training of informatics nurses mainly occurs in hospital settings. In each hospital, nurses working on medical information are active in committees and working groups. Most of them are involved with not only nursing-related work but also medical-information-related work. Their lack of formal technical education often causes difficulties, and hence it is predicted that the importance of nurses with nursing informatics education will increase. The JAMI began an accreditation program for healthcare information technologists in 2003. Hospitals are looking for new healthcare staff with knowledge of both healthcare and information technology who can control information flow. Although a healthcare information technologist is a healthcare professional with such training, it is necessary to distinguish between the roles of the nursing informatics clinical nursing specialist and a healthcare information technologist. Informatics nurses will be expected to expand their activities in healthcare when both professions are introduced to hospitals.

Japanese Government Initiatives and Standards Development in Japan

An "e-Japan" strategy encompassing all Japanese ministries and related agencies is progressing now in Japan. The standardization of medical information is one of the main themes in the healthcare sector. The Ministry of Health, Labor, and Welfare announced a grand design for healthcare, and set the following achievement goals for 2006 (Panel on Healthcare and Medical Information Systems, 2002): (1) electronic health records will be introduced into 60% of hospitals with more than 400 beds, and into 60% of clinics; and (2) the electronic health expenditure payment system will be introduced into 70% of all hospitals. Standardization of the terminology used in electronic health records is a requirement for achieving this goal, and the Ministry of Health, Labor, and Welfare has begun a project for developing a national standard, which is publicly available on the Internet (The Medical Information Systems Development Center, 2004). This is especially useful for hospitals introducing hospital information systems for the first time. The following 5 standards have already been completed: (1) 581 facilities now perform medical diagnoses using the ICD-10; (2) 330 facilities have surgical and medical treatment standards; (3) 5,700 clinical tests have been registered in the clinical laboratory test standard; (4) about 38,000 drug names have been registered by 203 enterprises; and (4) about 210,000 medical supplies have been registered by 336 enterprises. Standardized symptoms, physiologic function examinations, imaging tests, dental terminology, and nursing terminology are currently under development, and nursing actions and observation items in nursing terminology will be available to the public by the middle of 2004. The terminology used in nursing practice have been collected, analyzed, and redesigned. About 260 fundamental nursing practices have been identified and named in Japan. They have been categorized into daily-life care, family support, guidance and education, interorganizational coordination, care in the usage of equipment, and care for the terminally ill and the bereaved family, and others. The are two hospitals where electronic health records use this nursing terminology, which was developed utilizing the terminology describing nursing care plan and nursing order, and in the implementation of care; differences in the nursing care offered to patients became clear. Continuous 24-hour observation of nursing care can be shared, indicating that the use of such a system is very useful for the medical profession.

NURSING INFORMATICS IN TAIWAN

History of Nursing Informatics in Taiwan

The term *nursing informatics* (NI) was first used in Taiwan in 1990. At that time, the focus was on hospital information systems providing nursing data such as nursing personnel information, care planning, and scheduling. Therefore, before 2000, our issues mainly emphasized clinical information systems (CISs), nurse scheduling, e-human resources, patient classification systems, PDA applications in the clinical area, and ICNP transformation. After 2000, NI development moved to foster NI skills in the nursing field, point-of-care models, nursing information system evaluations, e-learning in nursing, and evidenc-based practice in nursing informatics. The Taiwan Nursing Informatics Association (TNIA) was established on June 18, 2006, initiated by Dr. Polun Chang. It was the first national nursing informatics association in Asia. The TNIA operates for the purposes of promoting nursing informatics professional services, improving informatics-related academic research, upgrading the level of nursing informatics education, enhancing nursing informatics for all national organizations, and strengthening relationships with other international nursing and medical informatics organizations. The members are mainly nursing informatics specialists, clinical nurses interested in informatics, or nurse advocates from medical centers, hospitals, and universities in Taiwan.

The TNIA is composed of a Standing Board of Directors, a Standing Board of Supervisors, a Secretary General, and 4 committees (Members, Finance, International Affairs, and Education/Research). Since 2006, at least one national nursing informatics symposium was held by the TNIA, and many international nursing informatics experts and leaders have been invited, including Drs. Suzanne Bakken, Marion Ball, Robyn Carr, Connie Delaney, Patricia Dykes, Anneli Ensio, Scott Erdley, Brian Gugerty, Kathryn Hannah, Rosemary Kennedy, Jeongeun Kim, Judy Murphy, Peter Murray, Susan Newbold, Hyeoun-Ae Park, Virginia Saba, Kaija Saranto, Bonnie Westra, and Patricia Walker.

Since 2002, from a policy level, a national e-Taiwan program has been initiated by the Ministry of Health to promote the development of health informatics in Taiwan. The TNIA was granted U.S. \$550,000/year for the period between 2010 and 2012 to chair the Office of National EHR Interoperability for the Ministry of Health.

In June 2010, the Taiwan NI Roundtable Alliance was organized to bring together stakeholders from medical centers, regional hospitals, as well as academic and other key institutions. This alliance is intended to promote a more active national initiative for NI, and eventually build international participation through a platform in which all members are treated equally and with respect.

Use of Computers in Nursing Research

Based on the development of the TNIA, growing interest in NI has been reflected in nursing research. The number of studies related to NI has increased exponentially in the past 10 years. Nursing research, especially that pertaining to NI, can empower evidence-based practice. Knowledge building creates the expertise to conduct comparative studies of nursing care. And those NI research studies, presentations, and publications empower Taiwan to be visible in the international NI community.

Standardized terminologies such as existing nursing diagnosis classification systems and the ICNP have been translated for clinical use, and tested for their reliability and validity (Lu, 1998; Chiang, 1998). Users' perceptions and satisfaction toward computer use in daily practice also have been analyzed. Qualitative approaches such as interviews have been used to explore how well nurses will accept the change from manual charting to computerized documentation (Lee, Yeh, & Ho, 2002). Quantitative approaches such as surveys have been applied to investigate the attitude toward and satisfaction with the use of PDAs for charting and the storage of nursing records (Lai & Chen, 2003), along with factors affecting the use of nursing information (Lee, Lin, & Chang, 2005).

After 2006, more and more nursing personnel have joined in conducting NI research, and these research studies have been published in national and international nursing journals. Some of the NI research has focused on security (Hsu, Lin, & Tseng, 2009). Another research focus has been quality improvement in utilization of information technology in nursing care (Chang, 2007). including surveys of the factors related to nurses' acceptance of the use of mobile nursing stations in hospitals (Chang et al., 2008). The scope of NI studies included system development (Tai, Lin, Chang, Lin, Ko, & Chang, 2009), nursing continuing education (Liu, Chang, Hsu, & Lai, 2007), and literature review (Chu et al., 2010). Currently, studies are focused on radio-frequency identification (RFID) applications in medical and health industry pilot projects (Shao, 2010) and the feasibility of the role of nurse informatics specialists.

Use of Computers in Nursing Education

Computer-assisted instruction programs have been developed by the Ministry of Education for nursing vocational education programs since 1986. The content includes diet education for diabetic patients, biostatistics, maternal child health, stress management, and patient nutrition (Chen, 1992). Although a formal master's program focusing on NI was not available until 2001, the elective courses in baccalaureate and master's programs had started in the late 1990s. All baccalaureate programs included at least one or two computer courses. Currently, some nursing students act as assistants for faculty in designing distance-learning classes.

The growth of the Internet has led to the integration of distance education into nursing curricula. Online courses are available for baccalaureate programs in counseling, teaching principles and strategies, and long-term care. In addition, some schools provide multimedia self-testing systems. Students are videotaped when tested for nursing skills such as injections or enemas, and then the content is sent online to the instructor for grading. Schools provide an environment with simulated patients for students to practice before taking the test (Chang, Shu, & Chang, 2002).

At least 8 graduate programs in health or biomedical/medical informatics provide informatics training at the master's level for students with a nursing background, including the National Yang-Ming University, the National Taipei College of Nursing, the Chung-Cheng University, Taipei Medical University, Chang-Gung University, and Tzu-Chi University. A total of about 10 master's students with nursing backgrounds will graduate from these informatics programs every year. Among these 8 universities, the National Yang-Ming University, the Chung-Cheng University, Taipei Medical University, and Tzu-Chi University have doctoral programs with about 10 students with nursing backgrounds enrolled, although no PhDs have been awarded yet.

In mid-2003, the TNIA conducted a series of seminars and training courses in NI that have been run continuously since then by the National Yang-Ming University, the Taipei College of Nursing, the National Union of Nurses' Associations, and the Chang-Gung Institute of Technology. Therefore, nursing informatics programs have been integrated into more universities and hospital institutions. The clinical application of office tools and information skills were very helpful for solving unique problems within the nursing field.

Use of Computers in Clinical Practice

According to a recent survey, about 60% of healthcare organizations plan to set up a nursing information system. Every large healthcare organization in Taiwan already uses information systems in nursing environments. With the increasing popularity of mobile nursing stations, nursing information systems, barcode medication administration, and RFID, it is evident that nursing information systems are growing rapidly (Chang et al., 2008). Currently, many hospitals have already implemented nursing information systems.

Since 1992, computerized care plan systems have been used in clinical settings. Moreover, patient classification systems have been applied in patient assessments, nursing interventions, and staff workload assignments (Hsu et al., 1996), and, decision support systems have been integrated with medical and nursing diagnoses. Expert systems implemented on PDAs for the emergency room triage system have also been reported (Chang, Tzeng, & Sang, 2003; Lai et al., 2001). In addition, PDAs have recently been used by nurses in their daily practice. Nurses can input and output data including vital signs when caring for patients, as well as access patient laboratory results, medications, and medical records without having to go back to nursing stations (Li et al.,1998; Lin & Laio, 2003).

In 2005, about 79% of hospitals in Taiwan had 80% of their nursing documentation computerized, including 50% of documentation in the ICU; 82% of the nursing staff were able to input and retrieve patient data from the information system.

Computerized nursing systems have mainly been established to manage patient vital signs, care plans and medication administration records in acute units, the ICU, and in long-term care units. These systems also contain administrative functions like clinical classification systems, shift arranging (scheduling), personnel management, education and training, quality control, as well as assets and material management.

The Care Information Council was initiated in some hospitals' Departments of Nursing (DON) to develop and integrate the hospital information systems into the relevant nursing processes, including electronic medical record and care planning systems. The learning platform provides nurses with self-designed educational tools, and demonstrates how the nursing information system can apply to clinical and health education.

It is very common to use information technology in nursing practice in Taiwan. It provides wireless and laptop equipment to help nursing staff collect, save, transmit, and manage patient data faster and correctly. Especially after nurses became proficient in the wireless environment, many medical centers and big hospitals widely built mobile nursing stations to provide instant, convenient, and point-of-care nursing.

In 2005, Chang Gung Memorial Hospital Linkou Branch established an RFID operational care system in order to make the operations processes easier. The system includes functions to ensure patient data such as autochecking, proof of action, and other applications (Chang, Lin, & Lee, 2008). Based on the success of the Chang Gung system, other hospitals are expanding RFID technology into units like the emergency room, the delivery room, and the nursery.

Taichung Veterans General Hospital was the first hospital to combine CPOE and RFID into a barcode management administration (BCMA) system. Currently, many hospitals have already implemented BCMA systems.

The Taiwan Nursing Information Council, which is part of the TNIA, has invited 18 hospitals to set up a clinical nursing terminology and share experiences using the platform in an effort to promote nursing information systems and enhance clinical nursing information environments in Taiwan.

Professional Outreach

- The TNIA organized an international symposium and joined the Joint Conference of Medical Informatics in Taiwan (JCMIT) to conduct an annual national NI academic conference, in addition to conducting biannual NI congresses, seminars, and workshops.
- The TNIA initiated a Nursing Informatics (NI) Roundtable Alliance to discuss NI issues and share experiences and knowledge among institutions.
- The TNIA has played a very important role in disseminating informatics by including nursing informatics as a required course for

any continuing education programs that were accredited and offered by the TWNA in 2005. Since 2000, the TNIA has also offered educational programs for those who have no background in informatics.

- The TNIA played a leadership role in the development of the electronic medical record starting in 2010.
- The TNIA is proposing that an informatics nurse specialty be recognized as one of the clinical nursing specialties.

Future Directions

- Expand the role of the informatics nurse specialist to take a more active part in developing nursing information systems in health institutions.
- Establish the nursing terminology system and communication platform in Taiwan.
- Improve and upgrade the level of nursing informatics education to include nursing informatics and computer courses in nursing programs.
- Strengthen relationships with other international nursing informatics organizations.
- Establish the Chinese Nursing Terminology Center to develop computerized literature databases so that researchers can conduct searches at any time and in any place.

SUMMARY

The healthcare environment in Asian countries is becoming inhospitable due to high healthcare costs, increasing competition among healthcare organizations, decreased funding from the government, and consumers with more sophisticated demands. The introduction of information technology and information systems can help healthcare organization to survive under these difficult circumstances.

Healthcare informatics and the use of information technology has proceeded rapidly in Asian countries, with exciting development in the areas of clinical practice, informatics research, and informatics education over the past two decades. All of these developments have improved – either directly or indirectly – the productivity of healthcare professionals, the efficacy of the healthcare industry, and also the education of healthcare professionals.

It is clear that professional organizations play a major role in raising awareness, educating, and disseminating knowledge in health informatics. This is becoming increasingly complex with the proliferation of government initiatives spanning multiple government departments, which is a reflection of the multi-disciplinary nature of health informatics. Nurses, as the largest group of health professionals, have a major role to play. A sound knowledge of the many stakeholders will ensure that nurses can coordinate their efforts to ultimately benefit the healthcare consumer, communities, and society as a whole.

ACKNOWLEDGEMENTS

The author would like to thank InSook Cho for contributing the section on Korea; Satoko Tsuru for contributing the section on Japan; and Rung-Chuang Feng, Ming-Chuan Kuo, Li-Ping Fang, Xiang-Fen Lai, Ming-Xiang Tu, and Polun Chang for contributing the section on Taiwan.

REFERENCES

References for Nursing Informatics in Korea

Chae, Y. M. (2005). *Survey report on computerization rate of healthcare institutes in Korea*. Seoul, Korea: Health Insurance Review and Assessment Services.

Lee, M. K., & Park, H. A. (2009). *Research trends in nursing informatics in Korea*. Poster presented at APAMI 2009, Hiroshima.

Park, H. A., & Cho, I. (2009). Education, practice, and research in nursing terminology: Gaps, challenges, and opportunities. *IMIA Yearbook of Medical Information 2009*, 103–108.

Sneha, Sweta and Varshney, Upkar, "Ubiquitous Healthcare: A New Frontier in E-Health" (2006). *AMCIS 2006 Proceedings*. Paper 319. http://aisel.aisnet.org/amcis2006/319

Statistics Portal of Korean Ministry of Health and Social Welfare, (2010). Retrieved from http://stat.mw.go.kr.

References for Nursing Informatics in Japan

Ezumi, H., Sota, Y., & Ochiai, H. (1997). Teaching method and evaluation of information education in Shimane Nursing College. In U. Gerdin et al. (Eds.), *Nursing informatics* (p. 601). Amsterdam, The Netherlands: IOS Press.

Health and Welfare Statistics Association (Tokyo). (2009). *Journal of Health and Welfare Statistics, 56*(9). (Japanese).

Japanese Nursing Association Publishing (JNAP). (2010). Statistical data on nursing service in Japan. Tokyo: Japanese Nursing Association Publishing Company. (Japanese).

Japan Association of Medical Informatics. (1996). *Nursing information system workshop. Information system for nursing* (Japanese). Tokyo: Japanese Nursing Association Publishing Company.

Japan Association of Medical Informatics. (1980–2003). *Japan Journal of Medical Informatics Supplement* (Japanese).

Kamiizumi, K., & Ota, K. (2004). *Nursing information Management* (Japanese). Tokyo: Japanese Nursing Association Publishing Company.

Kanai-Pak, M., Hosoi, R., Arai, C., Ishii, Y., Seki, M., Kikuchi, Y., et al. (1997). Innovation in nursing education: Development of computer-assisted thinking. In U. Gerdin et al. (Eds.), *Nursing informatics* (pp. 371–375). Amsterdam, The Netherlands: IOS Press.

Kawaguchi, T., Azuma, M., & Ohta, K. (2004). Development of a telenursing system for patients with chronic disease. *Journal of Telemedicine and Telecare, 10*(4), 239–244.

Majima, Y. (1997). Application of the Internet for nursing education, in nursing informatics. In U. Gerdin et al. (Eds.), *Nursing informatics* (p. 587). Amsterdam, The Netherlands: IOS Press.

Ministry of Health, Labour and Welfare. (2004). *Welcome to Ministry of Health, Labour and Welfare*. Retrieved from http://www.mhlw.go.jp/english/index.html.

Muranaka, Y., Fujimura, R., Yamashita, K., Furuhashi, Y., Yamamoto, S., & Arita, K. (1997). Development of a CAI program entitled "Introduction to Nursing Process." Requirement for nursing education in Japan. In U. Gerdin, et al. (Eds.), *Nursing informatics* (pp. 487–491). Amsterdam, The Netherlands: IOS Press.

Ochiai, N., Sota, Y., & Ezumi, H. (1997). Self-study program on HTML browser—application to clinical nursing general remarks course. In U. Gerdin, et al. (Eds.), *Nursing informatics* (pp. 360–363). Amsterdam, The Netherlands: IOS Press.

Panel on Healthcare and Medical Information System. (2010). *Final report of grand design for informatization in healthcare and medical field*. Retrieved from http://www.medis.or.jp. (Japanese).

Supplement of National University Medical Information Processing Department Liaison Conference. (1995–2003). (Japanese).

The Medical Information System Development Center. (2004). *MEDIS-DC*. Retrieved from http://www.medis.or.jp. (Japanese).

Tokyo Academy. (2004). *Data of Nursing Educational Facility*. Retrieved from http://www.tokyo-ac.co.jp/med/index.html. (Japanese).

Tsuru, S., Aida, H., Takahashi, H., & Iizuka, Y. (2004). Design of assessment sheet to estimate risk of accidents depending on patient. *Supplement of 74th meeting for reading research papers of the Japanese Society for quality control.* (Japanese).

Tsuru, S., Nakanishi, M., Kawamura, S., et al (2009). Structuring Clinical Nursing Knowledge. *Japan Journal of Medical Informatics Supplement* 2009, 279–283. (Japanese).

Tsuru, S., Nakanishi, M., Kawamura, S., et al (2010). Nursing Function and Nursing Knowledge in Clinical Practice from Acute Care to Home Care. *Japan Journal of Medical Informatics Supplement* 2010, 219–224. (Japanese).

Yamanouchi, K., Nakano, M., & Nojiri, M. (1997). A small intranet for teaching how to use Internet. In U. Gerdin, et al. (Eds.), *Nursing informatics* (p. 585). Amsterdam, The Netherlands: IOS Press.

References for Nursing Informatics in Taiwan

Chang, M., Lin, J. S., & Lee, T. T. (2008). Applications of nursing Informwation systems: Sharing the experience of implementation in a hospital. *The Journal of Nursing, 55*(3), 75–80.

Chang, P. J, Shu, T. H., & Chang, C. B. (2002). Current status and future development of multimedia web-based learning in the nursing department of the National Taipei College of Nursing. *Journal of Health Science, 4*(3), 265–272.

Chang, P., Tzeng, Y. M., & Sang, Y. Y. (2003). The development of wireless PDA support systems for comprehensive and intelligent triage in emergency nursing. *Journal of Nursing, 50*(4), 29–40.

Chang, W. (2007). Information technology application and patient safety. *Journal of Healthcare Quality, 1*(4), 16–19. (Chinese).

Chen, W. L. (1992). Application of computer assisted instruction in nursing education. *Journal of Nursing, 39*(4), 118–123.

Chiang, L. C. (1998). Nursing diagnosis development in Taiwan: Now and future. *Journal of Nursing, 45*(2), 28–39.

Chu, K. C., Tsai, M. Y., Huaa, C. Y., & Chen, K. H.(2010). *Nursing informatics - Current state and future trends.* (Chinese). Retrieved from http://libir.tmu.edu.tw/bitstream/987654321/22253/1/23_S1616561.

Hsu, N. L., Feng, R. C., Lo, H. Y., & Wang, P. W. (1996). The establishment of factor type patient classification systems. *Journal of Nursing, 43*(3), 23–35.

Hsu, C. L., Lin, Y. C., & Tseng, K. C. (2009). A real-time interactive healthcare platform preserving security and privacy. *Journal of Taiwan Occupational Therapy Research and Practice.* 5(2)156–171. (in Chinese)

Lai, H., & Chen, L. (2003). Nurse satisfaction with the clinical use of personal digital assistant. *Tzu Chi Medical Journal, 15*(2), 97–103.

Lai, Y. H., Liu, L., Hsu, C. Y., & Chen, J. S. (2001). Medical diagnosis assisted nursing process support system. *New Taipei Nursing Journal, 3*(1), 67–78.

Lee, T., Lin, K. G., & Chang, P. (2005). Factors affecting the use of nursing information systems in Taiwan. *Journal of Advanced Nursing, 50*(2), 170–178.

Lee, T. T., Yeh, C. H., & Ho, L. H. (2002). Application of a computerized nursing care plan system in one hospital: Experiences of ICU nurses in Taiwan. *Journal of Advanced Nursing, 39*(1), 61–67.

Li, T. Z., Wang, R. H., Hsu, S. S., Chen, L. F., & Chang, H. Y. (1998). Information technology and nursing: Using PDAs in clinical nursing care. *Journal of Nursing, 45*(1), 69–76.

Lin, J. S., & Liao, Y. C. (2003). A study of nurses' attitude and satisfaction toward using personal digital assistant in nursing practice. *New Taipei Journal of Nursing, 5*(2), 3–12.

Liu, S. C., Chang, P., Hsu, C. L., & Lai, H. F. (2007). From analyzing the nursing informatics courses in schools to improving the nursing informatics competencies. *The Journal of Taiwan Association for Medical Informatics, 16*(1), 79–92. (Chinese).

Lu, Z. Y. (1998). Current status and future development of ICNP. *Journal of Nursing, 45*(2), 35–39.

Shao, K. N. (2010). *A government project research in Taiwan: RFID applications in the medical and health industry pilot project.* (Chinese, unpublished project).

Tai, H. L., Lin, H. W., Chang, C.C., Lin, S. A., Ko, S. H., & Chang, P. (2009). Nurses developing an end-user-computing process research of information system—taking the hemodialysis nursing information system as an example. *VGH Nursing, 26*(3), 244–253. (Chinese).

49

Nursing Informatics in South America

Heimar F. Marin

- OBJECTIVES
  1. Describe nursing informatics development in South America.
  2. Identify the use of information technology in clinical practice
  3. Describe educational and distance learning efforts.

- KEY WORDS

  nursing informatics
  clinical informatics
  training and education

Worldwide, several countries are using information and communication technology to improve quality of life, health conditions, and professional performance. These resources are transforming not only the daily lives and health conditions of the general population, but also the practice of healthcare professions. Among all healthcare providers across the world, nurses have progressively incorporated information systems and educational resources in their practice (Marin & Lorenzi, 2010).

South America is a subcontinent that comprises 13 countries in 3 territories, with a total area of 17,819,100 km^2 covering 12% of Earth's surface; it contains 6% of the world's population. Nursing informatics in South American countries has been based more on activities of individuals than on a global policy established by governments or national efforts. The levels of development and deployment of technological resources are varied across countries in South America; however, the use of technology has enabled a significant evolution in health and nursing education, practice, research, and administration. Among all regions of the world, South America has consistently seen the highest growth in information technology for the past 20 years. However, there are still significant factors that impact a broad adoption and deployment of health IT resources for consumers and professionals in certain countries and regions within South America.

In addition, it is important to emphasize that the use of technology is consistent with the evolution of technology in the region. Most developed regions of the country have better access and ability to implement health IT services and applications in nursing. In the last 3 years, governmental bodies and stakeholders have realized that additional investments are necessary to change this situation, and more activities are being implemented to optimize educational and health resources in underdeveloped regions.

The healthcare reforms currently occurring worldwide are closely related to the political and economic development of each country. However, the nature of these worldwide changes in healthcare delivery requires that nurses and allied professionals be prepared for leading and managing in a global healthcare environment, either in the redesign of nursing care delivery or by assuming new roles and positions. In any event, nurses must participate in this process of transformation by providing expertise and knowledge to planning, management, education, and care delivery (Marin & Lorenzi, 2010).

Computers are considered an important tool to help nurses take care of patients and to organize nursing service and nursing education. In addition, the use of the Internet and wireless communication is also a definitive trend in this field. Consequently, health institutes and universities are exploring ways to introduce new resources in order to facilitate the process of patient care and promote quality and safety.

The objective of this chapter is to present an overview of the development of nursing informatics in South America, identifying some initiatives and progress in the field, including discussion of the current use of distance education programs, and initiatives to disseminate nursing informatics resources in the region.

BACKGROUND

Nursing has been identified around the world as an emerging profession for over 100 years. In 2010, we commemorate the 100th anniversary of the death of Florence Nightingale, widely considered the pioneer who established nursing as a profession. Since her work in the Crimean War, the professional has been continuously evolving based on the influences of science and technology. There are several examples of the use and development of computer applications in healthcare impacting the nursing profession, and nurses can be considered the primary users of technology in healthcare (Safran, Slack, & Bleich, 1989).

Historically, nurses are accustomed to facing challenges, adapting new tools into their practice to improve performance, and creating new models to enhance patient care. Technology represents a unique opportunity for nurses to face further challenges, discover ways to innovate, and possibly redesign their methods of care (Marin, 1996).

Today's technology significantly modifies human activities and, consequently, the way we learn and work. The traditional methods of teaching, managing, and practicing the healthcare professions do not support the requirements of modern life anymore. Education is achieved through a continuous and diverse process, and its value is enduring. Teaching and learning are critical to maintaining a high quality of life and designing our future.

In the healthcare area, information is the key element for the decision-making process. The more specific information is available to support clinical decisions, the better care can be delivered to the patient. The quality of care is related to the scope of knowledge and information that health providers can access on which to base their clinical decisions. Thus, technology plays an important role in facilitating access to this information; for the information to be useful and meaningful, it has to be easily available.

Currently, health systems around the world face considerable challenges in providing healthcare services, and more systems in the global health sector are seeking improvement in the overall health situation, enhancing the operative capacity of the irnational health programs, decreasing mortality and morbidity rates, and improving the quality of life through informatics-based systems (Marin & Lorenzi, 2010).

Recognizing that computers and all IT resources are powerful instruments, each country is gradually becoming aware of the potential for applying IT to enhance the quality of care of clients and patients. While the lack of national policies delays the process, cultivating awareness of the capabilities of IT is the first step toward adopting these technologies.

There is a clear trend toward computerization of health records. In addition, more people are able to connect to the Internet, which is a telecommunication resource that has no comparison when it comes to fast exchange of data and information. As a result, we can expect to see better-informed healthcare providers and consumers (Pan America Health Association & World Health Organization, 2001).

Considering trends in healthcare informatics, and to facilitate the process in South American countries, the Pan American Health Organization (PAHO) has published guidelines and protocols to orient the development and deployment of information and communication technology in Latin America and the Caribbean (Pan America Health Association & World Health Organization, 1998, 2001, 2003).

It is also important to emphasize that the South American region ranks third in information technology expenditure. The Information Society Index (www.idc.com/groups/isi/main.html), which measures the use of information, computers, and social infrastructure, identified that countries in the region are rapidly evolving.

NURSING INFORMATICS INITIATIVES

In South American countries, as in any other country in the world, the initial motivation to develop computer systems in the healthcare area was driven by financial and administrative concerns. The hospital sector can be considered the area better served by information systems. Countries like Brazil, Mexico, Argentina, Colombia, Chile, and Paraguay have implemented clinical information systems in hospitals or health institutes.

Although clinical information systems are being used in some ways to support clinical care and management, a few hospitals or healthcare institutes have developed applications for nursing documentation where nursing data can be processed. In general, patient data that are also used for nursing administration are integrated in the system or nurses have to collect and analyze nursing data separately.

Hospitals have been working to design their own systems in order to attend to specific needs and policies. More recently, national and international software industry has become more represented in the South America healthcare market. Consequently, they provide a broader range of solutions with systems that address patient care documentation.

Many additional initiatives are spread throughout Latin American countries. It can be observed that the use of computers as an instrument to support nurses' activities in taking care of patients still needs considerable investment of human and material resources. Clinical systems based on the nursing process are not common in these countries.

Most of the computer systems implemented are intended to control administrative data. The most frequently implemented and used applications still are the nursing orders and some functionalities for documenting nursing notes, but with no structure or format. Using free-text documentation, it is more difficult to perform analysis and evaluation of nursing care. In one sense, we have a large amount of nursing data, but not necessarily a large amount of information to design nursing care plans to be delivered at the patient's bedside.

In spite of this, nurses are becoming even more involved with the design, implementation, and evaluation of clinical information systems. Vendors and developers recognize that the success of a computer system requires nursing input and collaboration.

In addition, as an open and evolving market, international developers are making investments to sell and implement computer systems in South America, because South America represents one of the most promising markets in the world of technology.

In Argentina, for instance, most of the health computer systems in use were acquired from the health software industry, although some applications were also locally developed. In both cases, there are only a small number of applications that include resources for nursing activities. Furthermore, Argentina was one of the first countries in South America to introduce topics related to health informatics in the formal education of physicians. It is estimated that the beginning of the formal organization of the nursing informatics movement in South America began in 1991. Since then, interest in nursing informatics has been growing, and it has become an important topic at congresses and conferences. In 2008, the II Argentine Symposium of Nursing Informatics was held within the II Latin American Congress of Medical Informatics with more than 100 participants from different South American countries (Leonzio & Barrios, 2010).

Recently, in Chile, the introduction of information and communication technology into healthcare was established by the Ministry of Health by the Digital Agenda Initiative. This initiative has the objective to contribute to healthcare development through the use of technology in order to increase competitiveness, equality of opportunities, quality of life, efficiency, and transparency to the public sector (Munoz, 2010).

In Brazil, the Brazilian Society of Health Informatics with the Federal Council of Medicine established a certificate program for software in healthcare. A manual was prepared and published (available at www.sbis.org.br) to inform vendors and developers about the process of certification. In parallel, the Federal Council of Medicine established national laws related to the use of electronic health records (EHRs), digital signatures, and privacy, security, and confidentiality of EHRs. Currently,, more than 11 vendors hold a certificate stamp for specific software developed and implemented in several healthcare institutes in the country. The Federal Council of Medicine is providing a professional card with the digital signature that can be used by physician to make electronic notes and orders. In May 2010, a partnership was also established between the Brazilian Health Informatics Society and the Federal Council of Nurses to guarantee the same process of digital signature for nurses and to ensure the inclusion of nursing components in the certification process of software in healthcare.

Although, even with growing initiatives in South America countries, it is necessary to emphasize that the inclusion of nursing elements of practice in the patient record is the responsibility of nurses. They need to be involved with the programmers, vendors, and developers to drive the professional requirements. Taking care of patients is the primary focus for nurses. Therefore, it is essential to ensure that all information required to perform nursing care is present in the health information systems.

Congresses, conferences, workshops, education, and training programs are being organized throughout South America to share experiences and information in nursing informatics and search for solutions that could enhance the delivery of patient care.

DISTANCE LEARNING AND EDUCATIONAL PERSPECTIVES IN NURSING INFORMATICS

Education is achieved through a continuous and diverse process, and its value is enduring. Although educational strategies have changed over time, the essence and fundamental principles remain; education is a process that cultivates the development of values and civilization as a whole.

Technology is transforming not only nursing practice, but also nursing training and educational models. With the introduction of computers into the healthcare area, nurses became primary users, responsible for data input. Consequently, they had to become computer-literate in order to use computer technology in an efficient manner. To meet educational and training needs, nursing schools and hospitals initiated programs to prepare nurses to use computers. In addition to instruction on how to use computer applications, course instructors also began to consider the use of computers to teach nursing content.

Computer applications in nursing education are also causing a shift from a passive teaching model to an active learning process. Computers enable students to work at the time that best meets their specific needs. Usually, the programs are very interactive and easy to use and offer immediate feedback about students' performance.

Formal educational programs in nursing informatics, such as a specific nursing informatics specialization and master's or doctoral courses, are also available. The Núcleo de Informática em Enfermagem at the Universidade Federal de São Paulo (NIEn/UNIFESP) was the first center to offer the specialization degree (certificate) in South America. NIEn/UNIFESP also provides, since 1989, the nursing informatics discipline in its graduate and undergraduate nursing programs. The research area in nursing informatics is attended by professionals from different regions of the country and has been responsible for the preparation of several master's and doctoral students in nursing informatics. After graduation, the students return to their own institutes to implement education and research programs and to participate in the development of patient care systems.

A retrospective search was performed in the electronic directory of the National Research Council for Science and Technology (CNPq) of Brazil, between 1922 and 2008. It was found that within the 323 research groups included in this directory, approximately 28 groups, corresponding to 42%, developed some type of study and research in ICT. More specifically, there are 16 research groups in nursing informatics in the country; the pioneer is the Nursing Informatics Research Group at the Federal University of São Paulo (NIEn-UNIFESP). However, there is a growing research movement in this field, which is evidenced by the several groups that have been established in the last 7 years across the country, such as the Research Group in Technology, Information, Health and Nursing Informatics at the Federal University of Santa Catarina, and the GEPETE at the Nursing School at São Paulo University, a research group in information technology and nursing work process (Sasso, Silveira, Peres, Marin, 2010).

Latin American countries are investing a significant effort to prepare professionals in health informatics. An example of this was recently implemented in Brazil. A 4-year grant from the Fogarty International Center of the National Institutes of Health (U.S.), promoted the establishment of a bilateral consortium of health informatics faculty. A program was designed to enhance training in Brazil by augmenting the teaching resources of local faculty. This training program was based on the experience of the Brazilian faculty and some lessons learned from an existing training program in Boston (U.S.), which involved faculty from Harvard University and its affiliated hospitals: Massachusetts Institute of Technology (MIT), Boston University, and Tufts University (Marin et al., 2004).

The program started in October 1999. Since then, it has sponsored 10 onsite courses in Brazil, which were subsequently made available on the Internet and CD-ROM, together with regular medical informatics courses taught yearly at Harvard and MIT. There were short courses in Brazil, which were taught by a mix of Brazilian and U.S. faculty, as well as support for faculty enrichment via participation in international scientific events. The training program was responsible for the organization of several scientific meetings in Brazil and continued to promote student and faculty participation in national and international conferences, short-term courses, and workshops.

During the development and implementation of this training program, different regions of Brazil were reached, delivering courses that were previously given in São Paulo or Rio de Janeiro. By the end of 2003, it was found that around 1,724 professionals were involved as either faculty members or students in the program.

The grant was renewed for 4 more years, from 2004 to 2009. The program continued to provide the certificate program, and the graduate program stimulated students to participate in national and international conferences. At the end of 2009, the grant was once again renewed to fund the program for 5 more years. The latest term of the grant is dedicated to support the certificate program based on distance education, where Maputo University (Mozambique, Africa) was involved. The program is coordinated and delivered by faculty of the Health Informatics Department at Universidade Federal de São Paulo, which also offers the graduate program (master's and doctoral) in health informatics. This program already graduated 39 professionals (doctors and masters), and has 66 students registered and over 105 waiting to be included.

In 2008, the Ministry of Education and the Universidade Aberta do Brasil created a program of distance learning provided by UNIFESP that offers a specialized degree in healthcare informatics for 500 professionals at 10 different centers throughout Brazil. It was decided to combine the Fogarty International Center of the National Institutes of Health (U.S.) grant with this distance education certificate program.

There has been a trend toward distance learning program development in South America. Computer technology is providing students living in distant regions and having difficulties in accessing the main educational centers the opportunity to improve their personal knowledge base. A contributing factor to the development and success of these programs is the distance between countries and cities due to the geographic characteristics of South America.

In 2006, an important information and communication technologies project named the RUTE network was deployed in Brazil. The infrastructure was developed by the University Network of Telemedicine and Telehealthcare of the Science and Technology Ministry (MCT), which is coordinated by the National Network of Teaching and Research and the National Program of Telehealthcare for primary healthcare. The RUTE network integrates teaching hospitals and basic healthcare networks. Currently, the RUTE network integrates approximately 131 healthcare institutions throughout the country and hundreds of basic healthcare units in their respective states, covering all Brazilian states. In addition, RUTE handles integrating multiprofessional healthcare into the community, and this infrastructure has improved access to healthcare and health information for the populations that live in regions that are remote and difficult to reach. (For additional information the RUTE network, see rute.rnp.br/sobre/instituicoes.)

The RUTE network also opened an ongoing channel for the development of research studies and interchange of specialized health knowledge. This has resulted in the growth of scientific collaboration, increased enrollment in healthcare training courses, and improved access to continuing education with the introduction of e-learning on a national level. (For addition information, see www.rnp.br/index.php)

Since its creation, the Rute network has been used by nurses across states to promote meetings and scientific discussions. The available telecommunication resources can also be used as a tool by nurses to support activities in patient care delivery such as monitoring medications, fluids, and feedings; documenting physiologic examinations; clarifying instructions; and helping patients understand medical procedures and treatments, thereby reducing anxiety and promoting better treatment adherence.

Currently, the infrastructure built by RUTE is being used only for meetings and scientific discussions, such as case studies. The development of a specific curricula for training in nursing domains is being considered, but has not been organized yet.

It is acknowledged that distance learning can be used to train large numbers of nurses in different geographic locations and work settings. To take advantage of the available resources in information technology, nurses should have a minimum of computer-based education established in their educational curriculum. Nurses with little or no previous experience in data standards and computer technology should receive basic training in the use of computer-supported nursing information systems or computer applications in nursing practice.

In February 2009, in an effort to stimulate participation of nurses within the country, the first online social network for nursing informatics and telenursing was created. It will be being an ongoing source for nurses and other professionals to share information and innovations, as well as network with specialists for the development of the nursing profession (Sasso, Silveira, Peres, & Marin, 2010).

NURSING TERMINOLOGY AND DOCUMENTATION

Sharing and communicating information is essential to make decisions and deliver care. Exchange of information requires the communicating parties to agree on a communicating channel, an exchange protocol, and a common language. The language includes an alphabet, words, phrases, and symbols that express and assign meaning, understood by all users (Pan America Health Association & World Health Organization, 1997).

Efforts have been made in this area, and various clinical vocabularies are available; however, building a vocabulary that standardizes the clinical nomenclature for use in clinical practice and that fulfills all requirements is a challenge.

In Brazil, the dissemination of the International Classification of Nursing practice (ICNP) started around 1996, when NIEn/UNIFESP became a sponsoring partner in the Telenurse Consortium, a project led by Randi Mortensen, director of the Danish Institute for Health and Nursing Research. The paper and electronic forms of the Brazilian version of the ICNP (www.epm.br/enf/nien/cipe) have been available since September 1997. Later, the ICNP Beta 2 became available in a Brazilian Portuguese version (Conselho Internacional de Enfermagem, 2003). In 2007, ICNP Version 1 was published in Brazil; Version 2 is currently being translated (CIPE, 2007).

Other terminologies are also being used in the country, including the Home Health Care Classification (HHCC) System developed by Virginia Saba (Saba, 1992), which is also available on the Internet (www.sabacare.com) in a Brazilian Portuguese version and the Clinical Care Classification (CCC) System, translated and published in Portuguese in 2008 (Saba, 2008). In 2008, during the National Congress in Health Informatics (CBIS2008) organized by the Brazilian Society of Health Informatics, the Nursing Informatics Special Group (SBIS-GIE) hosted a symposium on nursing informatics where Dr. Virginia Saba presented the Clinical Care Classification System. The symposium was attended by over 120 participants and was followed by a celebration to launch the CCC book, along with the third edition of Introduction to Nursing Informatics written by Marion Ball, Kathryn Hannah, and Margaret Edward, which was also translated by members of the SBIS-GIE.

The most frequently used vocabularies may not necessarily be the best ones, but they may reflect the demands of insurance companies and other payers. Although there are quantitative differences in terms of breadth of coverage and internal representational structure, no clinical vocabulary has been elected so far as the ultimate solution for clinical documentation, automated retrieval, and rapid communication. Several obstacles have yet to be surpassed before nursing communities embrace a standardized vocabulary that proves useful in a variety of tasks and settings: regional, national, and international (Marin & Machado, 1996).

The task is a challenge, and continuous studies must be done to reach the balance that will facilitate nursing practice documentation around the world.

Historically, nurses have faced several problems obtaining nursing documentation. Currently, with the expansion of health knowledge and information, the quantity of nursing documentation has certainly increased; however, the same cannot necessarily be said about the quality of the information documented. Health data rarely become health information.

SUMMARY

Nursing informatics as an integrated part of healthcare follows the progress that has been made in the whole sector of health informatics. Because of the significant variation among countries and even within larger countries, the development of nursing informatics is conducted on a case-by-case basis, taking into consideration the specific requirements of each region. Furthermore, the development and deployment of nursing informatics is dependent on national priorities and policies, human capabilities, and continuous efforts and research to optimize resources and discover new models to enhance the quality of care delivered.

Technological advances give nurses the opportunity to drive their own professional destinies. Adapting technological resources into practice helps nurses see emerging trends in the healthcare field as challenges and unique opportunities for career growth. There are new roles, new areas, and new jobs demanding experts in every country. There are a vast number of opportunities available for those who have decided to incorporate information technology into their daily practice and the process of taking care of patients.

REFERENCES

CIPE Versão 1. (2007). *Classificação Internacional para a Prática de Enfermagem* Conselho Internacional de Enfermeiros. Translated by Heimar F. Marin. São Paulo: Algol Editora.

Conselho Internacional de Enfermagem. (2003). *Classificação internacional para a prática de enfermagem beta 2*. tradução: Heimar de F. Marin, São Paulo, SP.

INFOTELEN. (n.d.). *Brazil's nursing and telenursing network*. Retrieved from http://www.infotelen.ning.com.

Leonzio, C. H., & Barrios, C.(2010) A historical account and current status of hursing informatics in Argentina. In C. A. Weaver, C. W. Delaney, P. Weber, & R. L. Carr (Eds.), *Nursing and informatics for the 21st century:Aan international look at practice, education and EHR trends* (2nd ed., pp.332–336). Chicago, Il: HIMSS. .

Marin, H. F. (1996). Nursing informatics applications. In N. Oliveri, M. Sosa-Iudicissa, & C. Gamboa (Eds.), *Internet, telematics and health* (p. 265). Amsterdam, The Netherlands: IOS Press.

Marin, H. F., & Lorenzi, N. M. (2010).International initiatives in nursing informatics. In: C. A. Weaver, C. W. Delaney, P. Weber, & R. L. Carr (Eds.), *Nursing and informatics for the 21st century: An international look at practice, education and EHR trends* (2nd ed.). Chicago, Il: HIMSS.

Marin, H. F., & Machado, L. O. (1996). Introduction to clinical vocabularies: What does the clinician need to know? In *Proceedings of the eight national conference on clinical computing in patient care: Capturing the clinical encounter*, Boston.

Marin, H. F., Massad, E., Marques, E. P., & Machado, L. O. (2004). International training in health informatics: A Brazilian experience. In *MEDINFO 2004*, San Francisco.

Mortensen, R. (1996). *The International Classification for Nursing Practice ICNP with TELENURSE introduction*. Copenhagen: Danish Institute for Health and Nursing Research.

Munoz, E. M. C. (2010). The electronic health record in Chile. In Weaver, C.A., Delaney, C.W., Weber, P., Carr, R.L (eds). In C. A. Weaver, C. W. Delaney, P. Weber, & R. L. Carr (Eds.), *Nursing and informatics for the 21st century:Aan international look at practice, education and EHR trends* (2nd ed.). Chicago, Il: HIMSS.

Pan America Health Association, & World Health Organization. (1997). *Health technology linking the Americas. Moving towards a vision: Implementing and using information systems and technology to improve health and healthcare in Latin America and the Caribbean*. Washington, D.C.: Series Health Services Information Systems.

Pan America Health Association, & World Health Organization. (1998). *Information systems and information technology in health: Challenges and solutions for Latin America and the Caribbean*. Health Services Information Systems Program. Washington, D.C.: Division of Health Systems and Services Development.

Pan America Health Association, & World Health Organization. (2001). *Building standard-based nursing information systems*. Washington, D.C.: Division of Health Systems and Services Development.

Pan America Health Association, & World Health Organization. (2003). *O Prontuário eletrônico do paciente na assistência, informação e conhecimento médico*. Washington, D.C.: Division of Health Systems and Services Development.

Saba, V. K. (2008). *Sistema de Classificação de Cuidados Clínicos – CCC*. Translated by Heimar F. Marin, São Paulo: Algol Editora.

Saba, V. K. (1992). The Classification of Home Healthcare Classification of nursing diagnoses and interventions. *Caring Magazine, 11*, 50–56.

Safran, C., Slack, W. V, & Bleich, H. (1989). Role of computing in patient care in two hospitals. *M.D. Computing, 6*, 141–148.

Sasso, G. T. M., Silveira, D. T., Peres, H. H. C., & Marin, H. M. (2010). Brasil: Case Study 14G. In C. A. Weaver, C. W. Delaney, P. Weber, & R. L. Carr (Eds.), *Nursing and informatics for the 21st century:Aan international look at practice, education and EHR trends* (2nd ed., pp.343–346). Chicago, Il: HIMSS.

50

Nursing Informatics in South Africa

Irene van Middelkoop / Susan Meyer

- OBJECTIVES
  1. Introduce the history of nursing informatics in South Africa.
  2. Identify the problems of implementing computerization in a resource-constrained environment.
  3. Describe the barriers to establishing a nursing informatics speciality.
  4. Describe nursing informatics from a South African perspective

- KEY WORDS
  nursing informatics
  South Africa
  computers
  history
  barriers

INTRODUCTION

South Africa, the most southern country at the tip of the African continent, has been through some dramatic changes in recent years. Historically, it has been a country characterized by numerous conflicts. In 1652, Dutch settlers arrived to establish a refreshment post for the ships travelling the route from Europe to the East around the African Continent. The British also arrived and conflict between the two resulted in the Boer War at the turn of the 20th century. However, animosity was put aside and by 1910, the Union of South Africa was established under joint rule. In 1961, South Africa became a republic. In 1948 the National Party implemented a policy of apartheid, which led to a period of fear and protests and culminated in the first multiracial election in 1994. This election resulted in the African National Congress coming in to power (CIA, 2010).

A number of imbalances that had evolved during the apartheid regime now had to be corrected, one of which was the provision of healthcare.

HEALTHCARE IN SOUTH AFRICA

Healthcare in South Africa consists mainly of a very large public sector and a smaller private sector (South Africa Info, 2010a). The public sector caters to those who have insufficient funds for treatment and those who do not have medical insurance, which is about 72% of the population (South Africa Info, 2010a). Nearly half of the state's expenditures are spent on health, catering to almost 80% of the population. This has created yet another imbalance: the public sector is understaffed and overutilized. During the 2007–2008 budget year, 8.5% of the gross domestic product (GDP) was spent on healthcare, of which 3.5% was spent on the 41 million people who attended public facilities, and 5% was spent on the 7 million people who attended private facilities (South Africa Info, 2010b).

Currently, there are a number of changes proposed to the health services in South Africa. The government is undertaking a change in the way healthcare is provided in the public sector by way of a national health insurance (NHI) program to which all taxpayers will contribute. The hope is that through better facilities and treatment opportunities, those who are currently unable to afford private healthcare, may at least access healthcare appropriately. It is a rather ambitious project, as the current state of public facilities will definitely require upgrading, and the number of doctors, nurses, and allied healthcare professionals will have to be increased in order to cater to the proposed changes. The year 2012 has been marked as the start of the project, and it is proposed that it will be implemented over a period of 14 years, with the required funding sourced from increased tax revenue (Pillay, 2010).

However, there is the additional burden of AIDS and tuberculosis. In a country already struggling to provide a quality health service to its people, the prevalence of the HIV pandemic has placed an enormous burden on government resources. There has been the "brain drain," whereby thousands of healthcare workers—mainly nurses—have departed for "greener pastures" in countries such as Australia, Canada, the United Kingdom, and even countries in the Middle East. It is appropriate to ask why they have left; some of the main reasons include crime, fear of degradation of the public health and education systems, general feelings of insecurity, as well as the lure of a better income in first-world countries.

All this has contributed to a dearth of nurses in a country that is crying out for more nurses in their (mainly) nurse-driven clinics as well as in hospitals (Douglas-Sweet, 2008). South Africa needs to determine how to better facilitate the remaining nurses' work by providing tools that can access information in the form of electronic patient data. This may also lure nurses back to South Africa.

In 1997, a White Paper was published on the proposed health system in South Africa. In addition, a national committee was established to look at developing a National Health Information System Strategy for South Africa (NHIS/SA) (Mbananga, 2003). As of 2010 this work is still in progress, but during this period certain hospitals have implemented their own hospital information systems including one paperless hospital in 2002 (Mbananga, 2003). However, despite the advances in hospital information systems, there has been no corresponding advances in the recognition of nursing informatics as a professional entity in South Africa.

THE HISTORY OF NURSING INFORMATICS

In 1978, an International Medical Informatics Association (IMIA) working conference was held in Cape Town on hospital information systems, led by Marion Ball (Safran, 2003). There after, in 1988, the first nursing informatics workshop was held in Rustenburg, which was attended by a number of nurses keen to take on the specialty of nursing informatics. The Western Cape province of South Africa was, at that time, the focus area for health informatics, with an informatics department being established at the Groote Schuur Hospital, which had active participation from its members.

At MEDINFO 95, a paper was presented titled Recognizing Nursing Informatics, which emphasized the need for nursing informatics to be separated from medical informatics (Babst, 1995). Sadly, the status quo remains, with no further advancement in the South African nursing informatics environment.

In 2003, South Africa submitted a country report to the IMIA Nursing Informatics Special Interest Group, which stated that a national committee had been established in 1995 to develop a National Health Information System Strategy for South Africa (NHIS/SA) (Mbananga, 2003). The White Paper for this was published in 1997 and the process is still ongoing (Khotu, 2010). One of the aims was to establish a centralized database for all the different systems currently in use in hospitals and clinics—an arduous task. The proposed National Health Insurance system will assuredly require this information for integration purposes.

NURSING EDUCATION

Currently, nursing education in South Africa offers 3 main programs: a 4-year nursing degree, a 4-year nursing diploma and then the 2-year enrolled nurse's course. Although the courses may provide some basic computer literacy classes, this is not compulsory and many nurses are computer-illiterate when embarking on their careers. This causes a problem in facilities where there is computer technology involved in nurses' work, which could take the form of a hospital information system or a simple database in a rural clinic. The number of personal computers in South Africa lags far behind the rest of the first-world countries. In 2002, South Africa was estimated to have 7.30 personal computers per 100 people (up from 0.70 in 1990) and was ranked #69 in the world. For the sake of comparison, the U.S. ranked #3 and had 65.90 personal computers per 100 people (Globalis, 2010). Frequently when new employees start work, they are confronted with a computer and are expected to be able to use it. Nurses are no different. Thus, the inclusion of even a basic computer course as a compulsory subject in all nursing education programs should be compulsory.

Needless to say, there are no courses available specifically for nursing informatics, although postgraduate qualifications in medical (or health) informatics and telemedicine are offered at certain universities.

NURSING INFORMATICS IN PRACTICE

Nurses have always had tools to work with. From Florence Nightingale with her lamp, to the modern day nurse who uses electronic tools to do all sorts of assessments when nursing a patient. The humble thermometer has now been replaced with the safer electronic one; nurses no longer have to squint to see the level of the mercury, the digits are clearly readable on the thermometer's display. So too are the charts that nurses fill in being replaced, slowly but surely, with computer input terminals. Some of them are now even able to do this data input at the bedside.

In Africa, and South Africa in particular, there is a dichotomy between those who are able to use some of the tools that are considered modern—and the computer is one of them—and those who do not have such access. Not all hospitals are computerized, but this is indeed changing. The need for rapid access to validated data is becoming a pressing need. However, it must not be assumed that hospitals with computers have indeed integrated all data.

It is often the practice that administration (i.e., patient registration) and medical information are separate entities. Therein lies the absurdity of having to do "double work." This is an important facet in that it is always up to nurses to bridge the gap—in this case, the information gap. Further, the aspects of patient care and the ever-increasing need to "show where the money is," or the billing aspect, are currently treated separately.

Nurses must never lose their identity when using this tool called a computer. The nurse is still the patient's advocate, and whether patient information is written with pen on paper or typed into a data entry system, the data must remain relevant and available in real-time.

Yes, data sets for nursing have been developed and applied so that data entries are kept standardized and data analysis can be expedited. However, free text entry must remain a part of this data collection. The nuances of nursing will be forever lost if this is not allowed.

Although patient information systems are readily available, a fully integrated hospital information system is not commonly seen in South Africa, certainly not within public hospitals. In the province of KwaZulu-Natal, there are 2 large public hospitals that have computerized hospital information systems in place, and neither are fully integrated at this point in time. One of these hospitals has had a system in place for 21 years now; the other has been in place for less than 10 years.

There is a marked difference between these two hospitals, and especially in how the nursing staff approaches the systems. The hospital that has had the system for 10 years requires nursing staff to attend a training course that lasts for a week in order to become familiar with the applied system. This same hospital has the benefit of an electronic medical record. When speaking to nurses who have worked at this institution, they lament the fact that data entry is not a seamless process. This does not foster ownership of the system by the nursing staff and for that matter, the medical staff frequently comments on the cumbersomeness of data entry. The system itself is said not to be very user-friendly.

The hospital that has had a computerized hospital information system for 21 years has the benefit of a system that has been designed by nurses and is reliant on user input to assist future development of the software. The only downside there is that the electronic medical record module, although available, has not yet been applied due to financial constraints. Despite this fact, the nursing staff is the biggest user group in the hospital and it has been shown that if it were not for the computerized hospital information system, the hospital would not cope. In addition, the nurses are in the places where they should be—the wards where the patients are.

There is no need for a nurse to run around and collect billing data for every patient activity that is done; nor do they need to physically hand write a nursing management report, which in turn must get delivered to nursing management, usually a fair distance away from the wards. This same data is now available electronically and is sent to nursing management, literally, at the push of a button.

There are many information systems being applied in South Africa, both in the public and private sectors. It seems that the decision makers, besides looking at cost, which often becomes the driving factor, would benefit from inviting nursing staff to be part of the decision-making process. A common outcry is that senior nursing management have "lost touch" with their nursing skills. This may be true in part, but there is a more serious aspect that must be addressed. Nursing informatics is a reality, and the nursing establishment needs to come to grips with this aspect of nursing. It is indeed a specialization within the wider field of nursing abilities. Nursing informatics is not mutually exclusive, nor is it something that can be taken for granted. There are certain skills required to understand nursing concepts and precepts as well as to be cognitive of how tools, and in this case computers, are best applied to foster and enhance the appropriate care of patients.

HOW NURSES USE TECHNOLOGY

When considering how most nurses approach technology, the words that come to mind are *with caution*! It seems that nurses have to inspect all elements of how the technology functions and can best be used in the actual clinical environment before they reach a level of comfort with it. And that is the correct approach. As with every tool applied, caution must be exercised.

The presence computers in the nursing environment is not a new concept, but it is still not quite fully accepted on a broad scale in South Africa. If you are a nurse in the private sector the presence of computers is almost expected, but this is not so in the often-poorer public sector hospitals.

The best way for nurses to become familiar with new tools and technologies is to use them. Herein lies the crux: if systems are not fashioned for nurses to use seamlessly in their natural working environment, they are simply not going to be used. The choice of systems is vital. The system must include the flexibility for customization to suit the needs of nurses as required. In so doing, nurses will utilize these tools far more readily. However, very little emphasis is being placed on introducing nursing informatics as a skill set during training. This means that nurses learn systems (often paper-based) they may not necessarily encounter once they enter the nursing profession.

Much emphasis is being placed on the workload burden nurses are facing. Furthermore, in Africa, South Africa, and in particular the province of KwaZulu-Natal, HIV, AIDS, and tuberculosis are spiraling out of control. Patients are severely ill. Nursing staff numbers are constantly decreasing. Every conceivable tool needs to be applied to assist nurses in doing their job in a manner that is conducive to smooth workflow processes and facilitates patient care. Patients are entitled to quality care. The tools that are employed to enable nurses to perform their functions must not put nurses or their patients in harms way, and must promote the wellbeing of both.

Regardless of which computerized system is implemented, it must be set up by nurses who are familiar with systems thinking. Nursing is an applied science. Nursing informatics is the blending of practical nursing and technology. The goal is to have information that is usable for decision-making purposes and that can be interpreted universally with consistency. The information must always have patient safety at its core and, although specific in nature, must have the flexibility to include nursing processes that make sense to both the patient and the nurse.

STANDARDS

Presently, standards for computerized hospital information systems in South Africa are very rare. This is still an emerging field. In fact, there is very little change since 2003 when the following was described: "However despite these problems the importance of Health Informatics, and specifically Nursing Informatics, is definitely not perceived as a priority and generally has not yet been embraced by the nursing profession as something necessary for improving quality of care or as a tool that could improve their lot!" (Mbananga, 2003).

The National Health Information System (NHIS) has proposed a Management Information System, which is expected to be fully compliant with "open systems" standards. The NHIS indicated that the system should have the following functionalities (Khotu, 2010):

1. Fully operable on a network

2. Preferably have been developed using a fourth generation applications software development tool, a relational database management system, and a data dictionary

3. Have interfaces to popular programming languages

4. Have a front-end graphical user interface (GUI) product

5. Support the main electronic data interchange (EDI) formats

The Council for Health Service Accreditation of Southern Africa (COHSASA) is the watch-dog group regarding standards for patient care in South Africa. Hospitals achieve their ratings through a process of accreditation that is based on defined standards.

The following excerpt is reprinted directly from the COHSASA's Web site (COHSASA, 2010):

> The Council for Health Service Accreditation of Southern Africa assists a range of healthcare facilities to meet and maintain quality standards. It does so by enabling healthcare professionals to measure themselves against these standards and monitor improvements using our quality improvement methods, internationally accredited standards and a web-based information system.
>
> Our work shows us that strictly applied quality improvement methods can improve patient safety and the quality of care by guiding interventions, monitoring progress and identifying improvements. We also identify impediments to improvement and develop strategies to overcome them.
>
> COHSASA provides data on the quality of health service provision to governing authorities so that it can be used for strategic decisions. In the past 15 years over 553 facilities have entered the COHSASA programme.

Accreditation is a continuous process and, if not maintained, just becomes another activity the institution does because it is mandated. However, the standards for computerized hospital information systems are still growing, and much of the documentation required by COHSASA is still paper-based. The use of the electronic signature is an area that has to be debated legally and until such time, the good old-fashioned written signature will remain firmly in place. This too is a stumbling block in integrating nursing informatics into the information age.

CONCLUSION

A concerted effort is required by the informatics community to bring nursing informatics to the attention of educators and to the nursing community at large. More information needs to be disseminated so that the importance of nursing informatics, especially concerning the use of systems for information and patient management, is directed to the right sectors. It is the way of the future, but without skilled and trained nurses who are able to use the tools available to provide optimum patient care, the benefit of having such first-class technology may be lost.

REFERENCES

Babst, T. A., & Isaacs, S. (1995). Recognizing nursing informatics. *Medinfo. 8*(2), 1313–1315.

The Council for Health Service Accreditation of Southern Africa (COHSASA). (n.d.). Retrieved from http://www.cohsasa.co.za/health-service-read-more

CIA. (2010). *CIA - The world factbook.* Retrieved from https://www.cia.gov/library/publications/the-world-factbook/geos/countrytemplate_sf.html.

Douglas-Sweet, V. (2008). The storm after the calm: South Africa moves to a primary healthcare model. *Advanced Practice Nursing eJournal*, Retrieved from http://www.medscape.com/viewarticle/572044.

Globalis. (2002). *Personal Computer in Use*. Retrieved from http://globalis.gvu.unu.edu.

Khotu, D. S. (n.d.). *National Healthcare Management Information System of South Africa NCH/MIS.* Retrieved from http://www.doh.gov.za/nhis/docs/nchmis.htm.

Mbananga, N. D. K. (2003). *Nursing informatics in South Africa: A country report.* IMIA.

Pillay, V. (2010, September 21). ANC aims to implement NHI in 2012. *Mail & Guardian Online.* Retrieved from http://www.mg.co.za/article/2010-09-21-anc-aims-to-implement-nhi-in-2012.

Safran, C. (2003). Presentation of Morris F. Collen Award to Dr. Marion J Ball. *J Am Med Inform Assoc, 10*(3), 287–288.

SOUTHAFRICA.INFO. (2010a). *Healthcare in South Africa.* Retrieved from http://www.southafrica.info/about/health/health.htm.

SOUTHAFRICA.INFO. (2010b). *NHI: 'Decent healthcare for all'.* Retrieved from http://www.southafrica.info/news/nhi-010709.htm

PART 9

The Future of Informatics

Kathleen A. McCormick

Future Directions

Kathleen A. McCormick

- ## OBJECTIVES

  1. Define the differences between personal health and personalized health.
  2. Provide a vision for a patient centric future.
  3. Discuss the information technology supports for personalized health.
  4. Define the translational health future and the benefits to healthcare.
  5. Understand nursing's role and the educational resources available for nursing informatics to embrace this exciting future.

- ## KEY WORDS

  Personal Health
  Personalized Health
  Translational HealthcAre
  Genetics/Genomic/Bioinformatics
  Ethical/Legal/Social Implications
  Educational Competencies

INTRODUCTION

Each preceding chapter looks at an aspect of the future of nursing informatics involved in improving patient care, improving quality, increasing safety, improving resource utilization, establishing effectiveness of care, accelerating knowledge diffusion, reducing variability of healthcare delivery and access, empowering consumers, protecting security of data and information, assuring privacy and protections, promoting public health, assuring appropriate responsiveness to biologic events, and focusing on efficiently delivering care in a cost-effective manner. This chapter focuses on the role of personal and personalized health moving forward. This can be considered the penultimate evidence in patient care leading to precise diagnosis and treatment for individuals. The emerging needs of translational healthcare that establishes a new

continuum of care for the patients requiring coordination of care in a new continuum driven by new policy frameworks adapting this individual personalize care to enterprises and populations with similar conditions will also be discussed. The chapter further describes the unique role in counseling that nursing has traditionally been involved in supporting the ethical, legal, and social concerns of the patient and family. New educational resources are described that stimulate all nurses whether in informatics or other areas of nursing care to seek advanced education to participate as educated consumers in this new future of the first half of the 21st century (American Association of Colleges of Nursing, 2006).

In 2003 when we were celebrating the 50th anniversary of James Watson and Francis Crick's Nobel Prize–winning description of the DNA double helix, Francis Collins, now the Director of the National Institutes of

Health (NIH) (2010) predicted that we would have about a dozen validated, predictive genetic tests for as many as a dozen common conditions (Collins, Green, Guttmacher, & Guyer, 2003). Now in 2011, the new path from genetics to the next era of genomic medicine has been described; taking the science from base pairs to bedside (Green, Guyer and NHGRI, 2011). McCormick and Hoffman predicted that nursing would be able to use genetic factors to predict symptoms, increase wound healing and postoperative responses based upon the genetics of inflammation and blood coagulation, and even prevent some of the symptoms associated with inflammation and fatigue (McCormick & Hoffman, 2006). Today, there are reported to be nearly 600 genome-wide association studies covering 150 distinct disease and traits that have been published. There are 800 single-nucleotide polymorphisms (trait associations) that merit more testing to determine if they are genetic predictors, biomarkers, or involved in a multiple genetic pathway to conditions and disease (Manolio, 2010). Those genetic studies that have direct correlation with health conditions and disease require nursing, medical, and basic research to determine the associations so that these tests can be routinely incorporated into the healthcare delivery of patient care. However, many of these associations are still uncertain and further basic research is necessary before the clinical practice area can determine if the genetic testing is going to predict a disease. Another possible use of knowledge of your genetics is to be able to prevent disease, conditions, and symptoms. A third area is to determine if after a diagnosis you can match the treatment to the genetics profile which is the hope for personalized health. A key to moving forward is for the consumer to participate in the design of their care. Even if the students of nurses are not going to pursue a future that involved genetic care to patients, we are all going to be consumers of the genetic information in planning, designing, treating and evaluating the outcomes of our own personal health. The next section will describe how we as consumers and caregivers for our clients and patients can participate in their personal health. But first, what are the challenges to nurses in informatics?

THE CHALLENGES TO NURSES IN INFORMATICS

As Walker says in her chapter on nursing informatics, "nurses must be strategists, leaders, great communicators, and engage stakeholders across the multiple spectrums to ensure patients, nursing, and technological needs are understood and met" (Walker, 2010). This chapter will present six main challenges that the nurse studying this

chapter should come away with. The main challenges for nurses in informatics are to: (1) learn where to get reliable data to become informed by attending conferences, getting on list services of genomic discoveries, become engaged on networks of communication related to specific preventions/diseases/conditions/medications; (2) obtain advanced education in genetics, genomics, or biotechnology and engineering; (3) become the impetus for the message shaping the policies that develop effective use of genomics in prevention, diagnosis, and treatment of persons; (4) participate in task forces or committees deciding on the selection and implementation of designing genomic content in health records; (5) expand evidence and develop design components for workflows of decision making that involve the inclusion of genomic content; (6) conduct research on the utilization of genomics in healthcare focused on patient care and health services research on costs, patient preferences, and consumer choice.

A DEFINITION OF PERSONAL HEALTH

The role of personal health in the future begins the patient centric focus to offer patients access to their personal health information. Some of the multifaceted ways of delivering personal health information are through services, systems, and host platforms that allow consumers to keep their information and manage their own healthcare (Friends of the National Library of Medicine, 2009). The content that has been collected in personal health information systems includes: medication profiles, allergies, immunization profiles, chief medical condition(s), recent procedures and laboratory results. Of note is the usual absence of nursing assessments, functional abilities, including feeding, mobility, continence, pain and other symptom management, and conditions in personal health records, except for the vital signs that are collected and observed by nurses.

Personal records are linked to device information to allow the practitioner to monitor basic health profiles such as weight, blood pressure, temperature, and pulse.

Newer systems include blood glucose monitoring and decision supports for managing activities of daily living, insulin levels, and weight.

Most of the personal health records have allowed users to opt in or opt out of sharing data with healthcare professionals or other individuals. This assumes a level of consciousness that allows decision making at the time of a health occurrence.

There are several companies engaged in providing a personal health record. Three of the major personal health record systems are those from the Veterans Administration, MyHealthyVet, the Microsoft Vault, and Google Health. Entering the market are large electronic health record (EHR) vendors such as EPIC systems with information directly from the patient with MyChart or Lucy (EPIC, 2010). Some of the primary personal health record system vendors are teamed with large providers, EHR vendors, private pharmacy companies, laboratory chains, healthcare consortia, and community healthcare networks. It is currently not known how many of the major personal health record system vendors employ nursing informatics experts.

INTERACTIVE VOICE RESPONSE (IVR)

Interactive voice response allows the consumer or health provider to get information on a subject 24 hours a day. They are either hosted call or on-demand. They are used in call centers to route callers to the correctly matched resource. It is a phone-based triage system. This telephone technology is increasing and users frequently ask questions to standard repetitive questions. The decision trees for IVR systems follow the workflow of the potential calls and have as many prerecorded responses as possible. Callers can opt out and speak to a person. It is similarly not known how many nurses are working in IVR centers and where they get their professional support.

A PATIENT-CENTRIC FUTURE

Direct-to-consumer testing (DTC) began to engage the patient in profiling genes of individuals. The developments of repositories of patients who have come forward to test their genes and allow their profiles to be anonymously shared have grown to some of the largest disease repositories internationally. Several companies such as 23andMe, Knome, Decode Genetics, and Navigenics are making genetic test results and positive and negative predictive risk results available to the consumers. Recently, the inconsistencies in tests have been reported in *Nature*, and the Food and Drug Administration (FDA) has questioned these as unapproved diagnostic devices (*Nature*, 2009). Another company, Illumina, has been questioned by the FDA because they provide the tools to the DTC companies. All of these organizations (companies, FDA, and NIH) are developing standards and guidelines for providing genetic test results and risk estimates. They all seek to develop validation of these tests and predictive values of these tests because that could lead to results common to all companies and have a positive impact on disease diagnosis and treatment in the future.

In additional to the genetic sequencing companies, networks are developing utilizing social networking and Web 2.0 technology. These are becoming the domain of social networks or participatory medicine (www.health2con.com). Personalized health also includes the capability to conduct personalized searches using intelligent tools to better integrate data and content to convert to knowledge about your personal health. LinkedIn, Flickr, Vimeo, YouTube, Zinger, Twitter, and Facebook are all additions to the informatics domain. But within these domains, millions of nurses and patients are getting connected with Blue Button that challenges not only the policies and governance of healthcare, but also prevention, diagnosis, and treatment. The Blue Button Challenge is sponsored by the Markle Foundation and Robert Wood Johnson Foundation. It calls for Web applications developers to demonstrate how they can help people manage their health by making use of data from Medicare and the Veterans Administration.

We know that at least 61% of people are on the Internet look for information related to their health (http://www.pewtrusts.org/news_room_detail.aspx?id=53352). The amount of information varies from sharing information with patients with a similar diagnosis and condition, to uploading evidence and information from valid sources of government and professional organizational information. Today's patient care even access drug–drug interaction and side effects with a unique system for medication checking called DoubleCheckMD (DoublecheckMD, 2010).

Baaken and colleagues (2008) predicted this shift would occur. What this means is that patients with a particular condition are getting together on the web and seeking information on their diagnosis and cure, advances in science and technologies. One example is a network of women who have breast cancer and/or want to prevent it. Beckman Research Institute at the City of Hope in combination with the Susan Love Research Consortium is developing a network study of one million women to examine the causes, treatment, and prevention of breast cancer (Love, 2010). The goal is to empower women to connect to the work of research to know what clinical trials are available to treat their type of breast cancer.

The Family Health History—A Window into Predicting Disease Risks

Capturing a family history is a window into the genetic profile of a person and their family tree. A family history helps clinicians determine the susceptibility and risks of disease and conditions. Formalized capturing of the family history became a recognized priority of the Public Health Service Surgeon General in November 2004 (Department of Health & Human Services, 2004). The Surgeon General recommended that family members record a family history of risks of heart disease, cancer, and diabetes at least once a year in the United States at Thanksgiving when most families get together. Providing that paternity is what persons believe to be true, the family history is also unraveling some of the epigenetic trends that are passed down from generation to generation in the genetic maps. With more frequent genetic tests for conditions, the data are revealing that a father is actually not the biological father of the patient 5% to 10% of the time (McCormick & Hoffman, 2006). Pedigree tools have been developed to be included into EHRs and personal health records so that persons can capture their family history in the EHR.

Personalized Health Defined

Personalized health allows the capture of information so that the diagnosis and treatment can be tailored to an individual's health condition, susceptibility to a condition, and prevention of a condition (Buetow, 2009). It is a paradigm shift for the nursing profession because it focuses on genomic healthcare, shifts the research from a pipeline of discovery to and adaptive clinical trials model. Biomarkers of disease are now showing promise in informing treatment choices in some conditions such as breast cancer, but validation of the biomarkers requires clinical trials that have routinely been long and expensive.

The concept of using advanced information technology (IT) to improve treatment and accelerate advances in disease management such as cancer, is applying the concept of a "rapid learning health system" (Institute of Medicine, 2010a). The goal of these systems is to improve information access to deliver the best care at the point of care and personalized for each patient.

The adaptive clinical trial utilizes a new design of clinical trials. The ultimate goal is to shorten the time and cost from bench genomic research to drug discovery and patient treatment (Ivy, Siu, Garrett-Mayer, Rubenstein, 2010). New trials are being designed by the National Cancer Institute that can more efficiently screen breast cancer patients for promising agents that would normally take 15 to 20 years for drug availability to only a few years. The study is considered an adaptive clinical trial in which the data is used in real time combining information from the EHR and research information to direct the course of treatment for cancer trial participants (http://ispy2.org). The statistics analyses necessary to conduct predictive probability science are evaluated simultaneously in these new trials.

The adaptive clinical trial supported by innovative IT is being demonstrated at the University of California, San Francisco and multiple cancer sites in the country. The focus is on breast cancer. The IT component, I-SPY2, allows the clinicians/researchers to stratify patient into different treatment options according to their genetic profiles and to predict the response to their treatment (Barker, Sigman, Kelloff, et al., 2009).

The development of personalized science is a paradigm shift in the way that we have classically approached diagnosis and treatment. The shift is toward subclassifying individuals based on genetic, environmental, and other factors of disease into tailored treatments for their specific condition. Advances in genomics and microbiology, proteomics, and metabolomics are beginning to identify molecular markers that occur in persons who have a disease, condition, susceptibility to a disease, or a different response to treatment (PricewaterhouseCoopers, 2009).

Clinical and populations studies also require massive data collection of biospecimens and biorepositories, as well as biomarker standardized data incorporating the advanced genetic and molecular analyses. Biomedical informatics is also required in personalized medicine. Advances in the new science require the development of service oriented architectures (SOAs), storage on CLOUDS, and computational analytic skills in biomedical informatics (White House, 2008). Demonstrating that the White House reports are realities are several national efforts. The Lance Armstrong Foundation is a federated collaboration focused on tissue biospecimen samples of individuals aged 15 to 39 who have been diagnosed with cancer. An entire state, Arizona, is entering into this model of personal health in establishing a statewide biospecimen repository (National Cancer Center Annual Report 2009; National Cancer Institute, 2010a). Large academic institutions entering into enterprise-wide research support include the Winthrop P. Rockefeller Cancer Institute at the University of Arkansas for Medical Sciences . They track patients from admission to scheduling treatment, monitoring adverse events and clinical laboratory results and accessing biospecimen data for molecular diagnosis.

Additionally, the University of Alabama at Birmingham has driven an enterprise-wide integrated platform. They are using open source molecular, tissue, and other tools to manage the large volumes of data linking research environment. Integrated databases are a hallmark of consortium science in linking large academic settings to aggregate data of patients with specific genetic-based diagnostic tests, to confirm disease by gender and ethnic groups, and recommend differential treatments. The next quest is the linkage of these personalized data with the patient's individual health records and the EHR (McCormick, 2009). By extending the new personalized health beyond the classic clinical trials, larger populations of patients can be studied, new treatments can be developed, and adverse reporting of treatments can be monitored from diverse populations. This new technology warrants the nursing and engineering scientist to be particularly vigilant to several policy areas, including technology development, regulations, rules, imaging transmission, interoperability of platforms, common data standards, reimbursement, intellectual property, privacy and security. New technologies are being invented for both nurses and engineers to become engaged in as the area of personalized health expands. (McCormick, K.A., Sensmeier, J, Delaney, C & Bickford, C, 2012).

TRANSLATIONAL HEALTHCARE

Translational research bridges the benefits of personal and personalized health to the consumer and the clinicians in hospitals, community healthcare environments, ambulatory care, the community at large, and homecare (National Center for Research Resources, 2010). The technological challenges of translational health offer nursing informatics research and practice challenges. The teams being established for translational research also engage multidisciplinary teams. Translational research also requires the coordination of public and private entities such as academic settings and pharmaceutical companies in order to transfer the bench finding to bedside application. This is another shift occurring which moves some of the developments for the consumer from the industry to large academic consortia. The integration of longitudinal data in order to study a health condition also becomes critical in translational research as the clinical conditions present themselves over time.

Information Technology for Personal, Personalized, and Translational Healthcare

The mobile digital technology advances that began over a decade ago have converged on computer power, miniaturization, touch screen technologies, and high bandwidth for telephones. The new powerful, low-cost platforms are allowing healthcare professionals and consumers to access health information via smart phone apps, such as for the iPhone and iPad, from almost anywhere. The integration of these devices with entertainment, reminders, monitors, and even avatars, is presenting new opportunities for the development of health applications for almost every major condition. Already these smart phones and tablet computers

are changing the ways that nurses can monitor patients with such chronic conditions as congestive heart failure, diabetes, obesity; monitoring adverse drug effects; monitoring pain management and many other chronic symptoms and conditions such as fatigue, nausea, vomiting, and hair loss among other symptoms. The integration of these devices with geographical locators allows consumers to find the nearest healthcare facility, hospital, or 24-hour pediatric clinic. Their application to biosurveillance and bioterrorism, and inventory management in healthcare is just beginning.

Benefits of Using Information Systems in Patient Care

The transformative changes in present day healthcare throughout the United States include: (1) a focus on population health with services and technologies to support wellness and disease prevention; (2) self-management for those with chronic disease and transitioning resources and services from acute care to community and home; (3) a person-centric focus in care delivery and services for patient empowerment; (4) healthcare system reform using EHRs and other technologies that extend across all levels of services and care settings, including the person's home; and (5) increased resource demands including capacity as well as challenges in the healthcare workforce's skills and preparedness for this new work environment.

The Institute of Medicine (IOM) report *To Err Is Human: Building a Safer Health System* (Institute of Medicine, 1999) served as a wakeup call to the American public by documenting the grave and prevailing deficiency in quality that characterizes healthcare in the United States. This first in a series of reports from the IOM's quality initiative spoke to the serious needs for improvement and reform. A second report followed, *Crossing the Quality Chasm: A New Health System for the 21st Century* (Institute of Medicine, 2001), which offered a blueprint for such improvement and urged all organizations, professional groups, policy makers, educators, and healthcare providers to engage in the organic change required to make healthcare safer, effective, timely, efficient, equitable, and patient centered. This report also called for the essential redesign of health professional education to prepare the numbers and the kinds of providers required to activate and grow a quality-centered healthcare system. A third IOM report entitled *Health Professions Education: A Bridge to Quality* (Institute of Medicine, 2003) offered a strategy for redesigning the education of healthcare professionals to promote and sustain a reformed and responsive healthcare system. Five essential health professional competencies were identified to support and sustain the healthcare system. Health professionals need to be able to (1) provide patient-centered care, (2) work in interdisciplinary teams, (3) employ evidence-based practice, (4) apply quality improvement and fundamental to the preceding four, and (5) make use of informatics. Fundamentally all of these IOM reports acknowledge the critical role of information. There is a clear synergy among the changes in national and international healthcare environments, huge shifts in nations' health policies, the essential characteristics of the transformative healthcare system, and the areas of essential competencies of healthcare professionals. Informatics is fundamental to enhancing the performance of the other four IOM health professional competencies. The understanding and application of informatics facilitates and augments patient or client-centered care, interdisciplinary teamwork, quality improvement, and the incorporation of evidence into practice. The extensive application of informatics is a critical component of healthcare practice for all professions, and needed to enhance the safety and effectiveness of care. In the next section, the education of nurses to participate in these seismic changes, as a healthcare professional or consumer, will be described.

EDUCATIONAL RESOURCES FOR NURSING IT IN GENOMICS

As Androwich and colleagues state, one of the important influences in understanding the future is to know what competencies are available and how to access them (Androwich Kraft, & Haas, 2008). These educators further state competencies need to be understood not only by faculty and students in education but also for all nurses as consumers of their own healthcare. Basic genomic education is needed by nurses in administration and practice settings to understand what is needed in IT going forward. It is cogent that our leaders in nursing will be continually updating information by learning, unlearning, and relearning—a strategy of lifelong learning. This chapter focuses on competencies and new educational resources defined for nursing involved in our genomic future whether they are nurse leaders, academicians, clinicians, researchers, public health practitioners, or patient advocates. Historically, genetic and genomic educational programs have been prominent at the National Institutes of Health from the National Human Genome Research Institute (NHGRI) (2010), the National Center for Biotechnology Information (NCBI, 2010) from the National Library of Medicine, and the National Cancer Institute (2010b). The Department of

Energy (2010) also provides excellent training materials for genetics and genomics. The NCBI has tutorial information and toolkits and databases. Among the popular products for genetics and genomics on the NCBI site are BLAST (for genomic sequence), GenBank, Gene, OMIM, dbSNP, dbGAP (for genes and human health) which link to PubMed; and deCODE, UniSTS and electronic PCR (maps and markers); and UniGene, GEO, DNA sequencing projects, and SAGEmap (for transcribed sequences); BAC resources and SKY/CGH (for cytogenetics); and HomoloGene and Homology Map (for comparative genomics). While these are toolkits for discovery, what nurses in IT might want to look at are the NCBI home page of human genome resources that include the NIH Epigenomics Roadmap which maps the studies that have identified genes and their association to disease (http://www.ncbi.nlm.gov/guide/training-tutorials).

Another excellent resource for educational products online is from the Department of Energy's Human Genome Project Information (2010). The resources include educational modules related to genetics, pharmacogenomics, genetic counseling, and disease information. Ethical, legal, and social issues include patenting, forensics, genetically modified food, and human migration in addition to other areas. The publications and teaching products include online modules, videos and Web casts, graphics, and even animations (www.ornl.gov).

Funded by the NHGRI, the National Coalition for Health Professional Education in Genetics (NCHPEG) is a national organization that has been developing competencies for nurses involved in genetics for many years (NCHPEG, 2010). These competencies include basic genetics, ethical, and legal counseling related to genetic diseases.

In 2009, the NHGRI announced a funded educational program based at the University of Virginia called the Genetics/Genomics Competency Center (G2C2) that can be accessed at www.genome.gov (NHGRI, 2009). This program is designed to provide educators online resources to teach nurses and physician assistants about genetics and genomics and the applications available in healthcare today. The site includes materials that are meant to help the healthcare professionals become familiar with new practice trends in personalized medicine. Provided in the center are cross-mapped learning activities and assessments, outcome indicators and professional competencies, such as the genomics nursing competencies, curriculum guidelines, and outcome indicators.

Another university-based genetics training center is the University of Utah (2010). Their site Learn Genetics includes basic genetics, DNA to protein, understanding heredity and traits, amazing cells, stem cells, cloning, gene therapy, and transgenic mice. In addition, three fascinating pages are called: (1) Build a DNA Molecule, (2) Cell Size & Scale, and (3) Lick your Rats. Lick your Rats is an interactive learning program on how maternal behavior shapes epigenomes.

In 2008, the National Cancer Institute announced the funding for six Knowledge Centers that provide knowledge articles, a forum for questions and answers, and a wiki for open communication specifically about advances in biomedical computing to support cancer genetics and genomics. These same resources are being expanded to support additional healthcare conditions, such as heart, lung, and blood diseases and conditions. The centers focus on the (1) architecture; (2) molecular analysis; (3) data sharing, informed consent, privacy and security issues; (4) tissue; (5) clinical trials; and (6) vocabulary and ontology (NCI, 2010b).

The Centers for Disease Control and Prevention (CDC) has published minimum genomic competencies in public health. The competencies include environmental, ethnic disparities, health policy, law, risk, maternal-child health with links to toxicology and teratology, preventative and behavioral conditions such as obesity, communicable diseases, and family history. Since diagnosis of hereditary genetics is a primary focus in public health for pediatric inherited diseases, such as phenylketonuria, the CDC recognized the importance of genetics as a priority in public health education. The priorities for genomic competencies for all public health professionals in clinical services evaluating individual or families describe the health professional able to:

- Apply basic genomic concepts including patterns of inheritance, gene-environment interactions, role of genes in health and disease, and implications for health promotion programs to relevant clinical services

- Demonstrate understanding of the indications for, components of, and resources for genetic testing and/or genomic-based interventions

- Describe ethical, legal, social, and financial issues related to genetic testing and recording of genomic information

- Explain basic concepts of probability and risk and benefits of genomics in health and disease assessment in the context of the clinical practice

- Deliver genomic information, recommendations, and care without patient or family coercion within an appropriate informed-consent process.

The CDC utilizes genetics to analyze the bacterial genomes that may be involved in suspected disease outbreaks to readily determine whether the cases have a common origin (they share a genomic pattern) or are of disparate origins. There are current 3500 genes that might enable microbes and toxins to harm cells and tissues. Likewise, the use of genomic technologies is increasingly being utilized in support of identifying the genetics of infectious agents and their transmission in such areas as hospital infection control practices, and the spread of infections and viruses, and reportable diseases.

The National Office of Public Health Genomics at the CDC has many excellent resources that link the genomics into public health research, policy, and practice to prevent disease and improve health (2010). The site has many valuable resources including the Genomic Applications in Practice and Prevention Network (GAPPNet). This is a collaborative initiative involving the CDC, NCI Division of Cancer Control and Population Sciences, and other stakeholders. The goals of the initiative are to use valid and useful genomic information and applications, such as genetic tests, technologies, and family history into clinical and public health practice (CDC, 2010). Another valuable resource from the CDC for genetic/genomic influences in public health is the Human Genome Epidemiology Network (HugeNet) (CDC, 2010). The navigator of HugeNet allows the user to help translate genetic research findings into opportunities for preventive healthcare and public health. The network provides a synthesis, interpretation, and dissemination of population-based data on human genetic variation in health and in disease. Persons doing collaborative population genetics are encouraged to use HugeNet.

Claudia Mikail (2008) has authored a book entitled *Public Health Genomics: The Essentials*. The book expands the competencies of the CDC and also includes a description of molecular genetics, discusses the relevancy to public health issues in environmental health, ethnic health disparities, health policy and law, research ethics, maternal and child health, clinical preventive medicine, health behavior, health economics, and communicable disease control.

More educational training and resources recommendations come from the recent Department of Health and Human Services (HHS) Secretary's Advisory Committee on Genetics, Health and Society (SACGHS) that has issued a new report to describe the proposals for enhancing *Genetics Education and Training for Healthcare Professionals, Public Health Providers, and Consumers* (NIH, 2010). The chair of the SACGHS task force was Barbara Burns McGrath who is a research associate at the School of Nursing at the University of

Washington. This report describes the new training and teaching models required, stressing the need for incorporating pedigree maps for family health histories in vendor services, and proposing innovative incentives for reimbursement of healthcare providers who begin to grasp the utilization of genetic information and family histories for patients. All of these new advances have the potential of widening the digital divide for those who are poor, disenfranchised, or culturally diverse. The report focuses on healthcare professionals, public health providers, and patients and consumers. Besides recommending a national workshop that identifies new educational and training guidelines, the HHS intends to make available new funding streams to pay for educational advances, advancing the educational content, offer ideas for developing new and relevant educational standards, develop an ongoing advisory panel, and develop a plan to monitor the outcome of national efforts. A focus on underserved populations will be a targeted training activity from HHS. Integrating genetics and genomics as core competencies in healthcare provider educational program should ultimately be incentivized by this HHS programs. Organized IT nursing and public policy groups need to support these further initiatives.

The need for specialized genetic education for healthcare professionals, engineers and consumers is being driven by the revolution in science occurring at the bench and the need to quickly transfer this information to those in the field, as well as to consumers who can benefit from the advanced genomic science. Advances in genomics and personalized medicine are quickly advancing into the practices of doctors and advanced nurses as well as the everyday reading of consumers. Therefore, steps have begun to keep these groups educated and prepared to understand the implications of these tests on their susceptibility to disease, prevention of disease, and diagnosis and personalized treatments that may be available (Mantas, et al, 2010).

SUMMARY

This chapter exposes the reader to advances occurring in personal, personalized, and translational healthcare. It provides the educational recourses that can be utilized as a beginning foundation in understanding this exciting future. The main challenges for nursing to become involved are: (1) learn where to get reliable data to become informed by attending conferences, getting on list services of genomic discoveries, become engaged on networks of communication related to specific preventions/diseases/conditions/medications; (2) obtain advanced education in genetics, genomics, or biotech-

nology and engineering; (3) become the impetus for the message shaping the policies that develop effective use of genomics in prevention, diagnosis, and treatment of persons; (4) participate in task forces or committees deciding on the selection and implementation or designing genomic content in health records; (5) expand evidence and develop design components for workflows of decision making that involve the inclusion of genomic content; (6) conduct research on the utilization of genomics in healthcare focused on patient care and health services research on costs, patient preferences, and consumer choice. It provides the nurses links to places to acquire basic information whether they are consumers of healthcare, or delivering healthcare in multiple environments. Several competencies have been previously identified by nurses involved in shaping this future.

REFERENCES

American Association of Colleges of Nursing. (2006). *The essentials of doctoral education for advanced nursing practice*. Retrieved June 1, 2010 fromhttp://www.aacn. nche.edu/dnp/pdf/essentials.pdf

Androwich, I. M., Kraft, M. R., & Haas, S. (2008). Information technology core competencies: From now to tomorrow. *Nursing Outlook, 56*(5), 189–190.

Baaken, S., Stone, P. W., & Larson, E. I. (2008). A nursing informatics research agenda for 2008-2018: Contextual influences and key components. *Nursing Outlook, 56*(5), 206–214.

Barker, A. D., Sigman, C. C., Kelloff, G. H., Hylton, M. N., Berry, D. A., Esserman, I. J. (2009). I-SPY2: an adaptive breast cancer trial design in the setting of neoadjuvant chemotherapy. *Clin Pharmacol Ther, 86*(1), 97–100.

Buetow, K. H. (2009). The Biomedical Informatics GRID (BIG). *A platform for 21st century biomedicine*. In Nationwide Health Information Network Advances: Foundation for Interoperable Health Information Exchange Established – Path to Nationwide Production Set. Retrieved June 4, 2010 from http://www.hhs.gov/ myhealthcare/news/phc_2008_report.pdf

Centers for Disease Control and Prevention. (2010). *National Office of Public Health Genomics*. http://www. cdc.gov/genomics/translation/competencies/index.htm

Collins, F. S., Green, E. D., Guttmacher, A. E., & Guyer, A. S. (2003). *A vision for the future of genomics research*. Retrieved June 4, 2010 from http://www.genome. gov/11007524

Collins, F. S. (2010). *The language of life*. New York: HarperCollins.

Department of Energy. (2010). *Human genome project information*. Retrieved June 4, 2010 from http:// www.ornl.gov/sci/techresources/Human_Genome/ education/education.shtml

Department of Health & Human Services. (2004). *HHS launches new family history initiative.* Retrieved July 2010 from http://www.hhs.gov/familyhistory

DoublecheckMD. (2010). Retrieved September 2010 from http://www.doublecheckMD.com

Friends of the National Library of Medicine. (2009). *Personal health record. Presentations from the Conference.* Retrieved June 2, 2010 from http://www.fnlm.org

Green, E.D., Guyer, M.S., and the National Human Genome Research Institute (February 10, 2011). Charting a course for genomic medicine from base pairs to bedside. *Nature, 470,* 204–213.

Institute of Medicine. (1999). *To err is human.* Washington, DC: National Academies Press.

Institute of Medicine. (2001). Committee on Quality of Healthcare in America, Institute of Medicine. *Crossing the quality chasm: A new health system for the 21st century.* Washington, DC: National Academies Press.

Institute of Medicine. (2003). *Health professions education: A bridge to quality.* Washington, DC: National Academies Press.

Institute of Medicine. (2010a). *A foundation for evidence-driven practice. A rapid learning system for cancer care.* Washington, DC: National Academies Press.

Institute of Medicine. (2010b). *The future of nursing: Acute care.* Washington, DC: National Academies Press.

Ivy, S. P., Siu, L. L., Garrett-Mayer, E., & Rubenstein, L. (2010). Approaches to phase 1 clinical trial design focused on safety, efficiency, and selected patient populations: a report from the clinical trial design task force of the national cancer institute investigational drug steering committee. *Clinical Cancer Research, 16*(6):1726–1736.

Love, Susan. (2010). *Army of women.* Retrieved July 4, 2010 from http://www.armyofwomen.org/

Manolio, T. (2010) Genomewide association studies and assessment of the risk of disease. *New England Journal of Medicine, 363,* 166–176.

Mantas, J. Ammenwerth, E., Demiris, G., Hasman, A., Haux, R., Hersh, W., et al. (2010). Recommendations of the International Medical Informatics Association (IMIA) on education in biomedical and health informatics. *Methods of Information in Medicine, 49,* 105–120.

McCormick, K. A., & Hoffman, M. (2006). Genomics and bioinformatics relationship to current day electronic health record. In Weaver, C.A., Delaney, C.W., Weber, P, Carr, Robyn, L., et al. (Eds.), *Nursing and Informatics for the 21st Century: An International Look at Practice, Trends and the Future.* Chicago: HIMSS.

McCormick, K. A. (2009). *Individualizing cancer care with interoperable information systems.* Helsinki, Finland: IMIA-NI.

McCormick, K. A., Sensmeier, J., Delaney, C., & Bickford, C. (2012). An update of informatics and nursing. In

J. Bronzino (Ed.), *Handbook of biomedical engineering* (4th ed.). Boca Raton, FL: CRC Press.

Mikail, C. N. (2008). *Public health genomics:* The essentials. San Francisco, CA: Jossey-Bass.

National Cancer Institute. (2010a). *Empowering collaboration across the cancer community.* 2009 Annual Report. NIH Publication No. 10-7603. June 2010. Retrieved July 2010 from http://cabig.cancer.gov/gettingconnected/caBIGresources/annualreport/2009/

National Cancer Institute. (2010b). *Knowledge Centers.* Retrieved June 4, 2010 from https://cabig-kc.nci.nih.gov/MediaWiki/index.php/Main_Page

National Coalition for Health Professional Education in Genetics. Retrieved July 2010 from http://www.nchpeg.org

National Center for Biotechnology Information. (2010). *Training & tutorials.* Retrieved June 4, 2010 from http://www.ncbi.nlm.nih.gov/guide/training-tutorials

National Center for Research Resources. (2010). *Translational Science and CTSA.* Retrieved June 6, 2010 from http://www.ncrr.nih.gov and http://www.ctsaweb.org

National Human Genome Research Institute. (2010). *The Genetics/Genomics Competency Center (G2C2) at the University of Virginia.* Retrieved June 5, 2010 from http://www.genome.gov

National Institutes of Health. (2010). The Secretary's Advisory Committee on Genetics, Health and Society. *Genetics Education and Training for Healthcare Professionals, Public Health Providers, and Consumers.* Retrieved June 6, 2010 from http://oba.od.nih.gov/oba/SACGHS/SACGHS%20Draft%20Genetics%20Education%20and%20Training%20Report.pdf

Nature. (2009, October 8). Editorial. Putting DNA to the test genetic testing companies lack regulation, and the list of guiding principles does not go far enough. *Nature, 461,* 697–698.

PricewaterhouseCoopers, LLC. (2009). *The new science of personalized medicine: Targeting the promise into practice.* Retrieved June 1, 2010 from http://www.pwchealth.com

Thompson, Pat, EPIC. (2010). Challenges with Implementing Personalized Health. Retrieved June 2010 from http://www.fnlm.org/Events-2010-Conf.html

University of Utah. (2010). *Learn genetics.* Retrieved July 2010 from http://learn.genetics.utah.edu

Walker, A. M. (2010). Shaping nursing informatics through the public policy process. In V. Saba & K. McCormick (Eds.), *Essentials of Nursing Informatics* (5th ed). New York: McGraw-Hill.

White House. (2008). *Priorities for personalized medicine.* Retrieved June 2, 2010 from http://www.ostp.gov

APPENDIX A

Clinical Care Classification (CCC) System Version 2.0[1]

CCC of Nursing Diagnoses and Outcomes and CCC of Nursing Interventions and Actions Classified by 21 Care Components

An Overview of the CCC System is highlighted in Chapter 14 "Overview of the Clinical Care Classification (CCC) System."[2,3,4] For additional information, visit the Websites: http://www.sabacare.com or http://clinicalcareclassification.com

APPENDIX TABLE A.1.	Clinical Care Classification System: Nursing Diagnoses and Nursing Interventions by Care Component.[2,3,4]

Table A.1 presents the CCC System concepts for the CCC of Nursing Diagnoses and Outcomes; the CCC of Nursing Interventions/Actions for each of the 21 Care Components that are indexed alphabetically with definitions and codes. Table A.1 is organized into three columns: (1) Care Components; (2) Nursing Diagnoses (Major and Subcategories), and (3) Nursing Interventions (Major and Subcategories). A description of the coding structure and codes can be found in Chapter 14.

Care Component	Nursing Diagnoses and Outcomes		Nursing Interventions/Actions
	Expected Outcomes	**Actual Outcomes**	**Nursing Intervention Action Types**
	To Improve (.1) or	Improved (.1)	Assess or Monitor (.1)
	To Stabilize (.2) or	Stabilized (.2)	Care or Perform (.2)
	To Support		Teach or Instruct (.3)
	Deterioration (.3) or	Deteriorated (.3)	Manage or Refer (.4)
	Example: *Activity Alteration, Improved A01.0.1*		Example: *Perform Activity Care A01.0.2*

(continued)

[1] The Clinical Care Classification (CCC) System Version 2.0 [previously known as the Home Healthcare Classification (HHCC) System, version 1.0, Copyright © 1994] Copyright © 2004 by Virginia K. Saba, EdD, RN, FAAN, FACMI, may be used only with written Permission by Dr. Saba (see Website for Permission Form).

APPENDIX TABLE A.1.	Clinical Care Classification System: Nursing Diagnoses and Nursing Interventions by Care Component. *(continued)*	
Care Component	**Nursing Diagnoses and Outcomes**	**Nursing Interventions/Actions**
A. Activity Component: *Cluster of elements that involve the use of energy in carrying out musculoskeletal and bodily actions.*	**Activity Alteration A01.0** *Change in or modification of energy used by the body.*	**Activity Care A01.0** *Activities performed to carry out physiological or psychological daily activities.*
	Activity Intolerance A01.1 *Incapacity to carry out physiological or psychological daily activities.*	**Energy Conservation A01.2** *Actions performed taken to preserve energy.*
	Activity Intolerance Risk A01.2 *Increased chance of an incapacity to carry out physiological or psychological daily activities.*	**Fracture Care A02.0** *Actions performed to control broken bones.*
	Diversional Activity Deficit A01.3 *Lack of interest or engagement in leisure activities.*	**Cast Care A02.1** *Actions performed to control a rigid dressing.*
	Fatigue A01.4 *Exhaustion that interferes with physical and mental activities.*	**Immobilizer Care A02.2** *Actions performed to control a splint, cast, or prescribed bed rest.*
	Physical Mobility Impairment A01.5 *Diminished ability to perform independent movement.*	**Mobility Therapy A03.0** *Actions performed to advise and instruct on mobility deficits.*
	Sleep Pattern Disturbance A01.6 *Imbalance in the normal sleep/wake cycle.*	**Ambulation Therapy A03.1** *Actions performed to promote walking.*
	Sleep Deprivation A01.7 *Lack of the normal sleep / wake cycle.*	**Assistive Device Therapy A03.2** *Actions performed to support the use of products to aid in caring for oneself.*
	Musculoskeletal Alteration A02.0 *Change in or modification of the muscles, bones, or support structures.*	**Transfer Care A03.3** *Actions performed to assist in moving from one place to another.*
		Sleep Pattern Control A04.0 *Actions performed to support the sleep and wake cycles.*
		Musculosketal Care A05.0 *Actions performed to restore physical functioning.*
		Range of Motion A05.1 *Actions performed to provide the active and passive exercises to maintain joint function.*
		Rehabilitation Exercise A05.2 *Actions performed to promote physical functioning.*
		Bedbound Care A61.0 *Actions performed to support an individual confined to bed.*
		Positioning Therapy A61.1 *Process to support changes in body positioning.*

(continued)

APPENDIX TABLE A.1.	Clinical Care Classification System: Nursing Diagnoses and Nursing Interventions by Care Component. *(continued)*	
Care Component	**Nursing Diagnoses and Outcomes**	**Nursing Interventions/Actions**

B. Bowel/Gastric Component:
Cluster of elements that involve the gastrointestinal system.
	Bowel Elimination Alteration B03.0
	Change in or modification of the gastrointestinal system.
	  Bowel Incontinence B03.1
	  Involuntary defecation.
	  Colonic Constipation B03.2
	  Infrequent or difficult passage of hard, dry feces.
	  Diarrhea B03.3
	  Abnormal frequency and fluidity of feces.
	  Fecal Impaction B03.4
	  Feces wedged in intestines.
	  Perceived Constipation B03.5
	  Belief and treatment of infrequent or difficult passage of feces without cause.
	  Unspecified Constipation B03.6
	  Other forms of abnormal feces or difficult passage of feces.
	Gastrointestinal Alteration B04.0
	Change in or modification of the stomach or intestines.
	Nausea B51.0
	Distaste for food/fluids and an urge to vomit.
		Bowel Care B06.0
		Actions performed to control and restore the functioning of the bowel.
		  Bowel Training B06.1
		  Actions performed to provide instruction on bowel elimination conditions.
		  Disimpaction B06.2
		  Actions performed to manually remove feces.
		  Enema B06.3
		  Actions performed to administer fluid rectally.
		  Diarrhea Care B06.4
		  Actions performed to control the abnormal frequency and fluidity of feces.
		Ostomy Care B07.0
		Actions performed to control the artificial opening that removes waste products.
		  Ostomy Irrigation B07.1
		  Actions performed to flush or wash out an ostomy.
		Gastric Care B62.0
		Actions performed to control changes in the stomach and intestines.
		  Nausea Care B62.1
		  Actions performed to control the distaste for food and desire to vomit.

C. Cardiac Component:
Cluster of elements that involve the heart and blood vessels.
	Cardiac Output Alteration C05.0
	Change in or modification of the pumping action of the heart.
	Cardiovascular Alteration C06.0
	Change in or modification of the heart or blood vessels.
	  Blood Pressure Alteration C06.1
	  Change in or modification of the systolic or diastolic pressure.
		Cardiac Care C08.0
		Actions performed to control changes in the heart or blood vessels.
		  Cardiac Rehabilitation C08.1
		  Actions performed to restore cardiac health.
		Pacemaker Care C09.0
		Actions performed to control the use of an electronic device that provides a normal heartbeat.

(continued)

APPENDIX TABLE A.1.	Clinical Care Classification System: Nursing Diagnoses and Nursing Interventions by Care Component. *(continued)*	
Care Component	**Nursing Diagnoses and Outcomes**	**Nursing Interventions/Actions**
D. Cognitive Component: *Cluster of elements involving the mental and cerebral processes.*	**Cerebral Alteration D07.0** *Change in or modification of thought processes or mentation.* **Confusion D07.1** *State of being disoriented (mixed-up).* **Knowledge Deficit D08.0** *Lack of information, understanding, or comprehension.* **Knowledge Deficit of Diagnostic Test D08.1** *Lack of information on test(s) to identify disease or assess health condition.* **Knowledge Deficit Dietary Regimen D08.2** *Lack of information on the prescribed food or fluid intake.* **Knowledge Deficit of Disease Process D08.3** *Lack of information on the morbidity, course, or treatment of the health condition.* **Knowledge Deficit of Fluid Volume D08.4** *Lack of information on fluid volume intake requirements.* **Knowledge Deficit of Medication Regimen D08.5** *Lack of information on prescribed regulated course of medicinal substances.* **Knowledge Deficit of Safety Precautions D08.6** *Lack of information on measures to prevent injury, danger, or loss.* **Knowledge Deficit of Therapeutic Regimen D08.7** *Lack of information on regulated course of treating disease.* **Thought Process Alteration D09.0** *Change in or modification of cognitive processes.* **Memory Impairment D09.1** *Diminished or inability to recall past events.*	**Behavior Care D10.0** *Actions performed to support observable responses to internal and external stimuli.* **Reality Orientation D11.0** *Actions performed to promote the ability to locate oneself in an environment.* **Wandering Control D63.0** *Actions performed to control abnormal movability.* **Memory Loss Care D64.0** *Actions performed to control a person inability to recall ideas and/or events.*

(continued)

APPENDIX TABLE A.1.	Clinical Care Classification System: Nursing Diagnoses and Nursing Interventions by Care Component. *(continued)*	
Care Component	**Nursing Diagnoses and Outcomes**	**Nursing Interventions/Actions**
E. Coping Component: *Cluster of elements that involve the ability to deal with responsibilities, problems, or difficulties.*	**Dying Process E10.0** *Physical and behavioral responses associated with death.* **Community Coping Impairment E52.0** *Inadequate community response to problems or difficulties.* **Family Coping Impairment E11.0** *Inadequate family response to problems or difficulties.* **Compromised Family Coping E11.1** *Inability of family to function optimally.* **Disabled Family Coping E11.2** *Dysfunctional ability of family to function.* **Individual Coping Impairment E12.0** *Inadequate personal response to problems or difficulties.* **Adjustment Impairment E12.1** *Inadequate adjustment to condition or change* *in health status.* **Decisional Conflict E12.2** *Struggle related to determining a course of* *action.* **Defensive Coping E12.3** *Self-protective strategies to guard against threats* *to self.* **Denial E12.4** *Attempt to reduce anxiety by refusal to accept* *thoughts, feelings, or facts.* **Post-trauma Response E13.0** *Sustained behavior related to a traumatic event.* **Rape Trauma Syndrome E13.1** *Group of symptoms related to a forced sexual* *act.* **Spiritual State Alteration E14.0** *Change in or modification of the spirit or soul.* **Spiritual Distress E14.1** *Anguish related to the spirit or soul.* **Grieving E53.0** *Feeling of great sorrow.* **Anticipatory Grieving E53.1** *Feeling great sorrow before the event or loss.* **Dysfunctional Grieving E53.2** *Prolonged feeling of great sorrow.*	**Counseling Service E12.0** *Actions performed to provide advice or instruction to help another.* **Coping Support E12.1** *Actions performed to sustain a person dealing* *with responsibilities, problems, or difficulties.* **Stress Control E12.2** *Actions performed to support the physiological response of the body to a stimulus.* **Crisis Therapy E12.3** *Actions performed to sustain a person dealing* *with a condition, event, or radical change in* *status.* **Emotional Support E13.0** *Actions performed to maintain a positive affective state.* **Spiritual Comfort E13.1** *Actions performed to console, restore, or* *promote spiritual health.* **Terminal Care E14.0** *Actions performed in the period surrounding death.* **Bereavement Support E14.1** *Actions performed to provide comfort to the* *family/friends of the person who died.* **Dying/Death Measures E14.2** *Actions performed to support the dying process.* **Funeral Arrangements E14.3** *Actions performed to direct the preparation for* *burial.*

(continued)

APPENDIX TABLE A.1.	Clinical Care Classification System: Nursing Diagnoses and Nursing Interventions by Care Component. *(continued)*	
Care Component	**Nursing Diagnoses and Outcomes**	**Nursing Interventions/Actions**

F. Fluid Volume Component:
 	
Cluster of elements that involve liquid consumption.
	Fluid Volume Alteration F15.0
	Change in or modification of bodily fluid
	
	   Fluid Volume Deficit F15.1
	   Dehydration
	
	   Fluid Volume Deficit Risk F15.2
	   Increased chance of dehydration
	
	   Fluid Volume Excess F15.3
	   Fluid retention, overload, or edema.
	
	   Fluid Volume Excess Risk F15.4
	   Increased chance of fluid retention, overload, or edema.
		Fluid Therapy F15.0
		Actions performed to provide liquid volume intake.
		
		   Hydration Control F15.1
		   Actions performed to control the state of fluid balance.
		
		   Intake/Output F15.2
		   Actions performed to measure the amount of fluid/flood and excretion of waste.
		
		Infusion Care F16.0
		Actions performed to support solutions given through the vein.
		
		   Intravenous Care F16.1
		   Actions performed to administer an infusion through a vein.
		
		   Venous Catheter Care F16.2
		   Actions performed to control the use of infusion equipment.

G. Health Behavior Component:
 	
Cluster of elements that involve actions to sustain, maintain, or regain health.
	Health Maintenance Alteration G17.0
	Change in or modification of ability to manage health related needs.
	
	   Failure to Thrive G17.1
	   Inability to grow and develop normally.
	
	Health-Seeking Behavior Alteration G18.0
	Change in or modification of actions needed to improve health state.
	
	Home Maintenance Alteration G19.0
	Inability to sustain a safe, healthy environment.
	
	   Noncompliance G20.0
	   Failure to follow therapeutic recommendations.
	
	   Noncompliance of Diagnostic Test G20.1
	   Failure to follow therapeutic recommendations on tests to identify disease or assess health condition.
	
	   Noncompliance of Dietary Regimen G20.2
	   Failure to follow the prescribed food or fluid intake.
	
	   Noncompliance of Fluid Volume G20.3
	   Failure to follow fluid volume intake requirements.
	
	   Noncompliance of Medication Regimen G20.4
	   Failure to follow prescribed regulated course of medicinal substances.
		Community Special Services G17.0
		Actions performed to provide advice or information about special community services.
		
		   Adult Day Center G17.1
		   Actions performed to direct the provision of a day program for adults in a specific location.
		
		   Hospice G17.2
		   Actions performed to support the provision of offering and/or providing care for terminally ill persons.
		
		   Meals-on-Wheels G17.3
		   Actions performed to direct the provision of community program of meals delivered to the home.
		
		Compliance Care G18.0
		Actions performed to encourage conformity in therapeutic recommendations.
		
		   Compliance with Diet G18.1
		   Actions performed to encourage conformity to food or fluid intake.
		
		   Compliance with Fluid Volume G18.2
		   Actions performed to encourage conformity to therapeutic intake of liquids.
		
		   Compliance with Medical Regimen G18.3
		   Actions performed to encourage conformity to physician plan of care.

(continued)

APPENDIX TABLE A.1.	Clinical Care Classification System: Nursing Diagnoses and Nursing Interventions by Care Component. *(continued)*	
Care Component	**Nursing Diagnoses and Outcomes**	**Nursing Interventions/Actions**
	Noncompliance of Safety Precautions G20.5 *Failure to follow measures to prevent injury, danger, or loss.* **Noncompliance of Therapeutic Regimen G20.6** *Failure to follow regulated course of treating disease or health condition.*	**Compliance with Medication Regimen G18.4** *Actions performed to encourage conformity to follow prescribed course of medicinal substances.* **Compliance with Safety Precaution G18.5** *Actions performed to encourage conformity with measures to protect self or others from injury, danger, or loss.* **Compliance with Therapeutic Regimen G18.6** *Actions performed to encourage conformity with the health team plan of care.* **Nursing Contact G19.0** *Actions performed to communicate with another nurse.* **Bill of Rights G19.1** *Statements related to entitlements during an episode of illness.* **Nursing Care Coordination G19.2** *Actions performed to synthesize all plans of care by a nurse.* **Nursing Status Report G19.3** *Actions performed to document patient condition by a nurse.* **Physician Contact G20.0** *Actions performed to communicate with a physician.* **Medical Regimen Orders G20.1** *Actions performed to support the physician plan of treatment.* **Physician Status Report G20.2** *Actions performed to document patient condition by a physician.* **Professional/Ancillary Services G21.0** *Actions performed to support the duties performed by health team members.* **Health Aide Service G21.1** *Actions performed to support care services by a health aide.* **Medical Social Worker Service G21.2** *Actions performed to provide advice or instruction by a medical social worker.* **Nurse Specialist Service G21.3** *Actions performed to provide advice or instruction by an advanced practice nurse or nurse practitioner.*

(continued)

APPENDIX TABLE A.1.	Clinical Care Classification System: Nursing Diagnoses and Nursing Interventions by Care Component. *(continued)*	
Care Component	**Nursing Diagnoses and Outcomes**	**Nursing Interventions/Actions**
		Occupational Therapist Service G21.4 *Actions performed to provide advice or instruction by an occupational therapist.*
		Physical Therapist Service G21.5 *Actions performed to provide advice or instruction by a physical therapist.*
		Speech Therapist Service G21.6 *Actions performed to provide advice or instruction by a speech therapist.*
H. Medication Component: *Cluster of elements that involve medicinal substances.*	**Medication Risk H21.0** *Increased chance of negative response to medicinal substances*	**Chemotherapy Care H22.0** *Actions performed to control and monitor antineoplastic agents.*
	Polypharmacy H21.1 *Use of two or more drugs together.*	**Injection Administration H23.0** *Actions performed to dispense a medication by a hypodermic.*
		Insulin Injection H23.1 *Actions performed to administer a hypodermic administration of insulin.*
		Vitamin B12 Injection H23.2 *Actions performed to administer a hypodermic administration of vitamin B12.*
		Medication Care H24.0 *Actions performed to direct the dispensing of prescribed drugs.*
		Medication Actions H24.1 *Actions performed to support and monitor the use of medicinal substances.*
		Medication Prefill Preparation H24.2 *Actions performed to ensure the continued supply of prescribed drugs.*
		Medication Side Effects H24.3 *Actions performed to control untoward reaction or conditions to prescribed drugs.*
		Medication Treatment H24.4 *Actions performed to administer drugs or remedies regardless of route.*
		Radiation Therapy Care H25.0 *Actions performed to control and monitor radiation therapy.*

(continued)

APPENDIX TABLE A.1.	Clinical Care Classification System: Nursing Diagnoses and Nursing Interventions by Care Component. *(continued)*	
Care Component	**Nursing Diagnoses and Outcomes**	**Nursing Interventions/Actions**

I. Metabolic Component:
 	
Cluster of elements that involve the endocrine and immunological processes.
	Endocrine Alteration I22.0
	Change in or modification of internal secretions or hormones.
	
	Immunologic Alteration I23.0
	Change in or modification of the immune systems.
	
	    Protection Alteration I23.1
	    Change in or modification of the ability to guard against internal or external threats to the body.
		Allergic Reaction Care I26.0
		Actions performed to reduce symptoms or precautions to reduce allergies.
		
		Diabetic Care I27.0
		Actions performed to support the control of diabetic conditions.
		
		Immunological Care I65.0
		Actions performed to protect against a particular disease.

J. Nutritional Component:
 	
Cluster of elements that involve the intake of food and nutrients.
	Nutrition Alteration J24.0
	Change in or modification of food and nutrients.
	
	    Body Nutrition Deficit J24.1
	    Less than adequate intake or absorption of food or nutrients.
	
	    Body Nutrition Deficit Risk J24.2
	    Increased chance of less than adequate intake or absorption of food or nutrients.
	
	    Body Nutrition Excess J24.3
	    More than adequate intake or absorption of food or nutrients.
	
	    Body Nutrition Excess Risk J24.4
	    Increased chance of more than adequate intake or absorption of food or nutrients
	
	    Swallowing Impairment J24.5
	    Inability to move food from mouth to stomach.
	
	Infant Feeding Pattern Impairment J54.0
	Imbalance in the normal feeding habits of an infant.
	
	Breastfeeding Impairment J55.0
	Diminished ability to nourish infant at the breast.
		Enteral Tube Care J28.0
		Actions performed to control the use on an enteral drainage tube.
		
		    Enteral Tube Insertion J28.1
		    Actions performed to support the placement of an enteral drainage tube.
		
		    Enteral Tube Irrigation J28.2
		    Actions performed to flush or wash out an enteral tube.
		
		Nutrition Care J29.0
		Actions performed to support the intake of food and nutrients.
		
		    Feeding Technique J29.2
		    Actions performed to provide special measures to provide nourishment.
		
		    Regular Diet J29.3
		    Actions performed to support the ingestion of food and nutrients from established nutrition standards.
		
		    Special Diet J29.4
		    Actions performed to support the ingestion of food and nutrients prescribed for a specific purpose.
		
		    Enteral Feeding J29.5
		    Actions performed to provide nourishment through a gastrointestinal route.
		
		    Parenteral Feeding J29.6
		    Actions performed to provide nourishment through intravenous or subcutaneous routes.
		
		Breastfeeding Support J66.0
		Actions performed to provide nourishment of an infant at the breast.
		
		Weight Control J67.0
		Actions performed to control obesity or debilitation.

(continued)

APPENDIX TABLE A.1.	Clinical Care Classification System: Nursing Diagnoses and Nursing Interventions by Care Component. *(continued)*	
Care Component	**Nursing Diagnoses and Outcomes**	**Nursing Interventions/Actions**
K. Physical Regulation Component: *Cluster of elements that involve bodily processes.*	**Physical Regulation Alteration K25.0** *Change in or modification of somatic control.* **Autonomic Dysreflexia K25.1** *Life-threatening inhibited sympathetic response to noxious stimuli in a person with a spinal cord injury at T7 or above.* **Hyperthermia K25.2** *Abnormal high body temperature.* **Hypothermia K25.3** *Abnormal low body temperature.* **Thermoregulation Impairment K25.4** *Fluctuation of temperature between hypothermia and hyperthermia.* **Infection Risk K25.5** *Increased chance of contamination with disease-producing germs.* **Infection Unspecified K25.6** *Unknown contamination with disease-producing germs.* **Intracranial Adaptive Capacity Impairment K25.7** *Intracranial fluid volumes are compromised.*	**Infection Control K30.0** *Actions performed to contain a communicable disease.* **Universal Precautions K30.1** *Practices to prevent the spread of infections and infectious diseases.* **Physical Healthcare K31.0** *Actions performed to support somatic problems.* **Health History K31.1** *Actions performed to obtain information about past illness and health status.* **Health Promotion K31.2** *Actions performed to encourage behaviors to enhance health state.* **Physical Examination K31.3** *Actions performed to observe somatic events.* **Clinical Measurements K31.4** *Actions performed to conduct procedures to evaluate somatic events.* **Specimen Care K32.0** *Actions performed to direct the collection and/or the examination of a bodily specimen.* **Blood Specimen Care K32.1** *Actions performed to collect and/or examine a sample of blood.* **Stool Specimen Care K32.2** *Actions performed to collect and/or examine a sample of feces.* **Urine Specimen Care K32.3** *Actions performed to collect and/or examine a sample of urine.* **Sputum Specimen Care K32.5** *Actions performed to collect and/or examine a sample of sputum.*

(continued)

APPENDIX TABLE A.1.	Clinical Care Classification System: Nursing Diagnoses and Nursing Interventions by Care Component. *(continued)*	
Care Component	**Nursing Diagnoses and Outcomes**	**Nursing Interventions/Actions**
		Vital Signs K33.0 *Actions performed to measure temperature, pulse, respiration, and blood pressure.* **Blood Pressure K33.1** *Actions performed to measure the diastolic and systolic pressure of the blood.* **Temperature K33.2** *Actions performed to measure the body temperature.* **Pulse K33.3** *Actions performed to measure rhythmical beats of the heart.* **Respiration K33.4** *Actions performed to measure the function of breathing.*
L. Respiratory Component: *Cluster of elements that involve breathing and the pulmonary system.*	**Respiration Alteration L26.0** *Change in or modification of the breathing function.* **Airway Clearance Impairment L26.1** *Inability to clear secretions/obstructions in airway.* **Breathing Pattern Impairment L26.2** *Inadequate inhalation or exhalation.* **Gas Exchange Impairment L26.3** *Imbalance of oxygen and carbon dioxide transfer between lung and vascular system.* **Ventilatory Weaning Impairment L56.0** *Inability to tolerate decreased levels of ventilator support.*	**Oxygen Therapy Care L35.0** *Actions performed to support the administration of oxygen treatment.* **Pulmonary Care L36.0** *Actions performed to support pulmonary hygiene.* **Breathing Exercises L36.1** *Actions performed to provide therapy on respiratory or lung exertion.* **Chest Physiotherapy L36.2** *Actions performed to provide exercises to provide postural drainage of lungs.* **Inhalation Therapy L36.3** *Actions performed to support breathing treatments.* **Ventilator Care L36.4** *Actions performed to control and monitor the use of a ventilator.* **Tracheostomy Care L37.0** *Actions performed to support a tracheostomy.*

(continued)

APPENDIX TABLE A.1.	Clinical Care Classification System: Nursing Diagnoses and Nursing Interventions by Care Component. *(continued)*	
Care Component	**Nursing Diagnoses and Outcomes**	**Nursing Interventions/Actions**
M. Role Relationship Component: *Cluster of elements involving interpersonal work, social, family, and sexual interactions.*	**Role Performance Alteration M27.0** *Change in or modification of carrying out responsibilities.* **Parental Role Conflict M27.1** *Struggle with parental position and responsibilities.* **Parenting Alteration M27.2** *Change in or modification of nurturing figure's ability to promote growth.* **Sexual Dysfunction M27.3** *Deleterious change in sex response.* **Caregiver Role Strain M27.4** *Excessive tension of one who gives physical or emotional care and support to another person or patient.* **Communication Impairment M28.0** *Diminished ability to exchange thoughts, opinions, or information.* **Verbal Impairment M28.1** *Diminished ability to exchange thoughts, opinions, or information through speech.* **Family Processes Alteration M29.0** *Change in or modification of usual functioning of a related group.* **Sexuality Patterns Alteration M31.0** *Change in or modification of person's sexual response.* **Socialization Alteration M32.0** *Change in or modification of personal identity.* **Social Interaction Alteration M32.1** *Change in or modification of inadequate quantity or quality of personal relations.* **Social Isolation M32.2** *State of aloneness, lack of interaction with others.* **Relocation Stress Syndrome M32.3** *Excessive tension from moving to a new location.*	**Communication Care M38.0** *Actions performed to exchange verbal information.* **Psychosocial Care M39.0** *Actions performed to support the study of psychological and social factors.* **Home Situation Analysis M39.1** *Actions performed to analyze the living environment.* **Interpersonal Dynamics Analysis M39.2** *Actions performed to support the analysis of the driving forces in a relationship between people.* **Family Process Analysis M39.3** *Actions performed to support the change and/or modification of a related group.* **Sexual Behavior Analysis M39.4** *Actions performed to support the change and/or modification of a person sexual response.* **Social Network Analysis M39.5** *Actions performed to improve the quantity or quality of personal relationships.*

(continued)

APPENDIX TABLE A.1.	Clinical Care Classification System: Nursing Diagnoses and Nursing Interventions by Care Component. *(continued)*	
Care Component	**Nursing Diagnoses and Outcomes**	**Nursing Interventions/Actions**
N. Safety Component: *Cluster of elements that involve prevention of injury, danger, loss, or abuse.*	**Injury Risk N33.0** *Increased chance of danger or loss.*	**Substance Abuse Control N40.0** *Actions performed to control substances to avoid, detect, or minimize harm.*
	Aspiration Risk N33.1 *Increased chance of material into trachea-bronchial passages.*	**Tobacco Abuse Control N40.1** *Actions performed to avoid, minimize, or control the use of tobacco.*
	Disuse Syndrome N33.2 *Group of symptoms related to effects of immobility.*	**Alcohol Abuse Control N40.2** *Actions performed to avoid, minimize, or control the use of distilled liquors.*
	Poisoning Risk N33.3 *Exposure to or ingestion of dangerous products.*	**Drug Abuse Control N40.3** *Actions performed to avoid, minimize, or control the use of any habit-forming medication.*
	Suffocation Risk N33.4 *Increased chance of inadequate air for breathing.*	**Emergency Care N41.0** *Actions performed to support a sudden or unexpected occurrence.*
	Trauma Risk N33.5 *Increased chance of accidental tissue processes.*	**Safety Precautions N42.0** *Actions performed to advance measures to avoid, danger, or harm.*
	Violence Risk N34.0 *Increased chance of harming self or others.*	**Environmental Safety N42.1** *Precautions recommended to prevent or reduce environmental injury.*
	Suicide Risk N34.1 *Increased chance of taking one life intentionally.*	**Equipment Safety N42.2** *Precautions recommended to prevent or reduce equipment injury.*
	Self-Mutilation Risk N34.2 *Increased chance of destroying a limb or essential part of the body.*	**Individual Safety N42.3** *Precautions to reduce individual injury.*
	Perioperative Injury Risk N57.0 *Increased chance of injury during the operative processes.*	**Violence Control N68.0** *Actions performed to control behaviors that may cause harm to oneself or others.*
	Perioperative Positioning Injury N57.1 *Damages from operative process positioning.*	
	Surgical Recovery Delay N57.2 *Slow or delayed recovery from a surgical procedure.*	
	Substance Abuse N58.0 *Excessive use of harmful bodily materials.*	
	Tobacco Abuse N58.1 *Excessive use of tobacco products.*	
	Alcohol Abuse N58.2 *Excessive use of distilled liquors.*	
	Drug Abuse N58.3 *Excessive use of habit-forming medications.*	

(continued)

APPENDIX TABLE A.1.	Clinical Care Classification System: Nursing Diagnoses and Nursing Interventions by Care Component. *(continued)*	
Care Component	**Nursing Diagnoses and Outcomes**	**Nursing Interventions/Actions**

O. Self-Care Component:
 	
Cluster of elements that involve the ability to carry out activities to maintain oneself.
	Bathing/Hygiene Deficit O35.0
	Impaired ability to cleanse oneself.
	Dressing/Grooming Deficit O36.0
	Inability to clothe and groom oneself.
	Feeding Deficit O37.0
	Impaired ability to feed oneself.
	Self-Care Deficit O38.0
	Impaired ability to maintain oneself.
	    Activities of Daily Living (ADLs) Alteration O38.1
	    Change in or modification of ability to maintain oneself.
	    Instrumental Activities of Daily Living (IADLs) Alteration O38.2
	    Change in or modification of more complex activities than those needed to maintain oneself.
	Toileting Deficit O39.0
	Impaired ability to urinate or defecate for oneself.
		Personal Care O43.0
		Actions performed to care for oneself.
		    Activities of Daily Living (ADLs) O43.1
		    Actions performed to support personal activities to maintain oneself.
		    Instrumental Activities of Daily Living (IADLs) 043.2
		    Complex activities performed to support basic life skills.

P. Self-Concept Component:
 	
Cluster of elements that involve an individual mental image of oneself.
	Anxiety P40.0
	Feeling of distress or apprehension whose source is unknown.
	Fear P41.0
	Feeling of dread or distress whose cause can be identified.
	Meaningfulness Alteration P42.0
	Change in or modification of the ability to see the significance, purpose, or value in something.
	    Hopelessness P42.1
	    Feeling of despair or futility and passive involvement.
	    Powerlessness P42.2
	    Feeling of helplessness, or inability to act.
		Mental Healthcare P45.0
		Actions taken to promote emotional well-being.
		    Mental Health History P45.1
		    Actions performed to obtain information about past or present emotional well-being.
		    Mental Health Promotion P45.2
		    Actions performed to encourage or further emotional well-being.
		    Mental Health Screening P45.3
		    Actions performed to systematically examine the emotional well-being.
		    Mental Health Treatment P45.4
		    Actions performed to support protocols used to treat emotional problems.

(continued)

APPENDIX TABLE A.1.	Clinical Care Classification System: Nursing Diagnoses and Nursing Interventions by Care Component. *(continued)*	
Care Component	**Nursing Diagnoses and Outcomes**	**Nursing Interventions/Actions**
	Self-Concept Alteration P43.0 *Change in or modification of ability to maintain one image of self.*	
	Body Image Disturbance P43.1 *Imbalance in the perception of the way one body looks.*	
	Personal Identity Disturbance P43.2 *Imbalance in the ability to distinguish between the self and the non-self.*	
	Chronic Low Self-Esteem Disturbance P43.3 *Persistent negative evaluation of oneself.*	
	Situational Self-Esteem Disturbance P43.4 *Negative evaluation of oneself in response to a loss or change.*	
Q. Sensory Component: *Cluster of elements that involve the senses, including pain.*	**Sensory Perceptual Alteration Q44.0** *Change in or modification of the response to stimuli.*	**Pain Control Q47.0** *Actions performed to support responses to injury or damage.*
	Auditory Alteration Q44.1 *Change in or modification of diminished ability to hear.*	**Acute Pain Control Q47.1** *Actions performed to control physical suffering, hurting, or distress.*
	Gustatory Alteration Q44.2 *Change in or modification of diminished ability to taste.*	**Chronic Pain Control Q47.2** *Actions performed to control physical suffering, hurting, or distress that continues longer than expected.*
	Kinesthetic Alteration Q44.3 *Change in or modification of diminished ability to move.*	**Comfort Care Q48.0** *Actions performed to enhance or improve well-being.*
	Olfactory Alteration Q44.4 *Change in or modification of diminished ability to smell.*	**Ear Care Q49.0** *Actions performed to support ear problems.*
	Tactile Alteration Q44.5 *Change in or modification of diminished ability to feel.*	**Hearing Aid Care Q49.1** *Actions performed to control the use of a hearing aid.*
	Unilateral Neglect Q44.6 *Lack of awareness of one side of the body.*	**Wax Removal Q49.2** *Actions performed to remove cerumen from ear.*
	Visual Alteration Q44.7 *Change in or modification of diminished ability to see.*	**Eye Care Q50.0** *Actions performed to support eye problems.*
	Comfort Alteration Q45.0 *Change in or modification of sensation that is distressing.*	**Cataract Care Q50.1** *Actions performed to control cataract conditions.*
	Acute Pain Q45.1 *Physical suffering or distress to hurt.*	**Vision Care Q50.2** *Actions performed to control vision problems.*
	Chronic Pain Q45.2 *Pain that continues for longer than expected.*	
	Unspecified Pain Q45.3 *Pain that is difficult to pinpoint.*	

(continued)

APPENDIX TABLE A.1.	Clinical Care Classification System: Nursing Diagnoses and Nursing Interventions by Care Component. *(continued)*	
Care Component	**Nursing Diagnoses and Outcomes**	**Nursing Interventions/Actions**
R. Skin Integrity Component: *Cluster of elements that involve the mucous membrane, corneal, integumentary, or subcutaneous structures of the body.*	**Skin Integrity Alteration R46.0** *Change in or modification of skin conditions.* **Oral Mucous Membranes Impairment R46.1** *Diminished ability to maintain the tissues of the oral cavity.* **Skin Integrity Impairment R46.2** *Decreased ability to maintain the integument.* **Skin Integrity Impairment Risk R46.3** *Increased chance of skin breakdown.* **Skin Incision R46.4** *Cutting of the integument/skin.* **Latex Allergy Response R46.5** *Pathological reaction to latex products.* **Peripheral Alteration R47.0** *Change in or modification of vascularization of the extremities.*	**Pressure Ulcer Care R51.0** *Actions performed to prevent, detect, and treat skin integrity breakdown caused by pressure.* **Pressure Ulcer Stage 1 Care R51.1** *Actions performed to prevent, detect, and treat Stage 1 skin breakdown.* **Pressure Ulcer Stage 2 Care R51.2** *Actions performed to prevent, detect, and treat Stage 2 skin breakdown.* **Pressure Ulcer Stage 3 Care R51.3** *Actions performed to prevent, detect, and treat Stage 3 skin breakdown.* **Pressure Ulcer Stage 4 Care R51.4** *Actions performed to prevent, detect, and treat Stage 4 skin breakdown.* **Mouth Care R53.0** *Actions performed to support oral cavity problems.* **Denture Care R53.1** *Actions performed to control the use of artificial teeth.* **Skin Care R54.0** *Actions to control the integument/skin.* **Skin Breakdown Control R54.1** *Actions performed to support tissue integrity problems.* **Wound Care R55.0** *Actions performed to support open skin areas.* **Drainage Tube Care R55.1** *Actions performed to support drainage from tubes.* **Dressing Change R55.2** *Actions performed to remove and replace a new bandage to a wound.* **Incision Care R55.3** *Actions performed to support a surgical wound.*

(continued)

APPENDIX TABLE A.1.	Clinical Care Classification System: Nursing Diagnoses and Nursing Interventions by Care Component. *(continued)*	
Care Component	**Nursing Diagnoses and Outcomes**	**Nursing Interventions/Actions**
S. Tissue Perfusion Component: *Cluster of elements that involve the oxygenation of tissues, including the circulatory and neurovascular systems.*	**Tissue Perfusion Alteration S48.0** *Change in or modification of the oxygenation of tissues.*	**Foot Care S56.0** *Actions performed to support foot problems.* **Perineal Care S57.0** *Actions performed to support perineal problems.* **Edema Control S69.0** *Actions performed to control excess fluid in tissue.* **Circulatory Care S70.0** *Actions performed to support the circulation of the blood (blood vessels).* **Neurovascular Care S71.0** *Actions performed to control problems of the nerves and vascular systems.*
T. Urinary Elimination Component: *Cluster of elements that involve the genitourinary systems.*	**Urinary Elimination Alteration T49.0** *Change in or modification of excretion of the waste matter of the kidneys.* **Functional Urinary Incontinence T49.1** *Involuntary, unpredictable passage of urine.* **Reflex Urinary Incontinence T49.2** *Involuntary passage of urine occurring at predictable intervals.* **Stress Urinary Incontinence T49.3** *Loss of urine occurring with increased abdominal pressure.* **Total Urinary Incontinence T49.4** *Continuous and unpredictable loss of urine.* **Urge Urinary Incontinence T49.5** *Involuntary passage of urine following a sense of urgency to void.* **Urinary Retention T49.6** *Incomplete emptying of the bladder.* **Renal Alteration T50.0** *Change in or modification of the kidney function.*	**Bladder Care T58.0** *Actions performed to control urinary drainage problems.* **Bladder Instillation T58.1** *Actions performed to pour liquid through a catheter into the bladder.* **Bladder Training T58.2** *Actions performed to provide instruction on the training care of urinary drainage.* **Dialysis Care T59.0** *Actions performed to support dialysis treatments.* **Urinary Catheter Care T60.0** *Actions performed to control the use of a urinary catheter.* **Urinary Catheter Insertion T60.1** *Actions performed to place a urinary catheter in bladder.* **Urinary Catheter Irrigation T60.2** *Actions performed to flush a urinary catheter.* **Urinary Incontinence Care T72.0** *Actions performed to control the inability to retain and/or involuntarily retain urine.* **Renal Care T73.0** *Actions performed to control problems pertaining to the kidney.*

(continued)

APPENDIX TABLE A.1.	Clinical Care Classification System: Nursing Diagnoses and Nursing Interventions by Care Component. *(continued)*	
Care Component	**Nursing Diagnoses and Outcomes**	**Nursing Interventions/Actions**
U. Life Cycle Component: *Cluster of elements that involve the life span of individuals.*	**Reproductive Risk U59.0** *Increased chance of harm in the process of replicating or giving rise to an offspring/child.*	**Reproductive Care U74.0** *Actions performed to support the production of an offspring/child.*
	Fertility Risk U59.1 *Increased chance of conception to develop an offspring/child.*	**Fertility Care U74.1** *Actions performed to increase conception of an offspring/child.*
	Infertility Risk U59.2 *Decreased chance of conception to develop an offspring/child.*	**Infertility Care U74.2** *Actions performed to promote conception of the infertile client of an offspring/child.*
	Contraception Risk U59.3 *Increased chance of harm preventing the conception of an offspring/child.*	**Contraception Care U74.3** *Actions performed to prevent conception of an	offspring/child.*
	Perinatal Risk U60.0 *Increased chance of harm before, during, and immediately after the creation of an offspring/child.*	**Perinatal Care U75.0** *Actions performed to support the period before, during, and immediately after the creation of an offspring/child.*
	Pregnancy Risk U60.1 *Increased chance of harm during the gestational period of the formation of an offspring/child.*	**Pregnancy Care U75.1** *Actions performed to support the gestation period of the formation of an offspring/child (being with child).*
	Labor Risk U60.2 Increased chance of harm during the period supporting the bringing forth of an offspring/child.	**Labor Care U75.2** *Actions performed to support the bringing forth of an offspring/child.*
	Delivery Risk U60.3 *Increased chance of harm during the period supporting the expulsion of an offspring/child.*	**Delivery Care U75.3** *Actions performed to support the expulsion of an offspring/child at birth.*
	Postpartum Risk U60.4 *Increased chance of harm during the time period immediately following the delivery of an offspring/child.*	**Postpartum Care U75.4** *Actions performed to support the time period immediately after the delivery of an offspring/ child.*
	Growth and Development Alteration U61.0 *Change in or modification of the norms for an individual age.*	**Growth and Development Care U76.0** *Actions performed to support normal standards of performing developmental skills and behavior of an individual of any age group.*
	Newborn Behavior Alteration (first 30 days) U61.1 *Change in or modification of normal standards of performing developmental skills and behavior of a typical newborn the first 30 days of life.*	**Newborn Care (first 30 days) U76.1** *Actions performed to support normal standards of performing developmental skills and behavior of an individual of a typical newborn for the first 30 days of life.*
	Infant Behavior Alteration (31 days through 11 months) U61.2 *Change in or modification of normal standards of performing developmental skills and behavior of a typical infant from 31 days through 11 month of age.*	**Infant Care (31 days through 11 months) U76.2** *Actions performed to support normal standards of performing developmental skills and behavior of a typical infant 31 days through 11 months of age.*

(continued)

APPENDIX TABLE A.1.	Clinical Care Classification System: Nursing Diagnoses and Nursing Interventions by Care Component. *(continued)*	
Care Component	**Nursing Diagnoses and Outcomes**	**Nursing Interventions/Actions**
	Child Behavior Alteration (1 year through 11 years) U61.3 *Change in or modification of normal standards of performing developmental skills and behavior of a typical child from 1 year through 11 years of age.* **Adolescent Behavior Alteration (12 years through 20 years) U61.4** *Change in or modification of normal standards of performing developmental skills and behavior of a typical adolescent from 12 years through 20 years of age.* **Adult Behavior Alteration (21 years through 62 years) U61.5** *Change in or modification of normal standards of performing developmental skills and behavior of a typical adult from 21 years through 64 years of age.* **Older Adult Behavior Alteration (65 years and older) U61.6** *Change in or modification of normal standards of performing developmental skills and behavior of a typical older adult from 65 years of age and over.*	**Child Care (1 year through 11 years) U76.3** *Actions performed to support normal standards of performing developmental skills and behavior of a typical child 1 year through 11 years of age.* **Adolescent Care (12 years through 20 years) U76.4** *Actions performed to support normal standards of performing developmental skills and behavior of a typical adolescent 12 years through 20 years of age.* **Adult Care U76.5 (21 years through 64 years)** *Actions performed to support normal standards of performing developmental skills and behavior of a typical adult 21 years through 64 years of age.* **Older Adult Care U76.6 (65 years and older)** *Actions performed to support normal standards of performing developmental skills and behavior of typical older adult 65 years and over.*

[2] Adapted with permission from: NANDA. *Taxonomy I - Revised 1990- With Official Nursing Diagnoses.* St Louis, Mo: NANDA.
[3] Adapted with permission from: NANDA (2003). *Nursing Diagnoses: Definitions & Classifications 2003-2004.* Philadelphia, PA: NANDA International.
[4] Revised 1992, 1994, 2002, 2004, 2006.

INDEX

Page numbers followed by *f* or *t* indicate figures or tables, respectively.